# FOOD SAFETY
# 1995

# FOOD SAFETY 1995

Food Research Institute

*Department of Food Microbiology and Toxicology*
*University of Wisconsin—Madison*
*Madison, Wisconsin*

*prepared by*

**Carol E. Steinhart**
**M. Ellin Doyle**
**Barbara A. Cochrane**

Marcel Dekker, Inc.                    New York • Basel • Hong Kong

ISBN: 0-8247-9624-1

The publisher offers discounts on this book when ordered in bulk quantities. For more information, write to Special Sales/Professional Marketing at the address below.

This book is printed on acid-free paper.

MARCEL DEKKER, INC.
270 Madison Avenue, New York, New York 10016

Current printing (last digit):
10 9 8 7 6 5 4 3 2 1

**PRINTED IN THE UNITED STATES OF AMERICA**

# Preface

The *Food Safety* series is a comprehensive annual summary of the literature on food safety and foodborne illness. *Food Safety 1995* covers literature published during the latter half of 1993 and the first half of 1994. Journals covered by the *Life Sciences* and *Agriculture, Biology & Environmental Sciences* editions of *Current Contents* were surveyed. Articles from more than 620 sources are included in this volume. Such comprehensive coverage would not have been possible without the extensive library resources and services of the University of Wisconsin–Madison.

We have included as broad a range of articles as we deemed possible. Some sections in Part I, Diet and Health, include primarily papers covering epidemiological, clinical, and intervention studies in humans and experimental studies with primates. The sheer volume of work on rodents precludes inclusion of any but a few of the more salient papers. Coverage of pesticides is limited for the same reasons. Because of the book's organization, individual food components (e.g., fiber or selenium) and particular diseases and disorders (e.g., cancer, birth defects) are likely to appear in more than one section. We attempt to present new information or insights gleaned from "methods" papers without providing details of the methods themselves, as readers interested in using the method would have to consult the original publication in any case.

While we have made every effort to assure accuracy, we encourage readers to consult the original publications for specific information.

Foodborne viruses are reviewed annually by Dr. Dean O. Cliver of the Food Research Institute. This information, presented in the Appendix, completes the subject matter coverage of the food safety literature.

# Contents

## 5   FOOD AND DIETARY ANALYSIS

# PART II:  SAFETY OF FOOD COMPONENTS

## 6   ASSESSMENT OF FOOD SAFETY

## 7   INTENTIONAL (DIRECT) ADDITIVES

## 8   INDIRECT ADDITIVES, RESIDUES, AND CONTAMINANTS

## 9   NATURALLY OCCURRING TOXICANTS AND FOOD CONSTITUENTS OF TOXICOLOGICAL INTEREST

# PART III: FOODBORNE MICROBIAL ILLNESS

## 10 MYCOTOXINS

## 11 FOODBORNE BACTERIAL INTOXICATIONS AND INFECTIONS

## 12 FOODBORNE PARASITIC INFECTIONS

**APPENDIX**

**FOOD- AND WATER-ASSOCIATED VIRUSES**   *Dean O. Cliver*

# FOOD
# SAFETY
# *1995*

# Part I: Diet and Health

# 1

# Overview

---

---

The evolutionary history of the Primate Order can be told in dietary terms. This is of more than passing interest because it explains much about today's cultures, including people's propensity to overindulge in calorie- and nutrient-dense foods. Milton illustrated two food-procurement strategies seen among contemporary arboreal primates and perhaps in the evolution of our species (*1*). Some primates have morphologic and physiologic adaptations that permit subsistence on ubiquitous but low-quality plant parts such as mature leaves. This minimizes the time and energy expended to obtain food; it also requires minimal mental ability. Other primates adopted the strategy of selective feeding on high-quality plant foods. Arguably, this course was associated with development of a large brain because foraging efficiency mandates remembering the sources and locations of preferred foods. For example, a howler monkey eats fruits when they are readily available but otherwise subsists on leaves. Food passes slowly through its gut, allowing maximum extraction of energy. Its smallish brain does not confer notable mental skills. The similar-sized spider monkey relentlessly searches out nutrient-dense foods at all seasons, passes food more quickly through its shorter, narrower colon, and has roughly twice the howler's brain capacity. In hominid evolution, small-brained *Australopithecus*—strong-jawed, with formidable molars—contrasts sharply with weak-jawed, big-brained *Homo*. Are these differences inseparably linked to diet because the price of intellect is the *requirement* for energy-dense foods for both development and maintenance of a big brain? Leonard and Robertson summarized data showing that relative to body size, our species is exceptional even among primates for its very high-quality diet and high resting metabolic requirement, 20–25% of which is accounted for by the needs of our brains (*2*). They argue that hominid evolution was characterized by increasing diet quality and amounts of animal foods eaten. Ironically, the pursuit of foods ever lower in fiber—a driving force in our evolution—is now causing us grief. Among contemporary hunter-gatherers and in undeveloped nations where overindulgence is usually impossible, the appetite for high-quality foods is still adaptive. In developed societies, however, the same innate preference has precipitated the scourge of "diseases of affluence," which are the subject of the first chapters in this book.

Kritchevsky reviewed various types of evidence for the role of lipids, calories, and fiber in cardiovascular disease and cancer (*3*). Based on current knowledge and the guidelines issued by a number of health-oriented organizations, the best dietary advice is still moderation, balance, and variety. Willett discussed evidence for associations of diet with cancer, coronary heart disease, birth defects, and cataract, commenting on the food pyramid recently developed by the USDA (*4*). He concluded that many people in the USA have suboptimal diets and that the potential for preventing disease by improved nutrition is substantial. While applauding the food industry's rapid response to concerns about diet and health, he cautioned that the long-term effects of changes such as substituting diacylglycerides and artificial sweeteners for fats and sugar are unclear and could be adverse. Again, the best recommendation is a plant-enriched diet. This can be made interesting and enjoyable by adopting healthful dishes from other cultures.

Zifferblatt raised the issue of dietary supplements—how to make nutritional recommendations when knowledge is not definitive and science is in transition (*5*). He urged that science, the media, health practitioners, and business and industry (the "four gatekeepers") be used constructively and in concert for health recommendations, and gave persuasive examples of the confusion that results when this does not happen. As a procedural model he discussed the NHLBI "Foods for Health" pilot program, a cholesterol education program for the consumer conducted in cooperation with Giant Foods. Supermarkets provided biweekly brochures that discussed known relationships between heart disease and nutrition; acknowledged the uncertainties and the transitional state of the science; recognized the existence of the cholesterol controversy; outlined the costs, risks, and benefits of available options; and told each consumer "you decide." Zifferblatt recommended a similar approach to the issue of dietary supplements. Although it is impossible to give definitive recommendations, it *is* possible to offer objective guidance so individuals can make their own informed decisions. Ellenbogen provided basic information on the functions, current RDA (recommended dietary allowance), chemistry, sources, metabolism, and toxicity of constituents found in nutritional supplements (*6*). He also summarized drug–nutrient interactions.

Meanwhile, American food choices have been changing in a healthful direction—more low-fat and nonfat products and leaner cuts of meat (*7*). The trend is countered, however, by growing consumption of high-fat convenience foods, fast foods, and snacks. The new food-label requirements are seen as key to providing necessary information for making rational food choices. Data on availability and consumption of eggs, dairy products, and red meat, poultry, and fish were presented for 1980–1983, 1991, and 1992. Daily per capita levels of cholesterol in the food supply decreased from 447 mg in 1980 to 414 mg in 1990. During the same period the proportion of calories from fat decreased from 42% to 40% and of this fat, the contribution of animal fat decreased from 59% to 52%. Total calories increased from 3400 to 3700.

The 1987 National Health Interview Survey found that fat intake is consistently associated with specific dietary patterns, with few differences among demographic subgroups (*8*). High fat intake was associated with reduced intake of vegetables, fruits, cereals, fish and chicken, low-fat milk, vitamin C, carbohydrates, carotenoids, folate, vitamin A, and dietary fiber. As the percentage of calories from fat increased, so did intake of salty snacks, peanuts, processed and red meats, whole milk and cheese, desserts, eggs, fried potatoes, vitamin E, sodium, protein, and total calories. Overall, when the intake of foods perceived as healthful increases energy intake from fat decreases.

## DIET AND HEALTH IN SPECIFIC POPULATION GROUPS

### Women

Volume 12 number 4 of the *Journal of the American College of Nutrition* was devoted to issues in women's health and nutrition. In this issue, Cummings discussed the background and elements of the USPHS Action Plan for Women's Health, including the controversial Women's Health Initiative (*9*).

### Vegetarians

Proceedings of a symposium on vegetarian nutrition held in July 1992 were published in *The American Journal of Clinical Nutrition* (*10*). Three presentations summarized the history of vegetarianism and discussed the global environmental impacts of meat consumption. Other groups of papers dealt with chronic diseases, vegetarian diets in relation to stage in the life cycle, protein nutriture, and practical aspects of vegetarianism. Several of these papers are summarized here (*11–14,16*).

In Norway, health effects of the Seventh-Day Adventist lifestyle, which advocates vegetarianism, were assessed by computer linkage of official church rosters with national health registries (*11*). Compared with matched controls, Adventist mothers gave birth to infants 99 g heavier, total cholesterol levels in Adventists were 33 mg/dL lower in men and 18 mg/dL lower in women, and total mortality was significantly lower in men, most of the difference being due to decreased

mortality from cardiovascular disease. The cancer rate was not significantly different from that in the general population. Benefits of the Adventist lifestyle decreased with age of joining the church until no benefit was seen in persons converting after the age of 35 y. This may reflect the influence of early diet on health late in life. It is also possible that older converts were less successful than life-long members in adopting the recommended lifestyle.

The Adventist Health Study in California was based on responses to a lifestyle questionnaire that included questions on diet, exercise, smoking, use of medications, and history of surgeries, chronic diseases, and allergies (*12*). Vegetarians reported significantly fewer overnight hospitalizations than nonvegetarians, and vegetarian women reported fewer surgeries. Vegetarians also reported fewer chronic diseases and allergies and roughly half the use of medications. Diseases that were significantly more prevalent in nonvegetarians included coronary heart disease, stroke, hypertension, diabetes, diverticulosis, and rheumatoid arthritis. There was no significant difference in prevalence of cancer.

Mean intake of animal protein in China is one-tenth of that in the USA and total protein intake is ~30% lower (*13*). Fat accounts for only 14.5 en% of the Chinese diet, yet total caloric intake is ~12% greater. Consumption of dietary fiber averages 33 g/d, compared to 11 g/d in the USA. Even so, regional dietary differences permitted an interesting analysis of diet and chronic degenerative diseases in 65 rural Chinese counties in 1983–1984. The diseases clustered geographically into two groups, one associated with poverty and one with affluence. Diseases of poverty included pneumonia, digestive disorders, infectious and parasitic diseases, and complications of pregnancy and birth. Diseases of affluence were coronary heart disease, diabetes, and several cancers. The chief correlate of diseases of affluence was plasma cholesterol concentration. Even at the prevailing low intake of fat and animal protein there was no evidence of a threshold for fat intake or plant-food enrichment beyond which no further effect on disease occurs. The applicability of ecologic data from rural China to an American setting was discussed.

Young and Pellett reviewed plant proteins in relation to human protein and amino acid nutrition (*14*). They discussed the ability of plant foods to supply adequate amounts of essential amino acids and dispelled several myths concerning the nutritive value of plant proteins, concluding that mixtures of plant foods can be nutritionally complete and well balanced. The position of the American Dietetic Association is that vegetarian diets are healthful and nutritionally adequate when properly planned, although vegans must take care to insure sufficient intake of vitamin $B_{12}$ (15). In the end, there are many health-promoting diets, both vegetarian and nonvegetarian, and there is general agreement on the goal of achieving health through diet (16). The controversy lies in how to achieve that goal. Although some arguments are self-serving, differences in opinion also reflect a clash of values rather than inadequacy or misuse of scientific information. To the extent that one's entire constellation of values, as well as taste and economics, is involved in dietary choices, science cannot help. The larger societal issues cannot be dismissed as "emotional" or "unscientific," but must be taken seriously.

## Smokers

A study in Great Britain documented major dietary differences between smokers and nonsmokers (17). The results indicated that smokers are at higher risk of chronic disease partly because of their dietary pattern and partly because of the extra demands placed on the nutrient supply by the effects of smoking. Compared with nonsmokers, smokers ate more white bread, sugar, cooked meat, butter, and whole milk and less whole-grain bread, high-fiber breakfast cereal, fruit, and carrots. Smokers had lower intakes of polyunsaturated fat, protein, carbohydrate, fiber, iron, carotene, and vitamin C. At the same dietary intake of carotenoids, smokers tended to have lower concentrations of β-carotene in their serum. There were no major differences between light and heavy smokers. The group of nonsmokers was not subdivided into "ex-smokers" and "never-smokers."

In September 1992 an international conference entitled "Tobacco Smoking and Nutrition: Influence of Nutrition on Tobacco-Associated Health Risks" was held in Lexington, Kentucky. Presentations and discussions were published by the New York Academy of Sciences (18). The purpose of the volume was to assemble information on the role of nutrition in the major diseases associated with smoking, including attempts to assess the scientific evidence related to the impact of nutritional factors on basic cellular and molecular mechanisms involved in reducing risks. Groups of presentations addressed free radical biology, cardiovascular disease, carcinogenesis and chemoprevention, lung disease, and dietary habits, all in relation to tobacco smoking. Some of the presentations are summarized (19–28). In his overview, Diana cited universally unsuccessful attempts to abolish smoking beginning in Constantinople in 1633, when Sultan Murad IV decreed the death penalty for smoking tobacco (19). Background information on the

prevalence of smoking and smoking-related illness and possible mechanistic links between them was presented. If it is not possible to eliminate the smoking habit, at least it appears possible to ameliorate the damage caused by it.

Studies in Scotland, where the incidence of coronary heart disease is very high, compared smokers and nonsmokers with respect to antioxidant intake and status, indexes of free-radical damage, and known risk factors for coronary heart disease and asked whether indexes of free radical–mediated peroxidation can be modified by increased intake of vitamin E (20). On the basis of classic risk factors, the entire study population was at high risk: there were no significant differences between smokers and nonsmokers in diet, blood cholesterol, body mass index, or blood pressure. However, the study confirmed that the Scottish diet is relatively poor in foods providing good sources of antioxidants. Roughly half of the subjects had plasma levels of vitamin E indicative of deficiency and >95% failed to meet the U.S. RDA for this vitamin. Average intake of vitamin C and carotenoids was also inadequate. Smokers had higher plasma concentrations of LDL cholesterol and triacylglycerides than nonsmokers, and smoking appeared to perturb specific components of the antioxidant defense system. Some of the changes in antioxidant status appear to be compensatory adaptations to a sustained oxidant load. Lipid peroxidation could be suppressed in both smokers and nonsmokers by pharmacologic doses of vitamin E (400 IU), but the effect of an increased nutritionally relevant intake (40 IU) is not known. In contrast, Bolton-Smith's summary of published work and new data on the intake of antioxidant vitamins in Scottish smokers and nonsmokers found significant differences between current smokers, ex-smokers, and never-smokers (21). Intakes of vitamin C, vitamin E, and carotene, but not retinol, were inversely related to the number of cigarettes smoked per day. With time, intakes of ex-smokers approached those of never-smokers, becoming equal 4 y after quitting. A study in England found that smokers had a substantially higher intake of saturated fat and lower intake of polyunsaturated fat than nonsmokers and ex-smokers (22). The food choices that lead to these differences may partly explain smokers' increased risk of coronary heart disease.

Bertram summarized mechanistic studies on the inhibition of chemically induced neoplastic transformation of C3H 10T1/2 cells by carotenoids (23). The action of carotenoids was qualitatively similar to that of retinoids, but 10- to 1000-fold higher concentrations of carotenoids were required. However, activity was not associated with conversion to retinoids. Like retinoids, carotenoids appear to inhibit transformation by up-regulating intercellular gap-junctional communication. In the C3H 10T1/2 model the gap junction is a conduit for growth-regulatory signals from normal to initiated cells, and these signals suppress transformation of the initiated cells.

Krinsky reviewed some of the evidence that carotenoids, tocopherols, and ascorbic acid can prevent mutagenesis and transformation and inhibit tumor cell growth in vitro (24). Some of these micronutrients are also anticarcinogenic in animal models. Relatively small doses of carotenoids are effective and again, it is the carotenoid structure and not provitamin A activity that is important. Although the three types of micronutrients lack structural similarity, they do have a functional similarity: all are antioxidants. Schwartz et al. briefly reviewed studies using the hamster buccal pouch model of DMBA-induced carcinogenesis in conjunction with β-carotene or α-tocopherol treatment (25). From these results they developed two schemes for the molecular and biochemical reprogramming of oncogenesis and the control of tumor cell growth, triggered by prooxidants and antioxidants. Both mechanisms invoked changes in phosphorylation and ultimately in gene transcription. β-Carotene treatment was thought to produce an oxidative stress resulting in induction of heat-shock proteins and phosphoproteins such as p53 (tumor suppressor form). Concomitantly, growth factors contributing to tumor cell growth and expression of the transcription factor c-fos were reduced. Other changes such as increased DNA fragmentation, accumulation of tumor cells in $G_0 \rightarrow G_1$, and morphologic alterations were consistent with programmed cell death. α-Tocopherol, bound to membrane-associated proteins, could inhibit development of peroxidation products that attack proteins, modifying their function and promoting their degradation.

Chung et al. reviewed their studies showing that phenethyl isothiocyanate and indole-3-carbinol (both found in cruciferous vegetables) inhibit formation of lung tumors induced by the tobacco-specific nitrosamine NNK (26). The effect of phenethyl isothiocyanate stems from inhibition of NNK-metabolizing enzymes, whereas indole-3-carbinol acts by inducing hepatic NNK-metabolizing enzymes. On a molar basis, phenethyl isothiocyanate is considerably more effective than indole-3-carbinol. The authors have also shown that the major polyphenol of green tea inhibits NNK-induced lung tumorigenesis, probably through antioxidant activity.

The "French Paradox" is that France, particularly southwestern France, has an anomalously low rate of mortality from coronary heart disease relative to the prevalence of common risk factors. The paradox is often discussed in terms of the apparent protection red wine affords against the toll of dietary indiscretion. However, smoking-related illness is also paradoxically low (27). Regular drinking of red wine appears to reduce the rates of both coronary heart disease and lung cancer in smokers.

While reiterating the view that cessation of tobacco use is the single largest cancer prevention and control measure, Subar and Harlan found evidence from the 1987 National Health Interview Survey that U.S. smokers are at a slight additional risk from low intake of critical food groups or nutrients (28). Except for intake of desserts (which are generally high in fat and low in fiber and micronutrients), current tobacco users always had dietary patterns contrary to current recommendations to consume less total fat, cholesterol, high-fat meat, and alcohol and more fruits, vegetables, and whole grains. In fact, the more cigarettes a smoker smoked the less he or she was likely to consume of the nutrients and foods considered protective against cancer. These dietary habits may also put smokers at increased risk of colon cancer and other illnesses not directly associated with tobacco, illustrating the potential for confounding in epidemiologic studies.

## Other

A telephone survey of 2706 adults considered representative for the USA demonstrated the need to correct carefully for confounding before coffee is blamed for illness (29). Results of the study supported the hypothesis that heavy coffee drinkers are least likely to practice other health-promoting behaviors. People in the top quartile of caffeine-containing coffee consumption (>5.6 cups/day) were more likely to smoke cigarettes and less likely to take vitamin supplements and to eat a healthful diet.

Data from the Honolulu Heart Program strengthened the case for a J-shaped curve relating alcohol consumption and mortality in middle-aged and elderly men (30). However, in view of the significantly increased risk of diseases of major public health importance attributable to high alcohol consumption and methodologic difficulties in establishing alcohol intake, the authors recommended caution in approving any population-wide increase in alcohol consumption. They discussed problems posed by a change in alcohol-drinking during a study and by misclassification of nondrinkers.

# HEALTH EFFECTS OF DIETARY COMPONENTS

## Lipids

FATTY ACIDS. Dannenberg and Reidenberg reviewed the pharmacologic effects of fatty acids and argued that these substances should be studied individually as drugs as well as energy sources (*31*). They considered regulation of eicosanoid metabolism, modification of carcinogenesis, effects on drug-metabolizing enzymes, cardiovascular effects, and regulation of membrane-protein function. Another review discussed the properties of lipids relevant to regulation of cell function, protein kinase C as a model for such regulatory studies, and the implications of the still-fresh realization that lipids function in diverse ways to modulate cell function (*32*).

Evidence is accumulating that *n*–3 fatty acids are essential nutrients for mammals, particularly for the developing mammalian brain and retina (*33*). Most data are from rodent studies and observations in preterm and full-term human infants, but some experiments have been done in monkeys. In humans, several neurologic disorders, including multiple sclerosis and polyunsaturated fatty acid lipidosis, are associated with *n*–3 fatty acid deficiency in specific brain sites and cellular fractions. As a guide for desirable fatty acid intakes, the diet of our Paleolithic ancestors is thought to have had a ratio of polyunsaturated to saturated fats of ~1.4 and an *n*–6/*n*–3 ratio of 5:1 or less. Fernandes et al. discussed the importance of *n*–3 fatty acids for normal growth and development, their beneficial effects for burn and surgical patients and in patients with autoimmune disease, and the protection they afford against cancer and cardiovascular disease (*34*). Sanders summarized the metabolic effects of marine *n*–3 fatty acids; their role in infant nutrition, reproductive function, immune function and inflammation, cancer, and cardiovascular disease; their interaction with antioxidant nutrients; and their pharmacologic use (*35*). Small amounts of marine oils may be important in meeting requirements for *n*–3 fatty acids. Larger amounts have pharmacologic effects that may be valuable in some situations so long as care is taken to prevent excessive lipid peroxidation. Evaluation of the short- and long-term safety of a fish oil (Pikasol®) for healthy volunteers and patients with various disorders found no adverse effects of likely clinical importance (*36*). Bleeding risk was minimal and the theoretical risk of immune incompetence remained theoretical. It is important, however, to insure an adequate dietary intake of antioxidants and/or to use fish oil products that have

antioxidants added. Muggli reviewed the literature in an attempt to determine how much vitamin E is required to compensate for the elevated demand caused by polyunsaturated fatty acids (*37*). Although there have been no systematic studies in humans and the "requirement" depends on the parameter selected to establish vitamin E deficiency, a ratio of 0.9 mg of vitamin E per gram of linoleic acid appears adequate and safe. A study in healthy men showed that, as expected, fish oil supplementation without additional vitamin E lowered plasma α-tocopherol concentrations (*38*). The data also hinted that both *n*–3 fatty acids and α-tocopherol modulate retinol and β-carotene concentrations in plasma and platelets.

Polyunsaturated fatty acids influence the transcription of some genes. In addition to this rapid and direct effect there is a long-term modulation of membrane composition that modifies hormonal signaling. Clarke and Jump discussed how *n*–6 and *n*–3 polyunsaturated fatty acids suppress hepatic lipogenesis, inhibit enzyme synthesis, regulate gene transcription, and influence the expression of stearoyl-CoA desaturase (*39*). The potency and structural requirements of fatty acid inhibitors were considered.

Studies in rats demonstrated diverse effects of *trans* fatty acids (*40*). Incorporation into phospholipids varied with the phospholipid species and was greater in rats fed soybean protein than in rats fed casein. Other interactions with dietary protein were also seen. There was some evidence that *trans* fat interfered with desaturation of linoleic acid.

In rats, qualitative differences in dietary fatty acids alter the fatty acid composition of subcellular fractions and these changes have a profound effect on activities of some key mitochondrial enzymes (ubiquinol-2-cytochrome *c* reductase, cytochrome oxidase, and ATPase) in the liver, heart, and brain (*41*). The extent of change depends on the duration of the diet and may reflect aging-related phenomena.

THE CHOLESTEROL CONTROVERSY. This year, the literature contained a paucity of new data (*42*), but there were several reanalyses and metaanalyses of old data, many analyses of the reanalyses, and a lot of opinions on the relationship between mortality and changes in serum cholesterol (*43–55*).

Pekkanen et al. reported on the association between past changes in serum cholesterol (1959–1974) and cause-specific mortality (1974–1989) in a cohort of Finnish men all of whom were free of symptomatic coronary heart disease in 1974 (*42*). There was a significant U-shaped association between change in serum cholesterol and coronary and all-cause mortality risk. The authors suggested that a decline in serum cholesterol and the high mortality associated with it may both be attributable to a third factor, such as increased prevalence of chronic diseases or other changes associated with aging. Upon combined analysis of various combinations of previously published data, using the entire statistical armamentarium, the small excess of noncardiovascular deaths associated with low or lowered cholesterol refused to go away but its explanation remained elusive.

Muldoon et al. pronounced the evidence linking low or lowered cholesterol with risk of death from suicide or trauma "suggestive but not conclusive" (*43*). A review of data from cohort studies, international studies, and randomized trials found no evidence that low or reduced serum cholesterol increases mortality from any cause other than hemorrhagic stroke (*44*). Marmot concluded that population-wide lowering of cholesterol levels "probably" isn't harmful and should substantially reduce deaths from coronary heart disease (*45*). LaRosa concluded that, even though attempts should still be made to resolve questions about the safety of low(ering) cholesterol, evidence linking high blood cholesterol with coronary atherosclerosis and cholesterol-lowering with its prevention is broad-based and definitive and concerns about lowering cholesterol should not interfere with public policy for reducing the prevalence of atherosclerosis (*46*). Simes considered confounding to be the most likely explanation for the persistent association between low cholesterol and noncoronary fatal events, although the possibility that the increased risk is directly due to low cholesterol has not been ruled out (*47*). MacMahon's analyses found that in cholesterol-reduction trials, the small excesses of cancer and trauma deaths among subjects allocated to active treatment were nonsignificant whether trials were analyzed singly or combined; moreover, the increases were neither specific to one agent nor consistent between trials of the same agent (*48*). This suggests that the results occurred by chance. Sullivan invoked basic science, examining the possible role of cholesterol metabolism in noncardiovascular disease (*49*). Although a variety of aberrant phenomena can be demonstrated in vitro at levels of cholesterol far below the physiologic range, in more naturalistic models low cholesterol is more favorable than high for most aspects of cell function. Cellular mechanisms for cholesterol homeostasis are generally adequate and there is no evidence in vivo for any catastrophic response when an organism is exposed to low cholesterol. However, inflammatory processes are consistently related to low cholesterol levels. This and other unrecognized con-

founders might explain much of the association between low cholesterol and noncardiovascular disease. Lewis and Tikkanen tried to find a causal or biologically plausible explanation for an inverse relationship between cholesterol and noncardiovascular, noncancer mortality and could not (*50*). Low cholesterol, however, is a fairly common consequence of disease. Stamler et al. concluded that reductions in mortality from coronary heart disease, major cardiovascular diseases, and all causes has paralleled favorable dietary trends in the USA (*51*). However, Allred concluded that dietary modification of serum cholesterol will confer minimal benefits in relation to risk of coronary heart disease for most people and even less benefit when all-cause mortality is considered (*52*). Grover reminded readers that an undisputed relationship between elevated serum cholesterol and the development of premature coronary heart disease exists only for middle-aged men (*53*). Beyond that the evidence is murky and consensus on all aspects of the cholesterol debate is still not possible. Roussouw and Gotto argued that observational data on low cholesterol and data from clinical cholesterol-lowering trials are unrelated (*54*). In the former, excess mortality is associated with cholesterol levels below 160 mg/dL, whereas minimum levels in clinical trials average ~230 mg/dL.

In May 1993 the British Hyperlipidaemia Association held a symposium to establish points of agreement in the cholesterol controversy and to develop guidelines for identifying individuals who might benefit from cholesterol-lowering therapy (*55*). The conclusions were that low cholesterol in itself is unlikely to cause increased mortality; that the benefits of lowering cholesterol are clearest for those with ischemic heart disease or those at high risk because of elevated cholesterol; that cholesterol lowering's lack of favorable effect on all-cause mortality in low-risk individuals remains unexplained; and that hypercholesterolemic persons who are clearly at high coronary risk should be treated. Shortcomings in the data were recognized, but there was better agreement on the benefit of lipid lowering than many recent reports would suggest.

## Fiber and Carbohydrates

Anderson et al. reviewed dietary fiber, emphasizing its sources and health benefits (*56*). They included practical suggestions for high-fiber diets and vegetarian meal plans.

Truswell provided another summary of the wide-ranging physiologic and health effects of dietary fiber (*57*). Insoluble fibers exert their major effects in the colon. They tend to produce the greatest increase in fecal weight and to shorten transit time. Viscous polysaccharides slow the emptying of fluids from the stomach and reduce the glycemic response to carbohydrate meals. Some soluble fibers such as pectin and guar gum are fermented efficiently so that little of the original material passes on to the feces; other fibers are fermented to differing extents. This fermentation has a number of consequences. Although soluble and viscous fibers tend to lower plasma LDL cholesterol without influencing HDL cholesterol or triacylglycerides, this property of oat fiber has been oversold. Cholesterol reduction is also possible with a large intake of vegetable foods. The direct effect is most likely due to pectin; indirect effects stem from the (usually) lower fat content of such diets. Although there are theoretical reasons why fiber should protect against gallstone disease, addition of bran to the diet may not prevent recurrence of stones. Dietary fiber was also discussed in relation to colon cancer, estrogens, and mineral metabolism.

In most diets, cereals are the major fiber source. Asp et al. discussed the physiologic effects of cereal fibers, which include fecal bulking, reduction of blood cholesterol levels, and decreasing postprandial glucose and hormone responses (*58*). Other properties of foods that can modify or simulate the effects of fibers were also mentioned. Soluble fiber in particular seems important for prevention and possibly treatment of diabetes and hyperlipidemia. Hopewell et al. reviewed the influence of soluble fiber on carbohydrate and lipid metabolism, the effects of specific fibers on glucose and insulin responses and possible mechanisms for these effects, and findings from some epidemiologic and clinical studies (*59*).

In the gastrointestinal tract of nonruminant mammals, microorganisms ferment plant fibers to short-chain (volatile) fatty acids. These products of microbial metabolism have a wide spectrum of biological effects, as reviewed by Bugaut and Bentéjac (*60*). The review focuses on digestion of bovine milk fat as a source of butyrate, the effects of propionate on cholesterol homeostasis, and the effects of butyrate on cell proliferation. It is notable that the daily production of short chain fatty acids in the human colon probably exceeds 300 mmol, yet fecal excretion averages only 10 mmol per day. Thus these substances are absorbed rapidly and nearly completely, by mechanisms that are discussed. Salvador et al. related the sugar composition of dietary fiber to the short-chain fatty acids produced during in vitro fermentation by a human fecal inoculum (*61*). The predominant sugars of the fibers tested (wheat bran, sugar beet, corn, pea, and cocoa) were arabinose, xylose, glucose, and uronic acids. The rate and more importantly the extent of

fermentation of a sugar, both absolute and relative to other sugars, varied considerably from fiber to fiber. Uronic acids were the principal source of acetic acid; propionic acid was derived principally from glucose but also from xylose and arabinose; and xylose was the major precursor of butyric acid. Thus it should be possible to predict the types and amounts of short-chain fatty acids produced by fermentation of any fiber whose structure and chemical composition are known.

Hazan and Madar compared the effects in rats of two different fiber blend supplements and corncobs, a previously untested fiber source (*62*). Their own dietary fiber mixture, compounded of apple pectin, orange pectin, locust bean gum, and corncob, was superior to the commercial supplement Fiber-Plus in its beneficial effects on intestinal function, blood glucose, and serum lipids. Corncob sharply reduced transit time and β-glucuronidase activity in the cecum, colon, and feces, suggesting its likely effectiveness in eliminating carcinogens. Corncob appears promising as a fiber source for enrichment or supplement.

The succinct position of The American Dietetic Association is that "the public be encouraged to increase consumption of dietary fiber from a variety of foods" (*63*). This is based on consideration of dietary fiber's beneficial and potentially adverse effects, studies of optimal intake, and fiber's potential in the management of disease. The Association found that "dietary fiber, incorporated into a balanced diet high in complex carbohydrates and low in fat, is an important part of a healthful lifestyle that emphasizes regular physical exercise and stress management... ."

Proceedings of a symposium on carbohydrates in human nutrition were published as a supplement to *The American Journal of Clinical Nutrition* (*64*). Introductory papers discussed the classification and analysis of food carbohydrates and carbohydrates as an energy source. Groups of papers and poster presentations dealt with the digestion, absorption, and elimination of carbohydrates, specific physiologic effects, diabetes, and product development.

A review by Stephen examined the benefits of increased dietary levels of complex carbohydrate (*65*). She noted dietary trends and recommendations in Canada and the USA and summarized benefits directly attributable to dietary starch (as separate from benefits of the increased fiber and decreased fat intake that tend to accompany a high-starch diet). In the small intestine, starchy foods reduce and delay the postprandial glycemic response. Some 8–10% of the starch consumed ("resistant" starch) escapes digestion and absorption in the small intestine and reaches the colon, where it is fermented by the colonic microflora. Compared to fiber, starch fermentation yields a higher proportion of butyrate, a preferred energy source for cells of the colonic mucosa. Butyrate is anticarcinogenic in vitro.

A supplement to *The American Journal of Clinical Nutrition* was devoted to health effects of dietary fructose (*66*). Sections covered the production, composition, and use of fructose; food sources and levels of intake in the USA; nutritional biochemistry and physiology; clinical aspects of fructose metabolism; the influence of fructose on food choice and physical performance; and the public health significance of dietary fructose.

## Vitamins and Antioxidants

Evidence from many sources is converging to reveal a dynamic interplay among antioxidant systems. Concomitantly, free radicals are being found at the root of a growing number of pathologic processes. According to Packer (*67*), if free radicals cause pathology and antioxidants neutralize free radicals, then higher levels of antioxidants should reduce pathology—and this is what epidemiologic and laboratory studies almost unanimously show. The evidence is strong for an oxidant–antioxidant balance in the body, which tilts toward disease when oxidants predominate and toward health when antioxidants predominate. Therefore, for economic reasons as well as to prevent unnecessary suffering, Packer makes three recommendations. First, an intensive campaign to educate the public about the role of antioxidants in nutrition, patterned after the program of information about the basic food groups. Second, he recommends antioxidant supplementation, especially for groups subject to high oxidant loads. This applies particularly to the fat-soluble antioxidants for people eating the recommended low-fat diet. Third, because people in greatest need of more antioxidants are frequently least able to afford them, he recommends subsidizing supplementation for low-income and certain ethnic groups and targeting educational efforts to these groups.

Ames et al. discussed the sources and effects of oxidants, concluding with the admonition to eat your five daily servings of fruits and vegetables (*68*). Four unavoidable endogenous sources account for most oxidants produced by the body. Hydrogen peroxide, hydroxyl radicals, and superoxide anion are by-products of aerobic respiration. Ames calculates that each cell of a rat processes $\sim 10^{12}$ oxygen molecules daily, and leakage of partially reduced reactive oxygen species is $\sim 2\%$. A second source is the activity of phagocytes, which destroy bacteria and virus-infected cells with an oxidative burst of nitric oxide, superoxide anion, peroxide, and

$OCl^-$. Third, hydrogen peroxide is a byproduct of the degradation of fatty acids and other molecules in peroxisomes. Finally, the induction of cytochrome P450 enzymes, one of the body's primary defenses against toxic foreign substances, also generates oxidant by-products. Exogenous sources of oxidants include tobacco smoke and diet. Because the body's allocation of resources favors reproduction at the expense of maintenance, cumulative unrepaired damage to somatic cells is thought to lie at the root of aging. Enhancing antioxidant defenses protects against disease and appears to retard some aspects of aging.

A review by Jackson asked whether dietary micronutrients influence the antioxidant capacity of body tissues (*69*). It concluded that manipulating the intake of vitamins E, A, and C and carotenoids can cause important changes in tissue antioxidant potential and noted that antioxidant nutrients also protect against cellular damage by processes not directly related to inhibition of free-radical reactions. However, inorganic cations associated with antioxidant enzymes or their synthesis (selenium, zinc, copper, manganese, and iron) are under close homeostatic control and, except in cases of deficiency, supplementation does not necessarily lead to enhanced antioxidant potential. Moreover, their potential for toxicity is considerable.

Bonorden and Pariza updated and augmented previous reviews of antioxidant nutrients, sources and biologic consequences of free radicals, and cellular mechanisms that protect aerobic organisms against oxidative damage (*70*). Summary tables and figures illustrated the sources, targets, and products of reactive oxygen species, the intracellular location of major antioxidant defense systems, and chemical aspects of the action of antioxidants. The toxicity (especially carcinogenic, mutagenic, and teratogenic potential) of carotenoids and $\alpha$-tocopherol was scrutinized and found to be negligible. However, supplemental $\alpha$-tocopherol is not recommended during anticoagulant therapy or for persons with an autoimmune disease. Vitamin C supplementation, though safe for most healthy persons, is not recommended for recurrent renal calcium oxalate stone-formers. Again, the authors found that supplementation with minerals poses the greatest risks. Nonnutritive antioxidants, antioxidant activity of peptides and amino acids, and the work of Pariza and his colleagues on conjugated linoleic acid were summarized. The safest and probably best way to improve one's antioxidant status is to—you guessed—eat fruits and vegetables.

A study in rats showed that multiple antioxidants provide better protection than a restricted number of antioxidants against oxidative damage (*71*). Groups of rats were fed diets deficient in vitamin E and selenium, supplemented with vitamin E and selenium, and supplemented with vitamin E and selenium plus additional fat-soluble antioxidants, water-soluble antioxidants, or both. After 6 weeks they were killed, slices of their livers were exposed to various oxidant challenges, and oxidation of heme proteins was measured. Although significant protection was conferred by vitamin E and selenium alone, in all cases inclusion of one or both of the additional supplements gave the greatest protection. The authors concluded that protection by vitamin E and selenium is significantly enhanced by increasing the diversity and amount of antioxidants in the diet.

Increasing the concentrations of antioxidants may not necessarily improve defense against oxidative stress. Cao and Cutler reported studies using an in vitro method developed in their laboratory to quantitate total oxygen-radical absorbance capacity (72). In this system, the hydroxyl radical absorbance capacity of Trolox (a water-soluble analogue of α-tocopherol) and uric acid decreased at high concentrations. These observations may have important implications for dietary supplementation and therapeutic use of antioxidants.

Rice-Evans and Diplock reviewed the status of antioxidant therapy for disease states associated with increased oxidative stress from endogenous sources (73). They emphasized coronary heart disease, reperfusion injury, and storage of organs for transplantation, examining the nature of the damaging radical(s), the mechanism of antioxidant protection, possible production and accumulation of harmful by-products of antioxidant action, and the antioxidant's ability to reach the relevant site of action. They concluded that a great deal of research is still necessary before effective antioxidant therapies can be designed. For optimal synergistic protection and health, evidence suggests that plasma levels of all antioxidants should exceed certain thresholds (74). Suggested threshold levels are 28–30 μmol/L for lipid-standardized vitamin E, 40–50 μmol/L for vitamin C, 0.4–0.5 μmol/L for carotene, and 2.2–2.8 μmol/L for lipid-standardized vitamin A. These values were determined from results of numerous epidemiologic, case–control, prospective, and intervention studies of cancer and cardiovascular disease. However, the efficacy of an optimal antioxidant status remains to be proved in randomized intervention trials. Meanwhile, the protective potentials of other antioxidant plant components await exploration.

In a thought-provoking paper, Reynolds highlighted some of the controversies surrounding use of vitamin supplements (75). He cites authors whose verdicts on the use of supplemental vitamins, based on virtually the same data, range from harmless to unnecessary to actually dangerous. The public needs clear guidelines, but advice is frequently confounded by political considerations, imprecise goals of supplementation, semantic disputes, and gaps in scientific knowledge. Reynolds discussed the concept of RDAs, noting that if and when a truly optimal level of intake for any vitamin can be agreed on it may be beyond the range of any reasonable *dietary* intake. "Perhaps the usefulness of the RDAs has diminished, disappeared, or needs modification...". He considered the case *for* supplements with reference to antioxidants and cancer and cardiovascular disease, vitamin B$_6$ and carpal tunnel syndrome, nicotinic acid and cardiovascular disease, and folic acid and neural tube defects. The case *against* supplements used as examples the masking of pernicious anemia in older people who take folate supplements and the toxicity that can result from over-aggressive supplementation. At present, the decision on whether to use supplements must be an informed individual decision, perhaps with advice from a personal physician. It should be based on evaluation of published data rather than on recommendations of groups that may use or interpret the data to promote their own agendas.

**VITAMIN C.** Rose and Bode described seven properties of an ideal free radical scavenger and reviewed the literature to evaluate ascorbic acid against these criteria (76). Ascorbate passed all tests. It accumulates in many body tissues, it is versatile, it can be compartmentalized in sites where protection is needed, it is widely available from plant foods, its redox state is precisely maintained under normal conditions, it is conserved by the kidneys, and under most conditions the toxicity of it and its products is minimal. Some exceptions to these general findings were mentioned. For example, ascorbate can have prooxidant activity in certain situations. Further, under experimental conditions, dehydroascorbic acid has some undesirable effects (it is oxidized ascorbic acid, or perhaps its degradation product, that is implicated in "ascorbic acid toxicity"). Nevertheless, ascorbic acid fills an important roll as free-radical scavenger because it is well suited chemically to react with oxidizing free radicals, it occurs at effective concentrations in the body, and it conforms well to the physiology of cellular transport and metabolism.

Gershoff reviewed studies of vitamin C in animal models, cell culture systems, and humans in an attempt to answer the question "How much vitamin C is enough?" (77). Protective effects against many cancers, cataract, cardiovascular disease, and infectious diseases have been demonstrated. The vitamin has multiple functions and its optimal intake is clearly greater than the ≤10 mg/d needed to prevent scurvy. But how much greater? Are megadoses beneficial? One approach to answering this is to determine the dietary intake necessary to achieve tissue saturation in adults. There is some evidence, not conclusive, that a body pool of 20 mg/kg would result in saturation. In most healthy nonsmoking adults this would result from an intake of 100–200 (certainly <500) mg/d. At higher intakes, absorption decreases (due to breakdown by intestinal bacteria) and urinary excretion increases. There seems to be little justification for recommending intakes higher than ~100 mg/d for the general public. This amount is readily available in any plant-rich diet.

Reduced glutathione (GSH) protects constituents in the cytosol and mitochondria against oxidative damage and helps maintain ascorbate and α-tocopherol in the reduced state. Because of interactions between glutathione and ascorbic acid, Johnston et al. examined the effect of supplemental vitamin C on erythrocyte glutathione in healthy adults (78). A daily supplement of 500 mg maintained GSH concentrations in the blood and improved the overall antioxidant capacity of the blood, but no additional benefit was seen with 2000 mg.

Ascorbic acid was shown to either increase or decrease the oxidative modification of LDL by macrophages, depending on whether the LDL preparation was initially unoxidized (fresh) or mildly oxidized (stored at 3°C for 10 wk) (79). In the absence of macrophages, ascorbic acid itself modified the mildly oxidized LDL to greatly increase its subsequent uptake by macrophages. The authors concluded that if mildly oxidized LDL is present in plasma or in atherosclerotic lesions, it cannot be assumed that ascorbate would protect it from further modification. This may explain why epidemiologic studies have yielded conflicting evidence on the protective effect of vitamin C against cardiovascular disease.

**B VITAMINS.** A short review discussed reports that riboflavin protects against oxidative damage by oxidized heme proteins (80). A scheme was proposed whereby exogenous riboflavin interacts with an NADPH-dependent methemoglobin reductase to protect tissues from damage resulting when peroxide reacts with heme proteins. Although flavin reduction by this enzyme is sluggish at normal erythrocyte levels of flavin, it is rapid at elevated levels. Riboflavin protects the isolated rabbit heart against reperfusion injury and protects against oxidative lung and brain injury in rat models. These observations raise interesting questions about a possible function for NADPH-dependent methemoglobin reductase in combating clinically relevant situations and about the nutritional and therapeutic implications of this function.

Folic acid has long been known to prevent the megaloblastic anemia of pregnancy, but only recently have its protective effects against cervical cancer, neural tube defects, and atherosclerosis been recognized (81). The rise and fall of folate concentrations in the rat uterus accompanying the estrus cycle suggested that folic acid was involved in proliferation of uterine cells and led to the finding that adequate daily intake of folate minimizes risk of cervical dysplasia and cancer. Various lines of evidence converged to reveal the association between poor maternal folate status and fetal neural tube defects. Cumulative evidence from other studies has gradually linked methionine metabolism and folate with atherosclerosis, homocysteinemia, and neural tube defects. Russell reviewed the case for fortifying foods with folate (82). Although ample dietary intake is easily possible without fortification or supplements, there is evidence of poor folate status in the elderly, and low-income women may have difficulty achieving adequate folate nutrition. Recognizing the importance of adequate folate intake, especially for women of child-bearing age, Zimmerman and Shane focused on potentially adverse effects of supplementation (83). Although most people tolerate folic acid supplements well up to the maximum recommended level of 4 mg, certain individuals may suffer adverse effects. Folic acid can mask signs of vitamin $B_{12}$ deficiency, antagonize the action of anticonvulsant drugs, elicit hypersensitivity reactions, and possibly interfere with zinc nutriture. Pharmacologic doses should thus remain available only by prescription.

Because vitamin $B_{12}$ (cobalamin) is not synthesized by any plant, there is continuing concern about the cobalamin status of persons eating a strict vegan diet. The issue has been complicated by disagreement over which indicator of cobalamin status to use as a criterion of deficiency. Herbert discussed the staging of vitamin $B_{12}$ status in vegetarians (84). He identified four stages of negative cobalamin status: serum depletion, cell depletion, biochemical deficiency, and clinical deficiency. Markers and consequences of each stage were summarized. Effects of folate and ascorbic acid, aging, and genetic factors were discussed.

**VITAMIN A AND CAROTENOIDS.** The subject of the Fifteenth Marabou Symposium was "Vitamin A: From Molecular Biology to Public Health" (85). Several of the presentations are summarized elsewhere in this volume.

Recent advances in understanding the actions of vitamin A, its active metabolite retinoic acid, and its dietary precursor β-carotene were summarized by Ross and Ternus (*86*). They reviewed the dietary and cellular forms of vitamin A, metabolism and activation of retinol, characteristics and functions of retinoid-binding proteins, regulatory and hormonal functions of retinoic acid and their mechanisms, therapeutic roles for retinoids, and the functions, metabolism, and health benefits of β-carotene. Approaches to determining an RDA for β-carotene have included estimating the β-carotene content of recommended diets. Not surprisingly, this value significantly exceeds actual intake determined from a continuing survey by the USDA. Recommended menus provided 10,000–11,000 IU of vitamin A per day and 5.2–6.0 mg of β-carotene. Actual consumption averaged 5500 IU of vitamin A and 1.5 mg of β-carotene.

Vitamin A and carotenoids show both similarities and differences in physiologic aspects of their antioxidant activity (*87*). Both can either accept or donate electrons and carotenoids can also quench singlet oxygen; thus theoretically, both can participate in a biological antioxidant network. However, retinol and its active metabolites are largely bound in clefts of specific retinoid-binding proteins and tend to be protected by other antioxidants rather than conferring protection. Carotenoids, in contrast, are widely distributed in lipoproteins, membranes, and the lipid phases of intracellular structures, usually together with vitamin E. In vitro they interact with other antioxidants; the situation in vivo is less clear. The structures, functions, actions, and interactions of carotenoids in biological systems were reviewed by Krinsky (*88*).

For historical reasons relating to early studies of vitamin A, there is a persistent idea that β-carotene (indisputably the major—though not the only—dietary precursor of vitamin A) is the only carotenoid of consequence (*89*). However, carotenoids have biologic activities unrelated to provitamin A activity. Differences in activity of various carotenoids are related to subtle structural differences and the localization of the molecules within tissues and cells. β-Carotene (and in plants, other carotenoids having 9 or more conjugated double bonds) are photoprotective as a consequence of their ability to quench excited singlet oxygen. Lutein is the carotenoid most strongly associated with oxidative resistance of LDL; β-carotene supplements improve protection only when initial levels are pathologically low. Lutein, lycopene, and β-cryptoxanthin all quench lipid peroxy radicals more efficiently than β-carotene, and in vitro they are more effective than α-tocopherol. Smoking reduces circulating levels of lutein, β-cryptoxanthin, and α-carotene as well as β-carotene (but not lycopene). Distributions of the carotenoids are qualitatively similar in

blood and most tissues, but xanthophylls predominate in the eye and HDL.

The singlet oxygen–quenching ability of naturally occurring carotenoids increases with the number of conjugated double bonds but also varies with chain structure and the presence and nature of functional groups (*90*). Acyclic compounds are more effective than cyclic. Conjugated keto groups and a cyclopentane ring stimulate quenching, whereas hydroxy, epoxy, and methoxy groups reduce effectiveness. The most effective singlet oxygen quenchers were acyclic carotenoids found in photosynthetic bacteria.

A volume in the *Annals of the New York Academy of Sciences* covered subjects relating to carotenoids and health (*91*). Oral and poster presentations addressed the chemical and physical reactions of carotenoids, absorption and tissue distribution of dietary carotenoids, molecular actions of carotenoids, and their role in preventing chronic disease.

**VITAMIN E.** Abstracts of presentations at the 2nd Vitamin E Symposium of the German Society for Fat Science were published in *Fat Science and Technology* (*92*). Groups of reports addressed vitamin E's metabolism in humans, protective actions, role in human disease and pathologic conditions, and therapeutic uses.

Two types of study demonstrated a prooxidant role for vitamin E in lipid peroxidation. In vitro, α-tocopherol in detergent suspension is rapidly oxidized when exposed to $Cu^{2+}$ (*93*). In dispersions containing phospholipids and traces of their hydroperoxide derivatives, $Cu^{2+}$ alone initiates lipid peroxidation but this reaction is strongly stimulated by α-tocopherol. Because the consumption of α-tocopherol is identical in the presence and absence of phospholipids, any antioxidant effect is ruled out. These observations suggest that vitamin E's prooxidant effect stems from its ability to reduce $Cu^{2+}$ to $Cu^+$, which produces reactive alkoxyl radicals from lipid hydroperoxides. Whereas α-tocopherol is the most active chain-breaking antioxidant in extracted LDL lipid, it can be a strong prooxidant for the LDL itself (*94*). In an aqueous dispersion, the induction of ROO· in LDL by an azo initiator of lipid peroxidation was faster in the presence of α-tocopherol than in its absence. It was inhibited by ascorbic acid, ubiquinol-10, and small phenolic antioxidants but not by uric acid. In a cell culture medium, LDL peroxidation induced by an azo initiator or by transition metals was accelerated by increasing the α-tocopherol content of the LDL. The authors proposed that a reaction between ROO· and α-tocopherol initiates LDL peroxidation, and the inability of α-tocopherol radicals to escape from the LDL particle propagates a radical chain via reaction with polyunsaturated fatty acids within the particle. The chain is terminated by capture of a second radical from the aqueous medium. The authors concluded that peroxidation of LDL can only be prevented by agents (such as ascorbic acid or BHT) that eliminate the α-tocopherol radical.

VITAMIN D. Wiseman reported studies of vitamin D as a membrane antioxidant (95). She showed that vitamin $D_3$, its active metabolite 1,25-dihydroxycholecalciferol, its precursor 7-dehydrocholesterol, and vitamin $D_2$ all inhibited iron-dependent liposomal lipid peroxidation. 7-Dehydrocholesterol was most effective; it was also more effective than cholesterol, but less effective than ergosterol, tamoxifen, and 4-hydroxytamoxifen. These relationships provided insight into structure–function relationships in this group of compounds. The anticancer action of vitamin D was discussed in the context of these results, with special reference to tamoxifen.

CONSTITUENTS OF TEA AND SPICES. Infusions of black tea containing theaflavins and thearubigin may inhibit lipid peroxidation in biological systems in the same way as green tea infusions containing epicatechins (96). In rat-liver homogenates, theaflavins and thearubigin inhibited *tert*-butyl hydroperoxide–induced lipid peroxidation more effectively than glutathione, ascorbic acid, α-tocopherol, BHT, and BHA and had roughly the same effectiveness as several epicatechins. When lyophilized tea infusions, rather than purified compounds, were tested, green and black tea were about equally potent.

Plasma levels of α-tocopherol were 87% lower in rats fed a diet containing 30% perilla oil than in controls fed red palm oil, and lipid peroxidation as measured by TBA-reactive substances was three times as great (97). Addition of tea catechins to these diets significantly increased α-tocopherol concentrations in both groups, compared with rats fed the same diet without catechins; there was a small but significant decrease in TBA-reactive substances when the perilla oil diet was supplemented with catechins. No dietary treatment altered the deformability of erythrocytes, indicating that the erythrocytes were not severely enough affected by lipid peroxidation to influence their deformability.

Chlorogenic acid occurs in tea leaves and coffee beans. When administered by stomach tube daily for three days, it suppressed lipid peroxidation induced in rat liver by carbon tetrachloride or cobalt-60 irradiation (98). A clear effect of chlorogenic acid dose was seen in the $CCl_4$ challenge, with the highest dose, 800 µmol per kilogram of body weight, providing nearly total protection. A dose of 200 µmol/kg gave complete protection against the irradiation challenge. Ellagic acid and α-tocopherol were effective at somewhat lower doses. In further studies, ellagic acid prevented radiation-induced lipid peroxidation in the placentas and fetuses of pregnant rats as well as in the serum, liver, spleen, and brain of the rats themselves (99).

A diet supplemented with 1% turmeric and fed to rats for 10 wk before challenge with 30 mg of $Fe^{2+}$ per kilogram of body weight reduced lipid peroxidation in liver homogenates and microsomes by roughly one third (100). The activities of superoxide dismutase, catalase, and glutathione peroxidase in liver homogenates of turmeric-fed rats were ~20% higher than in controls, indicating that dietary turmeric reduces lipid peroxidation by enhancing the activities of antioxidant enzymes. Other feeding experiments in rats demonstrated that a variety of dietary antioxidants and lipids modulate lipid peroxidation in the liver by influencing antioxidant defense systems (101). Polyunsaturated fatty acids reduced levels of vitamin E and activities of several antioxidant enzymes but did not influence levels of ascorbic acid and glutathione. Curcumin, eugenol, and vitamin E significantly enhanced antioxidant enzyme activity. In rat-brain homogenates, addition of curcumin (0.25–20.0 mM) caused a dose-dependent reduction in $Fe^{3+}$-stimulated lipid peroxidation, as measured by formation of TBARS (102). To a lesser extent at the lower concentrations, curcumin also inhibited peroxidation stimulated by $Fe^{2+}$ and $Fe^{3+}$–ADP-ascorbate. In all systems, inhibition was >90% at 10 mM. In intact mice and in rat-liver homogenates, monomeric and dimeric phenylpropanoid constituents of mace inhibited both enzymatic and nonenzymatic lipid peroxidation (103). These observations are consistent with a direct scavenging of free radicals or active oxygen species by the antioxidants. Investigations using several models revealed structure–function relationships in the effects of eugenol, isoeugenol, and dehydrozingerone on lipid peroxidation (104). In rat-brain homogenates, isoeugenol was the most active inhibitor of lipid peroxidation induced by $Fe^{2+}$, $Fe^{3+}$, and cumene-hydroperoxide. It was also a potent scavenger of superoxide anion generated by the xanthine–xanthine oxidase system, whereas eugenol acted in this system by inhibiting the enzyme. The authors postulated that the high antioxidant activity of isoeugenol is due to the presence of a conjugated double bond, which enhances the stability of the phenoxyl radical. An electron-withdrawing keto group at the *para* position in dehydrozingerone decreases the stability of this compound.

**ANTINUTRIENTS.** Thompson reviewed the beneficial and adverse health effects of "antinutrients" widely found in plant foods (*105*). These substances are particularly common in legumes and cereals. Some studies have shown that phytic acid, lectins, tannins, saponins, and amylase and protease inhibitors reduce the availability of nutrients and inhibit growth; phytoestrogens and lignans have been implicated in infertility problems. However other studies have shown that phytic acid, lectins, tannins, amylase inhibitors, and saponins reduce blood glucose and insulin responses to starchy foods and reduce plasma levels of cholesterol and triacylglycerides. Moreover, some of the substances are associated with reduced cancer risk. Perhaps antinutrients have received too much bad press. Perhaps they should be reevaluated and renamed.

## Minerals

Data from the Baltimore Longitudinal Study of Aging indicate that many people in this well-educated and presumably well-nourished population do not consume adequate amounts of calcium, iron, magnesium, and zinc (*106*). Even subjects who took supplements did not receive adequate amounts of some minerals. More women than men were at risk. Median intake of calcium was below the RDA for unsupplemented women and for supplemented women older than 60 y. About 25% of women under 50 and 10% of women over 50 consumed less than two-thirds of the RDA for iron. All age groups of both men and women had median intakes below the RDA for magnesium.

A number of minerals (copper, selenium, iron, manganese, and zinc) are contained in antioxidant enzymes and in this capacity may be considered biological antioxidants. Johnson and Fischer reviewed the role of minerals in protection against free radicals (*107*). The enzymes that require these minerals cannot entirely explain the minerals' role in disease processes. There are reliable markers of nutritional status for iron and selenium, but not for copper. Selenium is clearly protective against heart disease and cancer but the authors could find no definitive evidence for any relationships between copper and chronic diseases. Both iron-deficiency and iron-overload diseases were discussed. Bettger compared and contrasted the antioxidant functions of zinc and selenium (*108*). Selenium's major role is as an integral part of Se-dependent glutathione peroxidases, a group of enzymes that catalyze the destruction of water-soluble and in some cases membrane-bound hydroperoxides. In contrast, zinc acts as an antioxidant only at specific sites. Although it has a structural role in Cu,Zn superoxide dismutase, the enzyme's activity not only is not decreased by zinc deficiency but may actually be depressed when zinc intake is high. One way in which zinc exerts its site-specific effect is by competing with iron and copper for binding to cell membranes and certain proteins, thus displacing the redox-active metals. Another way is by binding the sulfhydryl groups in proteins, protecting them from oxidation. Thus unlike selenium, zinc does not directly control tissue peroxide levels but does protect specific molecules against oxidative and peroxidative damage.

Naghii reviewed the role of boron in nutrition and metabolism (*109*). The boron content of plants varies considerably with plant species and growth stage and agricultural practices. It is also influenced by soil geochemistry and such soil characteristics as texture, pH, temperature, and moisture content. Moreover, different analytic methods yield widely differing results. The concentration of boron in water also varies widely with geographic source, and boron sees some use as a food preservative. As a result, estimates of dietary intake of boron range from 0.2 to 41 mg/d. Boron appears to interact with other nutrients to regulate mineral (and bone) metabolism, perhaps through effects on testosterone and β-estradiol. Depressed growth and reduced concentrations of steroid hormones in the blood are signs of boron deficiency. Large amounts are generally well tolerated and interact favorably with calcium and vitamin D metabolism. Boron's wide-ranging effects, including association with chronic diseases, were discussed and postulated biochemical mechanisms for these effects were summarized.

## Nucleotides

There has been persistent interest in the importance of dietary nucleotides, particularly in infant nutrition. A roundtable symposium, "Nucleotides and Nutrition," was held in New Orleans in March 1993 (*110*). Topics ranged from nucleotide biochemistry, physiology, and metabolism to dietary sources of nucleotides to immune and nonimmune system responses and the role of nucleotides in adult nutrition. Human milk contains considerably greater amounts of nucleotides than cow's milk and unsupplemented infant formulas, and these nucleotides may have significant effects in infants (*111*). Moreover, the major nucleotide in cow's milk is orotic acid, which appears to be poorly salvaged by human infants. As new foods are added to an infant's diet, any that contain cellular elements will provide dietary nucleotides. The increase in urinary uric acid after consumption of organ meats, fish, and poultry is presumptive evidence that dietary nucleotides are absorbed. Plant foods and dairy products are poor sources of nucleotides. Jyonouchi summarized nucleotide actions on humoral immune responses (*112*). Observations in mice suggest that these actions reflect local immune responses, perhaps at sites of inflammation. Under conditions of relative nucleotide deficiency, dietary mononucleotides and nucleosides may be incorporated fairly rapidly into the tissue nucleotide pool and they appear to help restore T-cell–dependent humoral responses. Carver reported cellular immune effects of dietary nucleotides, as well as intestinal and hepatic system effects (*113*). She suggested that de novo synthesis and salvage of nucleotides is metabolically costly and that dietary nucleotides may optimize the function of rapidly dividing tissues. Supplemental dietary nucleotides may be particularly important for formula-fed infants, whose growth is rapid and whose diet is low in nucleotides relative to human milk. Mechanisms for the effects of dietary nucleotides and the importance of these effects are poorly understood. Many questions remain concerning effects of nucleotides on gut-associated lymphoid tissue, the metabolic fate of dietary nucleotides, nucleosides, and nucleic acids in humans (particularly neonates), the bioavailability of cellular nucleic acids in human milk to the breast-fed infant, and the contribution of individual nucleotides to the observed effects. Uauy reviewed nonimmune system responses to dietary nucleotides (*114*). Bifidobacteria predominate in the fecal flora of breast-fed infants and infants fed a nucleotide-supplemented commercial formula, whereas enterobacteria predominate in infants fed unsupplemented formula. Dietary supplementation with nucleotides also modulates lipoprotein metabolism in very young human infants and improves liver function in rats after liver damage. Evidence for the role of nucleotides in adult nutrition was reviewed by Van Buren et al. (*115*). It is noteworthy that most enteral and all parental nutrient solutions are nucleotide-free. In a clinical study of septic and other critically ill patients, nucleotide supplementation significantly improved immune function and non-significantly shortened hospitalization. Nucleotide supplementation also improved immune function postoperatively in a group of gastrointestinal cancer patients. The clinical manifestation of this improvement was a 70% reduction in infectious and wound complications and a consequent 22% reduction in length of hospitalization. In animal models, nucleotide supplementation has reduced graft-vs.-host disease and rejection of cardiac transplants, delayed cutaneous hypersensitivity, and improved resistance to bacterial and fungal infections. Dietary nucleotides can restore lost immune

function even under conditions of protein starvation and weight loss.

Dietary nucleotides influence lipoprotein metabolism in preterm human neonates (*116*) and the lipid composition of liver microsomes in weanling rats (*117*). In human infants, nucleotide supplementation increased concentrations of all plasma lipoproteins, primarily by increasing the apolipoprotein content (*116*). The plasma esterification rate also increased, but total cholesterol concentrations were unchanged. The effect was significantly smaller for term than for preterm infants. Weanling rats fed nucleotide-supplemented diets had higher levels of long-chain $n$–3 and $n$–6 polyunsaturated fatty acids in the phospholipids of their liver microsomes; the ratio of cholesterol to phospholipid phosphorus was relatively constant (*117*). The authors concluded that the nucleotides were acting through a decreased $\Delta 9$ desaturate activity and increased activities of $\Delta 5$ and $\Delta 4$ desaturases.

## Fermented Foods and Related Bacteria

Microorganisms or enzymes are used in the production of fermented foods to cause desired biochemical changes and modification of the flavor and nutrient content of the food. The history of this ancient technology, its importance in today's world, and challenges for the future were reviewed by Campbell-Platt (*118*).

Chandan and Shahani discussed the definition of yogurt, the taxonomy and production of yogurt starters, aspects of yogurt production, quality control, and the physicochemical, nutritional, and health properties of yogurt (*119*). Yogurt's primary prophylactic and therapeutic effects seem to stem from antibiosis attributed to fermentation products and bacterial enzymes. Undissociated organic acids are bacteriostatic or bactericidal to a variety of foodborne pathogens, including *Salmonella enteritidis, Escherichia coli,* and *Yersinia enterocolitica.* Antibiosis due to bacteriocins and other substances may be important in the gastrointestinal tract as well as in food systems, but this has not been demonstrated convincingly. However, antibiosis due to deconjugation of bile salts by lactic acid bacteria has been demonstrated, and these deconjugated bile salts suppress growth of foodborne pathogens. Hypocholesterolemic and anticarcinogenic effects of fermented milk products have also been reported. Lactose intolerance and immune modulation were briefly discussed.

In January 1992 an interdisciplinary panel was convened to attempt to reach a consensus on the health attributes of lactic cultures and their significance in fluid milk products (*120*). The panel discussed lactose digestion, diarrheal diseases, chronic kidney disease, bacterial adherence, stimulation of the immune system, reduction of cholesterol levels, constipation, and safety. For each of these the legitimacy of health claims and research needs were evaluated. Promising results have been reported with lactic cultures in relation to lactose digestion, some diarrheal illnesses, small bowel overgrowth associated with chronic kidney disease, and protection from colon cancer, but additional confirmatory research is needed.

A volume in the *Food Science and Technology* series reviewed recent developments in the study of lactic acid bacteria, bearing in mind important weaknesses of many such studies (*121*). Numerous health foods, "functional foods," and pharmaceutical products bear health claims based on characteristics of specific strains of lactic acid bacteria, many of which have been poorly identified and inadequately studied. Moreover, health benefits are too frequently judged by subjective criteria without regard for accepted standards of clinical investigation. This reference gives an overview of the taxonomy and general physiology of lactic acid bacteria and discusses the genetics of these bacteria and technologic aspects of manufacturing functional lactic acid starters. Other chapters discuss the effects of lactic acid bacteria in health and disease and their use as animal probiotics. Salminen et al. reviewed the properties and physiologic function of probiotic bacteria (*122*). Lactic acid bacteria have proven or putative benefits for prevention and treatment of some forms of bacterial diarrhea and related conditions such as lactose intolerance, constipation, *Helicobacter pylori* infection, irritable bowel syndrome, and antibiotic-associated diarrhea. They act mainly by preserving a normal intestinal flora and promoting resistance to colonization by pathogens. Specific adherence to the intestinal mucosa and production of antibacterial substances are probably involved. Limited data suggest that lactic acid bacteria can reduce the side effects of radiotherapy and have therapeutic potential for patients with hepatic encephalopathy. There is also some evidence of antitumor activity.

There is also active interest in the probiotic action and other potential benefits of the bifidobacteria, which (because they are indigenous to humans) are thought to have a better chance than lactobacilli of surviving passage through the upper digestive tract and colonizing the colon (*123–126*). Ballongue comprehensively reviewed this group of organisms from their discovery to recent studies of their benefits for health (*123*). Relevant aspects of *Bifidobacterium*'s morphology, physiology, antibiotic resistance, culture, cell wall composition, mechanisms of adhesion, and molecular biology were summarized. Implantation and colonization in the neo-

nate were given considerable attention. The identification of bifidobacteria is difficult at the species level, and phenotypic and genotypic methods of identification were reviewed at length. There was a general discussion of the composition of the human intestinal flora, factors affecting it, and its role and effects. Hoover briefly reviewed the activity and potential benefits of the bifidobacteria (*124*). Because bifidobacteria are indigenous and well adapted to the human gastrointestinal tract, Hoover considers the key question to be whether dietary strategies can result in a sustained above-normal population level of these organisms with consequent long-term benefits for health. The answer from one study in healthy young adults is a qualified "maybe" (*125*). Because diet-induced changes in the colonic microflora seem to play a role in colonic carcinogenesis, the effects of yogurt on the fecal flora and several indexes of colon cancer risk were evaluated. Subjects ate 500 mL/d of conventional yogurt or yogurt enriched with *Bifidobacterium longum* and 5 g of lactulose. After 3 wk both groups had significantly higher levels of fecal bifidobacteria; counts of aerobes and anaerobes were unchanged. The supplemented yogurt caused elevated breath hydrogen and accelerated mouth-to-cecum transit time, but there were no differences in mean mouth-to-anus transit time, stool weight and pH, or fecal concentrations of short-chain fatty acids, bile acids, and neutral steroids. The authors concluded that the human fecal flora is extremely resistant to this kind of dietary manipulation. Meanwhile, spurred by the establishment and efforts of the Japan Bifidus Foundation, Japan has conducted active bifidobacteria research and development and bifidus food products are widely used (*126*). Ishibashi and Shimamura summarized applied research findings and some aspects of bifidus product development.

Esaki et al. studied the antioxidative activity and associated chemical components of traditional fermented soybean products cultured with *Aspergillus oryzae* ("miso"), *Bacillus natto* ("natto"), and *Rhizopus oligosporus* ("tempeh") (*127*). Fermented products underwent virtually no lipid peroxidation during 20–30 days of storage, whereas steamed soybean products showed considerable lipid peroxidation. As demonstrated by HPLC analysis, tocopherol content was little changed during fermentation but the free isoflavones daidzein and genistein increased sharply in tempeh and miso, accompanied by a decrease in the isoflavone glucosides daidzin and genistin. In fermented natto there was an increase in the antioxidative activity of a water-soluble fraction. Eighteen *Aspergillus* strains were evaluated for their effects on the antioxidative activity of aqueous ethanolic extracts of fermented soybeans.

# DESIGNER FOODS AND BIOTECHNOLOGY

In discussing the genetic engineering of foods, Harlander ranged from specific successful applications to societal and international issues (*128*). The applications discussed were production of enzymes, food ingredients, starter cultures, and peptide growth hormones; modification of nutritional quality; "antisense" technology; gene transfer in production agriculture; and use of transgenic animals to produce pharmaceutical products. Unresolved regulatory and labeling issues were thoughtfully considered. Although the initial focus of applied biotechnology was on improving agricultural productivity and providing substitutes for traditional products, the potential exits to profoundly modify the food supply. A majority of consumers interviewed in a survey had little knowledge or understanding of the technology itself, but they were interested in learning more and believed that benefits from biotechnology were imminent. Younes et al. view biotechnology as a rapid, precise, and powerful extension of traditional breeding techniques (*129*). They reviewed applications of biotechnology and types of novel foods, emphasizing issues of safety and regulation for microbial, plant, and animal products. Stressing the differences between evaluating the safety of single chemicals or simple chemical mixtures and that of whole foods, they urged a decision-tree approach to safety evaluation of novel foods and presented a general scheme for such an approach. At the same time, they acknowledged the need to consider the public requirement for authentic and nutritionally adequate food that is subjected only to minimal necessary processing.

Berkowitz and Kryspin-Sørensen reviewed some safety issues (other than impacts on nutritional quality or the environment) that could arise in connection with transgenic fish (*130*). Because many food fish are occasionally associated with toxins and safe fish may have poisonous relatives, the possibility arises that transgenes might turn on unexpressed toxin genes in species that do not normally express them. The common toxins in fish, however, are of exogenous origin; their genes are not part of the fish genome. Moreover, toxin-producing organisms have a limited host range, making it unlikely that introduction or activation of a toxin-resistance gene in the fish would render additional species toxic to humans. The safety of the transgene product should also be evaluated in terms of its effect on the health of the fish because the safety of unhealthy animals is always suspect. The potential allergenicity of genetically engineered foods is well recognized. The authors concluded

that if the transgene and its product are safe and the fish are healthy, the transgenic fish will probably be as safe as its parent line.

Criteria similar to those above (*130*) were discussed with relation to the safety of genetically engineered plants (*131*). The effect of the transgene and its product on the health and agronomic traits of the plant and on the processing and sensory characteristics of the food product must be considered. The gene product must be safe for human consumption; again, the question of allergenicity is important. Possible effects of introduced marker genes and regulatory genes are also of concern. Nine safety criteria for a genetically engineered protein are the source of the gene coding for it; its functional and structural similarity to other food proteins; its structural similarity to known or suspected toxins and antinutrients; its biological activity in the source and host organisms; host-specific modifications (e.g., glycosylation); known or potential allergenicity; digestibility; effects of processing; and the anticipated human intake. Many of these considerations also apply to the safety of lipid and carbohydrate constituents altered as a result of genetic engineering. Finally, unintended untoward effects may result from perturbation of the transgenic plant's metabolism. Because many consumers have a healthy skepticism toward the "genetic revolution," it is crucial that safety issues be addressed promptly and thoroughly by scientists and developers together. Another review discussed techniques used in genetic engineering of plants and genetic engineering for enhanced quality and again reviewed the safety and public acceptance of transgenic plant products (*132*). Resolution of both narrow (safety) and broader (e.g., environmental) science-related concerns and science-nonrelated (e.g., societal or value-related) issues can only be achieved by frank and respectful communication among all concerned.

Teuber described genetic engineering techniques in food microbiology and enzymology, using the chymosin and baker's yeast systems as examples (*133*). He discussed general aspects of safety, regulation and labeling, and acceptance by both consumers of the products and the general public. The chief concerns about biotechnology are related to socioeconomic, environmental, health, and ethical questions and "trust." Some suggested rules to "calm public outrage" are to accept and involve the public as a legitimate partner, to plan carefully and evaluate performance, to listen to the audience, to be honest, frank, and open, to meet the needs of the media, and to speak clearly and with compassion.

Ulbricht reviewed a British Nutrition Foundation task force report and a UK government white paper, both relating to health and the food industry (*134*). He foresees a trend toward polarization between fast-food outlets and supermarkets selling more and more convenience foods, on the one hand, and specialty shops catering for those who desire minimally processed quality foods, on the other. He also suggests that the pharmaceutical giants will become increasingly involved in producing foods ("nutriceuticals") intended not only to prevent chronic diseases but to treat them. Hunt discussed a category of compounds called nutraceuticals, which has been proposed as a new regulatory category separate from foods or drugs (*135*). She reviewed the terminology related to the concept of nutraceuticals, and current FDA definitions and regulations pertaining to foods, drugs, medical foods, and food additives. Much of the debate centers around health claims and scientific criteria for them and involves issues of labeling and regulation. These issues should be resolved promptly, because sales of food products with health claims are expected to be a major area of growth in the food industry. From a historical and somewhat philosophical perspective, Fürst discussed food as medicine—the transition from nutrient to pharmacologic agent (*136*). He lists dietary fiber, fish oil, certain proteins, peptides, and amino acids, keto acids, vitamins and antioxidants, and phytochemicals as proposed nutraceuticals. He reviewed the functional foods, particularly as they are defined and marketed in Japan, and the pros and cons of nutritional supplements. Reilly recognized that functional foods are a reality in Japan and will almost certainly be approved for sale in the UK and other countries before long (*137*). Because possibilities for further development seem endless, he discussed functional foods in terms of consumer attitudes, the challenge for communications, safety, health claims, and implications for general nutrition in the community. He concluded that while functional foods may not be the "foods of the future," they are certain to figure prominently on supermarket shelves. Their commercial potential is clearly recognized by manufacturers, their presumptive health benefits are appreciated by many consumers, and governments are alert to the potential savings in health care that might accrue from them. Therefore regulatory issues are of utmost importance for consumer protection and to prevent the market from outpacing scientific understanding.

One food for a special medical purpose has already undergone a pilot test (*138*). A new oral supplement was compared with a standard formula in patients with HIV infection and early stages of AIDS. At comparable caloric intake, patients taking the new supplement had fewer hospitalizations over the 6-month study and gained more weight than controls. The benefits may be attributable to novel peptides used as the sole protein source, but there were other differences—such as fatty acid composition—between the formulas as well. A common thread connecting this and other clinical nutritional studies is that no single nutrient is responsible for the observed effects. Rather, the constituents of the "cocktail" work in concert. The authors discussed the results in terms of immune function and cytokine activity and urged that this kind of study be given high priority by those engaged in AIDS research.

A symposium was held in spring 1990 to consider the impact of biotechnology on the food supply (*139*). Among the presentations were discussions of recombinant-DNA technology, modification of maize proteins, prospects for genetic modification of edible plant oils, modification of milk composition, bovine somatotropin, and economic issues.

Teater reported on a conference titled "Symbol, Substance and Science: the Societal Issues of Food Biotechnology" sponsored by the USDA and the North Carolina Biotechnology Centre (*140*). Topics included public trust and acceptance, safety issues, allergenicity, labeling, and questions of ethics and morality. The distinction between useful and frivolous applications arose in connection with the "Flavr Savr" tomato. One speaker cited the transgenic low-fat pig as a clear abuse of technology that had disastrous consequences for the pigs. She argued that a technologic fix is not necessary in order for people to eat less fat: a person need merely choose to eat less fat.

Transgenic technology is increasingly being applied to food animals to make them, not food animals, but "bioreactors." Lee and de Boer reported their work aiming to produce biomedically useful proteins in dairy cattle (*141*). The products are then isolated from the milk. Other potential medical application of their techniques were discussed.

## LITERATURE CITED

1. Milton, K. Diet and primate evolution. *Sci. Am.* 269(2):86–93 (1993).

2. Leonard, W.R., and M.L. Robertson. Evolutionary perspectives on human nutrition: the influence of brain and body size on diet and metabolism. *Am. J. Human Biol.* 6:77–88 (1994).

3. Kritchevsky, D. The role of fat, calories, and fiber in disease. In *Nutritional Toxicology.* F.N. Kotsonis et al. (eds.). New York, Raven Press. *Target Organ Toxicology Ser.* Pp. 67–93 (1994).

4. Willett, W.C. Diet and health: what should we eat? *Science* 264:532–537 (1994).

5. Zifferblatt, S.M. Nutrition and fitness recommendations when science is in transition. In *Nutrition and Fitness in Health and Disease.* A.P. Simopoulos (ed.). Basel, Karger. *World Rev. Nutr. Diet.* 72:177–189 (1993).

6. Ellenbogen, L. Nutritional supplements. *Pharm. Forum* 19(1):4664–4687 (1993).

7. Putnam, J.J. American eating habits changing: part 1. Meat, dairy, and fats and oils. *Food Rev.* 16(3):2–11 (1993).

8. Subar, A.F., R.G. Ziegler, B.H. Patterson, et al. US dietary patterns associated with fat intake: the 1987 National Health Interview Survey. *Am. J. Public Health* 84:359–366 (1994).

9. Cummings, N.B. Women's health and nutrition research: US governmental concerns. *J. Am. Coll. Nutr.* 12:329–336 (1993).

10. P.K. Johnston (ed.). *Vegetarian Nutrition.* Proceedings of symposium, Arlington, VA, 28 June–1 July 1992. *Am. J. Clin. Nutr.* 59(5S) (1994).

11. Fønnebø, V. The healthy Seventh-day Adventist lifestyle: what is the Norwegian experience? *Am. J. Clin. Nutr.* 59(Suppl.):1124S–1129S (1994).

12. Knutson, S.F. Lifestyle and the use of health services. *Am. J. Clin. Nutr.* 59(Suppl.):1171S–1175S (1994).

13. Campbell, T.C., and C. Junshi. Diet and chronic degenerative diseases: perspectives from China. *Am. J. Clin. Nutr.* 59(Suppl.):1153S–1161S 1994).

14. Young, V.R., and P.L. Pellett. Plant proteins in relation to human protein and amino acid nutrition. *Am. J. Clin. Nutr.* 59(Suppl.):1203S–1212S (1994).

15. Havala, S., and J. Dwyer. Position of the American Dietetic Association: vegetarian diets. *J. Am. Diet. Assoc.* 93:1317–1319 (1993).

16. Dwyer, J.T. Vegetarian eating patterns: science, values, and food choices—where do we go from here? *Am. J. Clin. Nutr.* 59(Suppl.):1255S–1262S (1994).

17. Margetts, B.M., and A.A. Jackson. Interactions between people's diet and their smoking habits: the dietary and nutritional survey of British adults. *Br. Med. J.* 307:1381–1384 (1993).

18. Diana, J.N., and W.A. Pryor (eds.). *Tobacco Smoking and Nutrition. Influence of Nutrition on Tobacco-Associated Health Risks. Ann. N.Y. Acad. Sci.* 686 (1993).

19. Diana, J.N. Tobacco smoking and nutrition. *Ann. N.Y. Acad. Sci.* 686:1–11 (1993).

20. Duthie, G.G., J.R. Arthur, J.A.G. Beattie, et al. Cigarette smoking, antioxidants, lipid peroxidation, and coronary heart disease. *Ann. N.Y. Acad. Sci.* 686:120–129 (1993).

21. Thompson, R.L., S. Pyke, E.A. Scott, et al. Cigarette smoking, polyunsaturated fats, and coronary heart disease. *Ann. N.Y. Acad. Sci.* 686:130–139 (1993).

22. Bertram, J.S. Inhibition of chemically induced neoplastic transformation by carotenoids. Mechanistic studies. *Ann. N.Y. Acad. Sci.* 686:161–176 (1993).

23. Krinsky, N.I. Micronutrients and their influence on mutagenicity and malignant transformation. *Ann. N.Y. Acad. Sci.* 686:229–242 (1993).

24. Schwartz, J.L., D.Z. Antoniades, and S. Zhao. Molecular and biochemical reprogramming of oncogenesis through the activity of prooxidants and antioxidants. *Ann. N.Y. Acad. Sci.* 686:262–279 (1993).

25. Chung, F.-L., M.A. Morse, K.I. Eklind, and Y. Xu. Inhibition of the tobacco-specific nitrosamine-induced lung tumorigenesis by compounds derived from cruciferous vegetables and green tea. *Ann. N.Y. Acad. Sci.* 686:186–201 (1993).

26. Renaud, S., and M. de Lorgeril. The French Paradox: dietary factors and cigarette smoking–related health risks. *Ann. N.Y. Acad. Sci.* 686:299–309 (1993).

27. Subar, A.F., and L.C. Harlan. Nutrient and food group intake by tobacco use status: the 1987 National Health Interview Survey. *Ann. N.Y. Acad. Sci.* 686:310–322 (1993).

28. Bolton-Smith, C. Antioxidant vitamin intakes in Scottish smokers and nonsmokers. *Ann. N.Y. Acad. Sci.* 686:347–360 (1993).

29. Leviton, A., M. Pagano, E.N. Allred, and M. El Lozy. Why those who drink the most coffee appear to be at increased risk of disease. A modest proposal. *Ecol. Food Nutr.* 31:285–293 (1994).

30. Goldberg, R.J., C.M. Burchfiel, D.M. Reed, et al. A prospective study of the health effects of alcohol consumption in middle-aged and elderly men. *Circulation* 89:651–659 (1994).

31. Dannenberg, A.J., and M.M. Reidenberg. Dietary fatty acids are also drugs. *Clin. Pharmacol. Ther.* 55:5–9 (1994).

32. Merrill, A.H., Jr., and J.J. Schroeder. Lipid modulation of cell function. *Annu. Rev. Nutr.* 13:539–559 (1993).

33. Salem, N., Jr., and G.R. Ward. Are ω3 fatty acids essential nutrients for mammals? In *Nutrition and Fitness in Health and Disease.* A.P. Simopoulos (ed.). Basel, Karger. *World Rev. Nutr. Diet.* 72:128–147 (1993).

34. Fernandes, G., and J.T. Venkatraman. Role of omega-3 fatty acids in health and disease. *Nutr. Res.* 13(Suppl. 1):S19–S45 (1993).

35. Sanders, T.A.B. Marine oils: metabolic effects and role in human nutrition. *Proc. Nutr. Soc.* 52:457–472 (1993).

36. Schmidt, E.B., J.M. Møller, N. Svaneborg, and J. Dyerberg. Safety aspects of fish oils. Experiences with an *n*–3 concentrate of re-esterified triglycerides (Pikasol®). *Drug Invest.* 7:215–220 (1994).

37. Muggli, R. Vitamin E-Bedarf bei Zufuhr von Polyenfettsäuren. *Fett Wissenschaft Technol.* 96:17–19 (1994).

38. Nair, P.P., J.T. Judd, E. Berlin, et al. Dietary fish oil–induced changes in the distribution of α-tocopherol, retinol, and β-carotene in plasma, red blood cells, and platelets: modulation by vitamin E. *Am. J. Clin. Nutr.* 58:98–102 (1993).

39. Clarke, S.D., and D.B. Jump. Regulation of gene transcription by polyunsaturated fatty acids. *Prog. Lipid Res.* 32:139–149 (1993).

40. Koga, T., T. Yamato, J.Y. Gu, et al. Diversity in the incorporation into tissue phospholipids and effects on eicosanoid

production of *trans*-monoene fatty acid in rats fed with different dietary proteins. *Biosci. Biotechnol. Biochem.* 58:384–387 (1994).

41. Barzanti, V., M. Battino, A. Baracca, et al. The effect of dietary lipid changes on the fatty acid composition and function of liver, heart and brain mitochondria in the rat at different ages. *Br. J. Nutr.* 71:193–202 (1994).

42. Pekkanen, J., A. Nissinen, E. Vartiainen, et al. Changes in serum cholesterol level and mortality: a 30-year follow-up. *Am. J. Epidemiol.* 139:155–165 (1994.

43. Muldoon, M.F., J.E. Rossouw, S.B. Manuck, et al. Low or lowered cholesterol and risk of death from suicide and trauma. *Metabolism* 42(9 Suppl. 1):45–56 (1993).

44. Law, M.R., S.G. Thompson, and N.J. Wald. Assessing possible hazards of reducing serum cholesterol. *Br. Med. J.* 308:373–379 (1994).

45. Marmot, M. The cholesterol papers. *Br. Med. J.* 308:351–352 (1994).

46. LaRosa, J.C. Cholesterol lowering, low cholesterol, and mortality. *Am. J. Cardiol.* 72:776–786 (1993).

47. Simes, R.J. Low cholesterol and risk of non-coronary mortality. *Aust. N.Z. J. Med.* 24:113–119 (1994).

48. MacMahon, S. Cholesterol reduction and death from non-coronary causes: evidence from randomised controlled trials. *Aust. N.Z. J. Med.* 24:120–123 (1994).

49. Sullivan, D. Cholesterol and non-cardiovascular disease: basic science. *Aust. N.Z. J. Med.* 24:92–97 (1994).

50. Lewis, B., and M.J. Tikkanen. Low blood total cholesterol and mortality: causality, consequence and confounders. *Am. J. Cardiol.* 73:80–85 (1994).

51. Stamler, J., R. Stamler, W.V. Brown, et al. Serum cholesterol. Doing the right thing. *Circulation* 88:1954–1960 (1993).

52. Allred, J.B. Lowering serum cholesterol: who benefits? *J. Nutr.* 123:1453–1459 (1993).

53. Grover, S.A. Modifying serum lipids to prevent coronary heart disease: do we have a consensus? *Cardiovasc. Drugs Ther.* 7:761–765 (1993).

54. Rossouw, J.E., and A.M. Gotto, Jr. Does low cholesterol cause death? *Cardiovasc. Drugs Ther.* 7:789–793 (1993).

55. Durrington, P.N. Can any agreement be reached on cholesterol lowering? *Br. Heart J.* 71:125–128 (1994).

56. Anderson, J.W., B.M. Smith, and N.J. Gustafson. Health benefits and practical aspects of high-fiber diets. *Am. J. Clin. Nutr.* 59(Suppl.):1242S–1247S (1994).

57. Truswell, A.S. Dietary fiber and health. In *Nutrition and Fitness in Health and Disease.* A.P. Simopoulous (ed.). Basel, Karger. *World Rev. Nutr. Diet.* 72:148–164 (1993).

58. Asp, N.-G., I. Björck, and M. Nyman. Physiological effects of cereal dietary fibre. *Carbohydrate Polymers* 21:183–187 (1993).

59. Hopewell, R., R. Yeater, and I. Ullrich. Soluble fiber: effect on carbohydrate and lipid metabolism. *Prog. Food Nutr. Sci.* 17:159–182 (1993).

60. Bugaut, M., and M. Bentéjac. Biological effects of short-chain fatty acids in nonruminant mammals. *Annu. Rev. Nutr.* 13:217–241 (1993).

61. Salvador, V., C. Cherbut, J.-L. Barry, et al. Sugar composition of dietary fibre and short-chain fatty acid production during *in vitro* fermentation by human bacteria. *Br. J. Nutr.* 70:189–197 (1993).

62. Hazan, A., and Z. Madar. Preparation of a dietary fiber mixture derived from different sources and its metabolic effects in rats. *J. Am. Coll. Nutr.* 12:661–668 (1993).

63. Gorman, M.A., and C. Bowman. Position of The American Dietetic Association: health implications of dietary fiber. *J. Am. Diet. Assoc.* 93:1446–1447 (1993).

64. Asp, N.-B. (ed.). *Carbohydrates in Human Nutrition. The Importance of Food Choice, Especially in a High-Carbohydrate Diet.* Proceedings of symposium, Ystad, Sweden, 19–22 May 1992. *Am. J. Clin. Nutr.* 59(3S) (1994).

65. Stephen, A.M. Increasing complex carbohydrate in the diet: are the benefits due to starch, fibre or decreased fat intake? *Food Res. Int.* 27:69–75 (1994).

66. Forbes, A.L., and B.A. Bowman (eds.). *Health Effects of Dietary Fructose. Am. J. Clin. Nutr.* 58(5S) (1993).

67. Packer, L. Health effects of nutritional antioxidants. (Letter.) *Free Rad. Biol. Med.* 15:685–686 (1993).

68. Ames, B.N., M.K. Shigenaga, and T.M. Hagen. Oxidants, antioxidants, and the degenerative diseases of aging. *Proc. Natl. Acad. Sci. USA* 90:7915–7922 (1993).

69. Jackson, M.I. Can dietary micronutrients influence tissue antioxidant capacity? *Proc. Nutr. Soc.* 53:53–57 (1994).

70. Bonorden, W.R., and M.W. Pariza. Antioxidant nutrients and protection from free radicals. In *Nutritional Toxicology.* F.N. Kotsonis et al. (eds.). New York, Raven Press. *Target Organ Toxicology Ser.* Pp. 19–48 (1994).

71. Chen, H., and A.L. Tappel. Protection by vitamin E, selenium, trolox C, ascorbic acid palmitate, acetylcysteine, coenzyme Q, beta-carotene, canthaxanthin, and (+)-catechin against oxidative damage to liver slices measured by oxidized heme proteins. *Free Rad. Biol. Med.* 16:437–444 (1994).

72. Cao, G., and R.G. Cutler. High concentrations of antioxidants may not improve defense against oxidative stress. *Arch. Gerontol. Geriatr.* 17:189–201 (1993).

73. Rice-Evans, C.A., and A.T. Diplock. Current status of antioxidant therapy. *Free Rad. Biol. Med.* 15:77–96 (1993).

74. Gey, K.F. Prospects for the prevention of free radical disease, regarding cancer and cardiovascular disease. *Br. Med. Bull.* 49:679–699 (1993).

75. Reynolds, R.D. Vitamin supplements: current controversies. *J. Am. Coll. Nutr.* 13:118–126 (1994).

76. Rose, R.C., and A.M. Bode. Biology of free radical scavengers: an evaluation of ascorbate. *FASEB J.* 7:1135–1142 (1993).

77. Gershoff, S.N. Vitamin C (ascorbic acid): new roles, new requirements? *Nutr. Rev.* 51:313–326 (1993).

78. Johnston, C.S., C.G. Meyer, and J.C. Srilakshmi. Vitamin C elevates red blood cell glutathione in healthy adults. *Am. J. Clin. Nutr.* 58:103–105 (1993).

79. Stait, S.E., and D.S. Leake. Ascorbic acid can either increase or decrease low density lipoprotein modification. *FEBS Lett.* 341:263–267 (1994).

80. Christensen, H.N. Riboflavin can protect tissues from oxidative injury. *Nutr. Rev.* 51:149–150 (1993).

81. Butterworth, C.E. Folate status, women's health, pregnancy outcome, and cancer. *J. Am. Coll. Nutr.* 12:438–441 (1993).

82. Russell, R.M. *JAMA* 271:1687–1689 (1994).

83. Zimmerman, M.B., and B. Shane. Supplemental folic acid. *Am. J. Clin. Nutr.* 58:127–128 (1993).

84. Herbert, V. Staging vitamin B-12 (cobalamin) status in vegetarians. *Am. J. Clin. Nutr.* 59(Suppl.):1213S–1222S (1994).

85. *Vitamin A: From Molecular Biology to Public Health.* Fifteenth Marabou Symposium. *Nutr. Rev.* 52(2 Part II) (1994).

86. Ross, A.C., and M.E. Ternus. Vitamin A as a hormone: recent advances in understanding the actions of retinol, retinoic acid, and beta carotene. *J. Am. Diet. Assoc.* 93:1285–1290 (1993).

87. Olson, J.A. Vitamin A and carotenoids as antioxidants in a physiological context. *J. Nutr. Sci. Vitaminol.* 39:S57–S65 (1993).

88. Krinsky, N.I. Actions of carotenoids in biological systems. *Annu. Rev. Nutr.* 13:561–587 (1993).

89. Thurnham, D.E. Carotenoids: functions and fallacies. *Proc. Nutr. Soc.* 53:77–87 (1994).

90. Hirayama, O., K. Nakamura, S. Hamada, and Y. Kobayasi. Singlet oxygen quenching ability of naturally occurring carotenoids. *Lipids* 29:149–150 (1994).

91. Canfield, L.M., N.I. Krinsky, and J.A. Olson (eds.). *Carotenoids in Human Health. Ann. N.Y. Acad. Sci.* 691 (1993).

92. Symposium of the German Society for Fat Science (Abstracts). *Fett Wissenschaft Technol.* 95:268–278 (1993).

93. Maiorino, M., A. Zamburlini, A. Roveri, and F. Ursini. Prooxidant role of vitamin E in copper induced lipid peroxidation. *FEBS Lett.* 330:174–176 (1993).

94. Bowry, V.W., and R. Stocker. Tocopherol-mediated peroxidation. The prooxidant effect of vitamin E on the radical-initiated oxidation of human low-density lipoprotein. *J. Am. Chem. Soc.* 115:6029–6044 (1993).

95. Wiseman, H. Vitamin D is a membrane antioxidant. *FEBS Lett.* 326:285–288 (1993).

96. Yoshino, K., Y. Hara, M. Sano, and I. Tomita. Antioxidative effects of black tea theaflavins and thearubigin on lipid peroxidation of rat liver homogenates induced by *tert*-butyl hydroperoxide. *Biol. Pharm. Bull.* 17:146–149 (1994).

97. Nanjo, F., M. Honda, K. Okushio, et al. Effects of dietary tea catechins of α-tocopherol levels, lipid peroxidation, and erythrocyte deformability in rats fed on high palm oil and perilla oil diets. *Biol. Pharm. Bull.* 16:1156–1159 (1993).

98. Zhou, J., F. Ashoori, S. Suzuki, et al. Protective effect of chlorogenic acid on lipid peroxidation induced in the liver of rats by carbon tetrachloride or $^{60}$Co-irradiation. *J. Clin. Biochem. Nutr.* 15:119–125 (1993).

99. Nishigaki, I., H. Oku, M. Noguchi, et al. Prevention by ellagic acid of lipid peroxidation in placenta and fetus of rats irradiated with $^{60}$Co. *J. Clin. Biochem. Nutr.* 15:135–141 (1993).

100. Reddy, A.Ch.P., and B.R. Lokesh. Effect of dietary turmeric (*Curcuma longa*) on iron-induced lipid peroxidation in the rat liver. *Food Chem. Toxicol.* 32:279–283 (1994).

101. Reddy, A.Ch.P., and B.R. Lokesh. Alterations in lipid peroxides in rat liver by dietary *n*–3 fatty acids: modulation of antioxidant enzymes by curcumin, eugenol, and vitamin E. *J. Nutr. Biochem.* 5:181–188 (1994).

102. Sreejayan and M.N.A. Rao. Curcumin inhibits iron-dependent lipid peroxidation. *Int. J. Pharm.* 100:93–97 (1993).

103. Hattori, M., X.-W. Yang, H. Miyashiro, and T. Namba. Inhibitory effects of monomeric and dimeric phenylpropanoids from mace on lipid peroxidation *in vivo* and *in vitro*. *Phytother. Res.* 7:395–401 (1993).

104. Rajakumar, D.V., and M.N.A. Rao. Dehydrozingerone and isoeugenol as inhibitors of lipid peroxidation and as free radical scavengers. *Biochem. Pharmacol.* 46:2067–2072 (1993).

105. Thompson, L.U. Potential health benefits and problems associated with antinutrients in foods. *Food Res. Int.* 26:131–149 (1993).

106. Hallfrisch, J., and D.C. Muller. Does diet provide adequate amounts of calcium, iron, magnesium, and zinc in a well-educated adult population? *Exp. Gerontol.* 28:473–483 (1993).

107. Johnson, M.A., and J.G. Fischer. Role of minerals in protection against free radicals. *Food Technol.* 48(5):112–120 (1994).

108. Bettger, W. Zinc and selenium, site-specific versus general antioxidation. *Can. J. Physiol. Pharmacol.* 71:721–724 (1993).

109. Naghii, M.R., and S. Samman. The role of boron in nutrition and metabolism. *Prog. Food Nutr. Sci.* 17:331–349 (1993).

110. Walker, W.A. (ed.). *Nucleotides and Nutrition. J. Nutr.* 124(1S) (1994).

111. Barness, L.A. Dietary sources of nucleotides. *J. Nutr.* 124(Suppl.):128S–130S (1994).

112. Jyonouchi, H. Nucleotide actions on humoral immune responses. *J. Nutr.* 124(Suppl.):138S–143S (1994).

113. Carver, J.D. Dietary nucleotides: cellular immune, intestinal and hepatic system effects. *J. Nutr.* 124(Suppl.):144S–148S (1994).

114. Uauy, R. Nonimmune system responses to dietary nucleotides. *J. Nutr.* 124(Suppl.):157S–159S (1994).

115. Van Buren, C.T., A.D. Kulkarni, and F.B. Rudolph. The role of nucleotides in adult nutrition. *J. Nutr.* 124(Suppl.):160S–164S (1994).

116. Sánchez-Pozo, A., J. Morillas, L. Moltó, et al. Dietary nucleotides influence lipoprotein metabolism in newborn infants. *Pediatr. Res.* 35:112–116 (1994).

117. Núñez, M.C., M.V. Ayudarte, A. Gil, and M.D. Suárez. Effect of dietary nucleotides on the fatty acid composition of rat liver microsomes. *Arch. Int. Physiol. Biochim. Biophys.* 101:123–128 (1993).

118. Campbell-Platt, G. Fermented foods—a world perspective. *Food Res. Int.* 27:253–257 (1994).

119. Chandan, R.C., and K.M. Shahani. Yogurt. In *Dairy Science and Technology Handbook. 2. Product Manufacturing.* Y.H. Hui (ed.). New York, VCH. Pp. 1–56 (1992).

120. Sanders, M.E. Summary of conclusions from a consensus panel of experts on health attributes of lactic cultures: significance to fluid milk products containing cultures. *J. Dairy Sci.* 76:1819–1828 (1993).

121. Salminen, S., and A. von Wright (eds.). *Lactic Acid Bacteria.* New York, Marcel Dekker. *Food Science and Technology. A Series of Monographs, Textbooks, and Reference Books.* Vol. 58 (1993).

122. Salminin, S., M. Deighton, and S. Gorbach. Lactic acid bacteria in health and disease. In *Lactic Acid Bacteria.* S. Salminin and A. von Wright (eds.). *Food Sci. Technol. Ser.* 58:199–225 (1993).

123. Ballongue, J. Bifidobacteria and probiotic action. In *Lactic Acid Bacteria.* S. Salminin and A. von Wright (eds.). *Food Sci. Technol. Ser.* 58:357–428 (1993).

124. Hoover, D.G. Bifidobacteria: activity and potential benefits. *Food Technol.* 47(6):120–124 (1993).

125. Bartram, H.-P., W. Sheppach, S. Gerlach, et al. Does yogurt enriched with *Bifidobacterium longum* affect colonic microbiology and fecal metabolites in healthy subjects? *Am. J. Clin. Nutr.* 59:428–432 (1994).

126. Ishibashi, N., and S. Shimamura. Bifidobacteria: research and development in Japan. *Food Technol.* 47(6):126–135 (1993)

127. Esaki, H., H. Onozaki, and T. Osawa. Antioxidative activity of fermented soybean products. In *Food Phytochemicals for Cancer Prevention I. Fruits and Vegetables.* M.-T. Huang et al. (eds.). *ACS Symp. Ser.* 546:353–360 (1994).

128. Harlander, S. Genetic engineering of foods: a US perspective. *Trends Food Sci. Technol.* 4:301–305 (1993).

129. Younes, M., G.J.A. Speijers, and C.A. van der Heijden. Biotechnology-derived and novel foods: safety approaches and regulations. In *Nutritional Toxicology.* F.N. Kotsonis et al. (eds.). New York, Raven Press. *Target Organ Toxicology Ser.* Pp. 181–197 (1994).

130. Berkowitz, D.B., and I. Kryspin-Sørensen. Transgenic fish: safe to eat? *Bio/Technology* 12:247–252 (1994).

131. Olempska-Beer, Z.S., P.M. Kuznesof, M. DiNovi, and M.J. Smith. Plant biotechnology and food safety. *Food Technol.* 47(12):64–72 (1993).

132. Comai, L. Impact of plant genetic engineering on foods and nutrition. *Annu. Rev. Nutr.* 13:191–215 (1993).

133. Teuber, M. Genetic engineering techniques in food microbiology and enzymology. *Food Rev. Int.* 9:389–409 (1993).

134. Ulbricht, T. Health and the food industry. What lies ahead—'nutriceuticals'? *Food Policy* 18:379–380 (1993).

135. Hunt, J.R. Nutritional products for specific health benefits—foods, pharmaceuticals, or something in between? *J. Am. Diet. Assoc.* 94:151–153 (1994).

136. Fürst, P. Nahrung als Arznei—der Übergang vom Nährstoff zum Pharmkon. *Ernährungs-Umschau* 40:364–369 (1993).

137. Reilly, C. Functional foods—a challenge for consumers. *Trends Food Sci. Technol.* 5:121–123 (1994).

138. Blackburn, G.L., and S. Bell. Eutrophia in patients with HIV infection and early AIDS with novel nutrient "cocktail": is this the first food for special medical purpose? *Nutrition* 9:554–556 (1993).

139. Bier, D.M. (ed.). *Impact of Biotechnology on the Food Supply.* Proceedings of symposium, Washington, DC, 30 April–1 May, 1990. *Am. J. Clin. Nutr.* 58(2S) (1993).

140. Teater, B.D. Symbol, substance and science: the societal issues of food biotechnology. *Transgenic Res.* 3:70–73 (1994).

141. Lee, S.H., and H.A. de Boer. Production of biomedical proteins in the milk of transgenic dairy cows: the state of the art. *J. Controlled Release* 29:213–221 (1994).

# 2

# Diet and Cancer

# OVERVIEW

A summary report was published of the Ole Møller Jensen Memorial Symposium on nutrition and cancer, held in Lyon, France, in March 1993 (*1*). Symposium sessions addressed the topics of energy and energy balance, diet and stomach cancer, alcohol and cancer, fat and breast cancer (one session on epidemiology and one on mechanisms), and fat, carbohydrates, and colorectal cancer. Many aspects of the relation between energy intake, energy balance, and cancer in humans are still poorly understood. Nevertheless, energy intake is considered very important and dietary data are frequently analyzed on an isocaloric basis to correct for this factor. Various statistical and biological models relating to energy intake, diet composition, physical activity, and body weight have been proposed. Epidemiologic evidence that fruits and vegetables protect against stomach cancer is very strong; by contrast, the relationship between dietary fat and breast cancer was considered tenuous. One participant thought it reasonable to conclude that fat intake during adulthood is unlikely to be a major risk factor for breast cancer, and there are insufficient data to relate fat intake during childhood and adolescence to later breast cancer. For colon cancer, the participants felt that the data support a clear protective role of vegetables and a probable causal role of animal fat and perhaps meat. It was evident that mechanistic studies at the organ, cell, and molecular levels are increasingly explaining epidemiologic findings, which in turn are posing new mechanistic questions.

A task force convened by the European School of Oncology comprehensively reviewed the epidemiologic evidence relating diet, nutrition, and cancer. Miller et al. reported their conclusions and recommendations (*2*). The task force considered methodologic issues and weaknesses in the available data and recommended considerations in planning new epidemiologic research. Their dietary recommendations stressed ethical factors, the quality of the evidence, competing risks (e.g., the reciprocal relationship between cancers of the colon and stomach), and the ability to effect the recommended change. They distinguished between recommendations for the population and the individual. Their recommendations (including advice on exercise and alcohol consumption) were similar to those proposed by other groups. Perhaps most interesting was a summary table estimating the potential effects of specific actions on the incidence of cancers at various sites. Estimates of population-attributable risk were derived primarily from population-based case–control studies in which attributable risk could be determined. For most sites, this ranged from ~30 to ~70%. The potentially preventable fraction was derived from the highest and lowest incidences reported in European cancer registries. This ranged from 66% for ovarian cancer to 98% for kidney cancer. The possibly conservative nature of some estimates and barriers to achieving maximal effects were discussed.

Clifford and Kramer reviewed the causative and protective roles of fat, fiber, body weight, and micronutrients against cancers at specific sites (*3*). They discussed nutrients as cancer therapy and summarized results of some dietary intervention trials for prevention or adjunct therapy. Information from selected studies in laboratory rodents was reviewed by Rogers et al. (*4*). They concentrated on areas in which strong epidemiological data require explanation or in which research is yielding mechanistic information. In rodents, vitamin A and retinoids influence carcinogenesis in the bladder, skin, mammary gland, respiratory tract, and colon. Methionine and choline influence carcinogenesis in liver, mammary gland, pancreas, and colon. Selenium plays a role in the colon, liver, skin, stomach, and mammary gland; calcium and fiber, in the colon; zinc, in the esophagus; vitamin C, in skin and stomach; fat, in mammary gland, colon, pancreas, and skin; and whole foods and total calories influence carcinogenesis at many sites. Energy restriction was discussed in terms of carcinogenic mechanisms, but because of the degree of restriction needed to obtain the observed results, this strategy may have little practical importance.

The Delaney Clause, an amendment to the Federal Food Drug and Cosmetic Act prohibiting addition of cancer-causing substances to foods, was enacted into law in 1958. Weisburger reviewed the history of this controversial amendment in terms of the changes in scientific knowledge and thought that have occurred since the first hearings were held in the mid-1950s (*5*). Mechanisms of carcinogenesis and the role of cell duplication rates were discussed. Weisburger emphasized the need to distinguish between genotoxic and nongenotoxic carcinogens and the importance of the methodological and analytical procedures used to assess health risk as a function of dosage and chronicity of exposure. The major causes of cancer in humans, as they are currently understood, were discussed, along with what the author considers misuses of the Delaney Clause by some interest groups. In the light of all this Weisburger suggests that it is time to reconsider the Delaney Clause and to search for new science-based strategies to protect the public and prevent disease.

## Dietary Trends and Strategies

The USA has set two population-wide dietary goals for the year 2000: to reduce fat intake to no more than 30% of calories (en%) and to double the consumption of carbohydrate and fiber. To measure progress toward those goals, data on food supply and dietary intake during the last 20 years were compiled from national surveys and individual studies (6). Fat intake, both absolute and as a percentage of caloric intake, has declined slightly but remains near 35 en%. Fruit and vegetable consumption has increased but averages no more than 3.4 servings per day, short of the 5 recommended. There is a trend toward a widening socioeconomic gap, indicating a need to augment education and interventions for targeted populations. Although the U.S. diet has been improving, the rate of change is too slow to achieve the year 2000 objectives.

In a brief review of the basis for current dietary advice, Kritchevsky found no single causative or inhibitory factor to emerge from studies of diet and cancer (7). In summary tables he showed the American Cancer Society's dietary guidelines, summary recommendations from 12 health authorities, the relationship between relative body weight and breast cancer mortality, sources and actions of various anticarcinogens in foods, effects of dietary fiber in the colon, and effects of calorie restriction on chemically induced mammary tumorigenesis in rats. His dietary advice: moderation and variety.

Bal and Foerster emphasized technology transfer in their discussion of dietary strategies for cancer prevention (8). They decried the lack of organized effort, with clearly identified steps, to translate research into practical approaches for meeting dietary goals for the year 2000, pointing to similar delays in implementing other cancer-control measures such as Papanicolaou and mammographic testing and tobacco intervention. They concluded that unless additional resources are dedicated to population-wide dietary modification, dietary goals will not be met in the foreseeable future. They presented a "stages of change" model for cancer prevention through diet, using American Cancer Society programs as examples. Heimendinger summarized the National Cancer Institute (NCI) approach to translating research into behavioral change in the general population, with the National 5-a-Day for Better Health program as an example (9). She described the use of national health objectives, community channels, and theories of health-related behavior to develop community nutrition intervention strategies. Community channels include health departments, work sites, schools, supermarkets, restaurants, physicians' offices, community organizations, and the media. Relevant behavior theories include social cognitive theory, consumer information processing, health belief models, social marketing, and stages of change. Intervention components can be directed at awareness, knowledge, attitudes, skills, motivation, the environment, policy, and organizational structure. Dwyer elaborated on 10 guiding principles for decreasing cancer risks and maximizing the "nutritional quality of life" (10). It is important to place diet in the overall context of risk reduction strategies and to remember that recommendations for cancer risk reduction and cancer treatment often differ. Dietary change is not easy but can be facilitated by education, a supportive environment, and the ready availability of healthful foods and meals. Although people need specific advice about good eating choices, the author stressed that each and every food choice should not be cast as a good food–bad food dichotomy and treated as a moral event. The last word is not yet in; no dietary advice is forever. Some current programs and strategies for future programs were discussed.

A supermarket nutrition intervention study, "Eat for Health," has been completed and evaluated (11). A matched-pair design was used, with 20 stores in the intervention group and 20 controls. The evaluation involved in-store monitoring, consumer surveys, and analysis of sales data on selected foods. Elements of the intervention program were special shelf price labels and a food guide containing nutritional information on the specially labeled items, a monthly bulletin containing nutrition information and recipes, signs in the produce department, and a multimedia advertizing campaign. Although the intervention was implemented successfully, it had only marginal success in changing behaviors. The only impacts on knowledge and attitudes were a nonsignificant increase in awareness of the link between diet and cancer and a widespread awareness of the intervention program itself. There were small, nonsignificant program-related changes in choices of cooking method and food choices related to fat and fiber content. The authors believe that the limited impact of this single program was due to the widespread diffusion of nutrition messages throughout society.

Ferguson believes that further research on the beliefs, attitudes, diets, and behaviors of different groups is needed for the development of successful health-promotion strategies (12). For colorectal cancer, basic dietary research requires appropriate biomarkers of dietary exposures in humans and animals; new human and animal models may need to be developed.

## Mechanisms

Food and Cancer Prevention '92 was the third in a series of biennial international conferences exploring the interface of diet and health (*13*). Sections in the proceedings addressed diet–cancer relationships in humans; carcinogens in foods; the role of free radical reactions and antioxidant nutrients in carcinogenesis; tumor initiation and diet; tumor development and diet; food components as immunomodulators; dietary fiber; new research techniques; and dietary guidance. From 30 to 35% of cancer mortality in the USA is estimated to be diet-related (*14*). In western nations, nutritional excesses are thought to have the major impact although nutritional inadequacies are also important. Carcinogens formed in foods may also contribute, but food additives and contaminants are thought to have negligible impact. By contrast, all four of these factors are probably important in Asia and Africa.

Borek reviewed molecular mechanisms in the induction and prevention of cancer (*15*). The role of oxygen radicals, the arachidonic acid cascade, and dietary factors in multistep carcinogenesis was discussed. Although environmental factors undoubtedly underlie development of most cancers, Borek thinks the message is optimistic because dietary factors can modify responses to these environmental agents at cellular and molecular levels to prevent the onset and progression of cancer. Rosin reviewed genetic alterations in carcinogenesis and chemoprevention, describing the approach of using intermediate end points (biological markers) as surrogates for clinical lesions (*16*). The biological marker would be a sign for intervention. For example, the finding of micronuclei or aneuploidy indicates genetic change, for which radical scavengers, antioxidants, or inhibitors of carcinogen bioactivation are appropriate chemopreventive agents. Various markers such as enhanced ornithine decarboxylase activity and tritiated thymidine labeling indicate proliferative activity, against which retinoids, calcium, and wheat fiber may be chemopreventive. Inflammation is marked by indicators of oxidative stress or induction of protooncogenes, and dietary radical scavengers may be chemopreventive. Large-scale, long-term clinical trials are required to determine whether the responses of intermediate markers to chemoprevention will translate into reduced cancer incidence in the treated population.

Netter discussed interactions between nutrients and xenobiotic metabolism, including both detoxifying and activating mechanisms (*17*). Cytochrome P450 synthesis and function and the cytochrome P450 reaction cycle were illustrated showing potential points of interference by dietary factors. The cytochromes P450 are a diverse family of enzymes that do not react uniformly to the biochemical challenge exerted by nutrients. For example, food deprivation can have either a positive or a negative effect on the ability to chemically convert toxicants. Dietary lipids were discussed and a few examples were given to illustrate the effects of minor herbal constituents.

A discussion of micronutrients and oxidative stress in the etiology of cancer summarized mechanisms of DNA damage and repair (*18*). The demonstrated involvement of free radicals in disease leads to the antioxidant hypothesis and the molecular epidemiological approach to disease prevention. This approach was illustrated by a study of smoking and nonsmoking Scottish men, in whom exposure to antioxidants was precisely monitored and controlled and molecular biomarkers indicating the level of oxidative damage were assayed.

Recently discovered functions of vitamins A, C, D, and E, retinoic acid, and β-carotene have suggested that supplemental intake of these substances may reduce the risk of cancer (*19*). However, this idea can be tested only by intervention trials; prospective and retrospective case–control experimental designs are not suitable. Prasad et al. reviewed experimental data suggesting that the potential cancer-preventive effects of vitamins have both cellular and molecular bases. For example, vitamins influence the expression of certain oncogenes in vitro. Other mechanisms involve cell-signaling systems. Processes by which vitamins induce differentiation in transformed cell lines are being clarified. Vitamin A and retinoids are particularly important for differentiation of epithelial cells, and in this capacity are protective against skin cancer and perhaps certain other carcinomas as well (*20*). Four distinct epithelial phenotypes can be recognized. Each serves specific functions and is found at specific sites. All, however, are subject to regulation by hormonal cycles and dietary intake of vitamin A or provitamin A. Studies are in progress to reveal how one epithelial phenotype is converted to another or transformed to a malignant phenotype, and how hormones and retinoids are involved in this process. Lupulescu reviewed studies of how vitamins A, C, and E and β-carotene influence the growth and differentiation of cancer cells (*21*). These substances exert pleiotropic effects on cancer cells, which vary with cell type and the size and duration of the vitamin dose. The vitamins may have differing effects on cancer cells and normal cells, and in vitro effects may not be relevant in vivo. However, they appear to influence synthesis of DNA, RNA, protein, and collagen, membrane biogenesis, and the transformation of precancer into cancer cells. Postulated mechanisms for observed metabolic effects involve oncogene expression, growth factors, and growth factor receptors. Vitamin C's role in collagen synthesis, basement membrane integrity, and hyaluronidase inhibition has implications for cancer cell invasiveness and metastasis.

Davison et al. reviewed the putative anticarcinogenic actions of carotenoids and their nutritional implications, stressing what is not known as well as what is (22). Claims have been made for beneficial actions related to vitamin A sparing, photoprotection, genotoxicity, immunostimulation, anticarcinogenesis, cataract, heart disease, and neurotoxicity. The authors surveyed the nature and occurrence of carotenoids, showed that in mammalian cells these substances have functions distinct from provitamin activity, established an antioxidant role for carotenoids, and presented evidence for and against their antineoplastic role. They unequivocally recommended a diet rich in carotenoid-containing foods and suggested some priorities for research.

A review of dietary fiber considered the chemical composition and structure of plant cell walls, methods of analysis, and properties of fibers and mechanisms of action that could increase or decrease colon cancer risk (23). Although the chemistry and structure of dietary fibers are well understood, the review highlighted enormous gaps in knowledge about how protection against colorectal cancer is mediated. Effects of fiber may be direct or indirect—a result of the fiber's degradation by colonic bacteria. Anticarcinogenic effects may occur before a carcinogen produces DNA lesions or later, at any stage in the progression to a fully developed tumor. Numerous possible mechanisms were discussed. To date, wheat bran has the most evidence for a protective effect, but other dietary fibers equally good or better may be discovered. The authors believe that investigators must better define the fiber preparations they study and the way in which epidemiological data on fiber intake are collected.

Just as a portion of dietary fiber is fermented in the colon, about 10% of starch ("resistant starch") in a normal diet escapes digestion and absorption in the small intestine and is fermented by the colonic microflora (24). In fact, resistant starch is potentially a much larger source of fermentable substrate than dietary fiber and could contribute significantly to

prevention of colon cancer. The effects of the short-chain fatty acids produced during fermentation on colonic pH and bile acid metabolism and the role of bile acids in colonic carcinogenesis were summarized. A diagram illustrated some possible and probable mechanisms for the protection afforded by dietary fiber and resistant starch.

METHYL DEFICIENCY. DNA methylation is one mechanism by which gene activity is regulated. Hypomethylation of a gene is necessary for that gene's expression, and changes in a gene's methylation status allow its potential for expression to be altered in a heritable manner. Goodman and Counts discussed the hypothesis that hypomethylation of DNA is a nongenotoxic mechanism underlying the role of cell proliferation in carcinogenesis (25). In nondividing cells, methylation is symmetrical, involving both strands of the DNA. Immediately after DNA replication the newly synthesized strand is unmethylated, but a maintenance enzyme that specifically recognizes hemimethylated sites restores the normal pattern. A deficiency of methyl groups in dividing cells would lead to hypomethylation and could facilitate the aberrant expression of protooncogenes involved in carcinogenesis. Evidence for the role of hypomethylation and cell replication comes from studies of hepatocarcinogenesis in rodents fed a choline-free diet, which depletes the maintenance enzyme's cofactor *S*-adenosylmethionine while increasing the rate of hepatocyte proliferation. Such animals develop liver tumors even without exposure to a chemical carcinogen. The authors argued that the hypomethylation hypothesis of carcinogenesis is compatible with the mutation theory because in nearly all cases a mutated gene must be expressed in order to affect the phenotype of a cell, and hypomethylation is required for expression. Poirier reviewed studies of methyl deficiency in hepatocarcinogenesis, beginning with the "methyl deletion hypothesis" put forward by James and Elizabeth Miller in the early 1950s (26). Evidence for alterations in oncogenes during hepatocarcinogenesis by methyl deprivation has accrued from dietary studies and from experiments using hypomethylating antimetabolites. Alternate mechanisms and some observations in humans were briefly discussed. Two additional papers on hypomethylation in carcinogenesis discussed tumorigenesis, protooncogene activation, and other gene abnormalities in methyl deficiency (27) and reviewed chemical carcinogenesis in methyl-deficient rats (28).

Christman et al. asked how loss of methylation at specific sites in growth regulatory genes is related to the ability of altered hepatocytes to escape normal constraints on cell division (29). Rats were fed a methyl-deficient diet and the ability of liver nucleic acids to accept methyl groups in in vitro methyltransferase-catalyzed reactions was measured. The level of methyl acceptance in DNA from the deficient group was 3–4 times that of controls, and in tRNA was 5–10 times as great. The intracellular pool of *S*-adenosylmethionine was depleted but the activity of the DNA and tRNA methyltransferase enzymes was increased in these animals. There was a selective time-dependent loss of methylation at specific CCGG sites in the c-*Ha-ras*, c-*fos*, and c-*myc* genes, which was accompanied by an increase in their mRNA transcripts. There was also evidence of hypomethylation of a *p*53 gene. Thus methylation is better maintained at some sites than at others when the supply of *S*-adenosylmethionine is limiting. Feeding of the methyl-deficient diet consistently led to a 4-fold or greater increase in the number of proliferating liver cells after as little as 1 day. Overall, rates of proliferation returned to normal within a few days and levels of DNA and tRNA methylation were normalized within 1–2 wk when a methyl-sufficient diet was reinstated. However, hypomethylation at specific sites in the c-*myc* gene persisted for at least 9 wk. Methyl-deficient animals also showed fatty changes in their livers that were slow to resolve. These observations were discussed in terms of the ability of cells containing specific hypomethylated genes to escape normal constraints on cell division when exposed to low doses of carcinogen or to mitogenic stimuli. Although no human diet is as severely methyl-deficient as the experimental diet, many people have marginally deficient diets and are exposed to other conditions that could reduce *S*-adenosylmethionine pools and/or methyltransferase activity or modify DNA so as to make it a poor substrate for methylation. The authors suggest that cumulative hypomethylation of genes is a factor in the etiology of liver cancer.

Along these lines, a brief review emphasizing findings in the Nurses' Health Study suggested an intriguing link between intake of folate, methionine, and alcohol, the risk of colon cancer, and hypomethylation of DNA (30). Another review of animal, epidemiologic, and clinical data concluded that folate status can modulate carcinogenesis in the colon and that some effect may be achieved with changes within the normal range of vitamin status (31). Methyltetrahydrofolate provides the methyl group for methionine and thus ultimately for *S*-adenosylmethionine. In this way folate status may affect patterns of DNA methylation, thereby influencing gene expression. The only other known functions of folate are also related to its transfer of one-carbon units. Mecha-

nisms by which folate could modulate carcinogenesis are diverse and are under intense investigation.

**ENERGY RESTRICTION.** That energy restriction inhibits tumor growth in rodents has been known for nearly a century. Kritchevsky reviewed the effects of caloric restriction on tumor development and lifespan, examining the extent of restriction necessary to produce such results and the stage of life during which restriction is effective (32). Most of the data are from rodents subjected to conditions too severe to have population-wide relevance for people. However, total caloric intake has been linked to breast cancer in women and to colorectal cancer in men and women; women who were college athletes reportedly have a lower prevalence of certain cancers; and obesity is a risk factor for several cancers. This suggests that a realistic level of diet restriction and/or exercise would reduce cancer incidence in people, a conclusion Kritchevsky also reached in a review of the role of fat and caloric restriction in colorectal cancer (33). Studies of the relationship between dietary fat intake and risk of colon cancer have yielded conflicting results. However in animals, restriction of total (as opposed to fat-derived) calories reliably inhibits growth of spontaneous and experimentally induced tumors. Exercise also reduces the incidence of chemically induced tumors in rats, and vigorous physical activity reduces risk of colon cancer in men. Therefore reducing total caloric intake and/or increasing energy expenditure may be a relatively simple way for people to reduce their cancer risk.

A special issue of *Mutation Research* was devoted to the impact of diet restriction on genetic stability (34). Reviews discussed the modulation of chemical toxicity by macronutrient restriction, compared protein and caloric restriction in terms of effects on DNA damage, carcinogenesis, and oxidative damage, and compared fat and caloric restriction in terms of oxidative damage to DNA. Other papers discussed effects of diet restriction on drug metabolism and on aging and biomarkers of aging. Several papers considered mechanisms related to DNA synthesis, damage, and repair.

In mice, caloric restriction delayed and inhibited growth of a transplanted ascitic lymphoma and lengthened survival of the host (35). Inclusion of soybean in the diet enhanced the effect. Diet restriction, with or without soybean, improved the proliferative response of peripheral blood lymphocytes, increased the cytolytic activity of peritoneal macrophages, and elevated serum IgG and IgM. Without soybean, diet-restricted animals had lower levels of serum α-tocopherol and retinol than controls; with soybean, these levels were normal.

# EPIDEMIOLOGY

## General

Although epidemiologic research repeatedly finds associations between diet and cancer, the strength of these associations is extremely uncertain (*36*). In 1981, the confidence limits for the percentage of diet-related cancers were 10 to 70%; by 1991, the best estimate had been narrowed but slightly, to 20–60%. Kromhout et al. discussed strengths and weaknesses of observational epidemiologic studies, with attention to limitations of various study designs and dietary survey methods. The most consistent finding in dietary epidemiologic studies is an inverse association between consumption of fruits and vegetables and the occurrence of epithelial cancers. The elements responsible for this association and their relative importance are still in dispute. Both well known and lesser known constituents may be involved. For example, interest in protective effects of plant flavonoids has been growing. The authors cited findings from recent quantitative studies of the five major flavonoids in common foods (quercetin, kaempferol, myricetin, apigenin, and luteolin) as evidence that currently used food tables do not provide the information that epidemiologists need.

In a major epidemiologic study, cancer incidence was monitored from 1976 to 1982 in a population of 34,000 Seventh-Day Adventists in California; residents of Connecticut provided an external reference group (*37*). Almost half of the Adventists were ovolacto-vegetarians. About 3% were vegans and the rest ate varying amounts of animal flesh (but no pork). Several nondietary aspects of lifestyle also distinguished Adventists from the reference group. Adventist men had a slightly but significantly higher incidence of prostate cancer; incidence of melanoma and pancreatic, brain, lymphatic, and hematopoietic cancers did not differ from the expected; and incidence at all other sites and for total cancers was significantly lower than expected. Adventist women had significantly elevated incidence of melanoma, cancer of the uterine corpus, and all genital cancers; incidence of cervical and ovarian cancer was slightly elevated. Women's standardized morbidity ratios for most other sites were closer to 1.0 than men's. The most interesting observation came from the age-specific incidence curves. At ages up to 40 y, Adventists and people in Connecticut experience similar rates of cancer. For the next 40 y, Adventists have uniformly lower incidence rates. However, at ages ≥80 y, there is a crossover and Adventists of both sexes experience higher cancer rates than the comparison population. This may simply represent an exhaustion of susceptible people in the comparison population; or, it may reflect a true delay in cancer risk among Adventists. The Adventist lifestyle may afford protection to a certain advanced age, after which another factor (immunologic? genetic?) overwhelms the lifestyle effect. Within the Adventist group, a large intake of beans, lentils, peas, tomatoes, and dried fruits was associated with decreased risk of prostate cancer. Meat consumption was *not* associated with higher risk. For women, breast cancer was not related to consumption of animal fats or animal products in general. High fruit consumption protected against lung cancer even after adjusting for smoking. Colon cancer risk was directly related to consumption of saturated fats and inversely related to legume and fiber consumption. High meat intake doubled the risk of bladder cancer. Soy products reduced risk of pancreatic cancer.

Examination of the WHO mortality database for the past three decades cast doubt on the facile "Westernized diet" explanation for cancer trends in Japan (*38*). Although overall mortality rates for colorectal, breast, and prostate cancer have risen steadily, supporting the diet theory, the trends for colorectal cancer in both sexes and for prostate cancer have reversed in persons born since 1945. This reversal is not consonant with the idea that cancer risk is rising as younger cohorts increasingly adopt Western eating habits.

A study was conducted of cancer incidence and mortality among butchers who were born after 1880 and had shops in Geneva, Switzerland, and their wives (*39*). Wives had no excess overall mortality or excess risk from any specific cancer or noncancer cause of death. The butchers, however, had excesses in incidence and mortality from colorectal cancer, prostate cancer, and all cancers, in incidence of liver cancer, and in mortality from laryngeal cancer. There was an excess of deaths from leukemia among butchers born in 1880–1899. Risk of lung cancer was significantly elevated in pork butchers. This might be attributable to exposure to polycyclic aromatic hydrocarbons during meat smoking. The butchers also had significantly elevated mortality from ischemic heart disease. The authors cited another study showing that butchers eat more animal fat and probably more animal protein than the average male population of Geneva.

Changes have been observed in the pattern of cancer among hospitalized black cancer patients in Soweto, South Africa (*40*). Between 1966 and 1991 numbers of patients with cervical, esophageal, and liver cancer first increased, then decreased. During the same period, increasing numbers of cases of breast and prostate cancer were seen. These data may reflect increasing urbanization and improved socioeconomic status, with the associated dietary changes.

In the USA, blacks have a greater cancer risk than whites. However, a dietary study found that the common dietary assumptions may not explain this racial disparity (*41*). Food frequency data obtained by interview from 881 blacks and 1985 whites randomly selected from three areas of the USA showed that compared to their white counterparts, blacks ate more fruits and vegetables considered protective against cancer and had a slightly lower intake of both total and saturated fat.

Soybeans contain a number of anticarcinogens and are the primary dietary source of the isoflavone genistein, which has weak estrogenic activity and acts as an antiestrogen in some animal models. Genistein also inhibits protein tyrosine kinases and several critical enzymes involved in signal transduction. In vitro it suppresses growth of a wide range of tumor cells. Messina et al. reviewed the literature to investigate the hypothesis that consumption of soy foods decreases cancer risk (*42*). While they were unable to conclude definitively that soy foods reduce risk, they found enough evidence for a protective effect to warrant further investigation. The epidemiologic data show that consumption of non-fermented soy products is either protective or not associated with cancer risk. Protective effects were seen for both hormone- and nonhormone-related cancers. No pattern was evident for fermented soy products such as miso. Of 26 studies of experimental carcinogenesis in animals in which soybeans or soybean isoflavones were fed, 17 (65%) reported a protective effect; the rest showed no effect.

Willett reviewed the influence of micronutrients on cancer risk, emphasizing results from Harvard University's Health Professionals Follow-Up Study and Nurses' Health Study (*43*). Although abundant data demonstrate that a high intake of fruits and vegetables reduces the risk of cancers at many sites, questions remain. Which cancers are affected? Which fruits and vegetables have an effect? Which components of these foods are involved? How much is risk reduced? Almost certainly, vitamin A, the carotenoids, and folic acid are important. In another discussion, Willett et al. evaluated the relationship between vitamin A intake and risk of breast, colorectal, and prostate cancer (*44*). They considered the quality of the data in terms of study design, dietary assessment, and validity of biochemical markers and attempted to distinguish between associations with preformed vitamin A obtained from animal sources or supplements and associations with carotenoid precursors of vitamin A obtained largely from plant

sources. They consider the available data compatible with a modest inverse association between vitamin A intake and breast cancer risk, although it is not clear whether this is attributable to preformed vitamin A, carotenoids, or both. The evidence that vitamin A protects against colon cancer is unconvincing, and most data suggest that dietary vitamin A does not protect against prostate cancer.

Block summarized the epidemiologic evidence that vitamin C or high intake of foods rich in vitamin C protects against cancer at nearly every major site (*45*). She showed, further, that substantial numbers of people in the USA have an inadequate intake of this vitamin.

## Colorectal Cancer

A comprehensive review of the epidemiology of colon cancer included extensive summary data in tabular form (*46*). Nearly all ecologic studies have shown correlations of at least .7 between consumption of fat, meat, and protein and colon cancer incidence or mortality. Most ecologic studies have also found inverse associations between fiber and cereal intake and colon cancer. One report concluded that total fat and fiber consumption accounts for 67% of the intercountry variation in colon cancer mortality among men. For studies of particular nutrients, the authors considered associations to be misleading because of collinearity and because some constituents are well measured while others are overlooked entirely. Among specific foods, vegetables consistently appear protective; fruits, less frequently. Calcium and vitamin D were discussed separately and at length because this had not previously been done. Also, there is a specific mechanistic hypothesis to explain the observations, and these nutrients are the focus of intervention studies in patients with adenomatous polyps. Alcohol was discussed in detail and several other diet-related and diet-nonrelated factors were reviewed briefly. An interesting feature of this review was its presentation of mechanistic models at several levels: an epidemiologic model (the fat/fiber hypothesis); several physiologic/biochemical models (e.g., the bile acid/volatile fatty acid hypothesis); growth medium and physiologic cascade models of the colonic cell milieu; a cell/crypt model (adenoma → carcinoma sequence and the cell replication hypothesis); and molecular models based on genetic predisposition.

At the root of the injunction to eat a variety of foods is the assumption that dietary diversity increases the likelihood of choosing an adequate diet, helps ensure proper balance among nutrients, and reduces exposure to harmful components carried by specific foods. In a case–control study (Western New York Diet Study), McCann et al. tested the hypothesis that a varied diet reduces the risk of colon cancer (*47*). Diversity was calculated for total foods and for the categories fruits, vegetables, grains, meats and meat substitutes, dairy foods, and nutrient-nondense foods, based on the number of items reported as eaten more than once monthly. Overall, 114 foods were included, ranging from 6 in the dairy category to 38 in the vegetable category. For men, colon cancer risk was positively associated not only with diversity within the meat category, but, surprisingly, with total diversity—and this risk was independent of possible confounders. No significant associations were found for women.

A case–control study of alcohol and nutrients in relation to colon cancer in middle-aged adults in western Washington found no associations with fat, protein, or vitamin consumption (*48*). Calcium and fruit and vegetable fiber were protective in women; cereal fiber was protective in men. As in several other studies, alcohol consumption was strongly related to risk of colon cancer for both men and women. However, a case–control study in northern Italy found that moderate beer drinking is not associated with elevated risk for cancers of the colon or rectum (*49*). Moreover, examination of data from the Iowa Women's Health Study found no significant association between overall alcohol consumption and colonic or rectal cancer in postmenopausal women (*50*). In fact, consumption of wine was inversely associated with cancer of the distal colon. Because men and women differ in gut physiology and alcohol metabolism, the authors recommend further study of the association between alcohol and colon cancer in women.

After a 5-year follow-up the Iowa Women's Health Study also identified several protective associations between fruit and vegetable consumption and colon cancer (*51*). The strongest association was for garlic, which showed an age- and energy-adjusted relative risk of .68 (95% confidence interval [CI] .46–1.02) for the highest vs. the lowest quartile of consumption. Protective effects were also seen for intake of fiber and all vegetables, but the 95% CIs spanned 1.

Frentzel-Beyme and Chang-Claude assessed colon cancer and other mortality risks in a cohort of 1904 self-identified moderate and strict vegetarians in Germany and reviewed other studies of dietary fiber, fiber-containing foods, and colon cancer risk (*52*). All-cause mortality of vegetarians was about half the national rate; cancer mortality was reduced ~50% for men and ~25% for women. Vegetarian men and women had about half the national rate of all intestinal system cancers and men had a reduced rate of colon cancer. No rectal cancers

occurred in men or women, but few were expected. However, vegetarians also practiced other health-promoting behaviors that may have had stronger effects than nutrition.

The Netherlands Cohort Study is a prospective study involving >120,000 adults. Goldbohm et al. reported on the relation between meat consumption and the risk of colon cancer in this group after 3.3 y of follow-up (*53*). They found no evidence that greater consumption of total energy or energy-adjusted fat, protein, total fresh meat, or individual fresh meats increased risk for colon cancer. However, consumption of processed meat (mainly sausages) was associated with increased risk at a relative rate of 1.17 per 15 g/day. After 6 y of follow-up in the Health Professionals Follow-Up Study, intakes of total, saturated, and animal fat were unrelated to risk of colon cancer (*54*). However, intake of red meat was associated with colon cancer risk. The highest quintile of consumption had a relative risk of 1.71 (95% CI 1.15–2.55) compared to the lowest quintile. Men who ate beef, pork, or lamb as a main dish ≥5 times per week had a relative risk of 3.57 (95% CI 1.58–8.06) compared to men who ate these foods less than once per month. The association remained after correction for potential confounders. Vegetable fat and other sources of animal fat (dairy products, fish, poultry) were slightly inversely associated with risk.

In Japan, a case–control study of colorectal cancer in relation to diet, cigarette smoking, and alcohol consumption found that preference for salty foods was an independent risk factor for both colon and rectal cancer, whereas consumption of seaweed was protective (*55*). Alcohol intake showed a slight but significant inverse association with colon but not rectal cancer risk when drinkers were compared with those who never drank, but there was no dose–response relationship. Apparent protective effects of soybean products and nuts vanished upon multiple regression analysis.

An ecologic survey of diet and colon cancer mortality in 49 rural Chinese counties suggested that observations in Western societies may also apply to China (*56*). Increased mortality was associated with high consumption of animal foods, salt-preserved vegetables, and beer; high intake of green vegetables was protective. Serum levels of total cholesterol, urea nitrogen, and lipid peroxides were positively correlated with colon cancer mortality after adjustment for each other and for other blood nutrients. Serum levels of β-carotene, α-tocopherol, vitamin C, and selenium were not significantly related to colon cancer. Schistosomiasis infection increased risk. The authors concluded that schistosomiasis infection and dietary factors are major determinants for the sharp geographic variation in colon cancer mortality in rural China.

A large screening trial in Denmark provided subjects for a study of dietary risk factors for colorectal cancer and adenomas (*57*). Forty-nine persons with cancer and 172 with adenomas diagnosed at the screening were recruited as case-patients; 362 who tested negative were recruited as controls. Dietary fiber intake was inversely associated with risk of both cancer and adenomas. Neither risk was related to body mass or total energy intake. Vitamins A and E were inversely associated with occurrence of adenomas.

Caderni et al. compared mitotic activity in the colorectal mucosa of healthy subjects in two Italian cities having different dietary patterns (*58*). Residents of Trieste in northern Italy had significantly higher mitotic activity than residents of Florence in central Italy. As a group, subjects in Trieste also consumed significantly less starch, fiber, protein, and nitrite. However, no correlations were seen in individuals between intestinal proliferation and consumption of these nutrients.

A case–control study in Majorca of diet and colorectal adenomas found an elevated risk related to consumption of sugar and pastries (*59*). High consumption of vegetables, regardless of cooking procedures, was strongly protective. By nutrient analysis, protective factors were fruit and vegetable fiber, magnesium and zinc, and vitamins C, $B_6$, and folic acid. No excess risk was associated with consumption of alcohol, saturated fats, or animal protein.

When some dietary patterns are clearly associated with reduced colon cancer risk and others are associated with enhanced risk, why bother to settle the disputes over what factor or factors really underlie the differences? Aside from the satisfaction of *knowing,* a practical reason involves understanding the advantages and disadvantages of dietary supplements. Dwyer discussed a metaanalysis of 13 case–control studies, which indicated an inverse association between dietary fiber intake and colon cancer risk (*60*). Much weaker protective effects were seen for vitamin C and β-carotene. If a direct protective effect of dietary fiber is confirmed, questions still remain. What are the protective mechanisms? Which fibers are most effective? Does fiber also reduce risk of cancers and diseases other than colon cancer? What is the optimal dietary fiber intake? Furthermore, metaanalyses are subject to their own difficulties, as discussed by this reviewer and by others (*61*). Friedenreich et al. examined the influence of methodologic factors in this same metaanalysis. They evaluated the methods used in each of the 13 studies, estimated a quality score, and used random effects models to reestimate the pooled odds

ratio for the association between dietary fiber and colorectal cancer based on these data. The odds ratio for ≥27 g/day of dietary fiber and colorectal cancer was 0.46 (95% CI 0.34–0.64) for the 13 studies. Two factors explained some of this heterogeneity: risk estimates were closer to null for studies in which the diet questionnaire had been validated before use and in which qualitative data on dietary habits and cooking methods had been incorporated. Quality score did not explain any between-study heterogeneity, but random effects models explained a portion of the heterogeneity. The authors concluded that differences in dietary assessment methods and food composition tables contribute to heterogeneity in study results and that standardization in study methods would facilitate pooled analyses and permit more reliable conclusions about diet–disease relationships.

Bostick et al. analyzed data from the prospective Iowa Women's Health Study, to investigate whether high intake of antioxidant nutrients protects against colon cancer (*62*). Age-adjusted vitamin E intake was inversely associated with risk: the relative risk for the highest quintile of intake relative to the lowest was 0.32 (95% CI 0.19–0.54, *p* <.0001). Adjustment for total energy intake and other risk factors had little effect on this estimate. The protective effect of vitamin E diminished with age, there being little or no effect in persons ≥65 years old. Multivariate-adjusted relative risk among women with high total intakes of vitamins A and C and among those who used selenium supplements did not differ significantly from 1.0. Bostick et al. also used data from the Iowa Women's Health Study to examine the relation of calcium, vitamin D, and dairy food intake to the incidence of colon cancer among older women (*63*). After adjustment for age, intakes of calcium and vitamin D in the highest quintile were significantly protective. Although the 95% CIs for multivariate-adjusted intakes spanned 1.0 and were statistically nonsignificant, relative risks for both nutrients were ~0.7 and the authors consider this finding compatible with other reports suggesting a modest role for calcium and vitamin D in reducing colon cancer risk. Two other large cohort studies found no convincing association between calcium intake and risk of colorectal adenomas in men and women (*64*). Nor was consumption of milk or fermented dairy products related to adenoma risk. Vitamin D from supplements may have had a small nonsignificant protective effect among women but not men.

Cassidy et al. compared intakes of starch, nonstarch polysaccharides (NSPs), protein, and fat with colorectal cancer incidence in 12 populations worldwide (*65*). Starch consumption was significantly inversely correlated with cancer risk (*r* = –.76 for colon cancer and −.70 for total colorectal cancer). There was no significant relationship with NSPs, although when NSP was combined with resistant starch (an estimate of fermentable carbohydrate) the association remained significant: $r = −.60$ for colon and −.52 for colorectal cancer. These strong associations suggest an important role for starch in protecting against colorectal cancer and support the hypothesis that colonic fermentation provides a protective mechanism.

Data from a large case–control study in northern Italy were used to investigate the relationship between intake of refined sugar and the risk of colorectal cancer (*66*). Sugar added to coffee and other hot beverages was an indicator of taste for sugar and consumption of sugar outside main meals. Compared with subjects who added no sugar to their beverages, the multivariate relative risk of colon cancer was 1.4 for those adding one spoonful, 1.6 for those adding two spoonfuls, and 2.0 for those adding 3 or more. For rectal cancer the corresponding risks were 1.3, 1.5, and 1.4, and for total colorectal cancer they were 1.4, 1.5, and 1.8. All trends were significant. Results were consistent across strata of study center, sex, and age and were not modified by adjustment for major potential confounders. The study was large enough to yield reasonably precise risk estimates and clear trends in risk. The authors suggest two possible explanations for their findings. One implicates total sucrose intake as a factor in colon carcinogenesis, but because intake of sugar-sweetened beverages was used as the indicator of sugar intake, another possibility is that even small amounts of sugar ingested on an empty stomach have a specific role in colon carcinogenesis.

## Stomach and Esophageal Cancer

Despite years of speculation and investigation, the precipitous decline in incidence of gastric cancer in the USA between 1930 and the mid-1970s has not been entirely explained. Concomitantly, the proportion of gastric cancers in the cardia region increased sharply, due largely to an absolute decrease in cancers in the antrum and prepyloric area. Longmire summarized current thinking about gastric cancer in the USA (*67*). The development of gastric cancer is thought to involve sequential stages from chronic gastritis to atrophy, intestinal metaplasia, dysplasia, and finally carcinoma. Gastritis and atrophy are linked to excessive salt intake and *Helicobacter pylori* infection. Intermediate stages are associated with a balance between intake of vitamin C, which is protective, and nitrate, which promotes intragastric nitrosation. The final stages are linked to a balance between the protective effect of β-carotene and

the harmful effect of excess salt. Medication-induced suppression of gastric acid secretion may also be involved. A review of risk factors and preventive factors found a number that are diet-related and indicated diagrammatically where in the process of gastric carcinogenesis they exert their influence (*68*). Some positive results have been seen in chemoprevention trials using vitamin E and β-carotene supplements. High intake of fruits and vegetables and antioxidant nutrients may decrease risk. Consumption of large amounts of alcohol, nitrates, nitrites, and pickled, highly salted, fermented, or smoked foods appears to enhance risk. Improper food storage, *H. pylori* infection, and several other environmental factors may also increase risk. Refrigeration of food can be directly protective by reducing microbial production of carcinogens, or indirectly protective by reducing the need for methods of food preservation (such as salting or smoking) that have been linked to gastric cancer.

Hansson et al. conducted a study of dietary and lifestyle risk factors for gastric cancer in areas of Sweden with contrasting incidences of this cancer (*69,70*). Subjects, 338 gastric cancer patients and approximately 2 age- and sex-matched controls per patient, were interviewed concerning their food and lifestyle habits during adolescence and in the period 20 y before the interview. During both time periods, high consumption of wholegrain bread, fruits, and vegetables reduced risk (*69*). High cheese, fish, and tea consumption during adolescence was protective. Risk was positively associated with the age at which the subject started using refrigeration. No risk was associated with intake of meat, sausages, cold cuts, liver, salt, coffee, or fried, smoked, or grilled foods. There was significant interaction between tobacco use and fruit consumption, high fruit intake being more protective among tobacco users than nonusers (*70*). A similar but smaller interaction was seen between vegetable intake and tobacco use. High alcohol intake increased the risk associated with tobacco.

Two case–control studies of diet and gastric cancer in Spain were reported. One involved dietary interviews of 117 case-patients and 234 population controls in the Barcelona metropolitan area (*71*). Only vitamin C intake showed a significant protective effect in multivariate analysis. Compared with the lowest quintile of vitamin C intake, the highest quintile had an odds ratio (OR) of 0.3 (95% CI 0.1–0.8). There was a nonsignificant protective trend for vitamin A intake. The other study was conducted in selected areas of Aragon, Castille, Catalonia, and Galicia (*72*). Increased risk was associated with high intake of exogenous nitrosamines. Decreased risk was associated with high intake of fiber, vitamin C, and folate. High vitamin C intake reduced the risk related to ingestion of nitrosamines. No dietary associations were seen with the histologic type of tumor.

A case–control study of gastric cancer in Puerto Rico found a significant difference (OR 3.34, $p$ <.001) between case-patients and controls in dietary salt intake, estimated from the consumption of nine common highly salted food items (*73*). The dose response was also significant. The association remained significant after adjustment for sex, education, and cigarette smoking. The authors believe they probably underestimated the true salt intake by not considering other foods or salt added at the table or during cooking; this probably biased the result toward the null hypothesis.

China has a very high rate of gastric cancer. Results of a study of serum micronutrients in relation to precancerous gastric lesions in a region of China with a particularly high incidence of this cancer complemented findings from numerous dietary studies (*74*). Serum levels of retinol, β-carotene, ascorbic acid, α-tocopherol, selenium, ferritin, copper, and zinc were measured in ~600 adults with precancerous lesions. Concentrations of β-carotene and ascorbic acid were significantly lower in subjects with intestinal metaplasia than in those with less advanced lesions. These associations were strong and independent. The odds of chronic atrophic gastritis progressing to intestinal metaplasia were only 17% as high among subjects with β-carotene and ascorbic acid levels in the upper tertile as among those in the lower two tertiles. Risk of intestinal metaplasia was also somewhat higher in those with low serum ferritin, but no significant effects were found for the other substances assayed.

A Japanese study found that the influence of dietary and lifestyle factors on risk of gastric cancer varies with the subsite of the cancer—whether proximal (cardia and fundus) or distal (pyloric antrum) (*75*). High intake of fresh vegetables was protective at all sites and preference for salty food increased risk at all sites. Preference for greasy food or for Western-style breakfasts increased the risk of cancer of the gastric cardia relative to that of other subsites, but consumption of Western-style breakfasts decreased risk of antrum cancer. No significant effects were associated with rice, fruit, miso soup, or milk. The joint effect of smoking and drinking appeared important in development of gastric cancer, particularly in the cardia.

Muñoz reviewed the epidemiology of esophageal cancer world-wide, classifying these cancers according to their relatedness to alcohol and tobacco use (*76*). A common denominator in all esophageal cancers is a diet containing few fresh vegetables, fruits, and dairy products. Beyond this, the etiology of esophageal cancer is poorly understood for populations in which alcohol and tobacco play a minor role. Hypotheses invoking consumption of pickled vegetables, moldy foods, and nitrates have not been confirmed. A recent study in Hong Kong, however, identified eating pickled vegetables and drinking hot beverages as major risk factors. Although thermal injury from hot food and drink is difficult to measure, the habit of drinking maté tea affords an opportunity to assess the role of hot drinks. Maté is drunk through a tube that delivers it to the back of the tongue, from where it is promptly swallowed. Maté drinkers may consume more than a liter of this beverage each day. South America has well-defined exposed and unexposed groups, and data from these groups indicate that hot maté drinking is associated with both esophagitis and esophageal cancer. Although the effect could be due to carcinogenic components of the maté, no such activity has been found in vitro. Moreover, a recent study among young adults in a high-risk area of China identified the habit of drinking "burning hot" beverages as the strongest risk factor for esophagitis, and a case–control study in Hong Kong estimated that 14% of the esophageal cancers in this population were explained by the preference for consuming very hot soups and drinks. Weaker evidence pointing in the same direction has been found in studies from other parts of the world. The author concluded that alcohol, tobacco, poor nutrition, and thermal injury cause most esophageal cancers in the Americas, Europe, and parts of Africa and Asia, but major causes in China and some Asian populations have not yet been identified.

Franceschi reviewed nine studies exploring the role of diet in the etiology of esophageal cancer in affluent nations, emphasizing the sharp gradients in incidence that exist even within Europe and the USA (*77*). She concluded that a higher than average intake of vegetables and fresh fruit, particularly citrus, can reduce risk of this cancer by a factor of 2–3. Of specific micronutrients, vitamins C and E and β-carotene appear protective. High intakes of retinol (preformed vitamin A), fat, butter, eggs, starchy foods, and total calories frequently appeared as risk factors, the association of enhanced risk with retinol intake being most consistent. It is possible that this elevated risk is a consequence of a diet poor in micronutrients that can prevent esophageal cancer. In most high-risk groups studied, high alcohol intake (up to 1000 kg or more daily) was common. The impact of nutritionally deficient alcoholic beverages is aggravated by the limited diet that characterizes high-risk groups: the staple bacon and sausages among blacks in the USA, potatoes in northern France, and corn in the mountains of northern Italy.

In northern Italy, risk factors for esophageal cancer in women were found to be similar to those in men (78). The major risk factor was cigarette smoking, followed by high alcohol consumption. Fresh fruit was significantly protective and there was an inverse relationship with estimated β-carotene intake. There was no association with retinol.

Smoking and alcohol consumption were also the major risk factors for esophageal cancer in a low-risk area of northeast China (79). High temperature of food and beverages was another risk factor. Fresh vegetables, fruits, vitamin C, and possibly β-carotene were protective. A 100 mg per day increase in vitamin C consumption reduced the adjusted odds ratio by 39%. Salt, salt-preserved foods, and pickled vegetables were not significantly associated with risk. In Shanghai, the incidence of esophageal cancer declined by >50% between 1972 and 1989, the decline being greatest in younger age groups (80). In contrast, stomach cancer incidence decreased only 20% in men and not at all in women during this period. The reasons for these trends are not known but they appear to be partly related to dietary changes.

## Nasopharyngeal and Oral Cancer

Hildesheim and Levine reviewed the etiology of nasopharyngeal carcinomas, which account for 85–95% of nasopharyngeal cancers (81). These carcinomas are rare in Europe and North America, occur at intermediate rates in parts of southeastern Asia, northern Africa, and the Arctic and among African Americans, and are extremely common among Chinese from southeast Asia and their descendants. Nasopharyngeal carcinomas are also more common in men than women, suggesting varying levels of exposure to environmental agents. Consumption of citrus fruits, tomatoes, and carrots appears protective, suggesting a protective role for vitamin C and carotenoids. Frequent consumption of salted fish is the best-confirmed risk factor for nasopharyngeal carcinoma. The epidemiologic evidence is supported by data from animal and in vitro studies. The method of producing and preparing the salted fish may be important. Age of exposure is also involved: consumption of numerous other processed and preserved foods at a young age has been implicated. The specific food items involved have varied from study to study but include salted duck eggs, salted shrimp paste, salted mustard greens, chung choi, dried fish, fermented soybean paste, preserved plums, spiced dried meat stored in

oil, and a preparation of red pepper, olive oil, garlic, caraway, and salt.

A case–control study of nasopharyngeal carcinoma was conducted in the Guangxi Autonomous Region of China after a survey identified lifestyle factors that could be linked to this tumor (82). Guangxi has the second highest mortality rate from nasopharyngeal carcinoma of all Chinese provinces. Consumption of leafy vegetables significantly reduced risk. Again, age of exposure is important. Consumption of salted, dried, or canned meat, eggs, and vegetables was not linked with risk except for consumption of dried salted melon seeds during childhood. Consumption of salted fish in rice porridge during weaning, before the age of 2 y, and between the ages of 2 and 10 y was a major risk factor. After multivariate analysis, three variables remained significantly associated with risk: use of wood cooking fuel, consumption of salted fish in rice porridge before the age of 2 y, and drinking herbal tea during the year preceding diagnosis. The possible nature of the risk associated with herbal tea preparations was discussed.

Among white men in the USA, high consumption of salted or smoked foods was associated with elevated risk for cancers of the nasal cavity and paranasal sinuses and high consumption of vegetables was protective (83). Cigarette smoking and alcohol drinking were strong risk factors; passive smoking and certain occupational factors also appeared to increase risk.

A case–control study of nonviral risk factors for nasopharyngeal carcinoma in the Philippines found no association with consumption of salted fish (84). Moreover, consumption of processed meats appeared protective. Smoking, use of herbal medicines, and several other environmental and occupational exposures appeared to increase risk.

An Australian case–control study of oral and pharyngeal cancer in men found statistically significant protective effects of increasing dietary intakes of vitamin C, β-carotene, fruits, vegetables, and dietary fiber (85). Case-patients had significantly lower serum levels of β-carotene and retinol than controls. Smoking and alcohol consumption enhanced risk synergistically.

A study by Flagg et al. illustrated a general weakness of epidemiologic studies, which of necessity focus on a selected few of the many possible foods, food components, and nutrients (86). These authors found a suggestive association between dietary glutathione and reduced risk of oral and pharyngeal cancer in a case–control study conducted in areas of New Jersey, Georgia, and California. The relative risk of these cancers among subjects in the highest quartile of total glutathione intake was 0.5 (95% CI 0.3–0.7). When analyzed by dietary source, only glutathione from fruit and from vegetables commonly eaten raw was associated with reduced risk. The analysis was limited by the small numbers of subjects with extreme combinations of intakes, and the study did not distinguish effects of glutathione from effects of fruits and raw vegetables or other constituents of fruits and raw vegetables. However, a possible mechanism exists for an anticarcinogenic effect of glutathione: it may act as an antioxidant or may bind with cellular mutagens.

## Lung Cancer

Reports of an association between lung cancer and dietary fat and cholesterol have been persistent, if not consistent. Kolonel reviewed evidence for such an association in his editorial comments on findings of a recent case–control study (*87*). Collinearity of variables is a major problem in all such studies, making it difficult to pinpoint the foods or dietary constituents that are actually responsible for the general association seen with a high-fat diet, and Kolonel does not believe the statistical methods used adequately address this problem. He asks further whether the identification of secondary risk factors for lung cancer plays into the hands of the tobacco industry, and whether addition of lung cancer to the growing list of harmful health consequences of a high-fat diet notably strengthens the arguments for taking aggressive public health measures to reduce the average fat level in the American diet. The specific new study in question investigated the association between saturated fat intake and lung cancer risk among nonsmoking women in Missouri (*88*). Women in the top quintile of saturated fat consumption had a relative risk for lung cancer more than six times that of women in the lowest quintile. The effect was greater for adenocarcinoma than for other cell types. Weekly servings of beans and peas were significantly protective. Other somewhat protective foods were fruits other than citrus, and fish and chicken. Unexpectedly, citrus fruit and juice appeared to increase risk. Slightly elevated risk was also associated with weekly consumption of red meat and dairy products. The significant effects of total fat, oleic acid, red meat, percent of calories from fat, and percent of calories from saturated fat seen in univariate analysis disappeared when daily intake of saturated fat was included in the regression model. In contrast, the effect of saturated fat remained highly significant regardless of which other fat measure was included. The leading contributors of dietary saturated fat were hamburgers, cheeseburgers, meat loaf, cheeses and cheese spreads, hot dogs, ice cream, and sausages. By limiting their analysis to nonsmokers,

the authors believe they have revealed an association with dietary saturated fat that may have been masked in studies involving a high percentage of smokers.

Another study of dietary factors and lung cancer risk among nonsmokers in the USA found significant dose-dependent reduction in risk associated with consumption of greens, fresh fruits, and cheese (*89*). Use of vitamin E supplements was also protective. There was a dose-related increase in risk associated with whole-milk consumption. Protective factors differed slightly between men and women. Overall the results indicate that dietary β-carotene, raw fruits and vegetables, and vitamin E supplements reduce lung cancer risk in nonsmokers.

Investigators in Japan reported protective effects of lettuce and cabbage, raw vegetables, green vegetables, and fruit against lung cancer in current smokers and exsmokers (*90*). The effect varied with the food and the tumor's histologic type.

A prospective cohort study in the Netherlands investigated the relationship between selenium status and risk of lung cancer (*91*). The selenium content of toenails was measured as a long-term marker of selenium status. The adjusted rate ratio of lung cancer for subjects in the highest quintile of selenium (compared with the lowest) was 0.50 (95% CI 0.30–0.81), with a significant trend across quintiles. The protective effect was greatest in subjects with a relatively low dietary intake of β-carotene (rate ratio 0.45, 95% CI 0.22–0.92) or vitamin C (rate ratio 0.36, 95% CI 0.17–0.75). Protection was not restricted to a particular sex, smoking category, or histologic type of cancer.

## Breast Cancer

A thoughtful review of diet, body size, and breast cancer concluded that dietary factors are probably important determinants but found little definitive evidence for which factors or why (*92*). The fat hypothesis, once considered virtually proven, is now more elusive than ever. Increases in breast cancer mortality rates in Japan are consistent with a birth cohort effect: little increase has occurred among older women. The increase of colon cancer (which is clearly linked to fat intake) in this group suggests that fat intake during adulthood does not substantially alter breast cancer risk. Seventh-Day Adventists, who eat relatively small amounts of meat and other animal products, have substantially lower rates of colon cancer than population controls but only slightly lower rates of breast cancer; and breast cancer rates in British nuns who ate little or no meat were similar to rates in single secular women. These data do not support an important association between animal fat and breast cancer. There is a strong possibility that selection or recall bias influences the results of case–control studies, some of which support the fat hypothesis. Data from prospective studies, which should suffer from minimal selection bias and no recall bias, provide solid evidence *against* a relationship between fat intake and breast cancer in developed countries during follow-up periods of up to 10 years. Two variations of the dietary fat hypothesis have not been tested. One is that fat intake during childhood and adolescence influences risk of breast cancer decades later. However, any hypothesis relating early diet to later breast cancer will remain difficult to test without valid markers of breast cancer risk, novel data sources, or reliable methods of measuring childhood diet. The other hypothesis is that extreme reduction in fat intake to <20 en% may reduce risk. If this is true, the association between fat intake and breast cancer would be highly nonlinear with a distinct threshold, and ecologic comparisons do not suggest such a threshold. The Women's Health Initiative intends to test a very low-fat diet, but this trial will not distinguish between the effect of fat reduction and the effect of increased intake of fruits, vegetables, and grains. From a public health standpoint, such an extreme diet is not feasible anyway. One hypothesis that may explain much of the international variation in breast cancer rates is energy restriction during growth, but this does not suggest a practical intervention strategy either. Evidence for a relationship between body mass index and breast cancer depends on menopausal status and while fairly consistent in case–control studies has not been reproduced in prospective studies. Studies of vitamin A and other micronutrients have produced inconclusive and sometimes conflicting results. Evidence for a protective effect of fiber is tenuous at best. Epidemiologic evidence is not compatible with any substantial effect of coffee drinking on breast cancer risk. The best established dietary risk factor for breast cancer is high alcohol consumption, but even here it may be that the major risk is related to drinking during adolescence and early adulthood.

A brief review also revealed the controversy over the links between diet and breast cancer, pointing out that known risk factors explain the etiology of fewer than half of breast cancer cases (*93*). However, this reviewer emphasized that at least two established risk factors, early menarche and obesity, are diet-related and she took an optimistic view of the potential knowledge to be gained from the Women's Health Initiative.

A case–control study of breast cancer in Switzerland found significant direct trends in risk related to total energy intake and consumption of various meats, cheese, and alcohol (*94*). Significant reductions in risk (40–60%

between the highest and lowest tertiles of consumption) were found for total green vegetables, cucumbers, onions, pears, and β-carotene. In Denmark, a combined population-based case–control and follow-up study identified high fat and alcohol consumption, early menarche, and several nondietary factors as risk factors for breast cancer (*95*). It found no association with intakes of vegetables, tea, coffee, and sweeteners. Survival of case-patients was not related to any dietary variable, including alcohol consumption, although there may have been a complex relationship between survival and body mass index. Analysis of breast cancer incidence data for Denmark, 1943–1989, showed significant increases for recent time periods and birth cohorts (*96*). Only a small proportion of this could be attributed to changes in fertility rates, age at menarche, and exposure to exogenous hormones. Most of the variation in incidence by time period was attributable to dietary factors and alcohol. The most significant protective factor was carbohydrate intake; the greatest risk factor was alcohol. After adjustment for these, dietary protein and fat made little further contribution to the amount of variation explained.

**DIETARY FAT.** Boyd et al. conducted a metaanalysis of 23 independent case–control and cohort studies of fat intake and breast cancer risk (*97*). From the relative risk in each study comparing the highest and lowest level of total fat intake they calculated a summary relative risk. This was 1.01 (95% CI 0.9–1.13) for cohort studies, 1.21 (95% CI 1.10–1.34) for case–control studies, and 1.12 (95% CI 1.04–1.21) for all studies. Confidence intervals for summary estimates of risk for specific types of fat excluded 1.0 only for saturated fat. Summary risks of ~1.2, confidence intervals excluding 1.0, were also associated with high meat, milk, and cheese consumption. Studies done in Europe were more likely than studies done elsewhere to show increased risk related to dietary fat.

Wynder et al. weighed evidence for the dietary fat hypothesis against the criteria of consistency, strength, specificity, temporality, and biological coherence (*98*). They argued that the hypothesis is supported by evidence from animal, metabolic, and ecologic studies in which diverse methods have led to similar conclusions. Both animal and ecologic studies show evidence of a dose-related gradient. Specificity of the effect is more easily demonstrated in animal and in vitro experiments than in clinical or ecologic studies, whereas changes in disease risk following changes in exposure are evident in epidemiologic studies. Finally, plausible biologic mechanisms exist. The authors discussed weaknesses of the epidemiologic data, but concluded that these problems do not justify discarding the dietary fat hypothesis when it is supported by the overall mosaic of evidence. In a point-by-point response to these arguments, Willett countered that the authors were selective in their citations and uncritical of the indirect evidence (*99*). He considers the evidence supporting a link between dietary fat and breast cancer risk to be far less compelling than suggested by Wynder et al., pointing out that prospective studies specifically designed to examine this relationship have been uniformly unsupportive of the hypothesis. Although further investigation is warranted, other dietary factors should be examined as fat may be among the less promising. Wynder et al. responded to Willett's specific criticisms and invoked the conclusions of the National Academy of Sciences and the World Health Organization to support their view (*100*). Debate continues.

A prospective study of 590 postmenopausal women in California identified 15 new cases of breast cancer in 15 years of follow-up (*101*). Women with incident breast cancer had significantly higher age-adjusted intake of total fat and oleic, linoleic, and linolenic acids, and there was a stepwise increase in risk across tertiles of consumption. They also consumed more calories, protein, and carbohydrates than other subjects. After each nutrient variable was adjusted for body mass index, alcohol consumption, and several nondietary factors, the strongest risks for breast cancer were associated with total calories and total fat. Fat composition did not influence risk.

**DIETARY FIBER.** An Australian study of 451 women with breast cancer and 451 population-based controls evaluated the risk of breast cancer in relation to intake of dietary fiber and various fiber components (*102*). Risk was estimated for each quintile of fiber density (intake per megajoule of total energy) relative to a risk of 1.0 for the lowest quintile. Women in the highest quintile had a risk of 0.46, and the trend across quintiles was significant (*p* <.001). For fiber components defined by the Englyst method of analysis, the greatest risk reduction was associated with high densities of mannose from insoluble NSP and of glucose from soluble NSP. For many fiber components, point estimates of relative risk were similar for premenopausal and postmenopausal women, but had greater statistical significance in the postmenopausal group, which contained many more subjects.

**ANTIOXIDANT MICRONUTRIENTS.** Garland et al. reviewed epidemiologic evidence on the relationship between breast cancer risk and vitamins A, C, and E and selenium (*103*). Vitamin A appears somewhat protective, but it is

not clear whether this is due to retinol, carotenoids, or both. Another component of vitamin A–rich foods could also account for the association. Evidence for vitamins C and E is limited and inconsistent. Within the range of normal human diets, selenium probably does not influence risk. Ethical and logistic constraints preclude rigorous testing of micronutrient hypotheses in controlled randomized trials. Future studies of this nature should be prospective to minimize selection and recall bias and should address methodologic issues such as confounding and appropriate storage of blood samples. However, although recall bias has weakened some case–control studies, Friedenreich et al. failed to find such bias in a nested case–control study within the Canadian National Breast Screening Study (*104*). Dietary data collected in 1988 from 325 women with breast cancer and 628 matched controls were compared with similar data collected on enrollment in the study in 1982–1985, before disease diagnosis. Prospective and retrospective estimates of mean dietary micronutrient intake were very similar for both case-subjects and controls. Prospective and retrospective odds ratios estimated for the association between micronutrient intake and breast cancer were similar in magnitude and the 95% confidence limits overlapped considerably. Errors in reporting previous supplementary use of vitamins were identical for the two subject groups. Thus there was no evidence for recall bias in this study.

A prospective study of >89,000 women participating in the Nurses' Health Study evaluated the influence of intake of vitamins C, E, and A on breast cancer risk (*105*). Intakes of these vitamins from foods and supplements was assessed at the beginning of the study in 1984. During 8 y of follow-up, 1439 cases of breast cancer were diagnosed. High intakes of vitamins C and E offered no protection. There was some evidence that a low intake of vitamin A increased risk, but any benefit of vitamin A supplements was limited to women whose diets were low in this nutrient.

**BREAST MILK.** Because of suggestions that nutrition in early childhood influences subsequent risk of breast cancer, Freudenheim et al. tested for an association between breast cancer and having been breast-fed in a case–control study in western New York (*106*). The multivariate adjusted odds ratio for having been breast-fed was 0.74 (95% CI 0.56–0.99). Results for premenopausal and postmenopausal women were very similar.

**ALCOHOL.** Alcohol consumption is frequently considered an established risk factor for breast cancer. However, a review of the epidemiologic evidence for an association between alcohol consumption and breast cancer risk concluded that although positive associations have frequently been observed, confounding has not been ruled out as an explanation (*107*). According to these authors, the associations are weak and inconsistent, the causes of most breast cancer are still largely unknown, and lifestyle correlates of alcohol use are poorly defined. Nor are proposed biologic mechanisms convincing.

**DIET AND BENIGN BREAST DISEASE.** Fibrocystic breast disease has been of interest as a possible stage in the progression from a benign abnormality to malignancy. Vobecky et al. evaluated the nutritional profile of women with fibrocystic breast disease, using data from the Canadian National Breast Screening Study (*108*). Women 50 y old or older with fibrocystic breast disease had higher intakes of calories, fat, carbohydrate, fiber, vitamin D, free folacin, calcium, sodium, potassium, and magnesium but a lower intake of cholesterol than controls. In women younger than 50 y, lower intake of protein, niacin, and several minerals was associated with fibrocystic breast disease. In general, use of oral contraceptives, cholesterol intake ≥300 mg/d, saturated fat >10 en%, and body mass index ≥25 kg/m² were protective. No effect was very large.

**DIET AND MAMMOGRAPHIC PATTERNS.** A Swedish study evaluated dietary habits in relation to mammographic patterns in patients with breast cancer (*109*). Diagnostic mammograms were coded according to Wolfe's criteria, N1, P1, P2, and Dy patterns representing successively higher breast cancer risk. Women with the Dy pattern reported significantly higher intake of total fat, monounsaturated fat, and polyunsaturated fat (en%) and α-tocopherol. In addition, women with the Dy mammographic pattern whose cancers were rich in estrogen receptors had significantly lower intake of carbohydrate and calcium. Women with the N1 pattern had the lowest fat intake. The authors suggested that dietary habits can affect the mammographic parenchymal pattern in women with breast cancer and that a high-fat diet is associated with a high proportion of mammograms with the Dy pattern in these patients. A preliminary report of a study in England examined the relationship between diet and mammographic patterns in women who participated in a breast cancer screening program (*110*). This study found small and nonsignificant pattern-related differences between women in the adjusted geometric mean of intakes of energy, fat, saturated fat, fiber, and alcohol. Women with the N1 and P1 patterns consumed

significantly more carotene and vitamin C than women with the Dy pattern.

**DIET AND PROGNOSIS IN BREAST CANCER.** An association has been found between DNA ploidy and prognosis in breast cancer. Pursuing this lead, Fürst et al. studied the relationship between diet and the nuclear DNA content of breast cancer cells in 82 women aged 50–65 y (*111*). Patients with euploid tumors reported lower mean intake of total, saturated, and monounsaturated fat and higher intake of protein, vitamin D, and selenium than patients whose tumors had an aneuploid pattern. In stepwise logistic regression analysis, the odds ratio for having a tumor with aneuploid DNA was 1.16 (95% CI 1.04–1.28) for each 1-g increase in intake of total fat and 0.95 (95% CI 0.92–0.99) for each 1-mg increase in selenium intake per 10 MJ. The odds ratio associated with each 1-g increment in saturated fat was 1.30.

Ingram reported an update of a study showing that diet can influence the survival of breast cancer patients (*112*). Patients underwent dietary assessment 3 months after surgery. Six to 8 years later, 21 subjects had died of advanced breast cancer; 76 were still living. Only one death occurred among women in the highest tertile of β-carotene consumption, whereas 8 and 12 deaths occurred in the middle and lowest tertiles, respectively. The possible antiproliferative effects of β-carotene have been recognized for some time, and Ingram believes a clinical trial should be conducted to determine the effectiveness of β-carotene in reducing recurrence of breast cancer and preventing development of new cancers.

An Australian study found a small but suggestive influence of diet on survival from breast cancer in a population of patients followed for a median of 5.5 y (*113*). Risk of death was decreased by 25–40% in all quintiles of protein and calorie intake above the lowest, whereas there was a 40% increase in risk for the highest quintile of fat intake. Slightly reduced risk was associated with the upper quintiles of β-carotene and vitamin C intake. However, no dose-related variations in risk were noted.

## Prostate Cancer

In editorial comments related to reference *115*, Pienta and Esper reasoned that because histologic evidence of prostate cancer is considerably less variable from country to country than symptomatic prostate cancer, marked cross-cultural differences in death rates from this cancer reflect differences in the promotion of tumorigenesis (*114*). They reviewed cross-cultural and analytic studies of diet and prostate cancer, concluding that fairly uniform rates of histologically evident prostate cancer coupled with widely disparate rates of clinical disease implicate a promotional event linked to an environmental cause and dietary fat seems to be the most likely culprit. Using data from the prospective Health Professionals Follow-Up Study, Giovannucci et al. evaluated the relationship between dietary fat and risk of prostate cancer (*115*). Total fat consumption was directly related to risk of advanced disease (relative risk 1.79, 95% CI 1.04–3.07, $p = .06$ for the highest vs. lowest quintiles). This association was primarily due to the animal fat component, but high intake of $\alpha$-linolenic acid was an independent risk factor. Red meat was the food most strongly associated with increased risk (relative risk 2.64, 95% CI 1.21–5.77, $p = .02$). These results support the hypothesis that animal fat, especially fat from red meat, is associated with increased risk of advanced prostate cancer. However, the roles of $\alpha$-linolenic acid and carcinogens formed during cooking of animal fat need further exploration.

Franceschi commented on two recently reported cohort studies (*116*). She observed that epidemiologic surveys and prospective studies have yielded mixed results relating fat consumption to prostate cancer risk, but case–control studies generally support an association—particularly for animal (saturated) fat. Now two cohort studies, one based on a food-oriented dietary analysis (*117*) and one with a more nutrient-oriented approach (*115*), considerably strengthen the evidence that consumption of animal fat increases risk of symptomatic prostate cancer. Franceschi recommends that a population-wide decrease in animal fat consumption be one of the highest health priorities in the modern world for both men and women. The cohort study by Le Marchand et al. involved 20,316 men representing various ethnic groups in Hawaii, who were interviewed between 1975 and 1980 and followed through December 1989 (*117*). During this period 198 incident cases of invasive prostate cancer were diagnosed. Compared with the lowest tertile of consumption, relative risks associated with the highest tertile were 1.6 (95% CI 1.1–2.4) for beef, 1.4 (95% CI 1.0–2.1) for milk, and 1.6 (95% CI 1.0–2.4) for high-fat animal products. These associations were stronger in men diagnosed before the age of 72 y. These findings suggest that animal fat shortens the latency period of prostate cancer. Risk estimates for intake of raw vegetables, fresh fruits, and alcohol were close to 1.0, and smoking status did not influence risk.

To complement dietary information on the association between fat and prostate cancer risk, Gann et al. analyzed plasma lipids in a nested case–control study within the Physicians' Health Study (*118*). Compared to the lowest quartile of plasma $\alpha$-linolenic concentration, relative risks for men in successively higher quartiles were 3.0, 3.4, and 2.1. For the highest quartile the 95% CI was 0.9–4.9 ($p$ for trend = .03). For stearic acid the relative risks from lowest to highest quartile were 1.0, 0.9, 0.7, and 0.4 ($p$ for trend .07); for linoleic acid, 1.0, 0.7, 0.8, and 0.6 ($p$ for trend .24). Plasma eicosapentaenoic acid levels were unrelated to risk. These estimates were not notably altered by adjustment for exercise, body mass index, consumption of meat and dairy products, or plasma levels of other fatty acids. However, the association between plasma $\alpha$-linolenic acid and risk of prostate cancer was stronger in men with low plasma linoleic acid and low intake of red meat. The authors suggested that plasma $\alpha$-linolenic acid above some threshold value is an independent risk factor for prostate cancer and this effect may be intensified by low levels of plasma linoleic acid. The effects of dietary linoleic acid and marine fatty acids seen in animal models may not apply to humans. The authors discussed four biological mechanisms that might explain their observations.

Ross and Henderson discussed the idea that diet and androgens influence prostate cancer risk via a common etiologic pathway (*119*). They suggested a model of prostate cancer pathogenesis involving interactions between diet and hormones during various stages of life, beginning in utero. Adlercreutz et al. reported another diet–hormone link with prostate cancer risk (*120*). Japanese men have a low rate of advanced prostate cancer and the Japanese diet contains large amounts of phytoestrogens, particularly isoflavonoids. The authors assayed four isoflavonoids in plasma samples from 14 Japanese and 14 Finnish men. The Japanese men had geometric mean levels of total and individual isoflavonoids 7–110 times higher than the Finnish men. Because estrogen therapy suppresses growth of prostate tumors, it is reasonable to think that high levels of circulating phytoestrogens throughout life suppress development of symptomatic prostate cancers.

## Other Sites

A multicenter case–control study found an inverse relationship between moderate alcohol consumption and risk of endometrial cancer (*121*). The effect was seen mainly in women younger than 55 y, in whom relative risk compared with nondrinkers was 0.8 for women consuming <1 drink per week, 0.6 for 1–4 drinks, and 0.4 for >4 drinks. The greatest effect was associated with beer, and the effect was not substantially altered by adjustment for potential dietary and nondietary confounders.

Cramer and Xu argued that the relationship between worldwide ovarian cancer rates and the ability to digest lactose is not merely one of the peculiar chance relationships dredged up by statisticians but may have a biological basis (*122*). They cited evidence that galactose is toxic to oocytes and that lactose consumption in excess of 18 g/d increases risk of ovarian cancer, particularly in women who had not used oral contraceptives. Moreover, galactose transferase activity, a measure of the ability to metabolize the galactose component of lactose, was lower in ovarian cancer patients than in controls. Study of population estimates of hypolactasia, ovarian cancer rates, and fertility shows that populations with higher levels of hypolactasia have smaller age-related declines in fertility and lower rates of ovarian cancer. Because lactase deficiency would limit the amount of galactose made available from lactose digestion, these observations are compatible with the idea of a cumulative effect of galactose consumption on ovarian function. If hypolactasia is correlated with lower ability to metabolize galactose, perhaps lactase enzyme replacement needs to be reconsidered in terms of potential complications of galactose toxicity, including cataracts and ovarian dysfunction.

A case–control study of ovarian cancer in Greece found high consumption of dietary fiber and mono-unsaturated fat to be protective (*123*). No significant associations were seen for total energy, total protein, saturated fat, polyunsaturated fat, cholesterol, carbohydrates, sucrose, vitamin A or C, riboflavin, or calcium.

It has been hypothesized that high dietary intake of nitrates, nitrites, and nitrosamines increases risk for brain tumors and that vitamins C and E, which inhibit formation of nitrosamines from nitrate and nitrite, may be protective. A case–control study by Bunin et al. investigated the hypothesis that there is a relation between these factors in the maternal diet and the subsequent occurrence of primitive neuroectodermal brain tumors in young children (*124*). Although high intake of vegetables, fruits, and folate and use of multivitamin and iron supplements were protective, the results did not support the idea that a mother's intake of nitrosamines has a role in development of brain tumors in her young child. Foreman and Pearson commented that in the UK, a sharp decrease in incidence of medulloblastoma (the most common neuroectodermal tumor reported by Bunin et al.) accompanied the introduction of multivitamin preparations including folate and iron to prevent neural tube defects (*125*). Bunin et al. pointed out the need to examine the incidence of primitive neuroectodermal tumors by year of birth rather than by year of diagnosis, and to correlate this with supplement use (*126*). They

said that unlike the situation in the UK, the incidence of childhood brain tumors has increased in the USA since the early 1970s. Clearly, more dietary studies are needed.

A case–control study of melanoma in the state of Washington suggested that dietary factors have a role in this malignancy (*127*). Vitamin E obtained from food was inversely related to risk of melanoma: for the highest quartile of intake vs. the lowest, the adjusted odds ratio was 0.34 (95% CI 0.16–0.72, $p = .01$). Zinc from food and supplements was also associated with reduced risk: adjusted odds ratio 0.46 (95% CI 0.24–0.91, $p = .01$). Risk was not affected by dietary retinol, carotenoids, or polyunsaturated fat or by alcohol consumption. Case-patients were significantly more obese than controls.

## CLINICAL STUDIES

### Lipids

In a randomized double-blind crossover study in healthy volunteers, Bartram et al. investigated fish oil's effects on several factors thought to be related to colon cancer risk (*128*). Subjects ate a controlled basal diet and took fish oil and corn oil supplements each for 4-week periods during the trial. Cell proliferation, ornithine decarboxylase activity, and prostaglandin $E_2$ release measured in rectal biopsy specimens were significantly lower during the fish-oil period. Fatty acid composition of the cell membranes did not change. A short review discussed evidence that fish-oil supplementation reduces intestinal hyperproliferation in people at risk for colon cancer (*129*). In particular, a randomized double-blind study of patients with sporadic adenomatous colorectal polyps showed that in conjunction with a standard diet, supplementation with fish oil significantly reduced the labeling index of the high crypt compartments in rectal biopsy specimens after only 2 wk. The eicosapentaenoic acid content of the rectal mucosa increased throughout the 12-wk trial in the fish-oil group while levels of linoleic and arachidonic acid decreased.

van Faassen et al. measured bile acids and pH in total feces and fecal water from healthy omnivorous and vegetarian volunteers in the Netherlands (*130*). Fecal pH did not vary between groups and was significantly correlated to the intake of calcium ($r^2 = .30, p < .05$). Fecal wet weight and defecation frequency were higher in vegetarians. Bile acid concentrations in total feces were similar in the two groups, but concentrations in fecal water were significantly lower in vegetarians. In particular, the fecal water of omnivores had a higher concentration of deoxycholic acid (a predictor of colorectal cancer risk), which was explained by the intake of saturated fat and daily fecal wet weight ($r^2$ = .50). The lower concentration of deoxycholic acid in fecal water of vegetarians and its shorter time of contact with the colonic mucosa due to their higher defecation frequency may partly explain the lower colorectal cancer mortality in this group.

A crossover study conducted within the Nutrition Research Unit of the Western Human Nutrition Research Center, San Francisco, showed that consumption of cooked fish containing *n*–3 PUFAs increases the urinary excretion of both thiobarbituric acid reactive substances (TBARS) and malondialdehyde (measured as thiobarbituric acid–malondialdehyde [TBA–MDA] adduct) (*131*). Nine healthy men were placed on a stabilization diet containing <1% *n*–3 PUFAs (mostly as α-linolenic acid) for 20 days. Three of them then continued this diet for an additional 40 days while 6 were fed a diet isocaloric for total fat, saturated fat, and *n*–6 PUFAs but containing enough salmon to provide 7.5% *n*–3 PUFAs. Both diets contained 200% of the RDA for vitamin E. The groups then switched diets for the final 40 days of the experiment. Although an individual subject's daily output of TBARS and TBA–MDA adduct varied considerably, the mean output at the end of the salmon diet period was significantly higher. Measured as μmoles TBA–MDA equivalents per day it was, for TBARS, 7.05 ± 1.33 vs. 5.65 ± 1.09 (*p* <.05), and for the adduct, 7.07 ± 1.73 vs. 4.65 ± 0.76 (*p* <.01). The authors concluded that consumption of cooked fish can increase exposure to MDA and other autoxidation products that may be carcinogenic or mutagenic. However, during the study, none of the subjects showed any adverse effects ascribable to lipid oxidation.

To see whether the amount of dietary fat influences the incidence of actinic keratosis (a premalignant lesion indicative of sun-induced skin damage), 76 patients with nonmelanoma skin cancer were randomly assigned to continue their usual diet or to eat a diet with 20 en% fat (*132*). The usual diet of the intervention group contained 39 ± 3 en% fat; this decreased to 21 en% within 4 months and remained at or below this level for the rest of the 24-month study. The dietary fat level in the control group began at 40 ± 4 en% and was at least 36 en% throughout the study. The cumulative number of new actinic keratoses per patient for months 4–24 was 10 ± 13 for controls and 3 ± 7 in the intervention group (*p* = .001).

## Fiber

A trial was conducted to study the effect of fiber-rich foods on the composition of the intestinal microflora

(*133*). After a 2-month stabilization on the American Heart Association step 2 diet, subjects were randomized to a diet rich in either soluble or insoluble fiber. After 4 months on this diet they crossed over to the other diet for an additional 4 months. Both experimental diets resulted in a significant decrease in fecal pH, a transient increase in counts of fecal anaerobes and bifidobacteria, and a significant increase in the logarithmic ratio of anaerobes to aerobes from 2.08 at baseline to 2.40 in week 15. The authors concluded that although the composition of the human intestinal microflora is quite stable and normalizes after a short-term perturbation, fermentation activity (as indicated by fecal pH) can be enhanced in the long term by increased intake of dietary fiber.

## Vitamins, Antioxidants, and Chemoprevention

A supplement to the *Journal of Cellular Biochemistry* was devoted to chemoprevention of premalignant lesions of the upper aerodigestive tract (*134*). There was considerable emphasis on identification and assay of biomarkers for carcinogen exposure and carcinogenesis. Both natural and synthetic chemopreventive agents were discussed.

Clinical trials in cancer prevention may be based on diet modification, in which overall eating patterns are changed, or chemoprevention, which involves administration of vitamins, minerals, or pharmaceuticals reported to be anticarcinogenic. Greenwald discussed features and examples of both types of cancer prevention trial (*135*). The target site, study population, and study agent(s) in 40 National Cancer Institute (NCI) chemoprevention trials were summarized in a table. Natural agents that have reached the stage of clinical trials include β-carotene, folic acid, wheat bran, calcium, *n*–3 PUFAs, vitamin C, vitamin E, 13-*cis*-retinoic acid, and retinol. In another paper, Greenwald et al. reviewed the epidemiology and etiology of esophageal cancer worldwide and discussed NCI-sponsored studies on chemoprevention of this cancer (*136*). Some of these NCI-sponsored trials are summarized later in this section. The NCI has developed a staged system for preclinical screening of potential chemopreventive agents and for Phase I, II, and III clinical intervention trials.

van Poppel summarized the state of knowledge on the cancer-preventive potential of carotenoids (*137*). Numerous case–control and prospective studies on the relationship between dietary carotenoids and cancers of specific sites were summarized in tables. A carotenoid-rich diet is associated with decreased risk of several (but not all) common cancers in humans and animal models. Although this association does not establish a cause–effect relationship and the applicability of lab animal data to humans is nearly always questionable, there are plausible mechanisms to explain such a relationship. A multistage scheme for carcinogenesis involving multiple genetic and epigenetic events was presented and the points at which carotenoids could modify or modulate this process were discussed. Conversion to retinol permits effects on cellular differentiation and proliferation rates and on intercellular communication. Antioxidant activity could prevent free radical–induced damage to cellular macromolecules. Immunomodulatory effects could enhance immune surveillance. Several effects of carotenoids on carcinogen metabolism and intercellular communication that are not mediated by retinol have also been demonstrated. Another table summarized ongoing human intervention trials using β-carotene.

CARET is a multicenter randomized trial in five states to test whether oral administration of β-carotene and retinol can decrease the incidence of lung cancer in heavy smokers and asbestos workers (*138*). The pilot phase began in 1985 and involved 1845 participants. All together the study will involve 14,420 smokers, 4010 asbestos-exposed workers, and 114,100 person-years of surveillance through February 1998. It is expected to detect a 23% overall reduction in lung cancer incidence, a 27% reduction in smokers, 49% in female smokers, 32% in male smokers, and 35% in asbestos-exposed workers. It complements a β-carotene–α-tocopherol study in Finland (see reference *140*) and the β-carotene component of Harvard's Physicians' Health Study.

Retinoid chemoprevention trials in upper aerodigestive tract and lung carcinogenesis at the M.D. Anderson Cancer Center have focused on subjects who have premalignant lesions or a history of epithelial cancer (*139*). Lippman et al. summarized these investigations, which include studies to develop practical intermediate markers of carcinogenesis and Phase III trials to evaluate the retinoid isotretinoin in chemoprevention of second primary tumors in patients who have received definitive local therapy for a previous head and neck or lung tumor. Other relevant studies were also cited.

A randomized, double-blind, placebo-controlled study of >29,000 Finnish male smokers aged 50–69 y found no reduction in incidence of lung cancer after 5–8 y of supplementation with α-tocopherol (50 mg/d), β-carotene (20 mg/d), or both (*140*). There was no evidence of an interaction between α-tocopherol and β-carotene. There was a nonsignificant 2% reduction in lung cancer incidence among subjects who received α-tocopherol. Fewer cases of prostate cancer were diagnosed in this group, but there were more deaths from hemorrhagic stroke. Unexpectedly, there was an 18%

*higher* incidence of lung cancer (95% CI 3–36%, $p = .01$) in subjects who received β-carotene. This group also had more deaths from ischemic heart disease. β-Carotene had no effect on incidence of cancers at other sites. Overall, mortality was 8% higher in subjects who received β-carotene than in subjects who did not. Thus not only did this trial fail to show a chemopreventive effect of α-tocopherol and β-carotene against lung cancer in smokers, it raised the possibility that these substances may have harmful as well as beneficial effects. The authors concluded that public health recommendations about supplementation with these micronutrients would be premature until further information is available. In editorial comments on this report and a summary of related data, Hennekens et al. concluded that although the Finnish trial did not disprove the possibility of benefits from antioxidant vitamins it did provide timely support for skepticism and for a moratorium on unsubstantiated health claims (*141*). They felt that the Finnish trial was well designed but nevertheless suffered from several weaknesses. The observed differentials in mortality and cancer incidence could have been due to chance (even if "statistically significant") because of the very large number of observations made. After adjustment for multiple comparisons, neither supplement was associated with greater changes in any particular cause of death than could plausibly be due to chance. However, the results suggest that benefits seen in earlier studies may have been overestimated. How the surprising results of the Finnish trial have been received and may affect similar, currently ongoing trials was discussed in a commentary in *Science* (*142*). Perhaps the most chilling possibility is that β-carotene actually *is* carcinogenic and its apparently protective effects in epidemiologic studies are due to its serving as a marker for other, truly protective, substances in β-carotene-rich foods. Very few people are ready to believe this, however. And Harvard's Physicians' Health Study and Women's Health Study are slated to continue as planned.

In comparison to the Finnish study, whose subjects were generally well nourished, nutrition intervention trials in Linxian, China, have produced more encouraging results (*143–146*). Linxian has one of the world's highest morality rates from cancers of the esophagus and gastric cardia, and there was epidemiologic evidence that multiple chronic micronutrient deficiencies were involved (*143*). Two randomized trials were conducted to test the ability of vitamin and mineral supplements to lower rates of gastric and esophageal cancer. In the first, a 6-y trial, 3318 adults with cytological evidence of esophageal dysplasia were given placebo or supplements of 26 vitamins and minerals at levels 2–3 times the U.S.

RDA. The second was a 5.25-y trial in the general population using a one-half replicate of a $2^4$ factorial design to test the effects of four combinations of nutrients at levels 1–2 times the U.S. RDA: retinol and zinc, riboflavin and niacin, vitamin C and molybdenum, and β-carotene, vitamin E, and selenium. During the multiple-supplement trial there were 167 deaths in the placebo group and 157 in the treatment group (*144*). Of these, 54% were due to cancer, 18% to cerebrovascular disease, and 20% to other causes. Cumulative death rates from esophageal/gastric cardia cancer were 8% lower in the intervention group, a nonsignificant difference. Risk of mortality from all causes, total cancer, and cerebrovascular disease was nonsignificantly lower and from other diseases nonsignificantly higher in the intervention group. The authors concluded that there was no substantial short-term benefit of this intervention for adults with precancerous esophageal lesions. A longer follow-up would be more informative. In the general population trial, the group receiving supplements of β-carotene, vitamin E, and selenium had significantly lower total mortality than other groups (relative risk 0.91, 95% CI 0.84–0.99, $p = .03$) (*143,145*). The reduction was mainly due to lower cancer rates, especially stomach cancer. The reduced risk became apparent 1–2 y after the start of the trial. No significant results were seen with the other three combinations of supplements. These studies were the subject of a brief review (*146*). Although the study design did not permit evaluation of single nutrients or optimal dosages, the results suggested that areas such as Linxian are fertile ground for this type of investigation.

Kaugars et al. reviewed the use of antioxidant supplements in treatment of oral leukoplakia (*147*). Oral leukoplakia is a clinical term associated with histopathologic diagnoses ranging from hyperkeratosis through dysplasia to carcinoma. β-Carotene, or foods rich in it, appear to reduce risk for oral cancer. For therapeutic purposes, however, supplements are the only practical way to achieve markedly higher serum levels of this substance, as doubling the dietary intake would increase serum levels by <30%. Preliminary clinical trials with β-carotene have achieved clinical improvement in about 15–70% of patients. Results with retinol and other retinoids are impressive, but there are undesirable side effects—sometimes severe enough to cause a subject to discontinue treatment. The mechanisms by which various forms of vitamin A prevent and/or reverse formation of epithelial keratin are not known. The association between vitamin C and oral carcinoma is based on dietary assessments showing increased risk when intakes of fruits and vegetables are low; no trials of

ascorbic acid as the sole treatment for oral leukoplakia have been reported. One study evaluating the effects of 800 IU/d of α-tocopherol for 24 weeks reported clinical improvement in 20 of 31 evaluable patients with oral leukoplakia. However, there were a variety of mild side effects and 12 patients could not be evaluated. When 79 patients with histologically verified hyperkeratosis or epithelial dysplasia were treated for 9 months with a combined supplement of β-carotene (30 mg), ascorbic acid (1000 mg), and α-tocopherol (800 IU), 56% showed clinical improvement. Thus antioxidant treatment for oral leukoplakia appears to offer modest benefits. Garewal reviewed epidemiologic, laboratory, and pharmacologic evidence suggesting that β-carotene and vitamin E reduce risk of oral cancer (*148*). He reported that 5 clinical trials of β-carotene alone, one of vitamin E, and one of both found that these substances cause regression of oral leukoplakia. He concluded that these data, combined with lack of major side effects and evidence that these nutrients also protect against several other chronic diseases, strongly indicate an important disease-preventive role for β-carotene and vitamin E including a chemopreventive role in oral cancer.

Ornithine decarboxylase catalyzes the first (often rate-limiting) step in the synthesis of polyamines, which are intracellular mediators of cell proliferation. In animal models of colon carcinogenesis, enzyme activity is induced by tumor promoters, and specific inhibitors of the enzyme inhibit carcinogenesis. A prospective study in 20 men who had undergone resection of colonic adenocarcinoma evaluated the potential of β-carotene to inhibit proliferation of the rectal mucosa, as reflected by mucosal ornithine decarboxylase activity (*149*). Serum and mucosal β-carotene concentrations increased as expected during 6 months of treatment with 30 mg/d of β-carotene and were still elevated 6 months after treatment ended. Ornithine decarboxylase activity was reduced by 44% after 2 wk of treatment and by 57% after 9 wk; it was still below baseline 6 months after treatment ended. Another study evaluated the effects of vitamin supplementation on the cell kinetics of adults with colonic adenomatous polyps (*150*). Subjects were randomly assigned to 1-month treatment with 750 mg/d of vitamin C, 9 mg/d of β-carotene, 160 mg/d of vitamin E, or no treatment. Colonic biopsy specimens were taken at the beginning and end of the trial for assessment of crypt cell proliferation. Vitamin C supplementation significantly reduced proliferation in all crypt compartments. β-Carotene reduced proliferation at the base of the crypt only, and vitamin E was without effect. The authors suggested that short-term supplementation with vitamin C reduces the S-phase duration, which might reduce the recurrence of polyps and the risk of their progression to carcinoma.

Compared with a supplement providing the RDA, megadoses of vitamins A, $B_6$, C, and E and zinc significantly reduced recurrence of bladder tumors in patients receiving BCG immunotherapy (151). Estimated 5-year recurrence was 91% in the RDA group and 41% in the high-dose group ($p < .001$); overall recurrence was 80% in the RDA group and 40% in the high-dose group ($p < .001$). Which ingredient(s) provided this protection was not determined.

## Other

Alder et al. evaluated the effect of calcium supplementation on fecal risk factors for colorectal cancer in healthy men (152). Subjects were randomly assigned to receive a daily supplement of 3 g of calcium carbonate or placebo for 1 wk. Fecal samples were collected before supplementation and during the last 2 days of supplementation. Complete dietary records were kept throughout the study. Counter to expectations, deoxycholic acid and total soluble bile acids decreased in the placebo group and increased slightly in the calcium group. Thus the results did not support the hypothesis that calcium supplementation alters aqueous phase bile acids in a way thought to afford protection from colorectal cancer. An in vitro study of apparently normal colonic tissue from biopsy specimens suggested that certain luminal compounds whose concentrations can be affected by diet can influence colonic proliferation (153). Measurement of proliferation in tissue incubated with butyrate, calcium, or deoxycholate or combinations of these had complex influences on proliferation. The authors concluded that a low-fat, high-fiber, high-calcium diet could affect colonic proliferation in several positive ways so as to reduce risk of colon cancer.

A study in healthy women suggested that living *Lactobacillus* strain GG (contained in yogurt) can modify the colonic environment in health-promoting ways (154). Groups of women were given *Lactobacillus* GG yogurt, *Lactobacillus* GG yogurt and a rye fiber supplement, or pasteurized yogurt and fiber, and various fecal enzyme activities were measured before, during, and after 4 wk of supplementation. The two groups given "living" yogurt had significantly lower fecal β-glucuronidase, nitroreductase, and glycocholic acid hydrolase activities than the group given pasteurized yogurt. These activities returned to baseline levels during a 2-wk follow-up. β-Glucosidase and urease activities were unaffected. The fiber supplement had no effect on activity of any enzyme except urease, whose activity was decreased

nonsignificantly. Urinary excretion of *p*-cresol, a bacterial metabolite, decreased significantly in groups receiving *Lactobacillus* GG. A bacillus common in yogurt is *Lactobacillus casei*. Oral administration of live freeze-dried *L. casei* cells to healthy volunteers for 3 wk decreased the urinary mutagenicity derived from eating fried ground beef by 6–67% (mean, 48%) (155). The authors suggested that the effect may be related to changes in the intestinal microflora.

In a study of obese subjects, Steinbach et al. assessed the effect of body mass index, body composition, resting metabolic rate, and caloric restriction on rectal cell proliferation (156). Before caloric restriction, body mass index was $38 \pm 4$ $kg/m^2$ and percentage of body fat was $41 \pm 2\%$. Subjects reduced their caloric intake by $34 \pm 4\%$ and their weight by $8.6 \pm 1\%$. This resulted in a highly significant 39% reduction in whole-crypt labeling index without reduction in crypt depth. Labeling index was unrelated to body mass index, resting metabolic rate, or body composition. The authors concluded that caloric restriction reduced rectal cell proliferation—a biomarker of colon cancer risk—during the 16-wk study and may have a role in preventing colon cancer.

# LABORATORY AND ANIMAL STUDIES

## Lipids

Burns and Spector reviewed the biochemical effects of PUFAs on cancer cells to evaluate the potential clinical utility of fatty acid supplementation in cancer therapy (157). Substantial changes can be produced in the degree of unsaturation of cancer cell membrane phospholipids. This makes some malignant cells more susceptible to lipid peroxidation and increases their drug and radiation sensitivity. Enrichment with docosahexaenoic acid slows growth and promotes differentiation of some strains of leukemic cells. Findings such as these suggest that PUFA supplementation might make certain forms of cancer treatment more effective, but it is not known whether or to what extent lipid-based approaches will be selective for malignant cells.

To investigate the effect of *n*–6 and *n*–3 fatty acids on tumor metastasis, mice were fed antioxidant-matched diets with corn oil or fish oil for several weeks and then challenged with B16.F10 melanoma cells by injection into the tail vein (158). Mice fed fish oil had fewer lung tumors. The effect was also seen when the mice were injected with monoclonal antibodies that depleted natural killer cells, CD8+ T cells, or CD4+ T cells. In vitro generation of specific anti-B16.F10 cytotoxic cells by splenocytes from immunized mice was greater in mice fed fish oil. These findings suggest that even though host resistance to lung metastases by B16.F.10 cells is largely mediated by natural killer cells, the dietary fat may have affected the tumor cells themselves or other cells not tested in this experiment.

Haegele et al. developed an ex vivo assay for 8-hydroxy-2'-deoxyguanosine (8-OHdG) that makes it a useful marker for oxidative DNA damage in studies of the role of dietary lipids and antioxidants in carcinogenesis (*159*). 8-OHdG was measured in mammary tissue from tumor-bearing and tumor-free rats fed diets of varied fatty acid composition and vitamin E and selenium content. Even though raising vitamin E and selenium levels from deficient to "adequate" reduced oxidative DNA damage, a significant positive correlation between degree of unsaturation of dietary fat and 8-OHdG remained regardless of antioxidant status. The slopes of the lines describing the effect of deficient and adequate antioxidant conditions on concentrations of the marker suggest that oxidative damage might be further reduced by even higher concentrations of antioxidants. Perhaps levels of dietary antioxidants currently considered adequate are not optimal for an endpoint such as 8-OHdG.

Docosahexaenoic acid, docosapentaenoic acid, and eicosapentaenoic acid were shown to have anticlastogenic effects in cultured CHO cells treated with various cross-linking and alkylating agents (*160*). Because chromosomal damage was suppressed by posttreatment with these fatty acids, a desmutagenic mechanism was ruled out. Suppression occurred when cells were treated with fatty acids during the G2 phase, suggesting that G2 events were responsible for the bio-anticlastogenic effect. Saturated fatty acids with the same number of carbons had no effect on the induction of chromosome aberrations.

While dietary fish oil (menhaden oil) is generally thought to inhibit experimental tumorigenesis at the promotional stage, Schut reported that menhaden oil may also inhibit initiation by suppressing the initial rate of DNA adduct formation (*161*). Rats were adapted to diets with various fat compositions and then given a single oral dose of the food mutagen 2-amino-3-methylimidazo[4,5-*f*]quinoline (IQ). A diet with 19% menhaden oil inhibited formation of IQ–DNA adducts in some but not all organs tested. However, this diet also appeared to impair adduct removal in several organs, including the small and large intestine, which are target organs in IQ carcinogenesis. Thus menhaden oil might have both protecting and enhancing activities in

carcinogenesis. The authors stressed the organ-specific nature of the observed effects.

**BREAST CANCER.** Freedman performed a metaanalysis of animal experiments on dietary fat intake and development of mammary tumors (*162*). The experiments varied the proportion of dietary fat, the type of fat, the total energy consumed, or combinations of these. The analysis employed a fixed-effects model and differed from typical metaanalyses of clinical trials in that the nutrient effects could not necessarily be estimated from the individual experiments. The author discussed statistical problems in analyzing this type of data and observed that there is no completely satisfactory method for testing for heterogeneity of effects. Several conclusions were possible from the analysis. Substituting fat for nonfat calories had a substantial effect on mammary tumor development. Increasing the intake of nonfat energy while keeping fat calories constant increased the log odds of tumor incidence, but less than increasing fat intake while keeping nonfat calories constant. There was strong evidence for differences between the effects of various fat sources. Only fish oil was significantly protective against tumor development. The effect for rapeseed oil was also negative, but nonsignificant. Statistical problems in estimating effects of individual fatty acids were discussed.

In three strains of immune-deficient mice, dietary fish oil's suppression of growth of transplanted MDA-MB231 and MCF-7 human breast carcinomas is not mediated by immune mechanisms involving T or B lymphocytes or NK/LAK cells (*163*). When female athymic nude mice were implanted subcutaneously with MDA-MB231 cells and fed diets containing fish oil and corn oil in various proportions with and without antioxidants, tumor growth was suppressed by fish oil in a dose-related way in the absence of antioxidants (*164*). However, antioxidant supplementation reversed the effect of fish oil. Without antioxidant supplements, TBARS in the carcinomas increased in direct proportion to the amount of dietary fish oil; with antioxidants, levels of TBARS were reduced. The authors concluded that dietary fish oil can suppress growth of human breast carcinoma cells even in the presence of fairly large amounts of linoleic acid, and this is related to an accumulation of lipid peroxidation products in the tumor tissue.

Rose and his colleagues have published several papers on the effects of fatty acids on growth and metastasis of human breast cancer cells. Rose and Connolly showed that growth rates of MDA-MB-435 cells in nude mice were significantly greater in animals fed diets with 18% corn oil and 5% menhaden oil than in animals fed 11.5% or 5% corn oil with, respectively,

11.5% or 18% menhaden oil (*165*). The incidence of macroscopic lung metastases was significantly greater in mice fed 18% corn oil than in mice fed only 5% corn oil. The authors concluded that a high-fat diet rich in *n*–3 fatty acids suppresses growth and metastasis of human breast cancer cells in this mouse model. The clinical implication of this is that dietary interventions to reduce risk of breast cancer recurrence should take into account both the amount and the fatty acid composition of dietary fat. In other experiments, Rose et al. fed nude mice isocaloric diets containing 23% by weight of fat with different mixtures of safflower oil and coconut oil to provide 2, 8, and 12% linoleic acid (*166*). Weights of primary tumors in mice fed 12% linoleic acid were significantly greater than those in mice fed 2% linoleic acid but not significantly different from weights in controls fed 5% corn oil. The incidence of macroscopic pulmonary lesions and the mean total calculated volume of metastases per tumor-bearing mouse were significantly lower in the 2% linoleic acid group. Micrometastases were observed most frequently in the 5% corn oil and 2% linoleic acid groups, but these differences were nonsignificant. Diet had no effect on tumor concentrations of prostaglandin E, leukotriene $B_4$, or 5-hydroxy-eicosatetraenoic acid. The authors cautiously commented that in white American breast cancer patients, a relatively high consumption of polyunsaturated fat has been associated with finding regional or distant metastases at the time of diagnosis. Rose and Hatala reviewed the evidence that dietary linoleic acid and its metabolic derivative arachidonic acid enhance breast cancer metastasis (*167*). Clinical observations, mechanistic studies, and implications for therapeutic strategies were discussed. Connolly and Rose reported an in vitro assay system for examining the effects of fatty acids on the invasive capacity of breast cancer cells (*168*). Using a reconstituted basement membrane ("Matrigel") they showed that tumor cell invasion was stimulated by linoleic acid and inhibited by eicosapentaenoic and docosahexaenoic acids. Indomethacin completely blocked the stimulatory activity of linoleic acid, suggesting that the fatty acid effects are mediated through eicosanoid biosynthesis.

COLON CANCER. Perilla oil is rich in α-linolenic acid. In rats, a relatively small fraction of dietary perilla oil (25% of total dietary fat) afforded significant protection against chemically induced colon cancer (*169*). The effect was not substantially increased by feeding 50 or 100% of dietary fat as perilla oil. In another rat model of chemically induced colon carcinogenesis, intragastric gavage with docosahexaenoic acid significantly reduced the numbers of aberrant crypt foci and mean number of aberrant crypts per focus (*170*).

PANCREATIC CANCER. Dietary linoleic acid has been implicated as a promoter of pancreatic carcinogenesis. Appel et al. asked whether linoleic acid is the cause of pancreatic tumor promotion in the context of a high-fat diet (25% by weight), using rat and hamster models of chemical carcinogenesis (*171*). The strongest enhancing effect on growth of preneoplastic pancreatic lesions was achieved in rats and hamsters, respectively, with 4 and 2% of dietary linoleic acid. At higher levels the tumor response seemed smaller rather than greater. There was some evidence that prostaglandins were involved in development of ductular adenocarcinomas in hamsters. The effect of *n*–3 fatty acids in this system is under investigation. Meanwhile, Falconer et al. reported effects of eicosapentaenoic acid and other fatty acids on growth of cultured human pancreatic cancer cell lines (*172*). Albumin-bound fatty acids were tested at concentrations of 1.25–50 μM, simulating conditions likely to be found in plasma in vivo. All PUFAs tested were inhibitory; monounsaturated and saturated fatty acids were not. The action of eicosapentaenoic acid could be reversed with vitamin E or oleic acid but indomethacin and piroxicam had no effect. Thus the effect appeared to be related to the generation of lipid peroxides (see reference *164*), although the level of lipid peroxidation was not always directly correlated with cell death.

## Fiber

Lee et al. conducted a 3 × 3 factorial experiment in rats to examine the interactive and site-specific effects of dietary fat and fiber on proliferation of colonic cells (*173*). Fiber had its main effect in the proximal colon, where pectin stimulated proliferation in comparison to cellulose and a fiber-free diet ($p < .05$). However, the proliferative effect was seen only when the dietary fat was corn oil. The main effect of fat was in the distal colon, where beef tallow promoted proliferation more than fish oil and corn oil had an intermediate effect ($p < .05$). Another study in rats investigated the effect of dietary beet fiber on development of chemically induced aberrant crypt foci, using archived tissue from a study on incidence of colon tumors (*174*). There was a significant inverse relation between the duration of a high-fiber diet and the number of animals with aberrant crypt foci, the total number of aberrant crypt foci, and the number of small foci per affected animal. However, the earlier study had shown no effect of fiber at any stage of colorectal carcinogenesis. The authors concluded that the hypothesis that aberrant crypt foci are preneoplastic lesions needs further investigation. The effects of wheat bran and psyllium fiber, alone and in combination, on chemically induced colon cancer was also investigated in rats in the context of a high-fat, low-calcium diet (*175*). Increasing the concentration of either fiber from 1% to 8% significantly reduced the number of tumors per group; the two fibers were equally effective. However, at comparable total fiber levels, combinations of wheat bran and psyllium fiber had a greater protective effect than either fiber alone.

Zakhary et al. assessed the effect of *Vicia faba* beans and bran (unspecified) on the carcinogenicity of dibutylamine and nitrite, precursors of dibutylnitrosamine (*176*). When mice were fed the precursors, 60% developed hepatomas and 40% developed bladder papillomas after 9 months. Concurrent feeding of *V. faba* reduced the incidence of hepatomas and bladder papillomas to 20%; bran reduced incidence of hepatomas to 20% and prevented formation of bladder papillomas. In in vitro studies, *V. faba* and bran eliminated nitrite and diphenylnitrosamine from the reaction medium and reduced the rate of formation of diphenylnitrosamine from its precursors nitrite and diphenylamine.

One way in which dietary fibers protect against colorectal cancer is by adsorbing carcinogens and carrying them out of the digestive tract. In vitro studies of carcinogen binding can supplement information from in vivo studies. α-Cellulose is frequently used as a model insoluble dietary fiber. Ferguson et al. studied this mechanism by testing the ability of α-cellulose to adsorb a range of carcinogens found or created in heated foods (*177*). They showed that the adsorption of a carcinogen is strongly related to its hydrophobicity. The hydrophilic carcinogen *N*-nitroso-*N*-methylurea was adsorbed only weakly, the very hydrophobic carcinogen benzo[*a*]pyrene was adsorbed strongly, and carcinogens with intermediate hydrophobicities showed intermediate absorption. Maruyama and Yamamoto measured the binding of *N*-[methyl-$^{14}$C]-nitrosodimethylamine by cellulose and eight kinds of dietary fiber from algae (*178*). All in vitro binding rates were <1%. In in vivo experiments, rats were fed a diet containing 2% kelp or agar for 4 d before intragastric administration of the carcinogen. Both fibers significantly increased urinary excretion of the carcinogen and its metabolite and decreased their level in feces 3 h after dosing. Both fibers nonsignificantly reduced carcinogen levels in liver 3 h after dosing; this effect was significant for kelp 24 h after carcinogen administration but not for agar.

O'Neill et al. reported further dietary studies in rats, using magnetic microcapsules to monitor DNA-damaging agents (*179*). They have developed several types of microcapsules designed to capture alkylating agents, cross-linking agents, precursors of reactive oxygen species, carcinogens with planar molecular structures, and various endogenous agents. They fed rats typical British diets containing the normal range of NSP and fat and found that such diets increased or decreased several end-points relevant to carcinogenesis by a factor of 2 or more. These studies have demonstrated relationships between microcapsule trapping, hepatic DNA adducts from endogenous agents, colorectal mucosal cell mitoses and micronuclei, endogenous cross-linking agents, enzyme activities of the gut microflora, and epidemiologic evidence that provide the basis for use of microcapsules and systematically controlled diets to study gastrointestinal carcinogenesis in humans.

Camire et al. developed an in vitro digestion procedure to measure binding of bile acids to potato peels and other materials (*180*). In this system, bile acid binding by cholesterol, pectin, and cellulose was similar to levels reported from radioassays. Potato peels bound more deoxycholic acid than cholic acid, and extrusion-cooked peels bound more of these substances than nonextruded peels. Extrusion had no effect on binding of taurocholic acid but enhanced glycocholic acid binding. Deoxycholic acid binding was correlated with total and insoluble dietary fiber and iron content.

Fermentation of fiber and resistant starch by the gut microflora is thought to influence colon cancer risk. Lupton and Kurtz investigated the mechanism by which fermentable fibers may stimulate proliferation of colonic cells in rats fed fiber-free diets and diets containing highly fermentable pectin or less fermentable wheat bran (*181*). They measured concentrations of short-chain fatty acids (SCFA) in the proximal and distal colon and cecum and correlated these measurements with cell proliferation indexes at the same location. Compared to the fiber-free diet, pectin caused higher concentrations of propionate in the proximal and distal colon; wheat bran caused higher concentrations of butyrate at all sites. In the cecum, all three indexes of cell proliferation were strongly correlated with low pH. In the distal colon, butyrate concentration was significantly correlated with two of the proliferation indexes. Hague et al. studied the effects of butyrate on cultured colonic adenoma and carcinoma cells (*182*). At physiologic concentrations butyrate induced enhanced apoptosis (programmed cell death) in two adenoma cell lines, one having a relatively high frequency of spontaneous apoptosis and the other a low frequency. Apoptosis was also induced in a carcinoma cell line whose growth was previously shown to be inhibited by butyrate. Since the carcinoma and one of the adenoma cell lines do not contain a wild-type *p*53, this tumor-suppressor gene is apparently not required to mediate signals for apoptosis in these cells. Escape from the induction of programmed cell death may be important in colorectal carcinogenesis; this study may partly explain how a high-fiber diet, yielding butyrate upon bacterial fermentation, protects against colon cancer. Berggren et al. measured SCFA and pH in the ceca of rats fed 11 different fibers and indigestible carbohydrates (*183*). They found wide variation in the ability of these substances to lower cecal pH and to form SCFA.

## Vitamins and Antioxidants

In an attempt to define a role for lipid peroxidation in malignancy and for antioxidants in cancer prevention, Diplock et al. conducted experiments in a baby hamster kidney cell line and its virus-transformed malignant counterpart (*184*). In this system, MDA levels were higher and α-tocopherol levels lower in transformed cells. Oxidative stress by $Fe^{3+}$ and ADP caused similar increases in MDA in the two cell types. α-Tocopherol had no effect on MDA in unstressed cells but abolished the increase in stressed cells. It stimulated growth of transformed cells more than of nontransformed cells. Thus in this system the growth-stimulatory effect of α-tocopherol is unrelated to its ability to control lipid peroxidation and the level of peroxidation is increased in transformed cells.

Ramanathan et al. studied the cytotoxic and lipid peroxidative effects of γ-linolenic acid, flavonoids, and vitamins on suspension cultures of Raji lymphoma cells (*185*). γ-Linolenic acid promoted lipid peroxidation in a dose- and time-dependent manner and the peroxidative effect was correlated with cytotoxicity. Alone, the flavonoids (quercetin, luteolin, butein, rutin), retinoids, and α-tocopherol did not influence lipid peroxidation in this system, although quercetin, luteolin, retinol, and α-tocopherol significantly inhibited cell proliferation. Overall, the investigation indicated that the plant flavonoids and fat-soluble compounds tested do not exert their cytotoxic effects through an antiperoxidative mechanism.

RETINOIDS. The term tumor-induced angiogenesis refers to the ability of transformed cells to stimulate new blood vessel formation. All-*trans*-retinoic acid, 13-*cis*-retinoic acid, 9-*cis*-retinoic acid, and 1,25-dihydroxyvitamin D$_3$ were able individually to inhibit tumor-induced angiogenesis in immunosuppressed mice (*186*). Most importantly, combinations of a retinoid and vitamin D showed significant synergism. The authors claim this to be the first report that 1,25-dihydroxyvitamin D$_3$

inhibits tumor-induced angiogenesis. The synergistic effect provides a basis for combined use of retinoids and vitamin D to control growth and spread of malignant tumors.

In vitro studies of the highly metastatic mouse lung carcinoma cell line C87 suggested that inhibition of the malignant phenotype by retinoic acid is associated with a marked reduction in expression of the β4 integrin subunit (*187*). The integrins are a family of cell-surface receptors with a role in cell adhesion. The β4 subunit is particularly abundant in lung and colon carcinomas, and the high metastatic capacity of C87 cells is associated with high levels of β4 expression. Retinoic acid negatively modulates the expression of β4 at the molecular level in C87 cells, at the same time producing marked changes in cell shape, increasing the number of flat cells, suppressing the cells' clonogenic potential in soft agar, reducing their chemotactic and chemoinvasive capacity, and reducing their lung colony–forming ability upon injection into mice.

A report by Chen et al. convincingly demonstrated the need for caution in interpreting studies of vitamin A and skin carcinogenesis in animal models (*188*). The most important conclusion from findings in the current paper, together with earlier observations by the same research group, is that retinoic acid's effect on formation of skin papillomas and carcinomas is critically dependent on the carcinogenesis protocol and method of retinoic acid administration. Another conclusion is that vitamin A deficiency almost completely inhibits tumor formation, whereas dietary retinoic acid or retinyl palmitate permits tumor formation in mice. The same group measured retinol and β-carotene concentrations in skin, skin tumors, liver, and serum of mice fed retinoic acid or β-carotene to suppress skin tumorigenesis (*189*). They found that retinoic acid spares endogenous retinol and that β-carotene enhances levels of retinyl palmitate in the liver. Moreover, while metabolizing retinoic acid very rapidly, mouse epidermal cells respond functionally by the induction of transglutaminase activity. This enzyme is thought to be involved in apoptosis, and its induction may partly explain the inhibition of carcinogenesis in mice fed pharmacologic doses of retinoic acid.

1,2-Diacylglycerols with long-chain fatty acids related to nutritional fat enhance growth and urokinase secretion in human colonic tumor cells but not in normal mucosa. Kahl-Rainer and Marian identified a colon carcinoma cell line that responds to these diacylglycerols in the same way as primary tumor cells and used it as a model to search for inhibitors of colon carcinogenesis (*190*). In this system, they showed that the effects of the diacylglycerols are mediated by protein kinase C and are abolished by down-regulation of the enzyme. In nanomolar concentrations, retinol, retinoic acid, and β-carotene inhibit diacylglycerol-induced growth and urokinase secretion and block stimulation of protein kinase C. At higher concentrations retinol and retinoic acid are also stimulatory, but β-carotene is not. At physiologic concentrations, β-carotene reduces diacylglycerol-induced urokinase secretion by ~50%.

CAROTENOIDS. Lambert et al. found that dietary β-carotene and vitamin E can both significantly reduce the number of chemically induced skin tumors in mice (*191*). However, there was no evidence of an additive or synergistic effect. There was no significant difference in tumor number between groups of mice fed 0.5% β-carotene, 0.12% vitamin E, or 0.5% β-carotene plus 0.12% vitamin E.

Edes and Gysbers discussed carcinogen-induced depletion of vitamin A in tissues in the absence of systemic deficiency, with reference to lung cancer and smoking (*192*). A feeding study in rats showed that feeding a vitamin A–sufficient diet plus benzopyrene, a carcinogen found in cigarette smoke, resulted in reduced lung and liver content of vitamin A while serum levels remained normal. Feeding β-carotene with or without benzopyrene had no influence on serum retinol concentration but β-carotene prevented the tissue depletion of vitamin A caused by the carcinogen. In contrast, dietary retinyl palmitate significantly increased serum retinol concentrations but was less effective than β-carotene in preventing tissue depletion. Further studies suggested that neither utilization nor mobilization of tissue vitamin A is affected by exposure to the carcinogen, but tissue repletion is impaired. Studies on inhalation exposure to carcinogens and the effect of dietary β-carotene on the vitamin A status of lung tissue are needed.

Formation of active oxygen species has been invoked to explain the cytotoxic action of bleomycin, a common cancer chemotherapeutic agent. To evaluate the anticlastogenic effects of carotenoids, healthy adults were given oral supplements of β-carotene (provitamin A activity) and canthaxanthin (no provitamin A activity) for 32 wk (*193*). Blood samples were taken at intervals for 52 wk to monitor carotenoid levels and for in vitro assay of bleomycin-induced micronuclei in cultured leukocytes. The reduction in number of micronucleated cells was correlated with the donor's blood level of carotenoids. Carotenoid and micronucleus levels did not return to baseline until 20 wk after supplementation was discontinued. The authors hypothesized that the protective effect of carotenoids was due to their antioxidant properties. However, less straightforward

results were obtained in experiments on the anticlastogenic effects of β-carotene in CHO cells (*194*). In this system the effects of β-carotene on chemically induced clastogenesis depended critically on the type and mechanism of action of the clastogen and the timing of the clastogenic treatment in relation to β-carotene administration. β-Carotene had no effect on micronucleus induction by methanesulfonate; it reduced mitomycin C–induced micronuclei nonsignificantly only at low concentrations; and it potentiated the clastogenicity of bleomycin when administered before or simultaneously with the drug but had no effect when administered afterward. In cultured human hepatoma cells, pretreatment and simultaneous treatment with β-carotene had no influence on the clastogenicity of mitomycin C but significantly reduced the number of cyclophosphamide-induced micronuclei (*195*). These results indicated that β-carotene was influencing the activation of cyclophosphamide and showed the value of tests in cell lines such as this one that are able to metabolize chemical mutagens.

A study on survival of hamsters given intratracheal instillations of benzopyrene and ferric oxide and fed various levels of vitamin A and β-carotene produced surprising results (*196*). Benzopyrene treatment produced virtually no hyperplasia or metaplasia of the respiratory epithelium and the tumor response of the respiratory tract was <3%, so the effect of diet on carcinogenesis could not be evaluated. However, animals fed a high-β-carotene diet had a mortality rate of only 2% after 69 wk, compared with a 25% mortality rate in all other groups. The exact cause of death of most hamsters could not be determined. Nevertheless, a 40% reduction in lipid peroxidation was seen in livers of the high-β-carotene group and this group also had a smaller incidence and degree of nephrosis and focal mineralization of heart and kidneys.

Shklar et al. tried to confirm previous reports of a synergistic effect between antioxidants in the prevention of cancer (*197*). They used a hamster model of chemically induced oral cancer. The right buccal pouch of each animal was painted with 7,12-dimethylbenz[a]anthracene 3 times weekly. One group served as a control. Five groups were given antioxidants orally by pipet 3 times weekly, on alternate days from carcinogen treatment: a mixture of equal amounts (12.5 μg) of β-carotene, vitamin E, glutathione, and vitamin C, or 50 μg of each of these alone. Vitamin C alone had no effect on areas of leukoplakia or number of tumors; in fact, it nonsignificantly increased mean tumor volume and tumor burden. In reducing tumor burden, β-carotene and glutathione were more effective than vitamin E as single agents, but the mixture was most effective. The results indicate synergism among the antioxidants in this model.

OTHER ANTIOXIDANTS. A study in rats evaluated the effect of dietary vitamin E on activities of drug-metabolizing enzymes and on aflatoxin $B_1$ genotoxicity measured in vitro (*198*). At high levels, vitamin E protected microsomal membranes against peroxidation and influenced their structure. Its effect on hepatic microsomal P450 enzymes modified in vitro aflatoxin $B_1$ genotoxicity. Vitamin E deficiency inhibited genotoxicity.

The effects of long-term dietary administration of tocotrienols on chemical hepatocarcinogenesis in rats were assessed by morphologic examination and measuring activities of several enzymes considered to be tumor markers (*199*). All 10 rats exposed to carcinogen without tocotrienol supplementation had liver nodules after 9 months, whereas only 1 of 6 supplemented rats had such nodules. Throughout the experiment, carcinogen treatment alone significantly increased levels of alkaline phosphatase and γ-glutamyl transpeptidase activity in blood and liver and glutathione *S*-transferase activity in liver. Tocotrienol supplementation either reduced or prevented these effects. Another study of palm oil tocotrienols also suggested that tocotrienols may be an overlooked factor in the cancer-preventive properties attributed to fruits and vegetables (*200*). The inhibition of tumor promotion by α- and γ-tocopherols, γ- and δ-tocotrienols, and dimers of γ-tocotrienol and γ-tocopherol was evaluated in an in vitro assay based on activation of Epstein-Barr virus (EBV) early antigen expression in human lymphoblastoid cells carrying the EBV genome. γ- and δ-tocotrienols strongly inhibited expression of the EBV early antigen, whereas the other substances were inactive. The authors concluded that tocotrienols may be more important inhibitors of tumor promotion than tocopherols or carotenoids, and that the triunsaturated isoprenoid side chain and a less substituted chromanol moiety are essential structural features for tocotrienols to exhibit this activity. They suggest that use of palm oil as dietary fat might offer particular health benefits in Asia, with its high incidence of nasopharyngeal carcinoma caused by Epstein-Barr virus.

Saez et al. studied the modulation of mammary tumor cell growth by 1,25-dihydroxyvitamin $D_3$ (*201*). One purpose of the research was to evaluate the therapeutic potential of this compound, or related synthetic molecules less active in calcium metabolism, for breast cancer patients. The vitamin reduced proliferation of MCF-7 (hormone-dependent) and BT-20 (hormone-independent) cell lines regardless of their sex steroid receptor status and abolished the stimulatory effect of coculture with fibroblasts derived from breast tumors. It also reduced the epidermal growth factor–induced increase in proliferation of two immortalized epithelial cell lines from patients with benign fibrocystic mastopathy. In rats, nontoxic doses significantly reduced proliferation of 7,12-dimethylbenz[*a*]anthracene-induced mammary tumors.

Leung et al. tested the cytotoxic effect of ascorbic acid and numerous derivatives and related compounds against 5 malignant and 3 nonmalignant cell lines (*202*). Malignant cells were, in general, 10–100 times as sensitive as nonmalignant cells. D-Ascorbate and D-isoascorbate, with ~5% of the antiscorbutic potency of L-ascorbate, were just as cytotoxic as L-ascorbate. L-Dehydroascorbic acid and a number of other ascorbic acid derivatives also had considerable lethal activity. The authors concluded that the cytotoxic effect of ascorbate is not related to its metabolic or vitamin activities at the cellular level, but to its chemical properties.

## Minerals

Weisburger et al. examined how dietary corn oil (5% vs. 23.5%) and calcium modulate carcinogenesis induced in rats by heterocyclic amines (*203*). In a 12-month experiment, the high-fat diet increased IQ-induced liver carcinomas in males and mammary carcinomas in females. On the low-fat diet, males had more lip cancers and females had more ear duct cancers. Another heterocyclic amine, 2-amino-1-methyl-6-phenylimidazo[4,5-*b*]pyridine, induced foci of aberrant crypts in the lower intestinal tract of male rats after 9 wk. There were significantly more aberrant crypt foci in rats fed the high-fat diet. With the low-fat diet, the higher level of calcium afforded some protection. Another study found that rats fed a 20% butterfat, high-calcium diet had fecal bile acid concentrations similar to those in rats fed a 5% butterfat diet (*204*). However, this effect of calcium on fecal bile acids was not accompanied by substantive effects on indexes of colonic cell proliferation.

Another dietary study in rats compared calcium carbonate, calcium phosphate, and calcium from lactase-treated whole milk powder for their effects on colonic epithelial proliferation and other cancer-related variables (*205*). The diets did not differ significantly in their effects on fecal bile acid secretion, but fatty acid excretion was stimulated by the calcium supplements in the order calcium carbonate > calcium phosphate > milk mineral. All supplements sharply reduced the cytolytic activity of fecal water. In vitro incubation of fecal water from the control group with calcium phosphate also decreased the concentrations and cytolytic activity of surfactants. The colonic epithelium responded to these primary luminal effects of the calcium supplements with a decrease in cell damage and proliferation. The authors concluded that the antiproliferative effect of milk mineral is mediated by its calcium content and is not diminished by phosphate.

Ip and Lisk compared the tissue selenium profiles and anticarcinogenic responses of rats fed equivalent amounts of selenium as selenite, selenomethionine, naturally selenium-rich Brazil nuts, or experimental selenium-fertilized onion or garlic (206). It was known that dietary selenomethionine produces higher tissue levels of selenium than does selenite, particularly in skeletal muscle, whereas selenite elevates liver glutathione. In this experiment the selenium-rich foods had patterns of effects distinct from both selenite and selenomethionine. Like selenomethionine, Brazil nuts caused significantly elevated selenium levels in liver, kidney, muscle, mammary gland, and plasma, whereas the selenium-enriched *Allium* vegetables produced tissue levels similar to or lower than selenite. Only selenite increased hepatic levels of oxidized glutathione. Selenite and the selenium-rich foods significantly reduced incidence of chemically induced mammary tumors; all sources of selenium significantly reduced the total number of tumors. Garlic was nonsignificantly more protective than the other selenium sources, perhaps because of its additional anticarcinogenic constituents. These results emphasize the importance of chemically characterizing the selenium in foods, particularly in foods considered for selenium enrichment.

Because molybdenum supplementation reduces the incidence of esophageal, forestomach, and mammary tumors in rats, Seaborn and Yang evaluated the effect of graded doses of molybdenum on mammary carcinogenesis and excretion of molybdenum and copper (207). Rats were maintained on a diet containing 0.026 mg/kg of molybdenum for 15 d and then given a single subcutaneous injection of *N*-nitroso-*N*-methylurea. One week later supplementation of their drinking water with 0, 0.1, 1.0, or 10.0 mg/L of molybdenum began. Molybdenum had little effect on copper excretion. Analysis of urine and feces indicated that molybdenum absorption was not easily saturated as the dosage increased. The total number of palpable tumors and total number of carcinomas per group was lower in groups given water with 1.0 and 10.0 mg/L of molybdenum than in groups receiving water with 0 or 0.1 mg/L. Because supplementation began after carcinogen treatment, the results were

probably due to inhibition of the promotion and/or progression stages of carcinogenesis.

## Bacteria

There is epidemiologic and experimental evidence that fermented milk products and bacterial cultures used to produce them reduce risk of certain cancers. Kato et al. reported experiments testing the hypothesis that oral administration of *Lactobacillus casei* could inhibit tumor growth and modify the immune response in mice (208). BALB/c mice were preimmunized by resection of a colonic tumor mass grown intradermally, then rechallenged by injection of the same tumor into the footpad. Bacteria were then administered at a dose of 100 or 200 mg/kg/d for 7 days. Viable, but not heat-killed, bacteria slowed growth of the secondary tumor in immunized mice. Bacteria did not suppress tumor growth in nonimmunized mice. Further, live bacteria prevented the suppression of lymphoproliferative responses of splenocytes from secondary tumor–bearing mice. The authors concluded that living *L. casei* can potentiate immune responses and act as an immunomodulator through the intestinal tract in an immune-deficient host.

In male rats, feeding of viable, lyophilized *Bifidobacterium longum* cultures in conjunction with a high-fat diet prevented colon tumors, reduced the incidence of liver tumors by 80%, and significantly reduced the multiplicity of tumors in colon, liver, and small intestine (209). Females had reduced incidence of mammary and hepatic tumors (nonsignificant) and a significantly lower multiplicity of mammary tumors.

Zhang and Ohta measured the ability of microorganisms in the rat's gastrointestinal tract to prevent absorption of the mutagen/carcinogen 3-amino-1,4-dimethyl-5*H*-pyrido(4,3-*b*)indole (210). Animals were starved and the carcinogen was then administered by stomach tube, alone or in combination with a lyophilized culture of *Bacteroides fragilis, Eubacterium aerofaciens, Lactobacillus acidophilus, Streptococcus cremoris,* or *Saccharomyces cerevisiae.* Without microorganisms, absorption of the carcinogen from the stomach was slow but absorption from the small intestine was very rapid. All microorganisms reduced absorption from the small intestine by more than 50%, and blood levels by 40–65%. The authors observed that because heterocyclic amine carcinogens and microorganisms used to prepare fermented foods are likely to be consumed together during meals, binding by these microorganisms could significantly reduce the absorption of carcinogens in the small intestine and reduce the amount of carcinogen reaching the large intestine via the enterohepatic circulation.

## ANTIMUTAGENS AND ANTICARCINOGENS

Many species of lactic acid bacteria used or found in fermented milk products also occur in idly, a naturally fermented traditional cereal pulse product of southern India (*211*). Strains of a number of *Streptococcus, Pediococcus, Leuconostoc,* and *Lactobacillus* species isolated from idly were tested for antimutagenicity against a variety of food mutagens in *Salmonella* mutagenicity assays. Most of the organisms tested significantly inhibited the mutagenicity of spice extracts, amino acid pyrolysates, and aflatoxin.

A review of dietary cancer-preventive agents suggested that balanced use of antimutagens and anticarcinogens throughout life may be the most effective way to prevent cancer and even genetic disease (*212*). The author discussed how mutagens/carcinogens act and ways in which mutagenesis can be reduced or prevented. By examples she illustrated how antimutagenic effects are often specific to certain types of mutagen or restricted to certain test systems. Because of the chemical and mechanistic diversity of mutagens and carcinogens, only combinations of types of antimutagens and anticarcinogens can provide maximal protection. Porphyrins and some dietary fibers act against large planar and hydrophobic carcinogens, which are common in the typical Western diet. Formation of *N*-nitroso compounds, another common class of mutagens, can be reduced by increasing consumption of fruits and vegetables rich in vitamins C and E, or possibly by taking vitamin supplements. Carotenoids and related compounds counteract the effects of endogenous metabolism and other events that generate free radicals and reactive oxygen species. There are also smaller, nonplanar carcinogens, but these may be of minor importance in the Western diet. The needs of particular subpopulations or high-risk individuals may differ. The author recommended a structured testing strategy progressing from in vitro to in vivo antimutagenicity tests against a defined range of mutagens. Better-informed advice on diet and use of supplements could then be given.

Another review summarized recent developments in the search for antimutagens and anticarcinogens in foods (*213*). A table showed the most prominent chemopreventers and the categories of foods in which they occur, including not only the usual food groups but spices, tea, coffee, wine, and water (a source of selenium); these were also discussed individually in the text. Their mechanisms of action during food preparation and extracellularly and intracellularly within the body were

listed and discussed. Wattenberg listed and discussed the known dietary "non-nutrient" anticarcinogens under the categories blocking agents and suppressing agents (*214*). Blocking agents may reduce the genotoxic effects of carcinogens or block carcinogenesis at a later stage, frequently by inhibiting the arachidonic acid cascade or preventing attack by oxygen radicals. Suppressing agents can be distinguished from blocking agents by time relationships revealed in various tumor models. Suppressing agents are effective when given after the carcinogenic agent and may act by one or more of a variety of mechanisms. Distinctions between the two classes of agents are not always clear-cut.

Two volumes in the American Chemical Society's symposium series were devoted to food phytochemicals for cancer prevention. The first covers the chemistry, biological properties, and health effects of phytochemicals in fruits and vegetables (*215*). In addition to papers on phytochemicals generally, groups of papers are devoted to sulfur-containing compounds in *Allium* vegetables, limonoids and phthalides, and phytochemicals in soybeans. Subjects from purification and identification of the compounds to their modulation of tumor development at molecular to organismic levels are discussed. The second volume covers the chemical and biological properties of phytochemicals found in teas, spices, Oriental herbs, and food coloring agents and their modulation of carcinogenesis (*216*). Groups of papers are devoted to antioxidants, lignans, and phytochemicals from particular sources. Both volumes contain primarily original research reports and reviews and all papers are peer-reviewed.

In India, health-promoting herbs and spices, classified by their actions as "rejuvenating," "nourishing," "wound-healing," etc., are commonly added to foods. The Amrita Bindu supplement is compounded of six salts and salt mixtures derived from various sources and preparations of *Tribulus terrestris, Calatropis gigantea, Zingiber officinale, Piper longum, Piper nigrum, Plumbago zeylanica,* and *Cyperus rotundus* (*217*). When fed to rats it prevented the nitrosamine-induced depletion of glutathione, vitamins A, C, and E, and activity of glutathione peroxidase and superoxide dismutase and the increase in lipid peroxidation measured as MDA in plasma and liver.

Marine brown algae have reported anticarcinogenic effects. Knizhnikov et al. evaluated the effect of a dietary *Laminaria japonica* (kelp) supplement on long-term induction of tumors in rats irradiated with [131]I and [137]Cs (*218*). Supplemented rats had a lower frequency of tumors and a longer latent period to tumor development than nonsupplemented rats. Rates of radiation-induced mammary cancers and liver injury were the same as in nonirradiated controls, frequencies of leukemia and lung and uterine cancer were significantly reduced, and frequencies of "other" tumors were lower than in nonirradiated, nonsupplemented animals. Okai et al. studied the antimutagenic activity in hot-water extracts of *L. japonica* and *Undaria pinnatifida*, using a *Salmonella typhimurium* assay based on the *umu* gene expression system (*219*). They found activity in both polysaccharide and nonpolysaccharide fractions, but the major activity was in the nonpolysaccharides. When this fraction was further separated, stronger activity was seen in the fraction of low molecular weight. Activity of all fractions varied with the nature of the mutagen. The authors concluded that water-soluble fractions of brown seaweeds commonly eaten in Japan contain heterogeneous antimutagenic activities against typical genotoxic substances.

## Carotenoids and Retinoids

Gerster reviewed the occurrence and nature of carotenoids in food; their distribution, concentration, metabolism, and safety in humans; and evidence for their anticarcinogenicity (*220*). There is abundant evidence that β-carotene is protective against several cancers. β-Carotene, lycopene, lutein, α-carotene, cryptoxanthin, and zeaxanthin appear to be taken up and stored in organs where they could act as anticarcinogens. Nearly 600 carotenoids have so far been identified and described. Of the roughly 60 having provitamin A activity, most are of the hydrocarbon type rather than the oxygenated (xanthophyll) type. Provitamin A carotenoids are only partly transformed to retinol, the extent of conversion being determined by a homeostatic mechanism limiting the level of vitamin A and by the nature of the carotenoid. β-Carotene is also thought to be a precursor of retinoic acid in this anticancer agent's target tissue; the low rate of conversion may be related to the number of retinoic acid receptors, which may account for β-carotene's lack of retinoic acid toxicity. Lutein and zeaxanthin concentrate in the retina and high concentrations of lycopene have been found in testes, but much more needs to be learned about the organ specificity of uptake and storage of individual carotenoids. Ferrets show promise as an animal model because they resemble humans in the absorption and metabolism of β-carotene; rats and chicks may not be suitable because they convert most β-carotene to retinol and accumulate almost none in their tissues. Part of β-carotene's anticarcinogenicity is related to provitamin A activity, but it and many other carotenoids also have antioxidative properties. Fur-

ther, it and canthaxanthin enhance immune defense against tumor development and canthaxanthin is not converted to retinol. The main anticarcinogenic effect of β-carotene occurs during promotion; other carotenoids are more active than β-carotene during initiation or progression. At least 6 retinoids and carotenoids in addition to β-carotene stabilize initiated cells by increasing gap junction communication, their potency being unrelated to either vitamin A or antioxidant activity, thus suggesting yet a third mechanism of action. Intervention studies have shown β-carotene to be both photoprotective and chemoprotective against skin cancer, whereas canthaxanthin specifically protects against chemical carcinogens. This suggests that conversion to retinol is necessary for photoprotection but not for chemoprotection. The xanthophyll astaxanthin reduced the incidence of chemically induced transitional cell carcinomas (but not squamous cell carcinomas) in bladders of mice from 31% to 3% (*221*). Canthaxanthin caused a smaller, nonsignificant reduction. The xanthophylls were administered in drinking water beginning 1 wk after the 20-wk administration of carcinogen ended. Both xanthophylls also reduced the number of silver-stained proteins per nucleus in the nucleolar organizer region in carcinogen-exposed transitional epithelium. This is a new index of cell proliferation. Astaxanthin was slightly more potent than canthaxanthin.

A book on the chemistry, biology, and medical uses of retinoids contained 16 chapters, many of which are relevant to issues of diet and health or diet and cancer (*222*). These include public health considerations related to vitamin A nutrition, the metabolism of retinol and retinoic acid, plasma retinol-binding protein, cellular retinoid-binding proteins, retinoid receptors, the biochemistry and cell biology of retinoids, and actions of retinoids on the immune system. A chapter by Hong and Itri comprehensively reviewed the epidemiology of retinoids and human cancer, the safety of specific natural and synthetic retinoids, and results of therapeutic and chemoprevention trials (*223*). A chapter by Moon et al. reviewed the effects of retinoids in chemoprevention of experimental cancer in animals (*224*). Chemotherapeutic effects and combination chemopreventive regimens were also discussed.

## Phytochemicals

PHENOLS. Ohta reviewed laboratory studies of the effects of vanillin, cinnamaldehyde, and coumarin on mutagenicity (*225*). These studies aim to prevent genetic hazards from environmental mutagens or to elucidate the process of mutagenesis. The review brings into sharp focus the fact that a substance that suppresses mutagenicity in one situation sometimes enhances mutagenicity under other conditions or when a different endpoint is measured. The different, sometimes opposing effects of vanillin, coumarin, and cinnamaldehyde were discussed in terms of their proposed mechanisms of action. Ohta emphasized that tests of antimutagenic and comutagenic effects based on mixing different mutagens and putative antimutagens in never-ending combinations are meaningless if mechanisms are disregarded.

Phenolic antitumor agents have been found in edible plants from Thailand, including *Boesenbergia pandurata* (Zingiberaceae), whose rhizome is used as a condiment and in folk medicine (*226*). An active compound in *B. pandurata* was identified as cardamonin (2',4'-dihydroxy-6'-methoxychalcone). Sixteen phenolic compounds were isolated from the apple, nut, and nut shell of the cashew (*Anacardium occidentale*) (*227*). Four were anacardic acids, derivatives of salicylic acid; four were cardols, derivatives of resorcinol; four were 2-methylcardols, and four were 3-substituted phenols. The anacardic acids, cardols, and methylcardols were moderately cytotoxic against BT-20 breast carcinoma cells and HeLa cells.

An interesting study evaluated the effects of β-carotene, α-tocopherol, and the plant phenols eugenol, hydroxychavicol, catechin, and curcumin on carcinogen-induced DNA damage in target and nontarget organs in mice (*228*). Test compounds were administered in drinking water for 15 days, after which the carcinogen was administered by gavage and animals were killed 4 h later. β-Carotene and all the phenols but eugenol completely prevented carcinogen-induced single-strand breaks in DNA of the forestomach (target organ). α-Tocopherol was partially effective and eugenol was ineffective. However, α-tocopherol and β-carotene failed to protect against micronucleus formation in bone marrow (nontarget organ), whereas again, all phenols except eugenol offered significant or total protection and eugenol was nonsignificantly protective. Moreover, α-tocopherol significantly increased micronucleus formation when administered alone. Another study evaluated the effect of these substances on the carcinogen–DNA interaction in the presence of S9 fractions from mouse and rat liver (*229*). α-Tocopherol was ineffective with both mouse and rat S9 fractions, whereas β-carotene inhibited the mouse S9-mediated interaction but enhanced the rat S9-mediated interaction. In contrast, all four phenols strongly inhibited both S9-mediated interactions. The authors suggest that the phenols act at a different locus than α-tocopherol and β-carotene. Other authors concluded

that eugenol and also *trans*-anethole preferentially induce phase II biotransformation enzymes in rat liver in vivo (*230*). In addition, dietary curcumin inhibits azoxymethane-induced ornithine decarboxylase and tyrosine protein kinase activity, arachidonic acid metabolism, and formation of aberrant crypt foci in the rat colon (*231*).

In mice, chlorogenic acid, curcumin, and β-carotene afforded significant protection against γ-radiation-induced micronucleus formation in bone marrow (*232*). A single dose of chlorogenic acid or curcumin administered orally 2 h before or immediately after whole-body irradiation was effective, whereas β-carotene had to be fed for 7 d before irradiation in order to reduce micronucleus formation significantly. The ability of chlorogenic acid and caffeic acid to alter hepatic and intestinal xenobiotic phase I and phase II enzyme activities was also tested in mice (*233*). Against benzo[*a*]pyrene, the inhibitory effect of these phenols occurred primarily in the intestine, where carcinogen-induced activation of glucuronosyl transferase was abolished and carcinogen-induced activity of aryl hydrocarbon hydroxylase was sharply reduced. When fed to rats during the same period that the carcinogen 4-nitroquinoline-1-oxide was administered in drinking water, chlorogenic, caffeic, ferulic, and ellagic acids in concentrations of 250–500 ppm significantly reduced the incidence of tongue neoplasms and the number and area of silver-stained nucleolar organizer region proteins per nucleus (*234*). Chlorogenic and ellagic acids completely prevented formation of neoplasms. Another study in rats showed that several caffeic acid esters found in honey inhibit azoxymethane-induced preneoplastic colonic lesions and activity of several enzymes relevant to colon carcinogenesis (*235*). In mice, dietary ellagic acid inhibited lung tumorigenesis induced by 4-methylnitrosamino-1-(3-pyridyl)-1-butanone (NNK), a carcinogen present in tobacco and tobacco smoke (*236*). The inhibition was related to the $\log_{10}$ of the ellagic acid dose, whereas pulmonary levels of the substance were directly related to doses between 0.2 and 2.0 mmol per kilogram of body weight. Another study suggested that ellagic acid and capsaicin exert their inhibition of NNK-induced tumorigenesis through inhibition of liver microsomal cytochrome P450 activity and xenobiotic metabolism (*237*).

Tanaka et al. reported the chemoprevention of 4-nitroquinoline 1-oxide-induced oral carcinogenesis (*238*) and colon carcinogenesis (*239*) in rats by dietary protocatechuic acid.

**FLAVONOIDS.** Flavonoids are strong naturally occurring antioxidants that can inhibit carcinogenesis in rodents.

It is difficult to obtain good data on their consumption by humans. Using data from the Dutch National Food Consumption Survey, 1987–1988, Hertog et al. estimated the intake of five potentially anticarcinogenic flavonoids (quercetin, kaempferol, myricetin, apigenin, and luteolin) in a population of 4112 adults (*240*). The flavonoid content and composition of fruits, vegetables, and beverages was determined by HPLC. The average intake of flavonoids was 23 mg/d, of which quercetin accounted for 16 mg. Nearly half of the flavonoids were derived from tea; onions contributed 29% and apples, 7%. Flavonoid intake did not show seasonal variation, was not correlated with total energy intake, and was only weakly correlated with intake of vitamins A and C and dietary fiber. Although these results from up-to-date analytic technology indicate that flavonoid intake has been greatly overestimated in the past, on a weight basis the intake of antioxidant flavonoids still exceeds that of β-carotene and vitamin E. Thus the flavonoids are a major source of antioxidants in the human diet.

Flavonoids occur ubiquitously and in great variety in plants. However, isoflavones such as genistein and daidzein occur in only a few plant families because of the limited distribution of the enzyme chalcone isomerase, which is required for their biosynthesis. Soybeans are the major dietary source of these substances. Coward et al. reported a method for separating and analyzing isoflavone β-glycoside conjugates and aglucones from a variety of Asian and American soy products (*241*). Except for soy sauce and soy protein preparations, the products analyzed had total isoflavone concentrations similar to those in the intact bean. Asian fermented soy foods contain predominantly isoflavone aglucones, whereas β-glycoside conjugates predominate in nonfermented soy foods. The typical Asian diet has a much higher content of these isoflavones than the typical American diet. In fact, levels in the Asian diet are comparable to those that inhibit tumorigenesis in animal models of breast cancer, a factor that may account for the lower incidence and mortality rates of breast cancer in Asian women. Evidence for the mechanism of genistein's protective effect came from in vitro studies using a human hepatocarcinoma cell line (*242*). Genistein significantly increased production of sex hormone–binding globulin by Hep-G2 cells and also suppressed proliferation of the cells. A vegetarian diet is associated with high plasma levels of sex hormone–binding globulin and reduced incidence of breast and prostate cancer. Another way in which genistein and other isoflavonoid phytoestrogens may act is by inhibiting estrogen synthetase (aromatase) in peripheral cells or cancer cells (*243*). These substances bind competitively near the substrate region of the active site of the P450 enzyme. Although their affinity is much less than that of the natural substrates, they occur at high levels in vegetarians. They could thus reduce estrogen formation locally and inhibit growth of estrogen-dependent tumors.

Seven isoflavones (genistein, daidzein, genistin, biochanin A, prunectin, puerarin, and pseudobabtigenin) were tested for cytostatic and cytotoxic effects against 10 cancer cell lines of human gastrointestinal origin (*244*). Genistein and biochanin A strongly inhibited proliferation of 3 of 7 stomach cancer cell lines and moderately inhibited the esophageal, colon, and other 4 stomach cancer lines. They were cytostatic at low concentrations and cytotoxic at higher levels. DNA fragmentation was seen at cytotoxic doses of both compounds, indicating the apoptotic mode of cell death. The other isoflavones showed lesser, variable activity against the 10 cancer cell lines. Biochanin A also suppressed growth of two cell lines in athymic nude mice.

Using a *Salmonella typhimurium* test, Edenharder et al. evaluated 64 flavonoids for antimutagenic potency against several heterocyclic amine mutagens from cooked food (*245*). They found that a carbonyl group at C4 of the flavane nucleus was necessary for activity. Two flavanols, 4 anthocyanidines, and 5 isoflavones (all except biochanin A) were inactive. Within the flavone, flavonol, and flavanone groups the parent compound had the highest activity in each case. Introduction of hydroxyl groups increased polarity and reduced potency, whereas reducing the polarity of hydroxy flavonoids by methyl etherification increased their antimutagenicity. Nine of 11 flavonoid glycosides tested (all except apigenin- and luteolin-7-glucoside) were inactive or only weakly active. Rings C and A of the nucleus are not essential, but a planar structure near the carbonyl group may be important for activity. No clear influence of the mutagen's structure on antimutagenicity was seen. Lee et al. also investigated relationships between flavonoid structure and antimutagenic activity (*246*). Activity of flavonoids in interfering with cytochrome P450 isozymes and reducing formation of the major active metabolite of 2-amino-3-methyl-imidazo[4,5-*f*]quinoline (IQ) correlated well with antimutagenic activity in a *Salmonella* test. One or more of the following features were associated with activity: a C4 keto group; a C2 phenyl group; a double bond between C2 and C3; or hydroxyl groups at C4', C5, and C7. Flavonoid glycosides were much less active than the corresponding aglycones.

Sathyamoorthy et al. developed a rapid, specific tissue culture assay to screen for diet-derived compounds with estrogen-like activity (*247*). Using the estrogen receptor–positive breast cancer cell line MCF-7, they monitored expression of the estrogen-responsive protein pS2. Daidzein, equol, nordihydroguaiaretic acid, enterolactone, and kaempferol elicited an estrogen-like response, whereas quercetin and enterodiol did not.

Three previously unknown biflavonoids and the known flavone 4',5-dihydroxy-3,3',6,7-tetramethoxy-flavone were isolated from flowers of *Calycopteris floribunda* (*248*). These were characterized by chemical, chromatographic, and spectroscopic techniques. The new biflavonoids had considerable cytotoxic activity against 9 tumor cell lines. The activity of calycopterone, the major compound, was comparable to that of doxorubicin against a colon adenocarcinoma cell line and greater than that of doxorubicin against a multidrug-resistant ovarian adenocarcinoma cell line. The flavone had relatively little cytotoxic activity.

In mice, dietary quercetin and rutin modified or inhibited chemically induced colonic carcinogenesis even in the context of a high-fat (20% corn oil) diet (*249*).

**OTHER PHYTOCHEMICALS.** Abdullaev reviewed the cytotoxic, anticarcinogenic, and antitumor properties of saffron extract (*250*). The complex chemical composition of the extract makes it difficult to determine the mechanism of the observed antitumor effects. However, the inhibition of nucleic acid synthesis by saffron extract has been the most consistent observation suggesting a possible mode of action.

A critical review by Elson and Yu suggested that suppression of growth of chemically induced and transplanted tumors by dietary isoprenoids is a consequence of their inhibiting components of the mevalonate pathway (*251*). The review summarized evidence that the mevalonate pathway of tumor tissues is uniquely sensitive to dietary isoprenoids, which are secondary products of mevalonate metabolism in plants. Examples of substances with blocking, suppressing, or chemopreventive activity are carveol, carvone, geraniol, *d*-limonene, β-myrcene, and γ-tocotrienol. Many of them act as competitive or noncompetitive inhibitors of HMG-CoA reductase.

Several triterpenes isolated from species of Cucurbitaceae reportedly have cytotoxic activity, but Konoshima et al. may be the first to report anticarcinogenic activity of these compounds (*252*). The authors screened 21 cucurbitane triterpenoids in an in vitro assay. Five significantly inhibited 12-*O*-tetradecanoyl-phorbol-13-acetate-induced activation of Epstein–Barr virus. Two of them strongly inhibited tumor promotion in a mouse model of two-stage skin tumorigenesis.

Zani et al. analyzed the desmutagenic and antimutagenic effects of an ethanolic *Glycyrrhiza glabra* extract and several of its purified components using a *Salmonella*/microsome reversion assay, which avoided the problem of false-positive results due to toxicity (*253*). No desmutagenic activity was seen against ethyl methanesulfonate or *N*-methyl-*N'*-nitro-*N*-nitroso-guanidine, and only the extract had antimutagenic activity against ethyl methanesulfonate. With the ribose–lysine mutagenic browning mixture, *G. glabra* extract, glycyrrhizinic acid, and 18α- and 18β-glycyrrhetinic acid were desmutagenic. The extract was also antimutagenic in this system.

Various preparations and extracts of wild rice have high antioxidant activity (*254*). The active constituent of the extracts was identified as phytic acid. A pilot study suggested that phytic acid protects rats against chemically induced mammary tumors (*255*). Phytate also protected rats against chemically induced colon tumors, in a study designed to correlate the number and size of aberrant crypt foci with tumor formation (*256*). Treatment with phytate beginning one week after carcinogen injection significantly reduced the incidence of tumors and large foci (containing 4 or more aberrant crypts), but there was no effect on total number of foci.

Chlorophyllin also shows antimutagenic and anticarcinogenic activity. Intraperitoneal injection into γ-irradiated mice protected against radiation-induced damage in bone marrow cells (*257*). A dose of 100 μg per gram of body weight totally prevented the induction of sister-chromatid exchanges by 1.0 Gy of γ-rays. Another study tested whether chlorophyllin can inhibit carcinogen-induced morphologic transformation of cultured BALB/3T3 cells (*258*). At concentrations that did not significantly affect growth, a dose-related inhibition of transformation was induced by a variety of complex carcinogenic materials and purified carcinogens. In rats, chlorophyllin inhibited IQ–DNA binding in the liver, small intestine, and colon (*259*). Dose–response and time-course studies indicated that the mechanism of action involves in vivo formation of a complex between the inhibitor and the mutagen, suggesting that chlorophyllin is likely to be most effective when ingested simultaneously with the carcinogen. Hayatsu et al. discussed porphyrins (of which chlorophyll and chlorophyllin are examples) as potential inhibitors of mutagenesis and carcinogenesis (*260*). Porphyrins appear to have a strong affinity for polycyclic compounds such as mutagenic heterocyclic amines from food.

***BRASSICA* VEGETABLES.** A large body of epidemiologic data and laboratory tests of crude extracts and purified compounds indicate that the common varieties of *Brassica oleracea* have cancer preventive properties (*261*).

Beecher discussed biological activities relevant to cancer prevention, reports of antimutagenicity of *B. oleracea* extracts, the stimulation of detoxification mechanisms, and other relevant reports.

Nijhoff et al. used a diet containing 20% Brussels sprouts as a positive control treatment to evaluate the effects of 9 naturally occurring anticarcinogens on glutathione *S*-transferase activity at five digestive system sites in rats (*262*). Anticarcinogens were added to the diet at levels of 0.25–1.0%. Brussels sprouts, flavone, and coumarin stimulated activity to a similar degree in the proximal and middle small intestine and liver but had no effect in the distal small intestine or large intestine. $\alpha$-Angelicalactone was active at all five sites, whereas quercetin, ferulic acid, ellagic acid, tannic acid, and curcumin were inactive at most sites. After looking at effects on individual glutathione *S*-transferase isozymes, the authors concluded that most of the anticarcinogens acted by inducing class $\alpha$ and $\mu$ isozymes at various sites in the digestive system. Although the doses used here are not realizable in the human diet, it is still conceivable that dietary modulation of important detoxification systems might help to prevent gastrointestinal tumors.

Lyophilized extracts of Chinese radish were tested for mutagenic and antimutagenic activity against direct and indirect mutagens in *Salmonella typhimurium* (*263*). Methanol extracts were inactive in all tests. Hexane and chloroform extracts were nonmutagenic and had strong antimutagenic activity against several direct and indirect mutagens, although they were ineffective against benzo[*a*]pyrene. These extracts also markedly inhibited the activities of rat liver aniline hydroxylase and aminopyrine demethylase. The authors concluded that Chinese radish contains one or more nonpolar compounds with antimutagenic activity toward both direct and indirect mutagens, and the antimutagenic activity toward aflatoxin $B_1$ may be partly due to inhibition of enzymes necessary to activate this mutagen.

In vitro studies showed that allyl isothiocyanate, a constituent of *Brassica* vegetables, is selectively toxic to transformed cells of a human colorectal tumor line (*264*). Cells detransformed with sodium butyrate or dimethylformamide were much less sensitive. The authors suggested that this compound may protect in vivo against cancer by selectively inhibiting growth of transformed cell clones within the gastrointestinal mucosa.

There is considerable interest in indole-3-carbinol as a chemopreventive agent. Tiwari et al. reported that this compound inhibits growth of the estrogen-responsive MCF-7 human breast cancer cell line but has little effect on estrogen-nonresponsive MDA-MB-231 cells (*265*). Specific C2 hydroxylation of estrogen and induc-

tion of cytochrome P450 1A1 were enhanced in MCF-7 but not in MDA-MB-231 cells. The authors suggested that the inhibitory effects of indole-3-carbinol involve induction of estradiol metabolism and the related cytochrome P450 system that may be limited to estrogen-sensitive cells. Newfield et al. studied relationships between estradiol 16$\alpha$-hydroxylation and the malignant sequelae of papillomavirus infection in the larynx, suggesting a protective role for indole-3-carbinol (*266*). They first showed that 16$\alpha$-hydroxylation was greater in tissue from laryngeal papillomas than in normal laryngeal tissue. Estradiol and 16$\alpha$-hydroxyestrone stimulated proliferation in both kinds of cells, whereas 2-hydroxyestrone was antiproliferative. Indole-3-carbinol, which induces 2-hydroxylation, inhibited the proliferative effect of estradiol. When human papillomavirus-infected laryngeal tissue was implanted under the renal capsules of immunocompromised mice, mice fed indole-3-carbinol had a significantly lower incidence of formation of papillomas than mice fed a control diet (25% vs. 100%). Dietary indole-3-carbinol was also reported to reduce the incidence of spontaneous endometrial cancer and preoplastic lesions in Donryu rats (*267*). Again, this was attributed to the substance's induction of estradiol 2-hydroxylation. Another effect of indole-3-carbinol is induction of aflatoxin $B_1$ metabolism and the cytochromes P450 associated with bioactivation and detoxification of aflatoxin $B_1$ in rats (*268*). The synthetic flavonoid $\beta$-naphthoflavone has similar properties. It and indole-3-carbinol may share the mechanism of inhibiting aflatoxin $B_1$ carcinogenesis by enhancing production of less toxic hydroxylated metabolites of the carcinogen through elevated P450 activity. However, indole-3-carbinol oligomers may also directly inhibit P450 bioactivation or induce phase II enzymes. Further examination of the mechanism by which indole-3-carbinol protects rats against aflatoxin $B_1$–induced carcinogenesis demonstrated induction of a liver glutathione *S*-transferase isozyme with unusually high activity toward aflatoxin $B_1$ *exo*-epoxide, a genotoxic metabolic intermediate (*269*). Dietary indole-3-carbinol reduced aflatoxin $B_1$–DNA adduct formation in these rats by 68%. The authors concluded that the detoxication of aflatoxin $B_1$ is enhanced by increased efficiency of conjugation with glutathione, resulting from elevated levels of this particular isozyme. This mechanism participates to a lesser degree in the protection afforded by $\beta$-naphthoflavone.

***ALLIUM* VEGETABLES.** Diallyl disulfide (an organosulfur compound in garlic and onions) and the substituted dithiolethione anethole trithione both inhibit azoxymethane-induced colon carcinogenesis in rats (*270*).

This inhibition is associated with activation of the phase II enzymes glutathione *S*-transferase, NAD(P)H-dependent quinone reductase, and UDP-glucuronosyl transferase in the liver and colon. Other mechanisms may also be involved.

Three water-soluble and three oil-soluble organosulfur compounds from garlic were tested for effects on growth of cultured canine mammary tumor cells (*271*). The water-soluble substances had no significant effect at concentrations of 1.0 mM or less, whereas oil-soluble substances were markedly inhibitory. The dose-related inhibition by diallyl disulfide was reduced by prior addition of glutathione and enhanced by treatment with an inhibitor of glutathione synthesis, showing that the inhibitory effect is modified by intracellular glutathione.

Amagase and Milner tested several forms of garlic and their constituents for their influence on in vivo binding of 7,12-dimethylbenz[*a*]anthracene to rat mammary cell DNA (*272*). It was clear that high levels of dietary garlic inhibit in vivo formation of carcinogen–DNA adducts, but the preparations had variable effectiveness. One active constituent is *S*-allylcysteine. In another dietary study in rats, processed garlic powder reduced the occurrence of DNA adducts caused by *N*-nitroso compounds (*273*). The effect seemed to reflect a decrease in formation of *N*-nitroso compounds from precursors, and changes in the bioactivation and/or denitrosation of these compounds.

Reeve et al. reported that a lyophilized aged garlic extract fed to hairless mice afforded dose-responsive protection against the ultraviolet B radiation–induced suppression of contact hypersensitivity (*274*). The mechanism appears to involve antagonizing the mediation of this form of immunosuppression by *cis*-urocanic acid.

TEA. Yang and Wang critically reviewed the literature on tea and cancer (*275*). They discussed the basic chemistry and biological activities of tea, epidemiologic investigations, and laboratory research. In laboratory studies, the inhibitory effects of tea extracts and polyphenols against tumor formation and growth are generally attributed to the antioxidative and possibly antiproliferative activity of polyphenolic constituents. These substances may also block the endogenous formation of *N*-nitroso compounds, suppress the activation of carcinogens, and trap genotoxic agents. With respect to public health, the effect of tea drinking will depend on the causative factors of a particular cancer; a protective effect against one cancer in one population may not be seen for another cancer or in another population. Moreover, high tea consumption has been implicated as a risk factor for esophageal cancer in some Asian populations (but see reference *285*), and epidemiologic studies have reported positive relationships or no relationship as well as negative relationships between tea drinking and cancers of the bladder, breast, colon and rectum, kidney, liver, lung, nasopharynx, pancreas, and stomach. Some of the positive associations, however, may be due not to tea itself but to drinking it at a high temperature or salted. Drinking "excessive" amounts may also be harmful. In view of the generally favorable findings of laboratory studies, however, clinical studies appear warranted.

Mukhtar et al. reviewed the effects of green tea and its polyphenols on skin carcinogenesis (*276*). Collectively, various types of animal experiments indicate that green tea has significant chemopreventive effects during each stage of carcinogenesis and that it may be useful against inflammatory responses associated with exposure to chemical tumor promoters as well as to solar radiation. Some mechanistic studies were discussed. The same research group reported that dietary green tea polyphenols protect the skin of hairless mice against inflammatory responses to ultraviolet B radiation (*277*) and that in vitro, epicatechin derivatives of green tea inhibit spontaneous and photo-enhanced lipid peroxidation in mouse epidermal microsomes (*278*).

It was reported that a very low dose of green tea polyphenols in drinking water protects rats against *N*-methyl-*N*-nitrosourea-induced colon cancer (*279*) and that administration of green tea polyphenols by oral intubation protects mice against chemically induced forestomach and lung tumors (*280*).

An interesting experiment using a rat multiorgan carcinogenesis model showed both protective and enhancing effects of green tea catechins (*281*). Rats were fed 0.1 or 1.0% catechins during or after exposure to *N*-methylnitrosourea, or both during and after exposure. The catechins inhibited carcinogenesis in the small intestine regardless of when they were administered. However, numbers of glutathione *S*-transferase placental form–positive liver foci were significantly increased in groups treated with 1 and 0.1% catechins during carcinogen exposure, 1% catechins after exposure, or 1% during and after. There were no significant effects on the incidence or multiplicity of lung or colon tumors or tumors at minor sites.

In an assay using rat erythroblastic leukemia cells, a crude catechin extract of green tea inhibited induction of sister-chromatid exchanges by $CHCl_3$ and $CHBr_3$ but not by $CHCl_2Br$ or $CHClBr_2$ (*282*). The suppression was related to the dose of catechin. Suppression of $CHCl_3$-induced sister-chromatid exchanges might be due to inhibition of mixed-function oxidases, but this cannot explain the effect on CHBr$_3$, which is a direct-acting mutagen.

In mice, weekly stomach perfusions of catechin (1 or 2 mg/mouse) or (–)-epigallocatechin-3-gallate (2 mg/mouse) reduced the incidence of 1,2-dimethylhydrazine-induced large intestinal cancers by ~50% (*283*). The incidence of anal cancers was sharply reduced and there were no lung metastases in treated mice. Superoxide dismutase activity was enhanced in the large intestine of treated animals. Administration of 0.05 or 0.1% (–)-epigallocatechin-3-gallate in drinking water significantly reduced the incidence and multiplicity of spontaneous hepatomas in C3H/HeNCrj mice (*284*). This compound also inhibited growth of human hepatoma-derived PLC/PRF/5 cells and their secretion of α-fetoprotein, without decreasing their viability.

A population-based case–control study of esophageal cancer in Shanghai found a protective effect associated with consumption of green tea (*285*). After adjustment for known confounders, the OR was 0.50 (95% CI 0.30–0.83) for women and the decrease in risk was dose-related; the OR was also <1 for men but this was not statistically significant. Among people who neither smoked nor drank alcohol, the ORs were ~0.40 and were statistically significant for both men and women.

Yen and Chen compared the antimutagenic effects of extracts of green, oolong, pouchong, and black teas (*286*). None of the extracts were mutagenic or toxic in *Salmonella typhimurium* TA98 or TA100. All extracts had antimutagenic activity. However, the semifermented teas (oolong and pouchong) were more potent than unfermented (green) tea, which was generally more potent than fermented (black) tea. This suggests that antimutagenic substances are formed and also destroyed in tea during manufacturing processes.

The major polyphenolic components of green tea are catechins, whereas the major polyphenolic components of black tea are theaflavins and thearubigins. Shiraki et al. evaluated the antioxidative and antimutagenic effects of four theaflavins (*287*). Theaflavins inhibited in vitro lipid peroxidation in erythrocyte membrane ghosts and microsomal systems. They also inhibited H$_2$O$_2$-induced DNA single-strand cleavage and mutagenesis. These observations suggest a radical-scavenging mechanism. The gallic acid moiety is essential for antioxidative activity.

Sohn et al. studied the effects of green and black tea on hepatic xenobiotic metabolizing systems in rats (*288*). For drinking, the rats were given free access to a standard 2% solution of tea. Both teas significantly increased P450 1A1, 1A2, and 2B1 activities but did not change P450 2E1 or 3A4. Of the phase II enzymes, UDP-glucuronyltransferase activity was increased but glutathione *S*-transferase was not. Several changes in serum parameters were also measured.

Studies in the well-characterized C3H10T1/2 mouse embryo fibroblast cell line demonstrated a radioprotective effect of Rooibos tea (*Aspalathus linealis*) (*289*). Extracts of Rooibos tea suppressed X-ray-induced oncogenic transformation of the cells. The effect was both dose- and time-related. It was seen with a concentration of extract as low as 2%, equivalent to the daily ingestion of 60 mL of Rooibos tea by a tea drinker. Green tea extract at an equitoxic concentration (0.2%) had no effect.

**PROTEASE INHIBITORS.** Protease inhibitors, which used to be considered "antinutrients," are now being intensely studied for their cancer-preventive action. Kennedy reviewed her laboratory's investigations of protease inhibitors, particularly the Bowman–Birk inhibitor derived from soybeans (*290*). This work has demonstrated the potency of the Bowman–Birk inhibitor against several types of carcinogen, in three rodent species, in five different tissues or organs, with various routes of administration including dietary, against several tumor types, and in both epithelial cells and connective tissue. The results suggest that anticarcinogenic protease inhibitors can reverse the initiating event in carcinogenesis by stopping the process begun by exposure to the carcinogen. Among the researchers' relevant observations are effects on the expression of c-*myc* and c-*fos* oncogenes and reduction of carcinogen-induced elevation of certain proteolytic activities. This versatility—the ability to affect so many different kinds of carcinogenesis—may be the most important difference between the anticarcinogenic protease inhibitors and other cancer-preventive agents. The one type of cancer that protease inhibitors would not be expected to affect is stomach cancer, because the inhibitory activity of protease inhibitors is pH-dependent. However, epidemiologic data show that large amounts of soybean in the diet are associated with reduced risk of gastric cancer. Conceivably, protease inhibitors could be protective even here if they are internalized by cells lining the stomach.

A book on protease inhibitors as cancer chemopreventive agents, edited by Troll and Kennedy, contains 18 chapters broadly ranging over the field (*291*). There is background material and a general review of the anticarcinogenic activity of protease inhibitors. Other chapters discuss epidemiologic studies and laboratory studies of particular protease inhibitors, including some of microbial origin. Structure–activity relationships and various types of target enzymes are discussed.

## Polysaccharides

Waldron and Selvendran reviewed evidence that bioactive cell wall and related components from plant foods and herbal products have antitumor activity (*292*). While there is no doubt that many cell wall–derived polysaccharides can act as immunomodulators in vivo, proof of antitumor activity requires demonstration that they stimulate the immune system to act against spontaneous autochthonous tumors. Much of the "antitumor activity" reported in early studies may have been due to stimulation of the graft-rejection system rather than to a true antitumor effect; even syngeneic tumors are subject to genetic drift over time. Nevertheless, there is some evidence for antitumor activity of certain polysaccharide preparations from fungi and higher plants, and these materials are effective in doses likely to be encountered in a healthful diet. The various immune activities of these substances were discussed.

The medicinal fungus *Ganoderma lucidum* (Polyporaceae) produces polysaccharides reportedly having antitumor activity. Wang et al. fractionated polysaccharides from the fruiting body of another *Ganoderma* species, *Ganoderma tsugae* (*293*). Antitumor activity was evaluated by injecting the fractions intraperitoneally into mice bearing grafted sarcoma 180 cells and observing effects on tumor growth. Seven glycans with strong antitumor activity were characterized. Four water-soluble fractions comprised three protein-containing glucogalactans associated with mannose and fucose and a (1→3)-β-D-glucan with a very low protein content. The three most active fractions were water-insoluble protein-containing (1→3)-β-D-glucans. Another polypore, the edible mushroom *Grifola frondosa*, also produces polysaccharides reportedly having antitumor activity. The same research group developed an automated liquid cultivation process that permits continuous production of fruiting bodies, harvesting of mycelium, and study of metabolites released into the culture medium. Now they have reported the fractionation and antitumor activity of polysaccharides from *G. frondosa* mycelia (*294*). Antitumor effects were tested against grafted sarcoma 180 in mice. The most active fractions were heteroglycans or their protein complexes. *Pleurotus sajor-caju*, another mushroom cultivated in China for its delicious flesh and medicinal properties, also yielded protein-containing antitumor polysaccharides (*295*). Active fractions were characterized as a mannogalactan, a xylan, a glucoxylan, and two xyloglucans.

Low-molecular-weight fucans from the brown seaweed *Ascophyllum nodosum* inhibit the in vitro proliferation of some types of cells, but not all (*296*). In a sensitive fibroblast cell line they were rapidly internalized and were distributed and retained in the cytoplasm but not the nucleus. In a less sensitive human colonic adenocarcinoma cell line they were strongly fixed on the cytoplasmic membrane but were not internalized. They did not inhibit a human breast cancer cell line or murine leukemia cells.

Screening of 12 seaweeds of the sargassum group (Phaeophyceae) for antitumor activity showed such activity only in *Sargassum thunbergii*. In follow-up studies, the authors tested fractions of an extract of *S. thunbergii* for antitumor effects on grafted Ehrlich carcinoma cells in mice (*297*). The most active fraction extended median survival time beyond the survival time of mice treated with the moderately active reference drug 5-fluorouracil, and this fraction was further examined. The active material, characterized as a hexuronic acid containing L-fucan sulfate (fucoidan), was not cytocidal against tumor cells. It did enhance the phagocytic activity and chemiluminescence of macrophages and increase the proportion of complement-positive cells. The authors concluded that the antitumor activity was related to enhancement of immune responses.

Polysaccharides extracted from the root of *Achyranthes bidentata*, a Chinese medicinal herb, inhibited the growth of sarcoma 180 in mice (*298*). Again, the antitumor activity seemed to be related to potentiation of specific and nonspecific immune responses in the host.

## Lipids

CONJUGATED LINOLEIC ACID (CLA). Because linoleic acid has been clearly linked to enhancement of carcinogenesis in several animal models, the discovery that a mixture of conjugated dienoic isomers of linoleic acid can *inhibit* carcinogenesis was of great interest. Chin et al. reviewed the important food sources of CLA, its formation by the microbial flora of ruminants and nonruminants, and its anticarcinogenic, antioxidant, and related activities (*299*). The *cis*-9,*trans*-11 isomer is incorporated into cell-membrane phospholipids, where it may provide protection from oxidation-induced free-radical damage. It also reduces 12-*O*-tetradecanoyl-phorbol-13-acetate-stimulated ornithine decarboxylase activity, most likely by inhibiting protein kinase C. Pariza briefly reviewed studies of CLA and an anticarcinogen from soy sauce recently identified as 4-hydroxy-2(or 5)-ethyl-5(or 2)-methyl-3(2H)-furanone

(HEMF) (*300*). It appears that in mammals, formation of CLA normally accompanies ingestion and uptake of linoleic acid, thus providing the cancer antidote along with the poison.

Ip et al. discussed the potential for modifying foods to prevent cancer, using CLA-rich foods and selenium-enriched garlic as examples (*301*). They presented a rationale for delivering these two substances through the food system and argued the advantages of using foods to provide anticarcinogens as part of a cancer chemopreventive strategy. Animal research on CLA was summarized. Ip et al. also reported their recent studies of CLA's suppression of mammary carcinogenesis and proliferative activity of the mammary gland in rats (*302*). Dietary CLA, at levels relevant to the human diet, was protective in both 7,12-dimethylbenz[*a*]anthracene and methylnitrosourea models of carcinogenesis. With dimethylbenzanthracene, inhibition was dose-related for long-term CLA feeding. Feeding for 5 weeks during maturation of the mammary gland also offered significant protection against tumors induced by subsequent administration of carcinogen. Protection in the methylnitrosourea model suggests direct modulation of the target organ's susceptibility to neoplastic transformation. CLA reduced the bromodeoxyuridine labeling index of the lobuloalveolar compartment but not the ductal compartment of the mammary tree. This is consistent with data on tumor inhibition, since lobuloalveolar structures are derived from terminal end buds, the sites of neoplastic transformation.

Chin et al. found that substantial amounts of CLA are produced in conventional rats fed linoleic acid, but CLA concentrations in tissues of germ-free rats did not respond to dietary linoleic acid (*303*). This indicates that CLA is a metabolic product of the host microflora, not of the host. Comparison of diets containing free linoleic acid with diets containing corn oil (linoleic acid esterified in triacylglycerols) further showed that the intestinal flora of rats can only convert the free fatty acid to CLA. The authors noted that in ruminants, high levels of free fatty acids are produced in the rumen through microbial hydrolysis of triacylglycerols. The microflora of nonruminants has a more limited source of free linoleic acid, and as a consequence nonruminants have lower tissue concentrations of CLA. However, the normal diet of nonruminants also provides preformed CLA.

SPHINGOMYELIN. Although sphingolipids are important components of all eukaryotic cells, little is known about their physiologic effects when ingested. Dillehay et al. reported that feeding a sphingomyelin preparation from milk at levels of 0.025–0.1 g per 100 g of diet reduced the incidence of 1,2-dimethylhydrazine-induced colon tumors by ~50% in CF1 mice (*304*). Tumor multiplicity was nonsignificantly reduced. Dietary sphingomyelin also reduced the number of dimethylhydrazine-induced aberrant crypt foci. The authors concluded that sphingolipids may be another important class of nutritional modulators of carcinogenesis.

## Maillard Reaction Products

The Maillard reaction between carbonyl and amino compounds occurs in foods during processing and storage. Some of these reaction products have antimutagenic activity. Yen and Hsieh suggested a possible mechanism for the antimutagenic effect of xylose–lysine Maillard reaction products (*305*). In a bioantimutagenic test the substances did not reduce the mutagenicity of IQ for *Salmonella typhimurium* TA98 or TA100, indicating that the effect was not on DNA repair. Further study demonstrated a desmutagenic effect: the xylose–lysine Maillard reaction products did not interact directly with IQ itself or inhibit activation of hepatic microsomes, but appeared to interact with proximate metabolites of IQ to form inactive adducts.

## Proteins and Peptides

In the *Salmonella*/microsome and *Escherichia coli* DNA-repair tests, casein showed varying degrees of antimutagenic activity depending on the mutagen tested (*306*). Casein's antimutagenic potential increased with pepsin digestion. Since casein is the major protein in milk, the authors suggest that dairy products may also be antimutagenic.

An aqueous extract of Thai rice seedlings had potent cytotoxic effects on 4 of 17 transformed cell lines but not on the 4 untransformed cell lines tested (*307*). It was moderately toxic to 10 transformed cell lines. The active substance was characterized as a protein-containing molecule of 40 kDa, resistant to freezing, heating, and mild acidic and basic conditions, and sensitive to trypsin digestion. This substance had quite different biochemical and biological properties from a polysaccharide antitumor substance from rice bran that was previously described. Moreover, its activity was substantially lower in dormant rice seeds, increased sharply 3–7 days after germination, and then declined.

Kawamura and Ishikawa purified a potent antitumor protein of 105 kDa from matsutake mushroom (*Tricholoma matsutake*) (*308*). It was active against cell lines representing both mouse and human tumors.

## *LITERATURE CITED*

1. Riboli, E., and J.H. Cummings. Ole Møller Jensen Memorial Symposium on Nutrition and Cancer. *Int. J. Cancer* 55:531–537 (1993).

2. Miller, A.B., F. Berrino, M. Hill, et al. Diet in the aetiology of cancer: a review. *Eur. J. Cancer* 30A:207–220 (1994).

3. Clifford, C., and B. Kramer. Diet as risk and therapy for cancer. *Med. Clin. North Am.* 77:725–744 (1993).

4. Rogers, A.E., S.H. Zeisel, and J. Groopman. Diet and carcinogenesis. *Carcinogenesis* 14:2205–2217 (1993).

5. Weisburger, J.H. Does the Delaney Clause of the U.S. food and drug laws prevent human cancers? *Fund. Appl. Toxicol.* 22:483–493 (1994).

6. Byers, T. Dietary trends in the United States. Relevance to cancer prevention. *Cancer* 72:1015–1018 (1993).

7. Kritchevsky, D. Dietary guidelines. The rationale for intervention. *Cancer* 72:1011–1014 (1993).

8. Bal, D.G., and S.B. Foerster. Dietary strategies for cancer prevention. *Cancer* 72:1005–1010 (1993).

9. Heimendinger, J. Community nutrition intervention strategies for cancer risk reduction. *Cancer* 72:1019–1023 (1993).

10. Dwyer, J.T. Diet and nutritional strategies for cancer risk reduction. Focus on the 21st century. *Cancer* 72:1024–1031 (1993).

11. Rodgers, A.B., L.G. Kessler, B. Portnoy, et al. "Eat for Health": a supermarket intervention for nutrition and cancer risk reduction. *Am. J. Public Health* 84:72–76 (1994).

12. Ferguson, L.R. Diet and the prevention of colorectal cancer. *Mutat. Res.* 290:139–143 (1993).

13. Waldron, K.W., I.T. Johnson, and G.R. Fenwick (eds.). *Food and Cancer Prevention: Chemical and Biological Aspects.* Proceedings of an International Conference, Norwich, UK, 13–16 September 1992. Cambridge, England, Royal Society of Chemistry (1993).

14. Williams, G.M. Food: its role in the etiology of cancer. In *Food and Cancer Prevention: Chemical and Biological Aspects.* K.W. Waldron et al. (eds.). Cambridge, England, Royal Society of Chemistry. Pp. 3–9 (1993).

15. Borek, C. Molecular mechanisms in cancer induction and prevention. *Environ. Health Perspect.* 101(Suppl. 3):237–245 (1993).

16. Rosin, M.P. Genetic alterations in carcinogenesis and chemoprevention. *Environ. Health Perspect.* 101(Suppl. 3):253–256 (1993).

17. Netter, K.J. The role of nutrients in detoxification mechanisms. In *Nutritional Toxicology.* F.N. Kotsonis et al. (eds.). New York, Raven Press. *Target Organ Toxicology Ser.* Pp. 1–18 (1994).

18. Collins, A., S. Duthie, and M. Ross. Micronutrients and oxidative stress in the aetiology of cancer. *Proc. Nutr. Soc.* 53:67–75 (1994).

19. Prasad, K.N., J. Edwards-Prasad, S. Kumar, and A. Meyers. Vitamins regulate gene expression and induce differentiation and growth inhibition in cancer cells. Their relevance in cancer prevention. *Arch. Otolaryngol. Head Neck Surg.* 119:1133–1140 (1993).

20. De Luca, L.M., N. Darwiche, G. Celli, et al. Vitamin A in epithelial differentiation and skin carcinogenesis. *Nutr. Rev.* 52:S45–S52 (1994).

21. Lupulescu, A. The role of vitamins A, β-carotene, E and C in cancer cell biology. Review. *Int. J. Vit. Nutr. Res.* 63:3–14 (1993).

22. Davison, A., E. Rousseau, and B. Dunn. Putative anticarcinogenic actions of carotenoids: nutritional implications. *Can. J. Physiol. Pharmacol.* 71:732–745 (1993).

23. Harris, P.J., and L.R. Ferguson. Dietary fibre: its composition and role in protection against colorectal cancer. *Mutat. Res.* 290:97–110 (1993).

24. Van Munster, I.P., and F.M. Nagengast. The role of carbohydrate fermentation in colon cancer prevention. *Scand. J. Gastroenterol.* 28(Suppl. 200):80–86 (1993).

25. Goodman, J.I., and J.L. Counts. Hypomethylation of DNA: a possible nongenotoxic mechanism underlying the role of cell proliferation in carcinogenesis. *Environ. Health Perspect.* 101(Suppl. 5):169–172 (1993).

26. Poirier, L.A. Methyl group deficiency in hepato-carcinogenesis. *Drug Metab. Rev.* 26:185–199 (1994).

27. Lombardi, B., and M.L. Smith. Tumorigenesis, protooncogene activation, and other gene abnormalities in methyl deficiency. *J. Nutr. Biochem.* 5:2–9 (1994).

28. Rogers, A.E. Chemical carcinogenesis in methyl-deficient rats. *J. Nutr. Biochem.* 4:666–671 (1993).

29. Christman, J.K., M.-L. Chen, G. Sheikhnejad, et al. Methyl deficiency, DNA methylation, and cancer: studies on the reversibility of the effects of a lipotrope-deficient diet. *J. Nutr. Biochem.* 4:672–680 (1993).

30. Anonymous. Folate, alcohol, methionine, and colon cancer risk: is there a unifying theme? *Nutr. Rev.* 52:18–20 (1994).

31. Mason, J.B. Folate and colonic carcinogenesis: searching for a mechanistic understanding. *J. Nutr. Biochem.* 5:170–175 (1994).

32. Kritchevsky, D. Energy restriction and carcinogenesis. *Food Res. Int.* 26:289–295 (1993).

33. Kritchevsky, D. Colorectal cancer: the role of dietary fat and caloric restriction. *Mutat. Res.* 290:63–70 (1993).

34. Hart, R.W., and A. Turturro (eds.). *The Impact of Dietary Restriction on Genetic Stability.* Special Issue, *Mutat. Res.* 295(4–6) (1993).

35. Mukhopadhyay, P., J. Das Gupta, U. Senyal, and S. Das. Influence of dietary restriction and soyabean supplementation on the growth of a murine lymphoma and host immune function. *Cancer Lett.* 78:151–157 (1994).

36. Kromhout, D., H.B.B. de Mesquita, and M.G.L. Hertog. Contribution of epidemiology in elucidating the role of foods in cancer prevention. In *Food and Cancer Prevention: Chemical and Biological Aspects.* K.W. Waldron et al. (eds.). Cambridge, Royal Society of Chemistry. Pp. 24–36 (1993).

37. Mills, P.K., W.L. Beeson, R.L. Phillips, and G.E. Fraser. Cancer incidence among California Seventh-day

Adventists, 1976–1982. *Am. J. Clin. Nutr.* 59(Suppl.): 1136S–1142S (1994).

38. Boyle, P., R. Kevi, F. Lucchuni, and C. La Vecchia. Trends in diet-related cancers in Japan: a conundrum? (Letter.) *Lancet* 342:752 (1993).

39. Gubéran, E., M. Usel, L. Raymond, and G. Fioretta. Mortality and incidence of cancer among a cohort of self employed butchers from Geneva and their wives. *Br. J. Indust. Med.* 50:1008–1016 (1993).

40. Walker, A.R.P., B.F. Walker, F.I. Sookaria, and I. Segal. Changing patterns of admissions of black cancer patients to hospital in Soweto, South Africa. *Cancer J.* 6:180–183 (1993).

41. Swanson, C.A., G. Gridley, R.S. Greenberg, et al. A comparison of diets of blacks and whites in three areas of the United States. *Nutr. Cancer* 20:153–165 (1993).

42. Messina, M.J., V. Persky, K.D.R. Setchell, and S. Barnes. Soy intake and cancer risk: a review of the *in vitro* and *in vivo* data. *Nutr. Cancer* 21:113–131 (1994).

43. Willett, W.C. Micronutrients and cancer risk. *Am. J. Clin. Nutr.* 59(Suppl.):1162S–1165S (1994).

44. Willett, W.C., and D.J. Hunter. Vitamin A and cancers of the breast, large bowel, and prostate: epidemiologic evidence. *Nutr. Rev.* 52:S53–S59 (1994).

45. Block, G. Vitamin C, cancer and aging. *Age* 16:55–58 (1993).

46. Potter, J.D., M.L. Slattery, R.M. Bostick, and S.M. Gapstur. Colon cancer: a review of the epidemiology. *Epidemiol. Rev.* 15:499–545 (1993).

47. McCann, S.E., E. Randall, J.R. Marshall, et al. Diet diversity and risk of colon cancer in western New York. *Nutr. Cancer* 21:133–141 (1994).

48. Meyer, F., and E. White. Alcohol and nutrients in relation to colon cancer in middle-aged adults. *Am. J. Epidemiol.* 138:225–236 (1993).

49. La Vecchia, C., E. Negri, S. Franceschi, and B. D'Avanzo. Moderate beer consumption and the risk of colorectal cancer. *Nutr. Cancer* 19:303–306 (1993).

50. Gapstur, S.M., J.D. Potter, and A.R. Folsom. Alcohol consumption and colon and rectal cancer in postmenopausal women. *Int. J. Epidemiol.* 23:50–57 (1994).

51. Steinmetz, K.A., L.H. Kushi, R.M. Bostick, et al. Vegetables, fruit, and colon cancer in the Iowa Women's Health Study. *Am. J. Epidemiol.* 139:1–15 (1994).

52. Frentzel-Beyme, R., and J. Chang-Claude. Vegetarian diets and colon cancer: the German experience. *Am. J. Clin. Nutr.* 59(Suppl.):1143S–1152S (1994).

53. Goldbohm, R.A., P.A. van den Brandt, P. van 't Veer, et al. A prospective cohort study on the relation between meat consumption and the risk of colon cancer. *Cancer Res.* 54:718–723 (1994).

54. Giovannucci, E., E.B. Rimm, M.J. Stampfer, et al. Intake of fat, meat, and fiber in relation to risk of colon cancer in men. *Cancer Res.* 54:2390–2397 (1994).

55. Hoshiyama, Y., T. Sekine, and T. Sasaba. A case–control study of colorectal cancer and its relation to diet, cigarettes, and alcohol consumption in Saitama Prefecture, Japan. *Tohuku J. Exp. Med.* 171:153–165 (1993).

56. Guo, W., W. Zheng, J.-Y. Li, et al. Correlations of colon cancer mortality with dietary factors, serum markers, and schistosomiasis in China. *Nutr. Cancer* 20:13–20 (1993).

57. Olsen, J., O. Kronborg, J. Lynggaard, and M. Ewertz. Dietary risk factors for cancer and adenomas of the large intestine. A case–control study within a screening trial in Denmark. *Eur. J. Cancer* 30A:53–60 (1994).

58. Caderni, G., F. Bianchini, A. Russo, et al. Mitotic activity in colorectal mucosa of healthy subjects in two Italian areas with different dietary habits. *Nutr. Cancer* 19:263–268 (1993).

59. Benito, E., E. Cabeza, V. Moreno, et al. Diet and colorectal adenomas: a case–control study in Majorca. *Int. J. Cancer* 55:213–219 (1993).

60. Dwyer, J. Dietary fiber and colorectal cancer risk. *Nutr. Rev.* 51:147–148 (1993).

61. Friedenreich, C.M., R.F. Brant, and E. Riboli. Influence of methodologic factors in a pooled analysis of 13 case–control studies of colorectal cancer and dietary fiber. *Epidemiology* 5:66–79 (1994).

62. Bostick, R.B., J.D. Potter, D.R. McKenzie, et al. Reduced risk of colon cancer with high intake of vitamin E: the Iowa Women's Health Study. *Cancer Res.* 53:4230–4237 (1993).

63. Bostick, R.M., J.D. Potter, T.A. Sellers, et al. Relation of calcium, vitamin D, and dairy food intake to incidence of colon cancer among older women. *Am. J. Epidemiol.* 137:1302–1317 (1993).

64. Kampman, E., E. Giovannucci, P. van 't Veer, et al. Calcium, vitamin D, dairy foods, and the occurrence of colorectal adenomas among men and women in two prospective studies. *Am. J. Epidemiol.* 139:16–29 (1994).

65. Cassidy, A., S.A. Bingham, and J.H. Cummings. Starch intake and colorectal cancer risk: an international comparison. *Br. J. Cancer* 69:937–942 (1994).

66. La Vecchia, C., S. Franceschi, P. Dolara, et al. Refined-sugar intake and the risk of colorectal cancer in humans. *Int. J. Cancer* 55:386–389 (1993).

67. Longmire, W.P., Jr. A current view of gastric cancer in the US. *Ann. Surg.* 218:579–582 (1993).

68. Hwang, H., J. Dwyer, and R.M. Russell. Diet, *Helicobacter pylori* infection, food preservation and gastric cancer risk: are there new roles for preventative factors? *Nutr. Rev.* 52:75–83 (1994).

69. Hansson, L.-E., O. Nyrén, R. Bergström, et al. Diet and risk of gastric cancer. A population-based case–control study in Sweden. *Int. J. Cancer* 55:181–189 (1993).

70. Hansson, L.-E., J. Baron, O. Nyrén, et al. Tobacco, alcohol and the risk of gastric cancer. A population-based case–control study in Sweden. *Int. J. Cancer* 57:26–31 (1994).

71. Ramón, J.M., L. Serra-Majem, C. Cerdó, and J. Oromí. Nutrient intake and gastric cancer risk: a

case–control study in Spain. *Int. J. Epidemiol.* 22:983–988 (1993).

72. González, C.A., E. Riboli, J. Badosa, et al. Nutritional factors and gastric cancer in Spain. *Am. J. Epidemiol.* 139:466–473 (1994).

73. Nazario, C.M., M. Szklo, E. Diamond, et al. Salt and gastric cancer: a case–control study in Puerto Rico. *Int. J. Epidemiol.* 22:790–797 (1993).

74. Zhang, L., W.J. Blot, W.-c. You, et al. Serum micronutrients in relation to pre-cancerous gastric lesions. *Int. J. Cancer* 56:650–654 (1994).

75. Inoue, M., K. Tajima, K. Hirose, et al. Life-style and subsite of gastric cancer—joint effect of smoking and drinking habits. *Int. J. Cancer* 56:494–499 (1994).

76. Muñoz, N. Epidemiological aspects of oesophageal cancer. *Endoscopy* 25(Suppl.):609–612 (1993).

77. Franceschi, S. Role of nutrition in the aetiology of oesophageal cancer in developed countries. *Endoscopy* 25(Suppl.):613–616 (1993).

78. Tavani, A., E. Negri, S. Franceschi, and C. La Vecchia. Risk factors for esophageal cancer in women in northern Italy. *Cancer* 72:2531–2536 (1993).

79. Hu, J., O. Nyrén, A. Wolk, et al. Risk factors for oesophageal cancer in northeast China. *Int. J. Cancer* 57:38–46 (1994).

80. Zheng, W., F. Jin, S.S. Devesa, et al. Declining incidence is greater for esophageal than gastric cancer in Shanghai, People's Republic of China. *Br. J. Cancer* 68:978–982 (1993).

81. Hildesheim, A., and P.H. Levine. Etiology of nasopharyngeal carcinoma: a review. *Epidemiol. Rev.* 15:466–485 (1993).

82. Zheng, Y.M., P. Tuppin, A. Hubert, et al. Environmental and dietary risk factors for nasopharyngeal carcinoma: a case–control study in Zangwu County, Guangxi, China. *Br. J. Cancer* 69:508–514 (1994).

83. Zheng, W., J.K. McLaughlin, W.-H. Chow, et al. Risk factors for cancers of the nasal cavity and paranasal sinuses among white men in the United States. *Am. J. Epidemiol.* 138:965–972 (1993).

84. West, S., A. Hildesheim, and M. Dosemeci. Nonviral risk factors for nasopharyngeal carcinoma in the Philippines: results from a case–control study. *Int. J. Cancer* 55:722–727 (1993).

85. Kune, G.A., S. Kune, B. Field, et al. Oral and pharyngeal cancer, diet, smoking, alcohol, and serum vitamin A and β-carotene levels: a case–control study in men. *Nutr. Cancer* 20:61–70 (1993).

86. Flagg, E.W., R.J. Coates, D.P. Jones, et al. Dietary glutathione intake and the risk of oral and pharyngeal cancer. *Am. J. Epidemiol.* 139:453–465 (1994).

87. Kolonel, L.N. Lung cancer: another consequence of a high-fat diet? *J. Natl. Cancer Inst.* 85:1886–1887 (1993).

88. Alavanja, M.C.R., C.C. Brown, C. Swanson, and R.C. Brownson. Saturated fat intake and lung cancer risk among nonsmoking women in Missouri. *J. Natl. Cancer Inst.* 85:1906–1916 (1993).

89. Mayne, S.T., D.T. Janerich, P. Greenwald, et al. Dietary beta carotene and lung cancer risk in U.S. nonsmokers. *J. Natl. Cancer Inst.* 86:33–38 (1994).

90. Gao, C.-m., K. Tajima, T. Kuroishi, et al. Protective effects of raw vegetables and fruit against lung cancer among smokers and ex-smokers: a case–control study in the Tokai area of Japan. *Jpn. J. Cancer Res.* 84:594–600 (1993).

91. van den Brandt, P.A., R.A. Goldbohm, P. van 't Veer, et al. A prospective cohort study on selenium status and the risk of lung cancer. *Cancer Res.* 53:4860–4865 (1993).

92. Hunter, D.J., and W.C. Willett. Diet, body size, and breast cancer. *Epidemiol. Rev.* 15:110–132 (1993).

93. Hankin, J.H. Role of nutrition in women's health: diet and breast cancer. *J. Am. Diet. Assoc.* 93:994–999 (1993).

94. Levi, F., C. La Vecchia, C. Gulie, and E. Negri. Dietary factors and breast cancer risk in Vaud, Switzerland. *Nutr. Cancer* 19:327–335 (1993).

95. Ewertz, M. Breast cancer in Denmark. Incidence, risk factors, and characteristics of survival. *Acta Oncol.* 32:595–615 (1993).

96. Ewertz, M., and S.W. Duffy. Incidence of female breast cancer in relation to prevalence of risk factors in Denmark. *Int. J. Cancer* 56:783–787 (1994).

97. Boyd, N.F., L.J. Martin, M. Noffel, et al. A meta-analysis of studies of dietary fat and breast cancer risk. *Br. J. Cancer* 68:627–636 (1993).

98. Wynder, E.L., L.A. Cohen, D.P. Rose, and S.D. Stellman. Dietary fat and breast cancer: where do we stand on the evidence? *J. Clin. Epidemiol.* 47:217–222 (1994).

99. Willett, W. Response to Wynder *et al.*'s paper on dietary fat and breast cancer. *J. Clin. Epidemiol.* 47:223–226 (1994).

100. Wynder, E.L., L.A. Cohen, D.P. Rose, and S.D. Stellman. Response to Dr Walter Willett's dissent. *J. Clin. Epidemiol.* 47:227–230 (1994).

101. Barrett-Connor, E., and N.J. Friedlander. Dietary fat, calories, and the risk of breast cancer in postmenopausal women: a prospective population-based study. *J. Am. Coll. Nutr.* 12:390–399 (1993).

102. Baghurst, P.A., and T.E. Rohan. High-fiber diets and reduced risk of breast cancer. *Int. J. Cancer* 56:173–176 (1994).

103. Garland, M., W.C. Willett, J.E. Manson, and D.J. Hunter. Antioxidant micronutrients and breast cancer. *J. Am. Coll. Nutr.* 12:400–411 (1993).

104. Friedenreich, C.M., G.R. Howe, and A.B. Miller. Recall bias in the association of micronutrient intake and breast cancer. *J. Clin. Epidemiol.* 46:1009–1017 (1993).

105. Hunter, D.J., J.E. Manson, G.A. Colditz, et al. A prospective study of the intake of vitamins C, E, and A and the risk of breast cancer. *New Engl. J. Med.* 329:234–240 (1993).

106. Freudenheim, J.L., J.R. Marshall, S. Graham, et al. Exposure to breastmilk in infancy and the risk of breast cancer. *Epidemiology* 5:324–331 (1994).

107. Rosenberg, L., L.S. Metzger, and J.R. Palmer. Alcohol consumption and risk of breast cancer: a review of the epidemiologic evidence. *Epidemiol. Rev.* 15:133–144 (1993).

108. Vobecky, J., A. Simard, J.S. Vobecky, et al. Nutritional profile of women with fibrocystic breast disease. *Int. J. Epidemiol.* 22:989–999 (1993).

109. Nordevang, E., E. Azavedo, G. Svane, et al. Dietary habits and mammographic patterns in patients with breast cancer. *Breast Cancer Res. Treat.* 26:207–215 (1993).

110. Key, T., D. Forman, L. Cotton, et al. Diet and mammographic patterns: work in progress. In *Food and Cancer Prevention: Chemical and Biological Aspects.* K.W. Waldron et al. (eds.). Cambridge, Royal Society of Chemistry. Pp. 37–41 (1993).

111. Fürst, C.J., G. Auer, E. Nordevang, et al. DNA pattern and dietary habits in patients with breast cancer. *Eur. J. Cancer* 29A:1285–1288 (1993).

112. Ingram, D. Diet and subsequent survival in women with breast cancer. *Br. J. Cancer* 69:592–595 (1994).

113. Rohan, T.E., J.E. Hiller, and A.J. McMichael. Dietary factors and survival from breast cancer. *Nutr. Cancer* 20:167–177 (1993).

114. Pienta, K.J., and P.S. Esper. Is dietary fat a risk factor for prostate cancer? *J. Natl. Cancer Inst.* 85:1538–1540 (1993).

115. Giovannucci, E., E.B. Rimm, G.A. Colditz, et al. A prospective study of dietary fat and risk of prostate cancer. *J. Natl. Cancer Inst.* 85:1571–1579 (1993).

116. Franceschi, S. Fat and prostate cancer. *Epidemiology* 5:271–273 (1994).

117. Le Marchand, L., L.N. Kolonel, L.R. Wilkens, et al. Animal fat consumption and prostate cancer: a prospective study in Hawaii. *Epidemiology* 5:276–282 (1994).

118. Gann, P.H., C.H. Hennekens, F.M. Sacks, et al. Prospective study of plasma fatty acids and risk of prostate cancer. *J. Natl. Cancer Inst.* 86:281–286 (1994).

119. Ross, R.K., and B.E. Henderson. Do diet and androgens alter prostate cancer risk via a common etiologic pathway? *J. Natl. Cancer Inst.* 86:252–254 (1994).

120. Adlercreutz, H., H. Markkanen, and S. Watanabe. Plasma concentrations of phyto-oestrogens in Japanese men. *Lancet* 342:1209–1210 (1993).

121. Swanson, C.A., G.D. Wilbanks, L.B. Twiggs, et al. Moderate alcohol consumption and the risk of endometrial cancer. *Epidemiology* 4:530–536 (1993).

122. Cramer, D.W., and H. Xu. Lactase persistence, galactose metabolism, and milk consumption as risk factors for ovarian cancer. In *Common Food Intolerances 2: Milk in Human Nutrition and Adult-Type Hypolactasia.* S. Auricchio and G. Semenza (eds.). Basel, Karger. *Dynam. Nutr. Res.* 3:52–60 (1993).

123. Tzonou, A., C.-c. Hsieh, A. Polychronopoulou, et al. Diet and ovarian cancer: a case–control study in Greece. *Int. J. Cancer* 55:411–414 (1993).

124. Bunin, G.R., R.R. Kuijten, J.D. Buckley, et al. Relation between maternal diet and subsequent primitive neuroectodermal brain tumors in young children. *New Engl. J. Med.* 329:536–541 (1993).

125. Foreman, N.K., and A.D. Pearson. Maternal diet and primitive neuroectodermal brain tumors in children. (Letter.) *New Engl. J. Med.* 329:1963 (1993).

126. Bunin, G.R., P.A. Witman, and A.T. Meadows. Maternal diet and primitive neuroectodermal brain tumors in children. (Reply.) *New Engl. J. Med.* 329:1963 (1993).

127. Kirkpatrick, C.S., E. White, and J.A.H. Lee. Case–control study of malignant melanoma in Washington state. *Am. J. Epidemiol.* 139:869–880 (1994).

128. Bartram, H.-P., A. Gostner, W. Scheppach, et al. Effects of fish oil on rectal cell proliferation, mucosal fatty acids, and prostaglandin $E_2$ release in healthy subjects. *Gastroenterology* 105:1317–1322 (1993).

129. Anonymous. Fish-oil supplementation reduces intestinal hyperproliferation in persons at risk for colon cancer. *Nutr. Rev.* 51:241–243 (1993).

130. van Faassen, A., M.J. Hazen, P.A. van den Brandt, et al. Bile acids and pH values in total feces and in fecal water from habitually omnivorous and vegetarian subjects. *Am. J. Clin. Nutr.* 58:917–922 (1993).

131. Nelson, G.J., V.C. Morris, P.C. Schmidt, and O. Levander. The urinary excretion of thiobarbituric acid reactive substances and malondialdehyde by normal adult males after consuming a diet containing salmon. *Lipids* 28:757–761 (1993).

132. Black, H.S., J.A. Herd, L.H. Goldberg, et al. Effect of a low-fat diet on the incidence of actinic keratosis. *New Engl. J. Med.* 330:1272–1275 (1994).

133. Rao, A.V., N. Shiwnarain, M. Koo, and D.J.A. Jenkins. Effect of fiber-rich foods on the composition of intestinal microflora. *Nutr. Res.* 14:523–535 (1994).

134. Schantz, S.P., W.K. Hong, C.W. Boone, and G.J. Kelloff (eds.). *Chemoprevention of Premalignant Lesions of the Upper Aerodigestive Tract. J. Cell. Biochem.* Suppl. 17F (1993).

135. Greenwald, P. Experience from clinical trails in cancer prevention. *Ann. Med.* 26:73–80 (1994).

136. Greenwald, P., G. Kelloff, S. Kalagher, and S. McDonald. Research studies on chemoprevention of esophageal cancer at the United States National Cancer Institute. *Endoscopy* 25(Suppl.):617–626 (1993).

137. van Poppel, G. Carotenoids and cancer: an update with emphasis on human intervention studies. *Eur. J. Cancer* 29A:1335–1344 (1993).

138. Omenn, G.S., G. Goodman, M. Thornquist, et al. The β-carotene and retinol efficacy trial (CARET) for chemoprevention of lung cancer in high risk populations: smokers and asbestos-exposed workers. *Cancer Res.* 54(Suppl.):2038s–2043s (1994).

139. Lippmann, S.M., S.E. Benner, and W.K. Hong. Retinoid chemoprevention studies in upper aerodigestive tract and lung carcinogenesis. *Cancer Res.* 54(Suppl.):2025s–2028s (1994).

140. The Alpha-Tocopherol, Beta Carotene Cancer Prevention Study Group. The effect of vitamin E and beta carotene on the incidence of lung cancer and other cancers in male smokers. *New Engl. J. Med.* 330:1029–1035 (1994).

141. Hennekens, C.H., J.E. Buring, and R. Peto. Antioxidant vitamins—benefits not yet proved. *New Engl. J. Med.* 330:1080–1081 (1994).

142. Nowak, R. Beta-carotene: helpful or harmful? *Science* 264:500–501 (1994).

143. Taylor, P.R., B. Li, S.M. Dawsey, et al. Prevention of esophageal cancer: the nutrition intervention trials in Linxian, China. *Cancer Res.* 54(Suppl.):2029s–2031s (1994).

144. Li, J.-Y., P.R. Taylor, B. Li, et al. Nutrition intervention trials in Linxian, China: multiple vitamin/mineral supplementation, cancer incidence, and disease-specific mortality among adults with esophageal dysplasia. *J. Natl. Cancer Inst.* 84:1492–1498 (1993).

145. Blot, W.J., J.-Y. Li, P.R. Taylor, et al. Nutrition intervention trials in Linxian, China: supplementation with specific vitamin/mineral combinations, cancer incidence, and disease-specific mortality in the general population. *J. Natl. Cancer Inst.* 85:1483–1492 (1993).

146. Mobarhan, S. Micronutrient supplementation trials and the reduction of cancer and cerebrovascular incidence and mortality. *Nutr. Rev.* 52:102–105 (1994).

147. Kaugars, G.E., S. Silverman, J.G.L. Lovas, et al. A review of the use of antioxidant supplements in the treatment of human oral leukoplakia. *J. Cell. Biochem.* Suppl. 17F:292–298 (1993).

148. Garewal, H.S. Beta-carotene and vitamin E in oral cancer prevention. *J. Cell. Biochem.* Suppl. 17F:262–269 (1993).

149. Phillips, R.W., J.W. Kikendall, G.D. Luk, et al. β-Carotene inhibits rectal mucosal ornithine decarboxylase activity in colon cancer patients. *Cancer Res.* 53:3723–3725 (1993).

150. Cahill, R.J., K.R. O'Sullivan, P.M. Mathias, et al. Effects of vitamin antioxidant supplementation on cell kinetics of patients with adenomatous polyps. *Gut* 34:963–967 (1993).

151. Lamm, D.L., D.R. Riggs, J.S. Shriver, et al. Megadose vitamins in bladder cancer: a double-blind clinical trial. *J. Urol.* 151:21–26 (1994).

152. Alder, R.J., G. McKeown-Eyssen, and E. Bright-See. Randomized trial of the effect of calcium supplementation on fecal risk factors for colorectal cancer. *Am. J. Epidemiol.* 138:804–814 (1993).

153. Bartram, H.-P., W. Scheppach, H. Schmid, et al. Proliferation of human colonic mucosa as an intermediate biomarker of carcinogenesis: effects of butyrate, deoxycholate, calcium, ammonia, and pH. *Cancer Res.* 53:3283–3288 (1993).

154. Ling, W.H., R. Korpela, H. Mykkänen, et al. *Lactobacillus* strain GG supplementation decreases colonic hydrolytic and reductive enzyme activities in healthy female adults. *J. Nutr.* 124:18–23 (1994).

155. Hayatsu, H., and T. Hayatsu. Suppressing effect of *Lactobacillus casei* administration on the urinary mutagenicity arising from ingestion of fried ground beef in the human. *Cancer Lett.* 73:173–179 (1993).

156. Steinbach, G., S. Heymsfield, N.E. Olansen, et al. Effect of caloric restriction on colonic proliferation in obese persons: implications for colon cancer prevention. *Cancer Res.* 54:1194–1197 (1994).

157. Burns, C.P., and A.A. Spector. Biochemical effects of lipids on cancer therapy. *J. Nutr. Biochem.* 5:114–123 (1994).

158. Abbott, W.G.H., B. Tezabwala, M. Bennett, and S.M. Grundy. Melanoma lung metastases and cytolytic effector cells in mice fed antioxidant-balanced corn oil or fish oil diets. *Nat. Immun.* 13:15–28 (1994).

159. Haegele, A.D., S.P. Briggs, and H.J. Thompson. Antioxidant status and dietary lipid unsaturation modulate oxidative DNA damage. *Free Rad. Biol. Med.* 16:111–115 (1994).

160. Sasaki, Y.F., M. Sakaguchi, T. Yamagishi, et al. Bio-anticlastogenic effects of unsaturated fatty acids included in fish oil—docosahexaenoic acid, docosapentaenoic acid, and eicosapentaenoic acid—in cultured Chinese hamster cells. *Mutat. Res.* 320:9–22 (1994).

161. Schut, H.A.J. Effects of dietary menhaden oil on DNA adducts of the food mutagen 2-amino-3-methylimidazo[4,5-f]quinoline (IQ) in Fischer-344 rats. *Anticancer Res.* 13:1517–1524 (1993).

162. Freedman, L.S. Meta-analysis of animal experiments on dietary fat intake and mammary tumors. *Stat. Med.* 13:709–718 (1994).

163. Welsch, C.W., C.S. Oakley, C.-C. Chang, and M.A. Welsch. Suppression of growth by dietary fish oil of human breast carcinomas maintained in three different strains of immune-deficient mice. *Nutr. Cancer* 20:119–127 (1993).

164. Gonzalez, M.J., R.A. Schemmel, L. Dugan, Jr., et al. Dietary fish oil inhibits human breast carcinoma growth: a function of increased lipid peroxidation. *Lipids* 28:827–832 (1993).

165. Rose, D.P., and J.M. Connolly. Effects of dietary omega-3 fatty acids on human breast cancer growth and metastases in nude mice. *J. Natl. Cancer Inst.* 85:1743–1747 (1993).

166. Rose, D.P., M.A. Hatala, J.M. Connolly, and J. Rayburn. Effect of diets containing different levels of linoleic acid on human breast cancer growth and lung metastasis in nude mice. *Cancer Res.* 53:4686–4690 (1993).

167. Rose, D.P., and M.A. Hatala. Dietary fatty acids and breast cancer invasion and metastasis. *Nutr. Cancer* 21:103–111 (1994).

168. Connolly, J.M., and D.P. Rose. Effects of fatty acids on invasion through a reconstituted basement membrane ('Matrigel') by a human breast cancer cell line. *Cancer Lett.* 75:137–142 (1993).

169. Narisawa, T., Y. Fukaura, K. Yazawa, et al. Colon cancer prevention with a small amount of dietary perilla oil high in α-linolenic acid in an animal model. *Cancer* 73:2069–2075 (1994).

170. Takahashi, M., T. Minamoto, N. Yamashita, et al. Reduction in formation and growth of 1,2-dimethylhydrazine-induced aberrant crypt foci in rat colon by docosahexanoic [sic] acid. *Cancer Res.* 53:2786–2789 (1993).

171. Appel, M.J., A. van Garderen-Hoetmer, and R.A. Woutersen. Effects of dietary linoleic acid on pancreatic carcinogenesis in rats and hamsters. *Cancer Res.* 54:2113–2120 (1994).

172. Falconer, J.S., J.A. Ross, K.C.H. Fearon, et al. Effect of eicosapentaenoic acid and other fatty acids on the growth *in vitro* of human pancreatic cancer cell lines. *Br. J. Cancer* 69:826–832 (1994).

173. Lee, D.-Y.K., R.S. Chapkin, and J.R. Lupton. Dietary fat and fiber modulate colonic cell proliferation in an interactive site-specific manner. *Nutr. Cancer* 20:107–118 (1993).

174. Thorup, I., O. Meyer, and E. Kristiansen. Influence of a dietary fiber on development of dimethylhydrazine-induced aberrant crypt foci and colon tumor incidence in Wistar rats. *Nutr. Cancer* 21:177–182 (1994).

175. Alabaster, O., Z.C. Tang, A. Frost, and N. Shivapurkar. Potential synergism between wheat bran and psyllium: enhanced inhibition of colon cancer. *Cancer Lett.* 75:53–58 (1993).

176. Zakhary, N.I., A.A. El-Aaser, A.A. Abdelwahab, et al. Effect of *Vicia faba* and bran feeding on nitrosamine carcinogenesis and formation. *Nutr. Cancer* 21:59–69 (1994).

177. Ferguson, L.R., A.M. Roberton, M.E. Watson, et al. The adsorption of a range of dietary carcinogens by α-cellulose, a model insoluble dietary fiber. *Mutat. Res.* 319:257–266 (1993).

178. Maruyama, H., and I. Yamamoto. *In vitro* binding of the carcinogen N-[methyl-$^{14}$C]-nitrosodimethylamine by algal dietary fibers and their role in reducing its bioaccumulation. *J. Appl. Phycol.* 5:201–205 (1993).

179. O'Neill, I., O. Ridgway, A. Ellul, and S. Bingham. Gastrointestinal monitoring of DNA-damaging agents with magnetic microcapsules. *Mutat. Res.* 290:127–138 (1993).

180. Camire, M.E., J. Zhao, and D.A. Violette. *In vitro* binding of bile acids by extruded potato peels. *J. Agric. Food Chem.* 41:2391–2394 (1993).

181. Lupton, J.R., and P.P. Kurtz. Relationship of colonic luminal short-chain fatty acids and pH to in vivo cell proliferation in rats. *J. Nutr.* 123:1522–1530 (1993).

182. Hague, A., A.M. Manning, K.A. Hanlon, et al. Sodium butyrate induces apoptosis in human colonic tumour cell lines in a p53-independent pathway: implications for the possible role of dietary fibre in the prevention of large-bowel cancer. *Int. J. Cancer* 55:498–505 (1993).

183. Berggren, A.M., I.M.E. Björck, E.M.G.L. Nyman, and B.O. Eggum. Short-chain fatty acid content and pH in caecum of rats given various sources of carbohydrates. *J. Sci. Food Agric.* 63:397–406 (1993).

184. Diplock, A.T., C.A. Rice-Evans, and R.H. Burdon. Is there a significant role for lipid peroxidation in the causation of malignancy and for antioxidants in cancer prevention? *Cancer Res.* 54(Suppl.):1952s–1956s (1994).

185. Ramanathan, R., N.P. Das, and C.H. Tan. Effects of γ-linolenic acid, flavonoids, and vitamins on cytotoxicity and lipid peroxidation. *Free Rad. Biol. Med.* 16:43–48 (1994).

186. Majewski, S., A. Szmurlo, M. Marczak, et al. Inhibition of tumor cell–induced angiogenesis by retinoids, 1,25-dihydroxyvitamin $D_3$ and their combination. *Cancer Lett.* 75:35–39 (1993).

187. Gaetano, C., A. Melchiori, A. Albini, et al. Retinoic acid negatively regulates β4 integrin expression and suppresses the malignant phenotype in a Lewis lung carcinoma cell line. *Clin. Exp. Metastasis* 12:63–72 (1994).

188. Chen, L.-C., S. Kirchoff, and L.M. De Luca. Effect of excess dietary retinoic acid on skin papilloma and carcinoma formation induced by a complete carcinogenesis protocol in female Sencar mice. *Cancer Lett.* 78:63–67 (1994).

189. Jones, C.S., L. Sly, L.-C. Chen, et al. Retinol and β-carotene concentrations in skin, papillomas and carcinomas, liver, and serum of mice fed retinoic acid or β-carotene to suppress skin tumor formation. *Nutr. Cancer* 21:83–93 (1994).

190. Kahl-Rainer, P., and B. Marian. Retinoids inhibit protein kinase C–dependent transduction of 1,2-diglyceride signals in human colonic tumor cells. *Nutr. Cancer* 21:157–168 (1994).

191. Lambert, L.A., W.G. Wamer, R.R. Wei, et al. The protective but nonsynergistic effect of dietary β-carotene and vitamin E on skin tumorigenesis in Skh mice. *Nutr. Cancer* 21:1–12 (1994).

192. Edes, T.E., and D.S. Gysbers. Carcinogen-induced tissue vitamin A depletion. Potential protective advantages of β-carotene. *Ann. N.Y. Acad. Sci.* 686:203–211 (1993).

193. Bianchi, L., F. Tateo, R. Pizzala, et al. Carotenoids reduce the chromosomal damage induced by bleomycin in human cultured lymphocytes. *Anticancer Res.* 13:1007–1010 (1993).

194. Salvadori, D.M.F., L.R. Ribeiro, and A.T. Natarajan. Effect of β-carotene on clastogenic effects of mitomycin C, methyl methanesulphonate and bleomycin in Chinese hamster ovary cells. *Mutagenesis* 9:53–57 (1994).

195. Salvadori, D.M.F., L.R. Ribeiro, and A.T. Natarajan. The anticlastogenicity of β-carotene evaluated on human hepatoma cells. *Mutat. Res.* 303:151–156 (1993).

196. Wolterbeek, A.P.M., A.A.J.J.L. Rutten, and V.J. Feron. High survival rate of hamsters given intratracheal installations of benzo[a]pyrene and ferric oxide and kept on a high β-carotene diet. *Carcinogenesis* 15:133–136 (1994).

197. Shklar, G., J. Schwartz, D. Trickler, and S.R. Cheverie. The effectiveness of a mixture of β-carotene, α-tocopherol, glutathione, and ascorbic acid for cancer prevention. *Nutr. Cancer* 20:145–151 (1993).

198. Cassand, P., S. Decoudu, F. Lévêque, et al. Effect of vitamin E dietary intake on in vitro activation of aflatoxin B1. *Mutat. Res.* 319:309–316 (1993).

199. Rahmat, A., W.Z.W. Ngah, N.A. Shamaan, et al. Long-term administration of tocotrienols and tumor-marker enzyme activities during hepatocarcinogenesis in rats. *Nutrition* 9:229–232 (1993).

200. Goh, S.H., N.F. Hew, A.W. Norhanom, and M. Yadav. Inhibition of tumour promotion by various palm-oil tocotrienols. *Int. J. Cancer* 57:529–531 (1994).

201. Saez, S., N. Falette, C. Guillot, et al. 1,25(OH)₂D₃ modulation of mammary tumor cell growth in vitro and in vivo. *Breast Cancer Res. Treat.* 27:69–81 (1993).

202. Leung, P.Y., K. Miyashita, M. Young, and C.S. Tsao. Cytotoxic effect of ascorbate and its derivatives on cultured malignant and nonmalignant cell lines. *Anticancer Res.* 13:475–480 (1993).

203. Weisburger, J.H, A. Rivenson, G.C. Hard, et al. Role of fat and calcium in cancer causation by food mutagens, heterocyclic amines. *Proc. Soc. Exp. Biol. Med.* 205:347–352 (1994).

204. Lupton, J.R., X.-Q. Chen, W. Frølich, et al. Rats fed high fat diets with increased calcium levels have fecal bile acid concentrations similar to those of rats fed a low fat diet. *J. Nutr.* 124:188–195 (1994).

205. Govers, M.J.A.P., D.S.M.L. Termont, and R. Van der Meer. Mechanism of the antiproliferative effect of milk mineral and other calcium supplements on colonic epithelium. *Cancer Res.* 54:95–100 (1994).

206. Ip, C., and D.J. Lisk. Characterization of tissue selenium profiles and anticarcinogenic responses in rats fed natural sources of selenium-rich products. *Carcinogenesis* 15:573–576 (1994).

207. Seaborn, C.D., and S.P. Yang. Effect of molybdenum supplementation on *N*-nitroso-*N*-methylurea-induced mammary carcinogenesis and molybdenum excretion in rats. *Biol. Trace Elem. Res.* 39:245–256 (1993).

208. Kato, I., K. Endo, and T. Yokokura. Effects of oral administration of *Lactobacillus casei* on antitumor responses induced by tumor resection in mice. *Int. J. Immunopharmacol.* 16:24–36 (1994).

209. Reddy, B.S., and A. Rivenson. Inhibitory effect of *Bifidobacterium longum* on colon, mammary, and liver carcinogenesis induced by 2-amino-3-methylimidazo[4,5-*f*]quinoline, a food mutagen. *Cancer Res.* 53:3914–3918 (1993).

210. Zhang, X.B., and Y. Ohta. Microorganisms in the gastrointestinal tract of the rat prevent absorption of the mutagen–carcinogen 3-amino-1,4-dimethyl-5*H*-pyrido(4,3-*b*)-indole. *Can. J. Microbiol.* 39:841–845 (1993).

211. Thyagaraja, N., and A. Hosono. Antimutagenicity of lactic acid bacteria from "Idly" against food-related mutagens. *J. Food Protect.* 56:1061–1066 (1993).

212. Ferguson, L.R. Antimutagens as cancer chemopreventive agents in the diet. *Mutat. Res.* 307:395–410 (1994).

213. Stavric, B. Antimutagens and anticarcinogens in foods. *Food Chem. Toxicol.* 32:79–90 (1994).

214. Wattenberg, L.W. Inhibition of carcinogenesis by nonnutrient constituents of the diet. In *Food and Cancer Prevention: Chemical and Biological Aspects.* K.W. Waldron et al. (eds.). Cambridge, Royal Society of Chemistry. Pp. 12–23 (1993).

215. Huang, M.-T, T. Osawa, C.-T. Ho, and R.T. Rosen (eds.). *Food Phytochemicals for Cancer Prevention I. Fruits and Vegetables.* ACS Symp. Ser. 546 (1994).

216. Ho, C.-T., T. Osawa, M.-T. Huang, and R.T. Rosen (eds.). *Food Phytochemicals for Cancer Prevention II. Teas, Spices, and Herbs.* ACS Symp. Ser. 547 (1994).

217. Shanmugasundaram, K.R., S. Ramanujam, and E.R.B. Shanmugasundaram. Amrita Bindu—a salt–spice–herbal health food supplement for the prevention of nitrosamine induced depletion of antioxidants. *J. Ethnopharmacol.* 42:83–93 (1994).

218. Knizhnikov, V.A., V.A. Komleva, N.K. Shandala, et al. Influence of *Laminaria japonica* added to the diet on remote effects of radiation injuries. *J. Appl. Phycol.* 5:191–194 (1993).

219. Okai, Y., K. Higashi-Okai, and S.-i. Nakamura. Identification of heterogenous antimutagenic activities in the extract of edible brown seaweeds, *Laminaria japonica* (Makonbu) and *Undaria pinnatifida* (Wakame) by the *umu* gene expression system in *Salmonella typhimurium* (TA1535/pSK1002). *Mutat. Res.* 303:63–70 (1993).

220. Gerster, H. Anticarcinogenic effect of common carotenoids. *Int. J. Vit. Nutr. Res.* 63:93–121 (1993).

221. Tanaka, T., Y. Morishita, M. Suzui, et al. Chemoprevention of mouse urinary bladder carcinogenesis by the naturally occurring carotenoid astaxanthin. *Carcinogenesis* 15:15–19 (1994).

222. Sporn, M.B., A.B. Roberts, and D.S. Goodman (eds.). *The Retinoids. Biology, Chemistry, and Medicine. 2nd Ed.* New York, Raven Press. (1994).

223. Hong, W.K., and L.M. Itri. Retinoids and human cancer. In *The Retinoids. Biology, Chemistry, and Medicine. 2nd Ed.* M.B. Sporn et al. (eds.). New York, Raven Press. Pp. 597–630 (1994).

224. Moon, R.C., R.G. Mehta, and K.V.N. Rao. Retinoids and cancer in experimental animals. In *The Retinoids. Biology, Chemistry, and Medicine. 2nd Ed.* M.B. Sporn et al. (eds.). New York, Raven Press. Pp. 573–595 (1994).

225. Ohta, T. Modification of genotoxicity by naturally occurring flavorings and their derivatives. *Crit. Rev. Toxicol.* 23:127–146 (1993).

226. Murakami, A., A. Kondo, Y. Nakamura, et al. Possible anti-tumor promoting properties of edible plants from Thailand, and identification of an active constituent, cardamonin, of *Boesenbergia pandurata. Biosci. Biotechnol. Biochem.* 57:1971–1973 (1993).

227. Kubo, I., M. Ochi, P.C. Vieira, and S. Komatsu. Antitumor agents from the cashew (*Anacardium occidentale*) apple. *J. Agric. Food Chem.* 41:1012–1015 (1993).

228. Lahiri, M., G.B. Maru, and S.V. Bhide. Effect of plant phenols, β-carotene and α-tocopherol on benzo[*a*]pyrene-induced DNA damage in the mouse forestomach mucosa (target organ) and bone marrow polychromatic erythrocytes (non-target organ). *Mutat. Res.* 303:97–100 (1993).

229. Lahiri, M., and S.V. Bhide. Effect of four plant phenols, β-carotene and α-tocopherol on 3(H)benzopyrene–DNA interaction in vitro in the presence of rat and mouse liver postmitochondrial fraction. *Cancer Lett.* 73:35–39 (1993).

230. Rompelberg, C.J.M., H. Verhagen, and P.J. van Bladeren. Effects of the naturally occurring alkenylbenzenes eugenol and *trans*-anethole on drug-metabolizing enzymes in the rat liver. *Food Chem. Toxicol.* 31:637–645 (1993).

231. Rao, C.V., B. Simi, and B.S. Reddy. Inhibition by dietary curcumin of azoxymethane-induced ornithine decarboxylase, tyrosine protein kinase, arachidonic acid metabolism and aberrant crypt foci formation in the rat colon. *Carcinogenesis* 14:2219–2225 (1993).

232. Abraham, S.K., L. Asram, and P.C. Kesavan. Protective effects of chlorogenic acid, curcumin and β-carotene against γ-radiation-induced in vivo chromosomal damage. *Mutat. Res.* 303:109–112 (1993).

233. Kitts, D.D., and A.N. Wijewickreme. Effect of dietary caffeic and chlorogenic acids on in vivo xenobiotic enzyme systems. *Plant Foods Human Nutr.* 45:287–298 (1994).

234. Tanaka, T., T. Kojima, T. Kawamori, et al. Inhibition of 4-nitroquinoline-1-oxide-induced rat tongue carcinogenesis by the naturally occurring plant phenolics caffeic, ellagic, chlorogenic and ferulic acids. *Carcinogenesis* 14:1321–1325 (1993).

235. Rao, C.V., D. Desai, B. Simi, et al. Inhibitory effect of caffeic acid esters on azoxymethane-induced biochemical changes and aberrant crypt foci formation in rat colon. *Cancer Res.* 53:4182–4188 (1993).

236. Castonguay, A. Pulmonary carcinogenesis and its prevention by dietary polyphenolic compounds. *Ann. N.Y. Acad. Sci.* 686:177–185 (1993).

237. Zhang, Z., S.M. Hamilton, C. Stewart, et al. Inhibition of liver microsomal cytochrome P450 activity and metabolism of the tobacco-specific nitrosamine NNK by capsaicin and ellagic acid. *Anticancer Res.* 13:2341–2346 (1993).

238. Tanaka, T., T. Kawamori, M. Ohnishi, et al. Chemoprevention of 4-nitroquinoline 1-oxide-induced oral carcinogenesis by dietary protocatechuic acid during initiation and postinitiation phases. *Cancer Res.* 54:2359–2365 (1994).

239. Tanaka, T., T. Kojima, M. Suzui, and H. Mori. Chemoprevention of colon carcinogenesis by the natural product of a simple phenolic compound protocatechuic acid: suppressing effects on tumor development and biomarkers expression of colon tumorigenesis. *Cancer Res.* 53:3908–3913 (1993).

240. Hertog, M.G.L., P.C.H. Hollman, M.B. Katan, and D. Kromhout. Intake of potentially anticarcinogenic flavonoids and their determinants in adults in the Netherlands. *Nutr. Cancer* 20:21–29 (1993).

241. Coward, L., N.C. Barnes, K.D.R. Setchell, and S. Barnes. Genistein, daidzein, and their β-glycoside conjugates: antitumor isoflavones in soybean foods from American and Asian diets. *J. Agric. Food Chem.* 41:1961–1967 (1993).

242. Mousavi, Y., and H. Adlercreutz. Genistein is an effective stimulator of sex hormone–binding globulin production in hepatocarcinoma human liver cancer cells and suppresses proliferation of these cells in culture. *Steroids* 58:301–304 (1993).

243. Yanagihara, K., A. Ito, T. Toge, and M. Numoto. Antiproliferative effects of isoflavones on human cancer cell lines established from the gastrointestinal tract. *Cancer Res.* 53:5815–5821 (1993).

244. Adlercreutz, H., C. Bannwart, K. Wähälä, et al. Inhibition of human aromatase by mammalian lignans and isoflavonoid phytoestrogens. *J. Steroid Biochem. Molec. Biol.* 44:147–153 (1993).

245. Edenharder, R., I. von Petersdorff, and R. Rauscher. Antimutagenic effects of flavonoids, chalcones and structurally related compounds on the activity of 2-amino-3-methylimidazo[4,5-*f*]quinoline (IQ) and other heterocyclic amine mutagens from cooked food. *Mutat. Res.* 287:261–274 (1993).

246. Lee, H., W.-W. Wang, H.-Y. Su, and H.J. Hao. The structure–activity relationships of flavonoids as inhibitors of cytochrome P-450 enzymes in rat liver microsomes and the mutagenicity of 2-amino-3-methyl-imidazo[4,5-*f*]quinoline. *Mutagenesis* 9:101–106 (1994).

247. Sathyamoorthy, N., T.T.Y. Wang, and J.M. Phang. Stimulation of pS2 expression by diet-derived compounds. *Cancer Res.* 54:957–961 (1994).

248. Wall, M.E., M.C. Wani, F. Fullas, et al. Plant antitumor agents. 31. The calycopterones, a new class of biflavonoids with novel cytotoxicity in a diverse panel of human tumor cell lines. *J. Med. Chem.* 37:1465–1470 (1994).

249. Deschner, E.E., J.F. Ruperto, G.Y. Wong, and H.L. Newmark. The effect of dietary quercetin and rutin on AOM-induced acute colonic epithelial abnormalities in mice fed a high-fat diet. *Nutr. Cancer* 20:199–204 (1993).

250. Abdullaev, F.I. Biological effects of saffron. *BioFactors* 4:83–86 (1993).

251. Elson, C.E., and S.G. Yu. The chemoprevention of cancer by mevalonate-derived constituents of fruits and vegetables. *J. Nutr.* 124:607–614 (1994).

252. Konoshima, T., M. Takasaki, T. Tatsumoto, et al. Inhibitory effects of cucurbitane triterpenoids on Epstein–Barr virus activation and two-stage carcinogenesis of skin tumors. *Biol. Pharm. Bull.* 17:668–671 (1994).

253. Zani, F., M.T. Cuzzoni, M. Daglia, et al. Inhibition of mutagenicity in *Salmonella typhimurium* by *Glycyrrhiza glabra* extract, glycyrrhizinic acid, 18α- and 18β-glycyrrhetinic acids. *Planta Med.* 59:502–507 (1993).

254. Wu, K., W. Zhang, P.B. Addis, et al. Antioxidant properties of wild rice. *J. Agric. Food Chem.* 42:34–37 (1994).

255. Vucenik, I., K. Sakamoto, M. Bansal, and A.M. Shamsuddin. Inhibition of rat mammary carcinogenesis by inositol hexaphosphate (phytic acid). A pilot study. *Cancer Lett.* 75:95–102 (1993).

256. Pretlow, T.P., M.A. O'Riordan, G.A. Somich, et al. Aberrant crypts correlate with tumor incidence in F344 rats treated with azoxymethane and phytate. *Carcinogenesis* 13:1509–1512 (1992).

257. Morales-Ramírez, P., and M.C. García-Rodríguez. In vivo effect of chlorophyllin on γ-ray-induced sister chromatid exchange in murine bone marrow cells. *Mutat. Res.* 320:329–334 (1994).

258. Wu, Z.L., J.K. Chen, T. Ong, et al. Antitransforming activity of chlorophyllin against selected carcinogens and complex mixtures. *Teratogen. Carcinogen. Mutagen.* 14:75–81 (1994).

259. Guo, D., and R. Dashwood. Inhibition of 2-amino-3-methylimidazo[4,5-*f*]quinoline (IQ)–DNA binding in rats given

chlorophyllin: dose–response and time-course studies in the liver and colon. *Carcinogenesis* 15:763–766 (1994).

260.   Hayatsu, H., T. Negishi, S. Arimoto, and T. Hayatsu. Porphyrins as potential inhibitors against exposure to carcinogens and mutagens. *Mutat. Res.* 290:79–85 (1993).

261.   Beecher, C.W.W. Cancer preventive properties of varieties of *Brassica oleracea*: a review. *Am. J. Clin. Nutr.* 59(Suppl.):1166S–1170S (1994).

262.   Nijhoff, W.A., G.M. Groen, and W.H.M. Peters. Induction of rat hepatic and intestinal glutathione *S*-transferases and glutathione by dietary naturally occurring anticarcinogens. *Int. J. Oncol.* 3:1131–1139 (1993).

263.   Rojanapo, W., and A. Tepsuwan. Antimutagenic and mutagenic potentials of Chinese radish. *Environ. Health Perspect.* 101(Suppl. 3):247–252 (1993).

264.   Musk, S.R.R., and I.T. Johnson. Allyl isothiocyanate is selectively toxic to transformed cells of the human colorectal tumour line HT29. *Carcinogenesis* 14:2079–2083 (1993).

265.   Tiwari, R.K., L. Guo, H.L. Bradlow, et al. Selective responsiveness of human breast cancer cells to indole-3-carbinol, a chemopreventive agent. *J. Natl. Cancer Inst.* 86:126–131 (1994).

266.   Newfield, L., A. Goldsmith, H.L. Bradlow, and K. Auborn. Estrogen metabolism and human papillomavirus-induced tumors of the larynx: chemo-prophylaxis with indole-3-carbinol. *Anticancer Res.* 13:337–342 (1993).

267.   Kojima, T., T. Tanaka, and H. Mori. Chemoprevention of spontaneous endometrial cancer in female Donryu rats by dietary indole-3-carbinol. *Cancer Res.* 54:1446–1449 (1994).

268.   Stresser, D.M., G.S. Bailey, and D.E. Williams. Indole-3-carbinol and β-naphthoflavone induction of aflatoxin $B_1$ metabolism and cytochromes P450 associated with bioactivation and detoxication of aflatoxin $B_1$ in the rat. *Drug Metab. Dispos.* 22:383–391 (1994).

269.   Stresser, D.M., D.E. Williams, L.I. McLellan, et al. Indole-3-carbinol induces a rat liver glutathione transferase subunit (Yc2) with high activity toward aflatoxin $B_1$ *exo*-epoxide. Association with reduced levels of hepatic aflatoxin–DNA adducts *in vivo*. *Drug Metab. Dispos.* 22:392–399 (1994).

270.   Reddy, B.S., C.V. Rao, A. Rivenson, and G. Kelloff. Chemoprevention of colon carcinogenesis by organosulfur compounds. *Cancer Res.* 53:3493–3498 (1993).

271.   Sundaram, S.G., and J.A. Milner. Impact of organosulfur compounds in garlic on canine mammary tumor cells in culture. *Cancer Lett.* 74:85–90 (1993).

272.   Amagase, H., and J.A. Milner. Impact of various sources of garlic and their constituents on 7,12-dimethylbenz[*a*]anthracene binding to mammary cell DNA. *Carcinogenesis* 14:1627–1631 (1993).

273.   Lin, X.-Y., J.-Z. Liu, and J.A. Milner. Dietary garlic suppresses DNA adducts caused by *N*-nitroso compounds. *Carcinogenesis* 15:349–352 (1994).

274.   Reeve, V.E., M. Bosnic, E. Rozinova, and C. Boehm-Wilcox. A garlic extract protects from ultraviolet B (280–320

nm) radiation–induced suppression of contact hypersensitivity. *Photochem. Photobiol.* 58:813–817 (1993).

275.   Yang, C.S., and Z.-Y. Wang. Tea and cancer. *J. Natl. Cancer Inst.* 85:1038–1049 (1993).

276.   Mukhtar, H., S.K. Katiyar, and R. Agarwal. Green tea and skin—anticarcinogenic effects. *J. Invest. Dermatol.* 102:3–7 (1994).

277.   Agarwal, R., S.K. Katiyar, S.G. Khan, and H. Mukhtar. Protection against ultraviolet B radiation–induced effects in the skin of SKH-1 hairless mice by a polyphenolic fraction isolated from green tea. *Photochem. Photobiol.* 58:695–700 (1993).

278.   Katiyar, S.K., R. Agarwal, and H. Mukhtar. Inhibition of spontaneous and photo-enhanced lipid peroxidation in mouse epidermal microsomes by epicatechin derivatives from green tea. *Cancer Lett.* 79:61–66 (1994).

279.   Narisawa, T., and Y. Fukaura. A very low dose of green tea polyphenols in drinking water prevents *N*-methyl-*N*-nitrosourea-induced colon carcinogenesis in F344 rats. *Jpn. J. Cancer Res.* 84:1007–1009 (1993).

280.   Katiyar, S.K., R. Agarwal, and H. Mukhtar. Protective effects of green tea polyphenols administered by oral intubation against chemical carcinogen-induced forestomach and pulmonary neoplasia in A/J mice. *Cancer Lett.* 73:167–172 (1993).

281.   Hirose, M., T. Hoshiya, K. Akagi, et al. Effects of green tea catechins in a rat multi-organ carcinogenesis model. *Carcinogenesis* 14:1549–1553 (1993).

282.   Fujie, K., T. Aoki, Y. Ito, and S. Maeda. Sister-chromatid exchanges induced by trihalomethanes in rat erythroblastic cells and their suppression by crude catechin extracted from green tea. *Mutat. Res.* 300:241–246 (1993).

283.   Pingzhang, Y., Z. Jinying, C. Shujun, et al. Experimental studies of the inhibitory effects of green tea catechin on mice large intestinal cancers induced by 1,2-dimethylhydrazine. *Cancer Lett.* 79:33–38 (1994).

284.   Nishida, H., M. Omori, Y. Fukutomi, et al. Inhibitory effects of (−)-epigallocatechin gallate on spontaneous hepatoma in C3H/HeNCrj mice and human hepatoma-derived PLC/PRF/5 cells. *Jpn. J. Cancer Res.* 85:221–225 (1994).

285.   Gao, Y.T., J.K. McLaughlin, W.J. Blot, et al. Reduced risk of esophageal cancer associated with green tea consumption. *J. Natl. Cancer Inst.* 86:855–858 (1994).

286.   Yen, G.-C., and H.-Y. Chen. Comparison of antimutagenic effect of various tea extracts (green, oolong, pouchong, and black tea). *J. Food Protect.* 57:54–58 (1994).

287.   Shiraki, M., Y. Hara, T. Osawa, et al. Antioxidative and antimutagenic effects of theaflavins from black tea. *Mutat. Res.* 323:29–34 (1994).

288.   Sohn, O.S., A. Surace, E.S. Fiala, et al. Effects of green and black tea on hepatic xenobiotic metabolizing systems in the male F344 rat. *Xenobiotica* 24:119–127 (1994).

289.   Komatsu, K., K. Kator, Y. Mitsuda, et al. Inhibitory effects of Rooibos tea, *Aspalathus linealis,* on X-ray-induced C3H10T1/2 cell transformation. *Cancer Lett.* 77:33–38 (1994).

290. Kennedy, A.R. Prevention of carcinogenesis by protease inhibitors. *Cancer Res.* 54(Suppl.):1999s–2005s (1994).

291. Troll, W., and A.R. Kennedy (eds.). *Protease Inhibitors as Cancer Chemopreventive Agents.* New York, Plenum Press (1993).

292. Waldron, K.W., and R.R. Selvendran. Bioactive cell wall and related components from herbal products and edible plant organs as protective factors. In *Food and Cancer Prevention: Chemical and Biological Aspects.* K.W. Waldron et al. (eds.). Cambridge, England, Royal Society of Chemistry. Pp. 307–326 (1993).

293. Wang, G., J. Zhang, T. Mizuno, et al. Antitumor active polysaccharides from the Chinese mushroom *Songshan lingzhi*, the fruiting body of *Ganoderma tsugae. Biosci. Biotechnol. Biochem.* 57:894–900 (1993).

294. Zhuang, C., T. Mizuno, H. Ito, et al. Fractionation and antitumor activity of polysaccharides from *Grifola frondosa* mycelium. *Biosci. Biotechnol. Biochem.* 58:185–188 (1994).

295. Zhuang, C., T. Mizuno, A. Shimada, et al. Antitumor protein-containing polysaccharides from a Chinese mushroom *Fengweigu* or *Houbitake, Pleurotus sajor-caju* (Fr.) Sings. *Biosci. Biotechnol. Biochem.* 57:901–906 (1993).

296. Ellouali, M., C. Boisson-Vidal, P. Durand, and J. Jozefonvicz. Antitumor activity of low molecular weight fucans extracted from brown seaweed *Ascophyllum nodosum. Anticancer Res.* 13:2011–2020 (1993).

297. Itoh, H., H. Noda, H. Amano, et al. Antitumor activity and immunological properties of marine algal polysaccharides, especially fucoidan, prepared from *Sargassum thunbergii* of Phaeophyceae. *Anticancer Res.* 13:2045–2052 (1993).

298. Xiang, D.-B., and X.-Y. Li. Antitumor activity and immuno-potentiating actions of *Achyranthes bidentata* polysaccharides. *Acta Pharmacol. Sinica* 14:556–561 (1993).

299. Chin, S.F., J.M. Storkson, and M.W. Pariza. Conjugated dienoic derivatives of linoleic acid. A new class of food-derived anticarcinogens. In *Food Flavor and Safety. Molecular Analysis and Design.* A.M. Spanier et al. (eds.). Washington,

DC, American Chemical Society. *ACS Symp. Ser.* 528:262–271 (1993).

300. Pariza, M.W. CLA and HEMF: newly recognized anticarcinogenic antioxidants. In *Active Oxygens, Lipid Peroxides, and Antioxidants.* K. Yagi (ed.). Boca Raton, FL, CRC Press. Pp. 359–365 (1993).

301. Ip, C., D.J. Lisk, and J.A. Scimeca. Potential of food modification in cancer prevention. *Cancer Res.* 54(Suppl.): 1957s–1959s (1994).

302. Ip, C., M. Singh, H.J. Thompson, and J.A. Scimeca. Conjugated linoleic acid suppresses mammary carcinogenesis and proliferative activity of the mammary gland in the rat. *Cancer Res.* 54:1212–1215 (1994).

303. Chin, S.F., J.M. Storkson, W. Liu, et al. Conjugated linoleic acid (9,11- and 10,12-octadecadienoic acid) is produced in conventional but not germ-free rats fed linoleic acid. *J. Nutr.* 124:694–701 (1994).

304. Dillehay, D.L., S.K. Webb, E.-M. Schmelz, and A.H. Merrill, Jr. Dietary sphingomyelin inhibits 1,2-dimethyl-hydrazine-induced colon cancer in CF1 mice. *J. Nutr.* 124:615–620 (1994).

305. Yen, G.-C., and P.-P. Hsieh. Possible mechanisms of antimutagenic effect of Maillard reaction products prepared from xylose and lysine. *J. Agric. Food Chem.* 42:133–137 (1994).

306. van Boekel, M.A.J.S., C.N.J.M. Weerens, A. Holstra, et al. Antimutagenic effects of casein and its digestion products. *Food Chem. Toxicol.* 31:731–737 (1993).

307. Okai, Y., T. Eksttikul, O. Svendsby, et al. Antitumor activity in an extract of Thai rice seedlings. *J. Ferment. Bioeng.* 76:367–370 (1993).

308. Kawamura, Y., and M. Ishikawa. Anti-tumorigenic and immunoactive protein and peptide factors in foodstuffs (I)—anti-tumorigenic protein from *Tricholoma matsutake*. In *Food and Cancer Prevention: Chemical and Biological Aspects.* K.W. Waldron et al. (eds.). Cambridge, England, Royal Society of Chemistry. Pp. 327–330 (1993).

# 3

# Diet and Cardiovascular Disease

The American Heart Association (AHA) monitors data on the relationship between diet and cardiovascular disease (CVD) and regularly updates its recommendations based on the best available scientific evidence. A report of the Nutrition Committee of the AHA summarized the history of AHA diet statements since 1957, when a group chaired by Irvine Page concluded that diet, particularly its fat and caloric content and possibly the type of fat, is important in the pathogenesis of atherosclerosis (1). The report gave the rationale for the current AHA position on diet, providing background on cholesterol transport via lipoproteins and summarizing epidemiologic observations, intervention trials, genetic studies, and other information linking diet, plasma lipids and lipoproteins, and atherosclerosis and coronary heart disease (CHD). Relationships between diet, blood pressure, and CHD were discussed, emphasizing salt intake and obesity. After considering some objections to the AHA diet, from possible hazards to charges that it does not go far enough, the report asserted the nutritional adequacy, practicality, and potential benefit of the AHA diet for all persons older than 2 years.

## GENERAL EPIDEMIOLOGY AND DIETARY STUDIES

### Serum Cholesterol as a Risk Factor for Cardiocerebrovascular Disease

Evidence from five sources links elevated serum cholesterol to CHD: epidemiology, animal data, clinical studies of genetic conditions influencing serum cholesterol, pathologic investigation, and new understanding of biologic mechanisms. Rossouw reviewed angiographic studies and cholesterol-lowering trials for primary and secondary prevention, employing both narrative review and metaanalysis (2). The most direct and convincing evidence that lowering cholesterol reduces risk of CHD comes from clinical trials. Analysis of the combined trials showed that the clinical event rate can be lowered by ~20% if cholesterol levels are lowered by 10%. This applies to both primary and secondary prevention. In support of this, angiographic studies show that vigorous lipid-lowering therapy improves the angiographic appearance of coronary vessels and these improvements are accompanied by large reductions in CHD risk. Diet, drug, and combined therapy are all effective. Rossouw concluded that top priority should be given to intensive diet and combination drug therapy for patients with existing CHD because of their high risk of reinfarction

and the demonstrated success of treatment. However, treatment of high-risk but apparently healthy individuals should not be neglected. Calvert looked at the data on plasma cholesterol and CHD in terms of Hill's criteria for establishing causality (3). He concluded that the relationship between cholesterol level and CHD is causal based on the strength, graded nature, temporal sequence, consistency, and independence of the association, its predictive capacity, and the coherence of epidemiologic, laboratory, and clinical data and theory.

Law et al. analyzed data from 10 cohort studies, 3 international studies, and 28 randomized controlled trials to estimate how much and how quickly reduction in serum cholesterol concentration reduces the risk of ischemic heart disease (IHD) (4). For men, the cohort studies showed that a reduction of 23 mg/dL in cholesterol (~10%) was associated with a decreased incidence of IHD of 54% at age 40 y, 39% at age 50, 27% at age 60, 20% at age 70, and 19% at age 80. From the international studies for ages 55–64 y, the combined estimate for risk reduction with a similar decrease in cholesterol was 38%. In the intervention trials, a 10% decrease in cholesterol reduced risk by 7% in the first 2 y, 22% between 2 and 5 y, and 25% after 5 y. Data for women were limited, but indicated similar effects. Law et al. also analyzed data from the British United Provident Association (BUPA) cohort study, to evaluate the effect of statistical bias on estimates of the association between serum LDL cholesterol and mortality from IHD (5). After correction for regression dilution bias, which affects all regression analyses when the independent variable is subject to random variation over time due to errors in measurement and within-subject variation, the difference in IHD mortality associated with a difference of 23 mg/dL in total cholesterol increased from 17% to 24%. After further correction for the surrogate dilution effect (differences in total cholesterol reflect smaller differences in LDL cholesterol), a difference of 23 mg/dL in LDL cholesterol was associated with a 27% reduction in risk of IHD mortality. The association was greater at younger ages. No excess mortality from any cause was associated with low cholesterol concentration.

Readers of the papers by Law et al. (4,5) raised a number of critical points. One argument was that differences in cholesterol concentrations may explain international variation in IHD mortality but do not explain the variation within a population (e.g., middle-aged men employed in London) (6). These readers also pointed out that although a 27% decrease in IHD mortality seems high, this represents a 2.5–5.0 month increase in life expectancy. Moreover, most people do not prefer health at all costs and eat a hamburger and fries with full knowledge that raw veggies are more healthful. The readers suggested that health programs addressing smoking, hypertension, or reducing the range of socioeconomic differences might reach the same goals more efficiently. Other readers thought that the importance of excess deaths from hemorrhagic stroke in drug trials was treated too lightly (7) and that the excess noncoronary mortality in drug trials should not be dismissed (8,9). It was pointed out that cholesterol-reduction goals cannot be reached through the NCEP step 1 diet, the step 2 diet differs from step 1 only in altering the relative amounts of different fats and has not been tested adequately, and step 3 diets (which do work) are unpalatable and unfeasible (10). Handling of the dilution bias was questioned (11,12). Even if the reductions in IHD mortality claimed by Law et al. do occur, the importance of this was questioned. Readers asked how many would take a pill every day if told it would reduce their risk of fatal heart attack by 50%, and how many would take this pill to reduce their risk from 2/1000 to 1/1000 (a 50% reduction) (13). For the general population, absolute risk is more meaningful than relative risk. These readers suggest that the observed risk reduction may even be of trivial clinical importance. They do not challenge the cholesterol hypothesis, only the appropriateness of treating large numbers of asymptomatic patients without discussing the small magnitude of the potential benefit. Moreover, reduction of IHD death implies increases in other causes of death. A computer model showed that cancer would be the major beneficiary of reduced IHD mortality (14). The model further showed that a 10% population-wide reduction in cholesterol concentration, an achievable goal, would increase the median lifespan by only 1 year; reduction to the range of the lowest quintile (in Australia), not a practical goal, would add 3 years. Having generated a hypothesis with his computer model, the reader suggested that Law and his colleagues use their data to find changes in the causes of death and to show the effect of reduced cholesterol concentrations on lifespan. Muldoon and Manuck wrote that the papers by Law et al. contributed little to resolution of issues surrounding population-based dietary intervention to lower serum cholesterol concentrations (15). Whereas some risk is acceptable in treatment of patients known to have a serious illness, safety and efficacy must be clearly proven before preventive intervention in healthy people is considered. Muldoon and Manuck believe that neither the safety of long-term cholesterol reduction nor the efficacy of low-fat diets has been established. Law et al. responded briefly to some of these comments (16,17).

A follow-up study of men in the Russian Lipid Research Clinics is one of the few studies not to find a continuously increasing risk of CHD with increasing levels of cholesterol (18). Rather, a J-shaped function was observed for both total and LDL cholesterol. Men with the lowest cholesterol levels were characterized by lower LDL cholesterol and higher HDL cholesterol levels, greater alcohol consumption, leaner body mass, and less education than men with normal or high cholesterol levels. When data were analyzed by education level, the J-shaped function applied only to men with less than a high school education. When deaths were classified as rapid or nonrapid, the J-shaped function applied only to rapid deaths (<24 h). Thus there was a sizeable subset of *hypo*cholesterolemic men in this population who were at increased risk of cardiac death associated with lifestyle characteristics.

Atkins et al. conducted a metaanalysis of randomized controlled trials, to evaluate the effect of cholesterol reduction on men's risk for fatal and nonfatal stroke (19). Thirteen studies met their criteria for inclusion in the analysis. Heterogeneity among studies and overall effects of treatment were estimated by the Mantel–Haenszel–Peto method and the influence of various study designs and interventions was examined by using subgroup comparisons. For fatal stroke, the odds ratio (OR) associated with cholesterol-lowering interventions was ~1.3, although the 95% CI included 1; the OR for nonfatal stroke was ~0.9 and again, the 95% CI included 1. Treatment with clofibrate significantly increased the OR for fatal stroke. The authors concluded that reducing serum cholesterol through diet modification or drugs does not reduce stroke morbidity or mortality in middle-aged men and that clofibrate may increase risk of fatal stroke.

## Reviews and Epidemiologic Studies

Woodard and Limacher reviewed findings from cohort studies and clinical intervention trials evaluating the impact of diet on CHD (20). They mentioned important early studies, including pioneering work to develop animal models of atherosclerosis. Stein and Black reviewed the role of diet in the genesis and treatment of hypertension, with brief discussions of sodium, obesity, potassium, calcium, magnesium, fat, and alcohol (21). They recognized the heterogeneity of hypertension and acknowledged the difficulty of achieving good compliance with recommended dietary and lifestyle changes. Nevertheless, even though the benefit of diet modifications proposed for treating hypertension may be modest at best, many of the changes also have other well-established health benefits. The authors do not recommend widespread potassium supplementation.

Loss of endothelial cell integrity may occur early in the etiology of atherosclerosis. A review by Hennig and Alvarado discussed the properties and functions of endothelial cells (*22*). It then considered certain lipids that cause endothelial cell injury or dysfunction and nutrients that act as antioxidants or membrane stabilizers and thus may have antiatherogenic properties. Cells of the vascular endothelium are involved in platelet aggregation and adhesion, fibrinogenesis, coagulation, and regulation of vascular tone; nutrients interact with the endothelium in all of these processes. Roles of iron, copper, zinc, selenium, and magnesium were discussed.

There is strong evidence that transient events in early life can profoundly and permanently affect physiology and metabolism. Furthermore, recent differences in death rates from CVD in England and Wales parallel regional differences in neonatal mortality early in the 20th century. Therefore the UK Medical Research Council at Southampton has attempted to identify environmental effects in utero and during infancy that influence later risk of CHD and stroke. Barker reviewed evidence from animal, geographic, and follow-up studies (*23*). It is difficult not to conclude that CHD, stroke, non-insulin-dependent diabetes mellitus, hypertension, and abnormalities of serum lipids and hemostatic factors can be programmed during fetal life and are related to maternal nutrition. Thus research on nutritional and other influences that modulate growth of the fetus and permanently program its metabolism deserves high priority. It may provide the key to preventing CVD and other important disorders in adult life.

With reference to the Women's Health Initiative, Preuss discussed the lingering misperception that coronary artery disease (CAD) is primarily an affliction of men (*24*). One consequence of this idea is a lack of data for women, even though CAD is the leading cause of death among elderly American women. Gender does influence development of CVD, but many risk factors are the same for men and women and diet plays a major role. Although at the moment there is no justification for different approaches in treating men and women, investigators must be alert for possible differences in responses to lifestyle interventions.

Ortega et al. investigated the idea that dietary habits have cultural or genetic determinants that indirectly influence CVD risk (*25*). They assessed dietary and nutritional differences between noninstitutionalized elderly subjects who were classified according to the cause of death of their parents. Subjects with at least one parent who died of CVD had significantly higher diastolic blood pressure and less favorable nutrient intakes than subjects whose parents died of other causes. Specifically,

they had significantly greater intakes of total fat, animal fat, saturated fatty acids (SFAs), myristic acid, and palmitic acid. Their ratios of monounsaturated fatty acid (MUFA) to SFA intake were significantly lower. The authors suggested that the diets of the subjects may reflect the diets of their parents, and habits learned during childhood can predispose a person to follow a diet that favors development of CVD.

A dietary study of noninstitutionalized subjects 60–100 years old showed that dietary and plasma concentrations of vitamin A, body mass index, age, and sex are important determinants of plasma lipid profiles (*26*). The plasma lipoprotein profile becomes more favorable with age, perhaps because the oldest group represents "survivors"—a population at reduced risk of death from CHD.

Using WHO data on CHD death rates for men aged 55–65 y and UN-FAO dietary data, Artaud-Wild et al. showed that differences in intake of cholesterol and saturated fat can explain differences in CHD mortality in 38 countries but not in France and Finland (*27*). CHD mortality was anomalously high in Finland and anomalously low in France, whereas intakes of cholesterol and saturated fat were similar in the two countries. In all 40 countries, however, CHD mortality was positively associated with intake of milk and several components of milk. Consumption of milk, cream, cheese, and butter was higher in Finland than in France, whereas consumption of vegetables and vegetable oil was greater in France. This may help to explain the paradox. [The familiar version of the "French Paradox" cites the French consumption of red wine. This study, however, found no correlation between wine consumption and CHD mortality.]

Gartside and Glueck used data from NHANES II to assess the relationship between diet and hospital admission for CHD and CVD (*28*). After adjustment for confounding factors they found independent inverse relationships between hospitalization and intakes of linoleic acid and alcohol. Taking relative risk for hospitalization to be 1.0 for a linoleate intake of 0–5.9 g/d, it was 0.72 for 6.0–11.39 g/d and 0.49 for ≥11.6 g/d (*p* ≤.01). Dietary cholesterol was an independent positive predictor of serum total cholesterol. Intakes of vitamin C and alcohol were independent positive predictors of HDL cholesterol. Carbohydrate and oleic acid intakes were independent negative predictors.

A study was done to learn whether proposed dietary scores of atherogenicity and thrombogenicity predict IHD risk in a community sample of middle-aged men who participated in the Caerphilly study (*29*). Calculated scores were positively associated with LDL cholesterol and white cell count and negatively associated with antithrombin III. During a 5-y follow-up there were 21 new IHD events among 512 men who had no evidence of IHD at baseline. There was a consistent but nonsignificant tendency for men with higher atherogenicity or thrombogenicity scores at baseline to have higher risk of subsequent IHD. The authors concluded that the proposed indexes are weak predictors of IHD risk, no better than simpler measures such as intake of SFAs. Another study of the Caerphilly cohort investigated relationships between hemostatic factors and some dietary and lifestyle determinants (*30*). Smokers had higher levels of fibrinogen, greater plasma viscosity, higher white cell counts, and reduced bleeding times. Alcohol drinkers had reduced platelet activity and lower levels of fibrinogen, von Willebrand factor, and white cells. Men who took fish-oil supplements had increased bleeding times and lower levels of von Willebrand factor. Platelets from men who took garlic supplements showed reduced retention in a filter test of platelet activation.

The Israeli Ischemic Heart Disease study was begun in 1961 to investigate factors related to development of CHD, hypertension, and diabetes in a multicultural migrant nation (*31*). Subjects were 10,000 male civil service and municipal employees. Over 23 years, several established risk factors for CHD predicted long-term mortality. A single blood pressure measurement was highly predictive. Blood lipids, although significantly associated with coronary and all-cause mortality, made only a small contribution to predicting the latter compared to hypertension, smoking habits, and diabetes. Weak associations between long-term CHD mortality and baseline fat intake were entirely due to the effect of diet on serum cholesterol. Ethnic diversity in CHD risk persisted in this cohort despite changes in the occupational and social environment. Religious orthodoxy provided protection part of which appeared independent of other lifestyle correlates.

A case–control study in Athens investigated the association between diet and CHD (*32*). Case-subjects were patients admitted to a hospital with a confirmed first coronary infarct or a first positive coronary arteriogram. Controls were admitted for minor conditions considered unrelated to nutrition. Total energy intake was inversely related to CHD risk. After correcting for total energy, dietary fat was positively related and carbohydrates were negatively related to CHD risk. Type of fat (SFA, MUFA, PUFA) was unrelated to risk. However, intake of SFAs is low in the typical Greek diet. Moreover, cooking with margarine was associated with elevated risk, suggesting that the *trans* isomers formed during partial hydrogenation of vegetable oils enhance risk for CHD. Calculations of MUFA and PUFA intake included both *cis* and *trans* isomers, potentially obscuring beneficial effects of unsaturated fats in their natural form and masking harmful effects of *trans* isomers. Intakes of protein, cholesterol, and vitamin C were not related to risk. These observations support the idea that reduced energy intake increases CHD risk, probably because it reflects lack of exercise (after correcting for obesity).

Dramatic changes in the frequency and spectrum of disease have accompanied post–World War II social and economic changes in Japan. Toshima considers changes in eating patterns to account for much of the trend in diseases (*33*). Movement away from the former high-salt, low-fat, low-protein diet is associated with a reduced incidence of stroke but not with increased CHD mortality. The typical current diet includes 25 en% fat, 60 en% carbohydrate, 15 en% protein, and 12 g/d of salt. Toshima suggests that this may represent an optimal eating pattern to maintain health. However, trends should be monitored because the increased intake of fat is recent. Not only has CHD mortality in Japan not increased with the trend toward Westernization of diet, it actually declined between 1980 and 1989 (*34*). A study of changes in diet and risk factors between those years found that age-adjusted serum total cholesterol levels and prevalence of hypercholesterolemia ($\geq 220$ mg/dL) increased in both men and women. However, blood pressure declined in both sexes and prevalence of smoking decreased in men. Decreases in these risk factors may overshadow the increased risk from elevated serum cholesterol. Nutrition surveys in 1980, 1983, 1986, and 1989 document increasing intakes of cholesterol, fat, eggs, meat, and dairy foods and decreasing cereal consumption. Fish and bean consumption has changed little. Calculated dietary atherogenicity and thrombogenicity indexes have remained constant. Again, these changes are recent and require monitoring, especially as they may have occurred mainly in younger cohorts.

A comparison of food habits and serum lipid concentrations identified differences between Japanese adults living in Hiroshima prefecture and Japanese-American adults living in Hawaii and Los Angeles (*35*). Total energy intake was similar in all groups, but the Japanese in Hiroshima consumed less animal fat and simple carbohydrates and more complex carbohydrates than their Japanese-American counterparts. These differences were associated with lower concentrations of serum cholesterol and triacylglycerols and lower prevalence of types IIa and IIb hyperlipidemia.

In Australia and New Zealand, CHD mortality rates rose until the mid-1960s and then began a decline that still continues. Recent declines in IHD mortality and fatal and nonfatal myocardial infarction have also occurred in many other countries. Lloyd examined lifestyle and environmental factors contributing to the decline (36). Although the studies reviewed are dissimilar in type and design, some patterns are apparent. Increases in the PUFA/SFA ratio are common and are more strongly correlated with CHD mortality than are absolute changes in fat intake. Data on the role of other dietary constituents are very limited. After a lag period, changes in prevalence of smoking are correlated with changes in CHD mortality in some countries but not all, suggesting interrelationships between smoking and other factors. In most studies, moderate alcohol consumption lessens the CHD mortality risk. Overall, evidence does not implicate changes in body weight or the prevalence of obesity in CHD mortality trends. Caffeine consumption was not examined. Decreases in blood pressure appear directly related to falling CHD mortality. Hardness of drinking water helps explain regional differences in CHD mortality but cannot explain time trends.

Fraser reviewed evidence that numerous dietary substances in addition to the publicized medium-chain fatty acids, soluble fiber, and cholesterol can influence CHD risk, frequently by mechanisms not directly related to LDL cholesterol (37). He described the effects of phytosterols, tocotrienols, arginine, and antioxidant vitamins on HDL cholesterol concentrations, fasting and postprandial triacylglycerols, oxidation of LDL particles, prostaglandins, and endothelium-derived relaxing factor. All this demonstrates that formation of atherosclerotic plaques is much more complex than simple excess filtration of LDL particles through the arterial endothelium when the plasma LDL level is elevated. Fraser sees a need for epidemiologic and clinical investigation of effects of particular foods rather than the traditional list of macronutrients and micronutrients. This is not only because the list is incomplete but also because the effects of a particular dietary component are influenced by the presence or absence of other components. In this light, Gutteridge and Swain discussed CVD mortality in terms of the European "fruit and vegetable gradient" and lipoprotein oxidation (38). They described how macrophages accumulate massive amounts of cholesterol when exposed to oxidatively modified LDL, leading to formation of foam cells and atherosclerotic lesions. This led to the free radical hypothesis of atherosclerosis and its corollary dietary antioxidant hypothesis, which they reviewed.

A study of African-American Seventh-Day Adventists found a vegetarian diet to be associated with lower CVD risk than an omnivorous diet (39). Subjects were classified as vegetarian (strict vegetarians and ovolactovegetarians), semivegetarian (consumed flesh foods 1–3 times weekly), or nonvegetarian. Vegetarians had significantly lower concentrations of serum total cholesterol, LDL cholesterol, and triacylglycerols, and lower ratios of total and LDL cholesterol to HDL cholesterol than nonvegetarians. Semivegetarians had intermediate values. The lower values of risk factors in vegetarians were related to less central-body fat (lower waist-to-hip ratio), lower intake of saturated fat, and higher ratio of polyunsaturated to saturated (P/S) fat. A study in young Chinese Buddhist vegetarians and omnivorous Chinese medical students revealed benefits of the modern Buddhist diet for blood cholesterol concentration, ratio of apolipoprotein A-I (apoA-I) to apolipoprotein B (apoB), and blood glucose and uric acid levels but not for most hemostatic variables (40). Vegetarian men did have significantly higher concentrations of antithrombin III than nonvegetarian men. The modern Buddhist diet contains 60 en% carbohydrate and 25–30 en% fat, with rice and soybeans as the major protein sources. Beilin summarized the convincing evidence for a blood pressure–lowering effect of certain complex vegetarian and semivegetarian diets (41). These diets are characterized by a relatively low fat content (<30 en%), a P/S ratio >1.0, and large amounts of fruits and vegetables providing 20–50 g/d of fiber. Reduced sodium intake and total abstinence from flesh foods are not required for the beneficial effect. The benefits cannot be attributed to any single nutrient or type of nutrient.

## Public Health Policy and Educational Programs

Posner et al. compared data from the Framingham Offspring–Spouse study with earlier data from NHANES II and USDA food consumption surveys to see whether the population estimates differed, to determine whether nutrition recommendations to reduce CVD risk are appropriate, and to identify areas for future nutritional interventions (42). They concluded that nutritional goals remain appropriate. However, future programs need to emphasize weight reduction, reduced intake of all high-fat foods and sodium, and increased intake of fiber, complex carbohydrates, and micronutrients. This advice is particularly relevant for men. Research is needed on effective strategies to promote and sustain preventive dietary behaviors. In another study, Posner et al. compared the Framingham data with the objectives of Healthy People 2000 and projected the 10-year incidence of CHD with and without lowering serum cholesterol levels (43). Reduction of cholesterol to <200 mg/dL would lower the projected 10-year cumulative incidence of CHD by up to

25%. The authors concluded that lowering risk factors, with emphasis on preventive nutrition and on reducing CVD risk, is an important element of health care reform.

Data from four U.S. surveys (National Health Examination Survey [NHES I] and NHANES I–III) between 1960 and 1991 reveal a consistent decline in mean serum total cholesterol levels in adults aged 20–74 y (*44*). In 1960–1962 the population mean was 220 mg/dL; in 1988–1991 it was 205 mg/dL. The authors believe that the Healthy People 2000 goal of <200 mg/dL can be realized. The drop in cholesterol levels coincides with a continuing decline in CHD mortality. However, some of the reduced mortality may be attributable to changes in smoking habits. Furthermore, not all of the drop in cholesterol is necessarily due to dietary change; some may result from increased exercise and use of cholesterol-lowering drugs. Between the data collection periods of NHANES II (1976–1980) and NHANES III phase 1 (1988–1991), the proportion of adults with blood cholesterol levels ≥240 mg/dL fell from 26% to 20% and the proportion with levels <200 mg/dL rose from 44% to 49% (*45*). According to guidelines of the second Adult Treatment Panel of the National Cholesterol Education Program (NCEP), the proportion of adults who would be candidates for diet therapy decreased from 36% to 29%. Assuming that diet intervention would reduce LDL cholesterol concentrations by 10%, up to 7% of all adult Americans (nearly 13 million) might be candidates for drug therapy as well. The second report of the NCEP Adult Treatment Panel emphasized overall CHD risk status as a guide to the type and intensity of cholesterol-lowering intervention (*46*). In particular it stressed the importance of age, existing CVD, and differences in risk between men and women. It emphasized physical activity and weight loss as components of diet therapy. It recommended that drug therapy generally be restricted to high-risk patients. Persons with high blood cholesterol who are otherwise at low risk should be treated with diet and exercise, which are safer and less expensive.

Dowler discussed policy implications of the role of diet in CHD (*47*). Her article was directed at women for three reasons. First, CHD has only recently been acknowledged as a major cause of death and morbidity in women. Second, although the entire household may be involved in food choices, women still make most decisions about food and budgeting—particularly in single-parent families. Third, nutrition during the fetal and perinatal period may be more important than adult lifestyle in determining later CHD; it is therefore crucial to target nutrition intervention at women of child-bearing age. Dowler recommended that interventions be focused on women of lower socioeconomic status, those most likely

to produce babies of low birth weight, and those whose babies show poor fetal or early development. School lunches need to be evaluated in terms of the nutritional needs of girls, especially as they enter their child-bearing years. Kris-Etherton and Krummel discussed the role of nutrition in primary and secondary prevention of CHD in women (*48*). They reviewed CHD risk factors for women, which are somewhat different from those for men. Women's response to intervention may also differ. Research on these differences is needed.

The Stanford Five-City Project evaluated the effectiveness of community health education in reducing CVD risk population-wide (*49*). There were two "treatment" cities and two controls; a fifth city was included in morbidity and mortality surveillance. During the 6-year intervention, education programs in treatment cities addressed risk-related behaviors such as food intake, weight control, exercise, and smoking. After 5 years of the campaign, the average person in treatment cities had been exposed to nutrition education in >35 public service television announcements, up to 100 newspaper articles, >25 fact sheets, 3 booklets, and 2 television shows. At least 10% of adults also attended lectures, seminars, or work-site programs. Dietary data were analyzed for time trends and association with treatment and city. Diet and nutrition knowledge improved in all cities, but the community programs had minimal effect. Nutritional knowledge among women increased more in treatment cities than in control cities. The authors concluded that continued and greater change in nutrition requires different, more sustained approaches, including changes in the food supply itself.

Baer described a successful nutrition education program for management-level men at the work site (*50*). Thirty-three men with plasma triacylglycerol levels >199 mg/dL participated in the year-long program. They reduced their daily intake of energy from 2546 to 2246 kcal, cholesterol from 444 to 304 mg, and total fat from 38 to 31 en%. Consumption of carbohydrate increased from 38 to 45% and fiber increased from 8 to 23 g. These dietary changes were accompanied by significant reductions in plasma total cholesterol and triacylglycerols, body weight, and body fat. Changes in LDL cholesterol were nonsignificant.

## Clinical Studies and Intervention Trials

Little is known about the influence of nutrition on cholesterol synthesis and metabolism in infants. Cruz et al. conducted a 4-month study in healthy male babies born in Cincinnati-area hospitals (*51*). Groups of infants were breast-fed or randomized to receive a cow milk formula, a cholesterol-free soy formula, or a modified soy formula containing the same level of cholesterol as cow's milk. The authors hypothesized that the cholesterol fractional synthesis rate (FSR) would vary inversely with the cholesterol content of the diet, being lowest in breast-fed infants because human milk has a high cholesterol content (2.6–3.9 mmol/L). They further hypothesized that the phytoestrogen content of soy would inhibit cholesterol synthesis and thus reduce serum cholesterol concentrations in infants fed soy and modified soy formulas. The cholesterol FSR decreased in the order soy formula > modified soy formula > cow's milk >> human milk. Urinary isoflavone excretion (an index of phytoestrogen absorption) was inversely related to the FSR but independent of serum cholesterol concentration. Concentrations of total and LDL cholesterol were significantly higher in breast-fed infants. There were no significant differences between formula-fed groups, although LDL cholesterol was slightly lower in the cholesterol-free soy group. The authors concluded that an infant's response to dietary cholesterol is the major determinant of the endogenous rate of cholesterol synthesis.

In an Italian trial, 6 months of diet therapy alone reduced total and LDL cholesterol to acceptable levels in 56 of 65 hypercholesterolemic children (ages not specified) (*52*). In these 56, the mean total cholesterol level decreased from 221 to 179 mg/dL. Despite some improvement, the remaining 9 did not achieve the desired reduction and were further treated with cholestyramine, with satisfactory results. These subjects began the study with a mean total cholesterol level of 325 mg/dL; it was reduced to 268 mg/dL after 6 months of diet and to 200 mg/dL after 2 y of diet and drug treatment. At the beginning of the study carbohydrate consumption was generally low (48 en%), fat and cholesterol consumption relatively high (35 en% and 122 mg per 1000 kcal, respectively), and fiber consumption low. Compliance with dietary treatment was good, although problems with long-term compliance were anticipated, particularly for adolescents. The authors noted the importance of preliminary counseling, motivation, and training of both the patient and the family. In a Spanish trial, 451 hypercholesterolemic (>200 mg/dL) children and adolescents aged 2–18 y were treated with AHA step 1 and step 2 diets (*53*). Follow-up continued for 6 months to 2 y. Total and LDL cholesterol and apoB-100 levels and the LDL/HDL cholesterol ratio decreased significantly after 1 month and HDL cholesterol increased. Compliance was 100% at this time. After 12 months, 58 of the 189 subjects still in the study were no longer following the diet strictly. Subjects who were not in compliance had significantly higher levels of total and LDL cholesterol

and apoB-100. The authors concluded that diet therapy is effective for hypercholesterolemic children and adolescents but long-term compliance is a major problem.

Connor and Connor discussed in detail the role of diet in treating heterozygous familial hypercholesterolemia (*54*). The principal goal of dietary treatment is reduction of plasma LDL cholesterol, which is best accomplished by enhancing the activity of LDL receptors while depressing hepatic cholesterol synthesis. The authors considered the effects of individual dietary factors on plasma LDL cholesterol and their underlying mechanisms of action. They concluded that the optimal therapeutic diet contains 100 mg/d of cholesterol, 20 en% total fat, 6 en% saturated fat, 65 en% carbohydrate of which 67% is starch, 15 en% protein, and 35–50 g/d of fiber. This diet, phased in gradually over many months, can lower plasma cholesterol by 18–21%. The authors gave suggestions for how to achieve dietary goals and developed a cholesterol–saturated fat index to allow evaluation of any food for its potential to elevate LDL cholesterol.

Denke reviewed the lines of evidence supporting the diet–CHD theory (*55*). She discussed dietary cholesterol, various types of fatty acids, phytosterols, fiber, calcium, coffee, and body weight as they affect LDL cholesterol. She also summarized the impact of body weight, fatty acids, carbohydrates, and alcohol on triacylglycerol and HDL cholesterol levels. Although alcohol consumption raises levels of HDL cholesterol, she noted that current dietary recommendations do not advocate alcohol drinking for the purpose of reducing CHD risk. Dietary factors that alter known and suspected nonlipid risk factors for CHD (hypertension, diabetes, obesity, LDL oxidation, blood coagulation) were considered. It is important to recognize which abnormalities are amenable to diet modification and which require drug therapy. The final section of the review addressed aspects of diet related to the food industry: food labeling and manufacture, and modification of plant and animal products.

Ornish discussed the ability of lifestyle changes to reverse CHD, citing results of the Lifestyle Heart Trial (*56*). The rigorous program consisted of a low-fat (10 en%) vegetarian diet, aerobic exercise, meditation, stress management training, and group support. Smoking was not permitted. Significant improvement was evident after 1 y. Degree of compliance with the regimen was strongly related to regression of stenosis, whereas stenosis progressed in the "usual care" control group. Women had better results than men in both the treatment and control groups, suggesting that response was modified by sex. Ornish concluded that comprehensive lifestyle changes are necessary for improvement of existing CHD, and it is unlikely that such changes would be accepted or sustained in the long term by any but the most highly motivated individuals. Nevertheless, for those willing to make the necessary changes, this method is medically effective and cost-effective and its only side effects appear to be desirable ones. In contrast, the St. Thomas' Atherosclerosis Regression Study found that a moderate lipid-lowering diet (27 en% fat) by itself retarded or even reversed progression of CAD (*57*). Subjects were middle-aged men referred for coronary angiography because of angina pectoris or myocardial infarction. Patients were randomized to a lipid-lowering diet or usual care and reviewed at 3-month intervals for 39 months. Disease was measured by quantitative image analysis as change in minimum absolute width of coronary segments. When patients were grouped according to whether they showed progression (*n* = 10), no change (*n* = 32), or regression (*n* = 8), intakes of total, saturated, and monounsaturated fat, total energy, and cholesterol differed significantly between the progression and regression groups. Only saturated fat intake differed significantly between those showing regression and those showing no change. There were no significant associations with polyunsaturated fat, carbohydrate, protein, fiber, alcohol, or P/S ratio. Associations with total and saturated fat persisted after adjustment for plasma LDL cholesterol, weight, blood pressure, and several other factors. The authors concluded that in middle-aged men, progression of CAD is strongly influenced by intake of saturated fat and this is partly via mechanisms other than those affecting levels of plasma total and LDL cholesterol.

Anderson summarized three studies comparing responses of women and men to low-fat, low-cholesterol diets (*58*). He noted differences between men and women in their likelihood to undergo public cholesterol screening and subsequently enroll in a research study. However, hypercholesterolemic men and women responded similarly to modified diets. After 8 weeks on the AHA step 1 diet, total cholesterol was reduced by 8.8% in women and 7.3% in men. LDL cholesterol fell 9.4% in women and 8.8% in men. A 12-month trial on the AHA step 2 diet reduced total and LDL cholesterol by 10 and 14%, respectively. Corresponding reductions with a high-fiber step 2 diet were 13 and 18%.

A study in Italy compared the long-term effects of two diets for treating hyperlipidemia (*59*). Both diets contained 8 en% saturated fat and ~200 mg/d cholesterol. One was low in total fat and rich in carbohydrate and fiber; the other was rich in polyunsaturated fat and lower in carbohydrate and fiber. The latter differed from the control diet mainly in the proportions of saturated

and polyunsaturated fat. Relative to the control diet, the two test diets caused similar reductions in plasma LDL cholesterol and triacylglycerols without affecting fasting HDL cholesterol or postprandial glucose or insulin concentrations.

Leenen et al. evaluated the relative effects of weight loss and dietary fat modification on serum lipid levels in obese subjects (*60*). After stabilization on a diet high in total and saturated fat, subjects were given a diet low in total and saturated fat with a 1000 kcal/d energy deficit for 13 weeks or a weight-stable low-fat diet for 7 weeks followed by the calorie-restricted diet for 13 weeks. Weight loss itself was responsible for ~50% of the reduction in total cholesterol, ~60% of the reduction in LDL cholesterol, and ~70% of the reduction in triacylglycerols. Fat modification without weight loss reduced HDL cholesterol by 11% and the HDL/LDL ratio by 8%, whereas weight loss by itself led to increases in HDL cholesterol and HDL/LDL ratio of 12 and 24%, respectively. The authors concluded that the effects of fat modification and weight loss are additive, but weight loss has a more favorable effect than fat modification on the serum lipid profile of obese subjects.

Diet and exercise used separately can partially control major CVD risk factors, but much better results are achieved by their combined use (*61*). For example, diet alone may reduce both HDL and LDL cholesterol, whereas a program of diet and exercise increases HDL cholesterol while decreasing body weight and fatness. Exercise thus should be considered an adjunct to diet. The Oslo Diet and Exercise Study (ODES) should provide valuable data on the separate and combined effects of diet and exercise (*62*). A final report has not been published, but a preliminary report described the design and objectives of the study. Subjects are moderately obese, mildly hypertensive, hyperlipidemic, hypercholesterolemic middle-aged men and women. They have a sedentary lifestyle and low levels of HDL cholesterol. They have been randomized to receive no treatment, exercise, diet modification, or exercise and diet modification. Diets are adapted to the individual participant's risk profile. The primary aim of the trial is to evaluate treatment effects on coagulation and fibrinolytic components and activities, but lipid parameters, glucose metabolism, several clinical, physiologic, and anthropometric variables, and quality of life will also be assessed.

Denke and Grundy evaluated the individual responses of 50 moderately hypercholesterolemic men to a cholesterol-lowering diet (*63*). A 1-month diet high in total and saturated fat was followed by 4 months on the step 1 diet recommended by the AHA and NCEP. Dietary responsiveness was normally distributed but there was marked individual variation in response. Variability was due both to compliance and to biologic factors. Nevertheless, many men achieved levels of LDL cholesterol low enough to make drug therapy unnecessary. The authors concluded that the step 1 diet effectively lowers LDL cholesterol levels in many hypercholesterolemic men and some outpatients can achieve results predicted by inpatient metabolic studies.

Truswell reviewed dietary intervention studies to evaluate their effect on coronary events and total mortality (64). The trials were grouped into classical prevention trials with death or disease as the end points and secondary prevention trials with coronary angiographic measurements before and after the intervention period. Because the first group of 14 trials was a heterogeneous collection of studies differing in design, duration, size, and nature of dietary advice, data were analyzed for 8 combinations of these trials. Results gave no indication of excess all-cause mortality from cholesterol-lowering dietary interventions and showed a significant reduction in the odds ratio for coronary events. In four recent secondary prevention trials with angiographic end points, plasma cholesterol was reduced and coronary stenosis either regressed in the diet group or progressed less than in controls. Of 10 trials of fish oil after coronary angioplasty, 4 found a significant reduction in restenosis rate, 1 found a nonsignificant reduction, 4 found no difference, and 1 found a higher rate. Fish oil works by a different mechanism than a cholesterol-lowering diet and its effect is generally manifest in a shorter time. It is thought to reduce endothelial reactivity or the tendency to thrombosis. A small preliminary trial of high-dose vitamin E after coronary angioplasty found a nonsignificant reduction in restenosis rate. However, the editor-in-chief of *The American Journal of Cardiology* feels that the improvements in CVD risk attainable through diets acceptable to the general population are too small and too slow to be of practical value (65). Dietary therapy should generally be the primary therapy before an atherosclerotic event, reserving drugs for patients in whom diet does not produce the desired results. However, Roberts recommends lipid-lowering drugs as primary therapy for secondary prevention after an atherosclerotic event, with diet viewed as secondary therapy.

A study in hyperlipidemic patients with low HDL cholesterol levels showed that a triacylglycerol-lowering diet and bezafibrate have disparate effects on the HDL system (66). During the lipid-lowering diet HDL levels appeared to change in relation to the reduction of plasma triacylglycerols due to decreased transfer of cholesteryl ester between lipoproteins, but there was no overall change in HDL cholesterol. During combined diet and drug therapy, increased plasma lipoprotein lipase activity had a strong effect on HDL in most subjects, and HDL cholesterol increased. Thus drug therapy may be more beneficial than diet therapy for patients with the syndrome of high plasma triacylglycerols and low HDL cholesterol.

In a randomized crossover study, healthy middle-aged Danes were given a low-fat (28 en%), high-fiber (1.3 g per 100 kcal) diet and an average Danish diet for 2-week periods (67). The low-fat high-fiber diet caused favorable changes in several independent risk markers of IHD. Serum total and LDL cholesterol were lower, triacylglycerols were higher, factor VII coagulant activity was lower, and plasma fibrinolytic activity was higher. However, serum HDL cholesterol was also lower. The authors concluded that a low-fat high-fiber diet reduces both the atherogenic tendency and the thrombogenic tendency of an individual. The same authors studied the effect of dietary fat and fiber on factors related to thrombogenicity and fibrinolysis in a randomized cross-over study of 6 healthy men (68). Subjects ate isoenergetic diets differing in fat (20 or 50 en%) and fiber (0.8 or 1.7 g per 100 kcal) content for 2 days with at least 5 days separating diet periods. Dietary fiber content had no significant influence on any measured variable, nor were fibrinolytic variables affected by changes in fat. However, the high-fat diet augmented postprandial activation of factor VII. The authors concluded that by shifting hemostatic balance toward a prothrombotic state, a high-fat diet might promote acute ischemic episodes in people with preexisting CHD. In contrast, Rankinen et al. found that a small decrease in saturated fat intake (from 16 en% to 13–14 en%) in the context of a high-fat diet, with or without aerobic exercise 4 times weekly, had no effect on thrombogenic or fibrinolytic factors in middle-aged men (69). Nor did the exercise training program alone, individually prescribed and carried out 2, 4, or 6 times weekly, affect these parameters during the 6-month study.

As part of a larger trial investigating the effect of lean beef on plasma cholesterol, Sinclair et al. reported that diets rich in lean beef increase arachidonic acid (20:4n–6) and long-chain n–3 PUFAs in plasma phospholipids (70). Healthy adult volunteers ate 500 g/d (raw weight) of lean beef for 4 weeks. The beef provided the following daily amounts of PUFAs: 60 mg of 20:3n–6, 230 mg of 20:4n–6, 125 mg of 20:5n–3, and 20 mg of 22:5n–3. Grilling reduced these levels by 20–30% but frying caused no change. In a diet containing only 10 en% fat, the beef significantly increased both absolute and relative amounts of these PUFAs in the plasma phospholipids and decreased the content of 18:2n–6. Increasing the fat content of the beef diet to 20 or 30 en%

with beef fat or olive oil did not affect the fatty acid profile, whereas adding safflower oil to the beef diet decreased the 18:3n–3 and 20:5n–3 content of plasma phospholipids while maintaining the increase in 20:4n–6. Thus a high level of dietary linoleic acid in a beef-rich diet prevented the rise in plasma levels of two PUFAs that antagonize the effects of arachidonic acid on platelet aggregation. In the absence of large amounts of 18:2n–6, a diet containing lean beef can improve the plasma fatty acid profile while lowering circulating cholesterol levels (as these authors reported in a previous article).

Pyruvate, in the setting of a high-fat high-cholesterol diet, decreases serum total and LDL cholesterol in humans. Because diet therapy is the primary intervention for most hyperlipidemic patients, Stanko et al. investigated whether pyruvate supplementation is also effective with a low-fat, low-cholesterol diet (71). Thirty-four hyperlipidemic subjects were given a diet containing 165–180 mg of cholesterol and 22–24 en% fat for 4 weeks, during which time their plasma lipid concentrations decreased. They were then randomized to receive 22–44 g/d of pyruvate or 18–35 g/d of polyglucose placebo, isoenergetically substituted for part of the dietary carbohydrate, for 6 weeks. Subjects in the pyruvate group lost significantly more weight and fat, but their plasma concentrations of total, LDL, and HDL cholesterol and triacylglycerols did not differ from those of the placebo group.

Sciarrone et al. studied the mechanisms underlying the reduction of blood pressure by an ovolacto-vegetarian diet (72). Subjects were 20 normotensive male hospital employees 30–59 years old. They were randomly assigned to an omnivorous control diet (40 en% fat, 45 en% carbohydrate) or an ovolactovegetarian diet (30 en% fat, 55 en% carbohydrate) for 6 weeks, during which biochemical and neurohormonal variables and blood pressure were measured. Data were analyzed by multiple regression and factor analyses. Ambulatory blood pressures at work were lower in vegetarians than in controls. This difference was associated with a factor representing lower plasma catecholamine and renin activity throughout the study and also with a factor representing reduced plasma glucose and insulin levels in the first week of intervention. Plasma atrial natriuretic peptide (ANP) levels were significantly higher during the first week of the vegetarian diet. These findings suggest that the effect of a vegetarian diet on blood pressure is mediated by reduced sympatho-adrenal activity consequent to altered glucose and insulin handling. The early increase in plasma ANP may contribute to the effect.

Ramsay et al. reviewed the value of nonpharmacologic interventions to reduce blood pressure (73). Interventions thought to lower blood pressure include reducing alcohol, salt, and total fat intake and weight, increasing potassium, calcium, magnesium, and fiber intake and the P/S ratio, vegetarian diets, and various behavioral methods. Weight reduction, moderate sodium restriction, and reduced alcohol consumption all lower blood pressure significantly in the short term and appear feasible in the long term. Exercise may be helpful for some patients. However, the authors do not believe that any other nonpharmacologic approach warrants a place in routine hypertension management, based on present evidence. Moreover, the modest success of regimens combining weight loss and reduced salt and alcohol intake may merely shift hypertensive patients from just above to just below some arbitrary cutoff point for intervention, actually increasing their risk of complications related to suboptimal blood pressure control. The authors believe that nonpharmacologic measures should be viewed as adjuncts to drug therapy rather than as alternatives.

## ANIMAL MODELS

Mice can provide valuable models for studies of atherosclerosis. Lusis discussed their many advantages and reviewed relevant studies of atherosclerosis in mice (74). Complete and detailed linkage maps have been made for the mouse, elucidation of its complete genomic sequence is anticipated, and many mouse–human chromosomal homologies are known. Many inbred, congenic, and recombinant strains are available, some of which show genetic variations relevant to atherosclerosis. Techniques for in vivo gene manipulation are most advanced in the mouse. Application of these techniques has been particularly informative in the area of lipoprotein metabolism and atherosclerosis.

Daley et al. reported their studies comparing cholesterol-fed and casein-fed rabbit models of atherosclerosis. Casein-fed rabbits had a primarily LDL hypercholesterolemia, whereas cholesterol-fed rabbits had roughly equal levels of VLDL, LDL, and intermediate-density lipoprotein (IDL) cholesterol (75). At equivalent concentrations of total plasma cholesterol, cholesterol-fed animals had lesions covering twice the luminal surface area and having three times the volume as animals eating a cholesterol-free casein diet. The topographic distribution of lesions was the same in the two groups. Lesions were classified morphologically as early fatty streaks, advanced fatty streaks, fibrous plaques, or atheromatous lesions (76). At matched plasma cholesterol levels, lesions in casein-fed animals were about equally distributed among the categories, whereas lesions in cholesterol-fed rabbits were predominantly of the more advanced atheromatous type similar to those seen in humans.

Although plasma lipoprotein profiles in humans and rodents differ, more analogies are evident with hamsters than with rats. Bravo et al. discussed reasons why Syrian golden hamsters are preferable to Wistar rats for studies of lipoprotein metabolism (77). Like the rat, the hamster is an "HDL animal," (i.e., HDL is the major lipoprotein class), whereas people are "LDL animals." However, hamsters are closer to humans in the distribution of cholesterol between free and esterified forms and the distribution of phospholipid classes in the various lipoprotein fractions.

## GENE–DIET INTERACTIONS

Goldbourt discussed the rationale for identifying genetic subgroups at differing risk for CHD (78). Not only do classical risk factors fail to identify many people who will develop CHD while many high-risk individuals never develop CHD, but not all variation in risk factors results from differences in diet, physical activity, stress, or other environmental conditions. It is apparent that diet and other lifestyle factors act on a background of highly variable individual constitutions. The first evidence for genetic involvement was the recognition of familial aggregation of CHD in both high-incidence and low-incidence populations. Active areas of current research concern the mechanisms by which dietary factors control gene expression and the interaction between genetic factors and nutrition in general. Specific topics of interest include the genetics of obesity, heritable lipoprotein phenotypes that influence the response to dietary fat, the genetics of hyporesponse and hyperresponse to dietary cholesterol, and genetic control of energy expenditure and the response to prolonged exercise. Goldbourt argued that intervention strategies for CHD place insufficient emphasis on family history and genetics. He believes the evidence justifies a major effort to identify genetically characterized subgroups at different underlying risk and with different probabilities of benefitting from various interventions.

Eastern Finland has one of the world's highest rates of CHD mortality; the rate in western Finland, though still high, is substantially lower. A study in Finland found evidence that both genetic and dietary factors influence serum cholesterol concentrations in children (79). Children were classified according to their residence in eastern or western Finland and according to the eastern or western origin of their grandparents (which is related to genetic background because internal migration was very limited at the time the grandparents were born). At a survey in 1980, "eastern" children living in the west had higher serum cholesterol levels than children of western origin despite eating a similar diet. The number of grandparents from the east was directly associated with serum cholesterol levels. By 1986 the fatty acid content of the Finnish diet had become more favorable and there was a population-wide decrease in serum cholesterol. On follow-up in 1986, the east–west difference in cholesterol levels had disappeared. The authors concluded that both diet and genetics determine serum cholesterol levels in Finns, but that diet plays the greater role.

Several genetic polymorphisms are known to influence the response to changes in dietary fat. Dreon et al. reported a major difference in responses to high- and low-fat diets between subjects with "A" and "B" LDL subclass patterns (80). Pattern B is a genetically influenced lipoprotein profile characterized by a predominance of small dense LDL particles and associated with increased levels of triacylglycerol-rich lipoproteins, reduced HDL cholesterol levels, and increased risk of CAD. In a randomized crossover study, pattern A and B subjects were given a high-fat (46 en%) and a low-fat (24 en%, carbohydrate substituted for fat) diet for 6-week periods. After the low-fat diet pattern B subjects had reductions in LDL cholesterol more than twice as great as pattern A subjects, and their apoB levels decreased significantly whereas those of pattern A subjects did not change. Differences remained significant after adjustment for covariates. Thus LDL subclass pattern contributes significantly to interindividual variation in plasma lipoprotein responses to a low-fat, high-carbohydrate diet.

Humphries reviewed progress of genetic epidemiology toward identifying genetic variables that influence the risk of heart attack and determining the relative contribution of genes and lifestyle or environmental factors, as well as interactions between these factors (81). As an example he discussed apoB and polymorphism in the apoB protein. Citing his own studies and work of others, he showed how genetic variation not only directly determines the levels of plasma risk factors such as cholesterol or fibrinogen, but also determines an individual's response to interventions such as dietary change or drugs. Since the gene for apoB protein was cloned in 1985 many interesting associations have been found. However, no in vitro expression studies have yet proved a causal relationship between a specific change in the gene for apoB protein, a specific amino acid substitution, and an effect on the function of apoB protein. When such data are available they can be integrated with information on anthropomorphic, lifestyle, and biochemical risk factors to give a better estimate of an individual's IHD risk and how to reduce it.

From their work on apoE, Hegele et al. hypothesized that variation at candidate genes in lipoprotein metabolism was associated with variations in the individual response of plasma lipoproteins to dietary fiber (82). They selected DNA markers within the coding sequence of candidate genes (LDL receptor, apoB, and hepatic lipase) or within noncoding regions associated with lipoprotein phenotypes (apoB and apoA-I). Using these they analyzed the association between genotype and the response of plasma lipoprotein levels in a 2-week metabolic study involving wheat bran and oat bran supplements. Reductions in plasma apoB were significantly related to LDL receptor genotype but not to alleles of other genes tested. These results illustrate the principle that common genetic variants can alter responsiveness to dietary treatment. They show that attempts to reduce plasma lipoprotein levels with dietary fiber have variable effects partly because of structural differences in genes whose products are involved in lipoprotein metabolism.

Friedlander et al. reported suggestive evidence that a single mutation at the XbaI locus of the apoB gene has a modest effect on the plasma lipid response to diet (83). Subjects were adult offspring of Israeli patients hospitalized with myocardial infarction. Twenty X1X1 homozygotes, two X2X2 homozygotes, and fifteen X1X2 heterozygotes were randomized to a crossover study involving 5-week periods on a prudent diet and a diet high in saturated fat and cholesterol. Carriers of the X2 allele showed less change in LDL cholesterol levels in response to diet than X1X1 homozygotes. There was an indication that XbaI genotype interacts with baseline LDL cholesterol levels to determine individual dietary response. However, the differences between groups were nonsignificant in this small study and the apoB XbaI locus does not appear to be a major determinant of dietary response in this population.

A study of normolipidemic subjects with apoE1/– or apoE4/– genotypes found no evidence that apoE genotype is associated with cholesterol synthesis rates in people eating self-selected low- or high-cholesterol diets (84). The genotype was related to circulating cholesterol levels, however. Moreover, hyporesponders to a dietary cholesterol challenge had higher synthetic rates than hyperresponders. The authors suggested that cholesterogenesis is not the primary regulator of serum cholesterol levels, but responds only when other systems are not fully effective.

Diabetes mellitus and obesity are risk factors for CHD. However, the Mvskoke Indians in Oklahoma, who have a high prevalence of non-insulin-dependent diabetes and obesity, have a low incidence of CHD. Russell et al. studied the plasma lipids and diet of a random sample of Mvskoke, their spouses, and available first-degree relatives (85). Despite a nontraditional diet high in total fat, saturated fat, and cholesterol, the subjects had favorable plasma lipid profiles. Their total and LDL cholesterol levels were lower and HDL cholesterol higher than age- and sex-matched Lipid Research Clinics values, especially for subjects with diabetes. The authors speculated that the relatively low plasma lipid and lipoprotein concentrations resulted from differences in regulation of these concentrations. These Indians may have variants or beneficial polymorphisms in genes regulating lipid metabolism that are protective against CHD even in the presence of diabetes and obesity.

Cobb et al. performed a metaanalysis of five studies conducted by Jan Breslow and his colleagues (86). They found sex-related differences in lipoprotein responses of normolipidemic subjects to high P/S and low P/S diets. "Responsiveness" was calculated as the adjusted difference ($\Delta$ mg/dL) after each diet period. $\Delta$LDL-cholesterol was similar in men and women, whereas changes in triacylglycerols, VLDL cholesterol, and HDL cholesterol were sex-specific. In women, HDL-cholesterol lowering was directly related to increase in PUFA intake and baseline HDL cholesterol concentration and inversely related to change in triacylglycerols, and was greater than in men. The authors concluded that increasing the dietary P/S ratio may be less beneficial for normolipidemic women than for men due to HDL cholesterol lowering, and that sex and diet may both be pivotal considerations in strategies to achieve plasma lipid goals.

Roach et al. reported studies of the LDL receptor in human mononuclear cells isolated from polygenic hypercholesterolemic subjects whose receptor activity was not significantly different from normal (87). Treatment of these subjects with simvastatin increased their LDL receptor activity by 70% while lowering their plasma cholesterol concentrations by 26%. In the same subjects, reducing dietary fat from 38 to 20 en% decreased plasma cholesterol by 10% but had no effect on the LDL receptor. Thus simvastatin appears to act in this group by up-regulating the LDL receptor, but dietary intervention works by another mechanism.

Baboons are frequently used in investigations of diet and plasma lipid response. Rainwater studied the separate and combined effects of dietary cholesterol and saturated fat on serum lipoprotein(a) concentrations in baboons (88). He found that both dietary components significantly increased lipoprotein(a) concentrations. All changes occurred within the first 8 weeks of feeding the experimental diet. There was also an effect of sire group membership, indicating genetic control of the response to diet. The genetic factors have not been identified, but they appear to be different from those specifying basal lipoprotein(a) levels.

Selective breeding has produced lines of baboons whose plasma LDL cholesterol shows high or low response to a high-fat, high-cholesterol diet. Hasan and Kushwaha investigated differences in bile acid metabolism between low and high responders (89). On a high-fat, high-cholesterol diet, low responders had higher plasma and liver concentrations of 27-hydroxycholesterol (the most abundant oxysterol) than high responders. This was associated with an increase in hepatic sterol 27-hydroxylase activity. There were no differences between groups when they were fed the basal laboratory diet. The authors concluded that hepatic sterol 27-hydroxylase is induced by dietary cholesterol and this induction is greater in low-responding animals. Kushwaha et al. studied the association of cholesterol absorption and liver cholesterol concentration with the high and low responses to diet (90). Animals were fed chow or a diet supplemented with cholesterol and either corn oil or coconut oil. High responders had a higher percentage of cholesterol absorption than low responders on both basal and challenge diets regardless of fat type, but hepatic cholesterol concentration varied with the duration of challenge and type of fat. Thus both cholesterol absorption and hepatic cholesterol concentration regulate cholesterolemic responses to diet, but by different mechanisms. In further studies this group investigated metabolic mechanisms underlying the high and low response to dietary fat and cholesterol (91). Baboons were challenged with increasing levels of dietary cholesterol combined with either corn oil or coconut oil. The results suggested that genetic differences in the initial response of LDL cholesterol to dietary cholesterol and saturated fat are not due to differences in hepatic transcription of apoB. As dietary cholesterol increased plasma cholesterol (mostly LDL cholesterol) concentrations increased in both phenotypes and with both types of fat, but phenotypic differences were greater with coconut oil. Baboons and humans have a similar response to dietary cholesterol: linear at low to moderate levels, plateauing at high intakes. Differences in individual baboons' responses to saturated fat are also consistent with the variability observed in humans.

## EFFECTS OF DIETARY COMPONENTS

### Fiber

Dietary soluble fiber is well known to lower serum lipid levels against a background of a "normal" diet. Jenkins et al. asked whether eating foods rich in soluble fiber can further lower blood lipids in hyperlipidemic subjects whose intake of saturated fat and cholesterol is already very low (92). Subjects who had been following the NCEP step 2 diet for at least 2 months were given two metabolically controlled diets, each for 4 months, in a randomized crossover study design. Diets provided 20 en% fat, 20 en% protein, 60 en% carbohydrate, and 2.5–3.0 g of fiber per 100 kcal, with 50 mg/d of cholesterol. One diet contained abundant legumes and other foods rich in soluble fiber; the other was rich in wheat bran and other insoluble fiber, considered lipid-neutral. The experimental periods were separated by a 2-month return to the step 2 diet. Modest reductions in total, LDL, and HDL cholesterol were associated with both metabolic diets, but soluble fiber produced a significantly larger decrease. Men had greater reductions than women during the soluble fiber diet, but there were no significant differences related to lipid phenotype or apoE polymorphism. Concentrations of fecal bile acids increased in relation to decrease in plasma total cholesterol ($r = -.42$, $p = .005$). Plasma triacylglycerols did not change. The authors concluded that a high intake of foods rich in soluble fiber lowers blood cholesterol levels in hyperlipidemic subjects even when the major dietary lipid modifiers of these levels are greatly reduced.

Morgan et al. evaluated the effects of three nonstarch polysaccharide supplements and cholestyramine on levels of circulating bile acids, hormones, and metabolites in healthy nonobese volunteers (93). The nonstarch polysaccharides were guar gum (a soluble galactomannan), sugar-beet fiber (containing pectic substances and soluble hemicelluloses), and wheat bran. Supplements were added to a high-fat food. Postprandial circulating bile acid levels, triacylglycerols, and gastric inhibitory polypeptide concentrations were markedly attenuated by guar gum and cholestyramine but were unaffected by sugar-beet fiber and wheat bran. Liquid gastric emptying was slightly accelerated by guar gum. Glycocholic acid bound strongly to the soluble fraction of guar gum, whereas it did not bind to the soluble fraction of sugar-beet fiber or wheat bran and bound only slightly to the insoluble fraction. These results show that postprandial bile acids provide an indirect measurement of bile acid binding to nonstarch polysaccharide in vivo.

The authors concluded that the hypocholesterolemic action of guar gum is mediated by interruption of the enterohepatic bile acid circulation, but that of sugar-beet fiber is mediated by another mechanism.

Hunninghake et al. evaluated the hypocholesterolemic effects of a dietary fiber supplement containing guar gum, pectin, soy fiber, pea fiber, and corn bran (*94*). Subjects were healthy, mildly to moderately hypercholesterolemic adults. After stabilization on the AHA step 1 diet they were randomly assigned to a 15-week treatment with placebo or 10 or 20 g/d of the supplement while continuing their step 1 diet. Total and LDL cholesterol and the LDL/HDL cholesterol ratio were significantly reduced in both fiber groups. There was no difference between fiber treatments. The fiber supplement had no significant effect on HDL cholesterol or triacylglycerol levels. From these results the authors concluded that the use of fiber supplements in conjunction with dietary change is the logical next step in management of hypercholesterolemia. Added to the average American diet, which contains 10–15 g/d of fiber, such supplementation would also bring fiber consumption closer to the recommended level.

Ten healthy, normal young women participated in a randomized crossover study to determine the effects of a citrus fiber concentrate on serum cholesterol levels (*95*). Under strict dietary control, subjects ate a control diet and a diet containing the identical foods to which the supplement was added. Total dietary fiber intake was 21 and 45 g/d during the control and high-fiber periods. After 4 weeks on the control diet, mean total serum cholesterol remained unchanged but HDL cholesterol levels were 6.5% lower. After 4 weeks on the high-fiber diet, total and HDL cholesterol were significantly reduced by 10.6 and 14.5%, respectively, with no change in the total/HDL cholesterol ratio. The additional fiber was fermented completely. The authors concluded that citrus fiber can help to reduce serum cholesterol. Because of its energy contribution it may be less suitable in weight reduction, although it may reduce hunger and food intake by virtue of its swelling properties. This could not be determined in this study.

Hypercholesterolemia was established in microswine and the animals were then continued on the atherogenic diet for 270 days while half were also fed grapefruit pectin (*96*). Although cholesterol levels did not differ between groups at the end of the experiment, pectin reduced the extent of atherosclerosis in the aorta and coronary artery by roughly 50%. This suggests that pectin has a direct effect on atherosclerosis by a mechanism independent of cholesterol level.

Blends of pectin and wheat bran were tested for their effects on blood lipid levels and fecal responses in rats (*97*). A 1:1 blend markedly reduced cholesterol in both cholesterol-fed hypercholesterolemic animals and normocholesterolemic animals. It also produced desirable fecal responses in terms of weight, volume, and density and in hypercholesterolemic rats it significantly lowered liver cholesterol levels. When substituted for 20% of the wheat flour in a traditional muffin formula, this fiber blend yielded a product that a panel of tasters rated nearly as high as the control product. It contained four times as much total fiber, five times as much soluble fiber, and 14% fewer calories. The blend may be suitable for a variety of bakery products.

Psyllium fiber is a soluble fiber that, administered in granular form with meals, can reduce serum cholesterol levels in diabetic and hyperlipidemic subjects. Wolever et al. asked whether a psyllium-containing breakfast cereal would reduce blood lipids in hyperlipidemic subjects who were eating the AHA step 2 diet (*98*). Wheat-bran cereals were used as a control. After 2 weeks, the psyllium cereal significantly reduced total, LDL, and HDL cholesterol and the LDL/HDL ratio, with no effect on triacylglycerols. There were no important differences between the responses of men and women. Again, this study shows that soluble fiber can reduce cholesterol levels in the context of a low-fat, low-cholesterol diet and the effect is not one of substituting fiber for fat. The same research group showed that psyllium fiber must be taken with foods to be effective (*99*). Hypercholesterolemic subjects on the NCEP step 2 diet were studied for three 2-week periods, in random order, with 2-week washout periods between the tests. During the test periods they ate the psyllium-containing cereal or the wheat-bran cereal, or took the same type and amount of psyllium as in the test cereal between meals. Significant reductions in serum cholesterol were seen only when the psyllium cereal was eaten. In another trial of psyllium cereal, nonobese hypercholesterolemic men were randomly assigned to 5-week cereal sequences of psyllium–wheat bran–psyllium or wheat bran–psyllium–wheat bran while following the NCEP step 1 diet (*100*). Total and LDL cholesterol were significantly lower after the psyllium periods, whereas HDL cholesterol and triacylglycerols did not change significantly. Sprecher et al. compared psyllium's efficacy in hypercholesterolemic subjects on high- and low-fat diets (*101*). Participants were selected if their habitual diet contained either ≥40 or ≤30 en% fat, and they maintained their usual dietary habits throughout the study. Half of the subjects in each diet group were randomly assigned to receive placebo and half took 5.1 g of psyllium (as Metamucil) twice daily before breakfast and dinner. Psyllium produced modest but significant reductions in total and LDL cholesterol regardless of the fat content of the diet. However, in hypercholesterolemic children who were being treated with a low-fat diet (<30 en%), a psyllium-containing cereal did not further reduce serum cholesterol levels (*102*). Children 5–17 years old with LDL cholesterol levels >110 mg/dL ate two 1-ounce servings of cereal containing wheat fiber or psyllium daily for 4–5 weeks. Although there were no statistically or clinically significant changes in cholesterol parameters, triacylglycerol levels were significantly higher after the wheat-fiber period. A comparison of the effects of psyllium seed and psyllium husk in normal and ileostomy subjects suggested that seed is more effective than husk in reducing serum cholesterol (*103*). The husk had a 67:33 ratio of soluble to insoluble fiber; the ratio for seed was 47:53. Subjects maintained their customary diets but ingested the husk or seed supplement with milk at meal times. The data suggested that the effect of psyllium seed was not mediated by increased loss of fecal bile acids, and increased ileal loss of bile acids might be compensated for by enhanced reabsorption in the colon.

Another study in ileostomy patients showed that consumption of 32 g/d of sugar beet fiber with low-fiber meals increased cholesterol excretion and decreased bile acid excretion from the small intestine (*104*). This pattern differs from that associated with pectin and oat fiber. The authors concluded that the interaction between dietary fiber and sterol metabolism is mediated by different mechanisms according to the fiber source.

Basu et al. investigated the effect of rhubarb stalk fiber on plasma and liver lipids and activities of several hepatic microsomal enzyme activities in mice (*105*). Animals were fed a cholesterol-enriched diet containing 5% rhubarb fiber or cellulose. The rhubarb diet sharply lowered plasma cholesterol and triacylglycerol concentrations and hepatic cholesterol. It reversed the cholesterol-stimulated increase in cholesterol acyl transferase activity but did not affect β-hydroxy β-methyl CoA reductase activity, which is inhibited by dietary cholesterol. The authors concluded that rhubarb stalk fiber reduces lipids by a mechanism that may not be mediated through alterations in cholesterol synthesis and metabolism. Its profound lipid-lowering action and possible use in food products warrant further study.

Hassona fed Egyptian breads containing 10–25% milled brewer's spent grain to rats and measured their plasma lipid response (*106*). The spent grain, a major by-product of the brewing industry, contains most of the protein, lipid, and fiber of the original barley and has been considered as an ingredient of foods for human

consumption. The experimental breads reduced total lipids by 5.7–8.0% and total cholesterol by 6.0–8.3%. Sensory evaluation of three breads yielded acceptance scores of 70, 63, and 63, compared with 81 for a white pan-bread control. Lupton et al. studied the cholesterol-lowering effect of barley oil and barley bran flour in hypercholesterolemic adults who were following the NCEP step 1 diet (*107*). Supplements were taken in pure form at breakfast and dinner: oil was taken as capsules; flour and cellulose control fiber were mixed into a beverage. Both the oil and the bran flour significantly lowered serum total and LDL cholesterol after 30 days, whereas cellulose had no effect. HDL cholesterol decreased significantly in the control and bran flour groups but not in the barley oil group. Thus barley bran flour and barley oil augment the cholesterol-lowering effect of the NCEP step 1 diet in hypercholesterolemic subjects.

Flaxseed, which has a high content of α-linolenic acid and fiber, reduces serum cholesterol levels in elderly subjects. Bierenbaum et al. reported a preliminary study of its effects on atherogenic risk in hyperlipidemic adults 21 to 65 years old who had taken 800 IU/d of vitamin E for 3 months (*108*). Vitamin E supplementation was continued for an additional 3 months while flaxseed products were substituted for the usual bread and cereal in the otherwise self-selected diet. Serum total and LDL cholesterol levels decreased significantly during the flaxseed test while HDL cholesterol did not change. Thrombin-stimulated platelet aggregation decreased. Vitamin E alone had no effect on cholesterol levels.

Zhang et al. studied the effect of rye bran on plasma lipid concentrations and excretion of bile acids, cholesterol, nitrogen, and fat in subjects with ileostomies (*109*). Measurements were made after 3-week periods on a low-fiber diet with wheat bread and a high-fiber diet with rye bran bread. The rye bran had no significant impact on plasma cholesterol concentrations. It did increase the excretion of fat, nitrogen, and energy and decrease the deconjugation of bile acid conjugates in the ileostomy effluents. The biological importance of these observations requires further study.

Kahlon et al. reviewed studies of the cholesterol-lowering properties of rice bran in humans (*110*). Studies in hamsters, rats, mice, rabbits, chicks, and cynomolgus monkeys were also summarized. Various fractions have shown activity in animals and humans, including rice bran oil, unsaponifiable matter, and protein. However, intact full-fat rice bran is generally most effective. Reductions in cholesterol usually occur in the atherogenic (LDL) fraction. Possible mechanisms of action were discussed. The healthful properties of rice bran have generated commercial interest, and new rice bran products are generally popular. Marsono et al. compared plasma lipid levels and large bowel volatile fatty acids in pigs fed white rice, brown rice, rice bran, and rice bran plus rice oil (*111*). Plasma HDL cholesterol and triacylglycerols were unaffected by diet. The rice bran diet caused a nonsignificant reduction in total cholesterol compared to white rice and brown rice; rice bran plus rice oil significantly lowered total cholesterol compared to white rice and brown rice. Pools of total and individual volatile fatty acids in the proximal colon were uninfluenced by diet. Some diet-related differences in total and individual volatile fatty acids were seen in the median and distal colon.

Poulter et al. tested the effect of daily consumption of an oat-based cereal on lipid profiles of adults having plasma cholesterol concentrations typical for the UK (~230 mg/dL) (*112*). Subjects were randomly allocated to eat the oat cereal or an oat-free cereal for 4 weeks, after which they crossed over to the other cereal for a further 4 weeks. Otherwise they followed their customary diet. Small but significant reductions in total (2.23%) and LDL (4.55%) cholesterol occurred during the oat-cereal phase.

In rats fed cholesterol-free diets, a diet based on white wheat flour produced significantly lower plasma cholesterol concentrations than diets based on whole wheat or wheat bran (*113*). Digesta bile acids and neutral sterol pools were negatively correlated with plasma cholesterol, indicating that excretion was regulating plasma concentration. Data on cecal volatile fatty acids suggested that these are indicators rather than regulators of altered cecal steroid metabolism. The authors cited a study in human subjects for which white wheat flour was used as a control in a test of oat bran. When there was no difference between the effects of oat bran and white wheat flour it was concluded that oat bran had no effect. The authors argued from their data that it was equally possible that the control diet was also effective in lowering cholesterol in the humans.

## Carbohydrates

Truswell briefly reviewed studies on dietary carbohydrates and plasma lipids (*114*). Epidemiologically, high carbohydrate intakes are associated with low plasma cholesterol and variable plasma triacylglycerol concentrations. Increased consumption of carbohydrate generally leads to a transient increase in plasma triacylglycerols but does not affect cholesterol. Ordinary intakes of sucrose and fructose have no important effect on triacylglycerols in most normal and diabetic people so long as

energy balance is not changed. Although theoretically fructose should be more lipogenic than sucrose, most reports that sugars elevate plasma lipids in animals have been based on rat studies using diets unnaturally high in these sugars. In people, fasting triacylglycerols are elevated only with huge sugar intakes, and even then usually only in males when dietary fat is saturated. In a minority of subjects with type IV hypertriglyceridemia, triacylglycerols may be lowered by reducing intake of sucrose or fructose. Even in these subjects, reduction of carbohydrate intake is not generally recommended because this implies a higher percentage of energy from fat.

Unlike Truswell (*114*), Hollenbeck concluded from a review of the literature that dietary fructose *can* significantly increase fasting plasma triacylglycerol and cholesterol concentrations (*115*). The changes are associated with increases in VLDL and LDL particles with no apparent change in HDL particle concentrations. The size of the effect varies with age, gender, and baseline glucose, insulin, and triacylglycerol levels. Insulin resistance and the amount of fructose consumed also influence the effect. Although not all studies show an effect, Hollenbeck argued that the positive data cannot easily be dismissed and may be of substantial clinical importance as an indicator of increased risk of CAD.

A dietary survey using data from two large CHD screening studies in Scotland found that neither extrinsic sugar, intrinsic sugar, nor the fat/sugar ratio is a significant independent predictor of CHD in the Scottish population (*116*). These findings agree with the general consensus that total sugar intake is not an important marker of CHD. They extend knowledge by showing that effects of extrinsic sugar intake cannot be differentiated from the effects of intrinsic sugar or lactose. Moreover, obesity did not stand out as a major risk factor for CHD. Other factors such as cigarette smoking and antioxidant intake were much more important.

Preuss et al. tested whether sugar-induced increases in systolic blood pressure in rats occurs through a mechanism common to salt-induced hypertension—renal retention of water and salt (*117*). They found that salt and water retention occur during sugar-induced hypertension due to reduced renal excretion. The effects were not due to angiotensin II inhibition, but a decreased availability of vasodilatory prostaglandins may have been involved. The high-sugar diet in this study contained >50 en% of sugar.

## Protein and Amino Acids

Dietary protein's influence on plasma lipids has received relatively little public attention even though it has been established that replacement of animal protein with soy protein lowers blood cholesterol levels in humans and studies in rabbits have helped to explain how this occurs. Potter et al. studied the effects of soy protein with and without soy fiber on plasma lipids in mildly hypercholesterolemic men (*118*). They tested four dietary treatments in a randomized Latin square design corrected for residual effects. Baked products containing 50 g of soy or milk protein and 20 g of soy fiber or cellulose were incorporated into a low-fat, low-cholesterol diet. All baked products except fruit bars were well accepted. The rest of the diet comprised ordinary foods. Soy flour had a significant cholesterol-lowering effect only when total cholesterol was compared between the soy flour treatment and the milk plus cellulose treatment. Total and LDL cholesterol were lowered to a similar extent by isolated soy protein, compared to milk plus cellulose and baseline levels, whether the accompanying fiber was cellulose or soy cotyledon fiber. No treatment altered HDL or VLDL cholesterol. However, isolated soy protein with cellulose reduced plasma VLDL slightly and significantly reduced apoA-I and apoB compared with both baseline and soy flour. In a study of similar design, hypercholesterolemic men were given muffins providing 25 g of isolated soy protein or casein and 20 g of soybean cotyledon fiber or cellulose (*119*). Consumption of soy protein—again, regardless of the fiber source—was associated with reduced total cholesterol concentrations in subjects whose initial level was >220 mg/dL. This level of soy protein consumption is both reasonable and achievable. The same research group investigated the effects of soy protein and soy fiber on hormones involved in cholesterol metabolism (*120*). The experimental design was as described in reference *118*. Mean values of total thyroxine and the free thyroxine index were higher than baseline after all treatments, but the change was significant only for the two isolated soy protein treatments. The highest plasma insulin concentrations were associated with soy flour, but the difference was significant only between soy flour and isolated soy protein plus soy cotyledon fiber. This raises the possibility that soy flour contains insulin-enhancing phytochemicals that are lost in the processing of soy protein and fiber. There was a suggestive but nonsignificant reduction of thyroid stimulating hormone with all three soy treatments. These data are consistent with data from animal studies showing protein-dependent changes in thyroid hormones. Elevated total thyroxine levels may be involved in the hypocholesterolemic effect of soy protein.

Widhalm et al. replaced the animal protein in a standard low-fat, low-cholesterol diet with soy protein and measured the effect on plasma lipids of children with familial or polygenic hypercholesterolemia (*121*). A crossover design was used with two 8-week diet periods separated by an 8-week washout during which subjects ate their customary diet. The soy protein diet reduced total and LDL cholesterol levels more than the standard diet. The authors concluded that a low-fat diet substituting soy protein for animal protein has a more beneficial short-term effect than a standard low-fat diet on cholesterol levels in hypercholesterolemic children.

Although dietary replacement of animal protein by plant protein consistently lowers plasma cholesterol levels and inhibits atherogenesis in experimental animals, studies in humans have produced varying results. This is partly because diets in the clinical trials are less rigorous and less well defined. Huang et al. discussed interrelationships between dietary protein and PUFAs and the metabolism of *n*–6 PUFAs and cholesterol (*122*). Overall, plant proteins, particularly the undigested fraction, decrease intestinal absorption of cholesterol, increase fecal excretion of steroids, and enhance the catabolism of cholesterol-carrying lipoproteins by increasing the number or activity of LDL receptors. PUFAs reduce intestinal cholesterogenesis, which reduces the cholesterol content of VLDL particles. This facilitates the rapid removal of triacylglycerols. PUFAs also increase cell-membrane fluidity and LDL receptor activity and thus the removal of LDL by hepatic LDL receptors. Intracellularly, dietary protein influences the cholesterol/phospholipid ratio in microsomes and consequently the fluidity of the microsomal membrane. These changes affect both PUFA and cholesterol metabolism. The protein's content of specific amino acids can influence secretion of hormones that modify activity of enzymes involved in PUFA and cholesterol metabolism. Dietary PUFAs affect the synthesis of eicosanoids that modulate the activity of enzymes involved in cholesterol metabolism.

Some saponins decrease plasma cholesterol levels when added to the diet of rats. Because proteins also influence lipid metabolism, Potter et al. investigated chemical interactions between proteins and saponins (*123*). Electrophoretic studies showed that complexes of high molecular weight are gradually formed between quillaja saponins and caseins, β-casein being most susceptible. The resulting complexes differed markedly in charge and molecular weight. Soy protein did not respond in this way. Soy proteins formed insoluble aggregates that were retained in the stacking gel regardless of the presence of saponin. In experiments with gerbils, dietary saponin in conjunction with isolated soy protein did not influence the hypocholesterolemic effect of the protein, whereas feeding of saponin with casein reduced LDL cholesterol and LDL/HDL cholesterol ratios to levels typical of animals fed isolated soy protein. Thus the protein-related effect of saponins on serum lipid profiles might be explained by the finding that quillaja saponin reacts differently with different proteins. The reaction of casein with saponin may modify the protein's chemistry or structure so as to alter its influence on blood lipids.

Egg white protein and protein hydrolysate are hypocholesterolemic in rats and mice (*124*). The effect is at least as great as that of isolated soy protein when results are compared with data for casein-fed controls.

The hypercholesterolemic or hypocholesterolemic effects of certain proteins are related to their amino acid profiles. Kurowska and Carroll reported hypercholesterolemic responses of young rabbits fed selected groups of casein amino acids (*125*). The response was greatest when all essential amino acids except arginine or all ketogenic essential amino acids were fed at high levels. The hypercholesterolemic effect of lysine–leucine–methionine and lysine–methionine mixtures was confirmed. Differences in growth rates and ketogenic responses were not generally correlated with hypercholesterolemia. Thus the ketogenic properties of some essential amino acids present at high levels in several hypercholesterolemic diets did not appear to be important in the mechanism leading to elevated cholesterol. The authors suggested that hypercholesterolemic amino acids themselves (not their metabolites) act directly or indirectly to down-regulate hepatic LDL receptors.

Protein isolates from radish and spinach leaves decreased serum cholesterol levels and the atherogenic index in cholesterol-fed rats (*126*). Addition of methionine to the radish leaf isolate improved its nutritive value without making it hypercholesterolemic relative to casein. Compared to casein, spinach leaf protein with or without added methionine enhanced excretion of cholesterol and bile acids. The authors postulated that the spinach protein exerted its hypocholesterolemic action by inhibiting intestinal absorption of cholesterol and bile acids.

## Lipids and Fatty Acids

Zöllner reviewed the effect of PUFAs, MUFAs, and SFAs on serum lipids and lipoproteins, and the CHD risk associated with increments in serum cholesterol concentration (*127*). The equations of Keys and Hegsted have been modified and refined, but the original equations remain reasonable approximations for the change in total serum cholesterol effected by a specified change in saturated fat and PUFA intake. Examples of application of the Keys equation clearly demonstrated the predominant influence of the P/S ratio on cholesterol levels. Steps in the desaturation and elongation of α-linolenic

acid, linoleic acid, and oleic acid were illustrated in a summary diagram and a diagram showing the relevant chemical structures. Summary information on effects of n–3 and n–6 PUFAs on serum triacylglycerols and LDL cholesterol was presented. Dietschy et al. reviewed the liver's role in cholesterol and LDL homeostasis (*128*). They showed similarities and differences in cholesterol synthesis and metabolism among various rodent and primate species. Sections of this comprehensive review covered cholesterol synthesis and LDL cholesterol transport in the absence of dietary lipids, regulation of cholesterol synthesis and LDL cholesterol transport by dietary lipids, and genetic variability in the mechanisms of cholesterol and LDL cholesterol homeostasis.

The effect of dietary fat on serum lipid and lipoprotein levels was examined in older infants (*129*). Healthy infants 4–6 months old were randomly assigned to four feeding groups until they were 12 months old. In addition to normal table foods, they were given a cow's milk formula (~48 en% fat), a formula with a soy–coconut oil blend (~48 en% fat), or one of two similar formulas containing 36 en% of a blend of palm olein, corn oil, and safflower oil. The total dietary intake of linoleic acid of infants given cow's milk failed to meet current recommendations. These infants had the highest intakes of total, saturated, and monounsaturated fat and cholesterol and the highest serum total cholesterol levels. Infants given the lower-fat formulas had the lowest levels of serum LDL cholesterol and apoB. The authors concluded that the fat composition of cow's milk is inferior to that of commercial formulas, but that the optimal fat blend for older infants needs further definition.

In the first such population-based study, Tell et al. evaluated the relationships between dietary fat and cholesterol intake and thickness of the carotid artery wall (*130*). Subjects were adult blacks and whites from communities in North Carolina, Mississippi, Maryland, and Minnesota. Their habitual diet was assessed with a food frequency questionnaire and wall thickness was measured with B-mode ultrasound. Animal fat, saturated fat, monounsaturated fat, cholesterol, and Keys' score were positively related to wall thickness. Vegetable fat and polyunsaturated fat were inversely related to wall thickness. The associations were consistent for men and women and both racial groups. These results are consonant with the putative atherogenic and antiatherogenic properties of dietary lipids.

Epidemiologic surveys suggest that the type, rather than the quantity, of dietary fat is associated with mortality from severe cardiac arrhythmia. Charnock reported long-term feeding studies with marmoset monkeys (*Callithrix jacchus*), in which he measured mechanical performance of the cardiac muscle (*131*). Diets rich in saturated fat promoted arrhythmia when the heart was subjected to pharmacologic or ischemic stress, whereas diets rich in *n*–3 or *n*–6 PUFAs reduced pharmacologic dysrhythmia in vitro and ischemic arrhythmia in vivo. PUFA-rich diets also improved myocardial performance measured as left ventricular ejection fraction and end diastolic volume, and raised the threshold for electrical induction of ventricular fibrillation. These changes were accompanied by changes in the fatty acid composition of cardiac muscle membranes and myocardial eicosanoid synthesis. Both *n*–3 and *n*–6 PUFAs increased the prostacyclin:thromboxane ratio, but *n*–3 PUFAs were more potent in reducing levels of thromboxane. These data may explain epidemiologic findings of low rates of sudden cardiac death in populations whose diet contains low levels of saturated fat (either plant or animal), and even lower rates in populations having a regular intake of long-chain marine *n*–3 PUFAs. The data also reinforce findings from a post–myocardial infarction study suggesting that nutritional intervention can achieve reductions in sudden cardiac death unattainable with post hoc administration of antiarrhythmic drugs.

Sanders et al. studied the effects of changing from a typical Western diet to a very-low-fat vegetarian diet (10 en% fat) containing one egg per day (*132*). After 2 weeks the fat content of the vegetarian diet was increased to 20 en% by adding butter, olive oil, or safflower oil to replace an equivalent amount of carbohydrate. This diet was followed for an additional 2 weeks, with 10 subjects randomly allocated to each fat group. Each diet caused characteristic changes in the fatty acid profile of plasma lipids and lipoprotein lipids. In particular, the very-low-fat diet and diets rich in butter, olive oil, or safflower oil had different effects on plasma 20-carbon eicosanoid precursor fatty acids. The authors recommended that advice on plasma lipid–lowering take into account the effect of diet on the fatty acid profile of plasma lipids.

The long-term effects of three fat-modified diets were studied in 160 moderately hypercholesterolemic adults (*133*). The control diet contained approximately 35 en% fat representing ~14 en% saturated, ~10 en% monounsaturated, and ~4 en% polyunsaturated (35/14:10:4). The approximate corresponding compositions of the fat-modified diets were 32/10:8:8 (AHA-type), 34/11:11:5 (MUFA-enriched), and 30/12:8:3 (reduced fat). After 6 months, the AHA-type diet and MUFA-enriched diet were equally effective in improving the serum lipid profile and more effective than reducing fat intake without modifying fat type. The results suggest that MUFAs may, like PUFAs, reduce LDL cholesterol levels. However, the beneficial effect of MUFAs was seen

only in subjects of the apoE 3/3 phenotype, whereas the AHA-type diet decreased LDL cholesterol to a similar extent in phenotypes 3/3 and 4/3 + 4/4.

Cobb and Teitlebaum derived a series of equations to predict lipoprotein responsiveness to diet, based on responses of normolipidemic subjects to two metabolically controlled diets with high and low P/S ratios (*134*). Changes in total, LDL, and HDL cholesterol were significantly responsive to diet, whereas changes in triacylglycerols and VLDL cholesterol were not. ΔLDL cholesterol was predicted by age, extent of change in dietary saturated fat, and baseline LDL cholesterol level. ΔHDL cholesterol was predicted by extent of change in saturated and polyunsaturated fat and baseline HDL cholesterol level.

A controlled crossover study compared the effects of whole milk and skim milk on blood lipids in healthy young men against a background diet meeting AHA recommendations (*135*). During the two 6-week diet periods the subjects consumed 236 mL of milk per 1000 kcal. Plasma total and LDL cholesterol and apoB were significantly higher after the whole milk period. Plasma levels of HDL cholesterol, apoA-I, triacylglycerols, and fatty acids were not affected. Thus substitution of skim milk for whole milk produces a more favorable plasma lipid profile in normal men. In growing pigs, 13 weeks of feeding a diet with milk fat produced significantly higher total cholesterol levels than diets with unhydrogenated or partially hydrogenated vegetable oils (*136*). The difference was due mainly to increases in the $LDL_2$ cholesterol fraction, with some increase in HDL cholesterol. The authors concluded that milk fat caused a shift towards smaller LDL particle size, and the effects of dietary *trans* fatty acids did not differ from effects of *cis* polyunsaturated and monounsaturated fatty acids.

There have been reports that nuts have a cardioprotective effect. A reader of the paper by Sabaté et al. (see *Food Safety 1994*, chapter 3, reference *57*) offered additional hypotheses to explain beneficial effects of walnuts (*137*). One is that walnut oil is rich in α-linolenic acid (18:3*n*–3), which is slowly desaturated and elongated to 20:3*n*–3 and 22:3*n*–3. These longer-chain PUFAs competitively displace arachidonic acid in both plasma and membrane phospholipids. In addition, the PUFAs and MUFAs found in walnuts may reduce the oxidation of LDL cholesterol and thus its atherogenicity. Other readers looked at data from the Iowa Women's Health Study to confirm the findings of Sabaté et al. (*138*). CHD mortality was inversely associated with nut intake in these women, but the effect could have been due to some other characteristic of women who eat nuts rather than to the nuts. Sabaté et al.

responded to the comments of these and other readers (*139*). They agreed that walnuts contain high amounts of α-linolenic acid (6.3 g per 100 g) and could have an antiatherogenic effect in addition to their hypocholesterolemic effect—whereas the amount of α-linolenic acid in almonds, pistachios, and pecans is probably too low to measurably affect platelet function. However, although most nuts are rich in antioxidant tocopherols, their effect on LDL oxidation is speculative.

Range-fed American buffalo (*Bison bison*) have a lower total saturated fat content, including the damaging C12:0–C16:0 fatty acids, than range-fed or grain-fed beef cattle. Towle et al. studied the effect of meat from beefalo (a beef cattle–bison hybrid) on serum cholesterol in hypercholesterolemic men (*140*). A 12-week single-blind randomized crossover study was divided into two 4-week treatment periods with a 4-week washout between. During treatment periods the subjects ate 8 oz of lean ground beef or beefalo per day for 5 days each week. The total fat contents of the two ground meats were the same. Otherwise subjects maintained their normal diets and activities. Serum LDL cholesterol levels were significantly higher at the end of the beef period than at the beginning and were also significantly higher than at the end of the beefalo period. Levels did not change between the beginning and end of beefalo treatment. The authors suggested lean meat from a bison hybrid as an alternative for people who want to maintain or reduce their LDL cholesterol level.

**SATURATED FATS.** Statistical considerations and doubts concerning individual variation in the diet-responsiveness of serum cholesterol levels have complicated the interpretation of some cholesterol-lowering dietary trials. Denke and Frantz assessed the extent to which regression to the mean confounds apparent responsiveness in subgroup analysis and whether hypercholesterolemic subjects are more diet-responsive than normocholesterolemic subjects (*141*). Regression to the mean is the name given to the phenomenon that subjects who have an extremely high or low value for some variable based on a single measurement are likely to have a more moderate value if a second measurement is taken. Therefore, if subjects are grouped on the basis of one prestudy cholesterol measurement, the response to intervention is likely to be magnified—or there may appear to be a response when there really is none. The authors examined data from the Minnesota Coronary Survey Dietary Trial. When regression toward the mean was not taken into account, subjects in the top quintile of cholesterol concentration (mean 280 mg/dL) responded to a diet low in saturated fat with a 25% decrease in mean

cholesterol level, compared to a 5% decrease in subjects in the lowest quintile (mean 156 mg/dL). After correcting for regression toward the mean, these decreases were 18 and 11%, respectively. The authors concluded that the efficacy of a cholesterol-lowering diet for individuals can be overestimated or underestimated if single measurements are used to evaluate response. However, hypercholesterolemic subjects are more diet-responsive than subjects with lower cholesterol levels even after adjusting for regression toward the mean.

Glatz and Katan investigated the effects of dietary fat on cholesterol synthesis and fecal steroid excretion in healthy adults eating a high-fat diet (*142*). Subjects ate mixed, natural, high-fat (45 en%) diets, with P/S ratios of 1.9 and 0.2, for two 3-week periods. The classical balance technique and a cholesterol precursor method (measuring serum lathosterol and the ratio of lathosterol to cholesterol) were used to estimate rates of cholesterol synthesis. Both methods showed that the synthesis rate was significantly higher during the low P/S period than during the high P/S period, indicating that saturated fat stimulates whole-body cholesterol synthesis.

Emken et al. investigated the hypothesis that differences in the desaturation of palmitic and stearic acids can explain differences in their effect on serum cholesterol levels in healthy young men (*143*). They also evaluated the in vivo effect of dietary linoleic acid on Δ9-desaturase products. Subjects were fed diets containing 35 en% total fat with two different levels of linoleic acid (P/S ratio 0.3 or 0.8) for 12 days. Triacylglycerols containing 16:0 and 18:0 fatty acids labeled with deuterium at carbons number 9 and 10 were then used to follow the metabolism of these fatty acids. The percentage of 18:0 desaturated to 18:1*n*–9 was more than twice as great as the percentage of 16:0 desaturated to 16:1*n*–9. This could help explain why stearic acid (18:0) is less cholesterogenic than palmitic acid. The considerable between-subject variability suggests that some variation in the diet-responsiveness of serum cholesterol is related to the ability to desaturate saturated fatty acids. The twofold difference in the diets' linoleic acid content had little influence on desaturation or distribution of 16:0 and 18:0 among plasma lipid classes.

A double-blind crossover study with two 4-week test periods compared the effects of palmitic acid on serum cholesterol with those of lauric (12:0) plus myristic (14:0) acids (*144*). Subjects were 17 normocholesterolemic men in the Malaysian army who were sequestered in a training camp. They were given whole-food diets containing 30 en% fat and 200 mg of cholesterol, in which 5% of energy was exchanged between palmitic acid and lauric (12:0) plus myristic (14:0) acids while holding all other fatty acids constant. Serum total cholesterol levels were 9% lower and LDL cholesterol levels 11% lower after the palmitic acid period. This study adds to the evidence that not all saturated fatty acids are equally cholesterogenic.

Using data from two clinical studies examining the effects of specific saturated fatty acids on plasma total cholesterol, Kris-Etherton developed an equation to predict the effect of changes in dietary fat (*145*). The best-fitting linear regression model for change in plasma total cholesterol ($\Delta TC$) was:

$$\Delta TC = 2.3\ \Delta C14{:}0 + 3.0\ \Delta C16{:}0 - 0.8\ \Delta C18{:}0 - 1.0\ \Delta PUFA,$$

where change in intake of the fatty acid is expressed as percent of calories. The equation for change in LDL cholesterol ($\Delta LDL$) was:

$$\Delta LDL = 2.6\ \Delta C14{:}0 + 2.9\ \Delta C16{:}0 - 0.5\ \Delta C18{:}0 - 0.7\ \Delta PUFA.$$

For total cholesterol, the coefficients associated with $\Delta C14{:}0$ and $\Delta C16{:}0$ do not differ significantly from the Keys coefficient. However, Kris-Etherton's equation clearly separates stearic acid from the other long-chain saturated fatty acids and suggests that it has an independent cholesterol-lowering effect.

Elevated levels of plasma factor VII coagulant activity ($VII_c$) are associated with increased risk of CHD. The effects of fats high in stearic, palmitic, or lauric plus myristic acids on factor $VII_c$ were evaluated in a strictly controlled metabolic feeding study in healthy young men (*146*). Diets were assigned in random order for 3-week periods. Levels of total, LDL, HDL, $HDL_2$, and $HDL_3$ cholesterol, apoA-I, and apoB were lowest after the stearic acid phase and highest after the lauric plus myristic acid phase. Most differences were statistically significant. There was no effect on VLDL cholesterol. Factor $VII_c$ was significantly lower after the stearic acid phase. Another study comprised three dietary periods that maximized SFA, PUFA, and carbohydrate intake in random order for 4-week periods with a washout between (*147*). The two high-fat diets contained >50 en% fat; the high-carbohydrate diet contained <20 en% fat. Effects of the diets on factor $VII_c$ were evaluated. Compared with the low-fat phase, plasma factor $VII_c$ was 6.5% higher on the high-PUFA phase and 13.1% higher on the high-SFA phase. The plasma concentration of stearic acid was strongly associated with factor $VII_c$ ($r = .58$, $p < .0001$), an association that remained significant after adjusting for plasma concentrations of palmitic, oleic, and linoleic acids. Plasma factor VII antigen levels were higher after the saturated-fat diet than after the other two diets. The authors discussed mechanisms by which diets rich in saturated fat may shift hemostasis toward hypercoagula-

bility. Factor $VII_c$ is also associated with self-reported consumption of fatty food in middle-aged men (*148*). Among >4000 subjects, the 9% who reported avoiding fatty foods during the month before interview had factor $VII_c$ averaging 7.8% (95% CI 5.1–10.6%) lower than the rest of the subjects. The $VII_c$ difference between men who had eaten much less fatty food than usual in the last month and those who had eaten much more was 11%. This study adds to the evidence that dietary fat influences factor $VII_c$ and coagulability. Moreover, the effect is rapid, so that most of the thrombogenic risk reduction is achieved within a short time. The results suggest the value of a low-fat diet even for patients with advanced atheroma.

Morgan et al. used another approach to identify the hypercholesterolemic fat culprit (*149*). During the first week of a dietary study subjects ate their customary diets. During the next 2 weeks all subjects ate a very-low-fat diet (9 en%) including 500 g of fat-trimmed lean beef per day. For the next phase, subjects were randomly assigned to safflower oil and olive oil groups. In the 4th and 5th weeks the fat content of the diet was incrementally increased first to 20 en% and then to 30 en% by substituting the appropriate oil for carbohydrate. LDL and HDL cholesterol concentrations decreased by 13–14% and 20–25%, respectively, during the very-low-fat phase. LDL cholesterol concentrations remained low after addition of safflower oil or olive oil to the diet. The authors concluded that a reduction in saturated fat is necessary to decrease serum cholesterol and that substantial amounts of lean beef can be eaten so long as the total diet is low in saturated fat.

**MONOUNSATURATED FATS.** Abstracts of the Seventh Créteil Symposium on Lipids, Lipoproteins and Nutrition were published in *Annals of Nutrition and Metabolism* (*150*). The subject of this symposium was monounsaturated fatty acids and lipoproteins.

A dietary crossover study in Sweden found that MUFAs and PUFAs were equally effective in lowering serum cholesterol levels in hyperlipidemic adults (*151*). The diet was based on normal foods. It contained 30 en% total fat and 8% saturated fat; the P/S ratio was 0.54 in the MUFA diet and 1.39 in the PUFA diet. Both diets significantly lowered serum total, LDL, and HDL cholesterol, the LDL/HDL cholesterol ratio, apoB, apoA-I, and lipoprotein(a) [Lp(a)]. There were no significant differences between diets. Although subjects lost weight during both diet treatment periods, analysis of covariance indicated that the effects on serum lipids were caused by the qualitative dietary changes and not by weight loss. The same research group compared a diet rich in monounsaturated rapeseed oil with a diet rich in sun-flower seed oil, in a randomized study in hypercholes-terolemic adults (*152*). Again, diets were based on foods normally eaten in Sweden and contained ~30 en% fat. The two diets were equivalent for reducing concentra-tions of serum total, LDL, and HDL cholesterol, apoA-I, and apoB. However, the sunflower oil diet reduced serum triacylglycerols by 29%, compared to 14% for the rapeseed oil. On the rapeseed oil diet, 20:5*n*–3 and 22:5*n*–3 fatty acids in serum phospholipids increased; they decreased with sunflower oil.

Accelerated CAD is the major complication limit-ing long-term survival after heart transplantation. Be-cause increased platelet aggregation and lipid per-oxidation may be as damaging as hypercholesterolemia in these patients, the wisdom of a high-PUFA diet is questionable. A group of heart transplant recipients in France, who had already received dietary advice and were following a prudent diet, were advised to follow a "French" Mediterranean diet (*153*). This involved fur-ther reducing saturated fat intake while completely re-placing butter, cream, and PUFA-rich vegetable oils with olive oil or rapeseed oil. Subjects were also advised to drink moderate amounts of wine during meals. Intakes of oleic and linolenic acid were significantly increased with this diet—a beneficial change because these fatty acids reduce platelet aggregation and protect against lipid peroxidation. After 1 year on this diet platelet aggregation in response to thrombin was significantly reduced and there was an inverse correlation between linolenic acid intake and platelet aggregation ($r = -.44$, $p = .02$). A further benefit of the diet was that patients were able to reduce their immunosuppressive therapy. The authors postulated that the decrease in LDL, coupled with lack of increase in PUFAs, improved immunosup-pression by preventing induction of T-cell activation by oxidized lipoproteins. For ethical reasons this study did not include a control group.

Abbey et al. evaluated the effects of a daily supple-ment of nuts, provided against a common background diet, on serum cholesterol levels in normocholesterol-emic men (*154*). The basal diet contained 18 en% fat from meat, dairy products, vegetable oils, and fat spreads. An additional 18 en% (half the total fat intake) was provided by walnuts (PUFA-rich), almonds (MUFA-rich), or peanuts and coconut (SFA-rich). Each nut supplement was given for 3 weeks. Both almonds and walnuts sig-nificantly reduced serum total and LDL cholesterol: by 7 and 10%, respectively, for almonds and 5 and 9% for walnuts.

de Bruin et al. demonstrated differences in the postprandial metabolism of olive oil and soybean oil,

which may explain olive oil's HDL-conserving effect (*155*). They administered oral loads of vitamin A with the two fats to normolipidemic young men, using a randomized crossover study design. The slower removal of olive oil chylomicron remnants was highly correlated with hepatic lipase activity ($r = .84$, $p < .02$). HDL cholesterol concentration decreased significantly after ingestion of soybean oil, from an initial $33.5 \pm 6.5$ mg/dL to $25.4 \pm 3.8$ mg/dL after 5 and 7 h, but did not change significantly after olive oil ingestion. Soybean oil–induced decreases in HDL fractions were inversely correlated with hepatic lipase activity ($r = -.88$, $p < .02$). The authors postulated that competition between olive oil chylomicron remnants and HDL for hepatic lipase pre-vented a postprandial decrease in HDL cholesterol. Results for olive oil in this fat-loading challenge agree with results of long-term studies showing that dietary supplementation with olive oil conserves plasma HDL cholesterol and apoA-I concentrations.

Dietary studies in cynomolgus monkeys (*Macaca fascicularis*) suggested that MUFAs and PUFAs decrease LDL concentrations by different mechanisms (*156*). Ten monkeys were fed diets enriched in saturated, mono-unsaturated, or polyunsaturated fatty acids in a cross-over design comprising three 13-week periods. Both types of unsaturated fat significantly lowered plasma total and HDL cholesterol, apoA-I, and apoB. PUFAs had the greater effect, but the differences between PUFA and MUFA dietary periods were nonsignificant. Dur-ing the PUFA phase there was also a significant reduc-tion in LDL + VLDL cholesterol. The reduced levels of apoB observed during the MUFA phase could not be explained by changes in LDL apoB clearance but were probably due to decreased rates of LDL apoB produc-tion. However, enhanced LDL apoB catabolism did account for the greater reduction in LDL + VLDL cholesterol and apoB seen during PUFA, as compared to MUFA, feeding. The authors concluded that PUFAs decrease production and increase catabolism of LDL apoB.

Nestel et al. compared the effects of palmitoleic acid, a minor MUFA found in relatively large amounts in macadamia oil, with those of oleic and palmitic acids on plasma lipids in middle-aged hypercholesterolemic men (*157*). The fatty acids were taken as oil supplements in a milk beverage against a background diet containing <15 en% fat. Palmitoleic acid behaved as a saturated fatty acid, rather than a monounsaturated one, in significantly raising total and LDL cholesterol concentrations. HDL cholesterol was significantly lower with palmitoleic acid than with palmitic acid. This study did not address the possibility that higher intakes of palmitoleic acid (16:1) might increase formation of oleic acid (18:1), producing different results.

Kleinveld et al. studied the in vitro oxidation resistance, oxidation rate, and extent of oxidation of LDL from vitamin E–deficient patients and healthy controls (*158*). Unexpectedly, both the rate and extent of oxidation were greater in controls than in vitamin E–deficient patients. Lag time to oxidation, a measure of oxidation resistance, did not differ between groups and was not related to the LDL's content of vitamin E. However, the oleic/linoleic acid ratio was directly correlated with lag time and inversely correlated with oxidation rate and extent of oxidation. Thus LDL relatively rich in oleic acid and poor in linoleic acid is less susceptible to oxidative modification independently of its antioxidant content.

***TRANS* FATTY ACIDS.** A short review by Lichtenstein presented clinical and epidemiologic evidence that *trans* fatty acids resemble saturated fats in their effects on serum lipids and CHD risk (*159*). However, estimates of the *trans* fatty acid content of foods and typical diets are uncertain. Moreover, a high intake of *trans* fatty acids may be related to other elements of diet and lifestyle that increase CVD risk. The best way to limit intake of *trans* fatty acids is to reduce total fat intake and reduce or eliminate consumption of margarine and such high-fat processed foods as cookies, crackers, and fried fast-food. Applewhite argued that the food industry substitutes *trans*-containing fats for other solid (saturated) fats, not for liquid vegetable oils, and *trans* fats are not hypercholesterolemic relative to the saturated fats they replace (*160*). He feels that experiments should evaluate *trans* monoenes relative to saturated fats in the presence of *cis*-monoenes and *cis-cis* dienes. Mann hypothesized that *trans* fatty acids created during hydrogenation of polyunsaturated oils ("a mixture of isomers quite foreign to human metabolism") interfere with the function of LDL receptors (*161*). In this way they make genetically normal people resemble people with familial hypercholesterolemia, whose inherited defect in cell-surface lipoprotein receptors hampers internalization of circulating LDL cholesterol. If Mann is correct, heterozygotes for familial hypercholesterolemia may be especially helped by avoiding dietary *trans* fats. Mann suggested a number of experiments to test his hypothesis.

In a case–control study, Ascherio et al. evaluated the association between intake of *trans* fatty acids and myocardial infarction (*162*). Subjects were 239 case-patients admitted to Boston area hospitals with a first infarction and 282 community controls. After adjustment for age, sex, and energy intake, the relative risk for the highest quintile of *trans* fat consumption compared

with the lowest was 2.44 (95% CI 1.42–4.19, *p* <.0001). The association remained highly significant after further adjustment for established CHD risk factors, multivitamin use, and dietary intake of saturated fat, monounsaturated fat, linoleic acid, cholesterol, vitamin E, vitamin C, carotene, and fiber. Intake of margarine, the major source of *trans* isomers, was also significantly associated with risk of myocardial infarction. The authors pointed out that if the observed association is causal, persons in the top quintile of *trans* fat consumption could halve their risk of myocardial infarction—a benefit comparable to that expected from a 20% reduction in plasma cholesterol—simply by reducing their intake of these isomers.

Judd et al. investigated the effects of *cis* and *trans* MUFAs on plasma lipids and lipoproteins in healthy adults eating controlled diets (*163*). The study used a Latin square design and each diet was followed for 6 weeks. The four test diets, each containing 39–40 en% total fat, provided 16.7 en% oleic acid, 16.2 en% lauric + myristic + palmitic acids, 3.8 en% *trans* fatty acids, or 6.6 en% *trans* fatty acids. Compared with the high–oleic acid diet, the moderate-*trans*, high-*trans*, and saturated fat diets increased LDL cholesterol by 6.0, 7.8, and 9.0%, respectively. The moderate-*trans* diet did not affect HDL cholesterol but the high-*trans* diet lowered it by 2.8% and the saturated fat diet raised it by 3.5%. Changes in apoA-I and apoB corresponded with changes in the lipoprotein cholesterols. The authors concluded that dietary *trans* fatty acids adversely affect plasma cholesterol risk factors for heart disease, but their overall impact on health has not been adequately assessed.

**POLYUNSATURATED FATS.** Zevenbergen and Rudrum reviewed the role of PUFAs in preventing CHD and cancer (*164*). For the known physiological risk factors for CHD, PUFAs have either a neutral or a beneficial effect. Yet together these factors leave about half the risk for CHD unexplained. Dietary advice and interventions to reduce CHD are based on the impact of diet on blood lipids. However, plasma Lp(a) may be a better predictor of CHD than LDL; and dietary factors (with the possible exception of *trans* fatty acids) appear not to have an important influence on this. Lp(a) may be a link between blood lipids and the blood clotting system. Thrombosis and hemostasis are probably important in development of CHD; in fact, the rapid improvement in coronary health seen in some diet intervention trials may be better explained by an effect on hemostasis than by an effect on lipid deposition. As for fish oil, *n*–3 and *n*–6 PUFAs compete for many enzymes involved in production of prostaglandins, leukotrienes, and other lipidlike mediators. Therefore the *n*–3/*n*–6 ratio may be more important than the absolute amounts of these PUFAs that are consumed. Factor VII$_c$ and fibrinogen levels also influence CHD risk but diets high in linoleic acid or fish oil or with a high P/S ratio have little or no effect on these variables. The modified (oxidized) LDL theory of CHD could explain how LDL causes atherosclerosis and why high levels of LDL increase risk. However, there are problems with the relevance and interpretation of animal and in vitro studies on which this theory is based, and both animal and epidemiologic studies indicate a lesser rather than greater CHD risk when PUFAs are partly substituted for saturated fat. The authors also consider evidence for hypotensive and antiarrhythmic effects of PUFAs to be unconvincing. There is considerable evidence that moderate fish consumption is protective against CHD mortality, but no conclusive evidence that this is due to *n*–3 PUFAs. In connection with cancer risk, the authors briefly mentioned effects of PUFAs on lipid peroxidation, immunosuppression, and prostaglandin synthesis and again questioned the relevance of widely used animal models.

Lichtenstein et al. evaluated the effects of canola, corn, and olive oils on plasma lipids in mildly hypercholesterolemic middle-aged and elderly men and women (*165*). The oils provided two-thirds of the fat calories in diets meeting the NCEP step 2 criteria (total fat <30 en%, saturated fat <7 en%). Diets were given for 32-day periods in a randomized, crossover fashion. All three diets reduced plasma cholesterol levels. Although each diet had its own characteristic effects on some plasma lipid measures, none had a significant advantage in terms of altering the overall lipoprotein profile. Similar changes were observed in fasting and postprandial measures.

In humans, *n*–3 fatty acids show their greatest lipid-lowering effect on triacylglycerol-rich lipoproteins (*166*). Thus their therapeutic potential is greatest in patients with hypertriglyceridemia. Their effect is modified by the lipoprotein phenotype of the subject. Besides their effects on plasma lipids, *n*–3 fatty acids may have favorable effects on blood pressure, platelet function, and blood viscosity. Although all this suggests the use of *n*–3 PUFA supplements in selected patients with hypertriglyceridemia, the benefits of such therapy have not been proven.

Dietary *n*–3 and *n*–6 fatty acids undoubtedly play a role in regulating blood pressure, but the precise nature of this role in not clear. A review by Iacono and Dougherty focused on how dietary *n*–3 and *n*–6 PUFAs influence prostaglandin synthesis in humans and laboratory animals (*167*). This is important because prostaglandins are clearly involved in blood pressure regulation.

To compare the antiarrhythmic effects of *n*–3 and *n*–6 PUFAs, 10 retired breeding pairs of marmoset monkeys (*Callithrix jacchus*) were fed diets containing blends of sheep fat and fish oil or sheep fat and sunflower seed oil (*168*). After 16 weeks, ventricular fibrillation could be induced in 6 of the monkeys on each diet, using a standardized electrophysiologic protocol. The ventricular fibrillation threshold was significantly higher in the fish-oil group (33.3 ± 3.1 mA vs. 14.3 ± 4.9 mA). During myocardial ischemia, ventricular fibrillation was inducible in all animals and the threshold was lowered. Under these conditions, the threshold was also significantly higher in the fish-oil group: 22.0 ± 2.8 mA vs. 12.3 ± 3.5 mA. Topping reviewed the effects of dietary fatty acids on experimental cardiac arrhythmias in rats (*169*), citing mainly studies by McLennan et al. Fish oil is also protective against arrhythmia in rats. Sunflower seed oil confers less protection, and olive oil yields the same frequency of arrhythmia as saturated fat. Other studies using the rat model showed that the incidence and duration of cardiac arrhythmia was significantly less in animals fed α-linolenic acid–rich canola oil or eicosapentaenoic acid–rich fish oil than in animals fed sheep fat (*170*). Although beef phospholipids contain small amounts of eicosapentaenoic acid (EPA) and the amount can be enhanced by fish-oil feeding, feeding such meat did not reduce arrhythmia. However, large amounts of lean beef could be fed without compromising the antiarrhythmic effect of fish oil or canola oil.

Sanigorski et al. investigated whether eicosanoid changes seen in butter-fed rats resulted more from decreased arachidonic acid levels or increased long-chain *n*–3 PUFAs (*171*). Rats were fed high-fat diets containing hydrogenated beef fat alone or with ethyl arachidonate, safflower oil, or a safflower oil–linseed oil mixture. Serum thromboxane levels were highly responsive to *n*–3 PUFAs, whereas aortic prostacyclin levels were more influenced by the level of arachidonic acid in the tissue phospholipids. This study also illustrated that assessment of eicosanoid biosynthesis in vitro can be influenced by the sampling technique.

Kawashima and Kozuka determined the effects of perilla- and fish-oil feeding on hepatic lipids and peroxisomal β-oxidation in rats and mice (*172*). Fish oil increased the content of 20:5*n*–3, 22:5*n*–3, and 22:6*n*–3; perilla oil increased the content of 18:3*n*–3, 20:5*n*–3, and 22:5*n*–3. The 20- and 22-carbon 5*n*–3 PUFAs apparently increased the activity of peroxisomal β-oxidation, whereas elevated 22:6*n*–3 in hepatic lipids was associated with lower levels of circulating cholesterol. Peroxisomal β-oxidation is of interest because administration of peroxisome proliferators such as clofibric acid or perfluorooctanoic acid depresses the detoxification activities of glutathione-dependent enzymes and in the long term induces hepatomas and hepatocellular carcinomas. However, the increased activity produced by fish-oil feeding was only 20–30% of the maximum activities induced by peroxisome proliferators. Moreover, neither fish oil nor perilla oil inhibited glutathione peroxidase or glutathione $S$-transferase activity in this study. The authors concluded that the toxic risk associated with $n$–3-rich dietary oils is much lower than that of the artificial peroxisome proliferators. They speculated that the increased activity of peroxisomal β-oxidation produced by the dietary oils facilitates formation of 22:6$n$–3 to supply the requirement of the brain and retina.

The percentage of linoleic acid in adipose tissue is used to indicate long-term dietary intake. A population-based case–control study showed that the adipose-tissue content of linoleic acid is inversely related to the risk of sudden cardiac death (173). Case-subjects were 84 men who died of CAD within 24 h of the onset of symptoms and had no history of CHD or medically treated hyperlipidemia. Healthy age-matched male controls were drawn from records of the general practitioners with whom the cases were registered. In the control population, the estimated relative risk of sudden cardiac death was 5.7 (95% CI 1.8–17.9) for the lowest quintile of adipose-tissue linoleic acid and 4.0 (95% CI 1.2–12.9) for the next lowest quintile, compared with the highest quintile. The estimated adjusted proportionate increase in risk of sudden cardiac death was 1.14 (95% CI 1.03–1.23) for each 1% reduction in the percentage of linoleic acid. However, the adipose tissue concentration of linoleic acid was positively associated with the degree of CAD in a cross-sectional study of 226 patients undergoing coronary angiography (174). Platelet linoleic acid concentration was also positively associated with CAD. The authors hypothesized that high linoleic acid intake may be a risk factor for coronary atherosclerosis, whereas low intake may be a risk factor for coronary events. They did not elaborate on this apparent paradox. The EPA concentration in platelets was inversely associated with CAD in men; docosapentaenoic acid (DHA) concentration in platelets was inversely associated with CAD in women. These findings are consistent with other observations suggesting that fish, fish oil, and $n$–3 PUFAs derived from fish and fish oils have a beneficial influence on macrovascular disease.

A study by Davis et al. suggested the potential for using modified-fat cheese products to help reduce plasma cholesterol levels in specific individuals and perhaps in the general population (175). One hundred grams per day of a linoleate-enriched mozzarella cheese product,

substituted into the normal diet of hypercholesterolemic adults with no other changes in diet or habits, significantly reduced LDL cholesterol compared with both the baseline level (–11 mg/dL, 95% CI –5 to –16 mg/dL) and the level during consumption of partial skim-milk mozzarella (–15 mg/dL, 95% CI –8 to –27 mg/dL). HDL cholesterol, plasma triacylglycerols, apoA-I, and apoB-100 were unaltered. Men and women responded similarly.

Borage oil is a particularly rich source of γ-linolenic acid (18:3$n$–6), which is elongated to dihomo-γ-linolenic acid (20:3$n$–6). Interest in increasing the ratio of dihomo-γ-linolenic acid to arachidonic acid in human tissues is based on the expected increase in prostaglandin $E_1$ (thought to have platelet antiaggregatory potential) relative to the proaggregatory eicosanoids derived from arachidonic acid (20:4$n$–6). However, a 42-day borage oil–feeding experiment in healthy men resulted in increased platelet aggregation on days 22 and 43, despite a significant increase in the 20:3$n$–6/20:4$n$–6 ratio (176). There were no significant changes in thromboxane $A_2$ or prostaglandin $E_1$ or $E_2$ formation or in their ratios. The authors hypothesized that γ-linolenic acid, some other component of borage oil, or a noneicosanoid mechanism was responsible for this unexpected result.

Finnish investigators measured changes in plasma lipid parameters when olive or canola oil was substituted for margarine on bread (177). Subjects had serum total cholesterol levels ranging from 190 to 330 mg/dL and normally ate at least 3 slices of bread with margarine per day. Except for the substitute fats, which were used on bread in accordance with established habits, subjects maintained their usual diets throughout the 6-week fat substitution. The replacement accounted for 16% of total fat intake on average, but varied considerably among subjects. Canola oil produced dose-dependent increases in total plasma oleic and α-linolenic acids and an increase in EPA in plasma phospholipids, as well as a slight decrease in LDL cholesterol and increase in HDL cholesterol. Olive oil caused a dose-related increase in total plasma oleic acid and a decrease in linoleic acid. The results suggest competitive interactions among dietary fatty acids, particularly for α-linolenic acid. Rapeseed oil's effects were attributed to α-linolenic and linoleic acids and suggest that modest substitution of this oil for other fats can favorably influence lipid parameters, preventing an excessive reduction of linoleic acid in plasma phospholipids that might increase CHD risk. Other investigators reported that dietary α-linolenic acid alters tissue fatty acid composition but not levels of blood lipids or lipoproteins (178). Subjects in this crossover study were healthy young men who ate controlled diets for 8-week periods. The basal diet contained ~23 en% fat; the test diet contained ~29 en% fat providing 6.3 en% of α-linolenic acid from flaxseed oil. Flaxseed oil did not alter factors associated with risk of atherosclerosis—serum triacylglycerols, cholesterol, HDL, LDL, apoA-I, apoB, or coagulation status. However, plasma and peripheral blood mononuclear cell lipids were enriched in α-linolenic acid, EPA, and DHA.

Because of competitive interactions between fatty acids, the dietary α-linolenic/linoleic acid ratio is of interest. Chan et al. studied how the amount of 18:3*n*–3 and the 18:3*n*–3/18:2*n*–6 ratio influence the fatty acid profile of platelet and plasma phospholipids (*179*). Normolipidemic young men were given four diets consisting of conventional foods, identical except for the sources of added fat. A low level of α-linolenic acid was coupled with a low 18:3*n*–3/18:2*n*–6 ratio; intermediate levels were coupled with intermediate and high 18:3*n*–3/18:2*n*–6 ratios; and a high level was coupled with a high 18:3*n*–3/18:2*n*–6 ratio. Phospholipid levels of 18:1*n*–9, 18:2*n*–6, and 18:3*n*–3 reflected the fatty acid composition of the diet. However, levels of longer-chain *n*–3 PUFAs, particularly 20:5*n*–3, were influenced by both the absolute amount of 18:3*n*–3 and the 18:3*n*–3/18:2*n*–6 ratio. Significantly more 6-keto-PGF$_{1\alpha}$ was produced after the diet with the high linolenic acid content and high linolenic/linoleic ratio than after the low-content, low-ratio diet, although dietary fat did not affect bleeding time or thromboxane B$_2$ production. Thus prostanoid production was related to diet-induced differences in phospholipid fatty acid patterns. Another dietary study of healthy young men found that in vitro platelet aggregation decreases as the ratio of α-linolenic to linoleic acid increases, when the diet is rich in monounsaturated fat (*180*).

In African green monkeys (*Cercopithecus aethiops*), early dietary intervention may reduce later CHD risk (*181*). Females with nursing infants were fed one of two semipurified diets that provided 40 en% fat, 40 en% carbohydrate, 20 en% protein, and 0.8 mg/kcal of cholesterol. This mimics an American diet in fat content. One diet had a P/S ratio of 0.3 and the other had a P/S ratio of 2.5. Infants, after weaning, were assigned to the diet of their mother. Age, sex, and dietary fat type independently influenced plasma lipid and apolipoprotein concentrations in the offspring. Before weaning, plasma total cholesterol and apoB were lower in high-P/S animals; this pattern was maintained into young adulthood. Lower concentrations of plasma triacylglycerols, HDL cholesterol, and apoA-I in response to the high P/S diet appeared only after weaning, when animals were 6–60 months old. Implications of the findings for human families and public health were discussed.

Horrobin reviewed the metabolism of *n*–3 and *n*–6 essential fatty acids and how this is related to vascular disease (*182*). In relation to this he considered the relative dietary intake of essential and other fatty acids and factors influencing it. He discussed some biologic effects of essential fatty acids, which include lowering plasma cholesterol and triacylglycerol levels and blood pressure, inhibiting platelet aggregation and smooth muscle proliferation, and preventing fatal arrhythmias. The metabolites of linoleic and α-linolenic acid may be more important than the parent fatty acids themselves.

Conjugated linoleic acid (CLA), best known for its anticarcinogenic effects, also has antioxidant and antiatherogenic activity (*183*). One group of 6 rabbits was fed an atherogenic diet for 22 weeks; another group was fed this diet augmented with 0.5 g of CLA per rabbit per day. By 12 weeks total and LDL cholesterol, triacylglycerols, and ratios of LDL and total cholesterol to HDL cholesterol were substantially lower in the CLA-fed rabbits. These rabbits also had less severe aortic atherosclerosis.

Interest in the cardiovascular effects of the *n*–3 PUFAs in marine oils continues (*184–215*). Alaskan Eskimos who subsist on marine fish and mammals continue to have a death rate from circulatory diseases less than one-third that of the white U.S. population. Plasma concentrations of *n*–3 fatty acids are higher in coastal village than in river village Eskimos and are significantly higher than *n*–3 levels in urban non-native controls (*184*). Arachidonic acid concentrations, while lower than those in non-native controls, are within the normal range and do not result in abnormal bleeding times.

Subbaiah et al. studied the incorporation of 20:5*n*–3 and 22:6*n*–3 into plasma phosphatidylcholine and cholesteryl ester, in an attempt to explain differences in the biological effects of these two *n*–3 PUFAs (*185*). Whereas the time course of incorporation of 20:5*n*–3 showed a precursor–product relationship, the 22:6*n*–3 concentration was markedly lower in cholesteryl ester than in phosphatidylcholine and the 20:5*n*–3/22:6*n*–3 ratio was substantially higher in cholesteryl ester than in phosphatidylcholine at all times. In vitro experiments indicated that 22:6*n*–3 is a poor substrate for lecithin–cholesterol acyltransferase.

Rats were fed semipurified diets containing 15% corn oil or sea lion oil with and without cholesterol, and the effects on plasma lipids and liver histochemistry were determined (*186*). Relative to corn oil, sea lion oil reduced plasma lipid levels and caused histochemical changes associated with increased hepatic excretion of lipids. These differences were seen regardless of whether the diet contained cholesterol. Liver cholesterol concentrations were not influenced by the type of dietary oil. Although sea lion oil reduced plasma lipids, it is possible, according to histologic findings, that it had some potentially detrimental effects associated with degradation of lysosomes or activation of peroxisomes. Another study in rats showed that dietary *n*–3 fatty acids significantly reduce ischemic and excitotoxic brain damage (*187*). Because excitotoxic damage mediated by activation of NMDA receptors has been implicated in many neurodegenerative conditions, the authors suggest that modification of dietary fatty acids might benefit a variety of patients. Such dietary treatment does not provide instantaneous results and therefore would be useless in cases of acute stroke; but it could help persons with chronic and progressive neurodegeneration or high risk of stroke.

Kristensen et al. briefly reviewed effects of fish oil on IHD (*188*). They discussed the relationship between *n*–3 PUFAs and cardiovascular risk factors and clinical studies in IHD patients. They believe there is enough evidence that eating fish protects against IHD to justify large-scale trials in patients with acute myocardial infarction and unstable angina pectoris and also in patients undergoing coronary bypass surgery or percutaneous transluminal coronary angioplasty. Aucamp et al. reported a randomized, placebo-controlled, crossover trial of low-dose fish oil in treating elderly patients with stable angina pectoris (*189*). The number of angina attacks and the number of isosorbide dinitrate tablets required to abort an attack were significantly reduced during the fish oil phase. Moreover, in patients who received fish oil first, an after-effect of fish oil persisted throughout the subsequent 12-week placebo period.

Sassen et al. reviewed studies on fish oil and other factors affecting atherogenesis, emphasizing fish oil's potential to prevent atherosclerosis or promote its regression (*190*). The veno-arterial autograft model mimics the situation in patients after coronary bypass grafting. In this model, dietary fish oil is consistently effective in preventing accelerated graft intima proliferation. The authors consider studies on restenosis after percutaneous transluminal angioplasty and on regression of experimental atherosclerosis to be inconclusive. However, a metaanalysis of results of four studies that used angiography to define coronary restenosis indicated that supplemental fish oil does reduce restenosis after coronary angioplasty (*191*). The absolute difference in restenosis rates between treatment and control groups was 13.9% (95% CI 3.2–24.5%). Based on this pooled estimate, a physician would have to treat 7 patients to prevent restenosis in 1. There was a positive linear relationship between fish oil dose and the absolute differ-

ence in restenosis rates ($r = .99$, $p < .03$). However, possible harmful effects of prolonged high-dose fish oil treatment have not been adequately investigated. When data were included from three studies that used stress testing to determine restenosis, the risk difference was only 5.1% (95% CI –3.8 to 13.9%).

Frankel et al. studied the effect of fish oil supplementation on the oxidation of LDL (*192*). Blood samples were taken from hypertriglyceridemic subjects enrolled in a randomized clinical trial of fish oil. LDL samples were prepared by density ultracentrifugation and exhaustively dialyzed against deoxygenated phosphate-buffered saline. Fish oil intake did not alter the oxidative susceptibility of the LDL, but chemically modified LDL particles from the fish oil and placebo periods generated distinct patterns of volatile oxidation products that reflected differences in their fatty acid composition.

In an Italian study of 16 patients with primary hyperlipidemia, 30 days of low-dose supplementation with fish oil significantly reduced serum triacylglycerol (–43.4%) and total cholesterol (–5.6%) levels and increased HDL cholesterol (20.2%) (*193*). Another trial in hypertriglyceridemic patients found that plasma triacylglycerol levels were 37% lower after 4 wk of supplementation with *n*–3 fatty acid ethyl esters and $HDL_2$ cholesterol was 56% higher (*194*). However, LDL cholesterol was also increased (by 23%) and lipoproteins were more susceptible to oxidation during supplementation. These changes occurred rapidly, and values returned to baseline within 10 days after supplementation was stopped. Bleeding time did not change. The authors concluded that *n*–3 fatty acid ethyl esters are effective hypotriglyceridemic agents but their impact on atherogenesis is unclear, because some risk factors are affected favorably and others unfavorably.

Salvi et al. evaluated the effect of fish oil supplements on serum Lp(a) concentrations in patients with heterozygous familial hypercholesterolemia who were being treated with the HMG-CoA reductase inhibitor simvastatin (*195*). After 4 weeks serum total and LDL cholesterol and triacylglycerols were significantly reduced. However, there was no significant change in HDL cholesterol or Lp(a). Another study evaluated the effects of *n*–3 fatty acids and the HMG-CoA reductase inhibitor pravastatin on plasma lipids and lipoproteins in patients with combined hyperlipidemia (*196*). Pravastatin treatment significantly reduced plasma total and LDL cholesterol and apoB. The LDL Stokes' diameter did not change. Fish oil significantly reduced plasma triacylglycerols and increased the LDL Stokes' diameter. An increase in LDL cholesterol was nonsignificant. There were no changes in the placebo group. After 12 weeks of combined therapy with pravastatin and fish oil there were significant decreases in total and LDL cholesterol, triacylglycerols, and apoB. None of the treatments influenced HDL or apoA-I levels. Pravastatin nonsignificantly reduced IDL, fish oil significantly reduced VLDL, and combined treatment significantly reduced both IDL and VLDL.

Dagnelie et al. investigated possible mechanisms by which dietary fish oil might reduce serum triacylglycerol levels (*197*). Groups of subjects supplemented their diet with 30 g/d of either fish oil or olive oil placebo. Blood concentrations of triacylglycerols and free fatty acids were significantly reduced after only 1 d of fish oil supplementation. There were no significant changes in levels of insulin, glucose, or ketone bodies. However, after fish oil, free fatty acid levels were significantly correlated with levels of ketone bodies and triacylglycerols. These findings are consistent with the hypothesis that hepatic β-oxidation contributes to reduced triacylglycerol levels after *n*–3 fatty acid supplementation. Turnover studies are needed to quantify these processes. In another study, subjects took a single 20-g dose of fish oil or corn oil at their evening meal and the effect on plasma lipids and lipoproteins was evaluated 14 h later (*198*). Fish oil had a pronounced hypotriglyceridemic effect, which was directly related to the initial triacylglycerol level. Both *n*–3 and *n*–6 PUFAs reduced serum total cholesterol. VLDL and HDL cholesterol also decreased significantly after fish oil.

Kim et al. investigated the effects of fish oil on atherogenesis and thrombogenesis in swine fed a hyperlipidemic diet (*199*). Fish oil–supplemented animals had significantly fewer adherent monocytes over endothelial lesions and greatly reduced counts of platelet clumps (microthrombi) attached to adherent monocytes or directly to the endothelium. Surprisingly, however, lesion growth was not retarded despite the reduction in attached monocytes and platelet clumps. This suggests that plasma cholesterol is the major factor controlling lesion growth in this model.

Studies of the hypotriglyceridemic effect of EPA in rats revealed that the almost instantaneous hypolipidemia produced by this *n*–3 fatty acid might be explained by a sudden increase in mitochondrial fatty acid oxidation (*200*). This would reduce the availability of fatty acids for hepatic synthesis of lipids to be exported in forms such as VLDL. Continuing administration of EPA induced peroxisomal fatty acid oxidation and inhibited activity of various enzymes involved in triacylglycerol biosynthesis and lipogenesis.

Several research groups reported effects of fish oil on blood pressure in hypertensive and borderline-hypertensive subjects (*201–206*). Appel performed a metaanalysis of controlled clinical trials to answer the question "does supplementation of diet with fish oil reduce blood pressure" (*201*). Of 11 trials that enrolled normotensive subjects, 2 found a reduction in systolic pressure and 1 in diastolic pressure. Of 6 trials that enrolled untreated hypertensive subjects, 2 found significant reductions in systolic pressure and 4 in diastolic pressure. The duration of 13 of these 17 trials was <3 months. The magnitude of blood-pressure reduction was greatest when blood pressure was high but was not significantly associated with dose of fish oil. The authors concluded that supplementation with *n*–3 PUFAs can produce clinically relevant blood pressure reductions in subjects with untreated hypertension but long-term efficacy and patient compliance have not been demonstrated. Another metaanalysis, by Morris et al., concluded that fish oil has a dose-related hypotensive effect (*202*). The effect appears strongest in subjects with hypertension, clinical atherosclerosis, or hypercholesterolemia. A randomized, double-blind, crossover comparison of olive oil and fish oil found that a moderate dose of fish oil for 6 weeks reduced diastolic blood pressure, intracellular free platelet calcium, and plasma triacylglycerols in subjects with essential hypertension (*203*). The decrease in intracellular free platelet calcium was apparently not due to diminished responsiveness of the calcium messenger system to thrombin. A study of healthy 30- to 60-year-old men evaluated the effects of incorporating fatty fish or fish oil into reduced-sodium diets containing 30 and 40 en% fat (*204,205*). Addition of fish, fish oil, or both to the high-fat diet increased serum total, LDL, HDL, and $HDL_2$ cholesterol and reduced triacylglycerols. Fatty fish added to the 30% fat, reduced-sodium diet produced a more favorable plasma lipid profile than the "normal" 40% fat diet or the 40% diet supplemented with fish and/or fish oil. The 30% fat control diet reduced all plasma cholesterol parameters but did not influence triacylglycerols. Blood pressure effects of fish and fish oil were small but favorable. The fall in blood pressure was related to the increase in *n*–3 and decrease in *n*–6 PUFAs in platelet phospholipids, and lower heart rates in supplemented groups were related to changes in platelet *n*–3 and *n*–6 fatty acids. In phase I of the Trials of Hypertension Prevention, supplementation with 6 g/d of fish oil had no significant overall effect on blood pressure in normotensive adults (*206*). Nor was there a tendency of fish oil to reduce blood pressure more in subjects with baseline pressure in the highest quartile, with low habitual fish consumption, or low baseline levels of plasma *n*–3 fatty acids. Fish oil did significantly increase $HDL_2$ cholesterol in women, but not in men. The authors concluded that moderate amounts of fish oil are unlikely to lower blood pressure in normotensive people but may increase $HDL_2$ cholesterol in women.

Malle and Kostner reviewed the effects of fish oils on lipid variables and platelet function indexes (207). They discussed the function and requirements of n–3 fatty acids, their absorption and metabolism, their susceptibility to oxidation, and their effect on the fibrinolytic system. Several research groups reported work on fish oil and platelet function (208–211). Because fish oil tends to reduce platelet aggregability, a common side effect is prolongation of bleeding time. This is desirable in some situations, undesirable in others. Swails et al. conducted a prospective study of platelet aggregation in 16 surgical patients who were randomly assigned to usual care or a diet containing ~14 g/d of fish oil (208). No significant effect on platelet aggregability was seen after 1 week. The authors concluded that at this dose, short-term supplementation with fish oil does not alter platelet function in hospitalized surgical patients. Because docosahexaenoic acid (DHA) affects some platelet functions more potently than EPA, Scheurlen et al. tested supplements providing EPA and DHA at ratios of 1.33 and 0.54 for their effect on platelet aggregation in healthy men (209). Both supplements caused only a nonsignificant increase in bleeding time and neither significantly influenced collagen- or ADP-induced aggregation. However, the two supplements had very different effects on platelet responsiveness to the stable prostaglandin–endoperoxide analogue U 46619. At the high EPA/DHA ratio the concentration of U 46619 required for half-maximum aggregation was unchanged while the Hill coefficient decreased from 6.2 to 3.3. At the high DHA level, the U 46619 dose for half-maximum aggregation increased from 0.3 to 1.4 μM. The authors concluded that EPA and DHA have different effects on the platelet thromboxane/endoperoxide-amplifying system, DHA perhaps acting directly on the presentation of the endoperoxide receptor and/or on postreceptor events. The higher dose of DHA (low EPA/DHA ratio) also increased platelet sensitivity to iloprost. Some inconsistent results of fish oil studies might be due to use of materials differing in their EPA/DHA ratio. Mundal et al. hypothesized a synergistic effect of nifedipine (a calcium channel blocker) and fish oil on platelet function (210). They tested this in hypertensive, hyperlipidemic men who were otherwise healthy. In a double-blind, placebo-controlled design, subjects received n–3 supplements for 4-week periods with a washout period between. Nifedipine was then added to the n–3 PUFA or placebo treatment for an additional 4 weeks. The fatty acid treatment alone did not change platelet count, platelet volume, median plasma

β-thromboglobulin concentration, skin bleeding time, supine mean blood pressure, or heart rate. Nifedipine significantly increased plasma β-thromboglobulin and reduced supine mean blood pressure in all subjects. None of the other variables was affected. These results do not support the hypothesis. The effect of nifedipine on β-thromboglobulin release was unexpected. Finally, experiments in rats showed that fish oil supplementation for 8 weeks significantly reduces the size of experimental myocardial infarcts, whereas 1 week of supplementation does not (211). The reduction in infarct size is associated with altered platelet function and platelet content of EPA and DHA.

Chin reviewed the effects of marine oils on cardiovascular reactivity (212). Major topics were IHD, cardiac function, arrhythmias, blood pressure, blood rheology, and atherosclerosis. Chin concluded that n–3 PUFAs can lower blood pressure and prevent atherosclerosis, thus preventing the vascular occlusion that leads to myocardial infarction and ventricular arrhythmias. The ways in which marine oils exert their cardioprotective effects should be viewed as a web in which all relevant factors are linked. Underlying many observed effects is the incorporation of EPA and DHA at the expense of arachidonic acid and the alterations in prostanoid profile that follow.

In an interesting study, Shiina et al. compared the ability of EPA, DHA, oleic acid, and linoleic acid to inhibit the in vitro proliferation of PUFA-rich vascular smooth muscle cells (213). Only EPA and DHA inhibited incorporation of [$^3$H]thymidine into cultured cells. The effect was dose-related and EPA was more potent than DHA. However, the effect of EPA was suppressed by addition of antioxidants (vitamin E or BHT). This suppression was also dose-related, and 10 μM BHT virtually abolished the inhibitory effect of 80 μM EPA. The authors postulate that it was oxidized derivatives of EPA, produced at low levels, that inhibited proliferation of the vascular smooth muscle cells. This could partly explain the antiatherosclerotic action of marine lipids.

Lervang et al. evaluated the effect of very-long-chain n–3 PUFA supplementation on some CHD risk markers in healthy young adults (214). A randomized, placebo-controlled, double-blind design was used. Daily intake of 0.65 g of the supplement for 8 weeks had no significant effect on any risk factor evaluated: plasma level of lipids, fibrinogen, factor VII, or plasminogen activator inhibitor; whole-blood aggregation; or aggregability of neutrophil leukocytes.

Huff et al. attempted to define the mechanisms responsible for some of fish oil's effects (215). To do this they determined lipolytic enzyme activity, lipoprotein density gradient profiles, and LDL receptor activity in miniature pigs fed fish oil or corn oil. The results indicated that the increased conversion of VLDL apoB to LDL was not related to increased activity of postheparin plasma lipoprotein lipase or hepatic triacylglycerol lipase or to changes in the density distribution of VLDL. However, it could result from a decrease in LDL receptor activity.

CHOLESTEROL. Spady et al. reviewed data from humans and experimental animals on the regulation of plasma LDL cholesterol by dietary cholesterol and fatty acids (*216*). From mathematical models of the data, they concluded that steady-state plasma LDL cholesterol levels are determined largely by the rate of LDL cholesterol formation and the activity of LDL receptors, located mainly in the liver. Increased net delivery of cholesterol to the liver suppresses receptor activity, slightly increases LDL cholesterol formation, and modestly increases the level of LDL cholesterol. Dietary C12–C16 saturated fatty acids enhance all these changes. The *cis* isomers of dietary 18:1*n*–9 and 18:2*n*–9 fatty acids restore hepatic receptor activity, decrease the rate of LDL cholesterol formation, and modestly reduce plasma LDL cholesterol levels. Short-chain saturated fatty acids (C4–C10), 18:0, and the *trans* isomer of 18:1*n*–9 have no measurable effect on any parameter of LDL cholesterol metabolism; they will alter plasma LDL cholesterol levels only to the extent that they replace active saturated or unsaturated fatty acids. The authors maintain that all the effects of dietary cholesterol and fatty acids can be explained by their effects on the size of the regulatory pool of cholesterol in hepatocytes.

Lichtenstein et al. evaluated the hypercholesterolemic effect of dietary cholesterol in diets enriched in corn oil or beef tallow (*217*). Subjects were healthy hypercholesterolemic adults 46–78 years old. They ate 5 isocaloric diets in sequence, each for 32 days. A baseline diet (35 en% fat: 13 en% saturated, 12 en% monounsaturated, 8 en% polyunsaturated) was followed by four fat-reduced (29 en%) diets—one based on corn oil and one on beef tallow, each one with and without egg yolks to provide ~200 mg of additional cholesterol per 1000 kcal. Reducing the fat content of the diet lowered concentrations of total, LDL, and HDL cholesterol. LDL cholesterol decreased more in response to corn oil than to beef tallow. LDL apoB concentrations reflected total cholesterol. Diet had no significant influence on apoA-I. Addition of egg yolks to the corn oil diet elevated total, LDL, and HDL cholesterol, whereas egg yolk added to the beef tallow diet increased only total and LDL cholesterol. The authors concluded that even in a reduced-fat diet,

beef tallow has an unfavorable effect on plasma lipids—particularly when the diet also contains moderate amounts of cholesterol.

If 14:0 and 18:2 are the only fatty acids that influence plasma cholesterol when LDL receptor activity is not impaired, then when these fatty acids are held constant the exchange of 18:1 for 16:0 should have no effect on plasma cholesterol. The effects of exchanging up to 10% of dietary energy between oleic and palmitic acids, with and without 0.3 wt% dietary cholesterol, were evaluated in normocholesterolemic cebus monkeys (*Cebus albifrons*) (*218*). Palmitic acid raised plasma LDL cholesterol (relative to oleic acid) only when the intake of cholesterol was high. Although cholesterol levels and kinetics did not differ between the two cholesterol-free diets, the 16:0-rich diet produced significantly higher triacylglycerol concentrations. Addition of cholesterol to the 16:0-enriched diet increased total and LDL cholesterol and further elevated triacylglycerol concentrations. The higher LDL level was associated with an elevated pool of LDL apoB. The authors concluded that 16:0 is hypercholesterolemic only when LDL receptors are down-regulated by high levels of dietary cholesterol. Even then, the impact of 16:0 is less than that of the cholesterol itself—suggesting that the greatest improvement in LDL receptor activity and plasma LDL would stem from restricting dietary cholesterol. The authors suggest that these results apply to hypercholesterolemic people as well as to cebus monkeys.

A study in rabbits showed that the fatty acid composition of a high-cholesterol diet influences cholesterol peroxidation and accumulation of cholesterol and oxysterols in the aorta (*219*). Plasma cholesterol levels in cholesterol-fed animals rose to a similar extent whether the dietary fat was corn oil or beef tallow. However, cupric ion–induced peroxidation of lipoprotein cholesterol was significantly greater in the corn oil group and the difference persisted for 5 weeks after animals were switched to a basic chow diet. The aortic content of cholesterol and cholesterol oxides was also significantly higher in the corn oil group at the end of the experiment (after the chow diet period), and aortic content of malondialdehyde appeared higher in these animals. The effects of oxidized cholesterol on cholesterol absorption were studied in lymph-cannulated rats (*220*). When emulsified lipid containing a tracer amount of [$^{14}$C]cholesterol and 50 mg of either cholesterol or oxidized cholesterols was administered intragastrically, oxidized cholesterols simultaneously interfered with the lymphatic absorption of cholesterol and oleic acid as triolein. Although the reduction of lymph flow might partly account for this, the authors have observed that these two parameters are not necessarily related. These findings should be of interest because the consumption of oxidized cholesterols in processed foods is increasing.

A crossover study in Denmark tested whether addition of two boiled eggs to the usual daily diet would increase levels of HDL cholesterol in healthy adults (*221*). Blood was sampled before, during, and after 6 weeks of extra egg consumption. Serum HDL cholesterol increased by 10% and total cholesterol increased by 4%. LDL cholesterol, serum triacylglycerols, and the ratio of total to HDL cholesterol did not change significantly. The authors concluded that healthy people need not restrict a moderate egg intake. Another study produced different results (*222*). The cholesterolemic effect of eggs enriched in *n*–3 PUFAs was evaluated in male university students who added 2 regular or 2 PUFA-enriched eggs to their usual daily diet for 18 d. Plasma total and LDL cholesterol were increased by regular eggs but were unchanged by consumption of PUFA-enriched eggs. Moreover, regular eggs did not influence plasma HDL cholesterol or triacylglycerols, whereas PUFA-enriched eggs increased HDL cholesterol levels and decreased triacylglycerols. Regular eggs tended to decrease ratios of HDL cholesterol to LDL and total cholesterol, whereas PUFA-enriched eggs tended to increase these ratios. These results show that the cholesterolemic properties of hen's eggs can be modified by altering the fatty acid composition of yolk lipids.

Subjects with ileostomies are frequently enlisted for studies of absorption and excretion from the small bowel. In one such study, healthy ileostomy subjects were given [$^3$H]cholesterol and [$^{14}$C]β-sitosterol in the same meal in conjunction with controlled diets consisting of normal foods and containing 150 or 450 mg/d of cholesterol (*223*). Each diet was eaten for 3 d, with a 4-d washout period between. Fractional cholesterol absorption increased but absolute cholesterol absorption decreased with the low cholesterol intake. Endogenous cholesterol excretion did not change, but net cholesterol excretion (output minus intake) was 37% higher on the low-cholesterol diet. The authors concluded that the immediate response of net cholesterol excretion to a change in dietary cholesterol is mediated by rapid changes in absorption efficiency.

Duane reported a metabolic ward study of biliary and fecal steroid outputs during four randomly allocated treatments (*224*). The treatments were low- and high-cholesterol diets, each with and without lovastatin. Each treatment lasted 6–7 weeks. No significant interactions between lovastatin and dietary cholesterol were seen. The high-cholesterol diet significantly lowered cholesterol balance but increased systemic cholesterol input and fecal output of acidic sterols. The primary action of lovastatin appeared to be to lower cholesterol synthesis and systemic cholesterol input; the main compensatory response was reduced biliary cholesterol secretion.

Barness reviewed the nutritional requirements of infants and children for cholesterol and related compounds (*225*). He presented cholesterol as a series of enigmas. Cholesterol is an essential metabolite and human milk contains significant quantities of it, yet human infants seem to thrive on cholesterol-free diets. On the one hand, recommendations to lower serum cholesterol are widespread; on the other, low serum cholesterol is associated with poorly understood morbidity. It is widely known that high-fat diets increase serum cholesterol, whereas in most people dietary cholesterol has relatively little impact. Overall, the need for dietary cholesterol has not been established. Barness suggests that the Smith–Lemli–Opitz syndrome, which is characterized by extremely low levels of serum cholesterol, is similar to other inborn metabolic errors for which dietary supplements can compensate; it also might provide a human model for evaluating the absorption and metabolism of dietary cholesterol. Wong et al. studied the effect of dietary cholesterol on cholesterol synthesis in breast-fed and formula-fed infants (*226*). Breast-fed infants had significantly higher cholesterol intakes and plasma levels of total and LDL cholesterol. In both groups, the fractional synthesis rate of cholesterol was significantly inversely related to dietary cholesterol ($r = -.66$, $p = .002$). The data show that dietary cholesterol is the predominant factor affecting plasma total cholesterol concentrations and cholesterol synthesis in infants and suggest that cholesterol synthesis is efficiently regulated via HMG-CoA reductase when dietary levels are high. The authors contrasted the cholesterol intake of breast-fed infants (~18 mg/d per kilogram of body weight) with the recommended intake for an adult (4 mg/kg/d). They suggested the possibility that cholesterol synthesis is down-regulated in children and adults who were breast-fed.

## Vitamins and Antioxidants

Although experiments suggest that antioxidant vitamins protect against the development of atherosclerosis, risk factors for aortic and coronary atherosclerosis differ and coronary atherosclerosis is only one factor in CHD. Moreover, the interpretation and relevance of many animal and in vitro studies are debatable. Riemersma reviewed epidemiologic evidence for the theory that the prooxidant/antioxidant balance influences risk of CHD (*227*). Epidemiologic evidence from cross-cultural studies is equivocal. There is usually an inverse association between CHD mortality and plasma antioxidant status. This is fairly strong for vitamins C and E, weaker for carotene. In Scotland, however, *low* levels of plasma and adipose vitamin E are consistently related to low CHD risk. The case for antioxidant protection grows stronger as one moves from surveys of healthy subjects to case–control studies to longitudinal studies and finally intervention trials. However, intervention trials usually use antioxidant doses unachievable through dietary intake. Riemersma concluded that firm dietary recommendations for antibiotics to prevent CHD cannot be given on the basis of current evidence. Another review summarized the strong evidence from animal studies that antioxidants reduce atherosclerosis (*228*). Again, it found the epidemiologic evidence less convincing, but conclusive data are expected from several large studies that are planned or underway. It is particularly important to evaluate effects in men and women separately, because there are clear gender differences in CHD risk factors and mortality.

A multicenter European case–control study evaluated the relationship between α-tocopherol and β-carotene levels in adipose tissue and risk of a first myocardial infarction (*229*). α-Tocopherol concentration was not related to risk of infarction. β-Carotene concentration was significantly associated with risk only for smokers, for whom the multivariate odds ratio in the lowest β-carotene quintile was 2.39 (95% CI 1.35–4.25).

Waeg et al. (*230*) and Esterbauer et al. (*231*) discussed the oxidative modification of LDL and how this is thought to be involved in the pathogenesis of atherosclerosis. The ex vivo oxidation resistance of LDL depends partly on its content of α-tocopherol, carotenoids, and ubiquinol-10. One clinical trial has shown an inverse correlation between severity of myocardial infarction and the resistance of LDL to oxidation. However, little is known about processes leading to LDL oxidation in vivo.

A randomized study in healthy men evaluated the effect of antioxidant supplementation on ex vivo oxidation of LDL (*232*). The treatment group received capsules providing 1 g/d of vitamin C, 800 IU/d of vitamin E, and 30 mg/d of β-carotene for 3 months. Controls received a placebo. A third group was given 800 IU/d of vitamin E. Copper-mediated LDL oxidation was measured ex vivo as production of TBARS and conjugated dienes. Both vitamin E and the combination supplement doubled the duration of the lag phase and reduced the oxidation rate by 40%. The authors stressed that the ineffectiveness of vitamin C and β-carotene in this assay does not indicate absence of in vivo effects. A 6-month study of both men

and women evaluated supplementation with commercially available antioxidant tablets providing 900 mg/d of vitamin C, 18 mg/d of β-carotene, ~200 IU/d of vitamin E, and 12 mg/d of zinc (*233*). A control group received nothing. This level of antioxidant supplementation influenced neither the rate of ex vivo LDL oxidation nor the total amount of conjugated diene produced, but lag time was significantly increased. Changes in lag time and plasma α-tocopherol levels were significantly correlated. In a third study, men and women were given supplements providing 1 g/d of vitamin C and 800 IU/d of vitamin E, and ex vivo lipoprotein oxidation was measured (*234*). Some subjects were given only vitamin C or only vitamin E. In controls, copper-mediated oxidation of VLDL + LDL, measured as appearance of TBARS, showed a 2-h lag phase followed by a propagation phase. After vitamin supplementation lipoprotein oxidation proceeded nearly linearly, without a propagation phase. The maximum mean reduction in TBARS production, 57%, was seen after 10 days. Individually, both vitamin C and vitamin E reduced copper-catalyzed and cell-mediated TBARS formation but vitamin E was more potent. The effects were roughly additive. TBARS production showed a strong inverse correlation with the α-tocopherol content of the lipoprotein ($r = -.64$, $p < .0007$). In two subjects vitamin E levels remained low after supplementation, and supplementation had no effect on formation of TBARS in these subjects.

Mackness et al. compared the effects of antioxidant supplementation and autologous HDL on generation of conjugated dienes and lipid peroxides during the copper-mediated oxidation of LDL (*235*). The daily antioxidant supplement provided 200 mg of selenium, 18 mg of β-carotene, 180 mg of vitamin C, and 75 IU of vitamin E. Blood samples were obtained from the subjects before and after 20 days of supplementation. Antioxidant supplementation significantly reduced formation of conjugated dienes but did not affect formation of lipid peroxides. In contrast, autologous HDL inhibited formation of lipid peroxides by as much as 90% but did not affect formation of conjugated dienes. The effect of HDL was dose-related and was not due to chelation of the copper. The authors concluded that HDL is a potent antioxidant or inhibitor of ex vivo LDL oxidation. They discussed the possibility that it protects against atherosclerosis in vivo by inhibiting LDL oxidation in the artery wall.

A critical review of substudies in the Nurses' Health Study and the Physicians' Health Study (see *Food Safety 1994*, references *246, 247*) discussed the finding that vitamin E supplements reduce CHD risk (*236*). The authors of the two studies, while concluding that protection is achieved at vitamin E dosages obtainable only through supplements, hesitated to recommend such supplementation. The reviewers pointed out differences between the two analyses and some possibly serious shortcomings of both, yet felt that these studies provide the strongest evidence to date that vitamin E protects against CHD. Readers also commented on these studies (*237–240*). O'Keefe and Lavie consider evidence supporting the benefit of vitamin E supplements in CHD to be stronger than that supporting the benefit of coronary angioplasty, yet physicians seem reluctant to recommend the former while they increasingly sanction the latter (*237*). Steiner did not dispute the effectiveness of vitamin E but did question whether an antioxidant mechanism is involved (*238*). In ex vivo studies he has found that vitamin E inhibits platelet adhesion. He suggests that reduced platelet adhesiveness helped prevent cardiovascular complications in the two studies cited. Powell and Black faulted the studies for their treatment of data on vitamin E supplements (*239*). Sullivan argued that the prooxidant role of iron was not considered and could account for the very large amounts of vitamin E needed to confer protection if these subjects had high levels of stored iron (*240*). The authors of the controversial papers responded to these comments (*241*). Steinberg attempted to justify the hesitancy to endorse use of vitamin E supplements (*242*). He believes the strongest statements that can be made at present are "It probably won't hurt" and "It might help." Many people will decide in favor of supplements on this basis, but an objective demonstration of efficacy is necessary before supplements are formally sanctioned for the general public or for treatment of any stage of CHD.

Several components of LDL scavenge peroxyl radicals, breaking the chain of lipid peroxidation reactions. Smith et al. evaluated the total capacity of the LDL particle to scavenge these radicals, using an assay based on the peroxyl radical–dependent oxidation of luminol (*243*). They found that α-tocopherol accounted for ~80% of the antioxidant capacity of individual LDL samples from a number of donors. However, samples of LDL from different donors showed a wide range of susceptibility to oxidation by copper. These results suggest that variability in copper-mediated oxidation is unlikely to be due to differences in the ability of LDL particles to scavenge peroxyl radicals.

Ex vivo, heme can rapidly oxidize LDL, which is then cytotoxic to cultured vascular endothelial cells. Both LDL oxidation and endothelial cytotoxicity can be inhibited by incubation with α-tocopherol or ascorbic acid. To relate these findings to in vivo conditions, Blecher et al. gave volunteers daily supplements of 800 IU vitamin E and 1000 mg of vitamin C, individually or

in combination, for 2 weeks (*244*). Vitamin C supplementation, alone or in combination with vitamin E, did not alter LDL's susceptibility to ex vivo oxidation by heme. Vitamin E, alone and with vitamin C, doubled the lag time for heme-induced production of conjugated dienes and completely prevented toxicity to aortic endothelial cells when LDL was preconditioned with copper or heme plus $H_2O_2$. Measurements returned to baseline levels within 2 weeks after supplementation was stopped.

Abnormalities in endothelium-dependent arterial relaxation develop early in atherosclerosis. Keany et al. investigated the effects of α-tocopherol on endothelial vasodilator function in rabbits (*245*). Test diets contained 1% cholesterol and α-tocopherol at levels of 0, 1000, and 10,000 IU per kilogram. The control diet contained no cholesterol or α-tocopherol. Endothelium-dependent relaxations mediated by acetylcholine and A23187 were significantly impaired in the cholesterol-only group but preserved in animals fed cholesterol and low-dose α-tocopherol. However, compared to the control and cholesterol groups, animals fed high-dose α-tocopherol showed profound impairment of arterial relaxation and significantly more intimal proliferation. α-Tocopherol had no effect on endothelial function in normal vessels. Both low- and high-dose α-tocopherol increased LDL resistance to ex vivo copper-mediated oxidation. The lower dose produced plasma levels of α-tocopherol comparable to those in humans supplemented with 1200 IU/d of α-tocopherol. The high dose produced plasma levels exceeding those achievable in humans. Nevertheless, the results suggest that excess α-tocopherol is potentially harmful and that assay of ex vivo copper-mediated LDL oxidation is a poor indicator of in vivo protection.

In vitro studies of the effect of α-tocopherol on platelet ultrastructure produced different results in washed platelets and platelet-rich plasma (*246*). Spontaneous aggregation was induced by incubation of washed platelets with concentrations of α-tocopherol 0.5 mM and higher. Some platelet disruption was seen using electron microscopy, and this may have released substances that promoted aggregation. Between 0.005 and 0.1 mM, α-tocopherol facilitated the first phase of ferritin-induced aggregation of washed platelets but reduced the second phase. These effects were not seen in platelet-rich plasma. The authors concluded that the platelet membrane is a target for vitamin E.

Ascorbic acid and urate are major water-soluble antioxidants in human plasma. Urate occurs at concentrations up to 10 times higher than ascorbate. Although urate contributes 35–65% of the chain-breaking antioxidant activity of human plasma, compared to ascorbate's

0–24%, little is known about its ability to inhibit LDL oxidation. Ma et al. compared the ability of urate and ascorbate to protect human LDL from oxidation (*247*). The consumption of endogenous tocopherols and exogenous urate and ascorbate and the formation of lipid hydroperoxides were measured as a function of time in an in vitro oxidation system. After the lag phase, during which endogenous tocopherols were totally consumed, the rate of lipid hydroperoxide formation increased sharply. At a concentration of 50 μM (comparable to ascorbate's level in human plasma), urate extended the lag phase more effectively and was consumed more slowly than ascorbate. However, it was less effective than ascorbate in preventing formation of lipid hydroperoxides during the lag phase. An empirical mathematical model was developed to describe the consumption of α- or γ-tocopherol as a function of time in the presence or absence of water-soluble antioxidants. The curve represented a modified sigmoidal equation. The data indicate that urate delays the oxidation of tocopherols in LDL and thus prevents its conversion to a more atherogenic form.

In an in vitro system containing the strong iron chelator desferrioxamine, ascorbic acid completely protected guinea-pig cardiac microsomes from superoxide-initiated lipid peroxidation and protein changes (*248*). Superoxide dismutase was also protective in this system, but catalase, α-tocopherol, glutathione, uric acid, thiourea, mannitol, and histidine were ineffective. Only ascorbic acid protected against NADPH-initiated lipid peroxidation.

Jacques et al. evaluated the association between plasma levels of ascorbate and lipoprotein cholesterol fractions in adult volunteers (*249*). For men, each 0.5 mg/dL increment in ascorbic acid was associated with a 2.1 mg/dL increase in HDL cholesterol, a 4.8 mg/dL decrease in total cholesterol, a 5.6 mg/dL decrease in LDL cholesterol, a 5.4% decrease in the total:HDL cholesterol ratio, and a 5.2% decrease in triacylglycerols. Women, in contrast, demonstrated a two-phase curve. The graph of HDL cholesterol vs. plasma ascorbic acid rose steeply at first but reached a plateau at an ascorbic acid concentration of ~1.0 mg/dL. A similar cutoff point was seen in the relationship between the total:HDL cholesterol ratio and ascorbic acid. Simon et al. examined the relationship between dietary vitamin C and serum lipids in 9- and 10-year-old black girls and white girls (*250*). In the group as a whole, vitamin C intake was not related to serum lipid levels after multivariate adjustment. However, in girls whose serum total cholesterol was ≥200 mg/dL, each 100 mg increment in vitamin C intake was associated with a decrement in total cholesterol of 4 mg/dL in blacks and 13 mg/dL in whites.

Adjustment was made for intake of saturated, polyunsaturated, and monounsaturated fat, cholesterol, fiber, and energy and for body mass index.

Most investigations of plasma homocysteine concentrations have shown a positive association with CVD risk. Folic acid and vitamin $B_{12}$ participate in the recycling of homocysteine into methionine. In a case–control study of early-onset CAD in white men, the odds ratio for CAD per quartile increase in plasma homocysteine was 1.6 (95% CI 1.3–2.1) (*251*). Adjustment for age, HDL and LDL cholesterol, body mass index, smoking, hypertension, and diabetes did not change this substantially. Plasma homocysteine showed significant inverse correlations with plasma folate and vitamin $B_{12}$ in both patients and controls. The odds ratio for CAD per quartile increase in plasma folate concentration was 0.8 (95% CI 0.6–1.0). This change was nonsignificant after adjustment for homocysteine. Plasma $B_{12}$ concentration was not associated with CAD risk on univariate analysis or after correction for the standard CAD risk factors. However, when homocysteine was added to the risk factors adjusted for, $B_{12}$ was significantly associated with risk: the odds ratio increase per quartile increase in $B_{12}$ was 1.5 (95% CI 1.0–1.8). The authors concluded that plasma homocysteine concentration is independently associated with CAD risk and that the relationship between low plasma folate and elevated risk stems from folate's role in homocysteine metabolism. Therefore CAD risk might be decreased by interventions that lower homocysteine concentrations by increasing plasma folate. In another investigation of homocysteine, Haglund et al. conducted a double-blind crossover study in which healthy normolipidemic to moderately hyperlipidemic volunteers were given fish oil with and without pyridoxine and folic acid for 4-week periods (*252*). These B vitamins, in addition to their role in homocysteine metabolism, are involved in the metabolism of unsaturated fatty acids. Both fish-oil treatments lowered plasma triacylglycerols and increased HDL cholesterol levels. Atherogenic index and plasma fibrinogen decreased after both treatments, but the decrease was twice as great when the fish oil was supplemented with B vitamins. Plasminogen activator inhibitor-1 antigen increased after both treatments. Only the vitamin treatment reduced plasma homocysteine levels. Although the authors concluded that there is synergism between fish oil and B vitamins, they did not test folate and pyridoxine by themselves.

Flavonoids and other phenolic substances from plants have a variety of antioxidant activities and may reduce risk of CHD. The French paradox—the anomalously low CHD mortality rate in a population that, based on most risk factors, "ought" to have a much higher rate—has been tentatively explained by widespread regular consumption of red wine. A short review discussed evidence that phenolic substances in red wine inhibit LDL oxidation (*253*). In an ex vivo assay, 3.8 and 10.0 μM polyphenols from the nonalcoholic fraction of a California red wine inhibited copper-mediated oxidation of freshly prepared human LDL by 60 and 98%, respectively. α-Tocopherol was only 60% as potent as the wine fraction or the flavonol quercetin. The activity was not due to metal chelation. Measurement of levels of oxidized LDL in wine-drinking subjects and appropriate controls could confirm this theory of the association between moderate wine consumption and reduced CVD risk. In addition to reducing susceptibility of LDL to oxidation, plant phenols alter prostaglandin metabolism by inhibiting cyclooxygenase and lipoxygenase activity in platelets and macrophages. Another brief review discussed the relationship between dietary flavonoids and CHD risk (*254*). It also mentioned red wine as an important source of flavonoids in some cultures. General structures of flavones, flavonols, and flavonones were presented. Results of the Zutphen Elderly Study related to dietary flavonoids and risk of CHD were reviewed. The Zutphen Elderly Study, a longitudinal investigation of risk factors for chronic diseases in elderly men, is an extension of the Dutch contribution to the Seven Countries Study. Hertog et al. measured the content of the five major flavonoids in fruits, vegetables, and beverages common in the Netherlands; they then estimated subjects' baseline intakes of flavonoids and determined the relation between intake and subsequent myocardial infarction and CHD mortality (*255*). The major sources of flavonoids were tea (61%), onions (13%) and apples (10%). Flavonoid intake, analyzed by tertiles, was inversely associated with CHD mortality ($p = .015$) and incidence of myocardial infarction ($p = .08$). The relative risk of CHD mortality in the highest vs. the lowest tertile of flavonoid intake was 0.42 (95% CI 0.20–0.88). After adjustment for numerous potential confounders, including intakes of antioxidant vitamins, the relative risk was 0.32 (95% CI 0.15–0.71).

## Minerals

Presentations at a Paris symposium on hypertension were published as a supplement to *The American Journal of the Medical Sciences*. A number of these dealt with sodium and other electrolytes. Grobbee summarized results from recent studies of electrolytes and hypertension (*256*). From Dahl's report 35 years ago—that the average sodium intake in a population was related to the prevalence of hypertension—to the INTERSALT study, interpretation of epidemiologic and cross-cultural studies of salt and blood pressure has been fraught with controversy. Evidence suggests that the blood pressure of newborn infants responds to changes in sodium intake but this sodium sensitivity is usually lost in older children. A number of intervention trials have demonstrated small reductions in blood pressure through sodium restriction, with older and more severely hypertensive subjects benefitting most. The anion associated with sodium may also be important. Studies of potassium, calcium, and magnesium were briefly reviewed.

Simon et al. evaluated the relation of sodium, potassium, calcium, and magnesium intakes to blood pressure in 9- and 10-year-old black girls and white girls (*257*). Cation intake was not associated with blood pressure in black girls. In white girls, dietary magnesium showed a strong inverse association with diastolic blood pressure ($p < .01$). The range of intake in these subjects was 53–511 mg/d. After correction for other factors frequently associated with blood pressure, each 100 mg/d increment in intake was associated with a 3.22 mm Hg decrease in diastolic pressure (95% CI –0.75 to –5.70). However, the association vanished upon adjustment for dietary fiber. The authors concluded that body mass index and pulse rate are the strongest correlates of blood pressure in girls of this age and that studies examining the influence of magnesium on blood pressure should control for the effects of dietary fiber.

Ruilope et al. discussed relationships between sodium intake and electrolyte excretion in subjects with essential hypertension, with reference to blood pressure changes in salt-sensitive and salt-resistant individuals (*258*). They presented evidence that the effect of low doses of calcium depends on renal production of prostaglandins. Overall, the kidney is the principal target organ of changes in calcium concentration and a disturbance in calcium use will be expressed as a defect in volume regulation. Insight into blood pressure effects involving interactions among sodium, chloride, and calcium also came from a study in rats (*259*). Weanling Sprague-Dawley rats were fed diets based on dried salted or unsalted cottage cheese, with and without calcium supplementation. Tests of sodium, potassium, calcium, magnesium, and chloride utilization, blood pressure, and kidney function suggested numerous interactions. Overall, ingestion of excess NaCl adversely affected potassium and magnesium retention, and calcium supplementation partially compensated for the effect on potassium utilization. Calcium also ameliorated the hypertensive effect of NaCl.

**SODIUM AND SALT.** Cugini et al. investigated the 24-h blood pressure pattern in healthy representative adults from two industrialized countries with very different salt intakes, Italy and Japan (*260*). The Mediterranean diet contains about half as much salt as the traditional Japanese diet. Contrary to expectations, the 24-h blood pressure pattern, mean blood pressure, prevalence of hypertension, and urinary potassium excretion did not differ between the cultures. In fact, mean 24-h blood pressure was nonsignificantly higher in Italians than in Japanese. Urinary sodium excretion was twice as high in Japanese as in Italians. The authors postulated a racial resetting of salt sensitivity in the Japanese, resulting from a selective or adaptive process by which the Japanese became relatively resistant to excess dietary salt. The authors further suggested that accepting such a racial susceptibility (a "phyletic escape to dietary salt excess") would clarify some scientific disputes on the relation between salt intake and blood pressure. Madhavan and Alderman also examined the impact of race on the relationship between sodium intake and blood pressure (*261*). They measured 24-h urinary sodium excretion and blood pressure in blacks and whites who participated in a union-sponsored workplace hypertension control program in New York. In this socioeconomically homogeneous population, race and ethnicity did not influence the relationship between sodium intake and blood pressure after adjustment for confounding factors.

The value of salt restriction for hypertensive patients is still controversial. Ghooi et al. argued that the presence of salt-sensitive individuals in all populations guarantees that epidemiologic studies of salt intake and blood pressure will *always* show a positive relationship (*262*). By analogy with the use of salt licks by cattle and wild animals, they reasoned that increased salt intake may result from rather than cause increased salt loss. In hot climates particularly, salt restriction may be a bad idea even for hypertensive patients. The authors concluded that salt restriction is not very useful in most cases and would probably be harmful for some. In a randomized controlled study of overweight hypertensive women, Kawamura et al. showed that short-term calorie restriction (2 weeks) with no change in sodium and potassium intake or exercise significantly reduced systolic and diastolic blood pressure (*263*). Although all calorie-restricted subjects showed similar weight loss, the extent of blood pressure reduction varied widely, suggesting a "calorie-sensitive" phenomenon analogous to salt sensitivity.

The Trials of Hypertension evaluated the feasibility and efficacy of sodium reduction as part of a phase I study (*264*). Subjects were 30- to 54-year-old men and women whose diastolic blood pressure was 80–89 mm Hg. The mean net decrease in sodium excretion was 43.9 mmol per 24 h at 18 months. Dose–response analysis indicated an adjusted change in blood pressure of –1.4 mm Hg (systolic) and –0.9 mm Hg (diastolic) for a decrease in sodium excretion of 100 mmol per 24 h. The response appeared to be associated with sex and initial level of sodium intake. However, race- and gender-specific comparisons were not an aspect of the study design and the statistical power of these comparisons was inadequate to support definitive inferences. The authors concluded that sodium reduction is feasible as a public health strategy and discussed the importance of what appears to be a trivial blood pressure reduction in terms of its population-wide impact.

Zoccali et al. conducted a randomized crossover study of various levels of sodium intake in mildly hypertensive men with different habitual levels of sodium intake (*265*). Arterial blood pressure and 24-h urinary sodium excretion were measured twice during a 1-month run-in phase during which subjects maintained their customary sodium intake. Each subject's sodium intake was then varied for 1-week periods to provide at least one period with a higher than usual intake and one or more periods with a lower intake. Mean 24-h urinary sodium excretion, 24-h blood pressure (both systolic and diastolic), and casual systolic and diastolic blood pressures during habitual sodium intake were intermediate between those after the highest and lowest intake periods. For sodium excretion and 24-h diastolic blood pressure these differences were highly significant ($p \leq .01$); for 24-h and casual systolic blood pressure the differences between habitual intake and lowest intake were highly significant. Individual blood pressure responses ranged from 1.4 to 20 mm Hg per 100 mg of sodium, but there was a well-defined linear trend in all cases.

James et al. examined the effect of large changes in dietary sodium on average ambulatory blood pressure and its variability in patients with uncomplicated borderline hypertension (*266*). The results suggested that sodium restriction has a variable, sometimes marked, effect on blood pressure and that sodium balance may influence variability in ambulatory blood pressure. They also suggested that the method of measuring blood pressure can influence results and that sodium reduction can affect the response of systolic pressure to activity.

Nestel et al. evaluated the blood pressure response of elderly men and women to dietary sodium and dihomo-γ-linolenic acid, a longer-chain derivative of linoleic acid (*267*). It was postulated that the linoleic acid derivative might have a hypotensive effect similar to that reported for long-chain n–3 PUFAs. Women were more responsive than men to changing sodium intake. A second major determinant of blood pressure responsiveness, but only in women, was the waist:hip ratio, an index of central obesity. Daily supplements of the fatty acid increased its concentration in plasma but did not influence blood pressure.

Divergent hemodynamic and hormonal responses to varying salt intake were seen in a study of nonobese normotensive adults (268). Subjects were classified as salt-sensitive, salt-resistant, or counterregulating (i.e., their blood pressure rose in response to salt restriction). They were given low- and high-salt diets for 1 week each in a single-blind, randomized, crossover fashion. Salt sensitivity was more frequent in women, in older subjects, and in subjects with a lower body weight or a family history of hypertension. Counterregulators were more common among younger subjects and those with higher body weight or a negative family history of hypertension. Plasma renin activity and plasma aldosterone concentrations were lower in salt-sensitive subjects, whereas the increase in plasma renin activity during salt restriction was greatest in counterregulators. Plasma norepinephrine concentrations did not differ between groups. During the high-salt diet, plasma levels of atrial natriuretic peptide increased most in salt-sensitive subjects, suggesting that the ability of their kidneys to excrete a salt load may be impaired.

Haythornthwaite briefly reviewed the literature implicating acute and chronic behavioral stress and dietary factors in development of hypertension (269). Two of her own studies, in particular, point to an interactive or additive effect of sodium intake and exam-period stress in medical students. Although age, diet, daily experience, and the objective stressful event—the examination period—are similar for most medical students, the blood pressure responses are variable, suggesting that this model would also be instructive in evaluating the role of genetic, physiologic, and psychologic factors in blood pressure responses.

One week of severe sodium restriction has been reported to cause hyperlipidemia in clinically healthy, nonobese, normotensive subjects (270). After adjustment for hematocrit, the increases in total and LDL cholesterol and triacylglycerols were significant only in counterregulators. After moderate salt restriction, blood pressure and serum lipids did not change. Moreover, this effect was not seen in a study of obese subjects who completed a course of salt-restricted weight reduction at the Duke Diet and Fitness Center (271). The authors concluded that severe salt restriction serves no useful purpose in normal people and the (perhaps transient)

hyperlipidemia it may cause is not relevant to the problem of nonpharmacologic and diuretic treatment of obese hypertensive patients.

Studies in borderline hypertensive rats indicated that the window of developmental sensitivity to modulation of blood pressure regulation by high dietary salt occurs during the prenatal and early postnatal period (272). The effects of perinatal and adult exposure to a high-salt diet were additive.

**CALCIUM.** Hatton and McCarron reviewed animal experiments relating dietary calcium to blood pressure (273). Extensive data were summarized in a table citing the study and identifying the model and level of calcium used, time factors, effect on systolic blood pressure, and the prime focus of the study (e.g., diet–stress interaction, calcium balance). Possible sites of calcium's action suggested by these studies include the cell, vascular tissue, calcium-regulating hormones, calcium-sensitive hormones, the sympathetic nervous system, and the kidney. It appears that dietary calcium acts simultaneously through multiple physiologic mechanisms to influence blood pressure. The relative importance of a particular mechanism can vary depending on the experimental model and design.

Effects of a low-calcium diet and a calcium-fortified diet on lipid parameters were compared in moderately hypercholesterolemic men (274). Both diets provided 34 en% from fat (13 en% saturated fat) and 240 mg of cholesterol. The low-calcium diet provided 410 mg/d of calcium; the high-calcium diet provided 2200 mg/d. Fecal excretion of saturated fat increased from 6% of dietary saturated fat with the low-calcium diet to 13% with calcium fortification. The high-calcium diet significantly reduced serum total and LDL cholesterol and apoB. HDL cholesterol and apoA-I did not change. The authors concluded that calcium fortification could be a useful adjunct to cholesterol-lowering diet therapy.

**MAGNESIUM.** Orlov et al. reviewed the use of magnesium in cardiovascular pharmacotherapy and the protective role of magnesium against myocardial infarction and arrhythmias (275). Among their observations were that magnesium deficiency has been associated with multiple cardiovascular problems; and although low serum levels of magnesium indicate a deficiency, "normal" levels do not assure adequate stores. Vegetables, grains, and dairy products are rich dietary sources of magnesium.

Singh et al. reported their case–control study of dietary and serum magnesium levels in patients with CAD, acute myocardial infarction, and noncardiac diagnoses (*276*). Consumption of fat and cholesterol was significantly higher and of carbohydrate nonsignificantly lower in patients with definite or possible acute myocardial infarction or unstable angina than in controls with noncardiac chest pain. Magnesium intake was comparable in all groups. However, in the subset of acute myocardial infarction patients who had ventricular arrhythmias, magnesium intake was lower than in controls (270–280 mg/d vs. 317 mg/d). Serum magnesium levels in the cardiac patients were within normal limits but significantly lower than in controls. The authors attributed the lower serum levels in the cardiac patients to an increased demand during infarction; however, the possibility that the low levels in patients with arrhythmic complications resulted partly from lower magnesium intake requires further study. In editorial comments on this study, Seeling marshaled other evidence that low magnesium levels increase the risk of arrhythmias and discussed some possible mechanisms for this (*277*). However, Galløe al. found that long-term oral treatment of survivors of an acute myocardial infarction with 15 mmol/d of magnesium did not reduce the subsequent incidence of cardiac events (*278*). In fact, after 1 year the incidence of cardiac events was 55% higher in the treated group than in controls.

POTASSIUM. A review of potassium's role in the pathogenesis of hypertension briefly summarized findings in experimental animals and made the following points relating to humans (*279*). Potassium supplementation lowers blood pressure in hypertensive subjects. Potassium supplementation to ameliorate diuretic-induced hypokalemia enhances the hypotensive effect of diuretics. Potassium depletion induced by dietary potassium restriction while normal sodium intake is maintained elevates blood pressure in normotensive and hypertensive subjects. Potassium depletion is accompanied by sodium retention and calcium depletion. If sodium intake is restricted, no blood-pressure response to potassium restriction or supplementation is seen. Thus sodium retention, altered response to vasoactive hormones, direct vasoconstrictive effects of hypokalemia, and calcium depletion may all promote elevation of blood pressure during potassium depletion.

Because the foundation for essential hypertension is laid early in life, Sinaiko et al. evaluated the feasibility of long-term sodium reduction and the effect of the dietary sodium:potassium ratio on blood pressure in adolescents (*280*). Fifth- to 8th-grade students from the highest 15 percentiles of blood pressure were randomly allocated to a low-sodium diet, normal diet with potassium chloride supplementation, or normal diet with

placebo. Their blood pressure was measured every 3 months for 3 years. Compliance was estimated from 24-h urinary sodium and potassium excretion and the sodium:potassium ratio. The effect of intervention was assessed as the rate of increase of blood pressure over time. Compliance with the potassium supplement and placebo regimens was high but compliance with the low-sodium diet was poor, particularly among the boys. Curves for the three boys' groups and the girls' placebo groups had similar, significantly positive slopes. The curve for the girls' low-sodium group had a slightly negative slope that was significantly lower than the slope of the girls' placebo group. The girls' potassium group had a slightly positive slope. The authors concluded that changes in sodium and potassium intake during childhood and adolescence can reduce blood pressure in girls, but that the feasibility of long-term sodium reduction in the USA is limited, especially for boys.

COPPER. Medeiros et al. reviewed studies of copper deficiency and cardiomyopathy in rats and discussed their possible relevance to certain cardiomyopathies in humans (*281*). Weanling rats fed a copper-deficient diet develop a concentric hypertrophy, whereas in older animals copper deficiency produces cardiomyopathy without apparent hypertrophy. From experiments with these two models, the authors hypothesized a possible sequence of events leading to heart failure in young rats fed a copper-deficient diet. They suggested that studies in humans with cardiomyopathies of unknown etiology should consider aspects of copper nutriture and utilization. Apparent mitochondrial defects associated with some forms of cardiomyopathy could implicate a link with copper metabolism.

Klevay briefly reviewed the importance of trace elements in biology and the evidence that IHD is a copper-deficiency disease (*282*). He laments the propensity of physicians to treat symptoms or phenomena with drugs rather than searching for a nutritional cause. He points out that the Western diet, a major contributor to IHD risk, seems to be low in copper and that copper deficiency disrupts metabolism that influence cardiovascular health. Moreover, several drugs commonly used to treat aspects of IHD have links with copper metabolism that could help explain their effects. Another short review discussed how copper deficiency might impair vascular function by altering interactions between vascular smooth muscle cells and nitric oxide (*283*). Relationships between copper deficiency and levels of CuZn superoxide dismutase, prostacyclin, guanylate cyclase, and cGMP should also be investigated. A review by Bunce showed how the hypercholesterolemia induced by copper deficiency is linked to glutathione metabolism and regulation of hepatic HMG-CoA reductase activity (*284*).

**SELENIUM.** A study in northern Italy linked changes in the selenium content of the municipality's water supply to changes in CHD mortality (*285*). The selenium content of tap water averaged 7 μg/L from the early 1970s until August 1988, when the two major wells providing water for this area were disconnected from the public water supply. The selenium content then fell to <1 μg/L. Except for selenium, there were no significant changes in the chemical composition of the water. From January 1986 through August 1988 there were 3 deaths from CHD in a cohort of 4419 local residents. From September 1988 through December 1992 there were 31 coronary deaths in this group. These findings support the hypothesis that selenium protects against CHD mortality.

**CHROMIUM.** Hermann et al. evaluated the effects of chromium supplementation on plasma lipids, apolipoproteins, and glucose in a randomized placebo-controlled study of independently living elderly subjects (*286*). In the treatment group as a whole, chromium had no significant effects. However, in subjects whose initial total cholesterol level was ≥240 mg/dL, total and LDL cholesterol and apoB were reduced significantly. HDL cholesterol, triacylglycerols, and glucose (which were in the normal range) were unaffected. Dietary copper was inversely correlated with apoB; dietary magnesium was inversely correlated with apoA-I.

## Miscellaneous Foods and Dietary Factors

**FISH.** Epidemiologic evidence that fish reduces risk of CHD is strong (*287*). This evidence is based both on cross-cultural studies and on cohort studies in which there is an appropriate range of fish consumption. The relationship between fish consumption and the mortality rate from stroke is less consistent. For example, Eskimos have very low CHD mortality but relatively high mortality from stroke—whereas the Zutphen Study in the Netherlands found that fish consumption is inversely related to both CHD and stroke (*288*). However, most strokes among Eskimos are hemorrhagic, whereas most strokes in the Netherlands are thrombotic. In addition, consumption of marine foods is higher among the Eskimos than among the Dutch. This suggests that moderate amounts of fish protect against ischemic stroke but very large amounts increase risk of hemorrhagic stroke. Although understanding of the mechanisms behind the inverse association between fish consumption and CVD

is fragmentary, it appears that eating one or two meals of fish weekly is protective.

Burr reviewed the association between IHD risk and intake of fish or fish oil (*289*). Epidemiologic studies are based on fish consumption because fish is a food that people eat. Experimental studies, however, usually employ fish oil supplements because the dosage can be controlled precisely, the diet does not have to be altered, and trials can be double-blinded. Although the question of whether all observed effects of fish are attributable to *n*–3 PUFAs has not been answered to everyone's satisfaction, the reviewer believes there are sound reasons to assume that the protective effects of fish come from its long-chain *n*–3 fatty acids, particularly EPA and DHA. In general, people who eat fish are less likely to die of IHD than people who do not. The preventive mechanism may involve a lessened tendency of blood to clot, protection against ventricular arrhythmias, or both.

Findings in the Atherosclerosis Risk in Communities (ARIC) Study suggest that increases in fish consumption can modify blood levels of several coagulation factors (*290*). Possible dietary determinants of six hemostatic factors—fibrinogen, factor VII, factor VIII, von Willebrand factor, protein C, and antithrombin—were assessed in a large study of four population-based samples from different parts of the USA. Intakes of *n*–3 PUFAs and of fish, the major source of dietary *n*–3 PUFAs, were negatively associated with levels of fibrinogen, factor VIII, and von Willebrand's factor in both blacks and whites and positively associated with protein C in whites. Other dietary substances (cholesterol, animal fat, fiber, caffeine, alcohol) were variously associated with hemostatic factors.

Mori et al. examined the influence of fat intake on the response of serum lipids to fish oil or fish in men with high-normal values for lipids and blood pressure (*291*). Seven diets were evaluated. Five provided 40 en% fat with placebo, fish oil, fish, fish oil and fish, or double-dose fish oil. Two provided 30 en% fat with and without fish. With 40% fat, both fish and fish oil increased total, HDL, $HDL_2$, and LDL cholesterol and decreased triacylglycerols. With 30% fat and no fish, total, LDL, and HDL cholesterol decreased and triacylglycerols did not change; with fish, total and LDL cholesterol and triacylglycerols decreased and $HDL_2$ cholesterol increased. There were no effects on blood pressure. The authors concluded that the adverse effects of *n*–3 PUFAs on total and LDL cholesterol against the background of a high-fat diet are reversed in the context of a lower-fat diet. Moreover, one daily fish meal prevents the reduction in HDL cholesterol that usually accompanies a reduced-fat diet. From a nutritional and public health viewpoint, a diet reduced in total fat and including one fish meal daily should alter lipid profiles beneficially. The advantages might be greatest for people with abnormal lipid profiles.

It is generally thought that only fatty marine fish confer substantial cardiovascular benefits. Tidwell et al. compared effects of incorporating wild Alaskan salmon or farm-raised catfish into diets conforming to the *Dietary Guidelines for Americans* (U.S. Dept. of Health and Human Services, 3rd edition, 1990) (*292*). Subjects were healthy men 21–42 years old. They ate similar control diets for the first 20 days and then were randomly assigned to one of the fish diets for a second 20 days. Total cholesterol and triacylglycerols were lower after the control diet and there were no further changes when fish was added. LDL cholesterol did not change on the control diet but decreased after consumption of fish. HDL cholesterol did not change during the trial. Thus despite their considerable differences in *n*–3 PUFA content, catfish and salmon had similar positive effects on lipid profiles.

**MILK.** Although cow's milk contains cholesterol and predominantly saturated fats and is therefore considered to be atherogenic, there are many reports that milk or milk products have a hypocholesterolemic effect. Eichholzer and Stähelin evaluated the evidence for hypocholesterolemic factors in milk (*293*). They believe that a hypocholesterolemic effect of milk or milk products can be neither confirmed nor ruled out by evidence from studies in humans. There is some evidence from animal studies that whole milk as well as skim and fermented milk reduces serum lipids, but these results raise questions about the kind of product that is important, the relevance of the animal model, and the composition of the control diet. As for the identity of the postulated milk factor(s), several constituents have been suggested: products of bacterial fermentation, orotic acid, calcium, lactose or whey, and casein. In general, single substances tested separately have been less effective than the complex food, suggesting additive or interactive effects of multiple substances.

A roundtable discussion on the impact of milk fat on health, in the context of a balanced diet, was held in San Francisco in October 1992. Representatives from the California Dairy Research Foundation and the Dairy Council of Wisconsin planned and conducted the program. Final statements of the group were published in the *Journal of Nutrition* (*294*). Participants evaluated the impact of milk fat, dairy foods, and specific fatty acids on CHD risk and identified research questions that must be addressed to understand the role of dietary fats in general and milk fat in particular in varied diets. They

agreed that diets meeting contemporary guidelines for fat intake can accommodate standard-fat dairy foods. More research is needed to reveal the impact of milk fat in mixed-fat diets on blood lipid profiles and other indicators of disease risk. The group saw no advantage to very-low-fat diets (≤25 en%) for the general U.S. population.

Sharpe et al. compared the hypocholesterolemic and blood pressure effects of normal skim milk powder and a skim milk powder produced from dairy cows hyperimmunized with a multivalent bacterial vaccine (*295*). Hypercholesterolemic subjects reconstituted and drank 90 g of control or immune milk powder daily in a randomized, double-blind, crossover study. Otherwise they were encouraged to follow a prudent diet and healthful exercise habits. The immune milk caused significant reduction in total and LDL cholesterol levels, with no change in HDL cholesterol or triacylglycerols. Systolic blood pressure was reduced by 5 mm Hg and diastolic pressure by 4 mm Hg. There was no correlation between blood pressure and cholesterol changes, suggesting different mechanisms for the two effects.

**GARLIC.** After the initial enthusiasm over the hypolipidemic action of garlic, the disappointing news appeared that yes, garlic works, if you eat massive amounts of it and you're a rat. Some early clinical trials were inconclusive and many were poorly designed, but five met the criteria of Warshafsky et al. for a metaanalysis of the effect of garlic on serum cholesterol levels in subjects whose total cholesterol level was >200 mg/dL (*296*). The metaanalysis showed that subjects treated with garlic consistently had a greater decrease in total cholesterol than subjects treated with placebo. The estimated net cholesterol decrease attributable to garlic was 23 mg/dL (95% CI 17–29 mg/dL, $p$ <.001). The best estimate for the fresh garlic equivalent of the powdered and aqueous garlic preparations evaluated in these studies indicates that only one-half to one clove of garlic per day can reduce total serum cholesterol by ~9% in hypercholesterolemic persons. A controlled study by Jain et al. evaluated the hypocholesterolemic effects of a standardized garlic powder in healthy adults whose total serum cholesterol level was ≥200 mg/dL (*297*). The mean baseline cholesterol level of 262 ± 34 mg/dL decreased to 247 ± 40 mg/dL ($p$ <.01) after 12 weeks of treatment. Values for placebo were 276 mg/dL before and 274 mg/dL after treatment. LDL cholesterol was 11% lower after garlic and 3% lower after placebo ($p$ <.05). HDL cholesterol, triacylglycerols, serum glucose, and blood pressure did not change. The 900 mg/d dose of the garlic preparation delivered 0.6% allicin.

The effect of garlic on platelet aggregation was evaluated in young adults with increased risk of ischemic attack and increased levels of spontaneous platelet aggregation (298). Daily ingestion of 800 mg of powdered garlic for 4 weeks significantly decreased the pathologically elevated level of spontaneous platelet aggregation (from 41% to 18%) and the proportion of circulating platelet aggregates (from 1.17 to 1.05). These values returned to baseline within 4 weeks after the end of treatment. There were no significant changes in the placebo group. Srivastava and Tyagi investigated the mechanism by which garlic inhibits platelet aggregation (299). They studied the effects of ajoene, an active derivative of alliin formed during processing of garlic, on aggregation and arachidonic acid metabolism in human platelets. Ajoene irreversibly inhibited platelet aggregation induced by arachidonic acid, adrenaline, collagen, ADP, and the calcium ionophore A23187. It had a direct, dose-related inhibitory effect on enzymes of the arachidonic acid cascade in platelets. It inhibited incorporation of arachidonic acid into platelet phospholipids only at high concentrations and had no effect on the deacylation of platelet phospholipids.

Gebhardt reported multiple inhibitory effects of a water-soluble garlic extract on cholesterol biosynthesis in primary rat hepatocytes and human HepG2 cells (300). At low concentrations, garlic reduced sterol biosynthesis from [$^{14}$C]acetate by inhibiting HMG-CoA reductase. At high concentrations, garlic also inhibited later steps in the synthetic pathway, resulting in the accumulation of the precursors lanosterol and 7-dehydrocholesterol. Allicin, but not the native alliin, caused a similar shift in the proportions of cholesterol and the sterol precursors. Nicotinic acid and adenosine, two other garlic constituents, were also active; adenosine showed a biphasic concentration dependence similar to that of the complete extract. The mode of action of garlic was compared with that of several cholesterol-lowering drugs. The gap between the low concentrations of garlic that inhibit early biosynthetic steps and the high concentrations required to inhibit later steps suggests that garlic can reduce cholesterol biosynthesis without leading to accumulation of undesirable cholesterol precursors, as happens in some drug therapy. Also using primary cultures of rat hepatocytes, Yeh and Yeh studied the effects of petroleum ether, methanol, and water extracts of garlic on incorporation of [$^{14}$C]acetate and [2-$^{3}$H]glycerol into cholesterol, fatty acids, and glycerol lipids (301). The results confirmed that the hypocholesterolemic action of garlic is related to decreased hepatic cholesterogenesis. The hypotriacylglycerolemic effect seen in rats may stem from inhibition of fatty acid synthesis.

**HERBS AND MEDICINAL PLANTS.** Sutter and Wang described the pharmacology of some cardiovascular drugs derived from Chinese medicinal plants (302). The types of activity described for the various drugs include calcium antagonism, adrenoceptor antagonism, antagonism of platelet activating factor, and antioxidant activity. The plant sources for each group of drugs were indicated. Some of the genera represented are *Stephania, Menispermum, Berberis, Nelumbo, Lindera, Corydalis, Ligusticum, Uncaria, Ginkgo, Piper, Magnolia, Paeonia, Triptospermum, Sophora, Rhododendron, Cascara, Rheum, Polygonum, Artemisia,* and *Panax.*

Flavonoids isolated from licorice roots (*Glycyrrhiza inflata*) showed several effects on platelet aggregation and arachidonic acid metabolism (303). Licochalcones A and B and—at higher concentrations—isoliquiritigenin and liquiritigenin inhibited formation of 12-hydroxy-5,8,10-heptadecatrienoic acid and thromboxane B$_2$. The latter two compounds also increased formation of 12-HETE but had no effect on arachidonate metabolism. Of six flavonoids tested, only the licochalcones inhibited thrombin-induced platelet aggregation. The mechanism seems to involve inhibition of Ca$^{2+}$ influx from an extracellular medium and of thrombin-stimulated Ca$^{2+}$ mobilization from calcium pools.

Ginger (*Zingiber officinale*) has reported antiemetic activity, but large amounts of fresh raw ginger can cause platelet dysfunction. To verify the safety of effective antiemetic doses of dried ginger for surgical patients, a randomized crossover trial in healthy men assessed effects of 2 g of ginger powder and placebo on several parameters of platelet function 3 and 24 h after administration (304). No effects were seen on bleeding time, platelet count, thromboelastography, or whole-blood aggregation.

Javanese turmeric (*Curcuma xanthorrhiza*) is a traditional food and medicinal plant in Indonesia, but little attention has been paid to its role in lipid metabolism. Yasni et al. isolated and identified α-curcumene from *C. xanthorrhiza* and demonstrated its hypotriacylglycerolemic activity in rats (305). Rats fed the essential oil or the hexane-soluble fraction had lower levels of hepatic fatty acid synthase activity than controls.

**MUSHROOMS.** The oyster mushroom (*Pleurotus ostreatus*) has several effects on lipid metabolism (306–308). When fed to rats along with cholesterol it accelerated the plasma clearance of LDL and HDL by increasing the rate of their catabolism (306). The level of triacylglycerols in serum was not influenced by the mushroom, but was significantly reduced in the liver. Another activity in cholesterol-fed rats was the reduction of VLDL secretion and acceleration of the fractional turnover rate of VLDL (*307*). The result was a precipitous fall (45%) in serum cholesterol after 12 weeks of feeding 5% by weight of the dried mushroom. In cholesterol-fed hamsters, the whole fungus and aqueous and ethanolic extracts significantly reduced serum levels of total cholesterol and triacylglycerols and liver total cholesterol (*308*). The major portion of the effect was due to the reduced cholesterol content of the VLDL fraction.

Sugiyama et al. reported that the hypocholesterolemic action of the shiitake mushroom (*Lentinus edodes*) in rats results from alteration of the phospholipid composition of liver microsomes (*309*). The major effect was a reduction in the ratio of phosphatidylcholine to phosphatidylethanolamine.

ALCOHOL. Klatsky reviewed the epidemiology of CAD, emphasizing the influence of alcohol (*310*). Clinical manifestations of CAD include angina pectoris, nonfatal acute myocardial infarction, and death. Although alcohol may reduce or mask symptoms of angina, it has no proven favorable effect on pathophysiology. However, most epidemiologic studies show drinkers to be at lower risk for nonfatal myocardial infarction and demonstrate a J- or U-shaped curve for risk of CAD mortality, in which light drinkers are at lower risk than nondrinkers or heavy drinkers. The author discussed individual studies and problems inherent in such studies. The most likely mechanisms of a protective effect involve elevation of protective HDL subfractions and apoA-I. An antithrombotic effect has been suggested but not established. In evaluating the alcohol–CAD relation in terms of the usual epidemiologic criteria for causality, Klatsky found a causal relation to be supported by the criteria of consistency, biologic plausibility, specificity, and probably temporal sequence. By the criteria of independence, strength, and gradient of risk, causality is less certain. When giving advice on alcohol consumption it is important to emphasize individual risks.

A review by Srivastava et al. discussed the association between alcohol intake, lipoproteins, and CHD (*311*). The authors concluded that the protective effect of moderate alcohol consumption, if real, is most likely explained by the elevation of protective HDL subfractions. Heavy alcohol consumption, in contrast, may increase risk of atherosclerosis by impairing HDL synthesis. Benefits of light to moderate drinking extend beyond reduction of atherosclerotic risk to reducing stress, improving mood, and decreasing tension and anxiety; in the elderly it can also stimulate appetite and promote regular bowel function. Elevated risks that could cancel these benefits include stroke, motor vehicle accidents, cancer, adverse drug reactions, and birth defects.

Maclure used the epidemiologic evidence for and against a causal relationship between ethanol intake and risk of myocardial infarction to demonstrate the method of deductive metaanalysis (*312*). He argued that most "metaanalyses" are not analyses at all, but syntheses. These metasyntheses use an inductive approach, generalizing from a set of particular observations. Maclure believes a metaanalysis should be structured using deductive reasoning, beginning with competing hypotheses that are either supported or refuted by the data. He discussed and illustrated refutation of various types of bias. His deductive metaanalysis of evidence for and against more than 20 hypotheses concerning the relationship between ethanol consumption and incidence of myocardial infarction corroborated the preventive hypothesis by weakening competing hypotheses. It showed that a refutationist approach can solve the problem of overinterpreting metaanalysis in epidemiology.

Data from NHANES I and the NHANES I Follow-Up were used to evaluate the effect of moderate alcohol consumption on CHD mortality (*313*). For white men, accelerated time-to-failure models showed lifespans 3–4% longer for moderate drinkers than for nondrinkers or light drinkers. No effect was seen for white women. A case–control study confirmed an inverse association between moderate alcohol intake and risk of myocardial infarction (*314*). In multivariate analyses, the relative risk for subjects who consumed $\geq 3$ drinks per day was 0.45, compared to those who had <1 drink per day (95% CI 0.26–0.80). Levels of HDL, $HDL_2$, and $HDL_3$ cholesterol were strongly associated with alcohol intake ($p$'s <.001). Moreover, HDL and its subfractions were the only plasma lipid parameters that substantially reduced the relation between alcohol intake and risk in the multivariate model. This supports the view that the protective effect of alcohol is largely mediated by increases in $HDL_2$ and $HDL_3$.

Data from the INTERSALT study were used to assess the relation between alcohol intake and blood pressure (*315*). Heavy drinking (at least 3–4 drinks per day) was positively associated with blood pressure in both men and women. When men were grouped by age, the association was seen in both the 20- to 39- and the 40- to 59-year groups. The relation was independent of smoking, body mass index, and urinary excretion of sodium and potassium.

A study in Finland demonstrated a positive association between heavy alcohol intake (>300 g per week) and risk of ischemic stroke (OR 4.45, 95% CI 1.09–18.1) (*316*). However, risk was significantly reduced in regular light-to-moderate drinkers (≤150 g per week) (OR 0.12, 95% CI 0.02–0.65). A sporadic or occasional pattern of consumption attenuated this association: the odds ratio in the combined group of regular and irregular light-to-moderate drinkers was 0.54 (95% CI 0.28–1.05).

OTHER. The angiotensin I–converting enzyme is important in regulating both blood pressure and salt and water balance. It catalyzes the hydrolysis of angiotensin I to a potent vasoconstrictor. Kinoshita et al. have purified and identified an inhibitor of this enzyme from Japanese-style soy sauce (*317*). Oral administration of a high-molecular-weight fraction of soy sauce reduced the blood pressure of hypertensive rats. The active component was nicotianamine (*N*-[*N*-(3-amino-3-carboxypropyl)-3-amino-3-carboxypropyl]azetidine-2-carboxylic acid). The $IC_{50}$ value of this inhibitor, using a rabbit lung enzyme with hippuryl-L-histidyl-L-leucine as substrate, was 0.26 mM.

Populations whose major dietary fat is olive oil tend to have low levels of serum cholesterol and a low prevalence of CHD. However, olive oil is a rich source of squalene, a $C_{30}H_{50}$ carotenoid with 6 unconjugated double bonds and a cholesterol precursor. Little is known about the impact of dietary squalene on serum cholesterol levels. There are theoretical arguments for both desirable and undesirable effects. Miettinen and Vanhanen explored the impact of squalene on cholesterol metabolism (*318*). In a crossover study, middle-aged hypercholesterolemic men consumed diets containing rapeseed oil with and without added squalene. Substitution of 50 g/d of customary dietary fat with 50 g of rapeseed oil reduced serum cholesterol levels by 9%. Addition of 1 g/d of squalene to the rapeseed oil increased cholesterol by 15%, significantly enhanced production of LDL apoB, and decreased removal of LDL apoB. Addition of 0.5 g/d of squalene had virtually no impact on lipoprotein concentrations. The authors concluded that long-term use of low-squalene olive oil (2–7 mg of squalene per gram of oil) would have few or no undesirable squalene-related effects on serum cholesterol. Other biochemical and metabolic findings and their implications were discussed.

Nanjo et al. explored the effects of green tea catechins on blood rheology in rats fed a high-fat diet (*319*). The transit time of erythrocytes was measured in an apparatus that forms simulated capillaries when the substrate is mechanically pressed against an optically flat glass plate. The time taken for a 100-mL sample to pass through the capillaries was taken to indicate the flow properties of the erythrocytes. Tea catechins prevented the fat-induced increase in transit time of erythrocytes in plasma suspension but had no effect on transit time in buffer. The authors concluded that catechins protect the flow properties of erythrocytes by inhibiting an undesirable interaction with plasma. The catechins also prevented plasma triacylglycerol levels from increasing by blocking lipid absorption.

Glucobrassicin is abundant in cruciferous vegetables. During food preparation and chewing it is autolyzed to indole-3-carbinol, which undergoes acid condensation in the stomach to yield various oligomeric derivatives. Orally administered indole-3-carbinol significantly reduced serum total, LDL, and VLDL cholesterol levels in cholesterol-fed mice (*320*). The effect was apparently mediated by the inhibition of acyl-CoA:cholesterol acyltransferase activity. This is one possible mechanism by which cruciferous vegetables lower serum cholesterol levels.

Costa et al. evaluated the lipid response of hypercholesterolemic pigs to 0, 100, 200, and 300 g of baked beans (*Phaseolus vulgaris*) added to a Western-type diet (*321*). Consumption of 100, 200, and 300 g/kg of baked beans reduced plasma total cholesterol by 5.3, 20.2, and 35.6%, respectively. Only the 35.6% reduction was statistically significant (*p* <.05). The highest level of beans also significantly reduced LDL cholesterol by 48%. VLDL and HDL cholesterol and triacylglycerols did not change. At 200 and 300 g/kg, baked beans significantly reduced cholesterol deposition in the liver by ~50%. These findings suggest that the beans act either by increasing cholesterol excretion and/or turnover or by inhibiting cholesterol synthesis.

Chitosan is the name given to the dilute acid–soluble fraction of deacetylated chitin. Chitosan's chemical structure is similar to that of cellulose. Because it is not hydrolyzable by human digestive enzymes it is considered a dietary fiber of animal origin. However, the presence of an amino group in the cationic polymer distinguishes chitosan from other dietary fibers. Maezaki et al. evaluated the hypocholesterolemic effect of chitosan in healthy young men (*322*). A daily dose of 3–6 g was incorporated into biscuits and fed for 14 days. Similar control biscuits contained no chitosan. Chitosan significantly decreased total serum cholesterol. HDL cholesterol and fecal excretion of cholic acid and chenodeoxycholic acid increased significantly. Values returned to baseline after chitosan feeding was stopped. These data suggest that chitosan formed complexes with the bile acids, which were then excreted. The decreased resorption of bile acids reduced the body's cholesterol pool and consequently the level of serum cholesterol.

## *LITERATURE CITED*

1. Chait, A., J.D. Brunzell, M.A. Denke, et al. Rationale of the diet–heart statement of the American Heart Association. Report of the Nutrition Committee. *Circulation* 88:3008–3029 (1993).

2. Rossouw, J.E. The effects of lowering serum cholesterol on coronary heart disease risk. *Med. Clin. North Am.* 78:181–195 (1994).

3. Calvert, G.D. A review of observational studies on the relationship between cholesterol and coronary heart disease. *Aust. N.Z. J. Med.* 24:89–91 (1994).

4. Law, M.R., N.J. Wald, and S.G. Thompson. By how much and how quickly does reduction in serum cholesterol concentration lower risk of ischaemic heart disease? *Br. Med. J.* 308:367–372 (1994).

5. Law, M.R., N.J. Wald, T. Wu, et al. Systematic underestimation of association between serum cholesterol concentration and ischaemic heart disease in observational studies: data from the BUPA study. *Br. Med. J.* 308:363–366 (1994).

6. Bonneux, L., and J.J. Barendregt. Ischaemic heart disease and cholesterol. (Letter.) *Br. Med. J.* 308:1038 (1994).

7. Ravnskov, U. Ischaemic heart disease and cholesterol. (Letter.) *Br. Med. J.* 308:1038 (1994).

8. Ramsay, L.E., W.W. Yeo, and P.R. Jackson. Ischaemic heart disease and cholesterol. (Letter.) *Br. Med. J.* 308:1038–1039 (1994).

9. Sheldon, T.A. Ischaemic heart disease and cholesterol. (Letter.) *Br. Med. J.* 308:1039 (1994).

10. Millo, J. Ischaemic heart disease and cholesterol. (Letter.) *Br. Med. J.* 308:1039 (1994).

11. Sudlow, C.L.M., and M.R. MacLeod. Ischaemic heart disease and cholesterol. (Letter.) *Br. Med. J.* 308:1039–1040 (1994).

12. Heady, J.A., J.N. Morris, and M.F. Oliver. Ischaemic heart disease and cholesterol. (Letter.) *Br. Med. J.* 308:1040 (1994).

13. Vine, D.L., and G.E. Hastings. Ischaemic heart disease and cholesterol. (Letter.) *Br. Med. J.* 308:1040 (1994).

14. Dugdale, A. Ischaemic heart disease and cholesterol. (Letter.) *Br. Med. J.* 308:1041 (1994).

15. Muldoon, M.F. Ischaemic heart disease and cholesterol. (Letter.) *Br. Med. J.* 308:1104–1105 (1994).

16. Law, M.R., N.J. Wald, T. Wu, et al. Ischaemic heart disease and cholesterol. (Reply.) *Br. Med. J.* 308:1041 (1994).

17. Law, M.R., N.J. Wald, T. Wu, et al. Ischaemic heart disease and cholesterol. (Reply.) *Br. Med. J.* 308:1105 (1994).

18. Shestov, D.B., A.D. Deev, A.N. Klimov, et al. Increased risk of coronary heart disease death in men with low total and low-density lipoprotein cholesterol in the Russian Lipid Research Clinics Prevalence Follow-Up Study. *Circulation* 88:846–853 (1993).

19. Atkins, D., B.M. Psaty, T.D. Koepsell, et al. Cholesterol reduction and the risk for stroke in men. A meta-analysis of randomized, controlled trials. *Ann. Intern. Med.* 119:136–145 (1993).

20. Woodard, D.A., and M.C. Limacher. The impact of diet on coronary heart disease. *Med. Clin. North Am.* 77:849–862 (1993).

21. Stein, P.P. The role of diet in the genesis and treatment of hypertension. *Med. Clin. North Am.* 77:831–847 (1993).

22. Hennig, B., and A. Alvarado. Nutrition and endothelial cell integrity: implications in atherosclerosis. *Prog. Food Nutr. Sci.* 17:119–157 (1993).

23. Barker, D.J.P. The intrauterine origins of cardiovascular disease. *Acta Pædiatr.* Suppl. 391:93–99 (1993).

24. Preuss, H.G. Nutrition and diseases of women: cardiovascular disorders. *J. Am. Coll. Nutr.* 12:417–425 (1993).

25. Ortega, R.M., P. Andres, M. Azuela, et al. Parental death from cardiovascular disease and dietary habits in an elderly group. *Br. J. Nutr.* 71:259–270 (1994).

26. Lamon-Fava, S., J.L. Jenner, P.F. Jacques, and E.J. Schaefer. Effects of dietary intakes on plasma lipids, lipoproteins, and apolipoproteins in free-living elderly men and women. *Am. J. Clin. Nutr.* 59:32–41 (1994).

27. Artaud-Wild, S.M., S.L. Connor, G. Sexton, and W.E. Connor. Differences in coronary mortality can be explained by differences in cholesterol and saturated fat intakes in 40 countries but not in France and Finland. A paradox. *Circulation* 88:2771–2779 (1993).

28. Gartside, P.S., and C.J. Glueck. Relationship of dietary intake to hospital admission for coronary heart and vascular disease: the NHANES II national probability study. *J. Am. Coll. Nutr.* 12:676–684 (1993).

29. Fehily, A.M., J.E. Pickering, J.W.G. Yarnell, and P.C. Elwood. Dietary indices of atherogenicity and thrombogenicity and ischaemic heart disease risk: the Caerphilly Prospective Study. *Br. J. Nutr.* 71:249–257 (1994).

30. Elwood, P.C., A.D. Beswick, J.R. O'Brien, et al. Inter-relationships between haemostatic tests and the effects of some dietary determinants in the Caerphilly cohort of older men. *Blood Coagulation Fibrinol.* 4:529–536 (1993).

31. Goldbourt, U., S. Yaari, and J.H. Medalie. Factors predictive of long-term coronary heart disease mortality among 10,059 male Israeli civil servants and municipal employees. *Cardiology* 82:100–121 (1993).

32. Tzonou, A., A. Kaladidi, A. Trichopoulou, et al. Diet and coronary heart disease: a case–control study in Athens, Greece. *Epidemiology* 4:511–516 (1993).

33. Toshima, H. Coronary artery disease trends in Japan. *Jpn. Circ. J.* 58:166–172 (1994).

34. Okayama, A., H. Ueshima, M.G. Marmot, et al. Changes in total serum cholesterol and other risk factors for cardiovascular disease in Japan, 1980–1989. *Int. J. Epidemiol.* 22:1038–1047 (1993).

35. Egusa, G., F. Murakami, C. Ito, et al. Westernized food habits and concentrations of serum lipids in the Japanese. *Atherosclerosis* 100:249–255 (1993).

36. Lloyd, B.L. Declining cardiovascular disease incidence and environmental components. *Aust. N.Z. J. Med.* 24:124–132 (1994).

37. Fraser, G.E. Diet and coronary heart disease: beyond dietary fats and low-density-lipoprotein cholesterol. *Am. J. Clin. Nutr.* 59(Suppl.):1117S–1123S (1994).

38. Gutteridge, J.M.C., and J. Swain. Lipoprotein oxidation: the 'fruit and vegetable gradient' and heart disease. *Br. J. Biomed. Sci.* 50:284–288 (1993).

39. Melby, C.L., M.L. Toohey, and J. Cebrick. Blood pressure and blood lipids among vegetarian, semivegetarian, and nonvegetarian African Americans. *Am. J. Clin. Nutr.* 59:103–109 (1994).

40. Pan, W.-H., C.-J. Chin, C.-T. Sheu, and M.-H. Lee. Hemostatic factors and blood lipids in young Buddhist vegetarians and omnivores. *Am. J. Clin. Nutr.* 58:354–359 (1993).

41. Beilin, L.J. Vegetarian and other complex diets, fats, fiber, and hypertension. *Am. J. Clin. Nutr.* 59(Suppl.): 1130S–1135S (1994).

42. Posner, B.M., L.A. Cupples, M.M. Franz, and D.R. Gagnon. Diet and heart disease risk factors in adult American men and women: the Framingham Offspring–Spouse nutrition studies. *Int. J. Epidemiol.* 22:1014–1025 (1993).

43. Posner, B.M., A. Cupples, D. Gagnon, et al. Healthy People 2000. The rationale and potential efficacy of preventive nutrition in heart disease: the Framingham Offspring–Spouse study. *Arch. Intern. Med.* 153:1549–1556 (1993).

44. Johnson, C.L., B.M. Rifkind, C.T. Sempos, et al. Declining serum total cholesterol levels among US adults. The National Health and Nutrition Examination Surveys. *JAMA* 269:3002–3008 (1993).

45. Sempos, C., J.I. Cleeman, M.D. Carroll, et al. Prevalence of high blood cholesterol among US adults. An update based on guidelines from the second report of the National Cholesterol Education Program Adult Treatment Panel. *JAMA* 269:3009–3014 (1993).

46. Expert Panel on Detection, Evaluation, and Treatment of High Blood Cholesterol in Adults. Summary of the second report of the National Cholesterol Education Program (NCEP) Expert Panel on Detection, Evaluation, and Treatment of High Blood Cholesterol in Adults (Adult Treatment Panel II). *JAMA* 269:3015–3023 (1993).

47. Dowler, E. Diet and coronary heart disease in women. *Food Policy* 18:224–236 (1993).

48. Kris-Etherton, P.M., and D. Krummel. Role of nutrition in the prevention and treatment of coronary heart disease in women. *J. Am. Diet. Assoc.* 93:987–993 (1993).

49. Fortmann, S.P., C.B. Taylor, J.A. Flora, and M.A. Winkleby. Effect of community health education on plasma cholesterol levels and diet: the Stanford Five-City Project. *Am. J. Epidemiol.* 137:1039–1055 (1993).

50. Baier, J.T. Improved plasma cholesterol levels in men after a nutrition education program at the worksite. *J. Am. Diet. Assoc.* 93:658–663 (1993).

51. Cruz, M.L.A., W.W. Wong, F. Mimouni, et al. Effects of infant nutrition on cholesterol synthesis rates. *Pediatr. Res.* 35:135–140 (1994).

52. Gaburro, D., E. Gonfiantini, R. Piccoli, et al. Diet and drugs therapy of hypercholesterolemia in childhood. *Nutr. Res.* 13(Suppl. 1):S73–S82 (1993).

53. Sanchez-Bayle, M., A. Ganzalez-Requejo, J. Baeza, et al. Diet therapy for hypercholesterolemia in children and adults. *Arch. Pediatr. Adolesc. Med.* 148:28–32 (1994).

54. Connor, W.E., and S.L. Connor. Importance of diet in the treatment of familial hypercholesterolemia. *Am. J. Cardiol.* 72:42D–53D (1993).

55. Denke, M.A. Diet and lifestyle modification and its relationship to atherosclerosis. *Med. Clin. North Am.* 78:197–223 (1994).

56. Ornish, D. Can lifestyle changes reverse coronary heart disease? In *Nutrition and Fitness in Health and Disease.* A.P. Simopoulos (ed.). Basel, Karger. *World Rev. Nutr. Diet.* 72:38–48 (1993).

57. Watts, G.F., P. Jackson, S. Mandalia, et al. Nutrient intake and progression of coronary artery disease. *Am. J. Cardiol.* 73:328–332 (1994).

58. Anderson, J.W. Diet, lipids, and cardiovascular disease in women. *J. Am. Coll. Nutr.* 12:433–437 (1993).

59. Rivellese, A.A., P. Auletta, G. Marotta, et al. Long term metabolic effects of two dietary methods of treating hyperlipidaemia. *Br. Med. J.* 308:227–231 (1994).

60. Leenen, R., K. van der Kooy, S. Meyboom, et al. Relative effects of weight loss and dietary fat modification on serum lipid levels in the dietary treatment of obesity. *J. Lipid Res.* 34:2183–2191 (1993).

61. Rontoyannis, G.P. Diet and exercise in the prevention of cardiovascular disease. In *Nutrition and Fitness in Health and Disease.* A.P. Simopoulos (ed.). Basel, Karger. *World Rev. Nutr. Diet.* 72:9–22 (1993).

62. The ODES Investigators. The Oslo Diet and Exercise Study (ODES): design and objectives. *Controlled Clin. Trials* 14:229–243 (1993).

63. Denke, M.A., and S.M. Grundy. Individual responses to a cholesterol-lowering diet in 50 men with moderate hypercholesterolemia. *Arch. Intern. Med.* 154:317–325 (1994).

64. Truswell, A.S. Review of dietary intervention studies: effect on coronary events and on total mortality. *Aust. N.Z. J. Med.* 24:98–106 (1994).

65. Roberts, W.C. The ineffectiveness of a commonly recommended lipid-lowering diet in significantly lowering the serum total and low-density lipoprotein cholesterol levels. *Am. J. Cardiol.* 73:623–624 (1994).

66. Arnon, R., E. Sehayek, and S. Eisenberg. Disparate effects of a triglyceride lowering diet and of bezafibrate on the HDL system: a study in patients with hypertriglyceridaemia and low HDL-cholesterol levels. *Eur. J. Clin. Invest.* 23:492–498 (1993).

67. Marckmann, P., B. Sandström, and J. Jespersen. Low-fat, high-fiber diet favorably affects several independent risk markers of ischemic heart disease: observations on blood lipids, coagulation, and fibrinolysis from a trial of middle-aged Danes. *Am. J. Clin. Nutr.* 59:935–939 (1994).

68. Marckmann, P., B. Sandström, and J. Jespersen. Dietary effects on circadian fluctuation in human blood coagulation factor VII and fibrinolysis. *Atherosclerosis* 101:225–234 (1993).

69. Rankinen, T., R. Rauramaa, S. Väisänen, et al. Blood coagulation and fibrinolytic factors are unchanged by aerobic exercise or fat modified diet. *Fibrinolysis* 8:48–53 (1994).

70. Sinclair, A.J., L. Johnson, K. O'Dea, and R.T. Holman. Diets rich in lean beef increase arachidonic acid and long-chain ω3 polyunsaturated fatty acid levels in plasma phospholipids. *Lipids* 29:337–343 (1994).

71. Stanko, R.T., H.R. Reynolds, R. Hoyson, et al. Pyruvate supplementation of a low-cholesterol, low-fat diet: effects on plasma lipid concentrations and body composition in hyperlipidemic patients. *Am. J. Clin. Nutr.* 59:423–427 (1994).

72. Sciarrone, S.E.G., M.T. Strahan, L.J. Beilin, et al. Biochemical and neurohormonal responses to the introduction of a lacto-ovovegetarian diet. *J. Hypertens.* 11:849–860 (1993).

73. Ramsay, L.E., W.W. Yeo, I.G. Chadwick, and P.R. Jackson. Non-pharmacological therapy of hypertension. *Br. Med. Bull.* 50:494–508 (1994).

74. Lusis, A.J. The mouse model for atherosclerosis. *Trends Cardiovasc. Med.* 3:135–143 (1993).

75. Daley, S.J., E.E. Herderick, J.F. Cornhill, and K.A. Rogers. Cholesterol-fed and casein-fed rabbit models of atherosclerosis. Part 1: Differing lesion area and volume despite equal plasma cholesterol levels. *Arterioscler. Thromb.* 14:95–104 (1994).

76. Daley, S.J., K.F. Klemp, J.R. Guyton, and K.A. Rogers. Cholesterol-fed and casein-fed rabbit models of atherosclerosis. Part 2: Differing morphological severity of atherogenesis despite matched plasma cholesterol levels. *Arterioscler. Thromb.* 14:105–114 (1994).

77. Bravo, E., A. Cantafora, A. Calcabrini, and G. Ortu. Why prefer the golden Syrian hamster (*Mesocricetus auratus*) to the Wistar rat in experimental studies on plasma lipoprotein metabolism? *Comp. Biochem. Physiol.* 107B:347–355 (1994).

78. Goldbourt, U. Coronary heart disease prevention, nutrition, physical exercise and genetics: rationale for aiming at the identification of subgroups at differing genetic risks. In *Nutrition and Fitness in Health and Disease.* A.P. Simopoulos (ed.). Basel, Karger. *World Rev. Nutr. Diet.* 72:23–37 (1993).

79. Pesonen, E., J. Viikari, L. Räsänen, et al. Nutritional and genetic contributions to serum cholesterol concentration in a children's follow-up study. *Acta Pædiatr.* 83:378–382 (1994).

80. Dreon, D.M., H.A. Fernstrom, B. Miller, and R.M. Krauss. Low-density lipoprotein subclass patterns and lipoprotein response to a reduced-fat diet in men. *FASEB J.* 8:121–126 (1994).

81. Humphries, S.E. Life style, genetic factors and the risk of heart attack: the apolipoprotein B gene as an example. *Biochem. Soc. Trans.* 21:569–582 (1993).

82. Hegele, R.A., G. Zahariadis, A.L. Jenkins, et al. Genetic variation associated with differences in the response of plasma apolipoprotein B levels to dietary fibre. *Clin. Sci.* 85:269–275 (1993).

83. Friedlander, Y., N.A. Kaufmann, H. Cedar, and J.D. Kark. XbaI polymorphism of the apolipoprotein B gene and plasma lipid and lipoprotein response to dietary fat and cholesterol: a clinical trial. *Clin. Genet.* 43:223–231 (1993).

84. Jones, P.J.H., B.F. Main, and J.J. Frohlich. Response of cholesterol synthesis to cholesterol feeding in men with different apolipoprotein E genotypes. *Metabolism* 42:1065–1071 (1993).

85. Russell, M.E., K.M. Weiss, A.V. Buchanan, et al. Plasma lipids and diet of the Mvskoke Indians. *Am. J. Clin. Nutr.* 59:847–852 (1994).

86. Cobb, M., J. Greenspan, M. Timmons, and H. Teitelbaum. Gender differences in lipoprotein responses to diet. *Ann. Nutr. Metab.* 37:225–236 (1993).

87. Roach, P.D., J. Hosking, P.M. Clifton, et al. The effects of hypercholesterolaemia, simvastatin and dietary fat on the low density lipoprotein receptor of unstimulated mononuclear cells. *Atherosclerosis* 103:245–254 (1993).

88. Rainwater, D.L. Genetic effects on dietary response of Lp(a) concentrations in baboons. *Chem. Phys. Lipids* 67/68:199–205 (1994).

89. Hasan, S.Q., and R.S. Kushwaha. Differences in 27-hydroxycholesterol concentrations in plasma and liver of baboons with high and low responses to dietary cholesterol and fat. *Biochim. Biophys. Acta* 1182:299–302 (1993).

90. Kushwaha, R.S., K.S. Rice, D.S. Lewis, et al. The role of cholesterol absorption and hepatic cholesterol content in high and low responses to dietary cholesterol and fat in pedigreed baboons (*Papio* species). *Metabolism* 42:714–722 (1993).

91. Kushwaha, R.S., C.A. Reardon, G.S. Getz, et al. Metabolic mechanisms for responses to dietary cholesterol and fat in high and low LDL responding baboons (*Papio* sp.). *J. Lipid Res.* 35:633–643 (1994).

92. Jenkins, D.J.A., T.M.S. Wolever, A. Venketeshwer, et al. Effect on blood lipids of very high intakes of fiber in diets low in saturated fat and cholesterol. *New Engl. J. Med.* 329:21–26 (1993).

93. Morgan, L.M., J.A. Tredger, Y. Shavila, et al. The effect of non-starch polysaccharide supplementation on circulating bile acids, hormone and metabolite levels following a fat meal in human subjects. *Br. J. Nutr.* 70:491–501 (1993).

94. Hunninghake, D.B., V.T. Miller, J.C. LaRosa, et al. Hypocholesterolemic effects of a dietary fiber supplement. *Am. J. Clin. Nutr.* 59:1050–1054 (1994).

95. Wisker, E., M. Daniel, and W. Feldheim. Effects of a fiber concentrate from citrus fruits in humans. *Nutr. Res.* 14:361–372 (1994).

96. Cerda, J.J., S.J. Normann, M.P. Sullivan, et al. Inhibition of atherosclerosis by dietary pectin in microswine with sustained hypercholesterolemia. *Circulation* 89:1247–1253 (1994).

97. Ranhotra, G.S., J.A. Gelroth, and B.K. Glaser. Effect of pectin–wheat bran blends on rat blood lipid and fecal responses and on muffin quality. *Cereal Chem.* 70:530–534 (1993).

98. Wolever, T.M.S., D.J.A. Jenkins, S. Mueller, et al. Psyllium reduces blood lipids in men and women with hyperlipidemia. *Am. J. Med. Sci.* 307:269–273 (1994).

99. Wolever, T.M.S., D.J.A. Jenkins, S. Mueller, et al. Method of administration influences the serum

cholesterol–lowering effect of psyllium. *Am. J. Clin. Nutr.* 59:1055–1059 (1994).

100. Stoy, D.B., J.C. LaRosa, B.K. Brewer, et al. Cholesterol-lowering effects of ready-to-eat cereal containing psyllium. *J. Am. Diet. Assoc.* 93:910–912 (1993).

101. Sprecher, D.L., B.V. Harris, A.C. Goldberg, et al. Efficacy of psyllium in reducing serum cholesterol levels in hypercholesterolemic patients on high- or low-fat diets. *Ann. Intern. Med.* 119:545–554 (1993).

102. Dennison, B.A., and D.M. Levine. Randomized, double-blind, placebo-controlled, two-period crossover clinical trial of psyllium fiber in children with hypercholesterolemia. *J. Pediatr.* 123:24–29 (1993).

103. Gelissin, I.C., B. Brodie, and M.A. Eastwood. Effect of *Plantago ovata* (psyllium) husk and seeds on sterol metabolism: studies in normal and ileostomy subjects. *Am. J. Clin. Nutr.* 59:395–400 (1994).

104. Langkilde, A.M., H. Andersson, and I. Bosaeus. Sugar-beet fibre increases cholesterol and reduces bile acid excretion from the small bowel. *Br. J. Nutr.* 70:757–766 (1993).

105. Basu, T.K., B. Ooraikul, and M. Garg. The lipid-lowering effects of rhubarb stalk fiber: a new source of dietary fiber. *Nutr. Res.* 13:1017–1024 (1993).

106. Hassona, H.Z. High fibre bread containing brewer's spent grains and its effect on lipid metabolism in rats. *Nahrung* 37:576–582 (1993).

107. Lupton, J.R., M.C. Robinson, and J.L. Morin. Cholesterol-lowering effect of barley bran flour and oil. *J. Am. Diet. Assoc.* 94:65–70 (1994).

108. Bierenbaum, M.L., R. Reichstein, and T.R. Watkins. Reducing atherogenic risk in hyperlipemic humans with flax seed supplementation: a preliminary report. *J. Am. Coll. Nutr.* 12:501–504 (1993).

109. Zhang, J.-X., E. Lundin, G. Hallmans, et al. Effect of rye bran on excretion of bile acids, cholesterol, nitrogen, and fat in human subjects with ileostomies. *Am. J. Clin. Nutr.* 59:389–394 (1994).

110. Kahlon, T.S., F.I. Chow, and R.N. Sayre. Cholesterol-lowering properties of rice bran. *Cereal Foods World* 39.99-103 (1994).

111. Marsono, Y., R.J. Illman, J.M. Clarke, et al. Plasma lipids and large bowel volatile fatty acids in pigs fed on white rice, brown rice and rice bran. *Br. J. Nutr.* 70:503–513 (1993).

112. Poulter, N., C.L. Chang, A. Cuff, et al. Lipid profiles after the daily consumption of an oat-based cereal: a controlled crossover trial. *Am. J. Clin. Nutr.* 58:66–69 (1993).

113. Illman, R.J., G.B. Storer, and D.L. Topping. White wheat flour lowers plasma cholesterol and increases cecal steroids relative to whole wheat flour, wheat bran and wheat pollard in rats. *J. Nutr.* 123:1094–1100 (1993).

114. Truswell, A.S. Food carbohydrates and plasma lipids—an update. *Am. J. Clin. Nutr.* 59(Suppl.):710S–718S (1994).

115. Hollenbeck, C.B. Dietary fructose effects on lipoprotein metabolism and risk for coronary artery disease. *Am. J. Clin. Nutr.* 58(Suppl.):800S–809S (1993).

116. Bolton-Smith, C., and M. Woodward. Coronary heart disease: prevalence and dietary sugars in Scotland. *J. Epidemiol. Commun. Health* 48:119–122 (1994).

117. Preuss, H.G., S. Memon, A. Dadgar, and J. Gongwei. Effects of high sugar diets on renal fluid, electrolyte and mineral handling in rats: relationship to blood pressure. *J. Am. Coll. Nutr.* 13:73–82 (1994).

118. Potter, S.M., R.M. Bakhit, D.L. Essex-Sorlie, et al. Depression of plasma cholesterol in men by consumption of baked products containing soy protein. *Am. J. Clin. Nutr.* 58:501–506 (1993).

119. Bakhit, R.M., B.P. Klein, D. Essex-Sorlie, et al. Intake of 25 g of soybean protein with or without soybean fiber alters plasma lipids in men with elevated cholesterol concentrations. *J. Nutr.* 124:213–222 (1994).

120. Ham, J.O., K.M. Chapman, D. Essex-Sorlie, et al. Endocrinological response to soy protein and fiber in mildly hypercholesterolemic men. *Nutr. Res.* 13:873–884 (1993).

121. Widhalm, K., G. Brazda, B. Schneider, and S. Koh. Effect of soy protein diet versus standard low fat, low cholesterol diet on lipid and lipoprotein levels in children with familial or polygenic hypercholesterolemia. *J. Pediatr.* 123:30–34 (1993).

122. Huang, Y.-S., K. Koba, D.F. Horrobin, and M. Sugano. Interrelationship between dietary protein, cholesterol and n–6 polyunsaturated fatty acid metabolism. *Prog. Lipid Res.* 32:123–137 (1993).

123. Potter, S.M., R. Jimenez-Flores, J. Pollack, et al. Protein–saponin interaction and its influence on blood lipids. *J. Agric. Food Chem.* 41:1287–1291 (1993).

124. Yamamoto, S., T. Kina, N. Yamagata, et al. Favorable effects of egg white protein on lipid metabolism in rats and mice. *Nutr. Res.* 13:1453–1457 (1993).

125. Kurowska, E.M., and K.K. Carroll. Hypercholesterolemic responses in rabbits to selected groups of dietary essential amino acids. *J. Nutr.* 124:364–370 (1994).

126. Satoh, T., M. Goto, and K. Igarashi. Effects of protein isolates from radish and spinach leaves on serum lipids levels in rats. *J. Nutr. Sci. Vitaminol.* 39:627–633 (1993).

127. Zöllner, N. Die Fettsäuren in der Nahrung: ihre Bedeutung für Serumlipide, Lipoproteine und Atherosklerose. *Fett Wissenschaft Technol.* 95:437–441 (1993).

128. Dietschy, J.M., S.D. Turley, and D.K. Spady. Role of liver in the maintenance of cholesterol and low density lipoprotein homeostasis in different animal species, including humans. *J. Lipid Res.* 34:1637–1659 (1993).

129. Fuchs, G.J., R.P. Farris, M. DeWier, et al. Effect of dietary fat on cardiovascular risk factors in infancy. *Pediatrics* 93:756–763 (1994).

130. Tell, G.S., G.W. Evans, A.R. Folsom, et al. Dietary fat intake and carotid artery wall thickness: the Atherosclerosis Risk in Communities (ARIC) study. *Am. J. Epidemiol.* 139:979–989 (1994).

131. Charnock, J.S. Dietary fats and cardiac arrhythmia in primates. *Nutrition* 10:161–169 (1994).

132. Sanders, K., L. Johnson, K. O'Dea, and A.J. Sinclair. The effect of dietary fat level and quality on plasma lipoprotein

lipids and plasma fatty acids in normocholesterolemic subjects. *Lipids* 29:129–138 (1994).

133. Sarkkinen, E.S., M.I.J. Uusitupa, P. Pietinen, et al. Long-term effects of three fat-modified diets in hypercholesterolemic subjects. *Atherosclerosis* 105:9–23 (1994).

134. Cobb, M.M., and H. Teitlebaum. Determinants of plasma cholesterol responsiveness to diet. *Br. J. Nutr.* 71:271–282 (1994).

135. Steinmetz, K.A., M.T. Childs, C. Stimson, et al. Effects of consumption of whole milk and skim milk on blood lipid profiles in healthy men. *Am. J. Clin. Nutr.* 59:612–618 (1994).

136. Jauhiainen, M., A. Aro, S.M. Blomqvist, et al. Effects of milk fat, unhydrogenated and partially hydrogenated vegetables oils on serum lipoproteins in growing pigs. *Comp. Biochem. Physiol.* 106A:565–570 (1993).

137. Mogadam, M. Walnuts and serum lipids. (Letter.) *New Engl. J. Med.* 329:358–359 (1993).

138. Prineas, R.J., L.H. Kushi, A.R. Folsom, et al. Walnuts and serum lipids. (Letter.) *New Engl. J. Med.* 329:359 (1993).

139. Sabaté, J., and G.E. Fraser. Walnuts and serum lipids. (Reply.) *New Engl. J. Med.* 329:359–360 (1993).

140. Towle, L.A., E.A. Bergman, and E. Joseph. Low-fat bison-hybrid ground meat has no effects on serum lipid levels in a study of 12 men. *J. Am. Diet. Assoc.* 94:546–548 (1994).

141. Denke, M.A., and I.D. Frantz, Jr. Response to a cholesterol-lowering diet: efficacy is greater in hypercholesterolemic subjects even after adjustment for regression to the mean. *Am. J. Med.* 94:626–631 (1993).

142. Glat, J.F.C., and M.B. Katan. Dietary saturated fatty acids increase cholesterol synthesis and fecal steroid excretion in healthy men and women. *Eur. J. Clin. Invest.* 23:648–655 (1993).

143. Emken, E.A., R.O. Adlor, W.K. Rohwedder, and R.M. Gulley. Influence of linoleic acid on desaturation and uptake of deuterium-labeled palmitic and stearic acids in humans. *Biochim. Biophys. Acta* 1170:173–181 (1993).

144. Sundram, K., K.C. Hayes, and O.H. Siru. Dietary palmitic acid results in lower serum cholesterol than does a lauric–myristic acid combination in normolipemic humans. *Am. J. Clin. Nutr.* 59:841–846 (1994).

145. Kris-Etherton, P.M. Effects of chain length of saturated fatty acids on plasma total, LDL- and HDL-cholesterol levels. *Fett Wissenschaft Technol.* 95:448–452 (1993).

146. Tholstrup, T., P. Marckmann, J. Jesperson, and B. Sandström. Fat high in stearic acid favorably affects blood lipids and factor VII coagulant activity in comparison with fats high in palmitic acid or high in myristic and lauric acids. *Am. J. Clin. Nutr.* 59:371–377 (1994).

147. Mitropoulos, K.A., G.J. Miller, J.C. Martin, et al. Dietary fat induces changes in factor VII coagulant activity through effects on plasma free stearic acid concentration. *Arterioscler. Thromb.* 14:214–222 (1994).

148. Connelly, J.B., P.J. Roderick, J.A. Cooper, et al. Positive association between self-reported fatty food consumption and factor VII coagulant activity, a risk factor for coronary heart disease, in 4246 middle-aged men. *Thromb. Haemostasis* 70:250–252 (1993).

149. Morgan, S.A., A.J. Sinclair, and K. O'Dea. Effect on serum lipids of addition of safflower oil or olive oil to very-low-fat diets rich in lean beef. *J. Am. Diet. Assoc.* 93:644–648 (1993).

150. Seventh Créteil Symposium on Lipids, Lipoproteins and Nutrition: Monounsaturated Fatty Acids and Lipoproteins. (Abstracts.) *Ann. Nutr. Metab.* 37:272–288 (1993).

151. Nydahl, M.C., I.-B. Gustafsson, and B. Vessby. Lipid-lowering diets enriched with monounsaturated or polyunsaturated fatty acids but low in saturated fatty acids have similar effects on serum lipid concentrations in hyperlipidemic patients. *Am. J. Clin. Nutr.* 59:115–122 (1994).

152. Gustafsson, I.-B., B. Vessby, M. Öhrvall, and M. Nydahl. A diet rich in monounsaturated rapeseed oil reduces the lipoprotein cholesterol concentration and increases the relative content of *n*–3 fatty acids in serum in hyperlipidemic subjects. *Am. J. Clin. Nutr.* 59:667–674 (1994).

153. Salen, P., M. de Lorgeril, P. Boissonnat, et al. Effects of a French Mediterranean diet on heart transplant recipients with hypercholesterolemia. *Am. J. Cardiol.* 73:825–827 (1994).

154. Abbey, M., M. Noakes, G.B. Belling, and P.J. Nestel. Partial replacement of saturated fatty acids with almonds or walnuts lowers total plasma cholesterol and low-density-lipoprotein cholesterol. *Am. J. Clin. Nutr.* 59:995–999 (1994).

155. de Bruin, T.W.A., C.B. Brouwer, M. van L.-S. Trip, et al. Different postprandial metabolism of olive oil and soybean oil: a possible mechanism of the high-density lipoprotein conserving effect of olive oil. *Am. J. Clin. Nutr.* 58:477–483 (1993).

156. Brousseau, M.E., A.F. Stucchi, D.B. Vespa, et al. A diet enriched in monounsaturated fats decreases low density lipoprotein concentrations in cynomolgus monkeys by a different mechanism than does a diet enriched in polyunsaturated fats. *J. Nutr.* 123:2049–2058 (1993).

157. Nestel, P., P. Clifton, and M. Noakes. Effects of increasing dietary palmitoleic acid compared with palmitic and oleic acids on plasma lipids of hypercholesterolemic men. *J. Lipid Res.* 35:656–662 (1994).

158. Kleinveld, H.A., A.H.J. Naber, A.F.H. Stalenhoef, and P.N.M. Demacker. Oxidation resistance, oxidation rate, and extent of oxidation of human low-density lipoprotein depend on the ratio of oleic acid content to linoleic acid content: studies in vitamin E deficient subjects. *Free Rad. Biol. Med.* 15:273–280 (1993).

159. Lichtenstein, A. *Trans* fatty acids, blood lipids, and cardiovascular risk: where do we stand? *Nutr. Rev.* 51:340–343 (1993).

160. Applewhite, T.H. *trans*-Isomers, serum lipids and cardiovascular disease: another point of view. *Nutr. Rev.* 51:344–345 (1993).

161. Mann, G.V. Metabolic consequences of dietary *trans* fatty acids. *Lancet* 343:1268–1271 (1994).

162. Ascherio, A., C.H. Hennekens, J.E. Buring, et al. *trans*–Fatty acids intake and risk of myocardial infarction. *Circulation* 89:94–101 (1994).

163. Judd, J.T., B.A. Clevidence, R.A. Muesing, et al. Dietary *trans* fatty acids: effects on plasma lipids and lipoproteins of healthy men and women. *Am. J. Clin. Nutr.* 59:861–868 (1994).

164. Zevenbergen, J.L., and M. Rudrum. The role of polyunsaturated fatty acids in the prevention of chronic diseases. *Fett Wissenschaft Technol.* 95:456–460 (1993).

165. Lichtenstein, A.H., L.M. Ausman, W. Carrasco, et al. Effects of canola, corn, and olive oils on fasting and postprandial plasma lipoproteins in humans as part of a National Cholesterol Education Program step 2 diet. *Arterioscler. Thromb.* 13:1533–1542 (1993).

166. Schmidt, E.B., S.D. Kristensen, R. de Caterina, and D.R. Illingworth. The effects of *n*–3 fatty acids on plasma lipids and lipoproteins and other cardiovascular risk factors in patients with hyperlipidemia. *Atherosclerosis* 103:107–121 (1993).

167. Iacono, J.M., and R.M. Dougherty. Effects of polyunsaturated fats on blood pressure. *Annu. Rev. Nutr.* 13:243–260 (1993).

168. McLennan, P.L., T.J. Bridle, M.Y. Abeywardena, and J.S. Charnock. Comparative efficacy of *n*–3 and *n*–6 polyunsaturated fatty acids in modulating ventricular fibrillation threshold in marmoset monkeys. *Am. J. Clin. Nutr.* 58:666–669 (1993).

169. Topping, D. Dietary fatty acids and protection against experimental cardiac arrhythmias in rats. *Nutr. Rev.* 51:271–273 (1993).

170. Siebert, B.D., P.L. McLennan, J.A. Woodhouse, and J.S. Charnock. Cardiac arrhythmia in rats in response to dietary *n*–3 fatty acids from red meat, fish oil and canola oil. *Nutr. Res.* 13:1407–1418 (1993).

171. Sanigorski, A.J., K. O'Dea, and A.J. Sinclair. *n*–3 fatty acids reduce in vitro thromboxane production while having little effect on in vitro prostacyclin production in the rat. *Prostaglandins Leukotrienes Essential Fatty Acids* 50:223–228 (1994).

172. Kawashima, Y., and H. Kozuka. Dietary manipulation by perilla oil and fish oil of hepatic lipids and its influence on peroxisomal β-oxidation and serum lipids in rat and mouse. *Biol. Pharm. Bull.* 16:1194–1199 (1993).

173. Roberts, T.L., D.A. Wood, R.A. Riemersma, et al. Linoleic acid and risk of sudden cardiac death. *Br. Heart J.* 70:524–529 (1993).

174. Hodgson, J.M., M.L. Wahlqvist, J.A. Boxall, and N.D. Balazs. Can linoleic acid contribute to coronary artery disease? *Am. J. Clin. Nutr.* 58:228–234 (1993).

175. Davis, P.A., J.-F. Platon, M.E. Gershwin, et al. A linoleate-enriched cheese product reduces low-density lipoprotein in moderately hypercholesterolemic adults. *Ann. Intern. Med.* 119:555–559 (1993).

176. Barre, D.E., B.J. Holub, and R.S. Chapkin. The effect of borage oil supplementation on human platelet aggregation, thromboxane $B_2$, prostaglandin $E_1$ and $E_2$ formation. *Nutr. Res.* 13:739–751 (1993).

177. Seppänen-Laakso, T., H. Vanhanen, I. Laakso, et al. Replacement of margarine on bread by rapeseed and olive oils: effects on plasma fatty acid composition and serum cholesterol. *Ann. Nutr. Metab.* 37:161–174 (1993).

178. Kelley, D.S., G.J. Nelson, J.E. Love, et al. Dietary α-linolenic acid alters tissue fatty acid composition, but not blood lipids, lipoproteins or coagulation status in humans. *Lipids* 28:533–537 (1993).

179. Chan, J.K., B.E. McDonald, J.M. Gerrard, et al. Effect of dietary α-linolenic acid and its ratio to linoleic acid on platelet and plasma fatty acids and thrombogenesis. *Lipids* 28:811–817 (1993).

180. Freese, R., M. Mutanen, L.M. Balsta, and I. Salminen. Comparison of the effects of two diets rich in monounsaturated fatty acids differing in their linoleic/α-linolenic acid ratio on platelet aggregation. *Thromb. Haemostasis* 71:73–77 (1994).

181. Wolfe, M.S., J.S. Parks, T.M. Morgan, and L.L. Rudel. Childhood consumption of dietary polyunsaturated fat lowers risk for coronary artery atherosclerosis in African green monkeys. *Arterioscler. Thromb.* 13:863–875 (1993).

182. Horrobin, D.F. Omega-6 and omega-3 essential fatty acids in atherosclerosis. *Sem. Thromb. Hemostasis* 19:129–137 (1993).

183. Lee, K.N., D. Kritchevsky, and M.W. Pariza. Conjugated linoleic acid and atherosclerosis in rabbits. *Atherosclerosis* 108:19–25 (1994).

184. Parkinson, A.J., A.L. Cruz, W.L. Heyward, et al. Elevated concentrations of plasma ω–3 polyunsaturated fatty acids among Alaskan Eskimos. *Am. J. Clin. Nutr.* 59:383–388 (1994).

185. Subbaiah, P.V., D. Kaufman, and J.D. Bagdade. Incorporation of dietary *n*–3 fatty acids into molecular species of phosphatidyl choline and cholesteryl ester in normal human plasma. *Am. J. Clin. Nutr.* 58:360–368 (1993).

186. Lutz, M., G. Ahumada, and G. Ruiz. Plasma lipids and liver histochemistry of rats fed sea-lion or corn oil with or without cholesterol supplementation. *Food Chem. Toxicol.* 31:425–430 (1993).

187. Relton, J.K., P.J.L.M. Strijbos, A.L. Cooper, and N.J. Rothwell. Dietary *n*–3 fatty acids inhibit ischaemic and excitotoxic brain damage in the rat. *Brain Res. Bull.* 32:223–226 (1993).

188. Kristensen, S.D., R. De Caterina, E.B. Schmidt, and S. Endres. Fish oil and ischaemic heart disease. *Br. Heart J.* 70:212–214 (1993).

189. Aucamp, A.K., H.S. Schoeman, and J.H.J. Coetzee. Pilot trial to determine the efficacy of a low dose of fish oil in the treatment of angina pectoris in the geriatric patient. *Prostaglandins Leukotrienes Essential Fatty Acids* 49:687–689 (1993).

190. Sassen, L.M.A., J.M.J. Lamers, and P.D. Verdouw. Fish oil and the prevention and regression of atherosclerosis. *Cardiovasc. Drugs Ther.* 8:179–191 (1994).

191. Gapinski, J.P., J.V. VanRuiswyk, G.R. Heudebert, and G.S. Schectman. Preventing restenosis with fish oils

following coronary angioplasty. *Arch. Intern. Med.* 153:1595–1601 (1993).

192. Frankel, E.N., E.J. Parks, R. Xu, et al. Effect of *n*–3 fatty acid–rich fish oil supplementation on the oxidation of low density lipoprotein. *Lipids* 29:233–236 (1994).

193. Saba, P., F. Galeone, F. Giuntoli, et al. A pilot study of the effects of omega-3 polyunsaturated fatty acids on blood lipids in hyperlipidemic patients. *Curr. Ther. Res.* 55:408–415 (1994).

194. Harris, W.S., S.L. Windsor, and J.J. Caspermeyer. Modification of lipid-related atherosclerosis risk factors by ω3 fatty acid ethyl esters in hypertriglyceridemic patients. *J. Nutr. Biochem.* 4:706–712 (1993).

195. Salvi, A., O. Di Stefano, I. Sleiman, et al. Effects of fish oil on serum lipids and lipoprotein(a) levels in heterozygous familial hypercholesterolemia. *Curr. Ther. Res.* 53:717–721 (1993).

196. Contacos, C., P.J. Barter, and D.R. Sullivan. Effect of pravastatin and ω-3 fatty acids on plasma lipids and lipoproteins in patients with combined hyperlipidemia. *Arterioscler. Thromb.* 13:1755–1762 (1993).

197. Dagnelie, P.C, T. Rietveld, G.R. Swart, et al. Effect of dietary fish oil on blood levels of free fatty acids, ketone bodies and triacylglycerol in humans. *Lipids* 29:41–45 (1994).

198. Svaneborg, N., J.M. Møller, E.B. Schmidt, et al. The acute effects of a single very high dose of *n*–3 fatty acids on plasma lipids and lipoproteins in healthy subjects. *Lipids* 29:145–147 (1994).

199. Kim, D.N., J. Schmee, J.E. Baker, et al. Dietary fish oil reduces microthrombi over atherosclerotic lesions in hyperlipidemic swine even in the absence of plasma cholesterol reduction. *Exp. Molec. Pathol.* 59:122–135 (1993).

200. Willumsen, N., J. Skorve, S. Hexeberg, et al. The hypotriglyceridemic effect of eicosapentaenoic acid in rats is reflected in increased mitochondrial fatty acid oxidation followed by diminished lipogenesis. *Lipids* 28:683–690 (1993).

201. Appel, L.J., E.R. Miller, III, A.J. Seidler, and P.K. Whelton. Does supplementation of diet with 'fish oil' reduce blood pressure? A meta-analysis of controlled clinical trials. *Arch. Intern. Med.* 153:1429–1438 (1993).

202. Morris, M.C., F. Sacks, and B. Rosner. Does fish oil lower blood pressure? A meta-analysis of controlled trials. *Circulation* 88:523–533 (1993).

203. Passfall, J., T. Philipp, F. Woermann, et al. Different effects of eicosapentaenoic acid and olive oil on blood pressure, intracellular free platelet calcium, and plasma lipids in patients with essential hypertension. *Clin. Invest.* 71:628–633 (1993).

204. Beilin, L.J., T.A. Mori, R. Vandongen, et al. The effects of omega-3 fatty acids on blood pressure and serum lipids in men at increased risk of cardiovascular disease. *J. Hypertens.* 11(Suppl. 5):S318–S319 (1993).

205. Vandongen, R., T.A. Mori, V. Burke, et al. Effects on blood pressure of ω3 fats in subjects at increased risk of cardiovascular disease. *Hypertension* 22:371–379 (1993).

206. Sacks, F.M., P. Hebert, L.J. Appel, et al. Short report: the effect of fish oil on blood pressure and high-density lipoprotein–cholesterol levels in phase I of the Trials of Hypertension Prevention. *J. Hypertens.* 12:209–213 (1994).

207. Malle, E., and G.M. Kostner. Effects of fish oils on lipid variables and platelet function indices. *Prostaglandins Leukotrienes Essential Fatty Acids* 49:645–663 (1993).

208. Swails, W.S., S.J. Bell, B.R. Bistrian, et al. Fish-oil–containing diet and platelet aggregation. *Nutrition* 9:211–217 (1993).

209. Scheurlen, M., M. Kirchner, M.R. Clemens, and K. Jaschonek. Fish oil preparations rich in docosahexaenoic acid modify platelet responsiveness to prostaglandin–endoperoxide/thromboxane A$_2$ receptor agonists. *Biochem. Pharmacol.* 46:245–249 (1993).

210. Mundal, H.H., K. Gjesdal, and K. Landmark. The effect of *n*-3 fatty acids and nifedipine on platelet function in hypertensive males. *Thromb. Res.* 72:257–262 (1993).

211. Zhu, B.-q., R.E. Sievers, Y.-p. Sun, et al. Is the reduction of myocardial infarct size by dietary fish oil the result of altered platelet function? *Am. Heart J.* 127:744–755 (1994).

212. Chin, J.P.F. Marine oils and cardiovascular reactivity. *Prostaglandins Leukotrienes Essential Fatty Acids* 50:211–222 (1994).

213. Shiina, T., T. Terano, J. Saito, et al. Eicosapentaenoic acid and docosahexaenoic acid suppress the proliferation of vascular smooth muscle cells. *Atherosclerosis* 104:95–103 (1993).

214. Lervang, H.-H., E.B. Schmidt, J. Møller, et al. The effect of low-dose supplementation with *n*–3 polyunsaturated fatty acids on some risk markers of coronary heart disease. *Scand. J. Clin. Lab. Invest.* 53:417–423 (1993).

215. Huff, M.W., D.E. Telford, B.W. Edmonds, et al. Lipoprotein lipases, lipoprotein density gradient profile and LDL receptor activity in miniature pigs fed fish oil and corn oil. *Biochim. Biophys. Acta* 1210:113–122 (1993).

216. Spady, D.K., L.A. Woollett, and J.M. Dietschy. Regulation of plasma LDL-cholesterol levels by dietary cholesterol and fatty acids. *Annu. Rev. Nutr.* 13:355–381 (1993).

217. Lichtenstein, A.H., L.M. Ausman, W. Carrasco, et al. Hypercholesterolemic effect of dietary cholesterol in diets enriched in polyunsaturated and saturated fat. Dietary cholesterol, fat saturation, and plasma lipids. *Arterioscler. Thromb.* 14:168–175 (1994).

218. Khosla, P., and K.C. Hayes. Dietary palmitic acid raises plasma LDL cholesterol relative to oleic acid only at a high intake of cholesterol. *Biochim. Biophys. Acta* 1210:13–22 (1993).

219. Bhadra, S., S.D. Banavali, M. Agrawal, and M.T.R. Subbiah. Cholesterol peroxidation potential as influenced by dietary fat type. *Int. J. Vit. Nutr. Res.* 63:223–228 (1993).

220. Osada, K., E. Sasaki, and M. Sugano. Inhibition of cholesterol absorption by oxidized cholesterol in rats. *Biosci. Biotechnol. Biochem.* 58:782–783 (1994).

221. Schnohr, P., O.Ø. Thomsen, P.R. Hansen, et al. Egg consumption and high-density-lipoprotein cholesterol. *J. Intern. Med.* 235:249–251 (1994).

222. Jiang, Z., and J.S. Sim. Consumption of *n*–3 polyunsaturated fatty acid–enriched eggs and changes in plasma lipids of human subjects. *Nutrition* 9:513–518 (1993).

223. Ellegård, L., and I. Bosaeus. Cholesterol absorption and excretion in ileostomy subjects on high- and low-dietary-cholesterol intakes. *Am. J. Clin. Nutr.* 59:48–52 (1994).

224. Duane, W.C. Effects of lovastatin and dietary cholesterol on sterol homeostasis in healthy human subjects. *J. Clin. Invest.* 92:911–918 (1993).

225. Barness, L.A. Nutritional requirements of infants and children with respect to cholesterol and related compounds. *Am. J. Med. Genetics* 50:353–354 (1994).

226. Wong, W.W., D.L. Hachey, W. Insull, et al. Effect of dietary cholesterol on cholesterol synthesis in breast-fed and formula-fed infants. *J. Lipid Res.* 34:1403–1411 (1993).

227. Riemersma, R.A. Epidemiology and the role of antioxidants in preventing coronary heart disease: a brief overview. *Proc. Nutr. Soc.* 53:59–65 (1994).

228. Manson, J.E., J.M. Gaziano, M.A. Jonas, and C.H. Hennekens. Antioxidants and cardiovascular disease: a review. *J. Am. Coll. Nutr.* 12:426–432 (1993).

229. Kardinaal, A.F.M., F.J. Kok, J. Ringstad, et al. Antioxidants in adipose tissue and risk of myocardial infarction: the EURAMIC study. *Lancet* 342:1379–1384 (1993).

230. Waeg, G., H. Puhl, and H. Esterbauer. LDL-oxidation—results and relevance for atherogenesis and possible clinical consequences. *Fett Wissenschaft Technol.* 96:20–22 (1994).

231. Esterbauer, H., G. Wäg, and H. Puhl. Lipid peroxidation and its role in atherosclerosis. *Br. Med. Bull.* 49:566–576 (1993).

232. Jialal, I., and S.M. Grundy. Effect of combined supplementation with α-tocopherol, ascorbate, and beta carotene on low-density lipoprotein oxidation. *Circulation* 88:2780–2786 (1993).

233. Abbey, M., P.J. Nestel, and P.A. Baghurst. Antioxidant vitamins and low-density-lipoprotein oxidation. *Am. J. Clin. Nutr.* 58:525–532 (1993).

234. Rifici, V.A., and A.K. Khachadurian. Dietary supplementation with vitamins C and E inhibits in vitro oxidation of lipoproteins. *J. Am. Coll. Nutr.* 12:631–637 (1993).

235. Mackness, M.I., C. Abbott, S. Arrol, and P.N. Durrington. The role of high-density lipoprotein and lipid-soluble antioxidant vitamins in inhibiting low-density lipoprotein oxidation. *Biochem. J.* 294:829–834 (1993).

236. Byers, T., and B. Bowman. Vitamin E supplements and coronary heart disease. *Nutr. Rev.* 51:333–336 (1993).

237. O'Keefe, J.H., and C.J. Lavie. Vitamin E and the risk of coronary disease. (Letter.) *New Engl. J. Med.* 329:1424 (1993).

238. Steiner, M. Vitamin E and the risk of coronary disease. (Letter.) *New Engl. J. Med.* 329:1424–1425 (1993).

239. Powell, L.H., and H.R. Black. Vitamin E and the risk of coronary disease. (Letter.) *New Engl. J. Med.* 329:1425 (1993).

240. Sullivan, J.L. Vitamin E and the risk of coronary disease. (Letter.) *New Engl. J. Med.* 329:1425 (1993).

241. Stampfer, M.J., E.B. Rimm, and W.C. Willett. Vitamin E and the risk of coronary disease. (Reply.) *New Engl. J. Med.* 329:1425–1426 (1993).

242. Steinberg, D. Vitamin E and the risk of coronary disease. (Reply.) *New Engl. J. Med.* 329:1426 (1993).

243. Smith, D., V.J. O'Leary, and V.M. Darley-Usmar. The role of α-tocopherol as a peroxyl radical scavenger in human low density lipoprotein. *Biochem. Pharmacol.* 45:2195–2201 (1993).

244. Belcher, J.D., J. Balla, G. Balla, et al. Vitamin E, LDL, and endothelium. Brief oral vitamin supplementation prevents oxidized LDL–mediated vascular injury in vitro. *Arterioscler. Thromb.* 13:1779–1789 (1993).

245. Keaney, J.F., Jr., J.M. Gaziano, A. Xu, et al. Low-dose α-tocopherol improves and high-dose α-tocopherol worsens endothelial vasodilator function in cholesterol-fed rabbits. *J. Clin. Invest.* 93:844–851 (1994).

246. Dierichs, R., and U. Maschke. Effects of α-tocopherol (vitamin E) on the ultrastructure of human platelets in vitro. *Platelets* 4(3):129–134 (1993).

247. Ma, Y.-S., W.L. Stone, and I.O. LeClair. The effects of vitamin C and urate on the oxidation kinetics of human low-density lipoprotein. *Proc. Soc. Exp. Biol. Med.* 206:53–59 (1994).

248. Mukhopadhyay, M., C.K. Mukhopadhyay, and I.B. Chatterjee. Protective effect of ascorbic acid against lipid peroxidation and oxidative damage in cardiac microsomes. *Molec. Cell. Biochem.* 126:69–75 (1993).

249. Jacques, P.F., S.E. Sulsky, G.A. Perrone, and E.J. Schaefer. Ascorbic acid and plasma lipids. *Epidemiology* 5:19–26 (1994).

250. Simon, J.A., G.B. Schreiber, P.B. Crawford, et al. Dietary vitamin C and serum lipids in black and white girls. *Epidemiology* 4:537–542 (1993).

251. Pancharuniti, N., C.A. Lewis, H.E. Sauberlich, et al. Plasma homocyst(e)ine, folate, and vitamin B-12 concentrations and risk for early-onset coronary heart disease. *Am. J. Clin. Nutr.* 59:940–948 (1994).

252. Haglund, O., A. Hamfelt, L. Hambraeus, and T. Saldeen. Effects of fish oil supplemented with pyridoxine and folic acid on homocysteine, atherogenic index, fibrinogen and plasminogen activator inhibitor-1 in man. *Nutr. Res.* 13:1351–1365 (1993).

253. Anonymous. Inhibition of LDL oxidation by phenolic substances in red wine: a clue to the French paradox? *Nutr. Rev.* 51:185–187 (1993).

254. Anonymous. Dietary flavonoids and risk of coronary heart disease. *Nutr. Rev.* 52:59–61 (1994).

255. Hertog, M.G.L., E.J.M. Feskens, P.C.H. Hollman, et al. Dietary antioxidant flavonoids and risk of coronary heart disease: the Zutphen Elderly Study. *Lancet* 342:1007–1111 (1993).

256. Grobbee, D.E. Electrolytes and hypertension: results from recent studies. *Am. J. Med. Sci.* 307(Suppl. 1):S17–S20 (1994).

257. Simon, J.A., E. Obarzanek, S.R. Daniels, and M.M. Frederick. Dietary cation intake and blood pressure

in black girls and white girls. *Am. J. Epidemiol.* 139:130–140 (1994).

258. Ruilope, L.M., V. Lahera, A. Araque, et al. Electrolyte excretion and sodium intake. *Am. J. Med. Sci.* 307(Suppl. 1):S107–S111 (1994).

259. Greger, J.L., K. Murphy, G. MacNeil, et al. Hypertension in rats: interactions among chloride, sodium, and calcium. *J. Agric. Food Chem.* 41:1292–1296 (1993).

260. Cugini, P., T. Kawasaki, L. Di Palma, et al. Blood pressure 24-hour pattern in two industrialized countries (Italy and Japan) with a different culture in salt intake. *Am. J. Cardiol.* 72:58–61 (1993).

261. Madhavan, S., and M.H. Alderman. Ethnicity and the relationship of sodium intake to blood pressure. *J. Hypertens.* 12:97–103 (1994).

262. Ghooi, R.B., V.V. Valanju, and M.G. Rajarshi. Salt restriction in hypertension. *Med. Hypoth.* 41:137–140 (1993).

263. Kawamura, M., T. Akasaka, T. Kasatsuki, et al. Blood pressure is reduced by short-time calorie restriction in overweight hypertensive women with a constant intake of sodium and potassium. *J. Hypertens.* 11(Suppl. 5):S320–S321 (1993).

264. Kumanyika, S.K., P.R. Hebert, J.A. Cutler, et al. Feasibility and efficacy of sodium reduction in the Trials of Hypertension Prevention, phase I. *Hypertension* 22:502–512 (1993).

265. Zoccali, C., F. Mallamaci, D. Leonardis, and M. Romeo. Randomly allocated crossover study of various levels of sodium intake in patients with mild hypertension. *J. Hypertens.* 11(Suppl. 5):S326–S327 (1993).

266. James, G.D., M.S. Pecker, T.G. Pickering, et al. Extreme changes in dietary sodium effect [sic] daily variability and level of blood pressure in borderline hypertensive patients. *Am. J. Human Biol.* 6:283–291 (1994).

267. Nestel, P.J., P.M. Clifton, M. Noakes, et al. Enhanced blood pressure response to dietary salt in elderly women, especially those with small waist:hip ratio. *J. Hypertens.* 11:1387–1394 (1993).

268. Overlack, A., M. Ruppert, R. Kolloch, et al. Divergent hemodynamic and hormonal responses to varying salt intake in normotensive subjects. *Hypertension* 22:331–338 (1993).

269. Haythornthwaite, J.A. Behavioral stress, sodium intake, and blood pressure. *Homeostasis* 34:302–312 (1993).

270. Ruppert, M., A. Overlack, R. Kolloch, et al. Effects of severe and moderate salt restriction on serum lipids in nonobese normotensive adults. *Am. J. Med. Sci.* 307(Suppl. 1):S87–S90 (1994).

271. Schneider, K.A., M. Paland, M. Hamilton, et al. Influence of dietary sodium restriction on lipid metabolism. *Clin. Invest.* 71:990–992 (1993).

272. Hunt, R.A., and D.C. Tucker. Developmental sensitivity to high dietary sodium chloride in borderline hypertensive rats. *Hypertension* 22:542–550 (1993).

273. Hatton, D.C., and D.A. McCarron. Dietary calcium and blood pressure in experimental models of hypertension. A review. *Hypertension* 23:513–530 (1994).

274. Denke, M.A., M.M. Fox, and M.C. Schulte. Short-term dietary calcium fortification increases fecal saturated fat content and reduces serum lipids in men. *J. Nutr.* 123:1047–1053 (1993).

275. Orlov, M.V., M.A. Brodsky, and S. Douban. A review of magnesium, acute myocardial infarction and arrhythmia. *J. Am. Coll. Nutr.* 13:127–132 (1994).

276. Singh, R.B., S.S. Rastogi, S. Ghosh, and M.A. Niaz. Dietary and serum magnesium levels in patients with acute myocardial infarction, coronary artery disease and noncardiac diagnoses. *J. Am. Coll. Nutr.* 13:139–143 (1994).

277. Seelig, M.S. Magnesium, antioxidants and myocardial infarction. *J. Am. Coll. Nutr.* 13:116–117 (1994).

278. Galløe, A.M., H.S. Rasmussen, L.N. Jørgensen, et al. Influence of oral magnesium supplementation on cardiac events among survivors of an acute myocardial infarction. *Br. Med. J.* 307:585–587 (1993).

279. Krishna, G.G. Role of potassium in the pathogenesis of hypertension. *Am. J. Med. Sci.* 307(Suppl. 1):S21–S25 (1994).

280. Sinaiko, A.R., O. Gomez-Marin, and R.J. Prineas. Effect of low sodium diet or potassium supplementation on adolescent blood pressure. *Hypertension* 21:989–994 (1993).

281. Medeiros, D.M., J. Davidson, and J.E. Jenkins. A unified perspective on copper deficiency and cardiomyopathy. *Proc. Soc. Exp. Biol. Med.* 203:262–273 (1993).

282. Klevay, L.M. Ischemic heart disease: nutrition or pharmacology? *J. Trace Elem. Electrolytes Health Dis.* 7:63–69 (1993).

283. Anonymous. Decreased dietary copper impairs vascular function. *Nutr. Rev.* 51:188–189 (1993).

284. Bunce, G.E. Hypercholesterolemia of copper deficiency is linked to glutathione metabolism and regulation of hepatic HMG-CoA reductase. *Nutr. Rev.* 51:305–307 (1993).

285. Vinceti, M., S. Rovesti, C. Marchesi, et al. Changes in drinking water selenium and mortality for coronary disease in a residential cohort. *Biol. Trace Elem. Res.* 40:267–275 (1994).

286. Hermann, J., A. Arquitt, and B. Stoecker. Effects of chromium supplementation on plasma lipids, apolipoproteins, and glucose in elderly subjects. *Nutr. Res.* 14:671–674 (1994).

287. Kromhout, D. Epidemiological aspects of fish in the diet. *Proc. Nutr. Soc.* 52:437–439 (1993).

288. Keli, S.O., E.J.M. Feskens, and D. Kromhout. Fish consumption and risk of stroke. The Zutphen Study. *Stroke* 25:328–332 (1994).

289. Burr, M.L. Fish and ischaemic heart disease. In *Nutrition and Fitness in Health and Disease.* A.P. Simopoulos (ed.). Basel, Karger. *World Rev. Nutr. Diet.* 72:49–60 (1993).

290. Shahar, E., A.R. Folsom, K.K. Wu, et al. Associations of fish intake and dietary *n*–3 polyunsaturated fatty acids with a hypocoagulable profile. The Atherosclerosis Risk in Communities (ARIC) Study. *Arterioscler. Thromb.* 13:1205–1212 (1993).

291. Mori, T.A., R. Vandongen, L.J. Beilin, et al. Effects of varying dietary fat, fish, and fish oils on blood lipids in a

randomized controlled trial in men at risk of heart disease. *Am. J. Clin. Nutr.* 59:1060–1068 (1994).

292. Tidwell, D.K., J.P. McNaughton, L.K. Pellum, et al. Comparison of the effects of adding fish high or low in *n*–3 fatty acids to a diet conforming to the dietary guidelines for Americans. *J. Am. Diet. Assoc.* 93:1124–1128 (1993).

293. Eichholzer, M., and H. Stähelin. Is there a hypocholesterolemic factor in milk and milk products? *Int. J. Vit. Nutr. Res.* 63:159–167 (1993).

294. Berner, L.A. Roundtable discussion on milkfat, dairy foods, and coronary heart disease risk. *J. Nutr.* 123:1175–1184 (1993).

295. Sharpe, S.J., G.D. Gamble, and D.N. Sharpe. Cholesterol-lowering and blood pressure effects of immune milk. *Am. J. Clin. Nutr.* 59:929–934 (1994).

296. Warshafsky, S., R.S. Kamer, and S.L. Sivak. Effect of garlic on total serum cholesterol. A meta-analysis. *Ann. Intern. Med.* 119:599–605 (1993).

297. Jain, A.K., R. Vargas, S. Gotzkowsky, and F.G. McMahon. Can garlic reduce levels of serum lipids? A controlled clinical study. *Am. J. Med.* 94:632–635 (1993).

298. Kiesewetter, H., F. Jung, E.M. Jung, et al. Effect of garlic on platelet aggregation in patients with increased risk of juvenile ischaemic attack. *Eur. J. Clin. Pharmacol.* 45:333–336 (1993).

299. Srivastava, K.C., and O.D. Tyagi. Effects of a garlic-derived principle (ajoene) on aggregation and arachidonic acid metabolism in human blood platelets. *Prostaglandins Leukotrienes Essential Fatty Acids* 49:587–595 (1993).

300. Gebhardt, R. Multiple inhibitory effects of garlic extracts on cholesterol biosynthesis in hepatocytes. *Lipids* 28:613–619 (1993).

301. Yeh, Y.-Y., and S.-M. Yeh. Garlic reduces plasma lipids by inhibiting hepatic cholesterol and triacylglycerol synthesis. *Lipids* 29:189–193 (1994).

302. Sutter, M.C., and Y.-X. Wang. Recent cardiovascular drugs from Chinese medicinal plants. *Cardiovasc. Res.* 27:1891–1901 (1993).

303. Kimura, Y., T. Okuda, and H. Okuda. Effects of flavonoids from licorice roots (*Glycyrrhiza inflata* Bat.) on arachidonic acid metabolism and aggregation in human platelets. *Phytother. Res.* 7:341–347 (1993).

304. Lumb, A.B. Effect of dried ginger on human platelet function. *Thromb. Haemostasis* 71.110–111 (1994).

305. Yasni, S., K. Imaizumi, K. Sin, et al. Identification of an active principle in essential oils and hexane-soluble fractions of *Curcuma xanthorrhiza* Roxb. showing triglyceride-lowering action in rats. *Food Chem. Toxicol.* 32:273–278 (1994).

306. Bobek, P., E. Ginter, and L'. Ozdín. Oyster mushroom (*Pleurotus ostreatus*) accelerates the plasma clearance of low-density and high-density lipoproteins in rats. *Nutr. Res.* 13:885–890 (1993).

307. Bobek, P., L. Kuniak, and L. Ozdín. The mushroom *Pleurotus ostreatus* reduces secretion and accelerates the

fractional turnover rate of very-low-density lipoproteins in the rat. *Ann. Nutr. Metab.* 37:142–145 (1993).

308. Bobek, P., L. Ozdin, and L. Kuniak. Influence of water and ethanol extracts of the oyster mushroom (*Pleurotus ostreatus*) on serum and liver lipids of the Syrian hamsters. *Nahrung* 37:571–575 (1993).

309. Sugiyama, K., T. Akachi, and A. Yamakawa. The hypocholesterolemic action of *Lentinus edodes* is evoked through alteration of phospholipid composition of liver microsomes in rats. *Biosci. Biotechnol. Biochem.* 57:1983–1985 (1993).

310. Klatsky, A.L. Epidemiology of coronary heart disease—influence of alcohol. *Alcoholism: Clin. Exp. Res.* 18:88–96 (1994).

311. Srivastava, L.M., S. Vasisht, D.P. Agarwal, and H.W. Goedde. Relation between alcohol intake, lipoproteins, and coronary heart disease: the interest continues. *Alcohol Alcoholism* 29:11–24 (1994).

312. Maclure, M. Demonstration of deductive meta-analysis: ethanol intake and risk of myocardial infarction. *Epidemiol. Rev.* 15:328–351 (1993).

313. Coate, D. Moderate drinking and coronary heart disease mortality: evidence from NHANES I and the NHANES I Follow-up. *Am. J. Public Health* 83:888–890 (1993).

314. Gaziano, J.M., J.E. Buring, J.L. Breslow, et al. Moderate alcohol intake, increased levels of high-density lipoprotein and its subfractions, and decreased risk of myocardial infarction. *New Engl. J. Med.* 329:1829–1834 (1993).

315. Marmot, M.G. P. Elliott, M.J. Shipley, et al. Alcohol and blood pressure: the INTERSALT study. *Br. Med. J.* 308:1263–1267 (1994).

316. Palomäki, H., and M. Kaste. Regular light-to-moderate intake of alcohol and the risk of ischemic stroke. Is there a beneficial effect? *Stroke* 24:1828–1832 (1993).

317. Kinoshita, E., J. Yamakoshi, and M. Kikuchi. Purification and identification of an angiotensin I–converting enzyme inhibitor from soy sauce. *Biosci. Biotechnol. Biochem.* 57:1107–1110 (1993).

318. Miettinen, T.A., and H. Vanhanen. Serum concentration and metabolism of cholesterol during rapeseed oil and squalene feeding. *Am. J. Clin. Nutr.* 59:356–363 (1994).

319. Nanjo, F., Y. Hara, and Y. Kikuchi. Effects of tea polyphenols on blood rheology in rats fed a high-fat diet. In *Food Phytochemicals for Cancer Prevention II. Teas, Spices, and Herbs.* C.-T. Ho et al. (eds.). Washington, DC, American Chemical Society. *ACS Symp. Ser.* 547:76–82 (1994).

320. Dujin, O.C., and C.A. LeBlanc. Hypocholesterolemic properties of plant indoles. Inhibition of acyl-CoA:cholesterol acyltransferase activity and reduction of serum LDL/VLDL cholesterol levels by glucobrassicin derivatives. *Biochem. Pharmacol.* 47:359–364 (1994).

321. Costa, N.M.B., A.F. Walker, and A.G. Low. The effect of graded inclusion of baked beans (*Phaseolus vulgaris*) on plasma and liver lipids in hypercholesterolaemic pigs given a Western-type diet. *Br. J. Nutr.* 70:515–524 (1993).

322. Maezaki, Y., K. Tsuji, Y. Nakagawa, et al. Hypocholesterolemic effect of chitosan in adult males. *Biosci. Biotechnol. Biochem.* 57:1439–1444 (1993).

# 4

# Other Effects of Diet

# INFLAMMATION AND THE IMMUNE RESPONSE

Both ends of the spectrum of nutritional status—undernutrition and overnutrition—can adversely affect the immune system. Kumari and Chandra summarized evidence that excessive intake of most macronutrients and micronutrients can cause immunosuppression, increasing the risk of cancer and infection in both humans and experimental animals (*1*). They discussed effects of obesity, dietary lipids, and vitamin and mineral excesses. Dietary lipids alter immune cells structurally, functionally, or both. With few exceptions (e.g., vitamin C), each micronutrient exhibits an upper and a lower threshold beyond which immune responses may be impaired. For example, amounts of zinc slightly exceeding the recommended intake enhance the immune response, but higher amounts sharply reduce it. A small excess of vitamin E is slightly stimulatory; larger excesses cause a slight depression. All doses of vitamin A exceeding the recommended intake depress the immune response. The undesirable effects are dose-related.

Scott et al. discussed the role of food in development of autoimmune diseases (*2*). They briefly reviewed the bases of tolerance and autoimmunity, types of autoimmune disease, genetic factors involved, and animal models for studying nutritional aspects of autoimmune disease. They discussed the phenomenon of oral tolerance, by which initial oral presentation of an antigen produces systemic tolerance, whereas initial systemic exposure generates an immune response. This is an important adaptation because of the vast array of foreign antigens bombarding an animal via food. Cow's milk, wheat, soybeans, and alfalfa are of particular interest as sources of possible autoimmunogens related to type I diabetes mellitus, systemic lupus erythematosus, rheumatoid arthritis, and possibly celiac disease. Postulated mechanisms through which food autoimmunogens act include metabolic effects on hormones, mediators, cytokines, prostaglandins, and cell membranes. It is important to understand the autoimmunogenicity of individual foods and their constituents. As food autoimmunogens are identified, it may be possible to develop special foods that lack the harmful components.

A case–control study of dietary and reproductive factors in relation to risk of systemic lupus erythematosus was conducted among women in Miyagi Prefecture, Japan (*3*). Frequent intake of meat was associated with increased risk (relative risk [RR] 3.36, 95% CI 1.10–10.24, for "frequent" vs. "rare" consumption). Case-patients preferred fatty meats such as beef and pork.

Wienken discussed possible dietary influences on psoriasis (*4*), acne (*5*), and neurodermatitis (*6*). Certain foods and nutrients are believed to exacerbate or ameliorate symptoms of these disorders, but diet therapy has yielded disappointing results.

Juvonen et al. postulated that early diet influences subsequent macromolecular absorption and serum IgE (*7*). They randomly assigned 130 healthy, full-term neonates to receive human milk from the milk bank, a cow's milk formula, or a casein hydrolysate formula for the first 3 d after birth, after which all infants were exclusively breast-fed until the end of the study. Blood samples were obtained 1 h after a breast feeding when infants were 4 days, 2 months, and 4 months old, for determination of serum $\alpha$-lactalbumin and total IgE. Infants in the casein hydrolysate group had elevated values for $\alpha$-lactalbumin at 2 months and lower levels of serum IgE at 2 and 4 months. The importance of these differences and reasons for them are not known.

## Immunomodulation by Nonlipid Dietary Components

VITAMINS AND ANTIOXIDANTS. Vitamin $B_6$ deficiency affects both humoral and cell-mediated immune responses. Rall et al. reviewed relationships between $B_6$ status and immune competence, as demonstrated in various animal models and studies of human subjects (*8*). Deficiency alters lymphocyte differentiation and maturation, reduces delayed-type hypersensitivity responses, and may indirectly impair antibody production. These functions are restored upon repletion, but megadoses of the vitamin do not confer additional benefit. In humans, $B_6$ status may influence tumor growth and other disease processes and immunologic changes seen in the elderly and persons with uremia, rheumatoid arthritis, or HIV infection. Mechanisms of action and the requirement for optimal immune response at various ages need to be established.

Jyonouchi et al. have studied the immunomodulating actions of carotenoids. Astaxanthin, a carotenoid without provitamin A activity, enhances in vitro production of specific antibodies to T cell–dependent antigens in normal mice (*9*). The maximum effect was seen when astaxanthin was present during the initial period of antigen priming. The action appeared to require direct interactions between T and B cells. It was abolished by depletion of T cells. Neither astaxanthin nor β-carotene facilitated activation of polyclonal B cells or augmented total immunoglobulin production. In autoimmune-prone mouse strains the action of astaxanthin on in vitro antibody production was attenuated, although earlier studies by this research group had found significant benefits in vivo. The authors postulated that astaxanthin acts through mechanisms affecting the initial stage of antigen presentation and subsequent differentiation of B lymphocytes. Lutein, another carotenoid with no provitamin A activity, also enhanced in vitro antibody production in response to T-cell-dependent antigens (*10*). Depletion of helper T cells abolished the effect. β-Carotene was inactive in this system. However, in vivo antibody production in response to T cell–dependent antigens was significantly enhanced by intraperitoneal injections of β carotene as well as by injections of lutein and astaxanthin. The response was greater in young mice than in old. No carotenoid affected either in vivo or in vitro antibody production in response to T cell–independent antigen.

Oxygen free radicals are thought to mediate tissue damage in patients with rheumatoid arthritis. A case–control study in Finland evaluated the association between risk of rheumatoid arthritis and serum levels of antioxidants (*11*). Subjects had served as a control group for cancer case-patients in a study of micronutrients and cancer, for which serum levels of α-tocopherol, β-carotene, and selenium were determined. During a median follow-up of 20 years, 14 initially healthy subjects developed rheumatoid arthritis. Elevated risk of rheumatoid arthritis was associated with low levels of each of the micronutrients and of an antioxidant index calculated as the product of the molar concentrations of these micronutrients. The association was significant for the index but nonsignificant for the individual antioxidants. These findings support the hypothesis that a low antioxidant level is a risk factor for rheumatoid arthritis.

Tang et al. investigated the hypothesis that dietary intake of micronutrients influences the progression of HIV infection to AIDS (*12*). Subjects were homosexual HIV-infected men who completed a dietary questionnaire on entry into the study and were evaluated semiannually for a median period of 6.8 y. For vitamin C, vitamin $B_1$, and niacin, the highest quartile of intake was associated with a significantly reduced progression rate. The relative risk was 0.55 (95% CI 0.34–0.91) for vitamin C, 0.60 (95% CI 0.36–0.98) for vitamin $B_1$, and 0.52 (95% CI 0.31–0.86) for niacin. The relation between total vitamin A intake and progression to AIDS was U-shaped, progression being significantly slower in the middle two quartiles (RR 0.55, 95% CI 0.35–0.88). Zinc intake was directly and monotonically associated with risk of progression. For the highest vs. the lowest quartiles, relative risk was 2.06 (95% CI 1.16–3.64).

Wang and Watson reviewed the role of vitamin E as an immunostimulant and antioxidant, in relation to alcohol consumption and development of AIDS (*13*). Ethanol consumption broadly suppresses immune response, impairing the normal host defense to invading microbes and tumorigenesis. The overwhelming evidence supporting this suggests that alcohol consumption could hasten progression to AIDS. There is also evidence that vitamin E acts on various components of the immune system to repair ethanol-induced immune defects, normalize other nutrient deficiencies initiated by alcohol consumption, and decrease the alcohol-related burden of oxidative stress.

**TRADITIONAL MEDICINES.** A number of Ayurvedic herbal supplements are believed to enhance resistance to infection and disease. The immunomodulatory actions of one such supplement, Maharishi Amrit Kalash Ambrosia, were evaluated in feeding studies of C57BL/6J mice (*14*). In the presence of activators, lymphocytes and peritoneal macrophages from treated mice showed a variety of responses greater than responses of cells from untreated mice. Without activators, the supplement had no effect. The authors concluded that Maharishi Amrit Kalash Ambrosia enhances functions of both T cells and macrophages via constituents that induce in vivo priming of these cells.

Sheehan and Atherton reported results of a 1-y treatment and follow-up of 37 children with atopic eczema who had participated in a short-term double-blind, placebo-controlled trial of Chinese medicinal herbs (*15*). Of the 23 children who completed the study, 18 had reductions in eczema activity scores of ≥90% at the end of the year and the rest showed lesser improvement. Seven children were able to discontinue treatment without relapse; 12 were able to control their eczema with reduced treatment; and only 4 still required daily treatment. Ten children withdrew from the study due to lack of response. Four withdrew because the treatment was unpalatable or difficult to prepare. The authors concluded that Chinese medicinal herbs are a therapeutic option for children with extensive atopic eczema that is unresponsive to other treatments. However, the safety of long-term treatment requires further study. Two subjects, who discontinued therapy because their eczema was controlled, showed asymptomatic elevation of serum aspartate aminotransferase. However, results of liver function tests returned to normal within 8 weeks after treatment was discontinued.

**LACTIC ACID BACTERIA.** Many health claims have been made for "living food" (fresh uncooked food and some fermented foods). Some beneficial effects may stem from modification of the fecal flora by lactobacilli used to ferment vegetables and milk. A Finnish study determined the influence of a vegan diet rich in lactobacilli on the fecal flora and disease activity of patients with rheumatoid arthritis (*16*). Subjects in the treatment group had significantly higher fecal lactobacillus counts and fewer symptoms of disease than omnivorous controls after 1 and 2 months of treatment.

The ability of pathogenic bacteria to stimulate production of cytokines in vitro and in vivo is well established; there is less information on induction of cytokines by nonpathogens. Solis Pereyra and Lemonnier evaluated the ability of human intestinal bacteria and bacteria used to ferment dairy foods to induce cytokine production by blood mononuclear cells (*17*). In vitro, dairy cultures of *Lactobacillus, Streptococcus,* and *Bifidobacterium* induced production of interleukin-1β, tumor necrosis factor–α (TNFα), and interferon-γ but not interferon-α or interleukin-2. Cell walls of these organisms were also active, but the cytoplasmic fraction was not. Intestinal isolates of *E. coli, Streptococcus* sp., and *Lactobacillus* sp. also induced interleukin-1 production. *Streptococcus* induced interferon-γ and TNFα as well. In vivo interferon production was estimated by the 2',5'A synthetase activity of blood mononuclear cells after subjects ingested sterile milk or $10^{11}$ yogurt bacteria in yogurt. Enzyme activity in the yogurt group was 83% higher than in the milk group. The authors concluded that both dairy bacteria and normal intestinal bacteria induce cytokine production and in this way can contribute to resistance against pathogenic bacteria.

Lee et al. screened 27 food species of *Bifidobacterium, Lactobacillus, Lactococcus, Streptococcus, Kluyveromyces,* and *Candida* for immunopotentiating activity (*18*). Mitogenic activity was measured in spleen, thymus, and Peyer's patch cells from BALB/c mice. Murine lymph node cells immunized with hen's egg ovomucoid were evaluated for proliferative response and antibody production. All strains of *Bifidobacterium,* but particularly *B. adolescentis* M101-4, had strong mitogenic activity and enhanced antibody production by lymph node cells but did not induce growth of thymocytes. Similar results were obtained with germ-free mice. The authors concluded that immunopotentiation by *B. adolescentis* was due to direct or indirect intrinsic activity toward B cells and not to secondary stimulation of lymphocytes primed by bacteria in the gut or the environment. A corollary to this was that the immunopotentiating activity of the food microorganisms depended on the individual properties of each strain.

PEPTIDES. Yamauchi and Suetsuna compared the effects of feeding equivalent amounts of soybean- and casein-

derived peptides and the corresponding intact protein on immune responses of specific pathogen–free rats (*19*). Mitogenic activity and the phagocytosis of opsonized sheep erythrocytes were assessed. Peptides from both sources, but especially soybean, were significantly more active than the corresponding protein. The active peptides remain to be characterized.

## Immunomodulation by Dietary Lipids

Hummell reviewed the ways in which dietary lipids may influence immune-mediated processes and inflammatory states (*20*). She discussed the importance of the family of cellular phospholipases and their products and described the components of the immune system and their functions. Eicosanoids were considered in terms of their synthesis, metabolism, and effects on immune function. How dietary lipids affect all of this was then addressed, including examples of specific diseases. Diets rich in fat or linoleic acid are in most cases detrimental to host immune function as evaluated in vitro. Plant and marine *n*–3 PUFAs are predominantly antiinflammatory in vivo and in vitro. However, Hummell observed that some effects have been demonstrated only in animal models and few clear-cut effects on clinical outcome have been confirmed.

Meydani et al. evaluated the immunologic effects of NCEP step 2 diets with and without fish to provide *n*–3 PUFAs (*21*). Subjects were normotensive, normolipidemic adults over the age of 40. Long-term consumption of a low-fat diet enriched in plant-derived PUFAs increased some immune responses and had no effect on others. In contrast, the low-fat, high-fish diet significantly decreased the percentage of helper T cells and increased suppressor T cells. Mitogenic responses to concanavalin A, the delayed-type hypersensitivity skin response, and production of TNF, interleukin-1β, and interleukin-6 by mononuclear cells were significantly reduced. Thus an NCEP step 2 diet rich in fish significantly decreases various parameters of the immune response in comparison to a similar diet low in fish. These alterations may be beneficial for preventing and treating atherosclerosis and inflammatory disease but detrimental to host defense against pathogens.

A dietary study using a mouse model of systemic lupus erythematosus demonstrated antiinflammatory effects of ethyl esters of two purified *n*–3 PUFAs, eicosapentaenoic acid (EPA) and docosahexaenoic acid (DHA) (*22*). Moreover, the effect of EPA and DHA together appeared to be greater than the sum of their individual effects. The extent of renal disease was estimated by light microscopy and the prevalence of proteinuria.

Cooper et al. investigated the effect of *n*–3 PUFA supplementation on acute-phase responses in healthy young adults (*23*). The active-treatment group received 4.5 g/d of fish oil for 6–8 weeks before challenge with typhoid vaccine. In unsupplemented subjects, injection of the vaccine caused increases in white cell count, resting heart rate, metabolic rate, oxygen consumption, and oral temperature. Fish-oil supplementation appeared to reduce tachycardia and the increases in oral temperature and metabolic rate, although similar effects were seen in subjects injected with saline rather than vaccine. In vitro production of interleukin-1 and interleukin-6 from whole blood was suppressed by fish oil, but production of TNFα was unaffected. Inflammation and soreness around the injection site and general flu-like symptoms were milder in the fish-oil group. The authors concluded that fish oil attenuates several responses associated with injury and infection and this may be related to reduced cytokine production.

In a double-blind trial, patients with psoriasis or atopic dermatitis were randomly allocated to receive daily supplements of EPA and DHA ethyl esters or corn-oil placebo for 4 months (*24*). The *n*–3 PUFA esters significantly reduced the percentage of CD25-positive lymphocytes from 40.5 at baseline to 35.5 at the end of the trial. This may partly explain the antiinflammatory effect of these fatty acids and may be clinically important for some diseases in which high levels of CD25 are expressed.

A study in piglets found that substitution of menhaden oil for lard in a sow's late-gestation and lactation diet greatly increased the content of *n*–3 PUFAs in the nursling's immune cells (*25*). Except for ionophore-stimulated release of leukotriene B, basal and stimulated in vitro release of prostaglandin E (PGE), thromboxane B, and leukotriene B by alveolar macrophages was sharply reduced in these piglets.

Circulating TNFα is usually associated with pathologic change, and its synthesis is under control at several levels. Somers and Erickson investigated how fish oil affects TNFα production and its $PGE_2$-mediated regulation (*26*). Mice were fed diets containing either fish oil or safflower oil. Cultures of peritoneal macrophages from the fish-oil group had more TNFα activity than control macrophages 24 h after in vitro stimulation with lipopolysaccharide (LPS). Because the onset of synthesis and maximal synthesis of TNFα and down-regulation of TNFα mRNA were similar in the two groups, the authors postulated that macrophages from mice fed *n*–6 PUFAs had a higher capacity to remove TNFα from the culture medium. Indomethacin, at a dose inhibitory to cyclooxygenase activity and $PGE_2$ synthe-

sis, increased TNFα levels at 24 h in cultures from the *n*–6 group but not the *n*–3 group. When $PGE_2$ was added at several levels, a dose too low to inhibit TNFα production induced clearance of soluble TNFα from the medium from macrophages of the *n*–3 group. The authors concluded that dietary *n*–3 PUFAs cause a selective loss in the TNFα clearance mechanism, reflecting specific alteration of $PGE_2$-mediated regulation of macrophage-produced TNFα.

Ferretti et al. demonstrated a significant change in prostaglandin metabolism through manipulation of the *n*–6/*n*–3 ratio (*27*). Other results of the study were presented in reference *21*. Healthy adults ate a typical American baseline diet for 6 weeks and then were fed low-fat NCEP step 2 diets containing either large or small amounts of fish. The high-fish diet led to a 27% reduction in excretion of the PGE metabolite 11α-hydroxy-9,15-dioxo-2,3,4,5,20-pentanor-19-carboxyprostanoic acid. The other low-fat diet also reduced excretion of the PGE metabolite, but nonsignificantly.

Brouard and Pascaud evaluated the in vitro effect of free PUFAs and aspirin on primary cultures of rat and human lymphocytes and the ex vivo effect of dietary *n*–6/*n*–3 ratio on function of rat lymphocytes (*28*). Dietary *n*–3 was enriched by either fish oil or linseed oil. In vitro, stimulated proliferation was inhibited to the greatest extent by docosatetraenoic acid and DHA and to a lesser extent by EPA; arachidonic acid was slightly stimulatory. Acetylsalicylic acid also stimulated lymphocyte proliferation. Diet did not affect mitogen-induced lymphocyte proliferation ex vivo, but both *n*–3-enriched diets reduced proliferation of unstimulated lymphocytes by a factor of 4. Fish oil significantly increased the natural killer cell activity of rat splenic lymphocytes; linseed oil did not. The *n*–3-enriched diets reduced the stimulatory effect of acetylsalicylic acid (which depends on eicosanoid synthesis) on in vitro lymphocyte proliferation. The authors concluded that PUFAs have highly individual and sometimes strikingly different effects on lymphocyte proliferation and function.

A study of relationships between dietary linoleate and the levels of linoleic and arachidonic acids in neutrophil phospholipids, plasma triacylglycerols, and plasma cholesteryl esters verified that the linoleic acid content of tissue lipids is an indicator of dietary intake (*29*). In contrast, when healthy men consumed diets providing from 2.5 to 17.5 en% linoleic acid, arachidonic acid concentrations in the same neutrophil and plasma fractions were not associated with differences in dietary linoleate. However, arachidonic acid concentrations were reduced by fish-oil supplements.

A study in healthy elderly men evaluated the effects of dietary fat on plasma fatty acid composition and immune status (30). The amount and type of dietary fat modified several in vitro measures of immune function. Basal natural killer cell activity was significantly negatively correlated with fractions of plasma fatty acids representing total PUFAs ($r = -.68$), total $n$–6 PUFAs ($r = -.62$), and linoleic acid ($r = -.52$). Other significant correlations between plasma fatty acids and immune function were also found. The overall pattern suggested that a high intake of $n$–6 PUFAs is inadvisable—that from an immunologic point of view, a low-fat diet providing relatively low amounts of $n$–6 PUFAs should be recommended to elderly people.

Businco et al. analyzed the fatty acid composition of lipids in milk from mothers of children with newly developed atopic dermatitis (31). Compared with control breast milk, milk from mothers of affected children had increased proportions of linoleic acid and significantly decreased proportions of its long-chain polyunsaturated derivatives. The ratio of linoleic acid to the sum of its metabolites γ-linolenic, dihomo-γ-linolenic, and arachidonic acids was 11.8 in the atopic group and 9.0 in controls ($p < .01$). These findings are consistent with findings of an abnormal fatty acid status in atopic subjects and could account for some discrepant results from studies of the effect of breast-feeding on subsequent development of atopic dermatitis.

γ-Linolenic acid is found at relatively high levels in evening primrose oil and borage oil. It is rapidly converted to dihomo-γ-linolenic acid, the immediate precursor of $PGE_1$, which has antiinflammatory and immunoregulatory properties. A 24-week randomized, double-blind comparison of γ-linolenic acid and cottonseed oil placebo was conducted in patients with rheumatoid arthritis and active synovitis (32). Active treatment produced clinically and statistically significant reduction in the signs and symptoms of disease activity. The dosage was 1.4 g/d of γ-linolenic acid, far higher than is usually taken. However, no subject withdrew from treatment because of adverse reactions. The authors noted that γ-linolenic acid is not approved in the USA for treatment of any condition. Nevertheless, the promising results of this trial and the adverse effects associated with many established therapies for rheumatoid arthritis seem to warrant further controlled studies of γ-linolenic acid.

James et al. suggested dietary supplementation with eicosatrienoic acid ($n$–9) as a novel approach to inhibiting eicosanoid synthesis (33). Feeding studies in rats showed that eicosatrienoic acid inhibits synthesis of the inflammatory mediator leukotriene $B_4$, while synthesis of other products of 5-lipoxygenase metabolism is not affected. This pattern suggests inhibition of leukotriene A hydrolase. Dietary EPA inhibited not only leukotriene $B_4$ synthesis but also synthesis of its all-*trans* isomers; there was no inhibition of 5-HETE synthesis. This pattern indicates inhibition of leukotriene A synthase. The authors concluded that the antiinflammatory benefits of eicosatrienoic acid are comparable to those of essential fatty acid deficiency or supplemental fish oil. Moreover, because eicosatrienoic acid is less unsaturated than EPA it should have greater chemical stability—a practical advantage for substances used as dietary constituents or supplements.

Leukotriene $B_4$ is isolated in abnormally high amounts from psoriatic skin. Extracts of the fern *Polypodium decumanum* (calaguala) are used in some countries to treat psoriasis. Vasänge-Tuominen et al. tested calaguala extracts for their ability to inhibit leukotriene $B_4$ formation in an in vitro system using human leukocytes (34). Sulfasalazine was used as a positive control. Both calaguala and sulfasalazine caused concentration-dependent inhibition of A23187-stimulated leukotriene synthesis. The $IC_{50}$ values for various PUFAs were determined and the calaguala extracts were analyzed quantitatively for PUFA content. From this, it appears that fatty acid constituents of *P. decumanum* can contribute to the extracts' clinical effects.

Miller et al. evaluated the ability of conjugated linoleic acid (CLA) to prevent endotoxin-induced growth suppression in mice (35). Mice fed a basal diet or a diet with 0.5% fish oil lost significantly more weight after endotoxin injection than mice fed a diet with 0.5% CLA. Weight loss was similar in the three endotoxin-injected groups for the first 10 h. Animals in the basal-diet and fish-oil groups continued to lose weight until 24 h after injection, then regained about half of the lost weight between 48 and 72 h after injection. Weight loss in the CLA group virtually stopped after 10 h and the animals regained their lost weight between 48 and 72 h after injection. CLA reduced or prevented endotoxin-induced anorexia and significantly increased splenocyte blastogenesis. Fish oil increased splenocyte blastogenesis to a lesser extent.

## GLUCOSE METABOLISM, GLUCOSE TOLERANCE, AND DIABETES

Toeller discussed nutritional recommendations for patients with type I (insulin-dependent) and type II (non-insulin-dependent) diabetes mellitus (IDDM and NIDDM, respectively) (36). General dietary guidelines for diabetic patients are no different from those now recognized for the population as a whole. Moreover, they are very similar to dietary guidelines aimed at reducing the incidence of many chronic diseases. Guidelines for diabetics also include specific advice for people at high risk of cardiovascular disease and modifications that compensate for the metabolic abnormalities characteristic of IDDM and NIDDM. The rationale underlying recommendations for intake of energy, fat, protein, carbohydrate, fiber, alcohol, vitamins, and minerals and for the timing and distribution of meals was reviewed. One interesting observation was that physicians and healthcare teams with interest and experience in lifestyle modification approaches achieve particularly successful long-term results from nutritional counseling of IDDM and NIDDM patients. Comparable shifts to "healthy eating" in the general public and corresponding adjustments in the food and food service industries would assure the success of the diabetes diet. There appears to be no need for special "diabetic" foods.

Dahlquist provided an epidemiologic perspective on the etiology of IDDM (37). The β-cell destruction leading to IDDM is considered to be a cell-mediated autoimmune process that occurs in genetically susceptible individuals. Clearly, however, nongenetic factors are also very important because monozygotic twins have a concordance rate of only 30–50% for IDDM. Dahlquist proposed that some risk determinants (maternal–child blood group incompatibility, fetal viral infection, early exposure to cow's milk proteins, exposure to nitrosamines) can provoke the initial damage to the β-cell, leading to antigen release and initiating the autoimmune process. Other risk determinants could promote an already ongoing autoimmune process by inducing lymphokine release or increasing the β-cell's work load. A high growth rate, cold environment, infectious disease, or other stress could promote or unmask β-cell impairment, making the disease clinically overt. A different risk profile characterizes each age group. The author concluded that the etiology of IDDM is similar in complexity to that of many cancers, cardiovascular disease, and probably other autoimmune diseases. The incidence of IDDM has been rising in many countries. If the genetic prerequisites for IDDM are prevalent whereas only a small proportion of people develop the disease, it must be concluded that the rising incidence represents an increase in one or more nongenetic risk factors. These risk factors are the proper focus of attempts at primary prevention. Some of them appear to be dietary.

Although epidemiologic and experimental data suggest that dietary exposures during infancy influence IDDM risk, current data on infant diet are inadequate for developing studies to test specific hypotheses and alternative hypotheses should the primary hypothesis fail (38). Kostraba sees the next step for epidemiologic research as a prospective study that follows children at risk for IDDM from birth to early signs of diabetes. It should monitor qualitative and quantitative dietary components, the timing of sensitization and development of immune memory to dietary factors, and signs of early preclinical diabetes. She discussed problems in the design and interpretation of individual studies and metaanalyses purporting to identify dietary risk factors. For example, time-series analysis, which has linked decreasing breastfeeding rates with increasing IDDM incidence in Scandinavia, has also implicated viral outbreaks. Moreover, breast feeding has become more prevalent since the 1970s but the incidence of IDDM has not fallen. Data supporting the idea that children with diabetes were exposed earlier to cow's milk also support the idea that they were exposed earlier to nonhuman dietary proteins in general—from solid foods and wheat- or soy-based formulas as well as cow's milk. Experimental data confirm that diet is important in development of diabetes in rat and mouse models, but again the chemical identity of the diabetogen(s) is not clear. The importance of the timing of introduction of formulas, cow's milk, and solid foods into the diet makes it conceptually and statistically difficult to untangle the independent effects of dietary exposures. Perhaps the advantage of breast feeding is that it minimizes the infant's exposure to a vast array of food antigens during a critical period of development.

Vinceti et al. examined the relationship between diet and glucose tolerance in obese middle-aged subjects with normal glucose tolerance, impaired glucose tolerance, and newly diagnosed NIDDM (39). In men, an association between worsening of glucose tolerance and high caloric intake was linked to high intake of animal fat and animal protein; no dietary variables remained significant after adjustment for body mass index and total energy intake. In women, lower intakes of refined carbohydrate, fiber, potassium, and possibly calcium were associated with diabetes after adjustment for body mass index. Other dietary associations were revealed in the subgroup of subjects with no family history of diabetes. In men, after adjustment for body mass index and total energy intake, low intakes of total and complex carbohydrates and plant protein and high intake of animal protein were associated with impaired glucose tolerance. In women, after adjustment for body mass index, low intakes of total carbohydrates, fiber, protein, plant protein, calcium, and potassium were associated with NIDDM. These associations were not seen in subjects with a family history of diabetes.

Laitinen et al. examined obese patients with recently diagnosed NIDDM, comparing the effects of intensive and conventional diet and exercise education on metabolic control and cardiovascular risk factors (40). Weight reduction and a moderate intake of saturated fat were associated with improved glycemic control. Dietary data collected at 15 months showed that subjects in the intensive education group were consuming fewer calories, less total and saturated fat, and more carbohydrate and fiber than subjects in the conventional education group. They also had better glycemic control. A multiple regression model based on initial level of fasting blood glucose, weight loss, initial level of fasting plasma insulin, change in plasma insulin response to an oral glucose load, intake of saturated fat, and proportion of palmitic acid in serum triacylglycerols explained 73% of the decrease in fasting blood glucose level.

People of South Asian origin settled overseas have higher morbidity and mortality from coronary disease and NIDDM than other groups. This is associated with central obesity and insulin resistance. Sevak et al. studied South Asian and European men living in London to see whether these disturbances were diet-related (41). Subjects were normotensive, nondiabetic, had no history of heart disease, and had plasma cholesterol concentrations <310 mg/dL. The South Asians consumed less energy, less total fat, less protein, more starch, more fiber, more polyunsaturated fat, and more *n*–3 polyunsaturated fatty acids than the Europeans. However, when subjects were categorized by ethnicity and low, medium, or high insulin (fasting plasma insulin and response to a glucose load), mean nutrient intakes were unrelated to hyperinsulinemia. The authors concluded that insulin resistance and high coronary risk in South Asians are not explained by any unfavorable characteristic of South Asian diets.

In the short term, insulin production is controlled primarily by translation of preexisting mRNA. Over the longer term, control is via modulation of insulin mRNA levels through effects on rate of transcription of the insulin gene and changes in rate of decay of insulin mRNA. Docherty and Clark reviewed how nutrients regulate expression of the insulin gene (42). Glucose is the major physiologic regulator of insulin secretion but mannose, leucine, and ketone bodies are also important. The authors discussed glucose metabolism, genetic regulation of insulin production, and glucose-mediated changes in metabolites within β-cells that are linked to increased insulin secretion. They depicted a scheme whereby glucose, leucine, and hormones stimulate insulin production and secretion by β-cells.

A wide-ranging discussion of nutrition principles for managing diabetes and related complications considered the goals of medical nutrition therapy (43). It addressed proteins, fats, carbohydrates, sweeteners, and fiber separately, considering their metabolic effects in IDDM, NIDDM, and related conditions as well as problems specific to particular age groups or pregnancy. Sodium, alcohol, and micronutrients were covered briefly. Dietary issues for diabetics relating to obesity, hypertension, nephropathy, and dyslipidemia were reviewed. Unanswered questions to be addressed by future research were listed.

Smith reviewed the causes and possible consequences of insulin resistance, emphasizing effects of diet (44). Although a very high dietary ratio of carbohydrate to fat improves insulin sensitivity and diabetes control, some undesirable consequences may accompany such a diet—for example, elevated triacylglycerol and lowered HDL cholesterol levels. More moderate increases in the carbohydrate/fat ratio, while not associated with adverse changes in lipids, have smaller and variable effects on insulin sensitivity. Smith recommended thorough study of high-carbohydrate diets based on fiber-rich foods and foods with a low glycemic index. However, Milne et al. pointed out that most dietary studies have involved intervention periods of only 4–12 weeks, and some of the changes observed may have been transient (45). These authors conducted an 18-month randomized trial in NIDDM patients to compare the effects of three diets: a standard weight-management diet, a modified-lipid diet containing 36 en% fat with equal amounts of saturated, monounsaturated, and polyunsaturated fats, and a high-carbohydrate (55 en%) high-fiber (≥30 g/d) diet. The results were unexpected. No significant weight changes occurred during the study or 9 months of follow-up. Among the subjects as a group, levels of glycated hemoglobin, total and HDL cholesterol, and triacylglycerols decreased slightly between the time of recruitment and the time of randomization. This was attributed to the participants' motivation and dietary advice they received around the time they entered the study. Although these changes were sustained throughout the study and follow-up, further improvement was negligible and there was little difference between diet groups. Despite considerable effort, almost none of the participants achieved the recommended intakes of carbohydrates and unsaturated fat.

## Glycemic Index

The glycemic index rates foods on the basis of their acute glycemic impact. In one version, the glycemic response is compared to the response to glucose, which is set at 100. Its relevance and value in planning meals for diabetics have been hotly debated. Brand Miller reviewed her own studies of sucrose-containing foods and the findings of others from studies in which the glycemic index of the overall diet was manipulated (*46*). Of 11 studies using the glycemic index approach to diabetes or lipid management, 10 showed improvement in carbohydrate or lipid metabolism or both. Overall, diets with low glycemic indexes reduced glycosylated hemoglobin by 9%, fructosamine by 8%, urinary C-peptide by 20%, 24-h blood glucose by 16%, cholesterol by 6%, and triacylglycerols by 9%. Although the improvements were only modest, so were the changes in the "user-friendly" diets. The author found that sucrose has little or no impact on glycemic index, except when added to dairy products. She concluded that the glycemic index is a useful concept and tool and that sucrose in moderate amounts does not compromise diabetes control.

White bread, assigned an arbitrary value of 100, is another common standard for the glycemic index. Wolever et al. measured the glycemic index of 102 common foods, using white bread as a reference (*47*). Values ranged from 37 for bean thread noodles to 127 for Rice Chex cereal. The use of white bread as a standard was validated by the finding that the glycemic index of 14 commercial leavened wheat breads averaged 97, with no significant difference between products. Legumes and pasta generally had low index values. The index was negatively correlated with protein content ($r = -.407$, $p < .001$) and fiber content ($r = -.322$, $p < .001$). It was unrelated to fat. However, the index could not be accurately predicted from chemical analyses of foods given in food tables. The authors concluded that the glycemic index is a useful supplement to food tables in planning diets for patients with metabolic disorders such as diabetes and hyperlipidemia. The same research group discussed the glycemic index in terms of the effects of "lente" carbohydrates, specific enzyme inhibitors or antinutrients, and physiologic effects of altering meal frequency (*48*). Lente carbohydrates have a low glycemic index because they are digested and absorbed slowly, generally as a consequence of their resistance to gelatinization or their high content of viscous fiber. Increased meal frequency can mimic these effects and also reduce serum concentrations of LDL cholesterol and apolipoprotein B.

Comparison of the glycemic and insulinemic responses to white, brown, and germinated rice of the same botanical variety showed no differences between the types of rice (*49*). In nondiabetic subjects the glycemic indexes of rice and white bread were similar, but the peak glucose amplitude occurred earlier for white rice than for bread and the other rice types. However, the peak insulin response to white bread was twice as high as to any of the rices and the insulin curve for white bread remained elevated significantly longer.

Granfeldt et al. evaluated glucose and insulin responses to intact and milled barley from four genotypes (*50*). All barley products elicited smaller metabolic responses than white bread. The lente behavior of boiled barley flours was attributed to the viscous properties of their β-glucans. However, boiled flours elicited greater glucose and insulin responses than the corresponding boiled kernels. High-amylose products released starch more slowly from dialysis tubing during in vitro enzymic digestion of chewed samples, but the amylose/amylopectin ratio had only marginal impact on the metabolic responses. This may have been because the amylose content of the boiled barley flours ranged only between 33 and 42%.

Trout et al. attempted to predict the glycemic index of starchy foods by regression analysis of published values for the index and chemical components of the foods (*51*). The foods comprised 8 legumes and 10 grains and tubers. Overall, glycemic index was unrelated to fat content but was significantly correlated with total dietary fiber, protein, and phytate. However, these correlations lost their significance when calculated separately for legumes and for grains and tubers. Legumes had lower glycemic indexes than nonlegumes. The authors cited evidence from the literature that methods of food preparation and the characteristics of the starch and starch granules are more important predictors of glycemic index than is the content of specific food components.

## Dietary Fiber

Viscous guar gum lowers the glycemic response to a solid meal. A study in healthy subjects to whom test meals were administered orally or by instillation into the duodenum showed that part of the effect stems from inhibition of starch digestion by pancreatic α-amylase (*52*). However, most of the effect was due to slowed gastric emptying. Groop et al. showed that 15 g/d of guar gum has favorable long-term effects on glycemic control and lipid concentrations in NIDDM patients (*53*). The single-blind placebo-controlled study began with 8 weeks of placebo treatment, which was followed by 48 weeks of guar gum and another placebo period. Guar gum improved glycemic control, postprandial glucose tolerance, and lipid concentrations. The amount of C-peptide increased markedly throughout guar gum treatment and the ratio of insulin to C-peptide decreased. C-peptide measurements are considered a better estimate of insulin secretion than are peripheral insulin measurements. Therefore the increased C-peptide concentrations probably represent a true enhancement of insulin secretion even though insulin concentrations appeared not to change.

## Dietary Fat

The Second International Smolenice Insulin Symposium dealt with dietary lipids and insulin action. Presentations at this symposium were published by the New York Academy of Sciences (*54*). Sections of the symposium addressed topics related to nutritional epidemiology, metabolic effects of fats and carbohydrates, cellular mechanisms, aspects of atherogenesis, and nutritional recommendations for fat intake.

A review by Bianchi and Erkelens described NIDDM as a complex metabolic disease characterized by abnormalities in both glucose and fat metabolism (*55*). Peripheral insulin resistance and increased hepatic glucose production are important in generating the syndrome comprising obesity, hypertension, hypertriacylglycerolemia, low HDL cholesterol, increased small dense LDL, and elevated plasma uric acid. Diet and drug therapy were briefly discussed. The authors feel that future therapy should be directed at a common target because the various metabolic disturbances may be mediated through a common pathophysiologic pathway—perhaps insulin resistance.

The Normative Aging Study examined the relationship of body mass index, waist/hip ratio, and diet to fasting and postprandial insulin concentrations in men 43–85 years old who had no chronic medical conditions (*56*). Log-transformed fasting insulin was significantly related to body mass index ($r = .45$), abdomen circumference ($r = .44$), waist/hip ratio ($r = .31$), saturated fat intake ($r = .17$) and total fat intake ($r = .14$). In multivariate models, body mass index, waist/hip ratio, and saturated fat intake were significant independent predictors of fasting and postprandial insulin concentrations after adjustment for age, smoking, and physical activity. The models indicated that reduction of SFA intake from 14 en% to 8 en% would reduce fasting insulin by 18% and postprandial insulin by 25%.

The San Luis Valley Diabetes Study examined the relationship between dietary fat intake in subjects with impaired glucose tolerance and subsequent development of NIDDM (*57*). One to 3 y after the initial diet assess-

ment and oral glucose tolerance test, 20 subjects had developed NIDDM, 103 still had impaired glucose tolerance, and 60 had reverted to normal. The baseline fat intakes of these groups were 43.4, 40.6, and 38.9 en%, respectively. After adjustment for total energy intake, age, sex, ethnicity, and obesity, an increase of 40 g/d in fat intake was associated with a 3.4-fold increase in NIDDM risk (95% CI 0.8–13.6). Risk increased 6-fold (95% CI 1.2–29.8) after adjustment for fasting glucose, insulin, and 1-h insulin. Thus fat intake significantly predicts NIDDM risk in subjects with impaired glucose tolerance after obesity and markers of glucose metabolism are controlled for. Among 544 healthy women who participated in the second examination of the Kaiser Permanente Women Twins Study, a 20 g/d increase in total dietary fat was associated with significant increases in fasting insulin level of 9 and 6%, respectively, before and after adjustment for obesity variables (*58*). Higher intakes of saturated fat, oleic acid, and linoleic acid were individually related to higher fasting insulin values. The association between dietary fat and fasting insulin was significantly smaller in physically active women. Within monozygotic twin pairs, total fat intake was positively related to fasting insulin only before adjustment for obesity. The authors concluded that high intake of dietary fat is positively related to fasting insulin levels but obesity independently contributes more strongly than fat to the variation.

MONOUNSATURATED FATS. High-MUFA diets for control of diabetes have generated considerable interest (*59–62*). Garg reviewed the results of studies challenging the notion that high-carbohydrate diets improve glycemic control and insulin sensitivity in NIDDM patients (*59*; also see reference *67*). Furthermore, high-carbohydrate diets generally decrease HDL cholesterol and increase serum triacylglycerols—variables that are already unfavorably altered in diabetic subjects. Against this, Garg discussed advantages of a high-MUFA diet. Rasmussen et al. reported that compared with a high-carbohydrate diet, a high-MUFA diet improved glycemic control and lowered blood pressure in NIDDM subjects (*60*). There were no adverse effects on lipid profiles. Campbell et al. described guidelines for a high-MUFA diet that is practical and well accepted (*61*). They reported improved glycemic control and plasma triacylglycerol levels in a short-term trial in men with mild NIDDM, concluding that the high-MUFA diet is a palatable alternative to a high-carbohydrate diet and in some respects is metabolically superior to it. Lerman-Garber et al. found that a high-MUFA diet in which avocado and olive oil were the main fat sources reduced triacylglycerol levels in women with NIDDM (*62*). Subjects received the diet recommended by the American Diabetes Association during a 4-week baseline period. They were then assigned to a high-carbohydrate diet and the high-MUFA diet in random order. Partial replacement of complex digestible carbohydrates with MUFAs improved the lipid profile, maintained adequate glycemic control, and was considered a good management alternative.

POLYUNSATURATED FAT. Fish and *n*–3 PUFAs have been studied in relation to impaired glucose tolerance and NIDDM. Donnelly et al. measured lipid peroxides in NIDDM patients and controls before and after treatment with fish oil and related this to their degree of LDL glycosylation (*63*). Baseline levels of glycosylated LDL were significantly higher in patients than in controls, confirming patients' lack of glycemic control. Baseline levels of lipid peroxides were also higher in patients, but these were not correlated with LDL glycosylation. Placebo treatment had no effect. Fish oil increased lipid peroxidation in diabetics, as reported by others, but did not influence glycemic control or glycosylation. The results do not support the hypothesis that glycosylation of the LDL particle drives free radical–mediated damage of LDL's constituent fatty acids by autoxidation. Fish or small amounts of *n*–3 PUFAs appear not only safe for NIDDM patients, but potentially beneficial (*64*). These patients have a high risk of cardiovascular complications. Compared with safflower oil placebo, supplementation with 5 g/d of fish oil inhibited platelet aggregation and thromboxane $A_2$ production, reduced triacylglycerol levels and upright systolic blood pressure, and had only a small effect on glucose and cholesterol levels in subjects with moderately controlled NIDDM. However, evaluation of the cardioprotective effect of dietary fish in elderly normoglycemic and glucose-intolerant subjects suggested that fish confers less protection in glucose-intolerant than in normoglycemic subjects (*65*). This study used age- and sex-adjusted 17-year mortality for coronary heart disease as an endpoint. Adjusted for age, sex, body mass index, smoking, alcohol use, and intakes of total energy, polyunsaturated fat, and carbohydrates, the risk ratio for the normoglycemic fish-eating population was 0.34 (95% CI 0.16–0.72), whereas for glucose-intolerant subjects it was 0.80 (95% CI 0.31–2.05).

Hughes et al. evaluated the lipoprotein response to aerobic exercise, a low-fat diet, or both in glucose-intolerant subjects aged 50–78 y (*66*). Exercise alone had no significant effect on lipoprotein cholesterol

or triacylglycerol concentrations. However, exercise training augmented the beneficial effects of the low-fat diet.

## Carbohydrate

Garg et al. reported a randomized crossover trial of the effects of two diets on glycemic control and plasma lipids in NIDDM patients (*67*). One diet contained 55 en% carbohydrates and 30 en% fat (SFA/MUFA/PUFA = 1:1:1); the other contained 40 en% carbohydrates and 45 en% fat (SFA/MUFA/PUFA = 1:2.5:1). Each diet offered diverse foods and was provided for 6 weeks. To assess longer-term effects, subjects were offered the option of continuing whichever diet they received second for an additional 8 weeks. Compared with the high-MUFA diet, the high-carbohydrate diet caused deterioration of glycemic control, accentuation of hyperinsulinemia, and increased plasma levels of VLDL cholesterol and triacylglycerols. The effects of the diets were independent of order and persisted throughout the 14-week period of the second diet. Similar effects were observed in a very different type of study. Gonzaléz et al. compared the clinical and dietary characteristics of low-income Mexican NIDDM patients living in Mexico City and low-income Mexican-American NIDDM patients living in San Antonio (*68*). The average diet of NIDDM patients in Mexico City contained 62–63 en% carbohydrate and 18–20 en% fat, whereas the diet of Mexican-Americans in San Antonio contained ~47 en% carbohydrate and 30–33 en% fat. Plasma triacylglycerol levels were higher and HDL cholesterol levels lower in Mexico City. Insulin responses to glucose challenge were greater in Mexico City. Similarities and other differences between the two groups of NIDDM patients were also noted. The authors observed that the Mexican diet is generally associated with a low incidence of cardiovascular disease, but this is in populations with low rates of diabetes; the diet that is protective in nondiabetic individuals may be undesirable for NIDDM patients.

Fructose was advocated as a sweetener for diabetic patients before the discovery of insulin. A review of beneficial effects of fructose and some possible adverse side effects reported that fructose elicits lower glucose and insulin responses than sucrose in both normal and diabetic subjects (*69*). In the short term, substitution of fructose for sucrose improves glycemic control and does not appear to have any important side effects. In a balanced diet, reasonable amounts do not affect lipoprotein metabolism or produce gastrointestinal symptoms. Whether the benefits are sustained over the long term without deleterious side effects has not been established.

## Protein

Peters and Davidson evaluated the glucose response and insulin requirements of subjects with IDDM in response to three meals: a standard meal of diverse normal foods and a similar meal supplemented with either additional fat-rich or protein-rich foods (*70*). Addition of protein to the meal increased both the late postprandial glucose response and the insulin requirement, whereas addition of fat did not influence these values.

Issues of protein nutrition for diabetic patients have not been resolved. Protein-rich foods generally induce glomerular hyperfiltration and may accelerate renal failure in diabetic persons. A study in healthy volunteers and NIDDM patients compared the renal effects of two protein-rich foods, tuna fish (0.7 g protein per kilogram of body weight) and egg white (0.7 and 1.4 g/kg) (*71*). Responses of patients and controls to the acute protein loading were similar. Ingestion of egg white had no influence on glomerular filtration rate in either group, whereas ingestion of tuna fish significantly increased the glomerular filtration rate in both groups. Tuna fish protein caused significantly greater increases in total plasma amino acids than an equivalent amount of egg white protein: 1.4 g/kg of egg white protein caused elevations similar to those from half the amount of tuna protein. Plasma levels of glycine and alanine, which are known to induce glomerular hyperfiltration, increased significantly more after ingestion of tuna than after either amount of egg white. Excretion of urinary 6-keto-prostaglandin $F_{1\alpha}$ increased only after tuna ingestion. The authors concluded that egg white and tuna have different effects on the glomerular filtration rate independent of the amount of protein ingested. These differences could be explained by differences in renal vasodilatory prostaglandin secretion or by differential increases in plasma glycine and alanine.

Metabolic studies in normal volunteers and IDDM patients with intensively controlled disease showed that a protein-free energy-maintenance diet decreases insulin requirements in IDDM and decreases fasting hepatic glucose output and basal insulin levels in normal subjects (*72*). Protein deprivation decreased average preprandial and 24-h blood glucose concentrations by 30% at the same time that basal and bolus insulin doses were decreased by 25%. This was attributed partly to decreased hepatic gluconeogenesis but could also involve increased insulin sensitivity. The authors stressed that this diet was a study tool and did not suggest severe protein restriction as diet therapy.

COW'S MILK AND MILK PROTEINS. Genetic predisposition to IDDM may be necessary but is not sufficient for development of the disease; an environmental trigger is also required. Gerstein reviewed the clinical evidence relating very limited breast-feeding or early exposure to cow's milk to development of IDDM (*73*). In case–control studies, patients with IDDM were more likely than controls to have been breast-fed for <3 months (RR 1.43, 95% CI 1.15–1.77) and to have been exposed to cow's milk before the age of 4 months (RR 1.63, 95% CI 1.22–2.17). Ecological and time-series studies, in which the prevalence of IDDM was compared with extent of breast-feeding or cow's milk consumption in different populations or changes in these practices within a population over time, consistently showed a positive relationship between IDDM and either exposure to cow's milk or diminished breast-feeding. Overall there was some evidence that exposure to cow's milk before the age of 3–4 months is more relevant for IDDM than the total extent or duration of exposure. The ecological studies suggest that 74–94% of the intercountry variation in incidence of IDDM may be related to differences in consumption of cow's milk. However, from these studies there is no way of knowing whether the people who drank the cow's milk were the ones who developed diabetes. Other criticisms can be leveled at the case–control studies, but Gerstein claims to have restricted his analysis to those that minimized the potential for bias. The design and findings of the 15 studies analyzed were summarized in two tables.

Dosch discussed IDDM as an autoimmune disease and reviewed the long and frustrating search for its environmental triggers (*74*). He described a large international clinical trial, centered in Finland, that when completed will determine whether avoidance of cow's milk during the first 9 months after birth will prevent IDDM. Phase I of the trial is underway, with pilot studies in Helsinki, Finland, and Hamilton, Ontario. Follow-up will be for 10 years.

Virtanen et al. reported findings of the Childhood Diabetes in Finland Study Group (*75,76*). This was a nationwide study of 690 IDDM patients <15 years old and age- and sex-matched population controls. IDDM patients had been exclusively breast-fed for a shorter time than controls and had started receiving dairy products sooner (*75*). There was no difference in the age at which solid foods were introduced. IDDM risk was doubled in infants who had been exclusively breast-fed for <2 months or had been introduced to dairy products before they were 2 months old. Multivariate analysis indicated that early introduction to dairy products was the more important of these two variables. Adjustment for birth order, birth weight, and mother's age and education did not influence the results. Immunologic studies showed that early introduction of dairy products and high milk consumption during childhood increased titers of cow's milk antibodies in newly diagnosed diabetic children (*76*). High levels of IgA antibodies to cow's milk formula were independently associated with elevated risk of IDDM.

Diet, temperature, cultural practices, viral infections, and genetic factors are among the variables that partially account for latitude-related cross-country differences in IDDM incidence. Sardinia, with its geographically well defined and ethnically homogeneous population, has a very high (second only to Finland) and rising incidence of IDDM (*77*). It is the most striking exception to the positive associations between IDDM risk and latitude or cow's milk consumption. The Sardinians are genetically different from other European populations, including Italians, and a genetic basis for IDDM susceptibility has been described. However, the increasing incidence of IDDM in Sardinia implicates an as-yet unidentified environmental trigger—perhaps one to which Sardinians are uniquely exposed.

A 17-amino-acid region in bovine serum albumin (BSA, a constituent of the whey fraction of cow's milk) is homologous with a surface protein on human pancreatic β-cells. Thus an immune response directed at milk protein could react with self-antigens, leading to IDDM. Monte et al. assayed 9 infant formulas popular in the USA for BSA (*78*). They also tested 2% cow's milk and pooled human milk. One formula was soy-based. The rest, including all of the powdered formulas, were based on cow's milk. Three of the 4 powdered formulas tested positive for BSA, whereas all five of the liquid formulas and human milk tested negative. The positive formulas contained 0.47–1.14 µmol/L of BSA, compared with 1.14 µmol/L for 2% cow's milk. Because the protein content of cow's milk is more than twice that of the formulas, its content of BSA as a percentage of protein is the same as that in the formulas, or less. The negative powdered formula contained enzymatically hydrolyzed whey. Although the digestion step may have produced nonimmunogenic peptides, the radial immunodiffusion procedure employed in this study was not sensitive enough to detect the BSA fragment homologous with β-cells. Therefore all of the BSA-"free" formulas may still have contained this fragment. The authors encouraged manufacturers of infant formulas to develop processing procedures to destroy BSA and its immunogenic subunit. This

could be a simple matter of altering the processing temperature. Strand argued that BSA is denatured at 85°C, and raising processing temperatures from the current level of 60–72°C to 85°C or above could destroy the trigger molecule for IDDM (*79*). In addition to reducing the incidence of IDDM, the author postulated that high-temperature treatment of milk could also reduce the incidence of other autoimmune diseases whose cause has not been determined but which also might result from BSA-triggered attacks by the immune system. These diseases include arthritis, multiple sclerosis, and systemic lupus erythematosus. Strand recommended developing more sensitive assays for BSA and trials of BSA-free milk products in IDDM-prone mice and humans.

## Vitamins

Cabalero briefly reviewed the effects of vitamin E in NIDDM (*80*). Vitamin E supplementation for 4 months produced significant improvement in glucose utilization and hepatic response to insulin in both normal and diabetic subjects. The major part of the increased glucose disposal was by the nonoxidative route. Although the dose employed was pharmacologic, it was within the range of doses reported to decrease risk of cancer and cardiovascular disease. There is evidence that the mechanism by which vitamin E improves insulin responsiveness is related to its antioxidant activity. Gerster discussed vitamin E in terms of its effects on platelet function and potential for preventing platelet dysfunction in the atherosclerosis associated with diabetes (*81*). Factors contributing to premature atherosclerosis and other vascular disorders in diabetics were reviewed, simplified lipid-hypothesis and reaction-to-injury models of atherogenesis were diagrammed, and steps in the synthesis of vasoactive prostanoids were presented. Several studies have found that moderate supplementation with vitamin E significantly decreases platelet activation and lipid peroxidation in IDDM and NIDDM patients, whereas even high-dose supplementation may have no effect in normal subjects. Vitamin E supplementation has also decreased the nonenzymatic glycation of proteins in diabetic subjects. So far the data are merely encouraging. Much additional work is required at both clinical and biochemical levels to verify that vitamin E protects patients with diabetes and other disorders against platelet adhesion and aggregation.

Like vitamin E, vitamin C appears to improve nonoxidative glucose metabolism. Paolisso et al. confirmed that diabetic subjects have reduced plasma levels of vitamin C (*82*). When they infused pharmacologic doses of vitamin C into elderly NIDDM patients and healthy age-matched controls, both groups showed improved insulin action and glucose homeostasis. The response was related to the rate of vitamin C infusion. The authors postulated that the infusion restored more favorable plasma levels of reduced glutathione, which would improve the physical state and function of plasma membranes.

## Alcohol

Facchini et al. conducted a study of healthy adults characterized as nondrinkers or light-to-moderate drinkers (10–30 g/d of alcohol) to evaluate the effects of alcohol on insulin sensitivity (*83*). Moderate drinkers had lower plasma glucose and insulin responses to oral glucose challenge, enhanced insulin-mediated glucose uptake, and higher plasma HDL cholesterol concentrations than nondrinkers. These changes may also be related to the lower risk of coronary heart disease associated with light to moderate alcohol consumption. Although alcohol-induced hypoglycemia is a dreaded complication of IDDM, Christiansen et al. showed that when taken in moderate amounts with a meal, alcohol causes no adverse serum glucose, insulin, free fatty acid, or triacylglycerol responses in subjects with NIDDM (*84*).

## Calorie Restriction

Wing et al. evaluated the effects of caloric restriction, independent of weight loss, on glycemic control, fasting insulin levels, and insulin sensitivity in obese NIDDM patients (*85*). Subjects were randomly assigned to two levels of calorie restriction: 400 or 1000 kcal/d. The 400-kcal diet was limited to lean meat, fish, and poultry and liquid formula, to be consumed in any desired combination as long as the calorie limit was not exceeded. The 1000-kcal diet was based on normal foods providing 30 en% fat, 55 en% carbohydrate, and 15 en% protein. Subjects were studied at the beginning of the diet and again when they had lost 11% of their initial body weight. At the time of equivalent weight loss, subjects on the very-low-calorie diet had lower fasting glucose levels and greater insulin sensitivity than those in the more moderately calorie-restricted group. When subjects increased their caloric intake from 400/d to 1000/d their glycemic control worsened despite continued weight loss. The authors concluded that calorie restriction and weight loss have independent effects on improvements in glycemic control and insulin sensitivity.

Dietary restriction also increases insulin sensitivity and lowers blood glucose in rhesus monkeys (*86*). These animals normally show an age-related decline in insulin sensitivity and glucose tolerance. Ad libitum food intake was measured in a group of adult monkeys, after which half of them were gradually restricted to 70% of their individually determined intake. Animals were monitored for 30 months. Basal glucose, basal insulin, and insulin responses to glucose and tolbutamide increased in the control group and decreased in the diet-restricted group. Insulin sensitivity decreased in controls and increased in restricted animals. Mechanistic studies are underway.

## Other

A diet containing 4% oyster mushroom (*Pleurotus ostreatus*) improved glycemic control in cholesterol-fed rats with streptozotocin-induced IDDM (*87*). Cellulose was substituted for dried mushroom in the control diet. After two months animals in the mushroom group had significantly lower basal and postprandial glucose levels than controls. Moreover, cholesterol concentrations were >40% lower and the lipoprotein profile was more favorable in the mushroom group. Insulin levels were unaffected.

The hypoglycemic activity of fenugreek (*Trigonella foenum-graecum*) in humans and experimental animals is well documented, but mechanistic details of this activity are unclear. Raghuram et al. conducted a metabolic crossover study of the effect of fenugreek seeds (25 g/d) in NIDDM patients (*88*). Fenugreek seeds significantly reduced the area under the plasma glucose curve in the glucose tolerance test and increased the metabolic clearance rate. It also increased the level of erythrocyte insulin receptors. These results suggest that fenugreek improves glucose tolerance by enhancing peripheral glucose utilization and exerts its effect systemically at the insulin receptor level. Other studies have demonstrated local action at the gastrointestinal level, attributed to the fiber content of the ground seeds.

# ENDOCRINE SYSTEM AND REPRODUCTION

## Fertility, Maternal Nutrition, and Fetal Development

A demographic study has contributed to the evidence that galactose has deleterious effects on ovarian function. Cramer et al. examined relationships between age-specific fertility, prevalence of hypolactasia (inability to digest lactose) in adults, and milk consumption (*89*).

The enzyme lactase, which hydrolyzes milk sugar to glucose and galactose, disappears in most mammals after weaning, but lactase persistence arose long ago as an autosomal dominant trait in certain human populations that practiced dairying. Contemporary populations vary widely in both milk consumption and prevalence of adult hypolactasia. Populations with the highest milk consumption and highest prevalence of lactase persistence have the greatest exposure to galactose; if galactose is toxic to the ovary and germ cells and the effect is cumulative, this exposure should have an impact on fertility and the impact should be greatest later in the reproductive period. That is what the authors found. For example, in Denmark the prevalence of hypolactasia is only 4% and per capita milk consumption is >400 g/d; fertility plummets by 87% between the ages of 30 and 40 years. In Thailand, where the prevalence of hypolactasia is 98% and per capita milk consumption is ~20 g/d, fertility decreases by only 26% during this period. Overall, in 36 countries for which data were available, the percentage decline in fertility at ages 30–40 was strongly correlated with both milk consumption ($r = .60$, $p \leq .0003$) and prevalence of hypolactasia ($r = -.68$, $p \leq .0001$).

Proceedings of a symposium on maternal nutrition held in 1993 in New Harmony, Indiana, were published as a supplement to *The American Journal of Clinical Nutrition* (*90*). The symposium updated information on nutrition during pregnancy and its effect on the health of the mother, fetus, and neonate. Some of the research is basic and still far from clinical application; some has advanced to the point where clinical recommendations could be made. A session was devoted to vitamin and mineral supplementation.

The severe famine that befell the western Netherlands during the wartime winter of 1944–1945 was a fertile source of data on prenatal and postnatal effects of maternal nutrition. Susser and Stein reviewed the findings from the Dutch Famine Study and discussed time-related effects of prenatal nutrition as revealed by this study and others in humans and laboratory animals (*91*). Because the famine was sharply delimited—it lasted from the November 1944 embargo to liberation in May 1945—its impact on successive developmental stages could be discerned. Exposure during the periconceptional period sharply reduced fertility. Organic brain defects (principally neural tube defects) increased in children conceived during the famine, and the subsequent incidence of schizophrenia and schizoid and antisocial personalities also increased. Exposure to famine somewhat later during gestation caused an increase in number

of preterm births, stillbirths, and first-week deaths and in the later prevalence of obesity. During the third trimester, maternal weight and infant birth weight were reduced, mortality at 0–3 months increased, and subsequent obesity decreased. The reduction in birth weight carried over to the second generation, suggesting that environmentally induced changes in maternal birth weight are transmitted to offspring with the same force as any other birth-weight determinants, including genetic ones.

In rats, the dam's protein nutriture during pregnancy has long-term effects on her offspring (*92*). Rats were fed diets containing 6, 9, 12, or 18% by weight of protein for 14 d before mating and throughout pregnancy. Lactating mothers and their offspring were fed standard chow (20% protein). Litter size and neonatal death rates were unaffected by diet. All offspring were grossly normal except that pups of dams fed 6% protein were smaller than the others. Offspring from all three low-protein groups had significantly elevated systolic blood pressure (15–22 mm Hg) when they were 9 weeks old. Blood pressure was still elevated after 21 weeks in the 6 and 9% protein groups. Hypertension was associated with elevated pulmonary angiotensin-converting enzyme activity. These data are consistent with the idea that poor maternal nutrition during pregnancy can irreversibly impair some aspects of fetal physiological and biochemical function, with adverse consequences for later health.

It is unclear whether periconceptional folic acid supplementation prevents neural tube defects by correcting a nutritional deficiency or by overcoming a metabolic block in folate metabolism, and studies of vitamin $B_{12}$ status and neural tube defects have produced negative or inconclusive results. Kirke et al. designed a case–control study large enough to resolve questions of folate and $B_{12}$ status in relation to neural tube defects (*93*). Maternal levels of folate and vitamin $B_{12}$ were independently related to risk. Plasma and erythrocyte folate levels were strongly correlated in both case-subjects and controls and plasma folate was not correlated with plasma $B_{12}$. Plasma $B_{12}$ and erythrocyte folate were significantly correlated, but only in case-subjects; this relationship was independent of plasma folate. Levels of folate and $B_{12}$ associated with increased risk were greater than those considered indicative of deficiency. Although an argument can be made for a purely nutritional etiology of neural tube defects, it is difficult to explain the correlation between erythrocyte folate and plasma $B_{12}$ in case-subjects on this basis. The authors favor a role for some metabolic abnormality that interacts with maternal levels of folate and $B_{12}$. The only factor independently influenced by both folate and $B_{12}$ is the activity of methionine synthase, which suggests direct or indirect involvement of this enzyme in the etiology of neural tube defects. The authors suggested that recommended daily allowances (RDAs) of folate and vitamin $B_{12}$ be reevaluated and $B_{12}$ supplementation be considered in programs to prevent neural tube defects. The FDA is proposing to require folic acid fortification of certain cereal grain products and to allow limited health claims on labels of folate-rich foods (*94*).

A British case–control study found no association between neural tube defects and levels of zinc in maternal serum (*95*). Nor was there any relationship between periconceptional folic acid supplementation and zinc status. (This was considered because a zinc-dependent enzyme is necessary to hydrolyze dietary folate in its usual polyglutamate form.) Because the study population was generally well nourished, this study could not exclude the possibility that zinc levels outside the range observed might influence risk of defects. In a case–control study in a poor, urban New Jersey community, a low zinc intake ($\leq 6$ mg/d) was associated with higher risk of very preterm delivery, preterm delivery, and low birth weight (*96*).

Olsen reviewed evidence that marine PUFAs in the maternal diet influence birth weight (*97*). Plausible mechanisms and rat studies relevant to them were discussed. Controlled trials and the strengths and weaknesses of the epidemiologic evidence were summarized. It has been suggested that marine *n*–3 PUFAs regulate processes that initiate parturition, and the strongest evidence from epidemiology is that *n*–3 marine fatty acids prolong gestation. Higher birth weight would be a corollary of this. However, these observations cannot be extrapolated to the occurrence of preterm and low-birth-weight deliveries. Moreover, associations with postterm deliveries and their related problems have not been evaluated. Olsen et al. looked for a dose–response effect of maternal seafood consumption on birth weight in the Faroe Islands (*98*). Women were placed into 7 groups according to the average number of seafood dinners (fish or pilot whale) they ate per week during pregnancy. Babies born to women who ate 3 seafood meals per week were on average 0.2 kg heavier and 1 cm longer than babies of women who ate none. The effect leveled off with further seafood consumption. Mean gestational age and placental weight also increased with seafood intake in some statistical models. After discussing possible sources of bias and error, the authors concluded that their study supports the hypothesis that maternal consumption of marine foods during pregnancy is related to

the baby's size at birth and the dose–response relationship has a saturation level.

Children of atopic parents are at increased risk of developing allergy. Lovegrove et al. evaluated the effects of a milk-free diet during late pregnancy and lactation on incidence and severity of atopic eczema in infants (*99*). Atopic mothers were randomly allocated to an unrestricted-diet group and a group instructed to avoid all dairy foods from the 36th week of gestation through lactation. Infants of mothers from these groups were compared with infants of nonatopic mothers on an unrestricted diet. Maternal serum levels of β-lactoglobulin IgG antibodies fell during the milk-free diet. Maternal and cord serum levels of these antibodies and α-casein antibodies were significantly correlated. The incidence of allergy was recorded when infants were 6, 12, and 18 months old. Children of atopic parents had a greater incidence and severity of atopic eczema than children of nonatopic parents, but a maternal milk-free diet during late pregnancy and lactation afforded some protection.

Vitamin D, calcium, and vitamin $B_{12}$ nutrition are of particular concern to lactating women who follow vegetarian diets. Nutritional inadequacies could affect the mother, the infant, or both. A review of studies on women in the northeastern USA who ate macrobiotic diets indicated that supplemental vitamin D is unnecessary if exposure to sunlight is adequate (*100*). Findings for calcium were inconclusive. Although calcium intake was relatively low in vegetarian mothers and differences in calcium-regulating hormones were apparent, adaptation may have been sufficient to prevent bone demineralization. The concentration of calcium in milk of these mothers was normal. However, vegetarian women and their infants both excreted elevated amounts of methylmalonic acid, a frequent finding in cases of vitamin $B_{12}$ deficiency. Infants who excreted high levels of methylmalonic acid were consuming milk low in vitamin $B_{12}$.

## Menstrual Cycle

Because age at menarche is associated with breast cancer risk, Merzenich et al. conducted a prospective study of German girls to evaluate effects of physical activity and dietary fat on menarche (*101*). A multivariate and several univariate models were developed. A girl's age at menarche was unrelated to her mother's age at menarche or to socioeconomic factors. In the multivariate model, the relative risk of early menarche was positively related to energy-adjusted fat intake (RR 2.1, 95% CI 1.10–3.95, $p = .03$) for the highest quartile vs. lowest quartile and negatively related to hours per week of physical activity

(RR 0.3, 95% CI 0.12–0.51, *p* <.0001). The strongest risk factor was percent of body fat (RR 4.0, 95% CI 2.11–7.47, *p* <.0001). Univariate effects were accentuated in the multivariate model, an example of negative confounding. The authors concluded that fat intake during childhood and puberty affects breast cancer risk by influencing hormonal events such as age at menarche.

Phipps et al. reported effects of flaxseed lignans on the menstrual cycle (*102*). In a randomized crossover study, 18 normally cycling women followed their usual omnivorous diet and the usual diet supplemented with 10 g/d of flaxseed powder, each for 3 cycles. Data were gathered for the 2nd and 3rd cycles on each diet. Three anovulatory cycles occurred during the 36 control cycles, none during the 36 flaxseed cycles. Flaxseed cycles were associated with a longer luteal phase, a higher luteal-phase ratio of progesterone to estradiol, and slightly higher midfollicular-phase testosterone concentrations. These data demonstrate that lignans contribute to the effect of diet on action of sex steroids and possibly on risk of breast and other hormonally dependent cancers.

Factors that influence endogenous postmenopausal estrogen levels are of interest because they may relate to risk of osteoporosis and coronary heart disease. Body fat mass and the presence of the ovaries have long been known to affect estrogen levels; moderate alcohol consumption has been recognized as a contributing factor only recently. Gavaler reviewed the effects of these three determinants of postmenopausal estrogen levels, with emphasis on alcohol (*103*). Levels of pituitary hormones (luteinizing hormone, follicle-stimulating hormone, prolactin) in postmenopausal women are the same in abstainers and moderate drinkers, but strikingly different in women with alcoholic cirrhosis. The situation for sex steroids contrasts sharply: estradiol levels are significantly higher in moderate drinkers than in nondrinkers and still higher in alcoholics, whereas testosterone levels fall as drinking increases. The estradiol:testosterone ratio, an estimate of aromatization, increases from 44 ± 6 in nondrinkers to 74 ± 4 in moderate drinkers to 169 ± 43 in alcoholics. Further analysis suggested a fourth determinant of postmenopausal estrogen levels: nationality. However, nationality may be a surrogate marker for dietary influences that include wine consumption and alcohol drinking. In addition to effects attributable to alcohol itself, phytoestrogens are found in beer and wine.

## Other

Thissen et al. comprehensively reviewed the nutritional regulation of insulin-like growth factors (*104*). Many observations have been made in human subjects, and animal models have been developed to investigate mechanisms. Both energy and proteins are key regulators of serum IGF-I concentrations, but energy may be the more important. The regulation of IGF-I by nutrients links diet and growth, showing how nutrients and hormones jointly stimulate growth and illustrating the role of nutrients in control of gene expression. The biological activity of circulating IGF-I is also regulated by nutrients—an observation with major clinical implications.

At high latitudes, vegetarians may be at risk of poor vitamin D status during the winter. Lamberg-Allardt et al. evaluated the prevalence of wintertime vitamin D deficiency in Finland and how it affects calcium metabolism (*105*). Subjects were middle-aged and were classified as strict vegetarians, lactovegetarians, ovolactovegetarians (including fish-eaters), and vegetarians who took vitamin D supplements or had been exposed to abundant sunlight during the preceding 6 months. A control group of omnivores was included. Compared with controls, strict vegetarians had lower intakes of vitamin D, lower serum concentrations of 25-hydroxyvitamin D, and significantly higher levels of serum intact parathyroid hormone. Intact parathyroid hormone levels correlated negatively with serum 25-hydroxyvitamin D and dietary calcium intake. The authors concluded that white strict vegetarians are at risk of vitamin D deficiency, at least during winter, primarily because of a low dietary intake. Normal sunlight exposure during summer cannot maintain satisfactory vitamin D status. However, vitamin D supplements and sunlight exposure during winter normalize vitamin D status in strict vegetarians. The relevance of vitamin D deficiency and the accompanying secondary hyperparathyroidism for bone health has not been evaluated.

## KIDNEY DISEASE AND FUNCTION

King and Levey discussed modulation of renal function by dietary protein and renal responses induced by changes in habitual protein intake (*106*). They examined the pattern and magnitude of changes in glomerular filtration rate and creatinine clearance and discussed the importance of variability of these measurements among individuals and populations, especially in interpretation of clinical studies. In the USA and other developed countries, average protein intake far exceeds the RDA. Nevertheless, wide variations in protein intake are associated with age, gender, body size, and dietary preferences. Differences in glomerular filtration rate and creatinine clearance reflect these dietary differences.

Possible mechanisms of protein-induced hyperfiltration were illustrated, classifying them according to their systemic or direct renal mode of action. Both the habitual level of protein intake and transient changes in it have multiple effects on renal function in healthy people and patients with kidney disease. For the most part, effects on the glomerular filtration rate and the generation and tubular secretion of creatinine appear to be homeostatic adjustments.

Gentile et al. confirmed that a vegetarian soy-based diet has long-term beneficial effects on hyperlipidemia and proteinuria in nephrotic patients (107). Because fish oil has had favorable effects in some experimental studies, they evaluated fish-oil supplements (5 g/d) in conjunction with the vegetarian diet in these patients. Although fish oil induced a small but significant decrease in diastolic blood pressure, it had no further effect on lipid abnormalities in this dietary regimen. However, in kidney transplant recipients who followed a diet unrestricted except for sodium, 6 g/d of fish oil during the first postoperative year had beneficial effects on both renal hemodynamics and blood pressure (108). Fish-oil recipients also had fewer rejection episodes than controls, although graft survival at one year did not differ between groups.

Glomerulonephritis and diabetic nephropathy are characterized by excessive proliferation of mesangial cells. Therefore, any factors that might inhibit this proliferation are of intense interest. Yokozawa et al. assessed the effects of green tea tannins on [$^3$H]thymidine uptake by primary cultures of mouse glomerular mesangial cells (109). A mixture of green tea tannins suppressed thymidine uptake by 55% at a concentration of 12.5 µg/mL and by 99% at 25 µg/mL; 6.25 µg/mL had no effect. (−)-Epigallocatechin 3-O-gallate, which accounted for 18% of the tannins in the mixture, decreased thymidine uptake by 19% at 6.25 µg/mL, 72% at 12.5 µg/mL, and virtually completely at higher levels. (−)-Epicatechin 3-O-gallate (4.6% of the mixture) was less effective at 6.25 µg/mL but similarly active at higher concentrations. These findings complement in vivo observations that green tea inhibits progression of renal failure.

# DIGESTIVE SYSTEM

## Ulcers

Many factors are involved in the etiology of ulcer disease. One of them appears to be diet, and one of the precipitating factors may be dietary exposure to particular patterns of staple foods. Tovey summarized historical and geographical evidence implicating the balance between ulcerogenic and protective foods in the prevalence of peptic and duodenal ulcer (110). In Asia and Africa, dietary staples where prevalence is high include rice, refined wheat and/or maize, cassava, and sorghum. Dietary staples in low-prevalence areas include unrefined wheat and/or maize, millets, pulses, and sorghum. Some proposed effects of diet were considered. Fiber appears protective, but its buffering capacity cannot account for this. The idea that diets requiring a lot of chewing induce a greater output of saliva, which is protective, is not supported by epidemiologic observations. There is no evidence supporting the notion that peppers and spices are ulcerogenic; nor do coffee, tea, and alcohol consumption reflect the distribution of ulcer disease in Africa. There is no geographical association with protein or vitamin deficiency or meal frequency. Experimental models of ulceration have yielded clues to a number of cytoprotective factors. In arguing for balance as the key, Tovey concluded that in southern India the ulcerogenic properties of stored refined polished rice and a paucity of protective foods explain the high prevalence of ulcers, whereas in northern India unrefined wheat is protective and fewer ulcerogenic foods are eaten. In other settings an unfavorable intake of n–3 and n–6 PUFAs has an adverse effect on prostaglandin metabolism and promotes ulcers. Further evidence that no single dietary factor explains ulcer occurrence or recurrence came from a study of patients with healed duodenal ulcers (111). Subjects were randomly allocated to receive 11 g/d of concentrated wheat fiber or placebo for one year. They continued to follow a traditional Norwegian diet. Ulcers recurred in 31 of 37 subjects in the active treatment group and in 30 of 36 controls.

The antiulcer properties of quercetin are not mediated through an effect on gastric acid or pepsin production. Therefore de la Lastra et al. studied the cytoprotective effects of quercetin in a rat model of ethanol-induced mucosal injury (112). The results indicated that the cytoprotection is complex, involving stimulation of prostaglandin production and inhibition of leukotriene production, mediated by quercetin's antioxidant properties and stimulation of mucus secretion. Potent antioxidant properties are also thought to account for the antiulcer actions of traditional Japanese Kampo medicines (113).

## Pancreatitis

Alcohol abuse is a major factor in chronic and acute pancreatitis. Horne and Tsukamoto reviewed dietary modulation of alcohol-induced pancreatic injury as revealed by studies in the rat intragastric infusion model (*114*). Use of this model helped identify key histopathologic and cellular pathophysiologic features leading to alcohol-induced pancreatic injury. Ethanol in conjunction with a high-fat diet caused acinar atrophy, brought about by a diminished trophic effect of cholecystokinin on pancreatic acini. Observations supporting the idea that a high-fat diet exacerbates alcohol-induced injury were summarized.

Noel-Jorand and Bras studied 58 variables related to diet, alcohol consumption, and tobacco use to determine their relationship to development of calcifying chronic pancreatitis or cirrhosis in southern France (*115*). The ratio of animal to vegetable protein was high for all subjects and did not differ between groups (normal controls and alcoholic subjects with digestive diseases, pancreatitis, or cirrhosis). However, subjects in all three alcoholic groups consumed more protein and fat (particularly saturated fat) than controls and these amounts were highest in the pancreatitis group. Carbohydrate and caloric intake from both food and alcohol were greater in chronic alcoholics than in normal controls. Overall the study found that the nutritional profile of alcoholics with chronic pancreatitis differs significantly from that of alcoholics with cirrhosis.

## STONE DISEASES

### Urinary Tract Stones

Diet has a role in both the origin and the treatment of nephrolithiasis, a disorder that occurs in 1–20% of the U.S. population. Brown and Wolfson reviewed the metabolic causes of kidney stones and the dietary management of nephrolithiasis and other renal disease (*116*). Bladder stones have been associated with protein malnutrition and economic deprivation, whereas upper urinary tract stones are associated with diets high in animal protein. These associations hold between and within countries. Excess intake of purines, oxalate, vitamin C, sodium, or calcium can stimulate stone formation in susceptible persons. General dietary recommendations for management of nephrolithiasis are fluid intake to maintain a urine output of at least 3 L/d, modest sodium restriction to inhibit calciuria, moderate protein intake, and avoidance of oxalate-rich foods and large doses of vitamin C. Specific advice considers dietary and metabolic idiosyncrasies of the individual. Goldfarb examined the role of diet in various forms of

nephrolithiasis and the effectiveness of diet therapy in preventing new stone formation (*117*). He discussed the roles of dietary protein and sodium in the pathogenesis of hypercalciuria, the role of dietary calcium in calcium-stone formation, the role of dietary oxalate in enteric hyperoxaluria and formation of calcium oxalate renal stones, and dietary factors in hyperuricosuria. Difficulties in evaluating the efficacy of pharmacologic therapy and the paucity of information from dietary trials were mentioned. Heckers et al. discussed dietary prevention and treatment of renal calcium oxalate stones (*118*). They discussed the metabolism of ascorbic acid, whose oxidation has been proposed as a major source of urinary oxalate. Chocolate and black tea were also considered as sources of oxalic acid and the effect of dietary fiber on intestinal absorption of oxalic acid was discussed.

Hesse et al. investigated the influence of foods and beverages on urine composition and its circadian fluctuations (*119*). Subjects ate a standardized diet consisting of ordinary foods. The same menu was provided every day during the study. On exposure days, one beverage or food was exchanged for the item to be tested. Orange juice significantly increased urinary pH and excretion of citric acid. Black tea raised oxalic acid excretion by 8%. Beer was diuretic in the short term, but then caused a compensatory antidiuresis that increased risk of stone formation. The effect of various mineral waters on urinary constituents depended on their composition. Milk and cocoa increased calcium excretion, and cocoa also increased oxalic acid excretion. Sodium chloride sharply increased calcium excretion. Spinach and rhubarb caused large oxalate peaks in the circadian excretion curve. Cheese increased calcium excretion and decreased urine pH and citrate excretion. Purine-rich foods increased uric acid excretion over a period of several days. Depending on their phytic acid content, brans bound calcium but increased oxalic acid excretion. From these observations the authors concluded that the average diet in Germany entails a high risk of urinary stone formation. Risk can be reduced by change to a balanced mixed or vegetarian diet.

In Brazil, a dietary case–control study of calcium-stone-formers found a low calcium intake in both case-patients and controls (*120*). Stone-formers had a higher body mass index than controls. Although nutrient intakes of the two groups were similar during the week, stone-formers ate more total and animal protein during weekends. These data demonstrate the importance of the quantity and type of dietary protein for a group of stone-formers whose intake of calcium is relatively low and show that habits of both the individual and the population need to be considered in dietary recommendations for stone-formers.

Calcium metabolism shows aberrations at the molecular, cell, and organ levels in essential hypertension. The kidney is frequently implicated. Strazzullo and Mancini pointed out that there is also evidence of deranged calcium metabolism in kidney stone disease and that kidney stones are associated with essential hypertension more often than can be explained by chance (121). They reviewed evidence for an increased incidence of nephrolithiasis in the hypertensive population and discussed the importance of diet in preventing and treating both of these widespread conditions. They hypothesized a renal calcium leak, resulting in hypercalciuria, as the mechanism linking hypertension to nephrolithiasis and suggested particular attention to intake of electrolytes for individuals at risk.

Massey et al. reviewed the effect of dietary oxalate and calcium on urinary oxalate levels and risk of calcium oxalate kidney stone formation (122), and Massey and Sutton reported that modification of dietary oxalate and calcium reduces urinary oxalate levels in hyperoxaluric stone-formers (123). Most urinary oxalate is derived from endogenous synthesis, but dietary intake of oxalate and calcium can be important, especially in subjects with a high rate of oxalate absorption (122). In normal subjects, oxalate-rich foods enhance excretion of urinary oxalate but not in proportion to the foods' oxalate content. Eight foods causing significant increase in urinary oxalate were identified: spinach, rhubarb, beets, nuts, chocolate, tea, wheat bran, and strawberries. Calcium restriction enhances oxalate absorption and urinary excretion, whereas increased calcium consumption may reduce urinary oxalate by binding more oxalate in the gut. As initial diet therapy for stone formers, an appropriate calcium intake and restriction of foods that demonstrably increase urinary oxalate can be recommended. A dietary study was conducted in subjects who were hypercalciuric when following their usual diets (123). They were tested on a low-oxalate low-calcium diet, a low-oxalate moderate-calcium diet, and a high-oxalate moderate-calcium diet. Oxalate excretion was highest during the high-oxalate diet and lowest during the low-oxalate moderate-calcium diet. Urinary calcium levels did not vary significantly between diets.

A study in normal volunteers evaluated the crystallization of stone-forming salts in urine in response to low- and high-sodium diets (124). A high sodium intake significantly increased urinary sodium, calcium, and pH and decreased urinary citrate. Serum bicarbonate levels also decreased. These changes were accompanied by increased urinary saturation of calcium phosphate and monosodium urate and decreased inhibition of calcium oxalate crystallization. Thus the net effect of the high-sodium diet was an increased propensity for crystallization of calcium salts in the urine. This increases the risk for kidney stone formation.

Singh et al. assessed the effects of ascorbic acid on lithogenesis in normal, hypercalciuric, and hyperoxaluric guinea pigs (125). Added to a basal diet at levels of 10, 40, and 60 mg per 100 g of body weight, ascorbic acid did not induce crystalluria, calcification, or stone formation. However, when hypercalciuria was induced by calcium carbonate feeding, or hyperoxaluria by sodium oxalate feeding, renal calcification was intensified. The authors postulated that large doses of ascorbic acid increase risk of renal calcification and stone formation only under conditions of preexisting hypercalciuria or hyperoxaluria, possibly as a consequence of metabolic conversion of ascorbate to oxalate.

In rat and clinical studies, Rothwell et al. investigated the hypothesis that dietary fish oil reduces calcium excretion and enhances protective mechanisms against urolithiasis (126). In rats, fish oil inhibited nephrocalcinosis induced by intraperitoneal administration of calcium gluconate. There were no significant changes in urinary biochemistry. A clinical study found that fish oil significantly decreased urinary excretion of calcium. However, beneficial decreases in calcium excretion were counterbalanced by decreases in magnesium and citrate excretion, so that the overall impact on stone-forming tendency calculated as $\Delta G$ for the major crystalline species was minimal. Oxalate excretion and urinary fibrinolytic activity were unchanged. Based on these results, fish oil supplementation cannot be recommended to reduce risk of stone formation.

## Gallstones

Duane reported studies of the effects of lovastatin and dietary cholesterol on bile acid kinetics and bile lipid composition in healthy men (127). The test diets provided cholesterol at levels approximating the range of cholesterol in typical Western diets. The data gave no evidence that under these conditions dietary cholesterol has an important role in the pathogenesis of cholesterol gallstone disease. However, normal subjects and persons predisposed to develop gallstones may respond differently to dietary cholesterol. It is also possible that stringent elimination of dietary cholesterol could have a more important influence on the cholesterol saturation index than the diets tested.

## BONES AND TEETH

### Bone Health

Heaney reviewed the role of nutritional factors in osteoporosis (*128*). A brief overview of osteoporosis discussed the interplay of injury, bone strength and fragility, and bone mass and density. How calcium nutrition relates to this was covered in more detail. Reasons for conflicting and confusing results of epidemiologic and clinical studies were discussed. It is ironic that so much effort has been expended to insure the accuracy, sensitivity, and specificity of bone mass measurements in view of the low accuracy of dietary calcium assessment—the usual independent variable in the hypothesis being tested. Adequate calcium nutrition permits acquisition of genetically programmed bone mass and conservation of acquired bone mass; it is also a component in treating established osteoporosis. Interactions of dietary calcium with dietary fiber, phosphorus, protein, and sodium were summarized. Roles of vitamin D, vitamin K, and trace minerals in bone health were covered briefly. In another review, Heaney summarized important recent studies on the effect of nutrition and lifestyle factors on bone mass (*129*). These studies indicate that the optimal calcium intake is 1000 mg/d for ages 2–8 years, 1600 mg/d for ages 9–17, 1100 mg/d for ages 18–30, and ≥1500 mg/d for postmenopausal women. Again, vitamin D nutrition and metabolism and the possible importance of vitamin K were summarized. Although alcohol abuse is a risk factor for low bone mass and fractures in both men and women, the dose–response curve may be J-shaped.

A review by Nilas emphasized the impact of physical activity on bone mass, calcium metabolism, and age-related bone loss (*130*). Wardlaw put osteoporosis into perspective, considering bone physiology and all known nutritional and non-nutritional determinants of bone mineral density (*131*). Results of various types of therapy for osteoporosis were summarized. Wardlaw made recommendations for preventing osteoporosis and stated some questions that remain to be answered. Harward discussed the epidemiology and pathogenesis of osteoporosis and some nutritive strategies for preventing and treating it (*132*).

Lauritzen et al. reviewed risk factors for hip fractures (*133*). The exponential increase in risk of fracture with aging fits a mathematical model based on age-specific bone mineral content and risk of falls. It is a typical Gompertzian function, influenced by multiple factors and determined by pathophysiologic processes that begin early in life and progress silently for many years before clinical manifestation. However, even in elderly and severely osteoporotic persons, risk can be reduced, as for example by vitamin D and calcium supplementation. A case–control study in Australia evaluated risk factors for hip fracture in the elderly (*134*). Consumption of dairy products—particularly at the age of 20 but also at age 50 and the current age—was directly related to multivariate-adjusted risk. This finding is certainly counterintuitive. The only mechanistic explanation the authors could suggest is that dairy products are protein-rich and consumption of dairy products is correlated with consumption of other protein-rich foods. There is some evidence linking catabolism of dietary protein with breakdown of bone and increased urinary excretion of calcium. However, recall bias and poor data quality could also explain the results.

CALCIUM. Nilas reviewed the relationship between calcium intake and osteoporosis (*135*). Epidemiologic data suggest that peak adult bone mass is related to calcium intake during childhood and adolescence. Maintenance of skeletal mass before menopause depends mainly on the integrity of ovarian function. Trials of supplemental calcium after menopause have raised more questions than they have answered. Calcium supplements cannot prevent perimenopausal bone loss. Moreover, many reported effects of calcium supplementation may be transient; knowledge about long-term adaptation and responses to variations in calcium intake is limited. Several studies suggest a critical threshold for calcium intake, which would indicate that supplementation when intake is already adequate confers no additional benefit. For most postmenopausal women, estrogen deficiency, not calcium deficiency, is the primary cause of osteoporosis.

The relationship between calcium intake and bone mineral content has been studied during various stages of life. Lee et al. assessed the long-term calcium intake of Chinese children in Hong Kong and its relationship to bone mineral content at the age of 5 years (*136*). The mean daily calcium intake in 5-year-olds was 546 mg/d, nearly half of which was provided by milk. Bone mineral content was not correlated with current intake of calcium, energy, or protein but was positively correlated with cumulative calcium intake since birth ($r = .235$, $p = .013$). Intake during the second year of life was most strongly correlated with bone mineral content at 5 years. These correlations remained significant after correction for weight, height, birth weight, sex, and cumulative intakes of energy and protein. Lloyd et al. reported a randomized placebo-controlled study of the effect of calcium supplementation on bone mass and bone density in adolescent girls of northern European descent in Pennsylvania (*137*). Subjects had a mean age of 11.9 ± 0.5 y at entry into the study. Their calcium intake from food sources averaged 960 mg/d. The supplement provided, on average, an additional 354 mg/d of calcium as calcium malate citrate for 18 months. Compared with the placebo group, girls in the supplemented group had greater increases in lumbar spine bone density (18.7% vs. 15.8%, $p = .03$), lumbar spine bone mineral content (39.4% vs. 34.7%, $p = .06$), and total-body bone mineral density (9.6% vs. 8.3%, $p = .05$). Thus increasing calcium from 80% to 110% of the RDA resulted in an additional 1.3% increase in skeletal mass per year in this age group. This could provide protection against future osteoporotic fracture. In 24- to 28-year-old women in North Carolina, moderate physical activity and adequate recent calcium intake were positively correlated with radial bone measurements (*138*). Intakes of protein and phosphorus in excess of recommended amounts were negatively correlated with radial bone density. In 21- to 47-year-old British women, correlations between bone density and calcium intake were found at all femoral sites (neck, $r = .41, p < .01$; Ward triangle, $r = .40, p < .01$; trochanter, $r = .47, p < .001$) and spine ($r = .27, p < .05$) but not radius (*139*). Calcium intake was ≤500 mg/d in 27% of subjects, giving cause for concern.

Anderson and Metz reviewed the timing of peak bone mass development in white females and the dietary and lifestyle factors that influence this process (*140*). The peripubertal period seems most responsive to manipulation of environmental and lifestyle factors. During late adolescence and early adulthood, gains of bone mass can still be achieved through regular exercise and improved dietary calcium intake. The authors discussed the need for a national U.S. policy for primary prevention of osteoporosis targeted at strategic age groups. These ideas were strengthened by a British study assessing the impact of milk consumption during various stages of life on bone mineral density in women 44–74 years old (*141*). Milk consumption up to age 25 y was a significant independent predictor of bone mineral density at all sites. Effects of milk consumption at ages 25–44 and >44 were qualitatively similar but not statistically significant. The authors concluded that frequent milk consumption before age 25 favorably influences hip bone mass in middle-aged and older women. Similar conclusions could be drawn from a study of dietary calcium and bone density in 35- to 75-year-old women from five Chinese

counties with strikingly different dietary patterns (*142*). Within each age group, women in a pastoral county characterized by a high consumption of dairy products had ~20% more bone mass than women in nonpastoral areas with lower calcium intakes. Age-related percentage decreases in mean bone mass were similar in the 5 counties. This suggests that the observed differences in bone mass were due to differences in bone mass at younger ages rather than to different rates of bone loss in later life. Calcium from dairy sources was more highly correlated with bone variables than was calcium from nondairy sources.

In reviewing results of 6 controlled clinical trials of calcium supplements in postmenopausal women, Prince concluded that an intake of 1500 mg/d should be recommended for this age group (*143*). Results of the trials support the conclusion that increasing calcium intake can slow bone loss at appendicular and axial skeletal sites, particularly in women with a low calcium intake or when combined with an exercise program in women with low bone mass. Supplementation became more effective with increasing time since menopause. The effect of calcium was to reduce bone resorption. The absorbed (bioavailable) fraction of dietary calcium was negatively related to dietary fiber and positively related to circulating levels of calcitriol, the active form of vitamin D. A 3-year study of women who were 1.2–2.4 y past menopause at baseline compared effects of a calcium supplement, calcium supplement plus hormone replacement, and placebo on bone loss (*144*). The calcium supplement provided 1700 mg/d of calcium as the carbonate. Although less effective than hormones plus calcium, calcium supplementation clearly retarded early postmenopausal bone loss. The effect was significant for change in total body calcium and bone mineral density of the femoral neck but nonsignificant for changes in the lumbar spine, trochanter, Ward triangle, and radius.

**OTHER MINERALS.** Calvo reviewed the effects of dietary phosphorus on calcium metabolism and bone (*145*). The American diet is typically phosphorus-rich and marginal or low in calcium. Such a diet causes secondary hyperparathyroidism and bone loss in animal models. Whereas the desired dietary ratio of phosphorus to calcium is 1, the actual ratio averages ~1.6. Studies in humans suggest that prolonged high phosphorus intake can impair the homeostatic mechanisms normally evoked when dietary calcium is limited. A high-phosphorus, low-calcium diet can produce persistent changes in calcium-regulating hormones that are not favorable for optimizing peak bone mass or slowing subsequent rate of bone loss.

Phosphorus is broadly distributed in the food supply, but dairy foods provide an estimated 80% of calcium. Thus preference for phosphoric acid-processed soft drinks over milk has substituted a high-phosphorus beverage for the most important source of calcium. In addition, phosphorus-containing food additives may account for as much as 30% of adult phosphorus intake.

A review by Lemann et al. found that an increase in dietary potassium reduces 24-h and fasting urinary calcium excretion and produces a more positive calcium balance (*146*). This suggests that directly or indirectly, potassium promotes renal calcium retention and reduces net bone resorption. Potassium's natriuretic effect may contribute to this. As a result of increased renal phosphate retention, potassium also inhibits renal synthesis of calcitriol. This would inhibit intestinal calcium absorption, thus reducing urinary calcium excretion, and with time it would reduce positive calcium balances. However, the positive effect of potassium appears to be sustained, indicating that potassium-rich diets help to protect skeletal mass. Potassium bicarbonate is the most effective form of potassium for supplementation.

Several trace elements are cofactors for enzymes essential in bone metabolism. Saltman and Strause reviewed the role of trace minerals in osteoporosis and reported a trial of calcium and trace-element supplementation in postmenopausal women (*147*). Animal studies demonstrate the importance of adequate copper and manganese nutrition. Osteoporotic women tend to have lower serum manganese levels than controls, and there is evidence that manganese deficiency affects bone remodeling. One study found a significant positive correlation between serum copper concentration and bone mineral density in postmenopausal women. The authors' study in elderly women showed the following changes in bone mineral density after 2 y of supplementation: placebo, –2.23%; copper, zinc, manganese supplement, –1.66%; 1000 mg/d of calcium as calcium citrate malate, –0.50%; calcium plus trace elements, +1.28%.

Boivin et al. reviewed fluoride metabolism and the use of fluoride in treating osteoporosis (*148*). Although the "therapeutic window" is narrow, low to moderate doses of fluoride can increase bone density, particularly in the lumbar spine, and increase osteoblastic bone formation. With careful selection of dose and formulation, the rate of vertebral fracture can also be reduced. The most common side effects of fluoride therapy are gastrointestinal or osteoarticular. Ewes and lambs, whose bone remodeling activity is similar to that of humans, provide a model for evaluating the

effects of fluoride on bone tissue. Studies on bone explants and cultured bone cells also yield information.

**VITAMIN D.** Hofeldt reviewed the importance of vitamin D deficiency in metabolic bone disease (*149*). He discussed vitamin D metabolism and aging-related changes in vitamin D–regulating hormones. Although there is general agreement that supplemental vitamin D should be used only to treat vitamin D deficiency because of potentially adverse effects on renal function and calcium metabolism, deficiency frequently goes unrecognized—particularly in the elderly. Promising results have been obtained in the treatment of postmenopausal osteoporosis with vitamin D analogues. The concept that aging and osteoporosis disrupt the dynamic relationships among parathyroid hormone, vitamin D metabolites, and calcium was discussed and evidence presented that supplementation with vitamin $D_3$ and calcium prevents hip fractures in very old women (*150*).

**OTHER DIETARY FACTORS.** Das summarized how cytokines mediate the process of osteoporosis and how estrogen blocks production of the implicated cytokines in peripheral blood monocytes, osteoblasts, and stromal cells (*151*). 1,25-Dihydroxyvitamin $D_3$ blocks interleukin-1 production and thus may fit into the scheme outlined by Das. Corticosteroids also block cytokine production, but instead of protecting against osteoporosis, they induce it. Das speculates that a second messenger is involved, through which cytokines, alcohol, and corticosteroids affect bone remodelling. He argues that essential fatty acids meet the requirements for second messengers in this system and proposes that a relative deficiency of essential fatty acids exacerbates osteoporosis. Support for the theory came from a study showing that eicosapentaenoic acid (EPA) inhibits bone loss in ovariectomized rats (*152*). Ovariectomized animals were fed a control diet or a low-calcium diet, each with and without EPA. After 35 days the femurs and tibias were weighed and the breaking force of the femurs was determined. EPA supplementation of the control diet did not influence these measurements. The low-calcium diet led to significant reductions in bone weight and breaking force, but addition of EPA to this diet prevented the reductions. This study was performed in Japan, where it is assumed that the antiosteoporotic effect of dietary fish stems from calcium in the bones that are eaten. The authors think it likely that EPA confers at least part of the benefits.

A prospective study of elderly white women compared changes in radial bone mineral density between ovolactovegetarians and omnivores (*153*). There was little change in calcium intake between 1983 and 1988: it averaged roughly 1000 mg/d in omnivores and 735 mg/d in ovolactovegetarians. In both groups, bone mineral density decreased at both radial sites by ≈1% per year during this period. Loss of bone mineral density was significantly correlated with loss of lean body mass but was independent of calcium intake within the range of intakes represented by these subjects. The authors concluded that some bone loss is inevitable, but maintenance of lean body mass through exercise may be an excellent strategy for retarding such loss in the elderly. Consideration of dietary sources of bioavailable calcium indicated that lactovegetarians have no greater risk of osteoporosis than omnivores, but vegans are at increased risk of not meeting their calcium needs (*154*). A table summarized the calcium content, fractional absorption rate, and estimated absorbable calcium per serving for 22 common foods and milk. Careful planning is necessary to ensure adequate calcium intake from a strict vegetarian diet, particularly during rapid growth. Calcium supplements or calcium-fortified juices would provide a margin of safety. Interactions among dietary components affecting calcium balance were discussed.

## Dental Health

Although sucrose consumption is unquestionably related to development of dental caries, it cannot explain the prevalence of caries. Navia presented a model for caries in which numerous host and environmental factors interact (*155*). Relevant host factors include age, race, behavior, and genetics. Dietary patterns and components have their influence in the setting provided by the host's mineral status (including trace elements and fluoride), saliva flow and composition, and the species distribution of the plaque bacteria. Diet also influences these factors. Navia summarized statistics on per capita sugar consumption (or disappearance or availability) in various countries, prevalence of decayed, missing, and filled teeth, levels of mutans streptococci in selected populations, and field studies of sugar substitutes, dietary sugars, and caries. He concluded that preventive programs in oral health must transcend the simplistic focus on sugar and pay attention to the bacterial components of plaque and the hygienic and general dietary behaviors that influence them.

Serra Majem et al. evaluated dietary habits in Spanish school-children with a low rate of dental caries (*156*). Although the decline in caries in Catalonia reflects the widespread use of fluorides after 10 years of preventive programs, improved dental education or changes in eating habits could have contributed. Subjects in this study were 893 school children aged 5–14 y, evenly distributed by age. They were categorized as having caries (*n* = 482) or caries-free (*n* = 411). There was a positive relationship between caries and frequency of consuming ice cream, cakes, pastries, sliced bread, sugar-free gum, and sugar-free candies. There was a negative relationship between caries and frequency of consuming skim milk and artificial sweeteners. Caries was not significantly related to consumption of sugar, sugared hard candies, sugared chewing gum, soft candies, chocolate, sugared or sugar-free soft drinks, fruit juice, citrus or non-citrus fruits, or a wide range of other common foods. Nor was it related to meal frequency, tooth-brushing habits, or consumption of fluoride supplements during the previous year. Children who had more caries visited the dentist more often. Some weaknesses and difficulties in this type of study were discussed.

Littleton and Frohlich analyzed dental pathology in skeletons from the Arabian Gulf to trace differences in diet and subsistence patterns (*157*). The conditions evaluated were attrition (dental wear), caries, calculus, abscessing, and antemortem tooth loss. Four basic but overlapping patterns of dental disease, corresponding to four different subsistence patterns, were identified. Dependency on marine foods was associated with severe attrition, low caries rate, wear-caused abscessing, and lack of antemortem tooth loss. Subsistence on a combination of agriculture with pastoralism or fishing was associated with moderate attrition and calculus, low caries rate, wear-caused abscessing, and low to moderate rates of antemortem tooth loss. A mixed-farming pattern was associated with low to moderate attrition, high rates of caries and calculus, abscessing due to caries, and severe antemortem tooth loss. Populations practicing intensive gardening experienced slight attrition, a high caries rate, a low rate of calculus, and severe antemortem tooth loss.

Polyphenols from green (unfermented) tea have proven anticaries effects, but other teas have been less intensively studied. Ooshima et al. reported that oolong (partially fermented) tea polyphenols also inhibit caries formation in *Streptococcus sobrinus*– and *Streptococcus mutans*–infected rats fed a cariogenic diet (*158*). The tea extract and its chromatographically isolated polyphenols were administered via both diet and drinking water. Although they had no effect on bacterial growth in vitro, they did inhibit synthesis of insoluble glucan from sucrose by the glucosyltransferases of both species and also sucrose-dependent bacterial adherence. In vivo, they significantly reduced development of plaque and caries in streptococcus-infected rats.

# NERVOUS SYSTEM AND BEHAVIOR

## Performance

In October 1993 the Institute of Medicine's Food and Nutrition Board sponsored a meeting at which participants reviewed and discussed the literature on diet and cognitive, physical, and emotional performance (159). While unanimously concluding that diet's effect on performance is a timely and important topic, they found the literature inconsistent and incomplete. Many studies on cognitive performance were not well controlled and did not employ well standardized tests. For improved physical performance, only carbohydrate loading, carbohydrate supplementation, and fluid replacement are demonstrably effective. Under certain conditions and for specific types of exercise, caffeine in doses of 500 mg enhances performance. There is some evidence that tyrosine reverses stress-induced deficits in performance and mood.

Fernstrom discussed the two groups of amino acids that reputedly can influence brain function when ingested in food (160). The aromatic amino acids tryptophan, tyrosine, and phenylalanine are the respective biosynthetic precursors for the neurotransmitters serotonin, dopamine, and norepinephrine. A meal's protein content can rapidly influence uptake of these amino acids into the brain and directly modify their conversion to neurotransmitters. However, the acidic amino acids glutamate and aspartate, although they are themselves brain neurotransmitters, do not have ready access to the brain from the circulation or the diet. Therefore ingestion of glutamate- and aspartate-rich proteins does not affect the level of acidic amino acids in the brain. Moreover, despite claims to the contrary, most published evidence clearly indicates that the brain is not affected by ingestion of aspartame and is affected by glutamate only when the amino acid is administered alone in enormous doses. Aspartame contains both aspartate and phenylalanine; both components were initially suspected and then exonerated. For all except a few sensitive individuals, both aspartame and monosodium glutamate are considered safe when consumed as a component of the diet.

Sucrose and aspartame both reportedly induce hyperactivity and other behavioral problems in children. Wolraich et al. conducted a double-blind controlled dietary trial with 25 normal 3- to 5-year-old children and 23 children 6–10 years old described by their parents as sugar-sensitive (161). The experimental diets were a high-sucrose diet with no artificial sweeteners and two low-sucrose diets, one containing aspartame and the other containing saccharin. Each experimental diet was provided for 3 weeks, using a Latin-square design. Within each experimental period, "sham" diets were distributed randomly for periods of 1 week each. Major components of the three sham diets were red and orange foods; beef and pork, with only raw fruits and vegetables; and chicken and fish, with only cooked fruits and vegetables. Each sham diet was thus provided in conjunction with each experimental sweetener. All diets were virtually free of artificial food coloring, preservatives, and other additives. In the "sugar-sensitive" school children, there were no significant differences among diets in any of 39 behavioral and cognitive variables evaluated. In the normal preschool children, only 4 of 31 measures differed significantly among the diets and there was no consistent pattern in these differences. The authors concluded that even when intake exceeds typical dietary levels, neither sucrose nor aspartame affects children's behavior or cognitive function.

Bernstein et al. investigated the effects of caffeine on learning, performance, and anxiety in normal prepubertal children 8–12 years old (162). A double-blind randomized crossover design was used. Children were evaluated at baseline and after ingestion of placebo, 2.5 mg/kg of caffeine, and 5.0 mg/kg of caffeine administered in caffeine-free Pepsi. Dependent measures were tests of attention, manual dexterity, short-term memory, processing speed, and anxiety rating. In the Test of Variables of Attention, caffeine improved two performance measures (variability of response and errors of omission) and had no effect on the other two (commission errors and reaction time). Caffeine also improved performance of the dominant hand (but not the nondominant hand) in a pegboard test of manual dexterity. Children reported feeling less sluggish but slightly more anxious after caffeine. Because caffeine is widely available and frequently consumed by children, these findings of mood changes and enhanced performance in a motor task and a test of attention are important and suggest the need for further research.

Most evidence that specific foods or food components have an adverse effect on behavior is anecdotal or comes from open, unblinded trials that do not rule out the effect of expectation and suggestion. In a carefully designed experiment, Carter et al. confirmed results of an open test using a controlled double-blind challenge (163). The original subjects were 78 children aged 3–12 who were referred to a diet clinic because of hyperactive behavior. Besides behavioral problems, 64 subjects had one or more physical symptoms (asthma, hay fever, eczema, skin rashes, headaches, gastrointestinal symptoms, or seizures). With a restricted few-foods diet, 59 children improved behaviorally and physically. On reintroduction of suspected foods, 47 relapsed and were considered responders. No relapse could be induced in 3 (nonresponders), and 9 withdrew from the study during this phase. Foods most commonly implicated in the open phase were (in decreasing order of reaction rate, from 70 to 18%) additive-containing foods, chocolate, cow's milk, oranges, cow's-milk cheese, wheat, other fruits, tomatoes, and eggs. Of the responders, 19 entered and completed the controlled double-blind phase of the trial in which placebo and foods implicated in the open trial were disguised in an excipient and fed in random order. For example, artificial colors and placebo were given in opaque capsules and chocolate was disguised in a carob confection. Neither parents nor children could identify which was the active food and which the placebo. Parents' global behavioral rating favored the placebo in 14 children, the active food in 3 children, and neither in 2 children. The latter 5 were considered treatment failures. There were fewer failures than predicted by chance ($p = .03$). Differences in scoring at the end of each phase were greatest for "restless," "disturbs others," "cries often," and "temper outbursts," suggesting a greater effect on irritability than on attention deficit. There was also a difference in latency and errors for the matching familiar figures test ($p < .01$). The psychologist's behavioral observations also showed differences for the scale of hyperactive behavior ($p < .01$), the greatest difference being for "fidgetiness." Children who responded to the few-foods diet were more likely than nonresponders to have already reported food reactions or food cravings and less likely to come from homes where there were discordant marital relations. These results support the idea that diet can directly influence behavior but do not rule out the possibility that behavioral effects stem from diet-related physical symptoms, which were also reduced in the absence of suspected foods.

The effects of dietary fat on performance have been investigated using rodent models. Winocur and Greenwood showed that high-fat diets impair conditional discrimination learning in rats (164). In addition to demonstrating adverse effects on learning and memory, the results also suggested that saturated fatty acids were specifically associated with these effects. Yehuda and Carasso investigated how free α-linolenic and linoleic acids modulate learning, pain threshold, and thermoregulation in adult rats and defined the optimal $n$–3/$n$–6 ratio (165). Test oils and saline placebo were administered daily by intraperitoneal injection. In this model, the most favorable effects on all measures were observed at an $n$–3/$n$–6 ratio of 1:4 (optimal range, 1:3.5–1:5). Wainwright et al. assessed the effects of dietary fat and

environmental enrichment on brain and behavior in mice (166). The test diets were a saturated fat diet deficient in essential fatty acids, a diet deficient in $n$–3 fatty acids only, and a diet containing $n$–3 and $n$–6 fatty acids in a ratio of 0.27. Females were fed these diets during pregnancy and lactation, and after weaning the pups were continued on the diet of their dam. At weaning, two female pups from each litter were randomly assigned to enriched and standard environments. The brain's fatty acid composition was determined 1, 9, 17, and 25 days and 3 months after birth. Adult percentages of 22:6$n$–3 were attained within the first week. They were reduced by 80% in the saturated-fat group and 50% in the $n$–3-deficient group. Several learning and behavioral deficits were noted in the saturated-fat group. Effects of diet and environment were additive; mice in all dietary groups benefitted from the enriched environment.

## Mood and Emotion

Wallin and Rissanen reviewed the relationships between food, serotonin (5-hydroxytryptamine), and affective disorders (167). Relationships between food, eating, and mood are complex and have broad clinical implications. Patients showing a relationship between food and behavior are found in a range of diagnostic categories, and serotonergic dysfunction occurs in conditions as diverse as seasonal affective disorder (SAD), atypical depression, premenstrual syndrome, and eating disorders. Serotonin deficiency in the central nervous system seems important in "food and mood" disorders, and eating behavior can be seen as the body's self-healing attempt. However, the attempt frequently fails and sometimes creates a vicious circle. Silverstone discussed the link between food, mood, and serotonin in bulimia nervosa and SAD (168). The former is considered an eating disorder with a high frequency of depressive symptoms, whereas the latter is a mood disorder frequently associated with disturbed eating behavior. Hypothalamic serotonin levels normally peak during autumn and reach their nadir during December and January; binge eating and mood disturbances are also most prevalent during winter. Evidence that serotonin acts selectively on carbohydrate intake is inconsistent, and a role of "carbohydrate craving" in bulimia and SAD is unconfirmed. Pharmacologically, however, serotonin agonists reduce bingeing and improve mood in patients with bulimia nervosa and improve mood and reduce eating in patients with SAD. Because the seasonal variation in hypothalamic serotonin parallels seasonal patterns of illness in these disorders, the two may be related pathophysiologically.

Smith et al. studied the effects of morning and evening meals and caffeine on cognitive performance, mood, and cardiovascular function in healthy adults. Subjects were tested after an overnight fast, after which they were given no breakfast, a breakfast of bacon, eggs, and toast, or a breakfast of corn flakes and toast (*169*). This was followed by regular or decaffeinated coffee and a repetition of the baseline tests. Breakfast did not affect performance of sustained-attention tasks. It did increase pulse rate and influence mood: the bacon-and-egg group felt more contented, interested, sociable, and out-going than the other groups. Caffeine did not affect mood but it improved performance of sustained-attention tasks and increased blood pressure and mental alertness. Breakfast improved performance on memory tests of recall and recognition, had no effect on a semantic memory task, and impaired accuracy in a logical reasoning task. Caffeine, in contrast, improved performance on all these tasks. To study the effects of the evening meal, subjects were tested before eating, after which they were given no meal or were allowed to select a three-course meal from a varied menu (*170*). In each group, half of the subjects were given regular coffee and half were given decaffeinated coffee. They were then tested again. Compared with subjects in the no-meal group, subjects given the meal felt stronger, more interested, and more proficient. They performed a logical reasoning task more quickly but did not differ in performance on other tests. Caffeine improved alertness and performance on sustained attention tasks. The authors concluded that the effects of the evening meal on mood and performance differ from those of breakfast. Effects of meals also differ from those of caffeine, which are fairly consistent throughout the day.

Farooqui et al. studied regional changes of dopamine and its metabolites in the brains of rats fed diets containing 8, 20, and 50% casein (*171*). No consistent response to protein level was seen in the midbrain or brainstem. In the substantia nigra, striatum, and dentate gyrus, dopamine concentrations were directly related to dietary protein. Similar but nonsignificant trends were seen in several forebrain nuclei. The authors concluded that in the rat brain, only discrete dopaminergic neuronal circuits are sensitive to quantitative changes in dietary protein and that selective modulation of dopaminergic activity in the forebrain may be a mechanism through which dietary protein influences locomotor behavior.

Tantalizing reports associating aggressive behavior with cholesterol metabolism have not been supported by biological data demonstrating a mechanism. Specifically, the identity of the lipoproteins responsible for the differences in cholesterol concentrations is not known. Gray et al. examined the relationship between violent behavior and plasma levels of lipoproteins and apolipoproteins (*172*). Subjects were 15 men who were serving prison sentences for violent offenses and 25 age-matched men who had no criminal records. The groups did not differ in any measure of plasma cholesterol or HDL subfractions. However, offenders had significantly different percentages of apoprotein A-IV (3.62 vs. 0.85, $p < .000001$), apoprotein E (7.70 vs. 5.19, $p = .0002$), and apoprotein A-I (39.2 vs. 44.5, $p = .006$). Possible implications of these findings were discussed.

## Nervous System Diseases and Disorders

**DEMENTIA.** The relationship between incidence of dementia and consumption of animal foods was examined in two cohort substudies within the Adventist Health Study in California (*173*). Subjects in one were matched for age, sex, and zip code in 68 quartets comprising 1 vegan, 1 ovolactovegetarian, and 2 "heavy" meat-eaters. Subjects who ate meat (including poultry and fish) were more likely than their vegetarian counterparts to become demented (RR 2.18, $p = .065$). When past history of meat consumption was accounted for, the difference between groups widened (RR = 2.99, $p = .048$). However in the larger substudy that included 2984 unmatched subjects, there was no significant difference between vegetarians and meat-eaters in risk for dementia. In both substudies there was a trend toward delayed onset of dementia in vegetarians. The authors believe these data increase the credibility of the hypothesis that meat intake influences the incidence of dementia, and that particular attention should be paid to the relationship in the age range of 60–80 years.

Sparks et al. reported the induction of Alzheimer-like β-amyloid immunoreactivity in brains of cholesterol-fed rabbits (*174*). Whereas control animals showed no accumulation of intracellular immunolabeled β-amyloid, cholesterol-fed animals showed progressive accumulation after 4, 6, and 8 weeks on the experimental diet. The biochemical and clinical implications of this observation were discussed.

**PARKINSONISM.** Diet can have adverse effects on the pharmacokinetics of L-dopa. Kempster and Wahlqvist reviewed dietary strategies to improve responsiveness of parkinsonism patients to pharmaceutical L-dopa treatment and the potential of diet itself to supply L-dopa (*175*). Dietary factors that affect the clinical response to L-dopa are the timing of medication in relation to meals, meal size and caloric density, food viscosity, and competition between neutral amino acids and L-dopa for absorption across the intestinal mucosa and active transport across the blood–brain barrier. Dietary sources of L-dopa include *Vicia faba* beans, the Georgia velvet bean (*Stizolobium deeringianum*), pods and seeds of the Indian medicinal legume *Mucuna pruriens*, and a few other legumes. The advantages and disadvantages of these foods were compared with those of pharmaceutical preparations.

**MULTIPLE SCLEROSIS.** The risk for multiple sclerosis (MS) in Gorski Kotar, the mountainous region of western Croatia, is one of the highest in Europe. Dietary staples include boiled potatoes, a cream soup of potatoes, beans, and barley, fresh and smoked pork, fresh and pickled cabbage and turnips, and full-fat milk. The cooking fat is lard. Dormouse (*Myoxus glis*) is the only unusual food in the diet. Large amounts of apple, plum, and juniper brandy are consumed. Cereal consumption is very low. Obesity is prevalent. Because the traditional diet is simple and unvaried, a dietary study of 46 MS patients and 92 controls was conducted (*176*). Compared with controls, case-patients consumed significantly more full-fat milk (RR 21.7, $\chi^2$ 42.34) and potatoes with lard and fresh or smoked meat (RR 20.7, $\chi^2$ 15.52). These are considered nutritional risk factors that could influence the severity of primary demyelinization in subjects at high risk for MS.

# EYE DISORDERS

Bunce reviewed nutrition's role in cataract and age-related macular degeneration (*177*). After summarizing the pathogenic roles of oxidant stress, phototoxicity, osmotic stress, and glycosylation the review discussed the protective role of nutrients in these processes. Diabetic retinopathy received particular attention, both as a model and as a problem in its own right. In vitro, experimental animal, and epidemiologic studies were reviewed. Bunce concluded that both cataract and macular degeneration are outcomes of the multiple processes of deterioration that accompany aging. Clearly nutrition is one factor that influences the rate of progression from senescence to disease, as signaled by loss of vision.

The National Cancer Institute and the Cancer Institute of the Chinese Academy of Medical Sciences have been conducting two collaborative trials in Linxian, China, to see whether multiple vitamin–mineral supplements can reduce the incidence of cancer of the

esophagus and gastric cardia in this poorly nourished population. The supplements under investigation include vitamins and minerals that also have the greatest potential for affecting age-related cataracts. Sperduto et al. reported findings from eye examinations after 5–6 y of supplementation (*178*). The placebo-controlled trial evaluated effects of a 9-constituent supplement. The factorially designed trial evaluated various combinations of these 9 constituents. In the first trial there was a significant reduction in prevalence of nuclear cataract in subjects 65–74 years old who received the supplement (RR 0.57, 95% CI 0.36–0.90). In the second trial, subjects who received a combination of riboflavin and niacin had significantly fewer nuclear cataracts than subjects given combinations not including these vitamins. However, the riboflavin–niacin combination was associated with a significant increase in number of posterior subcapsular cataracts (RR 2.64, 95% CI 1.31–5.35), although the number of these cataracts was very small. In neither trial was the prevalence of cortical cataracts influenced by supplementation. The antioxidant hypothesis could explain the beneficial effect of the multiple supplement and of riboflavin–niacin because riboflavin's active derivative is the cofactor for glutathione reductase. The authors suggested no biological explanation for the increased risk of posterior subcapsular cataract with use of the riboflavin–niacin supplement; they thought the association could have been due to chance, given the small number of these cataracts that were found. Bunce reviewed the background and findings of these studies with reference to the diet of Linxian residents (*179*). The importance of riboflavin as a protective factor was reviewed. It was also pointed out that flavins are light-sensitive, and exposure of unbound flavins to light can generate active oxygen species.

Schoenfeld et al. reported three case–control studies in India, the USA, and Italy that evaluated nutritional risk factors for each cataract type (*180*). Nutritional information came from blood analysis and a food frequency questionnaire. From blood data, a high antioxidant status was protective against mixed cataract and posterior subcapsular cataract in the Indian study but a high level of ascorbic acid increased risk of mixed cataract. In the Italian study, high levels of lactic dehydrogenase increased risk for posterior subcapsular cataract, high levels of glutamyl transpeptidase increased risk for mixed cataract, and high levels of glucose-6-phosphate dehydrogenase increased risk for nuclear and mixed cataracts. In the U.S. study, high values of α-tocopherol decreased risk for nuclear cataract, a high albumin/globulin ratio decreased risk for mixed cataract, and high blood iron decreased risk for cortical cataract. From dietary data in the Indian study, good nutritional status (using protein intake as an indicator) decreased risk for posterior subcapsular, nuclear, and mixed cataract types. In the USA, a high dietary antioxidant index was protective. The Italian study found no associations between diet and cataract. Several other risk factors, including exposure to sunlight and use of medications, were also evaluated. The major conclusion was that it is very difficult to conduct and compare parallel studies of the same disease in different countries. The findings do suggest nutritional components of cataract risk, but these are not consistent between studies or for the different cataract types.

Aging and diabetes have many physiopathologic similarities, including the relationship between lactose absorption and cataract formation. Birlouez-Aragon et al. investigated the mechanism by which sugar damages the lens in vivo and in vitro, and the metabolism of galactose in elderly and diabetic subjects (*181*). An oral galactose test showed significantly higher maximal galactose levels in elderly than in younger subjects. For a particular age group, levels were significantly higher in diabetic than in nondiabetic subjects and nonsignificantly higher in subjects with cataract. Incubation of clear postmortem cortex with 25 mM galactose induced significantly greater fluorescence than incubation without sugar or with 25 mM glucose. The results demonstrated that aging is associated with an increasing disturbance of galactose metabolism and that IDDM and NIDDM patients also have impaired galactose metabolism, but at younger ages. They further suggest the possibility that high levels of plasma galactose induce accumulation of fluorescence in long-lived lens proteins. The age at which dietary galactose begins to be cataractogenic is not known, but the authors suggest that galactose-free milk be made available to elderly and diabetic lactase-persistent individuals to reduce their risk of cataract.

Yokoyama et al. showed that a physiological level of ascorbate inhibits formation of galactose cataracts in guinea pigs by decreasing accumulation of galactitol in the lens epithelium (*182*). Interestingly, however, the mechanism is prooxidant, not antioxidant. It involves a preferential consumption of NADPH in the reduction of dehydroascorbic acid and $H_2O_2$.

Fryer reviewed the biochemical and biophysical mechanisms by which $\alpha$-tocopherol protects cell membranes from damage (*183*). He examined the evidence that vitamin E protects against light-induced cataractogenesis and retinal deterioration as well as several skin conditions that are mediated by photooxidative damage to cell membranes. In these situations, vitamin E may act as a biochemical antioxidant, a UV-B photoprotective sunscreen, and a physicochemical stabilizer. However, protective effects have not been demonstrated conclusively.

Relationships between age-related macular degeneration and fasting plasma levels of retinol, ascorbic acid, $\alpha$-tocopherol, and $\beta$-carotene were evaluated as part of the Baltimore Longitudinal Study of Aging (*184*). Overall the subjects were well nourished; $\alpha$-tocopherol was the only antioxidant that showed truly low levels in some subjects. High plasma levels of $\alpha$-tocopherol and a high antioxidant index based on ascorbic acid, $\alpha$-tocopherol, and $\beta$-carotene were significantly protective; a high level of ascorbic acid or $\beta$-carotene was nonsignificantly protective. Use of vitamin supplements did not reduce risk of macular degeneration. The authors emphasized that stronger relationships might be found in a study population showing a wider range of levels of plasma antioxidants.

Evaluation of the effects of vitamin A supplementation and dietary vitamin A on risk of xerophthalmia in Sudanese children showed only small benefit from supplementation (RR 0.88, 95% CI 0.72–1.07) (*185*). In contrast, total dietary vitamin A intake was strongly associated with risk. The multivariate relative risk for children in the highest quintile of intake compared with the lowest was 0.38 (95% CI 0.19–0.74, $p$ = .002). The authors interpreted this to mean that factors modifying the bioavailability of vitamin A supplements need further investigation. Meanwhile, increased consumption of fruits and vegetables will reduce risk of nutritional blindness.

# GROWTH, DEVELOPMENT, AND AGING

## Lipids and Development

The brain of a newborn human weighs about 350 g. By the end of the first year this increases by about 750 g. During this time the brain uses more than half of the infant's energy intake—much of which, along with crucial building blocks, comes from dietary fat. Thus fat is qualitatively and quantitatively a critical component of the infant's diet. Cockburn discussed some studies of early infant nutrition and the consequences of the habit, introduced about 130 years ago, of feeding infants various formulas as a substitute for human milk (*186*). Innis reviewed the pathways of *n*–3 and *n*–6 fatty acid metabolism and approaches to determining essential fatty acid requirements (*187*). Levels of 18:2*n*–6, 18:3*n*–3, and

22:6$n$–3 and the $n$–6/$n$–3 ratio in human milk vary considerably as a consequence of the lactating mother's diet. The effect of the mother's diet on 20:4$n$–6 is uncertain. There is evidence that very premature infants benefit from a dietary source of preformed 22:6$n$–3 and possibly also 20:4$n$–6. However, high intakes of $n$–3 fatty acids may have pharmacologic effects or negative effects on growth and development. It is possible that the fatty acid requirements of premature infants, term infants, and children—for whom the goal is to realize the genetic potential for growth and development—differ from those of adults, who wish to minimize morbidity and mortality from chronic disease. Involved in the uncertainty is incomplete knowledge about fatty acid metabolism in infants, particularly those born preterm. Van Aerde and Clandinin concluded that even though circulating levels of $n$–3 and $n$–6 PUFAs do not necessarily reflect the situation in specific organs and tissues, they are the only objective parameter available for assessing effects of dietary lipids on fatty acid status in neonates (*188*). They believe available information indicates that the optimal ratio of linoleic to linolenic acids for infant formulas is closer to 5, the lower end of the currently recommended range, than to 15, the higher end. They suggest that the ratio of $n$–6 to $n$–3 long-chain PUFAs be in the range of 1.1–1.4. Because the composition of dietary lipids alters both the function and the composition of membranes, manipulating the fatty acid composition of infant formulas could become a therapeutic tool as well as a way to optimize growth and development. Decsi and Koletzko summarized metabolic pathways of C18 fatty acids of the 1$n$–9, 2$n$–6, and 3$n$–3 series, which compete for the same microsomal enzyme system for further desaturation and elongation (*189*). They discussed the supply of long-chain PUFAs for the fetus and for breast-fed and formula-fed newborns. Environmental factors and characteristics of the neonate that affect PUFA metabolism were considered. Functional differences in term and preterm infants were related to differences in fatty acid status.

Farquharason et al. studied the effect of diet on the fatty acid composition of subcutancous fat in perinatal surgical patients and in term and preterm infants who died of sudden infant death syndrome (SIDS) (*190*). In formula-fed infants, the mean weight percentage of DHA fell rapidly from 0.4% at birth to undetectable levels (<0.05%) at 2 months, while arachidonic acid fell from 0.7 to 0.1%. Nonessential fatty acids were incorporated into fatty tissue in about the same weight percentages at which they were supplied. The results suggest that the enzyme systems involved in digestion and absorption of fatty acids are mature even in preterm infants,

whereas desaturase and elongase systems are not. The authors argued that since evolution has assured that arachidonic acid and DHA acid are supplied to the infant through breast feeding, it is probably unwise to feed formulas that don't do the same. A minimum daily requirement of 30 mg of DHA was suggested for term infants to prevent cerebral cortical deficiency of this fatty acid.

Visual acuity depends on development of the retina and visual cortex, both of which are highly enriched in DHA. Accumulation of DHA is most rapid during the last intrauterine trimester and the first 6 months of infancy. A study of preterm infants weighing 748–1398 g at birth compared the effects of standard formula and formula supplemented with marine oil on development of visual acuity (*191*). Binocular visual acuity was tested at the corrected ages of 0, 2, 4, 6.5, 9, and 12 months (postconceptional weeks 38, 48, 57, 68, 79, and 93, ±2). Infants fed supplemented formula had better visual acuity at 2 and 4 months. After 4 months, only birth weight and gestational age were consistently related to visual acuity.

Winter et al. fractionated the triacylglycerols in human milk and determined their compositions and structures (*192*). The two major fractions (16:0/18:1/18:1 and 16:0/18:1/18:2) were nearly twice as abundant as expected from random distribution of fatty acids. When the triacylglycerols were placed into structural groups according to the order of fatty acids with 0 (S), 1 (M), 2 (D), or 3–4 (T) double bonds, SMM, SMD, and SDD structures were more abundant than expected whereas SSS, SSM, MMM, MMD, SST, and SMT structures were less abundant. The apolarities of 16:0 and 18:0 seemed to be influenced by 18:1, 18:2, and 8:0–12:0 fatty acids. Optimal triacylglycerol structure and the importance of medium-chain fatty acids were discussed in terms of stereospecific substrate requirements of lingual and gastric lipases. These findings have important implications for the structuring of triacylglycerols in infant formulas. A similar study was conducted by Brühl et al., who determined the structures of 106 triacylglycerols that accounted for 81% by weight of the triacylglycerols in human milk (*193*). Fourteen triacylglycerols, each accounting for >1%, together contributed 42 wt%. These authors, too, commented on the nonrandom distribution of palmitic acid (16:0)—particularly its predilection for the 2-position, which is seen to a similar extent only in lard, of all the other fats and oils examined. They discussed these findings in terms of optimal structure of triacylglycerols in infant formulas and the suitability of lard as a raw material for infant formulas.

## Other Nutrients and Development

A study in New Zealand examined the association between breast-feeding and risk of SIDS (*194*). It included 485 infants who died of SIDS and 1800 randomly selected controls. Initially, 92% of controls and 86% of SIDS infants were breast-fed. When the criterion was "any" breast feeding rather than "exclusive" breast feeding, 67% of controls were breast-fed at 13 weeks, compared with 49% of SIDS infants. About 60% of controls were exclusively breast-fed at 16 weeks, compared with only 25% of SIDS infants. A significantly reduced risk of SIDS in breast-fed infants persisted throughout the first 6 months after control for confounding demographic, maternal, and infant factors.

Although strict vegetarian diets have certain health benefits for adults, their adequacy for children has been questioned. Sanders and Reddy reviewed the adequacy of vegan and vegetarian diets for children and identified the conditions that can give rise to nutritional deficiency (*195*). Hazards of vegetarian diets are iron deficiency anemia, vitamin $B_{12}$ deficiency, rickets, and a bulky diet that can restrict energy intake in the very young. However, these known problems can be avoided. Although there may be subtle differences between vegetarian and omnivorous children in their general health and development, vegetarian children appear to be completely normal. The authors recommended that vegans and vegetarians use oils with a low ratio of linoleic to linolenic acid, because of the importance of DHA in visual development. However, a detailed study in the Netherlands identified multiple nutritional deficiencies in infants and children reared on a macrobiotic diet (*196*). The study had a longitudinal design and included a matched omnivorous control group. The authors have systematically studied macrobiotic children, and this paper summarizes salient findings from their earlier investigations. On average, macrobiotic children have birth weights significantly lower than the Dutch average. For the first 6 months their growth rate is close to the median of the Dutch reference. However, macrobiotic infants between 6 and 18 months old showed important deficiencies of energy, protein, vitamin $B_{12}$, vitamin D, calcium, and riboflavin. Fiber intake increased from 6 g/d to 19 g/d, compared to 5 g/d to 8 g/d in controls; at the same time, fat intake decreased from 37 en% to 17 en%. This resulted in retarded growth, fat and muscle wasting, and slower psychomotor development. Despite a higher iron intake, 15% of macrobiotic infants showed iron deficiency; no controls were iron-deficient. In summer, 45% of macrobiotic infants had subclinical or clinical rickets; prevalence of rickets was 90% in winter. Milk from macrobiotic mothers contained less vitamin $B_{12}$, calcium, and magnesium. It is noteworthy that the educational level of the macrobiotic parents was higher than the Dutch average. Moreover, 97% of these mothers had attended general macrobiotic lectures and 92% had attended courses or consultations on macrobiotic child nutrition. The authors discussed features of the macrobiotic diet that contribute to nutritional deficiencies. For example, dietary seaweed contains vitamin $B_{12}$ analogues that can interfere with metabolism of the already low amount of dietary $B_{12}$; and the high-fiber diet decreases the bioavailability of mineral nutrients.

Since the establishment of taurine as an essential nutrient for cats, its importance in early human nutrition has been of interest. The issue of whether to supplement purified human infant formulas with taurine has been resolved in practical terms, but no official requirement has been established. Palackal et al. studied the effect of dietary taurine on development of the visual cortex in 6- and 12-month-old rhesus monkeys (*Macaca mulatta*) (*197*). From birth, infants were fed a taurine-free soy-based formula developed for human infants or the same formula fortified with taurine at the level found in rhesus monkey milk. Infants in a reversal group were switched from the taurine-free diet to the taurine-supplemented diet when they were 6 months old. Combined with results of a similar study of 3-month-old monkeys and with studies of visual acuity, the results confirmed the significant disadvantages of a taurine-free infant formula. Some qualitative differences in neuronal arborization noted at 3 months persisted in the older infants. Quantitative differences in astrocytes, microglia, and oligodendrocytes in various layers of the visual cortex were also noted. There was evidence in the reversal group that early taurine deficiency has some permanent effects on the visual cortex.

L-Carnitine is an acyl carrier involved in fatty acid synthesis and oxidation. In healthy people it is synthesized endogenously in adequate amounts; it is also obtained from dietary sources, predominantly animal flesh. Schek reviewed the sources, biosynthesis, physiology, and functions of carnitine (*198*). She discussed myopathies resulting from primary and secondary defects in carnitine metabolism and the importance of carnitine in infant nutrition. Human milk provides 3.5–7.0 μmol/dL of L-carnitine; cow's milk, 16–20 μmol/dL; cow's milk–based infant formulas, 5.0–23.0 μmol/dL; and soy-based formulas, none. In a companion paper she discussed some suggested, questionable, and senseless uses of carnitine supplementation (*199*). Supplemental carnitine has been suggested for athletes because of its importance in muscle physiology and for dieters because of claims that it enhances oxidation of fats and interferes with building up of fat depots, but there is no good evidence that it helps either athletic performance or weight loss. Several hypotheses for beneficial effects of carnitine supplements were presented and refuted.

Chhabra et al. studied hepatic xenobiotic metabolizing enzymes in suckling mouse pups and their dams when the lactating dams were given garlic at levels of 0, 200, or 400 mg per kilogram of body weight for 21 days (*200*). A number of effects were observed, depending on the dose of garlic and the age of the pups. Overall, early postnatal exposure to garlic via the transmammary route inhibited the neonatal detoxication system. The higher dose of garlic increased the hepatic sulfhydryl content of dams and pups. Implications of this for later life have not been investigated.

The general research interest of Mennella and Beauchamp is the flavor world of the breast-fed infant and how exposure to various flavors in the mother's milk influences later food preferences, food habits, and willingness to accept new foods. They have reported further studies of the effects of garlic-flavored milk on a human infant's feeding behavior (*201*; also see *Food Safety 1993*, reference *212*). Infants with no exposure to garlic volatiles in their mother's milk during a pretest experimental period spent significantly more time breast-feeding after their mother ingested garlic capsules than after she ingested placebo. Infants whose mothers had ingested garlic capsules at some time during the pretest experimental period spent equivalent time breast-feeding during the test whether their mother had ingested garlic or placebo. Unexposed infants whose mothers ingested garlic before the test also breast-fed longer than previously exposed infants.

Szylit and Andrieux reviewed the composition of the human fecal microflora at various stages of development from premature birth to adulthood and discussed the physiological and pathophysiological effects of carbohydrate fermentation by colonic microorganisms (*202*). They emphasized the importance of gnotobiotic models in such studies. Much can be learned about the role of specific organisms or communities of organisms by inoculating germ-free animals with components of the human fecal microflora and comparing results in these gnotobiotic animals with comparable observations in germ-free and conventional animals.

## Nutrition and Aging

Feldman summarized the areas of active research on nutrition in aging and areas in which important gaps in knowledge remain (*203*). Russell and Suter updated their earlier literature review of the vitamin requirements of elderly people (*204*). Although a poor diet causes much of the vitamin malnutrition in the elderly, aging itself affects requirements for certain vitamins. The 1989 RDAs for vitamins $B_6$, $B_{12}$, D, and riboflavin appear to be too low for persons older than 50 y. The RDA for vitamin A may be too high. The RDAs for thiamin, vitamin C, and folate seem appropriate for older persons but there are not enough data to make judgments for vitamin K, niacin, biotin, and pantothenic acid. Hoffman discussed nutritional topics important for the elderly (*205*). Aging-related changes relevant to nutrition include decrements in olfactory and taste perception, xerostomia (dry mouth), and need for dentures, but these do not appear to have a significant impact on nutritional status. Physical activity, caloric intake, and lean body mass decrease with aging; body fat increases. Changes in nutrient absorption may occur, but there are few data on this subject. Studies of vitamin, trace elements, and protein requirements in the elderly were reviewed. Multivitamin supplements are considered unnecessary for healthy persons, but calcium supplementation is suggested for postmenopausal women. Risk factors for malnutrition in the elderly were discussed.

Posner et al. described the development of the Nutrition Screening Initiative Checklist, a short questionnaire designed to identify free-living older persons at risk for low nutrient intake and health problems (*206*). The checklist was tested and evaluated in a random sample of Medicare beneficiaries, aged ≥70 years, in six New England states. A score of 6 or more defined subjects at high nutritional risk. According to this, 24% of the Medicare population was estimated to be at high risk. Among these, 56% perceived their health as fair or poor and 38% had dietary intakes below 75% of the RDA for at least 3 nutrients. Problems of nutritional excesses were also identified. Further study of nutritional risk in elderly New England residents involved telephone interviews and in-home assessments of oral health, anthropometrics, and completion of a 24-h dietary recall questionnaire (*206,207*). This revealed widespread and diverse nutrition-related problems. Mean dietary lipid intakes were considerably above recommended levels. More than 40% of the subjects were overweight and 16% were underweight. Calcium intake was low and 28% of subjects consumed <75% of the RDA for three or more key nutrients. Advanced age, gender, living situation, smoking, educational level, and dental health were associated with nutritional risk.

Morley reviewed the major nutritional problems of older women, stressing where they differ from those of men (*208*). Management of hyperglycemia and diabetes in the elderly was discussed.

Joosten et al. provided metabolic evidence that vitamin $B_{12}$, folate, and vitamin $B_6$ deficiencies are common in the elderly (*209*). They measured serum concentrations of the vitamins and of homocysteine, cystathionine, methylmalonic acid, and 2-methylcitric acid—metabolites that accumulate when enzymatic reactions that depend on these vitamins are impaired—in groups of healthy young subjects, healthy elderly subjects, and hospitalized elderly patients. Depending on the vitamin, low serum levels of vitamin were found in 5–9% of healthy older subjects and in 5–51% of hospitalized subjects. However, elevated levels of one or more metabolites were found in 63% of the healthy elderly and 83% of the hospitalized elderly. This suggests that the prevalence of tissue deficiencies of vitamins $B_6$, $B_{12}$, and folate is substantially higher than estimated by serum concentrations of these vitamins.

Yu reviewed how diet influences the aging process in rats (*210*). Restriction of total calories was compared with restriction of specific dietary components. The involvement of free radicals in aging and age-related diseases and how this is modulated by calorie restriction was discussed.

Ingram et al. described the design and early phases of a longitudinal study of aging, and how diet restriction affects it, in rhesus and squirrel monkeys (*211*). Because the lifespan of a rhesus monkey is about 40 y and a squirrel monkey may live 25 y, it was important to identify intermediate biomarkers that show whether a treatment is having an effect. In the 5 y since the study began, the investigators have established a model of diet restriction in long-lived nonhuman primates and have begun to identify parameters that will allow mechanistic hypotheses to be tested.

## ANTIMICROBIAL EFFECTS OF FOOD CONSTITUENTS

Kubo et al. have been studying plant-derived compounds that are bactericidal for *Streptococcus mutans*. They have shown that activity depends on a balance between hydrophobic and hydrophilic parts of the molecule. Now they report the anti–*S. mutans* activity of a series of long-chain aliphatic alcohols (*212*). The minimum inhibitory and minimum bactericidal concentrations (MIC and MBC) were determined. Because the hydrophilic hydroxyl group was common to all compounds, only the hydrophobic alkyl groups were of interest. The most active alcohols were 1-tridecanol and 1-dodecanol, with MICs of 6.25 μg/mL. Longer-chain alcohols were inactive (MIC >800 μg/mL), whereas activity decreased gradually as chain length decreased—e.g., MICs for 1-decanol, 1-octanol, and 1-hexanol were 50, 400, and >800 μg/mL, respectively. A similar pattern was seen for MBC values. Tests of series of secondary alcohols also suggested the importance of the chain length counted from the hydroxyl group. The alcohols were more active than the corresponding aldehyde or acid. These data were used to interpret previous measurements of the activity of more complex natural compounds such as isoprene long-chain alcohols. The same research group reported detailed studies of the anti–*S. mutans* activity of key flavor compounds in green tea (*213*). They demonstrated a dramatic synergism between indole and several sesquiterpenes and terpene alcohols. For example, the minimum inhibitory and bactericidal concentrations of β-caryophyllene alone were >1600 μg/mL and of δ-cadinene alone were 800 μg/mL. In combination with half the MIC of indole, these values were 6.25 μg/mL for both compounds. In combination with indole the MICs of linalool, geraniol, and nerolidol were halved. Synergistic antibacterial effects were also demonstrated between indole and (*E*)-2-hexenal, the most active of the 10 most abundant flavor compounds in the cashew apple (*Anacardium occidentale*) (*214*). (*E*)-2-Hexenal was active against all 14 microorganisms tested, including *S. mutans*.

Nakayama et al. found that the tea polyphenols (–)-epigallocatechin gallate and theaflavin digallate inhibit the infectivity of influenza virus (*215*). They agglutinated influenza A virus and influenza B virus as effectively as antibody, prevented the viruses from adsorbing to MDCK cells in vitro, and inhibited virus-induced hemagglutination of chicken erythrocytes. They lost their effectiveness in inhibiting plaque formation when added after adsorption of virus to MDCK cells. Thus the polyphenols can block the virus's adsorption and entry into cells but not its multiplication within cells. The concentrations of polyphenols active in these tests are realistic in terms of amounts that are ingested by tea-drinkers.

A study in elderly women indicated that popular beliefs about the effects of cranberry juice on the urinary tract may have microbiologic justification (*216*). Subjects were randomly assigned to drink 300 mL/d of a commercial cranberry beverage or an indistinguishable cranberry-free synthetic placebo beverage for 6 months. Urine samples were obtained at baseline and approximately monthly throughout the study. Samples were tested quantitatively for bacteria and white blood cells.

Compared with controls, subjects drinking the cranberry beverage had an odds ratio for bacteriuria ($\geq 10^5$ organisms per milliliter) with pyuria of 0.42 ($p = .004$). Their chance of remaining bacteriuric and pyuric for a second consecutive month was roughly one-quarter that of controls. Subjects in the cranberry group also had a nonsignificant trend toward less bacteriuria regardless of pyuria. The authors believe this to be the first large-scale placebo-controlled clinical trial to document an in vivo effect of cranberries on bacteriuria with pyuria. The effect appeared only after 4–8 weeks of use of the cranberry beverage, a time course compatible with modification of the gut flora, which contains the typical pathogens in urinary tract infections among women. The effect was not due to acidification of the urine—median pH was nonsignificantly higher in the cranberry group (6.0 vs. 5.5).

The meat, seeds, and pulp of unripe papaya (*Carica papaya* L.) are bacteriostatic against a variety of enteropathogens and papaya has traditionally been used to treat a variety of gastrointestinal disorders. Osato et al. correlated this antibacterial activity with the ability of the same papaya parts to quench superoxide and hydroxyl radicals (*217*). However, the antioxidant activity is much stronger than the antimicrobial activity: the concentration of papaya required to eliminate 50% of the generated free radicals is less than one-tenth of the MIC.

The malaria parasite is exceptionally sensitive to oxidative stress. Levander and Ager discussed the possibility of a nutritional prooxidant–antioxidant approach to controlling malaria (*218*). They reviewed the action of prooxidant antimalarial drugs and the effects of depleting dietary antioxidants or increasing the unsaturation of dietary lipids. A mouse model of malaria has been very useful in working out nutrient–disease interactions. However, the clinical complexity of the relationship between malaria and antioxidant status was illustrated in a short report by Davis et al. (*219*). In this study, low serum retinol in malaria patients could have been due to impaired hepatic function, but these patients also had low levels of serum carotene, which probably resulted from low intake of carotene-containing foods. The relationship between vitamin E status and development of malaria or response to therapy was unclear. Although the antioxidant picture is murky, ajoene (a substance derived from garlic) suppressed development of parasitemia in a mouse model of malaria when given by intraperitoneal injection at a level of 50 mg/kg (*220*). The level of suppression was comparable to that of 4.5 mg/kg of chloroquine (a subcurative dose). A combination of 4.5 mg/kg of chloroquine and 50 mg/kg of

ajoene completely prevented development of parasitemia. The combined effect appears to be synergistic, as further indicated by the appreciable antimalarial activity of an even lower subcurative dose of chloroquine (2.8 mg/kg) with a very low dose of ajoene (12.5 mg/kg). The mechanism of ajoene's action may reside in its effect on the platelet membrane.

Portier et al. showed that orally administered fermented milks increase the antibody responses of mice against cholera (*221*). Heated and unheated yogurt fermented by *Lactobacillus bulgaricus* and *Streptococcus thermophilus* and milk fermented by *Lactobacillus casei* were equally effective.

## MISCELLANEOUS EFFECTS OF DIET

### Respiratory System

Data from the Zutphen Study in the Netherlands were used to evaluate the association between diet and the 25-year incidence of chronic nonspecific lung diseases in middle-aged men (*222*). The incidence of new cases was 14.1 per 1000 man-years. Incidence was positively related to linoleic acid intake (RR 1.55 for highest vs. lowest quartile, 95% CI 1.11–2.16). Alcohol drinkers had less risk than nondrinkers (RR 0.72, 95% CI 0.55–0.95). There was no association with intake of several antioxidants, although a high intake of total fruits or solid fruits was protective (RRs 0.73 and 0.63, respectively). There was no association with intake of $n$–3 PUFAs. However, a review by Katz et al. suggested that $n$–3 PUFAs improve bronchodilation, reduce inflammation, prevent pulmonary hypertension, and protect against vascular remodeling and lung fibrosis (*223*). Supplementation with $n$–3 PUFAs thus may benefit patients with chronic inflammatory respiratory diseases such as COPD and cystic fibrosis. Benefits are likely the result of effects on eicosanoid metabolism. Recent animal studies indicate that $n$–3 PUFAs may also be a useful adjunct in treating sepsis and associated adult respiratory distress syndrome.

Knox speculated on why a high-salt diet may make asthma worse in men but not in women (*224*). Carey et al. reported a placebo-controlled randomized crossover study of asthmatic men showing that a large increase in dietary sodium leads to deterioration of lung function and reactivity, worsens symptom scores, and increases use of bronchodilators (*225*). A preliminary controlled crossover study supported the hypothesis that asthmatic subjects are salt-sensitive (*226*). Quantitative salt loading worsened clinical and functional measurements in asthmatics and salt restriction improved them. Moreover, it was sodium—not chloride or the sodium-chloride combination—that was responsible for these effects, as sodium chloride and sodium citrate had comparable effects. The small number of subjects did not permit data for men and women to be analyzed separately, but no sex-related differences in response to salt loading were apparent.

Schwartz and Weiss evaluated the relationship between dietary vitamin C and pulmonary function, using data from the first National Health and Nutrition Examination Survey (NHANES I) (227). To ensure that the assessment was not confounded by any correlations with smoking, they first meticulously developed several smoking models. Vitamin C intake was positively and significantly associated with the forced expiratory volume in 1 s ($FEV_1$). There were no significant interactions between vitamin C and smoking or respiratory disease.

Based on 4 placebo-controlled studies reported before 1971, Linus Pauling concluded that vitamin C reduces the incidence and severity of the common cold. This idea has remained controversial. Hemilä reviewed the 21 placebo-controlled studies reported since 1971, in which $\geq 1$ g/d of vitamin C was tested (228). Vitamin C had no obvious effect on incidence. Results of 17 studies were symmetrically grouped around 0, and the 4 outliers had serious shortcomings. Nevertheless, it is possible that vitamin C might reduce cold incidence in specific subgroups or under certain circumstances: military troops undergoing Arctic exercises and students at a ski school were subjects in 2 studies that found a significant effect. However, all 21 studies showed a decrease in the duration or severity of symptoms. The probability of this occurring by chance is .0000005. The decrease in morbidity ranged between 5 and 35%, averaging 23%. This may reflect the heterogeneity of the studies: they varied in type of subject, geographical location and climate, types of respiratory viruses involved, size of the vitamin C supplement, and definition and measurement of disease. One of the more important variables may have been the vitamin C intake of the controls. Overall, Hemilä believes that the role of vitamin C in treatment of the common cold should be reconsidered.

## Other

Rackett et al. reviewed the effects of dietary modification in preventing and treating skin disorders (229). For nonmelanoma skin cancer, there is some evidence that carotenoids, retinoids, selenium, and vitamin C may be protective. The clinical evidence is strongest for retinoids.

For melanoma, epidemiologic data are inconsistent although in vitro studies suggest that dietary factors are relevant. Deficiencies in dietary protein, zinc, and vitamins A, C, and K can delay wound healing. Nutritional supplementation may promote wound healing even in patients who do not appear nutritionally depleted. However, high zinc levels can have a detrimental effect on wound healing and there are conflicting reports on the role of vitamin E. For patients with atopic dermatitis, the commonest dietary strategy is avoidance of food allergens. However, beneficial results have been reported for unconventional treatments such as fish oil, evening primrose oil, and Chinese herbal tea. Modest improvements in psoriasis have been achieved with fish oil supplements. Dietary treatment of dermatitis herpetiformis was reviewed. Additional study of dietary manipulation and the effects of nutritional supplements on these and other skin diseases and disorders is required.

Patients with Wilson's disease (hepatolenticular degeneration) are unable to excrete excess copper. Therefore anti-copper therapy is key to the management of this disease. Brewer et al. reported two cases of Wilson's disease in which the subjects followed ovolactovegetarian diets (230). The first case was identified in an asymptomatic sister of a Wilson's disease patient during a family workup. She had followed an ovolactovegetarian diet by choice since adulthood. After 14 years of noncompliance with anti-copper therapy she remained asymptomatic with no trace of liver disease. The second case was diagnosed in a 14-year-old girl who became noncompliant with therapy over the next 4 years in an effort to let her disease kill her. After 2 years of virtually complete noncompliance she switched from an omnivorous diet to an ovolactovegetarian diet. Her motive for this was unclear but it was not an effort to treat her disease. Serum transaminase levels improved during the following year and at age 23, two years after initiating the diet, she remained clinically well. The authors commented that the typical American diet contains little copper in excess of the requirement, and although mixed and vegetarian diets may provide similar amounts, copper is less bioavailable from a vegetarian diet. While these case reports suggest that vegetarian diets may be effective in managing Wilson's disease, they also emphasize the marginal copper intake of most Americans and suggest that some apparently healthy people, particularly vegetarians, may have subclinical copper deficiency.

Koch et al. purified several fructans from fresh garlic cloves and demonstrated their competitive in vitro inhibition of adenosine deaminase (231). Adenosine regulates a variety of important physiologic processes, and the authors postulate that molecules that bind in vitro to the enzymes responsible for adenosine metabolism exert similar pharmacologic effects in vivo. Thus fructans may contribute to the diverse clinical effects of garlic. The active compounds were of medium size, containing 10–14 sugar moieties per molecule.

# NUTRIENT INTERACTIONS AND DRUG METABOLISM

## Interactions Among Nutrients

Calcium carbonate supplements may affect nitrogen excretion and nitrogen balance (*232*). Healthy adult volunteers were given a basal diet providing an adequate but relatively low level of protein and 325 mg/d of calcium. In one experiment, this diet was supplemented with calcium carbonate wafers taken at mealtime to provide an additional 0, 600, 1200, or 1800 mg/d of calcium. As levels of calcium carbonate increased, urinary and fecal nitrogen excretion increased and nitrogen balance decreased, becoming negative at the highest level of supplementation. A second experiment compared four types of calcium carbonate supplement (gum, caramel, tablet, and the wafer used in the first experiment) providing 600 mg/d of calcium. The wafer produced the lowest mean urinary and fecal nitrogen losses and the highest nitrogen balance. The authors concluded that excessive use of calcium carbonate supplements could impair protein nutriture in people with a marginal protein intake. They speculated that the effect of calcium carbonate on protein utilization depends on the timing of supplementation with respect to meals and the ease and speed of solubilization of the calcium. Theoretically, calcium carbonate might inhibit protein digestion in the stomach by raising pH and inhibiting conversion of pepsinogen to pepsin, whereas raising pH in the small intestine could enhance the action of pancreatic and intestinal digestive enzymes.

In a study in India, groups of healthy preadolescent girls of low socioeconomic status were tested on their habitual diet or their habitual diet supplemented with 34 g/d of pulses or 190 mL/d of milk (*233*). Supplementation with milk greatly improved the absorption and retention of trace minerals (zinc, iron, copper, and manganese). Intake of manganese from the habitual diet was high, but intake of copper and zinc was marginal. Iron intake just met the recommended allowance, but the actual requirement of girls in this age group could not be calculated.

Zheng et al. reported use of a whole-gut lavage technique in healthy adults to measure absorption of zinc in physiological doses from single foods (*234*). Their study confirmed that roughly three times as much zinc is available from beef as from a high-fiber breakfast cereal. Couzy et al. used a stable isotope technique to compare zinc absorption in young and old men (*235*). The $^{70}Zn$ isotope was added to test meals differing in zinc bioavailability mainly on the basis of their phytate content. No significant effect of age was seen. The authors concluded that healthy men retain their ability for zinc absorption at least until the age of 80 y.

Dietary zinc can suppress the bioavailability of copper, and the zinc/copper ratio may be near the maximum safe level in the American diet. Leung and Li measured concentrations of zinc and copper in gastric juice of chronic superficial gastritis patients, some of whom were receiving zinc replenishment therapy (*236*). They also measured zinc and copper levels in plasma of healthy subjects and in noncancerous tissue from cancer patients who were not taking zinc supplements. In plasma and normal tissue, zinc and copper concentrations were positively correlated. In gastric juice, zinc and copper were also positively correlated up to a concentration of 100 µmol/L of zinc. The authors concluded that under normal conditions, zinc and copper remain in balance. However, as the zinc concentration in gastric juice rose above 100 µmol/L copper concentrations fell. The mean copper concentration in gastric juice of zinc-supplemented gastritis patients was less than that in nonsupplemented patients.

In vitro and in vivo studies showed that copper bioavailability from a meal is enhanced by tea (*237*). The amount of dialyzable copper was determined after in vitro digestion of a meal containing white bread, margarine, strawberry jam, cheese, and water or black tea with or without milk. The percentage of dialyzable copper was markedly increased by tea. Milk had no significant effect. Whole-body $^{64}Cu$ retention studies in rats fed the same meals confirmed that tea leads to greater absorption and retention of copper, particularly in the liver. The authors concluded that inclusion of tea in a breakfast-type meal favors the formation of soluble copper compounds of low molecular weight, which are readily absorbed and retained by rats. Soluble tannins or flavonoids may be involved in this interaction.

Shackelford et al. examined mineral interactions in rats fed AIN-76A diets with and without excess calcium (*238*). They measured the mineral content of tissues from nonpregnant rats and from pregnant rats and their fetuses. Of the numerous interactions, those seen in fetuses were perhaps the most important. Fetuses from rats receiving calcium supplements had dose-related decreases in whole-body contents of phosphorus, iron, copper, and magnesium. In some cases these changes were reflected in maternal tissue.

Hurrell et al. reported the influence of NaFe³⁺EDTA and Na₂EDTA on zinc, calcium, and copper metabolism in rats fed zinc-deficient and zinc-sufficient diets (*239*). Their results indicated that using NaFe³⁺EDTA as a food fortificant would have no detrimental effect on mineral metabolism and could in fact improve zinc absorption and retention from a low-zinc diet. A study in Native American women, 38% of whom had iron deficiency, evaluated the effect of EDTA on absorption of iron from food (*240*). The results indicated that Na₂EDTA enhances absorption of intrinsic and added iron when the molar ratio of EDTA to iron is ≤1.00 and the meal contains appreciable amounts of phytate. In meals of high iron bioavailability EDTA had little effect.

## Bioavailability of Nutritional Supplements

Ip and Lisk evaluated the nutritional bioavailability of selenium from selenium-enriched garlic, using two hepatic selenoenzymes as biomarkers (*241*). Weanling rats were fed a selenium-deficient diet for 4 weeks to deplete activity of glutathione peroxidase and type I 5'-deiodinase. They were then fed nutritional levels of selenium as selenite or selenium-enriched garlic. The two supplements were equally effective in restoring enzyme activity.

Johansson and Westermarck compared the effects of inorganic selenium and a combination of organic and inorganic selenium on selenium status in healthy adults (*242*). One group of subjects was given 100 μg/d of selenium as selenite. Another received a combination of 50 μg/d of selenium as selenite plus 50 μg/d as L-selenomethionine, along with vitamins E, B₂, B₆, and B₁₂. The combination supplement produced significantly higher plasma and erythrocyte selenium levels and higher erythrocyte glutathione peroxidase activity than selenite alone. The groups did not differ significantly in activity of plasma glutathione peroxidase. McGuire et al. evaluated the selenium status of lactating and nonlactating women supplemented with selenomethionine, selenium-enriched yeast, or no selenium (*243*). Plasma selenium declined in unsupplemented lactating women but not in nonlactating women. Selenomethionine increased plasma selenium in all women, whereas selenium-enriched yeast was effective only in nonlactating subjects. Erythrocyte selenium was not influenced by lactation. Plasma glutathione peroxidase activity decreased during lactation in unsupplemented women; both supplements prevented

the decline. Selenium levels in milk of unsupplemented women declined during supplementation; selenium-enriched yeast prevented this decline, and selenomethionine significantly increased levels of milk selenium. Thus the influence of selenium supplementation on selected indexes of selenium status depends on lactation status and the form of the supplement.

Because of reports that β-carotene supplements can lower serum levels of α-tocopherol, possible interactions between supplemental vitamin C, vitamin E, and β-carotene were evaluated (*244*). Subjects were 505 patients participating in a clinical trial of antioxidant vitamin supplementation to prevent recurrence of colonic polyps. They were randomly assigned to receive 25 mg/d of β-carotene, 1 g/d of ascorbic acid plus 400 mg/d of α-tocopherol, all three agents, or placebo. Serum α-tocopherol and β-carotene were measured before and after 9 months of supplementation. Vitamin E levels changed very little in groups receiving placebo or β-carotene and rose substantially in both groups receiving vitamin E. Similarly, β-carotene levels did not change in the placebo and vitamin E plus ascorbic acid groups but rose sharply and equally in the groups receiving β-carotene or all three agents. The authors concluded that there is no significant interaction between these supplements with respect to serum concentrations of antioxidants.

The bioavailability of ascorbic acid from foods and supplements has received little attention because of limited data and the assumption that bioavailability is high (*245*). Now there is good experimental evidence that bioavailability from tablets with or without iron, orange juice, orange segments, and cooked broccoli is equivalent. Bioavailability from raw broccoli is 20% lower, but this probably has little nutritional importance in typical mixed diets.

## Interactions Between Nutrients and Drugs

Williams et al. discussed the influence of food on the absorption and metabolism of drugs (*246*). They provided a summary table showing specific drugs whose absorption may be enhanced, reduced, or delayed by food and the underlying mechanism(s) of the effect. Drug metabolism can be altered by dietary macronutrients or micronutrients or by particular foods or their components. The proportion of adverse drug reactions that are due to food–drug interactions is not known. Thomas and Tschanz discussed risk factors for nutrient–drug interactions and mechanisms by which foods or nutrients enhance or interfere with absorption of specific drugs (*247*). Alcohol–drug and vitamin–drug interactions and drug-induced lactose intolerance were reviewed. Certain disease states and other special conditions can interact with both nutrition and a drug's therapeutic efficacy. Neubert et al. reviewed the interactions between drugs and dietary carbohydrates, egg white, fat, and fiber (*248*). They summarized in vivo and in vitro methods for evaluating these interactions.

The absorption and disposition of paracetamol was investigated in healthy vegetarian and nonvegetarian Thai men (*249*). Plasma half-life, partial metabolic clearances, and fractional urinary excretion of the glucuronide, sulfate, cysteine, and mercapturic acid conjugates were not influenced by diet. However, absorption of the drug was significantly impaired in vegetarians, as indicated by lower peak plasma concentration, longer time to peak concentration, and lower 24-h urinary recovery of the drug and its metabolites.

## LITERATURE CITED

1. Kumari, B.S., and R.K. Chandra. Overnutrition and immune responses. *Nutr. Res.* 13(Suppl. 1):S3–S18 (1993).

2. Scott, F.W., J. Cui, and P. Rowsell. Food and the development of autoimmune disease. *Trends Food Sci. Technol.* 5:111–116 (1994).

3. Minami, Y., T. Sasaki, S. Komatsu, et al. Female systemic lupus erythematosus in Miyagi Prefecture, Japan: a case–control study of dietary and reproductive factors. *Tohoku J. Exp. Med.* 169:245–252 (1993).

4. Wienken, E. Psoriasis—durch Ernährung beeinflußbar? *Ernährungs-Umschau* 40:458–460 (1993).

5. Wienken, E. Akne—durch Ernährung beeinflußbar? *Ernährungs-Umschau* 40:385–386 (1993).

6. Wienken, E. Neurodermitis—durch Ernährung beeinflußbar? *Ernährungs-Umschau* 40:496–498 (1993).

7. Juvonen, P., M. Månsson, and I. Jakobsson. Does early diet have an effect on subsequent macromolecular absorption and serum IgE? *J. Pediatr. Gastroenterol. Nutr.* 18:344–349 (1994).

8. Rall, L.C., and S.N. Meydani. Vitamin $B_6$ and immune competence. *Nutr. Rev.* 51:217–225 (1993).

9. Jyonouchi, H., L. Zhang, and Y. Tomita. Studies of immunomodulating actions of carotenoids. II. Astaxanthin enhances in vitro antibody production to T-dependent antigens without facilitating polyclonal B-cell activation. *Nutr. Cancer* 19:269–280 (1993).

10. Jyonouchi, H., L. Zhang, M. Gross, and Y. Tomita. Immunomodulating actions of carotenoids: enhancement of in vivo and in vitro antibody production to T-dependent antigens. *Nutr. Cancer* 21:47–58 (1994).

11. Heliövaara, M., P. Knekt, K. Aho, et al. Serum antioxidants and risk of rheumatoid arthritis. *Ann. Rheum. Dis.* 53:51–53 (1994).

12. Tang, A.M., N.M.H. Graham, A.J. Kirby, et al. Dietary micronutrient intake and risk of progression to acquired immunodeficiency syndrome (AIDS) in human immunodeficiency virus type 1 (HIV-1)-infected homosexual men. *Am. J. Epidemiol.* 138:937–951 (1993).

13. Wang, Y., and R.R. Watson. Ethanol, immune responses, and murine AIDS: the role of vitamin E as an immunostimulant and antioxidant. *Alcohol* 11:75–84 (1994).

14. Dileepan, K.N., S.T. Varghese, J.C. Page, and D.J. Stechschulte. Enhanced lymphoproliferative response, macrophage mediated tumor cell killing and nitric oxide production after ingestion of an Ayurvedic drug. *Biochem. Arch.* 9:365–374 (1993).

15. Sheehan, M.P., and D.J. Atherton. One-year follow up of children treated with Chinese medicinal herbs for atopic eczema. *Br. J. Dermatol.* 130:488–493 (1994).

16. Ryhänen, E.-L., S. Mantere-Alhonen, M. Nenonen, and O. Hänninen. Modification of faecal flora in rheumatoid arthritis patients by lactobacilli rich vegetarian diet. *Milchwissenschaft* 48:255–259 (1993).

17. Solis Pereyra, B., and D. Lemonnier. Induction of human cytokines by bacteria used in dairy foods. *Nutr. Res.* 13:1127–1140 (1993).

18. Lee, J., A. Ametani, A. Enomoto, et al. Screening for the immunopotentiating activity of food microorganisms and enhancement of the immune response by *Bifidobacterium adolescentis* M101-4. *Biosci. Biotechnol. Biochem.* 57:2127–2132 (1993).

19. Yamauchi, F., and K. Suetsuna. Immunological effects of dietary peptide derived from soybean protein. *J. Nutr. Biochem.* 4:450–457 (1993).

20. Hummell, D.S. Dietary lipids and immune function. *Prog. Food Nutr. Sci.* 17:287–329 (1993).

21. Meydani, S.N., A.H. Lichtenstein, S. Cornwall, et al. Immunologic effects of National Cholesterol Education Panel step-2 diets with and without fish-derived *N*–3 fatty acid enrichment. *J. Clin. Invest.* 92:105–113 (1993).

22. Robinson, D.R., L.-L. Xu, S. Tateno, et al. Suppression of autoimmune disease by dietary *n*–3 fatty acids. *J. Lipid Res.* 34:1435–1444 (1993).

23. Cooper, A.L., L. Gibbons, M.A. Horan, et al. Effect of dietary fish oil supplementation on fever and cytokine production in human volunteers. *Clin. Nutr.* 12:321–328 (1993).

24. Søyland, E., T. Lea, B. Sandstad, and A. Drevon. Dietary supplementation with very long-chain *n*–3 fatty acids in man decreases expression of the interleukin-2 receptor (CD25) on mitogen-stimulated lymphocytes from patients with inflammatory skin diseases. *Eur. J. Clin. Invest.* 24:236–242 (1994).

25. Fritsche, K.L., D.W. Alexander, N.A. Cassity, and S.-C. Huang. Maternally-supplied fish oil alters piglet immune cell fatty acid profile and eicosanoid production. *Lipids* 28:677–682 (1993).

26. Somers, S.D., and K.L. Erickson. Alteration of tumor necrosis factor-α production by macrophages from mice fed diets high in eicosapentaenoic and docosahexaenoic fatty acids. *Cell. Immunol.* 153:287–297 (1994).

27. Ferretti, A., S.N. Meydani, A.H. Lichtenstein, et al. Prostaglandin E metabolite excretion in normolipidemic subjects is lowered by a moderate reduction of *n*–6/*n*–3 polyunsaturate ratio and total fat intake. *Nutr. Res.* 14:185–193 (1994).

28. Brouard, C., and M. Pascaud. Modulation of rat and human lymphocyte function by *n*–6 and *n*–3 polyunsaturated fatty acids and acetylsalicylic acid. *Ann. Nutr. Metab.* 37:146–159 (1993).

29. James, M.J., R.A. Gibson, M. D'Angelo, et al. Simple relationships exist between dietary linoleate and the *n*–6 fatty acids of human neutrophils and plasma. *Am. J. Clin. Nutr.* 58:497–500 (1993).

30. Rasmussen, L.B., B. Kiens, B.K. Pedersen, and E.A. Richter. Effect of diet and plasma fatty acid composition on immune status in elderly men. *Am. J. Clin. Nutr.* 59:572–577 (1994).

31. Businco, L., M. Ioppi, N.L. Morse, et al. Breast milk from mothers of children with newly developed atopic eczema has low levels of long chain polyunsaturated fatty acids. *J. Aller. Clin. Immunol.* 91:1134–1139 (1993).

32. Leventhal, L.J., E.G. Boyce, and R.B. Zurier. Treatment of rheumatoid arthritis with gammalinolenic acid. *Ann. Intern. Med.* 119:867–873 (1993).

33. James, M.J., R.A. Gibson, M.A. Neumann, and L.G. Cleland. Effect of dietary supplementation with *n*–9 eicosatrienoic acid on leukotriene $B_4$ synthesis in rats: a novel approach to inhibition of eicosanoid synthesis. *J. Exp. Med.* 178:2261–2265 (1993).

34. Vasänge-Tuominen, M., P. Perera-Ivarsson, J. Shen, et al. The fern *Polypodium decumanum*, used in the treatment of psoriasis, and its fatty acid constituents as inhibitors of leukotriene $B_4$ formation. *Prostaglandins Leukotrienes Essential Fatty Acids* 50:279–284 (1994).

35. Miller, C.C., Y. Park, M.W. Pariza, and M.E. Cook. Feeding conjugated linoleic acid to animals partially overcomes catabolic responses due to endotoxin injection. *Biochem. Biophys. Res. Commun.* 198:1107–1112 (1994).

36. Toeller, M. Diet and diabetes. *Diabetes Metab. Rev.* 9:93–108 (1993).

37. Dahlquist, G. Etiological aspects of insulin-dependent diabetes mellitus: an epidemiological perspective. *Autoimmunity* 15:61–65 (1993).

38. Kostraba, J.N. What can epidemiology tell us about the role of infant diet in the etiology of IDDM? *Diabetes Care* 17:87–91 (1994).

39. Vinceti, M., S. Rovesti, C. Pacchioni, et al. Diet as a risk factor for abnormal glucose tolerance in subjects with and without family history of diabetes mellitus. *Diabetes Nutr. Metab.* 7:21–28 (1994).

40. Laitinen, J., M. Uusitupa, I. Ahola, et al. Metabolic and dietary variables associated with glycaemic control in patients with recently diagnosed Type II diabetes mellitus. *Diabetes Nutr. Metab.* 7:77–87 (1994).

41. Sevak, L., P.M. McKeigue, and M.G. Marmot. Relationship of hyperinsulinemia to dietary intake in South Asian and European men. *Am. J. Clin. Nutr.* 59:1069–1074 (1994).

42. Docherty, K., and A.R. Clark. Nutrient regulation of insulin gene expression. *FASEB J.* 8:20–27 (1994).

43. Franz, M.J., E.S. Horton, J.P. Bantle, et al. Nutrition principles for the management of diabetes and related complications. *Diabetes Care* 17:490–518 (1994).

44. Smith, U. Carbohydrates, fat, and insulin action. *Am. J. Clin. Nutr.* 59(Suppl.):686S–689S (1994).

45. Milne, R.M., J.I. Mann, A.W. Chisholm, and S.M. Williams. Long-term comparison of three dietary prescriptions in the treatment of NIDDM. *Diabetes Care* 17:74–80 (1994).

46. Brand Miller, J.C. Importance of glycemic index in diabetes. *Am. J. Clin. Nutr.* 59(Suppl.):747S–752S (1994).

47. Wolever, T.M.S., L. Katzman-Relle, A.L. Jenkins, et al. Glycaemic index of 102 complex carbohydrate foods in patients with diabetes. *Nutr. Res.* 14:651–669 (1994).

48. Jenkins, D.J.A., A.L. Jenkins, T.M.S. Wolever, et al. Low glycemic index: lente carbohydrates and physiological effects of altered food frequency. *Am. J. Clin. Nutr.* 59(Suppl.):706S–709S (1994).

49. Noriega, E., O. Buix, J.F. Brun, et al. Glycaemic and insulinaemic responses to white, brown and germinated rices in healthy subjects. *Diabetes Nutr. Metab.* 6:215–221 (1993).

50. Granfeldt, Y., H. Liljeberg, A. Drews, et al. Glucose and insulin responses to barley products: influence of food structure and amylose–amylopectin ratio. *Am. J. Clin. Nutr.* 59:1075–1082 (1994).

51. Trout, D.L., K.M. Behall, and O. Osilesi. Prediction of glycemic index for starchy foods. *Am. J. Clin. Nutr.* 58:873–878 (1993).

52. Leclére, C.J., M. Champ, J. Boillot, et al. Role of viscous guar gums in lowering the glycemic response after a solid meal. *Am. J. Clin. Nutr.* 59:914–921 (1994).

53. Groop, P.-H., A. Aro, S. Stenman, and L. Groop. Long-term effects of guar gum in subjects with non-insulin-dependent diabetes mellitus. *Am. J. Clin. Nutr.* 58:513–518 (1993).

54. Klimeš, I., B.V. Howard, L.H. Storlien, and E. Šeböková (eds.). *Dietary Lipids and Insulin Action. Second International Smolenice Insulin Symposium. Ann. N.Y. Acad. Sci.* 683 (1993).

55. Bianchi, R., and D.W. Erkelens. Diabetes mellitus, lipids and insulin resistance. *Diabetes Nutr. Metab.* 7:43–51 (1994).

56. Parker, D.R., S.T. Weiss, R. Troisi, et al. Relationship of dietary saturated fatty acids and body habitus to serum insulin concentrations: the Normative Aging Study. *Am. J. Clin. Nutr.* 58:129–136 (1993).

57. Marshall, J.A., S. Hoag, S. Shetterly, and R.F. Hamman. Dietary fat predicts conversion from impaired glucose tolerance to NIDDM. The San Luis Valley Diabetes Study. *Diabetes Care* 17:50–56 (1994).

58. Mayer, E.J., B. Newman, C.P. Quesenberry, Jr., and J.V. Selby. Usual dietary fat intake and insulin concentrations in healthy women twins. *Diabetes Care* 16:1459–1469 (1993).

59. Garg, A. High–monounsaturated fat diet for diabetic patients. Is it time to change the current dietary recommendations? *Diabetes Care* 17:242–246 (1994).

60. Rasmussen, O.W., C. Thomsen, K.W. Hansen, et al. Effects on blood pressure, glucose, and lipid levels of a high–monounsaturated fat diet compared with a high-carbohydrate diet in NIDDM subjects. *Diabetes Care* 16:1565–1571 (1993).

61. Campbell, L.V., P.E. Marmot, J.A. Dyer, et al. The high–monounsaturated fat diet as a practical alternative for NIDDM. *Diabetes Care* 17:177–192 (1994).

62. Lerman-Garber, I., S. Ichazo-Cerro, J. Zamora-González, et al. Effect of a high–monounsaturated fat diet enriched with avocado in NIDDM patients. *Diabetes Care* 17:311–315 (1994).

63. Donnelly, J.P., L.T. McGrath, and G.M. Brennan. Lipid peroxidation, LDL glycosylation and dietary fish oil supplementation in type II diabetes mellitus. *Biochem. Soc. Trans.* 22:34S (1993).

64. Axelrod, L., J. Camuso, E. Williams, et al. Effects of a small quantity of ω–3 fatty acids on cardiovascular risk factors in NIDDM. *Diabetes Care* 17:37–44 (1994).

65. Feskens, E.J.M., C.H. Bowles, and D. Kromhout. Association between fish intake and coronary heart disease mortality. Differences in normoglycemic and glucose intolerant elderly subjects. *Diabetes Care* 16:1029–1034 (1993).

66. Hughes, V.A., M.A. Fiatarone, C.M. Ferrara, et al. Lipoprotein response to exercise training and a low-fat diet in older subjects with glucose intolerance. *Am. J. Clin. Nutr.* 59:820–826 (1994).

67. Garg, A., J.P. Bantle, R.R. Henry, et al. Effects of varying carbohydrate content of diet in patients with non–insulin-dependent diabetes mellitus. *JAMA* 271:1421–1428 (1994).

68. Gonzélez, C., M.P. Stern, B.D. Mitchell, et al. Clinical characteristics of type II diabetic subjects consuming high versus low carbohydrate diets in Mexico City and San Antonio, Texas. *Diabetes Care* 17:397–404 (1994).

69. Gerrits, P.M., and E. Tsalikian. Diabetes and fructose metabolism. *Am. J. Clin. Nutr.* 58(Suppl.):796S–799S (1993).

70. Peters, A.L., and M.B. Davidson. Protein and fat effects on glucose responses and insulin requirements in subjects with insulin-dependent diabetes mellitus. *Am. J. Clin. Nutr.* 58:555–560 (1993).

71. Nakamura, H., S. Ito, N. Ebe, and A. Shibata. Renal effects of different types of protein in healthy volunteer subjects and diabetic patients. *Diabetes Care* 16:1071–1075 (1993).

72. Larivière, F., J.-L. Chiasson, A. Schiffrin, et al. Effects of dietary protein restriction on glucose and insulin metabolism in normal and diabetic humans. *Metabolism* 43:462–467 (1994).

73. Gerstein, H.C. Cow's milk exposure and type I diabetes mellitus. A critical overview of the clinical literature. *Diabetes Care* 17:13–19 (1994).

74. Dosch, H.-M. The possible link between insulin dependent (juvenile) diabetes mellitus and dietary cow milk. *Clin. Biochem.* 26:307–308 (1993).

75. Virtanen, S.M., L. Räsänen, K. Ylönen, et al. Early introduction of dairy products associated with increased risk of IDDM in Finnish children. *Diabetes* 42:1786–1790 (1993).

76. Virtanen, S.M., T. Saukkonen, E. Savilahti, et al. Diet, cow's milk protein antibodies and the risk of IDDM in Finnish children. *Diabetologia* 37:381–387 (1994).

77. Muntoni, S., S. Loddo, M. Stabilini, et al. Cow's milk consumption and IDDM incidence in Sardinia. *Diabetes Care* 17:346–347 (1994).

78. Monte, W.C., C.S. Johnston, and L.E. Roll. Bovine serum albumin detected in infant formula is a possible trigger for insulin-dependent diabetes mellitus. *J. Am. Diet. Assoc.* 94:314–316 (1994).

79. Strand, F.T. Primary prevention of insulin-dependent diabetes mellitus: simple approaches using thermal modification of milk. *Med. Hypoth.* 42:110–114 (1994).

80. Cabalero, B. Vitamin E improves the action of insulin. *Nutr. Rev.* 51:339–340 (1993).

81. Gerster, H. Prevention of platelet dysfunction by vitamin E in diabetic atherosclerosis. *Z. Ernährungswiss.* 32:243–261 (1993).

82. Paolisso, G., A. D'Amore, V. Balbi, et al. Plasma vitamin C affects glucose homeostasis in healthy subjects and in non-insulin-dependent diabetics. *Am. J. Physiol.* 266:E261–E268 (1994).

83. Facchini, F., Y.-D.I. Chen, and G.M. Reaven. Light-to-moderate alcohol intake is associated with enhanced insulin sensitivity. *Diabetes Care* 17:115–119 (1994).

84. Christiansen, C., C. Thomsen, O. Rasmussen, et al. Effect of alcohol on glucose, insulin, free fatty acid and triacylglycerol responses to a light meal in non-insulin-dependent diabetic subjects. *Br. J. Nutr.* 71:449–454 (1994).

85. Wing, R.R., E.H. Blair, P. Bononi, et al. Caloric restriction per se is a significant factor in improvements in glycemic control and insulin sensitivity during weight loss in obese NIDDM patients. *Diabetes Care* 17:30–36 (1994).

86. Kemnitz, J.W., E.B. Roecker, R. Weindruch, et al. Dietary restriction increases insulin sensitivity and lowers blood glucose in rhesus monkeys. *Am. J. Physiol.* 266:E540–E547 (1994).

87. Chorváthová, V., P. Bobek, E. Ginter, and J. Klvanová. Effect of the oyster fungus on glycaemia and cholesterolaemia in rats with insulin-dependent diabetes. *Physiol. Res.* 42:175–179 (1993).

88. Raghuman, T.C., R.D. Sharma, B. Sivakumar, and B.K. Sahay. Effect of fenugreek seeds on intravenous glucose disposition in non-insulin dependent diabetic patients. *Phytother. Res.* 8:83–86 (1994).

89. Cramer, D.W., H. Xu, and T. Sahi. Adult hypolactasia, milk consumption, and age-specific fertility. *Am. J. Epidemiol.* 139:282–289 (1994).

90. Allen, L.H. (ed.). *Recent Developments in Maternal Nutrition and Their Implications for Practitioners. Am. J. Clin. Nutr.* 59(Suppl.) (1994).

91. Susser, M., and Z. Stein. Timing in prenatal nutrition: a reprise of the Dutch Famine Study. *Nutr. Rev.* 52:84–94 (1994).

92. Langley, S.C., and A.A. Jackson. Increased systolic blood pressure in adult rats induced by fetal exposure to maternal low protein diets. *Clin. Sci.* 86:217–222 (1994).

93. Kirke, P.N., A.M. Molloy, L.E. Daly, et al. Maternal plasma folate and vitamin B$_{12}$ are independent risk factors for neural tube defects. *Q. J. Med.* 86:703–708 (1993).

94. Nightingale, S.L. Proposals for folic acid fortification and labeling of certain foods to reduce risk of neural tube defects. *JAMA* 270:2283 (1993).

95. Hambidge, M., A. Hackshaw, and N. Wald. Neural tube defects and serum zinc. *Br. J. Obstet. Gynaecol.* 100:746–749 (1993).

96. Scholl, T.O., M.L. Hediger, J.I. Schall, et al. Low zinc intake during pregnancy: its association with preterm and very preterm delivery. *Am. J. Epidemiol.* 137:1115–1124 (1993).

97. Olsen, S.F. Consumption of marine *n*–3 fatty acids during pregnancy as a possible determinant of birth weight. A review of the current epidemiologic evidence. *Epidemiol. Rev.* 15:399–413 (1993).

98. Olsen, S.F., P. Grandjean, P. Weihe, and T. Viderø. Frequency of seafood intake in pregnancy as a determinant of birth weight: evidence for a dose dependent relationship. *J. Epidemiol. Commun. Health* 47:436–440 (1993).

99. Lovegrove, J.A., S.M. Hampton, and J.B. Morgan. The immunological and long-term atopic outcome of infants born to women following a milk-free diet during late pregnancy and lactation: a pilot study. *Br. J. Nutr.* 71:223–238 (1994).

100. Specker, B.L. Nutritional concerns of lactating women consuming vegetarian diets. *Am. J. Clin. Nutr.* 59(Suppl.):1182S–1186S (1994).

101. Merzenich, H., H. Boeing, and J. Wahrendorf. Dietary fat and sports activity as determinants for age at menarche. *Am. J. Epidemiol.* 138:217–224 (1993).

102. Phipps, W.R., M.C. Martini, J.W. Lampe, et al. Effect of flax seed ingestion on the menstrual cycle. *J. Clin. Endocrinol. Metab.* 77:1215–1219 (1993).

103. Gavaler, J.S. Alcohol and nutrition in postmenopausal women. *J. Am. Coll. Nutr.* 12:349–356 (1993).

104. Thissen, J.-P., J.-M. Ketelslegers, and L.E. Underwood. Nutritional regulation of the insulin-like growth factors. *Endocrine Rev.* 15:80–101 (1994).

105. Lamberg-Allardt, C., M. Kärkkäinen, R. Seppänen, and H. Biström. Low serum 25-hydroxyvitamin D concentrations and secondary hyperparathyroidism in middle-aged white strict vegetarians. *Am. J. Clin. Nutr.* 58:684–689 (1993).

106. King, A.J., and A.S. Levey. Dietary protein and renal function. *J. Am. Soc. Nephrol.* 3:1723–1737 (1993).

107. Gentile, M.G., G. Fellin, F. Cofano, et al. Treatment of proteinuric patients with a vegetarian soy diet and fish oil. *Clin. Nephrol.* 40:315–320 (1993).

108. van der Heide, J.J.H., H.J.G. Bilo, J.M. Donker, et al. Effect of dietary fish oil on renal function and rejection in cyclosporine-treated recipients of renal transplants. *New Engl. J. Med.* 329:769–773 (1993).

109. Yokozawa, T., H. Oura, M. Hattori, et al. Inhibitory effect of tannin in green tea on the proliferation of mesangial cells. *Nephron* 65:596–600 (1993).

110. Tovey, F.I. Diet and duodenal ulcer. *J. Gastroenterol. Hepatol.* 9:177–185 (1994).

111. Rydning, A., B. Børkje, O. Lange, et al. Effect of wheat fibre supplements on duodenal ulcer recurrence. *Scand. J. Gastroenterol.* 28:1051–1054 (1993).

112. de la Lastra, C.A., M.J. Martin, and V. Motilva. Antiulcer and gastroprotective effects of quercetin: a gross and histologic study. *Pharmacology* 48:56–62 (1994).

113. Takahashi, S., T. Yoshikawa, Y. Naito, et al. Antioxidant properties of antiulcer Kampo medicines. *Free Rad. Res. Commun.* 19(Suppl.):S101–S108 (1993).

114. Horne, W.I., and H. Tsukamoto. Dietary modulation of alcohol-induced pancreatic injury. *Alcohol* 10:481–484 (1993).

115. Noel-Jorand, M.C., and J. Bras. A comparison of nutritional profiles of patients with alcohol-related pancreatitis and cirrhosis. *Alcohol Alcoholism* 29:65–74 (1994).

116. Brown, W.W., and M. Wolfson. Diet as culprit or therapy. Stone disease, chronic renal failure, and nephrotic syndrome. *Med. Clin. North Am.* 77:783–794 (1993).

117. Goldfarb, S. Diet and nephrolithiasis. *Annu. Rev. Med.* 45:235–243 (1994).

118. Heckers, H., I. Wagner, E. Schmelz, and A. Trenkel. Zur diätetischen Therapie und Prävention von Calciumoxalat-Neirensteinen. *Ernährungs-Umschau* 40:416–420,429 (1993).

119. Hesse, A., R. Siener, H. Heynck, and A. Jahnen. The influence of dietary factors on the risk of urinary stone formation. *Scanning Microscopy* 7:1119–1128 (1993).

120. Martini, L.A., I.P. Heilberg, L. Cuppari, et al. Dietary habits of calcium stone formers. *Br. J. Med. Biol. Res.* 26:805–812 (1993).

121. Strazzullo, P., and M. Mancini. Hypertension, calcium metabolism, and nephrolithiasis. *Am. J. Med. Sci.* 307(Suppl. 1):S102–S106 (1994).

122. Massey, L.K., H. Roman-Smith, and R.A.L. Sutton. Effect of dietary oxalate and calcium on urinary oxalate and risk of formation of calcium oxalate kidney stones. *J. Am. Diet. Assoc.* 93:901–906 (1993).

123. Massey, L.K., and R.A.L. Sutton. Modification of dietary oxalate and calcium reduces urinary oxalate in hyperoxaluric patients with kidney stones. *J. Am. Diet. Assoc.* 93:1305–1307 (1993).

124. Sakhaee, K., J.A. Harvey, P.K. Padalino, et al. The potential role of salt abuse on the risk for kidney stone formation. *J. Urol.* 150:310–312 (1993).

125. Singh, P.P., R. Kiran, A.K. Pendse, et al. Ascorbic acid is an abettor in calcium urolithiasis: an experimental study. *Scanning Microscopy* 7:1041–1048 (1993).

126. Rothwell, P.J.N., R. Green, N.J. Blacklock, and J.P. Kavanagh. Does fish oil benefit stone formers? *J. Urol.* 150:1391–1394 (1993).

127. Duane, W.C. Effects of lovastatin and dietary cholesterol on bile acid kinetics and bile lipid composition in healthy male subjects. *J. Lipid Res.* 35:501–509 (1994).

128. Heaney, R.P. Nutritional factors in osteoporosis. *Annu. Rev. Nutr.* 13:287–316 (1993).

129. Heaney, R.P. Bone mass, nutrition, and other lifestyle factors. *Am. J. Med.* 95(Suppl. 5A):29S–33S (1993).

130. Nilas, L. Nutrition and fitness in the prophylaxis for age-related bone loss in women. In *Nutrition and Fitness in Health and Disease.* A.P. Simopoulos (ed.). Basel, Karger. *World Rev. Nutr. Diet.* 72:102–113 (1993).

131. Wardlaw, G.M. Putting osteoporosis in perspective. *J. Am. Diet. Assoc.* 93:1000–1006 (1993).

132. Harward, M.P. Nutritive therapies for osteoporosis. *Med. Clin. North Am.* 77:889–898 (1993).

133. Lauritzen, J.B., P.A. McNair, and B. Lund. Risk factors for hip fractures. A review. *Dan. Med. Bull.* 40:479–485 (1993).

134. Cumming, R.G., and R.J. Klineberg. Case–control study of risk factors for hip fractures in the elderly. *Am. J. Epidemiol.* 139:493–503 (1994).

135. Nilas, L. Calcium intake and osteoporosis. In *Osteoporosis: Nutritional Aspects.* A.P. Simopoulos and C. Galli (eds.). Basel, Karger. *World Rev. Nutr. Diet.* 73:1–26 (1993).

136. Lee, W.T.K., S.S.F. Leung, and S.S.H. Lui. Relationship between long-term calcium intake and bone mineral content of children aged from birth to 5 years. *Br. J. Nutr.* 70:235–248 (1993).

137. Lloyd, T., M.B. Andon, N. Rollings, et al. Calcium supplementation and bone mineral density in adolescent girls. *JAMA* 270:841–844 (1993).

138. Metz, J.A., J.J.B. Anderson, and P.N. Gallagher, Jr. Intakes of calcium, phosphorus, and protein, and physical-activity level are related to radial bone mass in young adult women. *Am. J. Clin. Nutr.* 58:537–542 (1993).

139. Ramsdale, S.J., E.J. Bassey, and D.J. Pye. Dietary calcium intake relates to bone mineral density in premenopausal women. *Br. J. Nutr.* 71:77–84 (1994).

140. Anderson, J.J.B., and J.A. Metz. Contributions of dietary calcium and physical activity to primary prevention of osteoporosis in females. *J. Am. Coll. Nutr.* 12:378–383 (1993).

141. Murphy, S., K.-T. Khaw, H. May, and J.E. Compston. Milk consumption and bone mineral density in middle aged and elderly women. *Br. Med. J.* 308:939–941 (1994).

142. Hu, J.-F., X.-H. Zhao, J.-B. Jia, et al. Dietary calcium and bone density among middle-aged and elderly women in China. *Am. J. Clin. Nutr.* 58:219–227 (1993).

143. Prince, R. The calcium controversy revisited: implications of new data. *Med. J. Aust.* 159:404–407 (1993).

144. Aloia, J.F., A. Vaswani, J.K. Yeh, et al. Calcium supplementation with and without hormone replacement therapy to prevent postmenopausal bone loss. *Ann. Intern. Med.* 120:97–103 (1994).

145. Calvo, M.S. Dietary phosphorus, calcium metabolism and bone. *J. Nutr.* 123:1627–1633 (1993).

146. Lemann, J., Jr., J.A. Pleuss, and R.W. Gray. Potassium causes calcium retention in healthy adults. *J. Nutr.* 123:1623–1626 (1993).

147. Saltman, P.D., and L.G. Strause. The role of trace minerals in osteoporosis. *J. Am. Coll. Nutr.* 12:384–389 (1993).

148. Boivin, G., J. Dupuis, and P.J. Meunier. Fluoride and osteoporosis. In *Osteoporosis: Nutritional Aspects.* A.P. Simopoulos and C. Galli (eds.). Basel, Karger. *World Rev. Nutr. Diet.* 73:80–103 (1993).

149. Hofeldt, F.D. Vitamin D deficiency: a culprit in metabolic bone disease. *Prog. Food Nutr. Sci.* 17:377–399 (1993).

150. Anonymous. Supplementation with vitamin $D_3$ and calcium prevents hip fractures in elderly women. *Nutr. Rev.* 51:183–185 (1993).

151. Das, U.N. Can essential fatty acids prevent osteoporosis? *Med. Sci. Res.* 22:163–165 (1994).

152. Sakaguchi, K., I. Morita, and S. Murota. Eicosapentaenoic acid inhibits bone loss due to ovariectomy in rats. *Prostaglandins Leukotrienes Essential Fatty Acids* 50:81–84 (1994).

153. Reed, J.A., J.J.B. Anderson, F.A. Tylavsky, and P.N. Gallagher, Jr. Comparative changes in radial-bone density of elderly female lactoovovegetarians and omnivores. *Am. J. Clin. Nutr.* 59(Suppl.):1197S–1202S (1994).

154. Weaver, C.M., and K.L. Plawecki. Dietary calcium: adequacy of a vegetarian diet. *Am. J. Clin. Nutr.* 59(Suppl.): 1238S–1241S (1994).

155. Navia, J.M. Carbohydrates and dental health. *Am. J. Clin. Nutr.* 59(Suppl.):719S–727S (1994).

156. Serra Majem, Ll., R. García Closas, J.M. Ramón, et al. Dietary habits and dental caries in a population of Spanish schoolchildren with low levels of caries experience. *Caries Res.* 27:488–494 (1993).

157. Littleton, J., and B. Frohlich. Fish-eaters and farmers: dental pathology in the Arabian Gulf. *Am. J. Phys. Anthropol.* 92:427–447 (1993).

158. Ooshima, T., T. Minami, W. Aono, et al. Oolong tea polyphenols inhibit experimental dental caries in SPF rats infected with mutans streptococci. *Caries Res.* 27:124–129 (1993).

159. Applewhite, M.P., G.R. Jansen, B.M. Marriott, and V. McC. Breen. The effects of diet on performance—an initial review. *JAMA* 271:98 (1994).

160. Fernstrom, J.D. Dietary amino acids and brain function. *J. Am. Diet. Assoc.* 94:71–77 (1994).

161. Wolraich, M.L., S.D. Lindgren, P.J. Stumbo, et al. Effects of diets high in sucrose or aspartame on the behavior and cognitive performance of children. *New Engl. J. Med.* 330:301–307 (1994).

162. Bernstein, G.A., M.E. Carroll, R.D. Crosby, et al. Caffeine effects on learning, performance, and anxiety in normal school-age children. *J. Am. Acad. Child Adolesc. Psychiatry* 33:407–415 (1994).

163. Carter, C.M., M. Urbanowicz, R. Hemsley, et al. Effects of a few food diet in attention deficit disorder. *Arch. Dis. Child.* 69:564–568 (1993).

164. Winocur, G., and C.E. Greenwood. High-fat diets impair conditional discrimination learning in rats. *Psychobiology* 21:286–292 (1993).

165. Yehuda, S., and R.L. Carasso. Modulation of learning, pain thresholds, and thermoregulation in the rat by preparations of free purified α-linolenic and linoleic acids: determination of the optimal ω3-to-ω6 ratio. *Proc. Natl. Acad. Sci. USA* 90:10345–10349 (1993).

166. Wainwright, P.E., Y.-S. Huang, B. Bulman-Fleming, et al. The effects of dietary fatty acid composition combined with environmental enrichment on brain and behavior in mice. *Behav. Brain Res.* 60:125–136 (1994).

167. Wallin, M.S., and A.M. Rissanen. Food and mood: the relationship between food, serotonin and affective disorders. *Acta Psychiatr. Scand.* Suppl. 377:36–40 (1994).

168. Silverstone, T. Mood, food and 5-HT. *Int. Clin. Psychopharmacol.* 8(Suppl. 2):91–94 (1993).

169. Smith, A., A. Kendrick, A. Maben, and J. Salmon. Effects of breakfast and caffeine on cognitive performance, mood and cardiovascular functioning. *Appetite* 22:39–55 (1994).

170. Smith, A., A. Maben, and P. Borckman. Effects of evening meals and caffeine on cognitive performance, mood and cardiovascular functioning. *Appetite* 22:57–65 (1994).

171. Farooqui, S.M., J.W. Brock, E.S. Onaivi, et al. Differential modulation of dopaminergic systems in the rat brain by dietary protein. *Neurochem. Res.* 19:167–176 (1994).

172. Gray, R.F., F.M. Corrigan, A. Strathdee, et al. Cholesterol metabolism and violence: a study of individuals convicted of violent crimes. *NeuroReport* 4:754–756 (1993).

173. Giem, P., W.L. Beeson, and G.E. Fraser. The incidence of dementia and intake of animal products: preliminary findings from the Adventist Health Study. *Neuroepidemiology* 12:28–36 (1993).

174. Sparks, D.L., S.W. Scheff, J.C. Hunsaker III, et al. Induction of Alzheimer-like β-amyloid immunoreactivity in the brains of rabbits with dietary cholesterol. *Exp. Neurol.* 126:88–94 (1994).

175. Kempster, P.A., and M.L. Wahlqvist. Dietary factors in the management of Parkinson's disease. *Nutr. Rev.* 52:51–58 (1994).

176. Sepčić, J., E. Mesaroš, E. Materljan, and D. Šepić-Grahovac. Nutritional factors and multiple sclerosis in Gorski Kotar, Croatia. *Neuroepidemiology* 12:234–240 (1993).

177. Bunce, G.E. Nutrition and eye disease of the elderly. *J. Nutr. Biochem.* 5:66–77 (1994).

178. Sperduto, R.D., T.-S. Hu, R.C. Milton, et al. The Linxian cataract studies. *Arch. Ophthalmol.* 111:1246–1253 (1993).

179. Bunce, G.E. Evaluation of the impact of nutrition intervention on cataract prevalence in China. *Nutr. Rev.* 52:99–101 (1994).

180. Schoenfeld, E.R., M.C. Leske, and S.-Y. Wu. Recent epidemiologic studies on nutrition and cataract in India, Italy and the United States. *J. Am. Coll. Nutr.* 12:521–526 (1993).

181. Birlouez-Aragon, I., P. Scalbert-Menanteau, L. Ravelontseheno, et al. Milk consumption and cataract formation. Impairment of galactose metabolism in elderly and diabetic subjects. In *Common Food Intolerances 2: Milk in Human Nutrition and Adult-Type Hypolactasia.* S. Auricchio

and G. Semenza (eds.). Basel, Karger. *Dynam. Nutr. Res.* 3:40–51 (1993).

182. Yokoyama, T., H. Sasaki, F.J. Giblin, and V.N. Reddy. A physiological level of ascorbate inhibits galactose cataract in guinea pigs by decreasing polyol accumulation in the lens epithelium: a dehydroascorbate-linked mechanism. *Exp. Eye Res.* 58:207–218 (1994).

183. Fryer, M.J. Evidence for the photoprotective effects of vitamin E. *Photochem. Photobiol.* 58:304–312 (1993).

184. West, S., S. Vitale, J. Hallfrisch, et al. Are antioxidants or supplements protective for age-related macular degeneration? *Arch. Ophthalmol.* 112:222–227 (1994).

185. Fawzi, W.W., M.G. Herrera, W.C. Willett, et al. Vitamin A supplementation and dietary vitamin A in relation to the risk of xerophthalmia. *Am. J. Clin. Nutr.* 58:385–391 (1993).

186. Cockburn, F. Neonatal brain and dietary lipids. *Arch. Dis. Child.* 70:F1–F2 (1994).

187. Innis, S.M. Essential fatty acid requirements in human nutrition. *Can. J. Physiol. Pharmacol.* 71:699–706 (1993).

188. Van Aerde, J.E., and M.T. Clandinin. Controversy in fatty acid balance. *Can. J. Physiol. Pharmacol.* 71:707–712 (1993).

189. Decsi, T., and B. Koletzko. Polyunsaturated fatty acids in infant nutrition. *Acta Pœdiatr.* Suppl. 395:31–37 (1994).

190. Farquharson, J., F. Cockburn, W.A. Patrick, et al. Effect of diet on infant subcutaneous tissue triglyceride fatty acids. *Arch. Dis. Child.* 69:589–593 (1993).

191. Carlson, S.E., S.H. Werkman, P.G. Rhodes, and E.A. Tolley. Visual-acuity development in healthy preterm infants: effect of marine-oil supplementation. *Am. J. Clin. Nutr.* 58:35–42 (1993).

192. Winter, C.H., E.B. Hoving, and F.A.J. Muskiet. Fatty acid composition of human milk triglyceride species. Possible consequences for optimal structures of infant formula triglycerides. *J. Chromatogr.* 616:9–24 (1993).

193. Brühl, L., E. Schulte, and H.-P. Thier. Zusammensetzung und Aufbau der Triglyceride von Muttermilch und einiger Rohstoffe für Säuglingsnahrung. *Fett Wissenschaft Technol.* 96:147–154 (1994).

194. Ford, R.P.K., B.J. Taylor, E.A. Mitchell, et al. Breastfeeding and the risk of sudden infant death syndrome. *Int. J. Epidemiol.* 22:885–890 (1993).

195. Sanders, T.A.B., and S. Reddy. Vegetarian diets and children. *Am. J. Clin. Nutr.* 59(Suppl.):1176S–1181S (1994).

196. Dagnelie, P.C., and W.A. van Staveren. Macrobiotic nutrition and child health: results of a population-based, mixed-longitudinal cohort study in The Netherlands. *Am. J. Clin. Nutr.* 59(Suppl.):1187S–1196S (1994).

197. Palackal, T., M. Neuringer, and J. Sturman. Laminar analysis of the number of neurons, astrocytes, oligodendrocytes and microglia in the visual cortex (area 17) of 6- and 12-month-old rhesus monkeys fed a human infant soy-protein formula with or without taurine supplementation from birth. *Dev. Neurosci.* 15:54–67 (1993).

198. Schek, A. L-Carnitin: Sinn und Unsinn der Substitution einer körpereigenen Substanz. Teil 1: Zur Physiologie und sinnvollen Substitution. *Ernährungs-Umschau* 41:9–15 (1994).

199. Schek, A. L-Carnitin: Sinn und Unsinn der Substitution einer körpereigenen Substanz. Teil 2: Zur fragwürdigen und unsinnigen Substitution. *Ernährungs-Umschau* 41:60–67 (1994).

200. Chhabra, S.K., and A.R. Rao. Transmammary exposure of mouse pups to *Allium sativum* (garlic) and its effect on the neonatal hepatic xenobiotic metabolizing enzymes of mice. *Nutr. Res.* 14:195–210 (1994).

201. Mennella, J.A., and G.K. Beauchamp. The effects of repeated exposure to garlic-flavored milk on the nursling's behavior. *Pediatr. Res.* 34:805–808 (1993).

202. Szylit, O., and C. Andrieux. Physiological and pathophysiological effects of carbohydrate fermentation. In *Intestinal Flora, Immunity, Nutrition and Health*. A.P. Simopoulos et al. (eds.). Basel, Karger. *World Rev. Nutr. Diet.* 74:88–122 (1993).

203. Feldman, E.B. Aspects of the interrelations of nutrition and aging—1993. *Am. J. Clin. Nutr.* 58:1–3 (1993).

204. Russell, R.M., and P.M. Suter. Vitamin requirements of elderly people: an update. *Am. J. Clin. Nutr.* 58:4–14 (1993).

205. Hoffman, N. Diet in the elderly. Needs and risks. *Med. Clin. North Am.* 77:745–756 (1993).

206. Posner, B.M., A.M. Jette, K.W. Smith, and D.R. Miller. Nutrition and health risks in the elderly: the Nutrition Screening Initiative. *Am. J. Public Health* 83:972–978 (1993).

207. Posner, B.M, A. Jette, C. Smigelski, et al. Nutritional risk in New England elders. *J. Gerontol.* 49:M123–M132 (1994).

208. Morley, J.E. Nutrition and the older female: a review. *J. Am. Coll. Nutr.* 12:337–343 (1993).

209. Joosten, E., A. van den Berg, R. Riezler, et al. Metabolic evidence that deficiencies of vitamin B-12 (cobalamin), folate, and vitamin B-6 occur commonly in elderly people. *Am. J. Clin. Nutr.* 58:468–476 (1993).

210. Yu, B.P. How diet influences the aging process of the rat. *Proc. Soc. Exp. Biol. Med.* 205:97–105 (1994).

211. Ingram, D.K., M.A. Lane, R.G. Cutler, and G.S. Roth. Longitudinal study of aging in monkeys: effects of diet restriction. *Neurobiol. Aging* 14:687–688 (1993).

212. Kubo, I., H. Muroi, and A. Kubo. Antibacterial activity of long-chain alcohols against *Streptococcus mutans*. *J. Agric. Food Chem.* 41:2447–2450 (1993).

213. Muroi, H., and I. Kubo. Combination effects of antibacterial compounds in green tea flavor against *Streptococcus mutans*. *J. Agric. Food Chem.* 41:1102–1105 (1993).

214. Muroi, H., A. Kubo, and I. Kubo. Antimicrobial activity of cashew apple flavor compounds. *J. Agric. Food Chem.* 41:1106–1109 (1993).

215. Nakayama, M., K. Suzuki, M. Toda, et al. Inhibition of infectivity of influenza virus by tea polyphenols. *Antiviral Res.* 21:289–299 (1993).

216. Avorn, J., M. Monane, J.H. Gurwitz, et al. Reduction of bacteriuria and pyuria after ingestion of cranberry juice. *JAMA* 271:751–754 (1994).

217. Osata, J.A., L.A. Santiago, G.M. Remo, et al. Antimicrobial and antioxidant activities of unripe papaya. *Life Sci.* 53:1383–1389 (1993).

218. Levander, O.A., and A.L. Ager, Jr. Malarial parasites and antioxidant nutrients. *Parasitology* 107:S95–S106 (1993).

219. Davis, T.M.E., P. Garcia-Webb, L.-C. Fu, et al. Antioxidant vitamins in acute malaria. *Trans. Roy. Soc. Trop. Med. Hyg.* 87:596–597 (1993).

220. Perez, H.A., M. de la Rosa, and R. Apitz. In vivo activity of ajoene against rodent malaria. *Antimicrob. Agents Chemother.* 38:337–339 (1994).

221. Portier, A., N.P. Boyaka, F. Bougoudogo, et al. Fermented milks and increased antibody responses against cholera in mice. *Int. J. Immunother.* 9:217–224 (1993).

222. Miedema, I., E.J.M. Feskens, D. Heederik, and D. Kromhout. Dietary determinants of long-term incidence of chronic nonspecific lung diseases. The Zutphen Study. *Am. J. Epidemiol.* 138:37–45 (1993).

223. Manner, T., D.P. Katz, B. Skeie, et al. Fish oils and the lung. *Clin. Nutr.* 12:131–146 (1993).

224. Knox, A.J. Salt and asthma. *Br. Med. J.* 307:1159–1160 (1993).

225. Carey, O.J., C. Locke, and J.B. Cookson. Effect of alterations of dietary sodium on the severity of asthma in men. *Thorax* 48:714–718 (1993).

226. Medici, T.C., A.Z. Schmid, M. Häcki, and W. Vetter. Are asthmatics salt-sensitive? A preliminary controlled study. *Chest* 104:1138–1143 (1993).

227. Schwartz, J., and S.T. Weiss. Relationship between dietary vitamin C intake and pulmonary function in the first National Health and Nutrition Examination Survey (NHANES I). *Am. J. Clin. Nutr.* 59:110–114 (1994).

228. Hemilä, H. Does vitamin C alleviate the symptoms of the common cold? A review of current evidence. *Scand. J. Infect. Dis.* 26:1–6 (1994).

229. Rackett, S.C., M.J. Rothe, and J.M. Grant-Kels. Diet and dermatology. The role of dietary manipulation in the prevention and treatment of cutaneous disorders. *J. Am. Acad. Dermatol.* 29:447–461 (1993).

230. Brewer, G.J., V. Yuzbasiyan-Gurkan, R. Dick, et al. Does a vegetarian diet control Wilson's disease? *J. Am. Coll. Nutr.* 12:527–530 (1993).

231. Koch, H.P., W. Jäger, U. Groh, et al. Carbohydrates from garlic bulbs (*Allium sativum* L.) as inhibitors of adenosine deaminase enzyme activity. *Phytother. Res.* 7:387–389 (1993).

232. Kandiah, J., and C. Kies. Calcium carbonate supplements may adversely affect protein nutriture. *Nutr. Res.* 14:177–184 (1994).

233. Randhawa, R.K., and B.L. Kawatra. Effect of dietary protein on the absorption and retention of Zn, Fe, Cu and Mn in pre-adolescent girls. *Nahrung* 37:399–407 (1993).

234. Zheng, J.-j., J.B. Mason, I.H. Rosenberg, and R.J. Wood. Measurement of zinc bioavailability from beef and a ready-to-eat high-fiber breakfast cereal in humans: application of a whole-gut lavage technique. *Am. J. Clin. Nutr.* 58:902–907 (1993).

235. Couzy, F., P. Kastenmayer, R. Mansourian, et al. Zinc absorption in healthy elderly humans and the effect of diet. *Am. J. Clin. Nutr.* 58:690–694 (1993).

236. Leung, P.L., and X.L. Li. The changes of metabolism balance of zinc and copper in gastric juice with widely varying dietary zinc intake. *Biol. Trace Elem. Res.* 39:33–39 (1993).

237. Vaquero, M.P., M. Veldhuizen, W. van Dokkum, et al. Copper bioavailability from breakfasts containing tea. Influence of the addition of milk. *J. Sci. Food Agric.* 64:475–481 (1994).

238. Shackelford, M.E., T.F.X. Collins, T.N. Black, et al. Mineral interactions in rats fed AIN-76A diets with excess calcium. *Food Chem. Toxicol.* 32:255–263 (1994).

239. Hurrell, R.F., S. Ribas, and L. Davidsson. NaFe$^{3+}$EDTA as a food fortificant: influence on zinc, calcium and copper metabolism in the rat. *Br. J. Nutr.* 71:85–93 (1994).

240. MacPhail, A.P., R.C. Patel, T.H. Bothwell, and R.D. Lamparelli. EDTA and the absorption of iron from food. *Am. J. Clin. Nutr.* 59:644–648 (1994).

241. Ip, C., and D.J. Lisk. Bioavailability of selenium from selenium-enriched garlic. *Nutr. Cancer* 20:129–137 (1993).

242. Johansson, E., and T. Westermarck. Studies of selenium supplementation with inorganic and combined inorganic–organic Se in humans. *J. Trace Elem. Electrolytes Health Dis.* 7:113–114 (1993).

243. McGuire, M.K., S.L. Burgert, J.A. Milner, et al. Selenium status of lactating women is affected by the form of selenium consumed. *Am. J. Clin. Nutr.* 58:649–652 (1993).

244. Nierenberg, D.W., T.A. Stukel, L.A. Mott, and E.R. Greenberg. Steady-state serum concentration of alpha tocopherol not altered by supplementation with oral beta carotene. *J. Natl. Cancer Inst.* 86:117–120 (1994).

245. Gregory, J.F. Ascorbic acid bioavailability in foods and supplements. *Nutr. Rev.* 51:301–303 (1993).

246. Williams, L., J.A. Davis, and D.T. Lowenthal. The influence of food on the absorption and metabolism of drugs. *Med. Clin. North Am.* 77:815–829 (1993).

247. Thomas, J.A., and C. Tschanz. Nutrient–drug interactions. In *Nutritional Toxicology*. F.N. Kotsonis et al. (eds.). New York, Raven Press. *Target Organ Toxicology Series.* Pp. 139–148 (1994).

248. Neubert, R., B. Fritzsch, and G. Dongowski. Wechselwirkungen zwischen Nahrungsbestandteilen und Arzneistoffen. *Pharmazie* 48:723–728 (1993).

249. Prescott, L.F., K. Yoovathaworn, K. Makarananda, et al. Impaired absorption of paracetamol in vegetarians. *Br. J. Clin. Pharmacol.* 36:237–240 (1993).

# 5

# Food and Dietary Analysis

# METHODS OF FOOD AND DIETARY ANALYSIS

## Food Constituents

Biosensors consist of a biological recognition element (e.g., an enzyme or antibody) coupled to an electrochemical, mass, optical, or thermal transducer. The use of biosensors is becoming a feasible alternative to conventional techniques for food analysis. A volume in the *Food Science and Technology* series summarizes the state of the art (*1*). General chapters on the types of biosensors and their potential use in the food industry and food research are followed by chapters on specific biosensor devices and their applications.

Petersson et al. have developed an HPLC method for quantitative separation of triacylglycerols in partially hydrogenated fats rich in oleic, elaidic, palmitic, and stearic acids (*2*). Triacylglycerols are described in terms of the number of carbon atoms and double bonds and the geometrical configuration (*cis* or *trans*) of their constituent fatty acids.

Al-Hasani et al. reported a rapid method for determination of cholesterol in single-component and multicomponent prepared foods (*3*). It involves saponification, hexane extraction, and injection into a gas chromatograph without prior derivatization. Recoveries of cholesterol from spiked oil and tomato vegetable soup average 100%, with coefficients of variation (CVs) of 1.5 and 1.6%, respectively. In the more than 300 samples tested, CVs ranged from 0.5 to 8.6%.

Nineteen German laboratories collaborated in a comparative evaluation of three methods for determining cholesterol in egg products (*4*). The methods (two gas chromatographic, one enzymatic) were comparable in precision and accuracy. The gas chromatographic method of Beyer et al. (*J. Assoc. Anal. Chem.* 72:746–748, 1989) required the least time and amount of reagents.

An improved method was reported for simultaneous determination of α-tocopheryl acetate, tocopherols, and tocotrienols in foods (*5*). It involves HPLC separation with fluorescence detection. Methods of sample preparation were developed for infant formulas, breakfast cereals, multivitamin juices, and isotonic beverages.

A new chromatographic method was developed for the separation and simultaneous determination of carotenoids (*6*). Separation of β-carotene, canthaxanthin, lutein, violaxanthin, and neoxanthin was accomplished by thin-layer chromatography (TLC) on Chromarods, followed by detection by flame ionization and a two-stage development technique. Results were highly repro-

ducible. There was no evidence of degradation during the analysis and up to 10 samples could be analyzed simultaneously within 2 h.

Kamal-Eldin et al. compared TLC, gas chromatography (GC), gas chromatography with mass spectrometry (GC/MS), and normal- and reversed-phase HPLC for separation of the lignans in four *Sesamum* species (*7*). Two-dimensional TLC was a valuable qualitative technique, whereas one-dimensional TLC was useful for preparative purposes. GC had many drawbacks as a quantitative tool. GC/MS was necessary to confirm the identity of the lignans. HPLC was simple and rapid for quantitative analyses but neither HPLC method permitted separation and elution of all lignans. A combination of methods was suggested.

Tsuda et al. reported a method for screening edible pulses for antioxidant activity (*8*). The method detected both polar and nonpolar substances. The authors also measured the individual tocopherols (α-, β-, γ-, and δ-) in the pulses.

One of the phenolic components of wines that may reduce CVD risk is *trans*-resveratrol. Mattivi developed a gradient reversed-phase HPLC method for determination of *trans*-resveratrol in wines (*9*). These studies revealed contents of *trans*-resveratrol in Italian wines much higher than those previously reported. Roggero and Archier surveyed the content of resveratrol and one of its glycosides in wines by a direct-injection HPLC method (*10*). They found the highest levels in wines made with mourverdre, pinot, and cabernet-sauvignon varieties and the lowest levels in wines made with gamay, cabernet franc, and grenache grapes.

A collaborative study evaluated an enzymatic–gravimetric method for determining total dietary fiber in foods (*11*). The laboratories analyzed duplicate samples prepared from turnips, wheat bran, canned beans in tomato sauce, rice, and whole wheat bread. Total dietary fiber was reported as the sum of soluble and insoluble fiber, which were determined separately. The method was adopted first action by AOAC International. Marlett and Vollendorf analyzed the dietary fiber of 12 types of vegetables (*12*). Total fiber was measured by both the AOAC method and a modification of the Uppsala method; fiber composition was measured by the Uppsala method. The results indicated that some vegetables that are frequently treated as similar foods in nutritional studies differ widely in fiber content and composition. For some vegetables the source, variety, method of preparation, and analytical method need to be considered in calculating daily intakes of total dietary fiber and fiber components. For example, peeled red potatoes contain 24–36% less fiber than peeled Maine or Wisconsin potatoes.

## Dietary Intake

**BIOMARKERS.** Nutritional exposures can be defined in terms of foods, nutrients, or biomarkers. van 't Veer discussed the overriding importance of appropriate measurement of nutritional exposures in a nutritional epidemiologic study (*13*). Choice of measurement depends on a clear statement of the hypothesis to be tested. This hypothesis will identify the period of time for which exposure should be measured. It will also help in selecting suitable populations for study and the most effective study design. A constant challenge in nutritional epidemiology is to reduce measurement errors in order to maximize the possibility of detecting weak associations. The author summarized principles of dietary assessment in retrospective studies, including use of biomarkers.

Sarkkinen et al. evaluated biomarkers of long-term adherence to fat-modified diets (*14*). Subjects were randomly assigned to a diet high in saturated fat, an AHA-type diet, a monoene-enriched diet, or a low-fat diet for 6 months. The fatty acid composition of erythrocyte and platelet membranes and serum cholesterol esters was measured. A decrease in the relative amount of palmitic acid in cholesterol esters reflected a reduced intake of saturated fat in the AHA and monoene groups. An increased proportion of linoleic acid reflected increased intake of this fatty acid on the AHA diet. The moderate increase in dietary monounsaturated fatty acids did not change any of the measurements, but increased intake of low-erucic-acid rapeseed oil was reflected in a relative increase of α-linolenic acid in cholesterol esters.

Rojas-Hidalgo and Olmedilla discussed the biochemical, functional, clinical, and dietary assessment of carotenoids (*15*). They concluded that methods for measuring carotenoids in humans are still relatively imprecise. Although it is assumed that plasma levels of carotenoids are a qualitative and quantitative index of dietary intake, many other factors associated with the host and the analysis also influence these measurements. Sowell et al. described a reversed-phase HPLC method with multiwavelength detection for the simultaneous determination of retinol, retinyl esters, α-tocopherol, and individual carotenoids in human serum (*16*). They analyzed serum samples from 3480 subjects who participated in several studies, including NHANES III. Bui described a highly sensitive isocratic liquid chromatographic method for the simultaneous quantitative determination of retinol, α-tocopherol, and individual carotenoids in human plasma (*17*). Epler et al. developed a liquid chromatographic method for measuring carotenoids, retinol, retinyl palmitate, and tocopherols in human serum (*18*). The same method is applicable for foods. Retinoids and carotenoids are monitored by a programmable ultraviolet–visible detector; tocopherols are monitored using a fluorescence detector. Lutein, zeaxanthin, β-cryptoxanthin, lycopene, α- and β-carotene, retinol, retinyl palmitate, and α-, γ-, and δ-tocopherol were measured quantitatively. Several polar carotenoids, 2',3'-anhydrolutein, α-cryptoxanthin, and geometric isomers of lycopene and β-carotene were also separated.

Contiero and Folin concluded that analysis of copper and zinc in hair can supplement information from conventional assessments of trace element status (*19*). However, they consider the method of questionable use for assessment of individuals because of wide individual variations, particularly for copper, and the variety of factors that influence concentrations in hair.

Studies of the digestibility of energy, protein, fat, and nonstarch polysaccharides in mixed diets evaluated rats as a model for this type of investigation (*20*). A low-fiber control diet and a variety of fiber-enriched diets were tested. Despite some dissimilarities between humans and rats in ability to digest nutrients, results for the two species were generally comparable. The major differences were that apparent digestibility of protein was slightly lower in humans than in rats, whereas rats had a lower capacity to digest fiber polysaccharides.

**DIET ASSESSMENTS.** Proceedings of the First International Conference on Dietary Assessment Methods, held in September 1992, were published as a supplement to *The American Journal of Clinical Nutrition* (*21*). Sessions at the conference addressed gaps in dietary survey methodology; gaps in epidemiologic research methods; assessment of diets of diverse populations, children, and the elderly; assessment of intake of specific food components; methodologic issues in use of international data sets; evaluating and interpreting dietary data; issues of concern to policy makers; and research priorities.

In investigations of the relationship between intake of fat (or some other nutrient) and disease, it is customary to adjust the data for total energy intake. Brown et al. discussed three statistical methods that have been proposed for doing this (*22*). When these methods are compared under circumstances in which intake of the nutrient of interest is measured as a continuous variable, they yield equivalent results. However, in practice, nutrient intakes are generally categorized into tertiles, quartiles, or quintiles. In this situation, the energy adjustment methods yield strikingly different risk estimates. The authors presented the statistical models that reveal these differences and discussed the importance of their findings for epidemiologic investigations.

Kaaks et al. presented a measurement error model defining the types of error that may occur in dietary intake measurements (23). They discussed how structural equation models can be used to estimate the magnitude of these errors. Dietary questionnaire assessments are usually validated against reference measurements based on weighed food records, although 24-h recalls have also been used. The correlation between questionnaire results and reference measurements is taken as an index of the accuracy of the questionnaire assessment, whereas the difference between group means indicates the average tendency to overestimate or underestimate dietary intake. Most approaches assume that random errors of repeated reference measurements are uncorrelated, so that the average of enough repeated measurements will permit ranking of individuals by their "true" intake level. Kaaks et al. showed how comparison with a third type of measurement (such as a biochemical marker) permits evaluation of the validity of dietary questionnaire measurements even when the random errors of repeat reference measurements cannot be assumed to be independent. A paper by Feunekes et al. illustrates the relative and biomarker-based validity testing of a food-frequency questionnaire (24). The relative validity of a new 104-item semiquantitative food-frequency method to assess intake of fat and cholesterol was tested against a previously validated dietary history interview. The food-frequency questionnaire overestimated mean intakes of total energy, cholesterol, and all types of fat by amounts ranging from 5% for total energy to 30% for linoleic acid. When individuals were classified into quintiles of consumption, the two methods placed 63–82% of subjects in the same category or an adjacent one. Fatty acid levels in adipose tissue and erythrocytes (biomarkers of consumption) showed similar correlations with intakes assessed by the two dietary methods. The authors concluded that the food-frequency questionnaire formed a suitable basis for dietary advice and checking dietary compliance.

A study by Howat et al. demonstrated the importance of using multiple assessment instruments on repeated occasions and comparing the results with an objective measure to determine the validity and reliability of data (25). The authors were determining the effect of training on the accuracy with which subjects estimated the size of food portions. Estimates from food diaries and 24-h recalls (the dietary assessment measures) were compared with objective measurements of total energy expenditure. Both dietary instruments were reliable, reproducible, and—by comparison with energy expendi-

ture measurements—not valid. Total energy intake was underreported by >20%.

Beerman and Dittus compared actual and reported food intakes to test the accuracy of 24-h dietary recall assessments (26). The subjects, students, were required to eat breakfast, lunch, and dinner at a campus dining facility on the first day of the study. All selected foods were recorded by the investigators, and foods not eaten were recorded when the trays were returned. This sort of direct observation is the "gold standard" against which to evaluate other methods of dietary assessment. The next morning, with no prior knowledge that they would be asked to do so, subjects were requested to list all food items eaten at the dining hall the previous day. No verbal prompts were given because the study was intended to show which items were most often omitted during recall. Except for condiments and some side dishes, recall was very accurate. The authors recommended that interviews be designed to assist recall of minor meal components, as they may be high in fat. This study shows that 24-h recall assessments, if carefully conducted, can be highly accurate. By a similar method, the same research group validated a 24-h semiquantitative food-frequency questionnaire. They then tested this questionnaire in a free-living population by comparing estimates of fat intake obtained by twelve questionnaires and twelve 24-h recalls (27). The results of the two methods agreed closely for men, but for women, fat-intake estimates by recall were significantly lower than estimates based on the questionnaire.

Horwath validated a short food-frequency questionnaire for estimating nutrient intake in the elderly (28). The mean age of the 53 subjects was 70 y. When subjects were grouped into quintiles of intake as assessed by the questionnaire and by five 2-d diet records, ≥70% fell into the same or an adjacent quintile.

A study based on food-frequency data from the 1987 National Health Interview Survey showed that classification of individuals into quantiles may be subject to a seasonal bias for some foods or nutrients (29). In general, however, seasonal bias is small and can be minimized if the food-frequency questionnaire is administered in all seasons.

Healthy twin sisters of breast cancer patients are probably well aware of their high-risk status. Richardson et al. used dietary information from a group of such women to answer questions about how accurately perceived dietary change reflects actual change (30). Subjects were aware of dietary guidelines for reducing cancer risk and had opinions about specific foods that increase or decrease risk. The authors found that self-reported perception of dietary change was not a reliable indicator of actual change in food frequency, as measured by differences between sequential food-frequency questionnaires. Moreover, prediction of past food frequency based on perceived change and current intake was less accurate than use of current intake alone. Perceived food intake seems to be biased in different ways for different foods, and is influenced by beliefs about the role of diet in cancer.

A new food-composition database for carotenoids was used to estimate carotenoid intake based on dietary information from 7-d food diaries and a food-frequency questionnaire (*31*). These results were then correlated with plasma carotenoid concentrations. Subjects were healthy nonsmoking men. After adjustment for energy intake, percentage of energy from alcohol, and plasma lipid concentrations, dietary carotenoid intakes were significantly associated with plasma carotenoids for all carotenoids when the questionnaire was used and for all except β-carotene when food diaries were used. The compounds evaluated were α- and β-carotene, β-cryptoxanthin, lycopene, and lutein.

## SOURCES OF FOOD CONSTITUENTS

Agriculture Canada has developed a computerized method to estimate current food sources of nutrients using household food-purchase data from Statistics Canada's family food expenditure survey (FOODEX) (*32*). Comparison of analyses based on 1986 and 1990 FOODEX compilations showed an apparent availability in 1986 of 2620 kcal/d, of which 15.2% was protein, 37.5% fat, and 47.3% carbohydrate. Distribution of the 2740 kcal/d available in 1990 was 14.7% protein, 36.0% fat, and 49.3% carbohydrate. Results based on food-purchase data from FOODEX were fairly consistent with food consumption data as reported from the Nova Scotia Nutrition Survey. Trends for specific nutrients and food groups were summarized.

### Fats

Moffat and McGill discussed the variability of the fatty acid composition of fish oils and the origins of this variability (*33*). It is important that differences in composition be recognized because of the proliferation of fish-oil products, the widespread advice to include more fish in the diet, expanding interest in therapeutic and prophylactic uses of fish oils, and the very specific pharmacological effects of individual fatty acids.

Conjugated linoleic acid (CLA), which has anticarcinogenic properties in animals and against malignant cells in vitro, has been identified in human tissues and fluids. Dairy products are a major dietary source of CLA. Huang et al. determined the CLA content in plasma of 9 ovolactovegetarian men who ate a quarter-pound of cheddar cheese daily for 4 weeks (*34*). Plasma CLA rose 35%, from $7.1 \pm 1.1$ μmol/L at baseline to $9.6 \pm 1.1$ μmol/L at the end of the intervention. Four weeks later it had fallen to $7.8 \pm 1.3$ μmol/L. Similar changes were seen in the plasma phospholipid fraction, in which changes in CLA incorporation were at the expense of linoleic acid at the *sn*-2 position. This corroborates other reports that dietary CLA directly influences CLA levels in humans.

Ratnayake et al. determined the fatty acid content and composition of 100 common items in 17 food categories from Canadian retail markets (*35*). Results were presented in a table, which showed by category, for each item, the source of fat as stated on the package and the percentages of total fat, total *trans* fatty acids, each major saturated and *trans* unsaturated fatty acid, oleic acid, 18:2*n*–3 fatty acids, 18:2*n*–6 fatty acids, and all others (odd and branched-chain fatty acids). The variation in fat content and composition was so wide even within a given category that it was not feasible to define the typical level or range for a category and not possible to reliably estimate the average intake of a particular fatty acid nationally.

*TRANS* FATTY ACIDS. Like the Canadian study (*35*), a survey of *trans* fatty acids in 196 German foods found a very wide range within food categories (*36*). For example, *trans* fatty acid content ranged from 0.6 to 23.5% in margarines and 5.8 to 32.8% in french fries. Except for hydrogenation, food processing had no notable effect on fatty acid composition. The authors pointed out that most *trans* fatty acids are listed in food composition tables under the category "monounsaturated fat," and that a distinction should be made between *cis* and *trans* isomers in this category. They ventured to estimate the average *trans* fat intake in Germany to be 3.4 g/d for women and 4.1 g/d for men. In Australia, Noakes and Nestel estimated mean *trans* fatty acid consumption using simulated diets and food-frequency intake data and established *trans* fat data for important foods (*37*). At present, mean *trans* fat intake is probably less than 2.0–2.5 en%. However, replacement of currently used commercial fats with more highly hydrogenated products would double consumption. The authors estimate that roughly half of the current *trans* fat intake is derived from margarines and the rest is from dairy and beef fats.

Litin et al. reported the *trans* fatty acid content of a variety of animal products, vegetable fats, and commercial and fast-food products analyzed by gas–liquid chromatography (*38*). They state that the intake of *trans* fatty acids from an average American diet can be great enough to thwart the dietary treatment of hypercholesterolemia.

An interesting study by Wolff estimated the contribution of *trans*-18:1 fatty acids from dairy fat to the European diet (*39*). The fatty acid composition of samples of 12 commercial French butters was determined by gas–liquid chromatography. Some small but highly significant differences between autumn and spring butters were seen. For example, the content of *trans*-18:1 was 3.22 ± 0.44% in autumn butter and 4.28 ± 0.47% in spring butter. Minimum and maximum values were 2.46% (in an autumn sample) and 5.10% (in a spring sample). From these data the authors calculated the average daily intake of *trans*-18:1 from dairy products by populations of member states of the EEC. It ranged from 0.57 g in Portugal to 1.66 g in Denmark. The mean for the 12 countries of the EEC was 1.16 g/d per person, comparable to published estimates for the USA. In France, dairy fat contributes more *trans*-18:1 to the average diet than does margarine (1.5 vs. 1.1 g/d).

The impact of dietary *trans* fatty acids in humans has not been clearly determined, but it is likely that the risk—if any—is greater for infants than for adults. Berra summarized data on food sources of *trans* fats and estimates of *trans* fat consumption in Europe and the USA (*40*). The amount of *trans* fat in infant foods and formulas is generally low—lower than in human milk. The metabolism of *trans* fatty acids was discussed. Although broad recommendations cannot be made, pending more specific data on risks it would seem prudent to avoid large intakes of *trans* fatty acids.

## Antioxidants

The list of potentially important dietary antioxidants and their sources is growing. Kanner et al. measured the concentrations of phenolic compounds in three grape varieties and two red wines, and determined their ability to inhibit oxidation of LDL (*41*). Tsuda et al. measured the antioxidative activity of pigments from seeds of *Phaseolus vulgaris* varieties with white, black, and red seed coats (*42*). Cuvelier et al. separated and identified the antioxidant components of oleoresin from sage (*Salvia officinalis*) and measured their antioxidative activity (*43*). Eiserich and Shibamoto reported the antioxidative activity of volatile heterocyclic compounds formed during Maillard reactions (*44*). Onyeneho and Hettiarachchy demonstrated strong antioxidative activity in phenolic

compounds (chiefly chlorogenic, protocatechuic, and caffeic acids) found in potato peels (*45*). Peels from red potatoes contained more polyphenols than peels from brown-skinned varieties. The authors also determined the fatty acid composition of potato peels. Hertog et al. determined the content of the flavonoids quercetin, kaempferol, myricetin, apigenin, and luteolin in fruit juices and other common beverages (*46*). None of the beverages contained detectable luteolin or apigenin. Total flavonoid levels in beer, coffee, chocolate milk, and white wine were low, 1 mg/L. Flavonoid levels in green and black teas were comparable and high; tea prepared from tea bags generally had higher levels than tea prepared from loose leaves. This study augments the database for epidemiologic studies investigating the relationship between intake of antioxidant flavonoids and risk of chronic diseases.

Block discussed nutrient sources of provitamin A carotenoids in the American diet (*47*). Using data from NHANES II she found that only 7 foods (carrots, vegetable soups, greens, spinach, green salad, orange juice, and sweet potatoes) account for half of dietary provitamin A. Beef stew, mixed vegetables, cantaloupe, peaches, broccoli, whole milk, and tomatoes each contribute more than 2%; 35 foods provide 90% of the provitamin A in the U.S. diet. She found that several major contributors of provitamin A are frequently omitted from questionnaires for assessing carotenoid intake (e.g., beef stew and milk) and several foods generally included are of minor importance (e.g., papaya and okra).

## Vitamin K

Lipsky reviewed the function of vitamin K, methods for vitamin K analysis, and the importance of dietary vitamin K in humans and animals (*48*). He argues that "The insistent belief that intestinal bacteria are an important source of vitamin K has led to erroneous conclusions about sources of vitamin K for human nutrition." His review indicated that humans can have nutritional deficiencies of vitamin K in the apparent presence of a normal intestinal microflora, and that dietary sources are crucial for maintaining adequate vitamin K status.

## Trace Elements

Gibson compared the content and major food sources of copper, manganese, selenium, and zinc in vegetarian and omnivorous diets (*49*). Cereals are the major source of copper, manganese, and selenium in most diets. They are also an important zinc source for vegetarians, whereas flesh foods are the primary source of zinc for omnivores.

Despite apparently lower bioavailability of trace elements in vegetarian diets, most adult vegetarians have adequate trace-element status. In fact, copper and manganese status may be higher in vegetarians than in their omnivorous counterparts. Vegetarian children, however, are vulnerable to suboptimal zinc status because of the high zinc requirement for growth and the failure of a child's body to adapt to a vegetarian diet by increased absorption of zinc.

Kumpulainen reported the selenium content of representative staple foods and diets in selected countries (50). The survey showed median intakes ranging from a low of 30 µg/d in Turkey to 130 µg/d in Japan. In many countries, the median intake is below the U.S. RDA. The selenium contents of wheat and potato samples from Sweden, the former Federal Republic of Germany, Switzerland, Scotland, and Norway were very low—except for Swiss wheat flour, which is mixed with imported high-selenium wheat before milling. The selenium content of staple foods in Finland increased sharply when selenium supplementation of fertilizers began in 1985 but has been stable since 1986. Zhang et al. measured the selenium contents of common meats, seafoods, and vegetables from Lubbock, Texas, and compared these with data for comparable local foods elsewhere in the USA and in Canada, France, England, and New Zealand (51). With few exceptions, the data were remarkably consistent. New Zealand, with its low-selenium soil, had the lowest selenium content in food samples.

Großklaus discussed the necessity and effectiveness of supplementing foods with iodine (52). He listed the iodine contents of some common German foods. Feasible vehicles for iodine supplementation include table and cooking salt, seasoning salts, nitrite pickling salt, and bottled infant formula.

## MODIFICATION OF FOOD CONSTITUENTS

Elevated serum cholesterol is a marker of increased risk of early-onset coronary heart disease, but not necessarily the cause. Sieber reviewed the rationale and methods for removing cholesterol from animal foods (53). A number of approaches based on biological, chemical, or physical processes have been successful and their application to animal foods—especially dairy products—is technically feasible. Sieber listed some patents granted for cholesterol removal from fats, to demonstrate the worldwide interest in these processes and their support by important

economic interests. However, Sieber concluded that the influence of dietary cholesterol on serum cholesterol is relatively weak and the extra costs to the consumer of removing it are unjustified. If the diet really contains too much cholesterol it almost certainly contains too much animal fat as well, and simply removing the cholesterol will not solve the problem.

Investigators in Switzerland found that milk from range-fed cows has a higher concentration of *n*–3 fatty acids than milk from cows fed corn and harvested grass (54). A similar relationship was seen in the *n*–3 fatty acid content of platelet-rich plasma from these cows. The authors suggest that milk from cows that graze on fresh grass is nutritionally superior to milk from conventionally fed cows.

In monitoring the content of CLA in cheese during processing, Garcia-Lopez et al. found that levels rose from 9.5 mg per gram of fat in the raw ingredients to 10.7 mg per gram of fat in the finished product (55). No change in the distribution of isomers was apparent. Thus although most of the CLA comes from the raw ingredients, some clearly originates during processing. The authors speculated on possible mechanisms for the formation of CLA during cheese-making.

Leeson discussed the potential for modifying the composition of poultry meat and eggs by dietary strategies (56). Protein content and composition and muscle growth are primarily influenced by genetic background and are refractory to dietary manipulation unless a deficiency is involved. In contrast, the fat content and composition of both meat and eggs is readily altered by diet modification. Higher intake of energy generally causes greater fat deposition, and the fatty acid profile of the tissues is strongly influenced by the fatty acid profile of the diet. Leeson considered the evolving attitudes and preferences of consumers, the particular case of linolenic acid, and the relative benefits and economic costs of implementing the changes that are possible. Hargis and Van Elswyk presented a similar but more comprehensive discussion of the potential for manipulating the fatty acid composition of poultry meat and eggs (57). They considered issues related to the stability and sensory quality of fat-modified eggs. Naber reviewed the potential for modifying the vitamin content of eggs (58). Levels of some vitamins respond rapidly to dietary change. At a modest level of dietary increase, the transfer efficiency to the egg is very high for vitamin A; high for riboflavin, pantothenic acid, biotin, and vitamin $B_{12}$; moderate for vitamins $D_3$ and E; and low for vitamin $K_1$, thiamine, and folacin. This information can guide growers in formulating diets for laying and breeding hens to enhance vitamin content and reduce the variability that has characterized the vitamin composition of eggs.

Although the cholesterol content of eggs strongly resists dietary modification, modest success has been achieved by administering a synthetic HMG-CoA reductase inhibitor to laying hens (*59*). Egg cholesterol content varied inversely with the amount of drug fed. At the highest level, cholesterol was reduced by ~30%, although hens produced significantly fewer eggs with this amount of drug.

Pursel and Solomon summarized methods for the production of transgenic farm animals (*60*). They discussed the particular case of introducing the cloned gene for bovine growth hormone into pigs. Although the resulting transgenic pigs grew faster than their conventional siblings, utilized feed more efficiently, and contained strikingly less fat and more lean tissue, the consequences for the health of the pigs were disastrous. This problem must be addressed in any further attempts to "improve" carcass quality.

Maehr et al. reported a method for enzymatic enhancement of the *n*–3 fatty acid content of fish oils (*61*). Commercially available fish oils with *n*–3 contents ranging from 29 to 34% yielded products with mixtures of acylglycerols containing ~50% *n*–3 fatty acids.

## LITERATURE CITED

1. Wagner, G., and G.G. Guilbault (eds.). *Food Biosensor Analysis.* New York, Marcel Dekker, Inc. *Food Science and Technology. A Series of Monographs, Textbooks, and Reference Books.* Vol. 60 (1994).

2. Petersson, B., O. Podlaha, and B. Jirskog-Hed. Triacylglycerol analysis of partially hydrogenated fats using high-performance liquid chromatography. *J. Chromatogr. A* 653:25–35 (1993).

3. Al-Hasani, S.M., J. Hlavac, and M.W. Carpenter. Rapid determination of cholesterol in single and multi-component prepared foods. *J. AOAC Int.* 76:902–906 (1993).

4. Littmann Nienstedt. Auswertung des Ringversuches der § 35-Arbeitsgruppe „Ei-Analytik" zur Bestimmung von Cholesterin in Eiprodukten. *Dtsch. Lebensm.-Rundsch.* 89:283–285 (1993).

5. Balz, M.K., E. Schulte, and H.-P. Thier. Simultaneous determination of α-tocopheryl acetate, tocopherols and tocotrienols by HPLC with fluorescence detection in foods. *Fett Wissenschaft Technol.* 95:215–220 (1993).

6. Rosas Romero, A.J., J.C. Herrera, E.M. De Aparicio, and E.A.M. Cuevas. Thin-layer chromatographic determination of β-carotene, cantaxanthin [sic], lutein, violaxanthin and neoxanthin on Chromarods. *J. Chromatogr. A* 667:361–366 (1994).

7. Kamal-Eldin, A., L.Å. Appelqvist, and G. Yousif. Lignan analysis in seed oils from four *Sesamum* species: comparison of different chromatographic methods. *J. Am. Oil Chem. Soc.* 71:141–147 (1994).

8. Tsuda, T., Y. Makino, H. Kato, et al. Screening for antioxidative activity of edible pulses. *Biosci. Biotechnol. Biochem.* 57:1606–1608 (1993).

9. Mattivi, F. Solid phase extraction of *trans*-resveratrol from wines for HPLC analysis. *Z. Lebensm. Unters. Forsch.* 196:522–525 (1993).

10. Roggero, J.-P., and P. Archier. Dosage du resvératrol et de l'un de ses glycosides dans les vins. *Sci. Aliments* 14:99–107 (1994).

11. Mongeau, R., and R. Brassard. Enzymatic-gravimetric determination in foods of dietary fiber as sum of insoluble and soluble fiber fractions: summary of collaborative study. *J. AOAC Int.* 76:923–925 (1993).

12. Marlett, J.A., and N.W. Vollendorf. Dietary fiber content and composition of vegetables determined by two methods of analysis. *J. Agric. Food Chem.* 41:1608–1612 (1993).

13. van 't Veer, P. Measuring nutritional exposures including biomarkers. *Proc. Nutr. Soc.* 53:27–35 (1994).

14. Sarkkinen, E.S., J.J. Ågren, I. Ahola, et al. Fatty acid composition of serum cholesterol esters, and erythrocyte and platelet membranes as indicators of long-term adherence to fat-modified diets. *Am. J. Clin. Nutr.* 59:354–370 (1994).

15. Rojas-Hidalgo, E., and B. Olmedilla. Carotenoids. *Int. J. Vit. Nutr. Res.* 63:265–269 (1993).

16. Sowell, A.L., D.L. Huff, P.R. Yeager, et al. Retinol, α-tocopherol, lutein/zeaxanthin, β-cryptoxanthin, lycopene, α-carotene, *trans*-β-carotene, and four retinyl esters in serum determined simultaneously by reversed-phase HPLC with multiwavelength detection. *Clin. Chem.* 40:411–416 (1994).

17. Bui, M.H. Simple determination of retinol, α-tocopherol and carotenoids (lutein, all-*trans*-lycopene, α- and β-carotenes) in human plasma by isocratic liquid chromatography. *J. Chromatogr. B* 654:129–133 (1994).

18. Epler, K.S., R.G. Ziegler, and N.E. Craft. Liquid chromatographic method for the determination of carotenoids, retinoids and tocopherols in human serum and in food. *J. Chromatogr. Biomed. Appl.* 619:37–48 (1993).

19. Contiero, E., and M. Folin. Trace elements nutritional status. Use of hair as a diagnostic tool. *Biol. Trace Elem. Res.* 40:151–160 (1994).

20. Bach Knudsen, K.E., E. Wisker, M. Daniel, et al. Digestibility of energy, protein, fat and non-starch polysaccharides in mixed diets: comparative studies between man and the rat. *Br. J. Nutr.* 71:471–487 (1994).

21. Buzzard, I.M., and W.C. Willett (eds.). *Dietary Assessment Methods. Am. J. Clin. Nutr.* 59(1S) (1994).

22. Brown, C.C., V. Kipnis, L.S. Freedman, et al. Energy adjustment methods for nutritional epidemiology: the effect of categorization. *Am. J. Epidemiol.* 139:323–338 (1994).

23. Kaaks, R., E. Riboli, J. Estève, et al. Estimating the accuracy of dietary questionnaire assessments: validation in terms of structural equation models. *Stat. Med.* 13:127–142 (1994).

24. Feunekes, G.I.J., V.A. Van Staveren, J.H.M. De Vries, et al. Relative and biomarker-based validity of a food-frequency questionnaire estimating intake of fats and cholesterol. *Am. J. Clin. Nutr.* 58:489–496 (1993).

25. Howat, P.M., R. Mohan, C. Champagne, et al. Validity and reliability of reported dietary intake data. *J. Am. Diet. Assoc.* 94:169–173 (1994).

26. Beerman, K.A., and K. Dittus. Sources of error associated with self-reports of food intake. *Nutr. Res.* 13:765–770 (1993).

27. Dittus, K.L., K.A. Beerman, and M.A. Evans. Testing the utility of a 24-hour semiquantitative food frequency questionnaire for estimating fat intake in a free living population. *Nutr. Res.* 14:807–815 (1994).

28. Horwath, C.C. Validity of a short food frequency questionnaire for estimating nutrient intake in elderly people. *Br. J. Nutr.* 70:3–14 (1993).

29. Subar, A.F., C.M. Frey, L.C. Harlan, and L. Kahle. Differences in reported food frequency by season of questionnaire administration: the 1987 National Health Interview Survey. *Epidemiology* 5:226–233 (1994).

30. Richardson, J.L., C. Koprowski, G.T. Mondrus, et al. Perceived change in food frequency among women at elevated risk of breast cancer. *Nutr. Cancer* 20:71–78 (1993).

31. Forman, M.R., E. Lanza, L.-C. Yong, et al. The correlation between two dietary assessments of carotenoid intake and plasma carotenoid concentrations: application of a carotenoid food-composition database. *Am. J. Clin. Nutr.* 58:519–524 (1993).

32. Robichon-Hunt, L., and L.G. Robbins. Food sources of nutrients available in the Canadian diet, 1990—an estimation based on food purchase data. *J. Can. Diet. Assoc.* 54:185–189 (1993).

33. Moffat, C.F., and A.S. McGill. Variability of the composition of fish oils: significance for the diet. *Proc. Nutr. Soc.* 52:441–456 (1993).

34. Huang, Y.-C., L.O. Luedecke, and T.D. Shultz. Effect of cheddar cheese consumption on plasma conjugated linoleic acid concentrations in men. *Nutr. Res.* 14:373–386 (1994).

35. Ratnayake, W.M.N., R. Hollywood, E. O'Grady, and G. Pelletier. Fatty acids in some common food items in Canada. *J. Am. Coll. Nutr.* 12:651–660 (1993).

36. Steinhart, H., and A. Pfalzgraf. *Trans*-Fettsäuren in Lebensmitteln. *Fett Wissenschaft Technol.* 96:42–44 (1994).

37. Noakes, M., and P.J. Nestel. *Trans* fatty acids in the Australian diet. *Food Aust.* 46:124–129 (1994).

38. Litin, L., and F. Sacks. *Trans*-fatty-acid content of common foods. (Letter.) *New Engl. J. Med.* 329:1969–1970 (1993).

39. Wolff, R.L. Contribution of *trans*-18:1 acids from dairy fat to European diets. *J. Am. Oil Chem. Soc.* 71:277–283 (1994).

40. Berra, B. *Trans* fatty acids in infantile nutrition. *Nutr. Res.* 13(Suppl. 1):S47–S59 (1993).

41. Kanner, J., E. Frankel, R. Granit, et al. Natural antioxidants in grapes and wines. *J. Agric. Food Chem.* 42:64–69 (1994).

42. Tsuda, T., K. Ohshima, S. Kawakishi, and T. Osawa. Antioxidative pigments isolated from the seeds of *Phaseolus vulgaris* L. *J. Agric. Food Chem.* 42:248–251 (1994).

43. Cuvelier, M.-E., C. Berset, and H. Richard. Antioxidant constituents in sage (*Salvia officinalis*). *J. Agric. Food Chem.* 42:665–669 (1994).

44. Eiserich, J.P., and T. Shibamoto. Antioxidative activity of volatile heterocyclic compounds. *J. Agric. Food Chem.* 42:1060–1063 (1994).

45. Onyeneho, S.N., and N.S. Hettiarachchy. Antioxidant activity, fatty acids and phenolic acids compositions of potato peels. *J. Sci. Food Agric.* 62:345–350 (1993).

46. Hertog, M.G.L., P.C.H. Hollman, and B. van de Putte. Content of potentially anticarcinogenic flavonoids of tea infusions, wines, and fruit juices. *J. Agric. Food Chem.* 41:1242–1246 (1993).

47. Block, G. Nutrient sources of provitamin A carotenoids in the American diet. *Am. J. Epidemiol.* 139:290–293 (1994).

48. Lipsky, J.J. Nutritional sources of vitamin K. *Mayo Clin. Proc.* 69:462–466 (1994).

49. Gibson, R.S. Content and bioavailability of trace elements in vegetarian diets. *Am. J. Clin. Nutr.* 59(Suppl.):1223S–1232S (1994).

50. Kumpulainen, J.T. Selenium in foods and diets of selected countries. *J. Trace Elem. Electrolytes Health Dis.* 7:107–108 (1993).

51. Zhang, X., B. Shi, and J.E. Spallholz. The selenium content of selected meats, seafoods, and vegetables from Lubbock, Texas. *Biol. Trace Elem. Res.* 39:161–169 (1993).

52. Großklaus, R. Jodierung von Lebensmitteln. *Ernährungs-Umschau* 41:55–59 (1994).

53. Sieber, R. Cholesterol removal from animal food—can it be justified? *Lebensm. Wiss. Technol.* 26:375–387 (1993).

54. Hebeisen, D.F., F. Hoeflin, H.P. Reusch, et al. Increased concentrations of omega-3 fatty acids in milk and platelet rich plasma of grass-fed cows. *Int. J. Vit. Nutr. Res.* 63:229–233 (1993).

55. Garcia-Lopez, S., E. Echeverria, I. Tsui, and B. Balch. Changes in the content of conjugated linoleic acid (CLA) in processed cheese during processing. *Food Res. Int.* 27:61–64 (1994).

56. Leeson, S. Potential of modifying poultry products. *J. Appl. Poultry Res.* 2:380–384 (1993).

57. Hargis, P.S., and M.E. Van Elswyk. Manipulating the fatty acid composition of poultry meat and eggs for the health conscious consumer. *World's Poultry Sci. J.* 49:251–264 (1993).

58. Naber, E.C. Modifying vitamin composition of eggs: a review. *J. Appl. Poultry Res.* 2:385–393 (1993).

59. Elkin, R.G., M.B. Freed, K.A. Kieft, and R.S. Newton. Alteration of egg yolk cholesterol content and plasma lipoprotein profiles following administration of a totally synthetic HMG-CoA reductase inhibitor to laying hens. *J. Agric. Food Chem.* 41:1094–1101 (1993).

60. Pursel, V.G., and M.B. Solomon. Alteration of carcass composition in transgenic swine. *Food Rev. Int.* 9:423–439 (1993).

61. Maehr, H., G. Zenchoff, and D.L. Coffen. Enzymic enhancement of *n*–3 fatty acid content in fish oils. *J. Am. Oil Chem. Soc.* 71:463–467 (1994).

# Part II: Safety of Food Components

# 6

# Assessment of Food Safety

A recent volume in the Target Organ Toxicology Series, *Nutritional Toxicology*, included chapters on a number of topics related to toxicological evaluation of food components and the impact of nutrition on disease (*1*). Among these topics were mechanistic considerations in the regulation of carcinogens, postmarketing surveillance in the food industry as exemplified by aspartame monitoring, threshold regulation, and the safety of biotechnology-derived foods.

Volume 7 of the *Handbook of Natural Toxins* comprehensively reviewed mushroom poisons, mycotoxins, seafood toxins, lectins, goitrogens, teratogens, and alkaloids in plants, nitrosamines in foods, and antibiotic residues in foods, in addition to toxins of bacterial origin (*2*). Each chapter described the structures and distribution of the important compounds found in foods, their biological effects, and methods for detection.

Biosensors have been developed for the detection of a variety of toxins, preservatives and compounds indicative of freshness in foods. A recent book (*3*) on this topic describes the rapid advances in the field of biosensors and discusses the need for biosensors in the food industry; the use of enzyme electrodes for food analysis; fiber-optic biosensors based on fluorimetric and on luminometric detection; whole cells and tissue sensors; and piezoelectric immunosensors. Such biosensors can detect compounds of interest with a great deal of specificity, speed, and accuracy.

# GENERAL DESIGN AND INTERPRETATION OF TOXICITY ASSAYS

Although toxicity tests in animals are still considered essential at some point in the evaluation process, the concern for animal welfare and the desire to reduce the cost and time required in toxicity testing has led to the development of a number of non-animal models for testing. A recent book edited by Kapis and Gad (*4*) reviewed such alternative techniques. Included were chapters on various in vitro methods currently in use, structure–activity approaches to predicting human toxicity, neurochemical indicators used in biological studies in psychiatry, network models in behavioral neuroscience, and computational modeling systems.

Proceedings of a 1992 Toxicology Conference on applications of recent innovations in toxicological methods in risk assessment have been published (*5*). Papers from different sessions in the conference considered alternatives to animals in toxicology research, pharmacokinetics in risk assessment, mechanisms in carcinogenicity, and advances in the assessment of toxicological end points.

A report by the British Toxicological Society presented a critical review of the optimum duration of chronic rodent testing studies for the determination of nontumorigenic toxic potential (*6*). A total of 81 reports on toxicity assays on pharmaceuticals, food additives/packaging material, agrochemicals, and industrial chemicals were examined to determine whether any new nontumorigenic, toxicological effects were observed after 3 months of testing in rodents. For 70% of the compounds considered, all toxicological findings in the two-year test were seen in, or predicted by, the 13-week tests. Although 6 months of repeated testing appeared to be adequate for pharmaceuticals, this test duration could not be recommended for all classes of chemicals. Further analyses utilizing confidential surveys of industrial data may aid in determining concordance between short- and long-term testing results for a larger group of chemicals.

A report has been published from a 1993 National Toxicology Program (NTP) workshop considering diets for Fischer 344 rats in long-term studies (*7*). Since 1980, the standard diet used in NTP studies has been the NIH-07 open-formula non-purified diet but there have been concerns that this diet may, by itself, be promoting toxic effects in the animals. A new diet has been proposed which contains about half the protein of the NIH-07 diet, increased levels of fat, fiber, and vitamin $B_{12}$, decreased levels of vitamin A, soybean, corn gluten, and fish meals, and eliminates dried skim milk.

Another aspect of experimental design, which may affect the outcome of testing, is the route of administration of test chemicals. Ashby (*8*) related that such a variation in testing caused the flavoring agent benzyl acetate to be classified as a carcinogen in 1986 when it was administered to rats and mice by gavage and as a noncarcinogen in 1993 when it was administered to these rodents mixed in their feed. Following gavage, peak blood levels of this compound were 300-fold higher than they were after consumption in the diet. This may explain the difference in carcinogenicity. But, as the author points out, most human exposures are through the diet and this route is therefore probably more relevant.

Compounds are often administered by gavage because they would be unstable if added directly to feed or drinking water. Microencapsulation in a medium of food-grade corn starch and sucrose was found to prevent the degradation of citral and permit its testing as a dietary additive. In experiments with mice, citral administered by gavage was found to be much more toxic than administration of the same compound by micro-encapsulation in feed (*9*).

Two recent reviews by Carman et al. (*10*) and by Roland et al. (*11*) discussed interactions between intestinal microflora and dietary components and their possible health consequences. An extremely complex and metabolically active group of microorganisms normally inhabit the colon. On the one hand, these microbes may be capable of detoxifying or toxifying various dietary components while, on the other hand, various foods consumed in different amounts by humans may selectively enhance or inhibit the growth of certain species. The first paper describes numerous microflora-associated characteristics (MACs) such as bile acids, fecal long-chain fatty acids, bacterial cellular fatty acids, short-chain fatty acids, cholesterol and copro-stanol, ratio of aerobes to anaerobes, fecal enzymes, and pH. Evaluation of new food components such as artificial fats and non-nutritive bulking agents should include a study of their effects on MACs. The latter paper reviews xenobiotic metabolizing enzymes and their activity in intestinal microflora. This was illustrated by a description of the effects of microflora on the toxicity of glucosinolates consumed in the diet.

Semi-permeable, magnetically recoverable, reactive microcapsules of various types have been synthesized for gastrointestinal monitoring of several kinds of genotoxic substances. O'Neill et al. (*12*) summarized and discussed data from numerous of their experiments utilizing capsules containing DNA-type substrates to detect the presence of alkylating agents, cross-linking agents, and reactive oxygen precursors. Use of these capsules demonstrated the importance of major dietary changes in intakes of fat and of fiber non-starch polysaccharides and the presence of genotoxic agents such as heterocyclic amines.

Although toxins are usually tested individually, there may be multiple toxic compounds in contaminated foods and water. An overview of a symposium addressing the biologic and toxicologic issues involved in risk assessment of chemical mixtures was presented by Mumtaz et al. (*13*). Mechanisms of toxicant interactions, physiologically based pharmacokinetic modeling of mixtures, and toxicology of chemical mixtures were discussed. Guidelines for risk assessment of chemical mixtures and current issues related to assessment procedures were also presented.

A new quantitative approach for analysis of binary toxic mixtures has been developed by Haas and Stirling (*14*). This method allowed ready assessment of the presence or absence of interactions between the test compounds and would enable regulatory agencies to more reliably estimate risks from mixtures of chemicals likely to be encountered in nature. Application of the proposed approach was illustrated using experimental data from studies on the joint administration of benzene and perchloroethylene to rats and on the joint administration of nickel, lead, and chromium to a copepod.

Papers from the 1991 International Biostatistics Conference on the Study of Toxicology have recently been published (*15*). Topics discussed included statistical issues in experimental design, multiple comparisons in long-term assays, statistical evaluation of mutagenicity test data from several assays, and predicting carcinogenicity using batteries of short-term tests.

Currently the NOAEL (no observed adverse effect level) is determined by identifying the highest administered dose of an agent which does not cause a response which is statistically significantly different from the control. However, Calabrese and Baldwin (*16*) contend that the NOAEL should be defined both in terms of the control and the LOAEL (lowest observed adverse effect level): the NOAEL is the highest dose that is not statistically significantly different from the control and yet is significantly different from the LOAEL. Adoption of this new definition would have implications for designing experiments for determining safety factors. These authors also proposed a new method for deriving the size of the interspecies uncertainty factor (*17*). They recommend that interspecies variation in susceptibility to toxic factors be quantified by the use of binary interspecies comparisons within 4 categories of phylogenetic relatedness. These 95% uncertainty factors would range from a low of 10 for species within a genus to a high of 65 for orders within a class. Since most mammalian toxicology studies use rodents, dogs, or cats, these would involve orders-within-a-class comparisons and have an uncertainty factor of 65.

The NOAEL for the most sensitive toxicological parameter for the most sensitive species forms the basis for estimating acceptable or tolerable daily intakes (ADI or TDI). The use of this animal-derived data for estimating human risks was discussed by Renwick and Walker (*18*) and Renwick (*19*). A number of factors must be considered in extrapolating risk from animal studies to humans. Among these are duration and route of exposure, species differences in toxicokinetics and toxicodynamics, and mechanism of action of the toxin. A scheme was proposed in which such biologically important data, relevant to safety assessment, could be used to calculate a data-derived safety factor.

# ACUTE TOXICITY

Acute toxicity of 50 priority chemicals of the Multicentre Evaluation of *In Vitro* Cytotoxicity was measured using 3 cyst-based standardized tests (using the rotifer *Brachionus calyciflorus* and the crustaceans *Artemia salina* and *Streptocephalus proboscideus*), the *Daphnia magna* test, and the bacterial luminescence inhibition test (20). Results from these assays, from rodent bioassays, and data on 5 physicochemical properties of the test compounds were compared with human oral lethal doses and concentrations derived from clinical cases. Although rodent bioassays were most accurate in predicting human acute toxicity, ethical and economic considerations have made them a less desirable choice for screening of large numbers of chemicals. Univariate regression analyses demonstrated that the in vitro bioassays, particularly those using crustacean species, were better predictors of human acute toxicity than physicochemical properties of the compounds.

In vitro assays using bovine (BE 12-6) and murine (NIH/3T3) embryonic cells were used to screen 17 mycotoxins for cytotoxic activity (21). Verrucarin A and roridin A were the most toxic and ergotamine tartrate was the least toxic. Results from these assays were significantly correlated with results from in vivo rodent bioassays ($LD_{50}$) in which the toxins were administered i.p. or i.v.

A microbial assay using *Klebsiella pneumonia*, used to test 12 chemicals, was found to generate 50% inhibitory concentration values which correlated well with $LD_{50}$ values when rats were dosed orally and mice were dosed i.p. (22). The bacteria were grown in a medium containing potassium citrate in which pH increased steadily as the bacteria grew. During a 15-hour period, pH was recorded automatically and this was used to determine inhibitory concentrations of the chemicals.

Although rodents may be more accurate predictors of acute toxicity in humans, there are differences between the physiological and behavioral responses of rodents and humans to xenobiotic compounds. Watkinson and Gordon (23) reviewed recent data on thermoregulatory responses of laboratory rats following acute exposure to toxic agents. In general, rats and mice respond to such challenges by lowering their core body temperatures by 1–4°C by decreasing their heart rates and arterial blood pressure. If given a choice of ambient temperatures, they will choose a temperature several degrees below their normal metabolic thermoneutral zone. If the exposed rodents are forced to remain at a higher temperature, toxicity of the compounds is increased. These physiologi-

cal changes in rodents may limit the ability to extrapolate results from one acute rodent study to another where ambient temperatures are unknown and should inject a note of caution into using rodent data for human risk assessment since similar adaptive responses have not been reported in humans.

Statistical evaluations of median effective doses ($ED_{50}$) and lethal doses ($LD_{50}$) are generally determined from tables published by Weil when data are available on the effects of 4 dose levels on 2, 3, 4, 5, 6, or 10 animals. These tables are based on the use of moving averages and interpolation. Schaper et al. (24) developed two computer programs, one written in BASIC and the other in FORTRAN, which may be used on personal computers for the calculation of median lethal and effective doses. The programs are easy and rapid to use and offer more flexibility that the previously published tables.

# MUTAGENICITY AND CARCINOGENICITY

## Overviews and Risk Assessment Considerations

Papers from a 1992 international conference on environmental mutagenesis in human populations at risk have been published (25). The conference addressed a range of issues, including screening tests for genotoxic effects, monitoring of populations exposed to different toxicants, mechanisms of mutagenesis and carcinogenesis, and hazard and risk assessment. Individual reports presented methods for investigation of these topics or data from research projects completed.

The significance of oxidative DNA damage caused by genotoxic and non-genotoxic carcinogens was reviewed by Clayson et al. (26). Available evidence indicates that oxidative damage to DNA can lead to base mispairing and mutation. Some compounds, however, are known to be oxidizing agents and yet are not carcinogenic and others are carcinogenic but not oxidizing agents. Therefore, other mechanisms are also important in inducing tumor formation.

In an attempt to determine whether short-term genotoxicity assays, chemical structures, and rodent toxicity tests can predict rodent carcinogenicity of untested compounds, several research groups predicted in 1990, based on their choice of the best experimental evidence available, the carcinogenicity of 44 compounds then in the process of evaluation by the U.S. National

Toxicology Program. Complete data are now available on 40 compounds and these data have been compared to the published predictions (27). For the 10 chemicals with an almost unanimous prediction of carcinogenicity, all were identified as carcinogens. For 9 chemicals almost unanimously predicted to be non-carcinogenic, 6 were designated as noncarcinogens and the other 3 had equivocal activity. For the remaining compounds, results were mixed. While no single short-term test was sufficient to predict every carcinogen, different combinations of these tests may be useful predictors.

Another prediction of rodent carcinogens from short-term assays was presented by Kitchin et al. (28). Data on the results of 11 possible predictors (including 4 biochemical assays, the Ames test, structural alerts, 3 in vitro mammalian cell genotoxicity assays, and the $k_e$ test) were compared with results from carcinogenicity assays for 111 chemicals. Although data were not available for all the chemicals on all the short-term tests, some useful observations were made. The test which gave the best prediction of carcinogenicity when used alone was DD (hepatic DNA damage by alkaline elution), with a concordance of 67%. Several combinations of tests gave higher levels of concordance with the carcinogenicity assays. With more complete data, this analysis may be able to suggest a combination of short-term tests with a high degree of predictivity.

Most of the participants in a workshop to evaluate the current guidelines which specify the use of two species and both sexes of rodents for carcinogenicity testing of chemicals agreed that the use of a reduced protocol may be sufficient for testing of some compounds (29). Such reduced protocols could involve testing of both sexes of rats or of mice or testing of female mice and male rats or vice versa. However, it was recognized that some chemicals or classes of chemicals may need to be tested more intensively than others.

Such reduced protocols would raise the question of how to treat data derived from different species, strains, and sexes on effects of the same chemical. Vater et al. (30) discussed various biological factors which affect whether carcinogenicity data from different experiments should be combined for analysis. These include pharmacokinetics of the test compound, mechanism of action of the agent, and any species/sex specificity of effect. Other important aspects of experimental design include dose selection and route of administration. Statistical analyses can also indicate whether data from different experiments can be described by the same multistage model and should therefore be combined.

One such biological factor to be considered in extrapolating carcinogenic risk from rodents to humans

is the case of male rat–specific nephropathy and carcinogenesis related to accumulation of $\alpha_{2u}$-globulin (31). Numerous chemicals have been shown to cause accumulation of this protein in kidney tubules, and chronic exposure leads to nephropathy and sometimes tumor formation. Although this protein is present in female rats, it accumulates only in the kidney of male rats and not in female rats, mice, or humans. Therefore, it is unlikely that chemicals which induce renal tumors in rats by this mechanism would pose a carcinogenic risk to humans.

Another varying biological factor which may differently affect the carcinogenetic process in rodents and humans is described by Sielkin and Stevenson as a difference in background transition rates (32). They point out that the majority of tumorigenic responses in mice and rats occur in organs with higher background levels of tumor incidence than are observed in humans. This implies that the rodents have higher background mutation rates, oncogene activation rates, and/or other forms of transition rates from one stage to another of the multistage carcinogenic process. Since the risk assessment calculations by federal agencies fail to account for such differences in rates of transition processes, they may be orders of magnitude in error.

The Carcinogenesis Working Group of the National Toxicology Program has recommended that the Program should shift its emphasis from hazard identification to the provision of the type of biological information needed in the risk assessment process (33). This information would aid in understanding the mechanisms of action of the chemicals involved and would permit a more rational approach to experimental design and to interpretation of results. The goal, of course, is to provide a reasonable assessment of the risk to humans of exposure to a particular agent.

Such knowledge of mechanisms of action of test compounds may allow the FDA to more realistically and appropriately interpret the Delaney Clause (which prohibits the addition of any known human or animal carcinogens to human foods). Picut and Parker (34) discuss this impending strategy of the FDA and explain why the FDA has the legal authority to consider such mechanistic information in its decision-making process. Formal guidelines or regulations should be issued to ensure consistent agency action in the evaluation of chemicals. An addendum to this paper reported that the U.S. Court of Appeals struck down the EPA's use of the negligible risk approach to interpret the Delaney Clause.

In another discussion of the appropriate interpretation of the Delaney Clause, Weisburger (35) pointed out that documented human carcinogens are DNA reactive or genotoxic. Therefore, he states that the Clause should be modified to emphasize the prohibition of proven genotoxins. Such genotoxins are those which reliably test positive in the Ames test, Williams test (induction of DNA repair in mammalian hepatocytes), and the use of $^{32}$P-postlabeling to detect DNA adducts.

Risk assessment of carcinogenic chemicals in the Netherlands was presented and discussed in a report from the Health Council of the Netherlands (*36*). Assessment criteria developed in 1978 were based on mechanistic considerations which distinguished two categories of carcinogens: (a) complete carcinogens and tumor initiators and (b) tumor promoters and substances which act as cocarcinogens. Substances in the first category are genotoxic and act by a stochastic mechanism with no threshold for the contribution to the carcinogenic affect. Promoters, on the other hand, act in a nonstochastic fashion and this implies a threshold dose. A recent reevaluation of this mechanistic method for assessment of carcinogenic risk concluded that it was still valid and appropriate.

## Physicochemical Properties and Structure–Activity Relationships

Because of the long time periods required for in vivo mammalian carcinogenicity studies, numerous lines of investigation have been undertaken to determine whether carcinogens have unique structural or physicochemical properties which could be used to predict the carcinogenicity of other, untested compounds. A special issue of *Mutation Research* was devoted to this topic of the use of structure–activity relationships (SAR) for prediction of rodent carcinogenicity (*37*). Importance of hydrophobic interactions, reactions of alkylating agents, and the use of the computer programs MULTICASE and TOPKAT were some of the topics discussed by the International Commission for Protection against Environmental Mutagens and Carcinogens (ICPEMC). ICPEMC has devised a hierarchical scheme, combining and weighting the results of many assays, for ranking chemicals according to their probable genotoxic effects. Rosenkranz and Klopman (*38*) compared these quantitative genotoxicity scores from the ICPEMC database with SAR analyses using CASE and MULTICASE and found that the scores were related to the presence of several structural determinants. Analyses of qualitative results from subsets of in vivo and in vitro genotoxicity assays as well as from the total database revealed that structural determinants could explain the scores of >95% of the chemicals.

In a review of current methods in genetic toxicology, Tennant and Zeiger (*39*) summarized information on the chemicals studied in the National Toxicology Program relating chemical structures to carcinogenicity. The values and limitations of various in vitro and short-term in vivo methods for detecting potential mutagens and carcinogens were discussed. Approaches to the complex study of nonmutagenic carcinogens were also considered.

Different families of mathematical models (classical regression, multivariate methods, neural networks) used in quantitative SAR studies were examined in a recent paper by Benigni and Giuliani (*40*). These mathematical models aid in determining important structural features of molecules but cannot be used simply to recognize patterns in chemical structures. There must also be a biological and chemical foundation to SAR analyses in order to provide predictive value and measure the degree of generalization found.

Structural determinants associated with the induction of unscheduled DNA synthesis (UDS) in isolated rat hepatocytes were investigated by Zhang et al. (*41*). Analyses of a series of 246 chemicals (including 114 known to induce UDS) used as the learning set identified 32 fragments which were significantly associated with UDS activity. Further analyses with 28 other chemicals revealed a concordance of >82% between prediction and experimentally determined UDS activity.

Since it has been suggested that some positive results in carcinogenicity assays occur because high, cytotoxic doses of test chemicals are used, two research groups have investigated and compared structural determinants associated with genotoxicity, cytotoxicity, and carcinogenicity. Using CASE/MULTICASE and several large databases of experimental results from different toxicology assays, Rosenkranz and Klopman (*42*) concluded that determinants of carcinogenicity could be separated into 2 groups: those associated with mutagenicity and electrophilicity and those associated with cell toxicity. The possible significance of these non-electrophilic (non-DNA-reactive) moieties was further investigated by Rosenkranz et al. (*43*). A great deal of overlap was found between structural determinants associated with cell toxicity and those associated with specific genetic effects. Whether this means that cytotoxic effects cause genotoxicity or whether this relationship is artifactual "noise" is unknown but should be further investigated because it may affect the assessment of risk from exposure to these chemicals.

On the other hand, Benigni and Andreoli (*44*) in an analysis of 297 chemicals found that there was no clear association between in vivo toxicity and the 5 physical–chemical properties considered. They also found that carcinogens tended to be more electrophilic and more hydrophobic than non-carcinogens and that bulkier molecules were less mutagenic than smaller molecules. Carcinogenicity and toxicity did not appear to be related.

The structures of 826 chemicals which had been tested for carcinogenicity were fragmented using a new computer program to produce all possible contiguous atom fragments with a size of 2–8 atoms (non-hydrogen) (45). Fragments from 80% of the chemicals were used as a training set and 20% were used as a test set. From the training sets, an average of 315 different fragments were significantly associated with either positive or negative results on carcinogenicity assays. Of the test set 23% lacked significant fragments. Using the significant fragments to analyze the remainder of the test set, the fragments were found to accurately predict carcinogenicity of 67.5% of the test compounds.

## Microbial Test Systems

A microcomputer program, AMESFIT, has been developed to fit a linear–exponential dose–response model to data on established mutagens from the widely used Ames-*Salmonella* assay (46). A linear term was used to describe effects of the test substance at low to moderate doses and an exponential attenuation factor was incorporated to account for downturns at high doses due to cytotoxic effects. The usefulness of this program was illustrated using data from a large-scale collaborative trial sponsored by the International Program on Chemical Safety.

Allele-specific oligonucleotide hybridization and DNA sequence analysis were used to examine the mutational specificity of 10 mutagens in *S. typhimurium* TA100 *his*G46 pKM101 (47). Five unique classes of reversion mutations induced by these mutagens in *his*G46 were identified. Since the mutational specificity observed in *his*G46 was similar to that seen in several eukaryotic gene targets, this *Salmonella* strain should be useful for investigating mechanisms of mutagenesis.

*S. typhimurium* strains carrying genes for human glutathione S-transferases alpha (GSTA1-1) and pi (GSTP1-1) were constructed to investigate the role of these enzymes in modulating the activity of several mutagens (48). GSTP1-1 had little effect on the activity of the mutagens tested except for a marginal depression of the mutagenicity of aflatoxin $B_1$. GSTA1-1 increased the mutagenicity of some compounds but significantly decreased that of aflatoxin $B_1$. These tester strains should be valuable in elucidating the role of GST enzymes in modulating the mutagenicity of various compounds.

Activation of promutagens before testing in the Ames assay is often accomplished using a rat liver microsomal preparation. Recent experiments demonstrated that the supernatant from human HEp G2 hepatoma cells, induced with hydrocortisone or benzanthracene, contains cytochrome P450 1A1 and 1A2 and other activating enzymes and therefore is suitable for activation of promutagens prior to testing with the Ames assay (49).

Quillardet and Hofnung (50) reviewed the performance of the SOS Chromotest as reported in over 100 publications with data on testing of 751 chemicals. The SOS-inducing abilities of these compounds span 8 orders of magnitude. For 452 compounds tested in both the SOS and the Ames assays, 82% gave similar responses in both tests. Of the remaining 18%, many were weakly positive in both assays and so the reported discordance may be simply a difference in interpretation of results. However, there are some compounds which are clearly positive in one assay and negative in the other. In comparing the ability of these two assays to identify carcinogens, the Ames test has a greater sensitivity while the SOS Chromotest has a greater specificity. Another paper comparing results from the SOS and the Ames tests for 330 compounds revealed an 86% concordance between the two tests (51). Of those which tested positive in the Ames test and negative in the SOS test, most exhibited a low level of mutagenicity.

SOS Chromotest bacteria exposed to complex mixtures may give inaccurate results because some components in the mixture are directly toxic to (inhibit the activity of) the enzymes being tested. A modified microplate procedure has been developed to circumvent these problems by challenging the test bacteria with the mixture (which previously gave positive results) just before enzymatic activities were estimated colorimetrically (52). This additional step eliminated the discrepancies between results from the standard and miniaturized procedures.

Ten compounds (including 8 known carcinogens) which are difficult to identify in the Ames assay were tested for genotoxicity in the *Saccharomyces cerevisiae* DEL assay (53). This assay was able to correctly identify 6 of the compounds as carcinogenic or not, while the Ames assay identified only 2 compounds correctly. Further evaluation and development of this assay should be undertaken since it appears to have a greater potential for identifying mammalian carcinogens.

The Mutatox® test (a bioluminescent bacterial genotoxicity test) has been evaluated in assays screening some compounds found in foods and feeds (54). Results from this assay correlate well with those from the

Ames test. Since Mutatox is much easier to conduct and can be completed in one day, it can serve as a rapid screening procedure for testing many samples.

## Genotoxicity Tests Using *Drosophila*

Two final reports presented data on the National Toxicology Program testing of an additional fifty (*55*) and seventy (*56*) compounds for mutagenic activity in post-meiotic and meiotic germ cells of male *Drosophila melanogaster* using the sex-linked recessive lethal (SLRL) assay. Eleven of the 50 chemicals, including urethane, tested positive in the SLRL assay and 5 of these also induced reciprocal translocations. Of the 70 compounds tested, 16 induced mutations in the SLRL assay and 7 of those also induced reciprocal translocations. Altogether 294 chemicals were tested in the SLRL assay and 88 of those have also been assessed for carcinogenicity in rodents and for genotoxicity in 4 in vitro assays: mutagenicity in *Salmonella* and mouse lymphoma cells and the induction of chromosomal aberrations and sister chromatid exchanges in Chinese hamster ovary cells. Of the 52 carcinogens, 14 were mutagenic in the SLRL assay, for a sensitivity of 27%, whereas 35 of the non-carcinogens were not mutagenic in the SLRL assay, for a specificity of 97%. Compared to the in vitro tests, the SLRL assay was less sensitive and therefore would not be useful as an initial screen for identifying potential mutagens. However, it might be useful in identifying probable carcinogens among known mutagenic compounds.

Genotoxicity of 16 pyrene, fluorene, and anthracene compounds was tested in Rec⁺ female *D. melanogaster* and in males of a strain of *Drosophila* carrying two meiotic recombination mutations on the X chromosome (Rec⁻) (*57*). DNA-damaging effects of the test compounds were manifested by a preferential killing effect on the Rec⁻ larvae. Of the 16 compounds, 3 tested negative, 11 were definitely positive, and 2 were weakly positive. Genotoxic effects of these compounds varied with their chemical structure as did mutagenic effects observed in *Drosophila* and carcinogenic effects observed in rodents. Therefore, this *Drosophila* DNA-repair assay could be a useful method for assessing genotoxicity of xenobiotic compounds.

A transgenic strain of *Drosophila* carrying a gene for canine hepatic cytochrome P450 1A1 was constructed and evaluated for its value in toxicology testing (*58*). Transgenic flies carrying the double recombination mutations (Rec⁻) were found to be sensitive to lower concentrations of 7,12-dimethylbenz[a]anthracene (enhanced mortality) than nontransgenic Rec⁻ flies. An inhibitor of P450 1A1 activity abolished this enhanced

mortality. Therefore, these transgenic *Drosophila* may be useful in screening for mammalian promutagens and procarcinogens.

## Bioassays in Mammals and Mammalian Cell Cultures

IN VITRO GENOTOXICITY ASSAYS. A review and evaluation of the sister-chromatid exchange (SCE) assay has been published as the second report of the Gene–Tox Program of the U.S. EPA (*59*). Literature reports through mid-1986 were considered, and the results of tests with numerous chemicals were summarized in 6 tables. A 7th table included information on the effects of specific chemicals on humans exposed in vivo. The SCE assay appears to be a useful indication of exposure although the mechanisms and biological significance of SCE formation are not completely understood.

An evaluation of the micronucleus assay in the Syrian hamster embryo (SHE) cells using 65 compounds with known carcinogenicity revealed that all 17 non-carcinogens tested negative while 41 of 48 carcinogens tested positive (*60*). Results also showed a high degree of concordance with results from in vivo micronucleus tests (89%) and with morphological SHE cell transformation assays (95%). These findings indicate that the in vitro SHE micronucleus assay does have a high predictive value.

In a further assessment of a micronucleus assay with Chinese hamster V79 cells modified to preferentially detect aneugens rather than clastogens, Seelbach et al. (*61*) tested 7 suspected aneugens. Five of these compounds gave positive results. So far the data produced by this assay appear to be quite reliable, and the reproducibility was also very good.

Use of Chinese hamster cells for genotoxicity assays has the drawback that these cells are not metabolically competent to activate promutagens. Therefore, V79 Chinese hamster cells have been genetically engineered to contain genes coding for different cytochrome P450 isoforms. The usefulness of these cell lines, which stably express xenobiotic metabolizing enzymes, in mutagenicity and metabolism studies has been reviewed (*62*). In a comparison of the performance of these genetically engineered cell lines with an S9 mix and primary Chinese hamster liver cultures in micronuclei assays, Ellard and Parry (*63*) observed that the engineered cells performed very well whereas the primary liver cell cultures suffered cytotoxic effects from the S9 mix which was required to activate the mutagens. However, some genetically engineered cell lines may have chromosomal instabilities as a result of the insertion of new genes and this should be investigated prior to using these strains for screening of genotoxins.

Advantages and drawbacks of the in vitro hepatocyte micronucleus assay were investigated by Müller et al. (*64*). Formation of micronuclei could be readily assessed by fluorescence microscopy. A fairly high number of micronuclei were observed in control cultures, probably as a result of disordered mitoses induced by mitogens used to stimulate growth. Two direct-acting mutagens produced dose-dependent positive results while a nonmutagen and a nonmutagenic carcinogen consistently tested negative. However, aflatoxin $B_1$, a known mutagen and carcinogen, also tested negative in this assay. It appeared that proliferating activity of hepatocytes in this assay was particularly susceptible to cytotoxic effects of chemicals.

Cytokinesis-blocked micronuclei and fluorescent in situ hybridization techniques were used to study aneuploidy in mouse splenocytes following in vitro/in vivo treatments with genotoxic compounds (*65*). Micronuclei can originate from chromosomal fragments caused by clastogenic agents which break chromosomes or from lagging chromosomes resulting from spindle malfunctions caused by aneugens. The mouse centromere satellite probe in conjunction with fluorescent in situ hybridization was used to distinguish these two types of micronuclei. Several known inducers of micronuclei were examined in this assay.

Difficulties in developing a relatively simple screening procedure for the detection of chemicals with aneugenic potential were discussed by Miller et al. (*66*). Both in vivo and in vitro systems were considered. The micronucleus assay appears to be the most suitable for detecting aneugenic effects. However, further developments in methodology are needed to test certain types of compounds more reliably.

One problem in accurately interpreting the results of in vitro mammalian genotoxicity assays is that some mutants and mutant progenitor cells grow more slowly during the expression period, and this would cause a decrease in the mutant to wild-type ratio. This would underestimate the actual number of mutational events which occurred. In order to more accurately quantitate the mutagenic response, Spencer et al. (*67*) developed an in situ procedure which segregated and immobilized cells during expression. This allowed slower growing cells to also produce colonies which could be scored as mutants. L5178Y *tk+/-* mouse cells were exposed to a mutagen and then plated on semisolid medium. As microcolonies were formed a selective agent was added as an overlay at specified times. In addition to more accurately scoring mutants, this procedure also

saved time and effort in the experimental evaluation process.

IN VITRO DETECTION OF NON-GENOTOXIC CARCINOGENS. Although numerous reliable genotoxicity assays have been developed, detection of non-mutagenic carcinogens (tumor promoters and co-carcinogens) remains problematic. An assay monitoring the transformation of BALB/c-3T3 cells was used to determine the carcinogenic effects of 84 carcinogens (49 mutagenic and 35 nonmutagenic), 77 noncarcinogens, and 7 other research chemicals (*68*). Multifactorial data analyses demonstrated that this assay could distinguish between nonmutagenic carcinogens and noncarcinogens: 64% of the carcinogens and only 26% of the noncarcinogens tested positive. In addition, most of the mutagenic chemicals were detected, including 94% of the carcinogens and 70% of the noncarcinogens. When compared with results from *Salmonella* mutagenicity assays and rodent bioassays, the transformation assay was found to complement the *Salmonella* assay in the identification of nonmutagenic carcinogens.

Since previous experiments have shown that tumor-promoting agents can induce the EBV (Epstein–Barr virus)-DR-promoter in Raji cells, Bouvier et al. (*69*) have undertaken a study to validate and quantitate the effect of a series of reference chemicals on this process and on the induction of the oxidative burst in human polymorphonuclear (PMN) cells as measured by chemiluminescence. A wide range of potent and potential tumor promoters was detected by one or both assays. Results of assays conducted in the presence of several potential inhibitory compounds provided information on the mechanisms of action of the tumor promoters. Both of these assays could be useful in screening for nongenotoxic carcinogens, and the PMN assay also has the potential for estimating individual sensitivity to environmental toxins.

Investigation of the effects of nongenotoxic carcinogens on liver cells has been difficult because liver cells in monolayer cultures show a rapid loss in viability and differentiation status and are not very useful after 3–4 days in culture. Hepatocyte spheroids, containing approximately 50–100 cells, were produced by Roberts and Soames (*70*) as a model to investigate the action of peroxisome proliferators in promoting rodent hepatocarcinogenesis. Hepatocytes inoculated onto culture plates coated with poly(2-hydroxyethyl methacrylate) attached to each other to form spheroids (since they could not attach to the plates), and these spheroids remained viable and capable of responding to peroxisome proliferators for up to 12 days. These spheroids should also be useful in the investigation of other non-genotoxic carcinogens.

Another approach to maintaining viable and metabolically competent hepatocytes in culture, described by Rogiers and Vercruysse (*71*), is the coculture of rat hepatocytes with epithelial cells. These cultures survive longer and maintain their phase I and phase II biotransformation capacities better than cultures containing only hepatocytes. Other factors in the medium which affect cell viability and metabolic competence were also reviewed.

An in vivo–in vitro replicative DNA synthesis (RDS) assay using rat hepatocytes was evaluated by Uno et al. (*72*) as an early prediction test for nongenotoxic hepatocarcinogens. Forty-seven compounds were tested, including 22 nongenotoxic hepatocarcinogens and 25 noncarcinogens. Compared to controls with an RDS incidence <1%, the RDS assay gave positive results for 18 of the known carcinogens and negative results for 20 of the known noncarcinogens, giving an overall concordance of 81%. This method appears to be very useful for the early detection of nongenotoxic carcinogens.

Another approach to the detection of nongenotoxic carcinogens as described by Kopponen et al. (*73*) is the assessment of a chemical's ability to induce expression of cytochrome P450 1A1 (CYP 1A1). Several complex mixtures from the environment, which were virtually nongenotoxic in a bacterial DNA repair test and in a mammalian SCE assay, were found to induce production of xenobiotic metabolizing enzymes. Thus, the compounds in these mixtures could act as co-carcinogens by stimulating the activation of procarcinogens.

**SHORT-TERM IN VIVO ASSAYS.** Several transgenic mouse strains are being intensively evaluated for their ability to detect chemicals which are genotoxic and/or carcinogenic to mammals. Gahlmann (*74*) reviewed the general features of these assay systems and discussed their advantages and disadvantages. The assays are expensive, with the test mice, the packaging mix used to generate infectious phage from isolated mammalian DNA, and the chromogenic substrate added to selection plates as the major costs. Some recent refinements in selection techniques should reduce costs, but the sensitivity, specificity, and reproducibility of these test systems must be confirmed.

An overview of reports from a symposium on Transgenic Animals in Toxicology held at the 32nd annual meeting of the Society of Toxicology has been published (*75*). Participants discussed construction of transgenic animals, use of transgenic mice in studies of in vivo mutagenesis, multistage carcinogenesis, and

tumorigenesis in *p*53-deficient mice, and implications of studies with transgenic animals for risk analysis.

Provost et al. (*76*) summarized results from their experiments exposing mice carrying the λ/*lac*I shuttle vector to several mutagens and described some recent modifications in their assay procedures which enhance the detection of mutations. Transgenic rats containing the same shuttle vector have also been developed and will provide a means of making interspecies comparisons of mutagenesis.

Results from published data on experiments with transgenic *lac*I mice have been compiled by Shephard et al. (*77*) and compared to literature data on the effects of these same compounds in long-term rodent bioassays and in in vivo micronucleus and chromosomal aberration assays. The sensitivity of the transgenic *lac*I assay was markedly improved by subchronic rather than acute administration of test chemicals. Compared to standard long-term carcinogenicity assays, the transgenic assay with a 250-day exposure period had approximately the same detection limit. When test compounds were administered subchronically to mice over a 3–4-month period, the sensitivity of the transgenic assay was about 1–2 orders of magnitude greater than that of the short-term genotoxicity assays. The authors concluded that a positive result in an assay with transgenic mice was highly predictive of carcinogenicity but that a negative result could not be completely trusted.

Experimental sources of variability in the *lac*I transgenic mouse mutation assay were investigated in detail by Piegorsch et al. (*78*). Several statistical methods were used to evaluate data from two laboratories to identify sources of variability. Little excess variability was observed in results on different plates made with a single λ-phage package reaction or in results obtained by treating a single DNA isolation with different packages of λ phage. However, excess package-to-package variability may occur if >3 months are allowed to elapse between isolation of genomic DNA and the packaging of that DNA into λ phage. A marginally excess variability was seen in comparing animal-to-animal results, and further study of the extent of this variability should be done.

One disadvantage of some transgenic mouse bioassays has been the tremendous amount of time and effort required to obtain reliable results. A modified selection procedure, utilizing a *gal*E⁻ bacterial host and a positive selection protocol which allows the growth of only *lac*Z mutant phage has been developed and tested (*79*). Up to 500,000 phage could be added to each selection plate with no loss in the recovery of *lac*Z mutants. Mutant frequency detected by this selection method was similar to that detected by the more time-consuming X-gal selection method.

Using this new selection procedure with the *lacZ* Muta™Mouse assay, Tinwell et al. (*80*) examined liver DNA from male mice gavaged with a single dose of dimethyl nitrosamine. A strong UDS (unscheduled DNA synthesis) response was observed in samples examined 2 hours after dosing, and a clear mutagenic response was observed in liver DNA isolated 7, 11, and 20 days after dosing. Compared to previous data from the Big Blue® (*lacI*) mutation assay, the selective Muta™Mouse assay was slightly more sensitive and was less time and resource consuming. However, the Big Blue assay system has the advantage of allowing access to a different strain of mice (B6C3F1) and to F344 rats.

Fenech (*81*) described and evaluated the use of mouse and human micronucleus assays for assessing the genotoxicity of whole foods in dietary intervention studies. Both the erythrocyte/reticulocyte and the lymphocyte assays appear to be capable of assessing the genotoxic potential of foods even though changes in the micronucleus index are usually quite small. Therefore, the scoring of several thousand cells is required and the development of automated procedures is important.

In an evaluation of the in vivo micronucleus assay in mouse splenocytes, a total of 14 compounds with different mechanisms of action were tested (*82*). All of the 3 direct alkylating agents, the 7 indirect alkylating agents, and the 2 intercalating agents significantly increased the binucleated micronucleated splenocyte rate, indicating that the assay could detect clastogenic compounds which cannot be detected by the bone marrow micronucleus assay. However, no increase was observed in tests with 2 spindle poisons, demonstrating that this assay would not reliably detect aneugenic compounds.

Tometsko et al. (*83*) rigorously evaluated and optimized experimental conditions for the use of flow cytometry for analyzing rare micronucleated cells in the total erythrocyte population. Use of a model clastogen, methyl methanesulfonate, in meticulously controlled and executed experiments demonstrated the importance of a suitable blood-sampling regimen, the advantages of obtaining an initial blood sample before dosing, the sex-linked difference in background micronucleus levels, and the clastogen-induced biological response in male and female mice. Careful attention to all experimental details can minimize experimental noise and provide results with high resolution and accuracy. This automated method can routinely score 1,000,000 cells for each blood sample.

A number of dietary variables, such as excess fat, insufficient fiber, and compounds in heated foods, have been epidemiologically associated with colorectal cancer. The potential carcinogenicity of several suspected food components to the colon has been tested using the in vivo aberrant crypt assay (*84*). Rats were gavaged with the test substances and their colons were examined 28 days later for evidence of aberrant crypt foci. Three new potential carcinogens were detected with these assays: 5-hydroxymethyl-2-furaldehyde in carmelized sugar, some factor in thermolyzed casein, and single bolus doses of sucrose and fructose. These substances should be further assessed in long-term carcinogenicity assays. Statistical analyses of data from aberrant crypt foci experiments were discussed by Minkin (*85*). In most cases, an estimate of the number of aberrant crypts per focus can be obtained by assuming a branching process with a gamma lifetime and a maximum likelihood estimation. A more robust analysis was based on experimental data which revealed that the relation between the variance of the number of aberrant crypts per focus and their mean was quadratic.

While many compounds testing positive in the Ames assay have later been shown to be rodent carcinogens, others are mutagenic non-carcinogens. In an attempt to identify these "false positives" without long-term carcinogenicity assays, Kitchin et al. (*86*) examined biochemical parameters in rats dosed with 28 such chemicals to determine whether one or more would be a reliable indicator of noncarcinogenicity. The specificity of 4 biochemical assays (in giving negative results for these 28 noncarcinogens) was 100% for hepatic DNA damage by alkaline elution, 89.3% for serum alanine aminotransferase activity, 85.7% for hepatic cytochrome P450 content, and 46.4% for hepatic ornithine decarboxylase activity. All except the last test could be useful in identifying mutagenic noncarcinogens.

The use of the restriction site mutation assay for the investigation of mutagenesis in rodent tissues has been reviewed by Myers and Parry (*87*). Analysis of base sequence changes resulting in altered restriction enzyme recognition sites in the *p*53 and α-hemoglobin genes of mice exposed to 1-ethyl-1-nitrosourea was described. DNA harvested from tissues 2–7 days after exposure was found to contain G→A transitions and G→T transversions in a number of different recognition sites. This procedure may be used to study mutation induction in any organ of any species for which DNA sequence information is available.

**MEDIUM- AND LONG-TERM ASSAYS.** The fifth plot of the Carcinogenic Potency Database, presenting results of carcinogenesis assays published in the general literature in 1987–88 and in technical reports of the National

Toxicology Program in 1987–89, has been published (*88*). This supplement includes data from 412 long-term experiments utilizing 147 test compounds, making a total of 4487 experiments and 1136 potential carcinogens included in all 5 plots. Updated results based on all 5 plots are given for the following: the most potent $TD_{50}$ value by species, reproducibility of bioassay results, positivity rates, and prediction between species. This report also provides a summary compendium of positivity and potency and an index to all chemicals included in the 5 plots.

Data from 32 years of long-term carcinogenesis assays in non-human primates (cynomolgus, rhesus, and African green monkeys) were recently summarized (*89*). Autopsies of 373 breeder and control monkeys demonstrated that cynomolgus and rhesus monkeys have a very low incidence of spontaneous tumors (1.5% and 2.8%, respectively) while spontaneous tumor incidence in African green monkeys is somewhat higher (8%). Among the compounds with potent carcinogenic effects were aflatoxin $B_1$, sterigmatocystin, the aglycone of cycasin, the heterocyclic amine IQ, and most of the *N*-nitroso compounds tested. Substances which were non-carcinogenic, even after >14 years' exposure, were saccharin, cyclamate, arsenic, and DDT.

Data on survival and spontaneous neoplasms in 1370 control Wistar rats from 10 carcinogenicity bioassays have been collated and summarized (*90*). Mean percentage survival at 104 weeks was 58–59%. Of a total of 1857 neoplasms observed, only 467 were malignant. The most common neoplasms (occurring in >7% of one sex) were pituitary adenoma, mammary fibroadenoma, mammary adenocarcinoma, adrenal cortical adenoma, and endometrial stromal polyp. These data should be useful in interpreting results of other carcinogenicity assays using Wistar rats and in choosing a strain of rat for testing other possible carcinogens.

Although more than 500 chemicals have tested positive in rodent carcinogenicity assays, these substances were often administered at much higher doses than humans would ordinarily encounter. A recent analysis by Munro and Davies (*91*) considered whether these high dose levels improve the detection of human carcinogens. Examination of data from rodent bioassays testing the effects of confirmed human carcinogens (as designated by IARC) revealed that all carcinogens to which humans are orally exposed could be detected in rodents at dose levels ≤43 mg/kg body weight or 880 ppm in the diet. Therefore, the maximum recommended levels of test substances in rodent assays (incorporating a safety factor of 10) were 500 mg/kg for gavage doses or 10,000 ppm (1%) in the diet.

In another approach to the question of adequate dose levels, Haseman and Lockhart (*92*) examined results from the NCI/NTP database on 216 rodent carcinogens to determine whether exposure to the maximum tolerated dose (MTD) was necessary to detect these carcinogens. Only 13 of these compounds produced increased tumor rates only at the MTD while about 67% would have been designated as carcinogens even without the MTD. However, of the latter group, some site-specific carcinogenic effects would have been missed. Of the chemicals which required the MTD to induce statistically significant carcinogenesis, a majority also produced numerically elevated rates of the same site-specific tumors at lower doses.

Dose–response relationships have been investigated in effects of genotoxic (*93*) and of nongenotoxic (*94*) carcinogens. Twelve rodent carcinogens, which damage hepatic DNA in female rats, were given to rats by gavage at several levels, down to 1/50,000 of the oral $LD_{50}$ value. Plotting of results (hepatic DNA damage) vs. log of the molar dose and vs. percent of the chemical's oral $LD_{50}$ produced dose–response curves which fit a linear model well and a quadratic model even better. Dose–response curves were also generated for 7 promoters of hepatocarcinogenicity. Analyses were not so straightforward in these data sets because of deficiencies and limitations in the data available and also because the different promoters are acting by different mechanisms which may result in different dose–response relationships. However, a number of interesting points emerged. There is evidence of a threshold of effect for several promoters and, for two of the compounds, there was some evidence that very low doses actually had antipromotional or protective effects.

Papers from an international symposium on Cell Proliferation and Chemical Carcinogenesis have recently been published (*95*). Topics included critical evaluations of cell proliferation methodologies, cell proliferation and modeling of organ-specific carcinogenesis, and cell proliferation and human carcinogenesis. Participants generally agreed that although cell growth and replication is an essential part of the carcinogenic process, the observation that a chemical enhances cell proliferation does not necessarily predict its carcinogenicity.

Five carcinogens with different target organs were examined for effects on cell proliferation in target and nontarget organs in rats during a multiorgan carcinogenesis bioassay (*96*). Cell proliferation, as measured by bromouracil deoxyriboside labeling indices, in urinary bladder, liver, and colon was elevated only by their respective carcinogens. But this was not true for the thyroid, lung, and kidney, where several carcinogens which did not induce tumors in these organs did elevate cell proliferation. Therefore, the specific carcinogenic potency of chemicals should be evaluated in terms of the appearance of preneoplastic or neoplastic lesions and not simply on the basis of induction of cell proliferation.

In experiments testing the reversibility of forestomach lesions induced by carcinogens, rats were exposed to one of 4 genotoxic or 4 nongenotoxic carcinogens for 24 weeks, followed by another 24 weeks of nonexposure and then examined for extent and severity of lesions (97). While lesions induced by genotoxic compounds did not regress after cessation of treatment, simple or papillary hyperplasia induced by nongenotoxic carcinogens clearly did regress. However, other types of hyperplasia (basal cell and atypical) induced by the nongenotoxins persisted even after discontinuing treatment. Thus, exposure to nongenotoxic carcinogens may also result in heritable changes in DNA during strong cell proliferation.

## Indices of Human Exposure

A recent special issue of *Drug Metabolism Reviews* contained several comprehensive reports on various aspects of biomonitoring of human populations to identify persons exposed to carcinogens. Among the topics considered were $^{32}$P-postlabeling methods for DNA adduct detection (98), protein adducts as biomarkers of human carcinogen exposure (99), and human exposure monitoring, dosimetry, and cancer risk assessment (100). Other articles in this issue concern metabolic activation of carcinogens and *p*53 mutations.

Some recent strategies for the development and validation of molecular biomarkers for human chemical carcinogen exposures were highlighted in an article by Groopman and Kensler (101). Validation of any biomarker requires specific knowledge of the metabolism, macromolecular adduct formation, and mechanism of action of the chemical agent derived from human and animal studies. Data from pilot human studies can then be used to assess intra- and interindividual variability, background levels, and the relationship of the marker to exposure or disease state. Few chemically specific exposure biomarkers have so far been rigorously validated.

In another recent review on biomarkers for carcinogenicity and toxicity, Chang et al. (102) focused on methods for studying macromolecular adducts, the molecular dosimetry of such adducts and carcinogenesis, and applications of macromolecular adduct research to human carcinogenesis. Examples are given of studies

with humans exposed to aflatoxins and to polycyclic aromatic hydrocarbons.

Non-destructive biomarkers detectable in vertebrates were the subject of a recent book (103). A variety of different biomarkers which may be indicative of different toxic effects were discussed. These included blood esterases as indicators of exposure to some insecticides; clinical biochemical tests; porphyrins as indicators of exposure to heavy metals, pesticides, and polyhalogenated compounds; genotoxic responses in blood; and hemoglobin adducts. Such markers may be useful in monitoring both human and animal populations for exposure to environmental toxins.

Human cancers commonly contain mutations in the tumor suppressor gene, *p*53. Examination of the specific base pair changes in this gene can yield several important pieces of information about the carcinogenic process, as discussed by Harris (104). Since different carcinogens are known to induce specific mutations, analyses of these mutations could identify the mutagen(s) to which a person or population has been exposed. Other specific mutations arise endogenously and may indicate that certain persons have an increased susceptibility to cancer.

Principles of physical methods for the detection of carcinogen–DNA adducts have been summarized by Weston (105) and the advantages and limitations of different methods for human biomonitoring studies were discussed. These methods include fluorescence spectroscopy, gas chromatography/mass spectrometry, electrochemical conductance, and atomic absorption spectroscopy. Depending on the type of adduct under study, the use of some methods is more appropriate than others.

Surface-enhanced Raman scattering spectroscopy, utilizing silver-coated microspheres deposited on glass as a special conductive surface, is capable of detecting DNA adducts in minute sample volumes (1 µL) and at extremely low sample concentration (femtomole) levels (106). This method can detect infrequent alterations or substitutions in DNA molecules treated with carcinogens (such as benzo[a]pyrene) in vitro, and experiments are currently underway to determine the level of DNA purity required for such analyses.

Detection and preparative concentration of carcinogen–DNA adducts by use of specific antisera was reviewed by Poirier (107). Methods for preparing immunogens, establishment of immunoassays, characterization of antisera, specific problems encountered with DNA isolated from biological samples, and the use of immunoaffinity chromatography for preparative concentration of adducts were discussed. Such specific antisera currently have wide applications in studies of carcinogen–DNA interactions and can be used for adduct preparation and quantitation.

Immunological techniques can also be used in the detection of DNA bases altered by carcinogen exposure. Bianchini et al. (*108*) used antibodies specific to 7-methyldeoxyguanosine in an immunoaffinity column to purify this base from human pancreatic DNA and from rat hepatic DNA. Adduct levels were then quantified using an ELISA or HPLC with electrochemical detection. The latter method had a lower detection limit of 0.5 pmol compared to 2 pmol for the ELISA. Between 2 and 7 pmol 7-methyldeoxyguanosine was detected in the tissues from healthy animals.

A method has been developed by Pfeifer et al. (*109*) for the detection of DNA adducts at the DNA sequence level by ligation-mediated PCR (polymerase chain reaction). Whenever it is possible to convert the adduct, either chemically or enzymatically, into a DNA strand break with a 5'-phosphate group, the PCR reaction can amplify the fragments containing the adducts. This method has been successfully used to detect pyrimidine dimers and alkylguanine adducts. The sensitivity of this method, its limitations, and its potential for mapping other DNA adducts in mammalian cells were discussed.

One of the major impediments in human biomonitoring studies is the need to obtain DNA from tissues. Garg et al. (*110*) evaluated a method for detection of adduct-forming metabolites in rodent serum as a possible means of circumventing this problem. Rodents were treated with benzo[a]pyrene (which is known to form adducts) and then animals were sacrificed at 4 hours (mice) and at ½–5 days (rats). Serum samples were examined for the presence of adduct-forming metabolites by reaction with exogenous DNA and detection by $^{32}$P-labeling. Large interstrain differences were observed in the serum level of these metabolites, and these differences correlated with previously reported variations in sensitivity to the carcinogenic effects of benzo[a]pyrene. These adduct-forming metabolites were detectable as late as 2 days and 5 days after dosing in C57Bl/6 mice and Sprague–Dawley rats, respectively.

Analyses of micronuclei in cytokinesis-blocked lymphocytes of 200 healthy volunteers with no known exposure to genotoxins revealed a large inter-individual variation in frequency, 9.87 ± 3.1/1000 cells (*111*). Neither age nor sex affected this variability, but smoking was found to increase the frequency of micronuclei by 25%. Mean micronuclei frequency in a sample of 33 male industrial painters was significantly higher (18.3 ± 7.39/1000 cells), indicating that the painters are occupationally exposed to genotoxin(s).

A new technique, employing fluorescence in situ hybridization (FISH), has been developed for the detection of micronuclei and aneuploidy in exfoliated human nasal, buccal, and bladder cells (*112*). Micronuclei levels in these cells ranged from 0.07 to 0.21% in samples from healthy volunteers. FISH was also successfully used for the detection of aneuploidy in exfoliated cells by use of a DNA probe specific for chromosome 9. These techniques may be useful for epidemiological studies and are currently being used to study some arsenic- and formaldehyde-exposed populations.

## REPRODUCTIVE AND DEVELOPMENTAL TOXICITY

Impact of the environment on reproductive health was the main theme of a 1991 international conference in Denmark. Participants discussed a range of topics, including the identification of environmental factors harmful to reproduction, transplacental transfer of genotoxins, exposure to chemicals in breast milk, evidence for increasing incidence of abnormalities of the human testis, and approaches to evaluating reproductive hazards and risks (*113*). Reports from another conference on reproductive health hazards were also published in the same issue of *Environmental Health Perspectives* (*114*). In addition to general environmental toxicants, reports from this conference focused on occupational hazards to reproductive health.

A recent book in the Target Organ Toxicology Series, edited by Kimmel and Buelke-Sam, was devoted to developmental toxicology (*115*). Contributors discussed normal developmental processes, abnormal development in several organ-systems (nervous, immune, cardiovascular, and renal systems), relationships between maternal and developmental toxicity, pharmacokinetics and pharmacodynamics, human studies, mathematical approaches to data evaluation, and regulatory aspects of developmental toxicology.

Status of the field of toxicology and contributions of the National Toxicology Program (NTP) were reviewed by Schwetz and Harris (*116*). More than 50 chemicals have been evaluated by the NTP, often in multiple species. Several caused developmental toxicity in the absence of maternal toxicity. Adverse effects observed at the LOAEL were usually reductions in body weight (rats and mice) and an increase in resorptions (rabbits). Although several in vitro or short-term assays appear promising as screening tools, only two have been rigorously tested and validated by the NTP: the human embryonic palatal mesenchymal cell growth inhibition assay and the mouse ovarian tumor cell attachment inhibition assay.

Approximately 160 published reports of adverse developmental effects resulting from concurrent exposure to more than one toxicant were reviewed by Nelson (*117*). Of these, about one-third each reported no interactive effects, antagonistic effects, and potentiative or synergistic effects. However, the quality of the research was highly variable. Often small numbers of animals and few dose levels were evaluated and maternal toxicity was rarely discussed. In addition, definitions of terms used to describe interactions were not consistent and differed from current usage. In order to obtain more useful and comparable data, aspects of experimental design were discussed and definitions were proposed for additivity, antagonism, potentiation, synergism, and interaction.

Expression of xenobiotic metabolizing cytochromes P450 in fetal tissues was reviewed by Raucy and Carpenter (*118*). Although numerous fetal biotransformation reactions have been observed, only a few fetal cytochrome P450s have been identified. One of these, P450 3A7 appears to be exclusive to human fetal tissues. This enzyme is structurally different from its adult counterparts, suggesting that other novel fetal enzymes may also be present. This review focuses primarily on xenobiotic-metabolizing enzymes present in human fetal tissues, with some studies demonstrating transplacental exposure in animals also described.

Failure of implantation (attachment and embedding of blastocyst in the uterine wall) is believed to be a common cause of pregnancy loss. Since this process, as it occurs in humans, can only be studied in vitro, several in vitro models have been developed to investigate different aspects of the process. A review by Genbacev et al. (*119*) provided essential background information on the preimplantation stage, the early development of the placenta, and the phases of implantation in humans and then critically evaluated various in vitro culture and coculture procedures for investigating these processes. Cell populations derived from available human tissues have provided considerable new data on mechanisms of cell–matrix interactions, antigenic characteristics of cytotrophoblast cell populations, and some aspects of extravillous cell differentiation. Human trophoblast cultures serve as useful models for studies of peri-implantation toxicology.

A rat embryo culture system was evaluated as a predictive test for human teratogens by exposure of the cultures to two known teratogens (valproic acid and captopril) and to two compounds which are not known to be embryotoxic (ibuprofen and diphenhydramine) (*120*).

Three drugs, ibuprofen, diphenhydramine, and valproic acid, exerted concentration-dependent decreases in growth and increases in anomalies. Captopril had no adverse effects. Since this assay produces both false-positive and false-negative results, it cannot be considered a sensitive indicator of human teratogens.

In vitro perfusion techniques as a tool for toxicity testing in the rat ovary were discussed by Jarrell et al. (*121*). A brief review of the development of the procedure, focusing on steroidogenesis and physiology of ovulation, was presented, and surgical procedures, perfusate, and criteria for viability were outlined. Advantages of the technique were outlined and applications of the model for toxicology testing were illustrated with data on exposure to hexachlorobenzene.

In vitro approaches to the study of testicular and germ cell toxicity were reviewed and discussed in terms of their ability to complement in vivo tests (*122*). Numerous cell culture systems, including Sertoli–germ cell cultures, Sertoli cell-enriched cultures, germ cell-enriched cultures, Leydig cell cultures, and Leydig–Sertoli cell cocultures, have provided important information on the relative toxicity of certain chemicals, cellular responses to toxicants, metabolic capabilities of the cells, and interactions of adjacent cell types. Although these in vitro methods cannot supplant in vivo assays, they are suited to the investigation of specific mechanisms of action of toxins.

Sensitivity of somatic and germ cells to 4 carcinogens (dimethylnitrosamine, diethylnitrosamine, 1,1-dimethylhydrazine, and β-propiolactone) was investigated in mouse bone marrow and spermatid micronucleus tests (*123*). None of the 4 tested positive in the bone marrow assay but all induced clastogenic effects in the spermatid micronucleus test. These results demonstrate that the bone marrow test cannot reliably detect compounds which can cause clastogenic effects in germ cells.

Among the recently developed in vitro tests for reproductive hazards is the micromass test (a culture of differentiating rat embryo limb and midbrain cells). Flint (*124*) described the most recent protocol for this assay and summarized validation and mechanistic studies confirming its usefulness. These cultures can be used to examine the effects of toxins on cell adhesion, movement, communication, division, and differentiation involving new synthesis of tissue-specific patterns of enzymes and structural proteins. Cells can be exposed directly in culture or transplacentally prior to culture in ex vivo experiments.

Primary cell culture models, in particular embryonic brain and retina cells in culture, were reviewed for their application in neurodevelopmental toxicity testing by Reinhardt (*125*). Both organ slice and aggregate cultures under constant gyratory movement as well as micromass cultures were considered robust in vitro systems. Of 16 known, possible, and unlikely human teratogens tested, all except 2 were classified correctly in assays with brain and retina cells. Preliminary data on the lowest effect levels of 4 potential neurotoxicants correlate surprisingly well with known human toxic plasma levels. A battery of in vitro tests was proposed as a screening procedure for neurodevelopmental toxins.

Teratogenic risk of low doses of the model compound methylnitrosourea to mice has been estimated by several different risk assessment procedures (*126*). Estimated risk was calculated by linear extrapolation to zero, by extrapolation by probit analysis, by establishment of a "virtually safe dose" by means of the NOAEL risk factor approach, and by determining adduct rates of $O^6$-methylguanine in DNA of the embryos. In the case of steep dose–response relationships (typical of most teratogenic effects), the NOAEL risk factor approach was more conservative than extrapolation based on probit analysis. Risk assessment at very low doses remains uncertain because even though small changes may be detected in parameters such as adduct levels, these minor effects may not be of biological significance.

Comparisons were made between data from animal teratogenicity studies and data on teratogenic effects in exposed humans for 4 well-known human developmental toxicants (valproic acid, isoretinoin, thalidomide, and methotrexate) (*127*). Results indicated that for these chemicals a margin of exposure of 1/100th the NOAEL for the most sensitive animal species tested provided adequate safety for the human conceptus. The lowest reported human exposures which were teratogenic were at least one log above the estimated safe dose based on the most sensitive animal species.

Analyses of dose–response relationships from an extensive historical database on teratology bioassays revealed that the benchmark dose (dose at which a chemical causes a small but measurable increase in frequency or severity of its effect) may serve as a good basis for risk assessment of toxic chemicals (*128*). Doses corresponding to 1 and 5% increases in lesions were calculated and compared to NOAEL values for the different toxins. Doses based on the 1% level could not be calculated accurately but those based on 5% could be calculated for most datasets and may be preferable to NOAEL levels for setting reference doses because they are based on data from all dose levels of the experiment.

Application of the Tukey trend test procedure to assess data from developmental and reproductive toxicity assays was described and discussed by Antonello et al.

(*129*). This procedure was recommended as a first-line statistical method in the evaluation of direct treatment effects in most conventional toxicological studies. Tukey's trend test has been found to be more likely to detect an adverse effect of a compound (if one exists) than any pairwise comparison approach. However, this procedure is not suitable for data where there is a nonmonotonic response to dose, such as with chemicals which induce effects, at extreme doses, that are opposite in direction from those observed at lower doses.

## ENDOCRINE TOXICOLOGY

In a recent review, van Leeuwen (*130*) discussed the application of endocrinology in experimental toxicology. Endocrine toxins may exert direct effects by interfering with hormone-receptor reactions and responses (for example, compounds which are structural analogs of natural hormones) or they may exert indirect effects by inhibiting hormone synthesis or release. Suggested procedures for detecting such toxins include determination of the weight and histology of endocrine organs; determination of circulating hormone levels; and tests to determine dysfunction of specific endocrine organs or cells. Further research into endocrine toxicology may aid in understanding mechanisms of action of a number of toxins.

In vitro methods for detecting compounds with hormonal activity include the use of human and animal cells that have been transfected with a specific hormonal receptor and a reporter gene. McLachlan (*131*) describes how such experiments could be used in screening for functional toxicology of xenobiotic compounds. Chemicals reacting with certain receptors would be expected to have certain toxic effects and could then be examined for those effects.

## NEUROTOXICITY AND BEHAVIORAL EFFECTS

The use of database programs to aid toxicological research was explained and demonstrated by Anger (*132*) in a review of 185 published studies on human behavioral toxicology. Specific information from each article was entered in a record form on a user-constructed database. Once the information has been entered, the program can be used to arrange information in a variety of ways and ask new questions. As new studies are published, they can be added to the database and newly important categories of information can be added by retrieving information from the original papers.

A cross-cultural assessment of the WHO-recommended neurobehavioral test battery was conducted in 10 countries of Europe, North and Central America, and Asia (*133*). Data were collected from >2300 men and women with no known occupational exposure to toxic chemicals. Performance on two of the tests (Simple Reaction Time, and Benton Visual Retention) was similar in a broad range of countries, while performance on 4 other tests (Santa Ana, Digit Symbol, Digit Span, and Aiming) was more variable from country to country. Data from very poorly educated males in one country revealed very low performance levels, suggesting that this test battery may not be appropriate for neurobehavioral testing in poorly educated subjects.

Several new in vitro assays for the assessment of neurotoxicity were discussed and the FRAME/EC-coordinated validation study of a tiered in vitro neurotoxicity test model was described by Atterwill et al. (*134*). A hierarchical assessment procedure has been proposed which involves testing in cell cultures with 3 levels of neural complexity: neuroblastoma cell lines, primary cultures of rat and chick midbrain, and organotypic, whole brain reaggregate cultures. This scheme is currently being validated in tests with 40 chemicals; preliminary results from testing of 6 chemicals are reported.

Reports from a conference on markers of neuronal injury and degeneration have recently been published (*135*). Topics discussed included changes in protein structure and function, altered gene expression, and non-neuronal markers of neuronal injury.

Another approach to the identification of neuronal damage, biochemical markers of neurotoxicity, was reviewed by Silbergeld (*136*). Neurochemical methods have a great potential for the sensitive and specific detection of early events in neurotoxicity and may therefore play an important role in the prevention of neurotoxic disease. However, a great deal of research remains to be done to elucidate the mechanisms of action of specific neurotoxicants and the specific neurochemical events in the pathogenesis of neurotoxic damage.

Two neurotoxic excitatory amino acids, kainate and β-*N*-methylamino-L-alanine (associated with amyotrophic lateral sclerosis in Guam), were found to modulate neurite outgrowth in mouse neuroblastoma cells (*137*). Low doses of both compounds decreased the concentration of two neurofilament proteins while high concentrations caused an apparent increase of these proteins. This in vitro assay may have broader applications in testing for neurotoxic substances.

A hybrid cell line (NSC-34) produced by fusion of embryonic mouse spinal cord neurons with mouse neuroblastoma cells was evaluated as a model for neurotoxicity testing (*138*). These cultures contain two populations of cells: small, undifferentiated cells which are capable of dividing and larger multinucleate cells which express many of the properties of motor neurons. These cultures were found to respond well to agents which affect voltage-gated ion channels, cytoskeletal organization, and axonal transport, but they were not a good model for the investigation of agents which affect synaptic transmission. The cell line was difficult to use because of its poor adhesion to substrates, requirement for routine subculture, and change in expression of neuronal phenotype with repeated subculture.

## IMMUNOTOXICITY

Risk assessment procedures for routine 28-day studies of chemicals with sensitizing or immunosuppressive properties were discussed by Basketter et al. (*139*). It was recommended that, in addition to tests for total and differential white blood cell counts and histopathological examination of the spleen, Tier 1 testing should include spleen and thymus weights and histopathology and draining and distal lymph node histopathology. Positive results in these tests would indicate immunotoxic effects, and these could be further investigated with appropriate Tier 2 tests.

A database comprising results from over 50 chemicals tested with a screening battery for immunotoxicity in mice has been used to develop statistical models of the relationship between immune function and host resistance (*140*). Such analyses may aid in identifying the most appropriate immune endpoints for establishing quantitative relationships between immune changes and impairment of host defenses. Good linear correlations were observed between changes in many of the tests and altered host resistance, but no single test was fully predictive for altered host resistance.

## BIOTECHNOLOGY AND FOOD SAFETY

Safety assessment of foods produced with the aid of biotechnology was discussed in depth in a recent book

*(141)*. Topics reviewed included clinical pharmacology of rDNA agents, in vitro and in vivo methods for the toxicological evaluation of biotechnology-derived foods, biotransformation of xenobiotics, safety evaluations of genetically engineered plants, and regulations regarding biotechnology-derived foods.

## LITERATURE CITED

1. Kotsonis, F.N., M. Mackey, and J.J. Hjelle (eds.). *Nutritional Toxicology.* New York, Raven Press. *Target Organ Toxicology Series* (1994).

2. Tu, A.T. (ed.). *Food Poisoning.* New York, Marcel Dekker. *Handbook of Natural Toxins.* Vol. 7 (1992).

3. Wagner, G., and G.G. Guilbault (eds.). *Food Biosensor Analysis.* New York, Marcel Dekker, Inc. *Food Science and Technology. A Series of Monographs, Textbooks, and Reference Books.* Vol. 60 (1994).

4. Kapis, M.B., and S.C. Gad (eds.). *Non-Animal Techniques in Biomedical and Behavioral Research and Testing.* Ann Arbor, Lewis Publishers (1993).

5. Mattie, D.R., D.E. Dodd, and H.J. Clewell III (eds.). *Applications of Advances in Toxicology to Risk Assessment.* Proceedings of the 1992 Toxicology Conference, Wright-Patterson Air Force Base, Ohio, 19–21 May 1992. *Toxicol. Lett.* 68(1–2) (1993).

6. Betton, G., A. Cockburn, E. Harpur, et al. A critical review of the optimum duration of chronic rodent testing for the determination of non-tumourigenic toxic potential: A report by the BTS Working Party on duration of toxicity testing. *Human Exp. Toxicol.* 13:221–232 (1994).

7. Rao, G.N. Diet for Fischer-344 rats in long-term studies. *Environ. Health Perspect.* 102:314–315 (1994).

8. Ashby, J. Benzyl acetate: from mutagenic carcinogen to non-mutagenic non-carcinogenic in 7 years? *Mutat. Res.* 306:107–109 (1994).

9. Dieter, M.P., T.J. Goehl, C.W. Jameson, et al. Comparison of the toxicity of citral in F344 rats and B6C3F₁ mice when administered by microencapsulation in feed or by corn-oil gavage. *Food Chem. Toxicol.* 31:463–474 (1993).

10. Carman, R.J., R.L. van Tassell, and T.D. Wilkins. Interactions between dietary compounds and the colonic microflora. In *Science for the Food Industry of the 21st Century. Biotechnology, Supercritical Fluids, Membranes and Other Advanced Technologies for Low Calorie, Healthy Food Alternatives.* M. Yalpani (ed.). Mount Prospect, IL, ATL Press. *Frontiers in Foods and Food Ingredients* 1:313–342 (1993).

11. Roland, N., L. Nugon-Baudon, and S. Rabot. Interactions between the intestinal flora and xenobiotic metabolizing enzymes and their health consequences. In *Intestinal Flora, Immunity, Nutrition and Health.* A.P. Simopoulos et al. (eds.). Basel, Karger. *World Rev. Nutr. Diet.* 74:123–148 (1993).

12. O'Neill, I., O. Ridgway, A. Ellul, and S. Bingham. Gastrointestinal monitoring of DNA-damaging agents with magnetic microcapsules. *Mutat. Res.* 290:127–138 (1993).

13. Mumtaz, M.M., I.G. Sipes, H.J. Clewell, and R.S.H. Yang. Risk assessment of chemical mixtures: biologic and toxicologic issues. *Fund. Appl. Toxicol.* 21:258–269 (1993).

14. Haas, C.N., and B.A. Stirling. New quantitative approach for analysis of binary toxic mixtures. *Environ. Toxicol. Chem.* 13:149–156 (1994).

15. Multiple authors. *The International Biostatistics Conference on the Study of Toxicology.* May 23–25, 1991. Tokyo, Japan. *Environ. Health Perspect.* 102(Suppl. 1) (1994).

16. Calabrese, E.J., and L.A. Baldwin. Improved method for selection of the NOAEL. *Regul. Toxicol. Pharmacol.* 19:48–50 (1994).

17. Calabrese, E.J., and L.A. Baldwin. A toxicological basis to derive a generic interspecies uncertainty factor. *Environ. Health Perspect.* 102:14–17 (1994).

18. Renwick, A.G., and R. Walker. An analysis of the risk of exceeding the acceptable or tolerable daily intake. *Regul. Toxicol. Pharmacol.* 18:463–480 (1993).

19. Renwick, A.G. Data-derived safety factors for the evaluation of food additives and environmental contaminants. *Food Addit. Contam.* 10:275–305 (1993).

20. Calleja, M.C., G. Persoone, and P. Geladi. Human acute toxicity prediction of the first 50 MEIC chemicals by a battery of the ecotoxicological tests and physicochemical properties. *Food Chem. Toxicol.* 32:173–187 (1994).

21. Terse, P.S., M.S. Madhyastha, O. Zurovac, et al. Comparison of in vitro and in vivo biological activity of mycotoxins. *Toxicon* 31:913–919 (1993).

22. Ishii, R., and K. Yoshikawa. Microbial bioassay of acute toxicity by the pH inhibition method and comparison of IC₅₀ (pHI) with LD₅₀ for rats and mice. *J. Ferment. Bioeng.* 76:361–366 (1993).

23. Watkinson, W.P., and C.J. Gordon. Caveats regarding the use of the laboratory rat as a model for acute toxicological studies: modulation of the toxic response via physiological and behavioral mechanisms. *Toxicology* 81:15–31 (1993).

24. Schaper, M.M., R.D. Thompson, and C.S. Weil. Computer programs for calculation of median effective dose (LD₅₀ or ED₅₀) using the method of moving average interpolation. *Arch. Toxicol.* 68:332–337 (1994).

25. Au, W.W., W.R. Anwar, and R.W. Tennant (eds.). *The First International Conference on Environmental Mutagenesis in Human Populations At Risk.* January 19–24, 1992. Cairo, Egypt. *Environ. Health Perspect.* 101(Suppl. 3) (1993).

26. Clayson, D.B., R. Mehta, and F. Iverson. Oxidative DNA damage — The effects of certain genotoxic and operationally non-genotoxic carcinogens. *Mutat. Res.* 317:25–42 (1994).

27. Ashby, J., and R.W. Tennant. Prediction of rodent carcinogenicity for 44 chemicals: results. *Mutagenesis* 9:7–15 (1994).

28. Kitchin, K.T., J.L. Brown, and A.P. Kulkarni. Complementarity of genotoxic and nongenotoxic predictors of rodent carcinogenicity. *Teratogen. Carcinogen. Mutagen.* 13:83–100 (1994).

29. Lai, D.Y., K.P. Baetcke, V.T. Vu, et al. Evaluation of reduced protocols for carcinogenicity testing of chemicals:

report of a joint EPA/NIEHS workshop. *Regul. Toxicol. Pharmacol.* 19:183–201 (1994).

30.  Vater, S.T., P.M. McGinnis, R.S. Schoeny, and S.F. Velazquez. Biological considerations for combining carcinogenicity data for quantitative risk assessment. *Regul. Toxicol. Pharmacol.* 18:403–418 (1993).

31.  Swenberg, J.A. $\alpha_{2u}$-Globulin nephropathy: review of the cellular and molecular mechanisms involved and their implications for human risk assessment. *Environ. Health Perspect.* 101(Suppl. 6):39–44 (1993).

32.  Sielken, R.L., Jr., and D.E. Stevenson. Another flaw in the linearized multistage model upper bounds on human cancer potency. *Regul. Toxicol. Pharmacol.* 19:106–114 (1994).

33.  Goodman, J.I. A rational approach to risk assessment requires the use of biological information: an analysis of the National Toxicology Program (NTP), final report of the Advisory Review by the NTP Board of Scientific Counselors. *Regul. Toxicol. Pharmacol.* 19:51–59 (1994).

34.  Picut, C.A., and G.A. Parker. Interpreting the Delaney Clause in the 21st century. *Toxicol. Pathol.* 20:617–627 (1992).

35.  Weisburger, J.H. Does the Delaney Clause of the U.S. Food and Drug Laws prevent human cancers? *Fund. Appl. Toxicol.* 22:483–493 (1994).

36.  Health Council of The Netherlands: Committee on the Evaluation of the Carcinogenicity of Chemical Substances. Risk assessment of carcinogenic chemicals in The Netherlands. *Regul. Toxicol. Pharmacol.* 19:14–30 (1994).

37.  Brusick, D.J. (ed.) *Use of SAR for the Prediction of Rodent Carcinogenicity. Mutat. Res.* 305:1–97 (1994).

38.  Rosenkranz, H.S., and G. Klopman. Structural implications of the ICPEMC method for quantifying genotoxicity data. *Mutat. Res.* 305:99–116 (1994).

39.  Tennant, R.W., and E. Zeiger. Genetic toxicology: current status of methods of carcinogen identification. *Environ. Health Perspect.* 100:307–315 (1993).

40.  Benigni, R., and A. Guiliani. Quantitative structure–activity relationship (QSAR) studies in genetic toxicology: mathematical models and the "biological activity" term of the relationship. *Mutat. Res.* 306:181–186 (1994).

41.  Zhang, Y.P., A. Van Praagh, G. Klopman, and H.S. Rosenkranz. Structural basis of the induction of unscheduled DNA synthesis in rat hepatocytes. *Mutagenesis* 9:141–149 (1994).

42.  Rosenkranz, H.S., and G. Klopman. Structural evidence for a dichotomy in rodent carcinogenesis: involvement of genetic and cellular toxicity. *Mutat. Res.* 303:83–89 (1993).

43.  Rosenkranz, H.S., Y.P. Zhang, and G. Klopman. Evidence that cell toxicity may contribute to the genotoxic response. *Regul. Toxicol. Pharmacol.* 19:176–182 (1994).

44.  Benigni, R., and C. Andreoli. Rodent carcinogenicity and toxicity, in vitro mutagenicity, and their physical chemical determinants. *Mutat. Res.* 297:281–292 (1993).

45.  Malacarne, D., R. Pesenti, M. Paolucci, and S. Parodi. Relationship between molecular connectivity and carcinogenic activity: a confirmation with a new software program based on graph theory. *Environ. Health Perspect.* 101:332–342 (1993).

46.  Leroux, B.G., and D. Krewski. AMESFIT: a microcomputer program for fitting linear-exponential dose-response models in the Ames *Salmonella* assay. *Environ. Molec. Mutagen.* 22:78–84 (1993).

47.  Koch, W.H., E.N. Henrikson, E. Kupchella, and T.A. Cebula. *Salmonella typhimurium* strain TA100 differentiates several classes of carcinogens and mutagens by base substitution specificity. *Carcinogenesis* 15:79–88 (1994).

48.  Simula, T.P., M.J. Glancey, and C.R. Wolf. Human glutathione S-transferase-expressing *Salmonella typhimurium* tester strains to study the activation/detoxification of mutagenic compounds: studies with halogenated compounds, aromatic amines and aflatoxin $B_1$. *Carcinogenesis* 14:1371–1376 (1993).

49.  Duverger-van Bogaert, M., P.J. Dierickx, C. Stecca, and M.-C. Crutzen. Metabolic activation by a supernatant from human hepatoma cells: a possible alternative in mutagenic tests. *Mutat. Res.* 292:199–204 (1993).

50.  Quillardet, P., and M. Hofnung. The SOS chromotest: a review. *Mutat. Res.* 297:235–279 (1993).

51.  Mersch-Sundermann, V., U. Schneider, G. Klopman, and H.S. Rosenkranz. SOS induction in *Escherichia coli* and Salmonella mutagenicity: a comparison using 330 compounds. *Mutagenesis* 9:205–224 (1994).

52.  Hoflack, J.C., J.F. Férard, P. Vasseur, and C. Blaise. An attempt to improve the SOS Chromotest responses. *J. Appl. Toxicol.* 13:315–319 (1993).

53.  Carls, N., and R.H. Schiestl. Evaluation of the yeast DEL assay with 10 compounds selected by the International Program on Chemical Safety for the evaluation of short-term tests for carcinogens. *Mutat. Res.* 320:293–303 (1994).

54.  Sun, T.S.C., and H.M. Stahr. Evaluation and application of a bioluminescent bacterial genotoxicity test. *J. AOAC Int.* 76:893–898 (1993).

55.  Foureman, P., J.M. Mason, R. Valencia, and S. Zimmering. Chemical mutagenesis testing in *Drosophila*. IX. Results of 50 coded compounds tested for the National Toxicology Program. *Environ. Molec. Mutagen.* 23:51–63 (1994).

56.  Foureman, P., J.M. Mason, R. Valencia, and S. Zimmering. Chemical mutagenesis testing in *Drosophila*. X. Results of 70 coded chemicals tested for the National Toxicology Program. *Environ. Molec. Mutagen.* 23:208–227 (1994).

57.  Fujikawa, K., F.L. Fort, K. Samejima, and Y. Sakamoto. Genotoxic potency in *Drosophila melanogaster* of selected aromatic amines and polycyclic aromatic hydrocarbons as assayed in the DNA repair test. *Mutat. Res.* 290:175–182 (1993).

58.  Komori, M., R. Kitamura, H. Fukuta, et al. Transgenic *Drosophila* carrying mammalian cytochrome P-4501A1: an application to toxicology testing. *Carcinogenesis* 14:1683–1688 (1993).

59.  Tucker, J.D., A. Auletta, M.C. Cimino, et al. Sister-chromatid exchange: second report of the Gene-Tox program. *Mutat. Res.* 297:101–180 (1993).

60.  Fritzenschaf, H., M. Kohlpoth, B. Rusche, and D. Schiffmann. Testing of known carcinogens and noncarcinogens in the Syrian hamster embryo (SHE) micronucleus test in vitro;

correlations with in vivo micronucleus formation and cell transformation. *Mutat. Res.* 319:47–53 (1993).

61. Seelbach, A., B. Fissler, and S. Madle. Further evaluation of a modified micronucleus assay with V79 cells for detection of aneugenic effects. *Mutat. Res.* 303:163–169 (1993).

62. Doehmer, J. V79 Chinese hamster cells genetically engineered for cytochrome P450 and their use in mutagenicity and metabolism studies. *Toxicology* 82:105–118 (1993).

63. Ellard, S., and J.M. Parry. A comparative study of the use of primary Chinese hamster liver cultures and genetically engineered immortal V79 Chinese hamster cell lines expressing rat liver CYP1A1, 1A2 and 2B1 cDNAs in micronucleus assays. *Toxicology* 82:131–149 (1993).

64. Müller, K., P. Kasper, and L. Müller. An assessment of the in vitro hepatocyte micronucleus assay. *Mutat. Res.* 292:213–224 (1993).

65. Farooqi, Z., F. Darroudi, and A.T. Natarajan. The use of fluorescence *in situ* hybridization for the detection of aneugens in cytokinesis-blocked mouse splenocytes. *Mutagenesis* 8:329–334 (1993).

66. Miller, B.M., S. Madle, and S. Albertini. Can a 'relatively simple' screening procedure for the detection of chemicals with aneugenic potential be recommended at the moment? *Mutat. Res.* 304:303–307 (1994).

67. Spencer, D.L., K.C. Hines, and W.J. Caspary. An in situ protocol for measuring the expression of chemically-induced mutations in mammalian cells. *Mutat. Res.* 312:85–97 (1994).

68. Matthews, E.J., J.W. Spalding, and R.W. Tennant. Transformation of BALB/c-3T3 cells: V. Transformation responses of 168 chemicals compared with mutagenicity in Salmonella and carcinogenicity in rodent bioassays. *Environ. Health Perspect.* 101(Suppl. 2):347–482 (1993).

69. Bouvier, G., M. Hergenhahn, A. Polack, et al. Validation of two test systems for detecting tumor promoters and EBV inducers: comparative responses of several agents in DR-CAT Raji cells and in human granulocytes. *Carcinogenesis* 14:1573–1578 (1993).

70. Roberts, R.A., and A.R. Soames. Hepatocyte spheroids: prolonged hepatocyte viability for *in vitro* modeling of nongenotoxic carcinogenesis. *Fund. Appl. Toxicol.* 21:149–158 (1993).

71. Rogiers, V., and A. Vercruysse. Rat hepatocyte cultures and co-cultures in biotransformation studies of xenobiotics. *Toxicology* 82:193–208 (1993).

72. Uno, Y., H. Takasawa, M. Miyagawa, et al. An in vivo-in vitro replicative DNA synthesis (RDS) test using rat hepatocytes as an early prediction assay for nongenotoxic hepatocarcinogens: screening of 22 known positives and 25 noncarcinogens. *Mutat. Res.* 320:189–205 (1994).

73. Kopponen, P., R. Törrönon, J. Mäki-Paakkanen, et al. Comparison of CYP1A1 induction and genotoxicity in vitro as indicators of potentially harmful effects of environmental samples. *Arch. Toxicol.* 68:167–173 (1994).

74. Gahlmann, R. Pros and cons of transgenic mouse mutagenesis test systems. *J. Exp. Anim. Sci.* 35:232–243 (1993).

75. Goldsworthy, T.L., L. Recio, K. Brown, et al. Transgenic animals in toxicology. *Fund. Appl. Toxicol.* 22:8–19 (1994).

76. Provost, G.S., P.L. Kretz, R.T. Hamner, et al. Transgenic systems for in vivo mutation analysis. *Mutat. Res.* 288:133–149 (1993).

77. Shephard, S.E., W.K. Lutz, and C. Schlatter. The *lacI* transgenic mouse mutagenicity assay: quantitative evaluation in comparison to tests for carcinogenicity and cytogenetic damage in vivo. *Mutat. Res.* 306:119–128 (1994).

78. Piegorsch, W.W., A.-M.C. Lockhart, B.H. Margolin, et al. Sources of variability in data from a *lacI* transgenic mouse mutation assay. *Environ. Molec. Mutagen.* 23:17–31 (1994).

79. Dean, S.W., and B. Myhr. Measurement of gene mutation *in vivo* using Muta™Mouse and positive selection for *LacZ⁻* phage. *Mutagenesis* 9:183–185 (1994).

80. Tinwell, H., P.A. Lefevre, and J. Ashby. Response of the Muta™Mouse lacz/galE⁻ transgenic mutation assay to DMN: comparisons with the corresponding Big Blue™ (lacI) responses. *Mutat. Res.* 307:169–173 (1994).

81. Fenech, M. Mouse and human micronucleus models for assessing genotoxicity of whole foods in intervention studies. *Mutat. Res.* 290:119–125 (1993).

82. Benning, V., D. Brault, C. Duvinage, et al. Validation of the *in vivo* CD1 mouse splenocyte micronucleus test. *Mutagenesis* 9:199–204 (1994).

83. Tometsko, A.M., D.K. Torous, and S.D. Dertinger. Analysis of micronucleated cells by flow cytometry. 3. Advanced technology for detecting clastogenic activity. *Mutat. Res.* 292:145–153 (1993).

84. Bruce, W.R., M.C. Archer, D.E. Corpet, et al. Diet, aberrant crypt foci and colorectal cancer. *Mutat. Res.* 290:111–118 (1993).

85. Minkin, S. Statistical analysis of aberrant crypt assays for colon cancer promotion studies. *Biometrics* 60:279–288 (1994).

86. Kitchin, K.T., J.L. Brown, and A.P. Kulkarni. Predicting rodent carcinogenicity of Ames test false positives by in vivo biochemical parameters. *Mutat. Res.* 290:155–164 (1993).

87. Myers, B., and J.M. Parry. The application of the restriction site mutation assay to the study of the induction of mutations in the tissues of rodents. *Mutagenesis* 9:175–177 (1994).

88. Gold, L.S., N.B. Manley, T.H. Slone, et al. The fifth plot of the Carcinogenic Potency Database: results of animal bioassays published in the general literature through 1988 and by the National Toxicology Program through 1989. *Environ. Health Perspect.* 100:65–135 (1993).

89. Thorgeirsson, U.P., D.W. Dalgard, J. Reeves, and R.H. Adamson. Tumor incidence in a chemical carcinogenesis study of nonhuman primates. *Regul. Toxicol. Pharmacol.* 19:130–151 (1994).

90. Walsh, K.M., and J. Poteracki. Spontaneous neoplasms in control Wistar rats. *Fund. Appl. Toxicol.* 22:65–72 (1994).

91. Monro, A., and T.S. Davies. High dose levels are not necessary in rodent studies to detect human carcinogens. *Cancer Lett.* 75:183–194 (1993).

92. Haseman, J.K., and A. Lockhart. The relationship between use of the maximum tolerated dose and study sensitivity for detecting rodent carcinogenicity. *Fund. Appl. Toxicol.* 22:382–391 (1994).

93. Kitchin, K.T., and J.L. Brown. Dose-response relationship for rat liver DNA damage caused by 49 rodent carcinogens. *Toxicology* 88:31–49 (1994).

94. Kitchin, K.T., J.L. Brown, and R.W. Setzer. Dose–response relationship in multistage carcinogenesis: promoters. *Environ. Health Perspect.* 102(Suppl. 1):255–264 (1994).

95. Multiple authors. *Chemical Proliferation and Chemical Carcinogenesis*. January 14–16, 1992. Research Triangle Park, North Carolina. *Environ. Health Perspect.* 101(Suppl. 5) (1993).

96. Yoshida, T., M. Tatematsu, K. Takaba, et al. Target organ specificity of cell proliferation induced by various carcinogens. *Toxicol. Pathol.* 21:436–442 (1993).

97. Kagawa, M., K. Hakoi, A. Yamamoto, et al. Comparison of reversibility of rat forestomach lesions induced by genotoxic and non-genotoxic carcinogens. *Jpn. J. Cancer Res.* 84:1120–1129 (1993).

98. Randerath, K., and E. Randerath. $^{32}$P-Postlabeling methods for DNA adduct detection: overview and critical evaluation. *Drug Metab. Rev.* 26:67–86 (1994).

99. Skipper, P.L., X. Peng, C.K. Soohoo, and S.R. Tannenbaum. Protein adducts as biomarkers of human carcinogen exposure. *Drug Metab. Rev.* 26:111–124 (1994).

100. Poirier, M.C. Human exposure monitoring, dosimetry, and cancer risk assessment: the use of antisera specific for carcinogen–DNA adducts and carcinogen-modified DNA. *Drug Metab. Rev.* 26:87–110 (1994).

101. Groopman, J.D., and T.W. Kensler. Molecular biomarkers for human chemical carcinogen exposures. *Chem. Res. Toxicol.* 6:764–770 (1993).

102. Chang, L.W., S.M.T. Hsia, P.-C. Chan, and L.-L. Hsieh. Macromolecular adducts: biomarkers for toxicity and carcinogenesis. *Annu. Rev. Pharmacol. Toxicol.* 34:41–67 (1994).

103. Fossi, M.C., and C. Leonzio (eds.). *Nondestructive Biomarkers in Vertebrates*. Ann Arbor, Lewis Publishers (1994).

104. Harris, C.C. p53: At the crossroads of molecular carcinogenesis and risk assessment. *Science* 262:1980–1981 (1993).

105. Weston, A. Physical methods for the detection of carcinogen–DNA adducts in humans. *Mutat. Res.* 288:19–29 (1993).

106. Helmenstine, A., M. Uziel, and T. Vo-Dinh. Measurement of DNA adducts using surface-enhanced Raman spectroscopy. *J. Toxicol. Environ. Health* 40:195–202 (1993).

107. Poirier, M.C. Antisera specific for carcinogen–DNA adducts and carcinogen-modified DNA: Applications for detection of xenobiotics in biological samples. *Mutat. Res.* 288:31–38 (1993).

108. Bianchini, F., R. Montesano, D.E.G. Shuker, et al. Quantification of 7-methyldeoxyguanosine using immunoaffinity purification and HPLC with electrochemical detection. *Carcinogenesis* 14:1677–1682 (1993).

109. Pfeifer, G.P., R. Drouin, and G.P. Holmquist. Detection of DNA adducts at the DNA sequence level by ligation-mediated PCR. *Mutat. Res.* 288:39–46 (1993).

110. Garg, A., A.C. Beach, and R.C. Gupta. Interception of reactive, DNA adduct-forming metabolites present in rodent serum following carcinogen exposure: implications for use of body fluids in biomonitoring. *Teratogen. Carcinogen. Mutagen.* 13:151–166 (1993).

111. Di Giorgio, C., M.P. De Méo, M. Laget, et al. The micronucleus assay in human lymphocytes: screening for inter-individual variability and application to biomonitoring. *Carcinogenesis* 15:313–317 (1994).

112. Moore, L.E., N. Titenko-Holland, P.J.E. Quintana, and M.T. Smith. Novel biomarkers of genetic damage in humans: use of fluorescence in situ hybridization to detect aneuploidy and micronuclei in exfoliated cells. *J. Toxicol. Environ. Health* 40:349–357 (1993).

113. Skakkebæk, N.E., A. Negro-Vilar, F. Michal, and K.M. Grigor (eds.). *International Workshop on the Impact of the Environment on Reproductive Health*. 30 September–4 October 1991. Copenhagen, Denmark. *Environ. Health Perspect.* 101(Suppl. 2) (1993).

114. Paul, M.E. Overview: conference on occupational and environmental reproductive hazards. *Environ. Health Perspect.* 101(Suppl. 2):171–174 (1993).

115. Kimmel, C.A., and J. Buelke-Sam. *Developmental Toxicology*. 2nd ed. New York, Raven Press. *Target Organ Toxicology Series* (1994).

116. Schwetz, B.A., and M.W. Harris. Developmental toxicology: status of the field and contribution of the National Toxicology Program. *Environ. Health Perspect.* 100:269–282 (1993).

117. Nelson, B.K. Interactions in developmental toxicology: a literature review and terminology proposal. *Teratology* 49:33–71 (1994).

118. Raucy, J.L., and S.J. Carpenter. The expression of xenobiotic-metabolizing cytochromes P450 in fetal tissues. *J. Pharmacol. Toxicol. Meth.* 29:121–128 (1993).

119. Genbacev, O., T.E.K. White, C.E. Gavin, and R.K. Miller. Human trophoblast cultures: models for implantation and peri-implantation toxicology. *Reproduct. Toxicol.* 7:75–94 (1993).

120. Guest, I., H.S. Buttar, S. Smith, and D.R. Varma. Evaluation of the rat embryo culture system as a predictive test for human teratogens. *Can. J. Physiol. Pharmacol.* 72:57–62 (1994).

121. Jarrell, J.F., M.L. Sevcik, D.C. Villeneuve, and P.O. Janson. Toxicity testing using the isolated in vitro perfused ovary. *Reproduct. Toxicol.* 7:63–68 (1993).

122. Lamb, J.C., IV, and R.E. Chapin. Testicular and germ cell toxicity: in vitro approaches. *Reproduct. Toxicol.* 7:17–22 (1993).

123. Cliet, I., C. Melcion, and A. Cordier. Lack of predictivity of bone marrow micronucleus test versus testis micronucleus test: comparison with four carcinogens. *Mutat. Res.* 292:105–111 (1993).

124. Flint, O.P. In vitro tests for teratogens: desirable endpoints, test batteries and current status of the micromass teratogen test. *Reproduct. Toxicol.* 7:103–111 (1993).

125. Reinhardt, C.A. Neurodevelopmental toxicity in vitro: primary cell culture models for screening and risk assessment. *Reproduct. Toxicol.* 7:165–170 (1993).

126. Platzek, T., G. Bochert, R. Meister, and D. Neubert. Embryotoxicity induced by alkylating agents: 7. Low dose prenatal-toxic risk estimation based on NOAEL risk factor approach, dose-response relationships, and DNA adducts using methylnitrosourea as a model compound. *Teratogen. Carcinogen. Mutagen.* 13:101–125 (1993).

127. Newman, L.M., E.M. Johnson, and R.E. Staples. Assessment of the effectiveness of animal developmental toxicity testing for human safety. *Reproduct. Toxicol.* 7:359–390 (1993).

128. Auton, T.R. Calculation of benchmark doses from teratology data. *Regul. Toxicol. Pharmacol.* 19:152–167 (1994).

129. Antonello, J.M., R.L. Clark, and J.F. Heyse. Application of the turkey trend test procedure to assess developmental and reproductive toxicity. I. Measurement data. *Fund. Appl. Toxicol.* 21:52–58 (1993).

130. van Leeuwen, F.X.R. Endocrine toxicology: a review of the application of endocrinology in experimental toxicology. *Comp. Haematol. Int.* 3:8–13 (1993).

131. McLachlan, J.A. Functional toxicology: a new approach to detect biologically active xenobiotics. *Environ. Health Perspect.* 101:386–387 (1993).

132. Anger, W.K. Database programs as a literature research tool for the 1990s scientist: surveillance of neurotoxicology data. *Environ. Res.* 62:71–75 (1993).

133. Anger, W.K., M.G. Cassitto, Y.-X. Liang, et al. Comparison of performance from three continents on the WHO-recommended neurobehavioral core test battery. *Environ. Res.* 62:125–147 (1993).

134. Atterwill, C.K., J. Davenport-Jones, S. Goonetilleke, et al. New models for the *in vitro* assessment of neurotoxicity in the nervous system and the preliminary validation stages of a 'tiered-test' model. *Toxicol. in Vitro* 7:569–580 (1993).

135. Johannessen, J.N. *Markers of Neuronal Injury and Degeneration. Ann. N.Y. Acad. Sci.* 679 (1993).

136. Silbergeld, E.K. Neurochemical approaches to developing biochemical markers of neurotoxicity: review of current status and evaluation of future prospects. *Environ. Res.* 63:274–286 (1993).

137. Abdulla, E.McF., and I.C. Campbell. Use of neurite outgrowth as an *in vitro* method of assessing neurotoxicity. *Ann. N.Y. Acad. Sci.* 679:276–279 (1993).

138. Durham, H.D., S. Dahrouge, and N.R. Cashman. Evaluation of the spinal cord neuron × neuroblastoma hybrid cell line NSC-34 as a model for neurotoxicity testing. *NeuroToxicology* 14:387–396 (1993).

139. Basketter, D.A., J.N. Bremmer, M.E. Kammuller, et al. The identification of chemicals with sensitizing or immunosuppressive properties in routine toxicology. *Food Chem. Toxicol.* 32:289–296 (1994).

140. Luster, M.I., C. Portier, D.G. Pait, et al. Risk assessment in immunotoxicology. II. Relationships between immune and host resistance tests. *Fund. Appl. Toxicol.* 21:71–82 (1993).

141. Thomas, J.A., and L.A. Myers (eds.). *Biotechnology and Safety Assessment.* New York, Raven Press (1993).

# 7

# Intentional (Direct) Additives

# OVERVIEW

A recent review by Taylor and Nordlee (*1*) summarized and discussed data on various chemical additives in seafood products. Over 70 such additives or ingredients are commonly found in processed seafood but only a few of these are likely to cause adverse reactions in sensitive persons. Probably the most important are sulfiting agents, which have caused life-threatening reactions in some sulfite-sensitive people. Other compounds discussed include MSG, hydrolyzed vegetable protein and other proteinaceous ingredients, modified food starch, BHA, sorbic acid and sorbitol, food colors, and vegetable gums.

Relatively few of the approximately 2700 chemical compounds and mixtures and plant extracts permitted as food additives by the U.S. FDA have been tested for mutagenicity (*2*). A recent review on this subject pointed out that, of those additives tested, about 15% induced mutations in the Ames test. A large proportion of these mutagenic additives generate oxygen- or free radicals. However, the potential hazard of these compounds is unknown because they are generally added to foods in very small amounts and the modifying effects of other food components are unknown.

Some common food additives, including vanillin, tartrazine, octyl gallate, and erythrosin B, were found to inhibit the sulfation of some xenobiotic compounds by human hepatic cytosolic sulfotransferases in vitro (*3*). Since the sulfation reaction can detoxify these compounds, these additives may enhance the toxicity of these xenobiotics. For example, vanillin inhibits sulfation of 17α-ethinylestradiol (used as a contraceptive) and, if this reaction occurs in vivo, it could greatly increase the absorption and bioavailability of this steroid. Vanillin also inhibits the in vitro metabolism of the neurotransmitter dopamine, and this could have neurotoxic effects if it occurs in animals.

A multicenter Danish study tested 335 children referred for allergy testing in an open challenge to determine whether they were allergic to food additives (colors, flavors, citric acid, preservatives) (*4*). Only 23 children reacted positively to the open challenge, and further testing of 16 of these children in a double-blind challenge showed only 6 had a positive reaction to one or more food additives. Therefore, the incidence of intolerance to food additives was estimated to be 2% based on the double-blind assay or 7% based on the open challenge.

# PRESERVATIVES

## Sulfiting Agents

Concentrations of sulfite in foods have become a concern lately because some steroid-dependent asthmatics have suffered life-threatening symptoms following consumption of sulfited foods. Analyses of 4 batches of shrimp purchased from different vendors in Spain revealed excessive amounts of sulfite in all of them (*5*). Although the maximum permitted level is 100 mg total $SO_2$ per kg food, mean sulfite concentrations in the edible portions of these shrimp ranged from 182–579 mg/kg and were even higher in the inedible portions (heads and shells), at 971–2399 mg/kg. Boiling of the shrimp reduced sulfite levels by about 33%, but levels were still higher than permitted levels in all batches. It appears that these shrimp were not treated according to the recommended protocol but were exposed to solutions with excessive amounts of sulfite and/or were immersed for very long periods of time.

A survey in Japan tested a wide variety of raw and processed foods for naturally occurring sulfites (*6*). Sulfite concentrations were generally <1 mg/kg, with just a few vegetables (onions, garlic, radishes, mushrooms) and other foods (algae, shrimp) having >1 mg/kg. None of the samples had sulfite concentrations close to 100 mg/kg.

Dried apricots are commonly sulfited to preserve their color and taste. A mathematical model has been devised to describe and predict the absorption of sulfur dioxide during treatment (*7*). The model assumes the existence of two diffusive species (aqueous $SO_2$ and $HSO_3^-$) and considers operating conditions such as temperature, pH, and sodium disulfite concentrations. This model may also be useful in describing the absorption of sulfur dioxide by other food products.

Several procedures have been described for the quantitative determination of sulfite: an HPLC method for total sulfites in foods (*8*); flow injection analysis with reductive amperometric detection and electrolytic cleanup for sulfur dioxide in wines and other beverages (*9*); fluorometric determination of total and bound sulfite in wine by *N*-(9-acridinyl)maleimide (*10*); and an HPLC method with electrochemical detection for sulfite and ascorbic acid in beer and other beverages (*11*).

## Organic Acids

Benzoic acid and sodium benzoate are employed as food preservatives (to control the growth of bacteria) in a number of different foods. Toxicity studies demonstrated that rodents had elevated liver and kidney weights and serum levels of albumin, total protein, and γ-glutamyl transpeptidase when fed diets containing 3% (mice) or 2.4% (rats) sodium benzoate (*12*). Enlargement and necrosis of hepatocytes was also observed.

A relatively simple HPTLC method, which does not require sample extraction or cleanup, has been developed for the determination of sorbic acid, benzoic acid, and dehydroacetic acid in beverages (*13*).

# NITRATE, NITRITE, AND *N*-NITROSO COMPOUNDS

Effects of nitrates, nitrites, and *N*-nitroso compounds on human health have been reviewed by Bruning-Fann and Kaneene (*14*). Particular attention was given to infant methemoglobinemia and gastric cancer, with some discussion of adult methemoglobinemia and toxicity, hypo- and hypertension, Balkan nephropathy, and slowing of motor reflexes in children. Sources of these nitrogenous compounds were detailed and the importance of endogenous nitrosation was discussed.

## Nitrates and Nitrites in Foods

Using data from 48-hour recall interviews, the dietary intake of nitrates and nitrites by 1212 Finns aged 9–24 years was estimated to average 54.0 and 1.4 mg/day, respectively (*15*). Vegetables, including potatoes, supplied about 86% of the daily intake of nitrates while meats, particularly sausages, provided 69% of the nitrites. Since drinking water supplied only 1–2 mg nitrate and 0–0.2 mg nitrite/day, foods were the major source of these nitrogenous compounds.

Excessive nitrate consumption induces methemoglobinemia in young infants and this most often occurs when a drinking water source is high in nitrates. To determine the potential for infant foods to cause this disorder, commercial, strained baby foods representing 3 national brands were purchased in grocery stores and analyzed for nitrates (*16*). Most cereals, fruits, and meats were low in nitrates. However, some samples of mixed vegetables, bananas, carrots, garden vegetables, spinach, green beans, and beets contained >45 ppm nitrate. Since some sources recommend starting infants on solid food as early as 3 months of age, baby foods high in nitrates could be potentially hazardous. No cases of infants developing methemoglobinemia from high nitrate baby foods have been described, but the

authors recommend that infants not be started on solid foods until 5–6 months of age when they would not be as sensitive to nitrate.

Samples of all the major vegetables grown in Queensland (Australia) were collected near peak harvest and analyzed for nitrate and nitrite (*17*). A small sample of hydroponic produce was also assayed. Nitrites were only found in lettuces and dwarf beans, at concentrations of 1–4 mg/kg. Nitrate concentrations varied a great deal in the same vegetables from different farms. Highest median concentrations were present in silver beet (570 mg/kg), beetroot (480 mg/kg), radish (392 mg/kg), and celery (295 mg/kg). Hydroponic lettuce and beetroot contained 465 and 785 mg nitrate/kg, respectively. The very high nitrate levels in some of these vegetables (higher than those reported in other surveys) may be a result of excessive use of nitrogen fertilizers and indicates a need for more careful management of nitrogen fertilization.

A survey of a wide variety of Japanese foods was conducted to determine naturally occurring levels of nitrates and nitrites (*18*). Nitrate concentrations were high in some leafy vegetables (>1000 mg/kg in some lettuce, cabbage, and mustard greens). Some preserved and processed vegetables and seaweeds also were very high in nitrates. Nitrite levels were also relatively high in some fresh (up to 7 mg/kg) and preserved (up to 38 mg/kg) vegetables.

Improved analytical procedures have been described for the determination of: nitrate in baby foods by a spectrophotometric method which was adopted first action by AOAC International following a collaborative study (*19*); nitrite in food and water by fluorimetric methods (*20,21*); and nitrite in food and water by a spectrophotometric method using Nile blue 2B (*22*).

## Biological Effects of Nitrates and Nitrites

An unusual incident of methemoglobinemia occurred in a 34-year-old woman who collapsed shortly after drinking a beverage made with water contaminated by the accidental addition of an anti-corrosive agent containing 30% sodium nitrite (*23*). Her initial gastrointestinal symptoms were succeeded by dizziness, weakness, and cyanosis. She was taken to a hospital where subsequent investigation revealed a methemoglobin concentration of 49%. The patient apparently ingested a near lethal dose of 0.7 g sodium nitrite but recovered rapidly after appropriate treatment.

At low doses nitrite is not obviously toxic but it may enhance the toxicity or carcinogenicity of other compounds. A compound highly toxic to cultured

Chinese hamster ovary cells is formed when low concentrations of BHA (butylated hydroxyanisole) and sodium nitrite react in an acidified physiological saline solution (24). The toxic compound, which induced statistically significant chromosomal damage, may be an intermediate involved in the induction of tumors in the rat forestomach.

In in vivo experiments with rats initiated with N-methyl-N'-nitro-N-nitrosoguanidine (MNNG), chronic administration of phenolic compounds significantly enhanced forestomach carcinogenesis. Coadministration of sodium nitrite did not further increase the development of tumors (25). However, in the absence of MNNG, nitrite did increase the hyperplasia induced by the phenolic compounds (catechol, t-butylhydroquinone, and gallic acid).

## Endogenous Nitrosation

In a study of factors related to endogenous nitrosation, a total of 457 fresh, fasting gastric juice samples were obtained from patients with various gastrointestinal conditions and analyzed for nitrite and N-nitroso compounds (26). The samples varied in pH from very acidic (1.13) to slightly basic (8.42) with nitrite concentrations higher in the more basic samples. N-nitroso compounds were significantly more abundant in the most acidic samples (average of 1.45 µmol/L at pH 1.13–2.99) and in the most basic samples (3.57 µmol/L at pH 6.0–8.42). However, there were great variations in both nitrite and N-nitroso concentrations at different pHs, indicating that both acid-catalyzed and biologically catalyzed nitrosation processes are markedly affected by factors other than pH and nitrite levels.

Numerous amine-containing compounds which are present in different foods may react with nitrite in the saliva or the stomach and be converted to N-nitrosamines. An unknown alkali-labile nitroso compound previously detected in nitrosated cocoa and dried tomatoes has been identified as N-nitroso-pyrrolidin-(2)-one (NPyrO) (27). A method was then developed to detect the precursor compound PyrO (pyrrolidinone) and was used to survey a variety of foods and beverages for this compound. Highest concentrations were found in cocoa powder (77 ppm), roasted coffee beans (50 ppm), instant coffee (42 ppm), and dried tomatoes (48 ppm). Although these foods did not contain any preformed NPyrO, in the presence of nitrite and acidic conditions (as in the stomach), PyrO is readily converted to NPyrO.

Reconstituted instant coffee, treated with 10 mmol nitrite under mildly acidic conditions (pH 3), was found

to form direct-acting compounds mutagenic in the Ames test (28). The mutagen(s) were extracted and partially purified and appeared to be different from other known mutagens in coffee (methylglyoxal and hydrogen peroxide). Exposure of the purified fraction to an S9 activating mixture abolished the mutagenicity of the compound(s).

Two new nitroso compounds, mononitrosocaffeidine (MNC) and dinitrosocaffeidine (DNC), produced when a widely consumed, salted alkaline tea from Kashmir is treated with nitrite, were tested for genotoxicity (29). MNC, with or without metabolic activation, did not induce mutations in any of the Salmonella typhimurium tester strains used nor did it induce single-strand chromosomal breaks in rat hepatocytes. DNC, on the other hand, was a direct-acting mutagen in 3 tester strains (but not in 2 others) and also exhibited cytotoxic effects and produced breaks in DNA in rat hepatocytes. MNC has only a single nitroso group while DNC has both nitrosamine and nitrosamide groups. DNC may play a role in the high incidence of esophageal and gastric cancer in Kashmir.

Mutagenic nitrosated compounds are also formed when red wine is incubated with sodium nitrite at pH 3 for 1 hour (30). Some of the nitrosatable compounds present in red wine, tyramine, quercetin, and malvidine-3-glucoside, were found to become direct acting mutagens in the Ames assay and the SOS chromotest after they were treated with nitrite. However, the concentration of these 3 nitrosatable precursors in wine is too low to account for most of the genotoxic activity found in the wine. Two other nitrosatable components of wine, histamine and phenylethylamine, tested negative in the Ames test after nitrosation.

Nitrosation of dietary components under gastric conditions is inhibited by ascorbic acid. In a recent review, Mirvish (31) summarized some of the older and the more recent literature on the inhibition of gastric nitrosation by ascorbic acid, discussed in vivo studies with humans given ascorbic acid to prevent nitrosation of proline, and considered the role of other substances in fruits and vegetables which might inhibit nitrosation.

Inhibition of nitrosation by tomato juice was investigated by testing phenolic and ascorbate fractions for their ability to prevent formation of N-nitrosomorpholine (NMOR) (32). Although the ascorbate fraction effectively inhibited nitrosation, several phenolic fractions, particularly those containing p-coumaric acid and chlorogenic acid, also exhibited substantial inhibitory action.

## Occurrence and Formation of *N*-Nitroso Compounds in Foods

A survey of 25 cured meats, 8 samples of smoked seafood, 15 smoked poultry products, and 17 smoked cheeses purchased in Canada was conducted to determine concentrations of two non-volatile *N*-nitroso compounds (NOC), 2-(hydroxymethyl)-*N*-nitrosothiazolidine-4-carboxylic acid (HMNTCA) and 2-(hydroxymethyl)-*N*-nitrosothiazolidine (HMNTHZ) (*33*). Neither compound was detected in the cheese and no HMNTHZ was present in any uncooked meats. Appreciable levels of HMNTHZ were formed in one cured meat sample after frying. HMNTCA was detected in 11 cured meats, 6 poultry products, and 2 smoked fish at concentrations of 10–260 µg/kg. The toxicological significance of the presence of these NOC is, at present, not clear.

With the interest in producing lower fat foods has come the suggestion that part of the meat in frankfurters be replaced with minced fish. However, there has been some concern that this would introduce amine precursors which could be nitrosated. In an investigation of the feasibility of using Atlantic menhaden mince and surimi to replace 15% or 50% of the meat in frankfurters, only one of 10 volatile NOC tested for was detected in any of the samples (*34*). Trace levels of *N*-nitrosodimethylamine (NDMA) were present in uncooked 15% and 50% samples (0.03–0.13 ppb and 0.03–0.28 ppb, respectively) with somewhat higher concentrations in broiled samples (0.25–0.76 ppb and 0.78–3.07 ppb, respectively). The highest concentrations, in all cases, were found in the frankfurters prepared with unwashed mince.

Volatile NOC were not formed in cooked cured meat or meat–fish products which were prepared without the use of nitrite as a preservative (*35*). As a replacement for nitrite, the pork and pork–fish products were treated with sodium ascorbate and preformed cooked cured-meat pigment. This appears to be a useful alternative method for producing cured meat products without NOC.

Fairly high levels of some NOC are formed in some cured pork products packaged in elastic rubber netting as a result of the reaction between the nitrite in the meat and the amine additives used in the curing of the rubber. A recent survey of 20 such pork products revealed that this problem has yet to be solved (*36*). Only one sample had no detectable NOC. Six samples contained one NOC, *N*-nitrosobenzylamine (NDBZA), at concentrations of 12–32 µg/kg and the remaining 13 samples had 18–520 µg NDBZA/kg and 0.6–48 µg NDBA (*N*-nitroso-*n*-butylamine)/kg.

A multiresidue method using supercritical fluid extraction has been developed for the efficient recovery and determination of 10 volatile nitrosamines in frankfurters (*37*).

Twenty types of vegetables, spices, and other foods purchased at retail markets in Nigeria were analyzed for volatile nitrosamines (*38*). Fifteen samples contained detectable levels of NDMA (0.4–4.6 ppb), with highest concentrations found in cabbage and amaranth.

## Biological Effects of *N*-Nitroso Compounds

In a epidemiological study in China involving approximately 4000 healthy men in 69 counties in the most highly populated areas of the mainland, geographic variations in urinary excretion of *N*-nitroso compounds were compared with mortality rates for esophageal cancer (*39*). A 350-fold variation in esophageal cancer mortality in these counties was observed in data collected in the 1970s. Positive and significant correlations were observed between cancer mortality and the excretion of *N*-nitrososarcosine (NSAR) and the excretion of *N*-nitrosoproline (NPRO) after a loading dose of proline. (NSAR is known to cause esophageal cancer in animals.) The results suggest that persons in certain counties who have a greater exposure to nitrosamines, either preformed in foods or produced endogenously with the aid of nitrite derived from nitrate-rich foods, have a greater risk for esophageal cancer. No correlations were observed between gastric cancer mortality and these measures of endogenous nitrosation.

Analyses of gastric juice samples from a total of 210 persons from Colombia (a high-incidence area for gastric cancer) and from the UK and France (with similar, lower incidences of gastric cancer), supported the role of endogenous nitrosation in gastric cancer etiology (*40*). Gastric nitrite concentrations were higher at higher pH values and were higher in patients with precancerous lesions of the stomach than in those with noncancerous conditions. Nitrite and NOC levels were significantly higher in the subjects from Colombia than in those from the other countries.

In order to exert their carcinogenic effects, nitrosamines are first activated by cytochrome P450-dependent monooxygenases. Examination of this activation process using *N*-nitrosodiethylamine (NDEA) and *N*-nitrosodimethylamine (NDMA) and hepatic microsomes from humans and mice revealed similarities between the two species (*41*). Two human enzymes, CYP2A6 and CYP2E1, metabolized these nitrosamines but evidence from studies using enzyme inhibitors revealed a great interindividual variation in the amounts and activity of the enzymes. It appeared that different CYP enzymes had different preferred substrates but some overlapping occurred in substrate specificity.

One mechanism by which nitrosamines may initiate carcinogenesis is by activation of oncogenes. A recent study of pancreatic cancer induced in hamsters by *N*-nitrosobis(2-hydroxypropyl)amine revealed that 10 of 16 pancreatic duct carcinomas and 3 of 12 cholangiocarcinomas had a G→A transition mutation in codon 12 of the K-*ras* oncogene (42). A similar point mutation has been observed at high frequency in human pancreatic adenocarcinomas.

Analyses of esophageal tumors induced in rats by *N*-nitrosomethylbenzylamine (NMBA) demonstrated the presence of mutations at codon 12 of the Ha-*ras* oncogene in about half of the 84 papillomas examined (43). Mutations in the rat *p*53 tumor suppressor gene also were detected in 36% of the papillomas. In contrast, only *p*53 mutations and no Ha-*ras* mutations have been found in human esophageal cancers. This suggests that either nitrosamines are not a major risk factor for human esophageal carcinogenesis or that the carcinogenic process differs in rats and humans.

Other environmental, including dietary, factors may modulate the carcinogenic effects of nitrosamines. Of 10 organosulfur compounds from onion and garlic tested in an in vivo assay with rats dosed with NDEA, 5 were found to enhance the hepatocarcinogenic process while 2 others inhibited it (44). This promoting effect appears to be a consequence of the stimulation of ornithine decarboxylase (ODC) activity. ODC is induced by most promoters of carcinogenesis and this induction is known to precede cell proliferation. In contrast, dietary protocatechuic acid (a natural component of many fruits and vegetables) reduced hepatic ODC levels in rats and also inhibited hepatocarcinogenesis induced by NDEA (45).

# FOOD PRESERVATION BY IRRADIATION

A recent review by Elias (46) covered the topic of food irradiation in a comprehensive manner. Physical and technological aspects of irradiation and methods for identification of irradiated food were described. Toxicological and food safety consequences of food irradiation, both positive and negative, were also discussed. Status and prospects for food irradiation were reviewed by Loaharanu (47). Regulatory approval of irradiation in different countries was described and

its practical applications and commercialization were discussed.

## Potentially Toxic or Antinutritional Effects

Data related to the wholesomeness of irradiated poultry was reviewed by Thayer (48). Both short- and long-term multigenerational feeding studies with rodents and dogs have demonstrated no toxic effects resulting from consumption of chicken irradiated at the currently approved level of 3 kGy. Although irradiation can cause losses of up to 8.6% of the thiamine in chicken, significant losses of this vitamin also occur if the meat is heat processed. Free radicals are generated in irradiated foods but because they are such active compounds, their lifetime is fairly short. The author concludes that irradiated poultry is a wholesome food.

A recent study on the effects of irradiation on safflower oilcake (the residue left after extraction of oil from safflower seeds) pointed out that irradiation can have other beneficial effects besides the destruction of food pathogens (49). Antinutritional factors in oilcakes have restricted their use as protein sources. However, irradiation of safflower oilcakes at 42 Gy was found to inactivate the trypsin inhibitor and significantly improve in vitro digestibility.

No statistically significant adverse effects in hematological parameters, histopathology of internal organs, or chromosomal structure in liver and bone marrow cells were observed in rats fed for 4 or 90 days on diets containing 70% freshly irradiated wheat (0.25, 0.75. or 2.25 kGy) (50). Minor changes in ploidy of liver cells and cell cycling of bone marrow cells were noted but these were qualitatively similar to those which occur after food restriction in animals. It may be that an altered composition of fatty acids in the irradiated wheat was responsible for these marginal effects.

One known adverse effect of irradiation on the nutritional value of some foods is the destruction of some vitamins. This topic has been reviewed by Kilcast (51). Published studies indicate that vitamins A, B₁, C, and E are the most sensitive to irradiation, with losses of up to about 50% occurring in some foods (depending on irradiation dose and type of food). However, at high irradiation doses, organoleptic changes occur which limit the palatability of foods, and the author concludes that vitamin losses caused by irradiation will not be of importance in Western countries.

Microbial contamination of foods is of particular concern to immunosuppressed patients, and therefore high irradiation doses may be used to sterilize their foods. Effects of 40 kGy irradiation on the vitamin A, amino acid, and fatty acid contents of some dairy foods were investigated (*52*). At this dose >93%, 75%, and 16% of the vitamin A was destroyed in cheese, yogurt bars, and nonfat dry milk, respectively. Amino acid and fatty acid concentrations were not substantially affected by this irradiation dose.

In other studies, chicken breasts irradiated at 3 kGy and 2°C, the radiation level approved by the FDA for processing poultry, a 6% decrease in α-tocopherol concentrations was observed (*53*). Thiamine losses from skeletal muscles of pork, chicken, and beef irradiated at 1.5–10 kGy were about three times as great as losses from liver from the same animals (*54*).

In terms of food safety, one must be concerned not only about the effects of irradiation on the food itself but also on the packaging material around the food. In a two-part series (*55,56*), Buchalla et al. addressed this question in a review of available information. In terms of effects on the structure of the packaging material, permeability of plastic films is generally not affected and deterioration of mechanical properties can often be controlled with stabilizers. However, effects of irradiation on multilayer structures and on some important materials such as polystyrene and poly(vinyl chloride) have not been well investigated. A variety of gaseous radiolytic products have been identified from irradiated plastics, including hydrocarbons, alcohols, aldehydes, ketones, carboxylic acids, hydrogen, methane, and hydrogen chloride. Migration of some of these compounds as well as of degradation products of phenolic antioxidants and organotin stabilizers into foods, particularly fatty foods, has been detected and should be further investigated.

## Detection of Irradiated Foods

Two recent articles discussed and evaluated various methods for the detection of irradiated foods. Glidewell (*57*) described the irradiation process with its production of free radicals and other chemical changes in foods. Detection methods include EPR (electron paramagnetic resonance) or ESR (electron spin resonance) which are sensitive to free radicals, histochemical methods which visualize changes in cellulosic or pectic materials or changes in mitochondrial activity in plants, and detection of radiation-resistant bacteria. It is likely that there will not be one simple method for the detection of irradiated foods but rather a battery of methods will be developed. Stevenson (*58*) described and evaluated two methods in particular, ESR and the detection of 2-alkylcyclobutanones which are formed in irradiated fats. Experiments to date suggest that this latter

method may be useful in analyses of meats, eggs, and some fruits.

Since contaminated eggs have been responsible for many recent outbreaks of food poisoning, there is much interest in irradiation as a means of sterilizing eggs. Helle et al (*59,60*) reported on several methods that have been developed for the detection of irradiated eggs. GC/MS analyses of fat components can detect irradiation-specific compounds such as 2-dodecylcyclobutanone (DCB), which is formed from palmitic acid. ESR can detect irradiated packaging materials (cellulose radicals) and also radiation-specific radicals in the calcite matrix of eggshells. HPLC analyses are useful for low-fat samples with a high protein content by detection of *o*-tyrosine. Microbiological tests are not as effective in determining if a sample has been irradiated because microbiological status is affected by many other factors such as storage conditions.

Another radiation-specific fatty acid derivative, 2-tetradecylcyclobutanone (TCB), which is formed from stearic acid, has been synthesized and characterized (*61*). This compound was detected by GC/MS in both raw and thermally processed liquid whole eggs which had been irradiated and was present at about 3 times less the concentration of DCB.

Electrophoretic analyses of egg white proteins have demonstrated that irradiation partially fragments some of the proteins. Immunoblotting analysis, using antibodies to egg white proteins, has been proposed as another useful procedure for detecting irradiated eggs (*62*). Some antigenic peptide fragments of mass ≤30 kDa were clearly detected in egg whites irradiated at 2 and 10 kGy. While no ESR signals are detectable in shells of unirradiated eggs, strong signals can be detected for up to 200 days after irradiation of whole eggs (*63*). The most intense signal increased linearly with a dose up to 6 kGy. About 20% of the signal decayed within the first 5 days but it remained fairly constant thereafter.

A method utilizing adsorption chromatographic column separation and gas chromatography has been developed to measure very low levels of cholesterol oxidation products in meat (*64*). Using this procedure increased levels of 6-ketocholestanol could be detected in samples of irradiated chicken meat. An irradiation dose of 10 kGy increased 6-ketocholestanol concentrations about 4-fold as compared to unirradiated meat.

Some irradiated plant materials can be detected by ESR signals from the "cellulosic" radical. An improved procedure optimizing experimental parameters for detection of this radical has produced signal intensities of up to 200% greater amplitude (*65*). Using an incident microwave power of ≤250 μW resulted in greater sensitivity and fewer false negatives.

Two methods have been described for the detection of irradiated spices. ESR analysis of irradiated cinnamon and allspice demonstrated the formation of two radicals, one of which appeared to be unique to irradiated samples (66). The other radical was also produced by heat and photo-exposure. Irradiation of some spices causes changes in viscosity after heat gelatinization at pH 12. Hayashi et al. (67) investigated the conditions for measuring viscosity and the applicability for using this method to detect irradiation of different spices. The method appears to be reliable for analyses of black and white peppers and other spices with a high starch content.

Irradiated and nonirradiated water can be distinguished by using an electronic sensor to detect hydrogen generated during irradiation (68). Since this hydrogen diffuses away within 12 hours if the container is open, this method for detecting irradiated foods would only be useful for packaged or solid foods which retain the characteristic hydrogen marker.

Irradiation of potatoes in Japan is legal although no reliable method has yet been developed to detect irradiated specimens. Procedures to detect treated potatoes by measuring electrical conductivity or impedance were investigated and the incubation conditions of potatoes prior to measurements were found to be critical to ensuring reliable results (69). Impedance ratios depended on the radiation dose applied and the potato cultivar. If the cultivar was known, tubers irradiated at 0.1 kGy could be distinguished from unirradiated tubers.

Irradiation of deep frozen foods can be detected by comparison of an aerobic plate count with a cell count obtained by direct epifluorescent filter technique (70). Irradiation kills bacterial cells, thereby drastically decreasing plate counts, but both live and dead cells fluoresce when stained with acridine orange. This method was capable of detecting irradiated parsley, mechanically deboned poultry meat, and liquid egg whites even after 12 months' storage.

## ANTIOXIDANTS

Although some evidence indicates that dietary antioxidants have a protective effect, other studies have documented carcinogenic effects. Further evidence for such equivocal effects comes from a multiorgan carcinogenesis model in which rats were given initiating doses of several different N-nitroso compounds and then fed diets containing 0.7–1.0% of one of four different anti-

oxidants (71). The experiment was terminated at 36 weeks with all surviving animals examined at this time and others examined at the time of death. Propyl gallate reduced the number of atypical tubules in the kidney. The other antioxidants had both positive and negative effects: butylated hydroxytoluene (BHT) enhanced the development of thyroid hyperplasias but reduced the incidence and multiplicity of colon adenocarcinomas and renal cell tumors. α-Tocopherol increased the incidence of atypical foci in the glandular stomach but decreased the incidence and multiplicity of kidney atypical tubules. TBHQ (tert-butylhydroquinone) significantly elevated the incidences of papillomas in the esophagus and forestomach but significantly reduced the multiplicity of colon adenocarcinomas.

A collaborative study involving 10 laboratories evaluated a liquid chromatographic method for the determination of 9 antioxidants [propyl, octyl, and dodecyl gallates, TBHQ, BHT, butylated hydroxyanisole (BHA), Ionox-100 (2,6-di-tert-butyl-4-hydroxy-methylphenol), nordihydroguaiaretic acid, and 2,4,5-trihydroxybutyrophenone] (72). This method was adopted first action by AOAC International as a modification of AOAC method 983.15.

Considerable experimental data is available on the adverse effects of BHA in laboratory rodents but the application of this data to human risk assessment remains controversial. Würtzen (73) utilized a method for the systematic weighting of information to calculate data-derived safety factors in an analysis of the toxicological and biochemical information on BHA. Safety factors based on the no-observed-effect-level (NOEL) for liver and body weight changes (which are relevant for humans) indicate that the acceptable daily intake of BHA for humans is 0.7 mg/kg body weight.

In a long-term study, high dietary levels of BHA (6000 and 12,000 ppm) caused a statistically significant increase in the time-related incidence of forestomach but not of glandular stomach or esophageal tumors in rats initiated with MNNG (74). This level of BHA required to enhance forestomach carcinogenesis is at least 1500-fold greater than ordinary human dietary exposures.

Previous experiments with rats have demonstrated that BHA and some other antioxidants can act as promoters of bladder carcinogenesis. However, recent studies with mice, initiated with N-butyl-N-(4-hydroxybutyl)nitrosamine indicated that dietary BHA (1%) and sodium ascorbate (5%) do not enhance the development of bladder tumors in this species (75). Neither does treatment with these antioxidants alone for 8 weeks significantly elevate DNA synthesis in bladder epithelial cells.

Treatment of rats and mice with BHA results in increased levels of hepatic glutathione (GSH) and it has been proposed that this increase along with an increase in GSH S-transferase activity forms the basis for the protective effects of BHA in carcinogenesis experiments. Recent experiments with mice fed diets containing 0.05–0.75% BHA for up to 14 days showed that BHA elevated hepatic activity of γ-glutamylcysteine synthetase, the rate limiting enzyme in hepatic GSH synthesis (76). It is not known whether this increased enzyme activity is a result of stabilization of existing enzyme molecules or enhanced transcription of the gene coding for this enzyme.

BHT is generally regarded as nonhazardous when used in low concentrations as a food preservative but in some assays it has been shown to cause chromosomal damage. Of several BHT metabolites tested, 2,6-di-*t*-butyl-*p*-benzoquinone (BHT-quinone) was found to cleave supercoiled DNA in vitro at concentrations as low as $1 \times 10^{-6}$ M (77). Two other metabolites caused lesser amounts of damage and 6 others had no effect on DNA structure. A solution of BHT-quinone produced superoxide radicals which may be the cause of the DNA breaks. TBHQ, a metabolite of BHA, has also been shown to generate superoxide radicals and to damage DNA in vitro (78).

## SWEETENERS

### Aspartame

Although numerous clinical trials have attested to the safety of aspartame, there continue to be reports of adverse reactions to this sweetener in some apparently sensitive individuals. To ascertain whether persons with mood disorders are particularly susceptible to such effects, 8 subjects with unipolar depression and 5 without any psychiatric history consumed 30 mg aspartame per kg per day for one week and placebo for another week in a blinded crossover design (79). The original protocol called for the testing of 40 patients with depression but the study was halted after some participants experienced severe reactions. No significant differences in symptoms during the aspartame and placebo weeks were reported by the control group (even though 3 of the controls believed they experienced headaches in response to aspartame ingestion). Three of the depressed subjects spontaneously reported that they felt they had been "poisoned." Two depressed patients suffered severe eye problems (retinal detachment and conjunctival hemorrhage) during or shortly after the aspartame

phase. Patients also more often reported symptoms of nervousness, dizziness, difficulty in remembering, nausea, and depression during the aspartame week. Because a significant pattern of adverse reactions to aspartame occurred in this group with mood disorders, they may be particularly sensitive to aspartame. The association of aspartame with eye problems should be further investigated.

An association of aspartame ingestion with seizures has been previously reported. A recent letter describes two more such cases (80). Two women, who ingested >40 mg aspartame/kg/day for a few weeks, were hospitalized with a first classic episode of a generalized seizure. A thorough examination revealed that EEG, brain CT, blood cytochemistry, and a lumbar puncture all were normal. The timing of the seizures and the lack of other probable causes suggests that the chronic high aspartame ingestion may have caused the seizures.

However, a randomized, double-blind, placebo-controlled crossover study with 10 children with known seizure disorders did not demonstrate significant differences in a standard EEG or a continuous 24-hour EEG following aspartame vs. placebo consumption (81). Each child received a single morning dose of 34 mg aspartame/kg for 2 weeks and placebo during another two weeks. No significant differences in symptoms or behavior were reported on the STESS or the Conners Behavior Rating Scale. It appears that this potentially vulnerable group of children was not sensitive to the possible neurological effects of aspartame.

Some other reports have implicated aspartame in allergy-hypersensitivity-type reactions. However, in a multicenter, placebo-controlled clinical study, 21 subjects who reported that they had experienced urticaria and/or angioedema following aspartame ingestion were found to be no more likely to develop these symptoms after aspartame than after placebo doses (82). On different days, subjects were challenged with placebo or with increasing doses (50, 300, 600 mg) of aspartame in capsules at 2-hour intervals. Two subjects had positive reactions following the aspartame doses while two others reacted positively following the placebo. Although the researchers attempted to recruit many more subjects for testing, these were the only subjects they were able to prescreen who met the criteria for probable reaction to aspartame and who had no other conditions (pregnancy, skin problems, etc) which prevented their participation.

Some anecdotal reports have also suggested that aspartame negatively affects cognitive performance or behavior. However, 3 recent controlled studies, in which subjects received daily doses of aspartame for 1–2 weeks, failed to confirm this effect of aspartame. Twelve healthy university students were assessed for performance in aviation-relevant cognitive tasks, using the SPARTANS cognitive test battery, following separate 9-day periods of chronic consumption of placebo, aspartame (50 mg/kg/day), and alcohol (positive control) (83). Although alcohol caused a pattern of impairment in certain specific visuospatial skills associated with the right parietal region of the brain, there was no evidence of a detrimental effect of aspartame on cognitive performance.

Fifteen unmedicated children with attention deficit disorder were observed by their parents and classroom teachers during two 2-week periods when they consumed a daily dose of placebo or of 34 mg aspartame per kg (84). The doses were administered in a randomized, double-blind, crossover pattern. No clinically significant differences were noted during the two test periods in the STESS, MIT, or Conners ratings or for the MFFT, CCT, WCST, or Airplane cognition tests. Neither were there any significant differences in blood chemistry (except for increases in plasma phenylalanine and tyrosine following aspartame doses) or urinalysis parameters tested. Thus it appeared that aspartame ingestion at 10 times the usual rate had no detrimental effects on behavior or cognitive function.

Because aspartame contains phenylalanine (phe), persons with phenylketonuria (PKU, an inability to metabolize phe) are advised not to consume this sweetener. Since parents and siblings of persons with PKU may be heterozygous for the "PKU" gene and possibly at risk if they consume aspartame, 10 PKU heterozygotes and 10 controls were challenged with 85 μmol aspartame/kg added to a noon meal already containing 303 μmol/kg phe (85). Other PKU heterozygotes and controls consumed the meal without the added aspartame. The meal plus aspartame significantly increased plasma phe levels and the ratio of plasma phe to large neutral amino acids in both the controls and the PKU heterozygotes. In no case did these elevated levels approach the high levels known to cause adverse effects in persons with PKU.

Aspartame was nitrosated under conditions which could occur in the stomach and the resultant products were tested for mutagenicity using the Ames test (86). Nitrosation of the primary amine in aspartame generated mutagenic compounds but it appeared that under stomach conditions nitrosation of some tryptophan peptides would form more mutagenic compounds than nitrosation of aspartame.

Metabolism of aspartame by human and pig intestinal microvillar peptidases was examined using intestinal membrane preparations in vitro (87). Selective peptidase inhibitors indicated that, in both species, the cell surface aminopeptidase A was the major enzyme involved in the hydrolysis of aspartame. The stimulation of hydrolysis by calcium chloride also pointed to aminopeptidase A as the primary enzyme.

At the normal pH of milk (6.6) aspartame is unstable and this limits the use of this sweetener in milk beverages. Therefore, experiments were conducted to determine the effects of different conditions of pH, holding temperature, and different buffer salts on the stability of aspartame in commercially sterilized skim milk beverages (88). Temperature and pH proved to be the most important variables. Decreasing pH from 6.7 to 6.4 approximately doubled the half-life of aspartame while decreasing holding temperature from 30°C to 4°C increased aspartame's half-life from 1 to 24 days (pH 6.6) and from 4 to 58 days (pH 6.4). Type and concentration of buffer (phosphate and citrate) had only a minor effect on stability, and the addition of vanilla had no effect. Therefore proper formulation, processing, and storage can ensure a long enough shelf life for aspartame-sweetened, reduced-calorie dairy beverages.

An enzymatic method, utilizing α-chymotrypsin and alcohol oxidase immobilized on a resin has been developed for the spectrophotometric determination of aspartame (89).

## Saccharin

When male rats are fed diets containing ≥3% sodium saccharin from birth, they incur significantly more bladder cancer than rats not consuming saccharin. Using data from numerous experiments testing the carcinogenicity of saccharin, Renwick (90) developed a data-derived safety factor to estimate the risk to humans consuming this sweetener. Based on this analysis, an overall safety factor of 50 was calculated, and this would indicate an acceptable daily intake of 0–10 mg per kg body weight. A large number of epidemiological studies have failed to demonstrate an association between bladder cancer and saccharin consumption in humans. It may be that humans are inherently less sensitive to saccharin than rats and that an even greater intake of saccharin is safe.

In tests to determine cocarcinogenicity of saccharin in female rats, these animals were treated with N-methyl-N-nitrosourea (MNU) to induce bladder tumors (91). They were also fed diets containing 0, 1.0, 2.5, or 5.0% sodium saccharin for 4 weeks before, during, or after carcinogen administration. Examination of rats after 580–790 days showed that only the 2.5% saccharin diet given after MNU exerted a consistent but statistically weak enhancement of tumor prevalence. Saccharin therefore appeared to be a weak promoter of bladder cancer.

## Stevioside

Leaves from a South American shrub, *Stevia rebaudiana*, have been used for sweetening beverages and foods for centuries. Commercialization of the intensely sweet compounds from this plant has raised the question of their possible toxic effects. Recent testing of stevioside and steviol revealed that neither compound had clastogenic effects on cultured human lymphocytes (*92*). Regardless of metabolic activation, steviol was not mutagenic to *S. typhimurium* strains TA98 and TA100. Stevioside induced mutations only in TA98 at concentrations ≥50 mg/plate.

Since previous experiments indicated that stevioside had nephrotoxic effects in some rodents, this was further investigated by injecting rats with 1.5 g stevioside/kg body weight (*93*). Nine hours after dosing the animals were sacrificed and it was found that stevioside significantly decreased the ability of excised renal cortex slices to accumulate *p*-aminohippurate (PAH) in vitro by 63.4% but had no effect on lipid oxidation in plasma. In vitro experiments confirmed these results: Both steviol and stevioside at a concentration of 100 µM, directly inhibited accumulation of PAH in renal cortical slices and did not induce the formation of lipid peroxides.

## Other Sweeteners

Sugar alcohols (polyols) are widely used as sweeteners because their energy level is low and they do not promote dental caries. To determine whether calciuria and oxaluria increase after consumption of these sweeteners as they do after an oral glucose load, 10 healthy volunteers consumed, on 5 different days, 20 g of glucose, lycasin (a hydrogenated glucose syrup), maltisorb (a hydrogenated disaccharide), sorbitol, and xylitol (*94*). Only the xylitol dose caused increases in both urinary calcium and oxalate. At this dose, glucose only increased urinary calcium. Neither xylitol nor sorbitol caused the increases in glycemia and insulinemia which occurred after ingestion of glucose, lycasin, and maltisorb. Polyols appear to have less of an effect on pancreatic secretions than glucose and the hydrogenated sugars.

An enzymatic method utilizing sorbitol dehydrogenase and diaphorase was evaluated by 19 labs in Germany and proved to be an efficient and reproducible method for the determination of D-sorbitol in dietetic bakery products (*95*).

Sucralose, an intensely sweet derivative of sucrose produced by a selective chlorination process was recently reviewed by Wallis (*96*). This sweetener is quite inert, and over 100 studies have reported that it has no toxic effects and does not promote dental caries. Very little sucralose is absorbed from the intestines and most of it is excreted virtually unchanged in the feces.

# FLAVORS AND FLAVOR ENHANCERS

Safety evaluation of flavoring substances, including the GRAS process and current evaluation criteria for safety assessment, was discussed by Emerson and Stone (*97*). Historically, many flavoring substances in common use were listed as GRAS (generally recognized as safe) shortly after passage of the 1958 Food Additives Amendment. Further evaluation of flavors is now done by the Flavor and Extract Manufacturers' Association Expert Panel, a group of independent scientists which investigates the safety of flavoring substances in foods under the conditions of intended use. Evaluations consider exposure levels, metabolism and pharmacokinetics, and toxicological studies.

## Synthetic Flavors

A new liquid smoke preparation, UTP, produced by refining of wood tar and used in manufacture of smoked meat, has been evaluated for genotoxic effects in mice (*98*). After 4 weeks' exposure to drinking water containing 0.1, 1, 10, or 100 mL UTP/L, bone marrow cells were examined for cytogenetic effects. UTP did not induce chromosomal aberrations nor did it affect the body weight of treated animals. At the highest dose level, mice were ingesting 2.5–3.8 mL UTP/day as compared to the predicted human intake of 40 mL UTP/year.

Protein hydrolysates, widely used as savoury flavorings, are commonly produced by HCl hydrolysis of vegetable proteins. This results in formation of some chlorinated compounds which may be present in the derived food products. Analysis of volatile constituents of traditionally manufactured soybean meal hydrolysates by GC and GC/MS revealed the presence of two new chlorinated esters derived from residual lipids and from saccharides (*99*). These compounds were present in concentrations of 0.6–1.1 mg/kg but were readily decomposed under alkaline conditions.

## Natural Flavors

Aryl sulfotransferases catalyze the conjugation of a sulfate group to a phenolic compound which generally inactivates the organic compound and makes it more easily excreted. Thus, these enzymes are important in detoxifying some xenobiotics. In vitro experiments demonstrated that vanillin inhibits rat liver aryl sulfo-transferases in a partial noncompetitive fashion (*100*). At present it is difficult to know whether this inhibition also occurs in vivo and, since there is no information available on the absorption and distribution of vanillin in the body, it is not possible to predict internal concentrations.

A thin-layer chromatography procedure with automated multiple development has been developed for determination of vanillin and other polar aromatic flavor compounds commonly found in natural and artificial extracts of vanilla flavors (*101*). This method was used to confirm the authenticity of natural vanilla extracts purchased in the USA and to detect some counterfeit "natural" vanilla extracts purchased in Puerto Rico and Mexico.

Safrole, a natural constituent of sassafras, basil, nutmeg, and other spices, has been shown to be a rodent carcinogen. Analysis of hepatic DNA from mice injected with 0.001–10 mg safrole/mouse revealed about a ten-fold increase in safrole–DNA adducts for each 10-fold increase in safrole dose (*102*). Adduct levels peaked two days after dosing and remained fairly constant thereafter (up to 30 days). Two major and two minor safrole–DNA adducts have been characterized, all involving deoxyguanosine (*103*). The possible effects of these adducts on protein–nucleotide interactions and implications for carcinogenesis were discussed.

Eugenol, a principal constituent of clove oil, has been tested for genotoxicity in the mouse bone marrow micronucleus assay (*104*). At high doses (injections of 400 and 600 mg eugenol/kg) a significant induction of micronuclei was observed. At a lower dose of 100 mg/kg, there was no evidence of genotoxicity.

Genotoxicity of some alkenylbenzenes used as flavorings was assessed in the UDS (unscheduled DNA synthesis) assay in rat hepatocytes (*105*). Elemicin (found in nutmeg and sassafras) and α- and β-asarone (found in oil of calamus) did induce UDS while myristicin (found in nutmeg, mace, black pepper, and carrots) did not. Neither myristicin nor elemicin is hepatocarcinogenic in rodents while the other compounds are.

β-Myrcene (MYR), a constituent of lemon grass, hop, bay, and other herbs, was tested for peri- and postnatal toxicity in rats (*106*). Female rats were gavaged from day 15 of pregnancy throughout the lactation period with 0.25, 0.5, 1.0, or 1.5 g MYR/kg. No adverse effects were observed on the offspring at the lowest dose but at the higher doses there was evidence of decreased birth weight, increased perinatal mortality, delay in the appearance of landmarks of postnatal development, and subsequent impairment of the fertility of the female offspring. These data indicate a no-obseved-adverse-effects level (NOAEL) of 0.25g/kg.

Acetaldehyde, widely used in artificial fruit flavors, is an extremely reactive, strong electrophile. Therefore, it has the potential to cross-link with proteins and to react with DNA. Using a newly developed derivatization method, followed by GC with a nitrogen–phosphorus detector, 14 commercial food and beverage items were analyzed for acetaldehyde (*107*). Concentrations ranged from 0.46 ppm (cola) to 101.9 ppm (whiskey).

## Flavor Enhancers

Previous investigations of the role of monosodium L-glutamate (MSG) in producing the symptoms associated with "Chinese Restaurant Syndrome" have yielded contradictory results. In a recent study by Tarasoff and Kelly (*108*) a true randomized, double-blind, crossover protocol which controlled for the strong taste of MSG was used to determine the effects of realistic but high doses of MSG in the presence of food on 71 healthy volunteers. On 3 different days, volunteers were given 6 capsules containing only placebo, 1.5 g MSG, or 3.0 g MSG while on two other days they were given a flavored drink containing 3.15 g MSG or a placebo. In each case the dose was followed by the same identical light breakfast. Two hours later the subjects were contacted and questioned about the taste of the drink or food and about any sensations they experienced since the meal. Most subjects (85–86%) reported no responses to either placebo or MSG. Of the sensations reported which were similar to those previously attributed to MSG, none were more frequent after MSG than after placebo consumption. These results demonstrate that food consumption can negate the effects of large MSG doses and call into question the common practice of extrapolating from food-free tests to actual "in use" situations. The authors pointed out that most previous studies were not truly blind because the strong taste of MSG was not disguised.

Fructooligosaccharides (FOS) are naturally occurring carbohydrates consisting of sucrose molecules to which 1, 2, or 3 additional fructose units have been added. In a recent review of these flavor enhancers, Spiegel et al. (*109*) pointed out that these compounds are virtually undigestible by human digestive enzymes and appear to have little effect on humans or laboratory animals except for softening of stools and diarrhea (if consumed at a concentration ≥5% of the diet). The no-observed-effect level in rats is 2.17 g per kg body weight per day. These compounds are about half as sweet as sucrose and are used to improve the flavor of more than 500 food products in Japan.

Methods for the simultaneous determination of 3 flavor enhancers, MSG, inosine 5'-monophosphate, and guanosine 5'-monophosphate, in foods by derivative spectrophotometry have been developed (*110,111*).

## FOOD COLORS

Erythrosine (FD & C Red No. 3) is a widely used, iodine-containing food color which is known to have effects on the thyroid gland. Data-derived safety factors calculated for erythrosine from data on long-term carcinogenicity assays in rodents, hormonal effects in rats, and hormonal changes in humans indicated acceptable daily intakes (ADIs) for humans of 0.25, 0.3, and 0.1 mg/kg body weight, respectively (*112*). The ADI based on human data is considered the most appropriate. Because of the uncertainty of the variability in human pharmacokinetics, further research should be done to elucidate this point.

Teratogenic potential of erythrosine was investigated in experiments with pregnant rats gavaged with 15, 30, 100, 200, 400, or 800 mg erythrosine/kg on gestation days 0–19 (*113*). On day 20, the animals were sacrificed and the fetuses examined. No dose-related adverse effects in maternal weight gain, implantations, fetal viability, fetal size, and fetal skeletal and visceral development were observed. Therefore, this food color is neither fetotoxic nor teratogenic when given, by gavage, at a dose of 800 mg/kg to rats.

Spectroscopic characterization of allura red (FD & C Red No. 40) was achieved using fast atom bombardment–mass spectrometry (FAB–MS), high resolution FAB–MS, and proton and carbon NMR (*114*). This data confirmed the structure of this compound. Reverse-phase HPLC analysis of 6 samples of allura red revealed the presence of the unsulfonated primary aromatic amine, *p*-cresidine, at concentrations of 0.08 to 1.9 μg/g (*115*).

Reproductive and neurobehavioral effects of the color additive amaranth were examined in mice provided with drinking water containing 0, 0.025, 0.075, and 0.225% amaranth from 5 weeks of age in the $F_0$ generation until weaning of the $F_1$ generation (*116*). Little effect was observed on litter sizes and weights. Some neurobehavioral parameters were adversely affected but the effects were often observed in only one sex or at one time point and not at later times. Therefore amaranth at these dose levels was considered to be only mildly toxic.

A carcinogenic aromatic amine, benzidine, which has been detected in some lots of tartrazine (FD & C Yellow No. 5), is limited to a concentration of 1 ng/g by FDA regulations. A survey of 53 samples of tartrazine from 12 different dye distributors revealed that 25 samples contained 7–83 ng combined benzidine/g (*117*). All other samples contained <5 ng/g (limit of quantitation for the analytical method). Of the positive samples, all except 2 were from the same manufacturer. Previous surveys indicated that a greater percentage of dye samples were contaminated with benzidine and greater concentrations were also found.

Three methods have been developed for the simultaneous determination of Sunset Yellow (FD & C Yellow No. 6) and Quinoline Yellow in foods (*118*). These methods do not require a separation step and involve first and second derivative spectrophotometry and the first derivative of the ratio spectra.

One component of Caramel Color III which is known to be responsible for lymphopenia in laboratory animals fed a vitamin $B_6$-deficient diet is designated THI. To determine the safety of Caramel Color III with a low THI content (<25 ppm), mice were provided with drinking water containing 2 or 10% of this food color and a diet high in vitamin $B_6$ for 9 weeks (*119*). Although the exposed mice did not develop lymphopenia, some lymphocyte populations were reduced in number and the proliferative response of spleen cells to mitogens was also decreased. These results indicate that Caramel Color III with a THI content within the specified limits may still affect the lymphoid system in mice with an adequate vitamin intake.

Phloxine is a food color additive permitted for use in Japan and some other countries but not in the USA. Recent experiments with mice which were fed diets containing 0, 0.1, 0.3, and 0.9% phloxine from 5 weeks of age of the $F_0$ generation to 8 weeks of the $F_1$ generation revealed that this compound produced a few adverse reproductive and neurobehavioral effects (*120*). Some measurements of surface righting, motor activity, and speed of movement differed in the experimental and control mice.

A combination of liquid chromatography and an electromigration technique, called pseudo-electrochromatography, was developed for the separation of food colors (sulfonated azo dyes) and aromatic glucuronides prior to detection with mass spectrometry (*121*). By applying voltages of differing polarity during chromatography, selective separation of different compounds can be achieved.

Natural food colors may contain residues of organic solvents used in their preparation. A simple headspace GC method was developed for the simultaneous determination of 7 solvents in natural color preparations (*122*). Of 35 food colors tested, methanol was detected in 20, acetone in 3, and isopropanol in 1, at concentrations exceeding limits set by the FDA.

## VITAMINS AND MINERALS

### Vitamin A

Concern has been raised about consumption of liver because of its high vitamin A content and the known teratogenic effects of large doses of this vitamin. A survey of 45 bovine and 141 pork liver samples in Finland revealed similar mean concentrations of retinol equivalents (RE) of 28.8 and 25.5 mg RE/100 g, respectively (*123*). While most of the livers contained <40 mg RE/100 g, a few samples had quite high levels of 80–90 mg/100 g. RE levels were quite variable for both types of liver, probably due to the varied nutritional background of these slaughterhouse animals. In addition, there appeared to be a seasonal variation in vitamin A levels in bovine liver. Occasional consumption of liver should be safe but frequent consumption, especially by children, should not be encouraged.

In an investigation of the teratogenic metabolites of vitamin A, 10 healthy female volunteers were given 4 oral doses of vitamin A: 50 and 150 mg as retinol palmitate and two portions of fried calf liver containing 50 and 150 mg of retinol equivalents (*124*). Peak plasma concentrations of all-*trans*-retinoic acid, the principal teratogenic metabolite of retinol, was approximately 21 times higher after the palmitate supplement than after the liver dose, and the area under the concentration–time curve was 7–15 times greater after the palmitate supplement. From these data it appears that liver and oral supplements, even though they contain equivalent amounts of retinol, are not of equal teratogenic potential. Therefore, moderate consumption of liver by pregnant women may not be a great risk to their offspring.

### Vitamin D

To prevent bone disease in premature infants, formulas designed especially for these infants contain more calcium and vitamin D than standard formulas. Hypercalcemia was diagnosed in a 16-month-old boy who had been fed for 15 months with a premature formula because of chronic lung disease and failure to thrive (*125*). This formula contained about 400% more vitamin D than a standard formula. Although no specific symptoms of hypercalcemia were observed (vomiting, hypertension, irritability), routine blood analysis at 16 months revealed a blood calcium level of 14.1 mg/dL (normal level is ≤11 mg/dL). Serum vitamin D levels were also elevated and this hypervitaminosis D was apparently responsible for the hypercalcemia.

### EDTA and Possible Adverse Effects of Iron Supplementation

Disodium and calcium disodium EDTA (ethylenediaminetetraacetate) are approved by the FDA for use as food supplements and, recently, nutritionists have become interested in sodium iron (III) EDTA as a means of supplementing foods with highly available iron. A recent review by Whittaker et al. (*126*) presented toxicological profiles of EDTA compounds, acceptable daily intakes and estimated daily intakes of EDTA, and regulatory issues related to the use of sodium iron EDTA for fortifying foods. Recent data on estimated exposure to EDTA in the USA suggests that it is much lower than previously assumed. Therefore, the authors conclude that it is probably safe to increase the use of EDTA as a food additive except in areas with known zinc deficiency.

However, experiments with rats fed zinc-deficient and zinc-sufficient diets supplemented with disodium EDTA or sodium iron (III) EDTA demonstrated that both forms of EDTA had a positive effect on zinc nutrition (*127*). Both zinc absorption and retention were increased, more so in rats on the zinc-deficient diet. EDTA supplements did not substantially affect absorption or retention of dietary calcium or copper.

A sensitive spectrophotometric method has been developed for the determination of EDTA in foods (*128*). No interference was encountered from the common ingredients of commercial foods.

Although iron is certainly an element essential to life, it is increasingly being recognized that more is not better because ferrous iron can produce oxygen radicals. A recent review of iron metabolism and toxicity summarized the various reactions of iron in the body, including the production of free radicals by the reduction of oxygen (*129*). These free radicals can initiate lipid peroxidation and DNA damage, processes which may be involved in many pathological conditions. While iron may not cause disease, excess iron in the body may exacerbate free radical–associated diseases. McCord (*130*) also discussed the production of free radicals by iron in the body and pointed out that iron stores in the body increase almost linearly with age in males and postmenopausal females.

This stored iron may become a liability in older people. Herbert et al. (*131*) also discussed the detrimental effects of excess iron in producing the toxic hydroxyl radical. Excess vitamin C can enhance the prooxidant effects of iron and thus supplementing generally adequate diets with iron and vitamin C may actually be harmful.

Effects of iron supplementation on the growth rate of 47 iron-sufficient Indonesian children (12–18 months old) were monitored over a 4-month period (*132*). The children received daily doses of 3 mg ferrous sulfate or a placebo. Before the experiment the length and weight measurements of the two groups were similar, but during the experiment the rate of weight gain was significantly greater in the placebo group than in the iron-supplemented group. No differences were noted in the rates of respiratory or gastrointestinal infections.

A recent article by Weinberg (*133*) reviewed experimental and epidemiological investigations relating excess iron stores or iron intake to colorectal cancer. Experiments with rats and mice, initiated with known carcinogens, demonstrated that diets fortified with high levels of iron increased the incidence and multiplicity of colorectal tumors. Some epidemiological studies with humans also suggest that high iron levels promote carcinogenesis while substances such as phytate, which bind iron and reduce its bioavailability, appear to have a protective effect.

A case–control study involving 333 subjects with fecal occult blood in the stool or possible colonic polyps was conducted to determine factors associated with colonic neoplasia (*134*). Serum ferritin levels, measured in sera obtained 5–8 years previously, ranged from 8 to 928 ng/mL. These iron levels were compared to results from colonoscopy. A total of 159 subjects were classified as normal (without neoplastic disease), 145 had adenomas, and 29 had colon cancer. Analysis of the data, controlling for known or suspected risk factors, revealed statistically significant increased risks for adenomas for those in the third and fourth quintiles of ferritin relative to the first quintile. The lower mean ferritin levels observed in patients with colon cancer were probably caused by the disease. The apparent dose–response relationship observed between ferritin levels and adenoma risk suggests that exposure to iron may be related to adenoma formation.

Serum iron, total iron-binding capacity (TIBC), and transferrin saturation levels in a cohort of 41,276 Finnish men and women were studied for their predictive ability for the development of cancer during a mean followup of 14 years (*135*). During this time a total of 2469 cases of cancer were diagnosed. Elevated risks for colorectal and lung cancers were observed in subjects with transferrin saturation levels exceeding 60%. An inverse relationship was noted between serum iron and transferrin saturation and the risk for stomach cancer, but these associations were weakened when cases occurring within 5 years of followup were excluded. These data suggest that high iron stores may increase the risk of colon cancer and that low iron stores may be an early sign of developing stomach cancer.

Analyses of data from the NHANES I (National Health and Nutrition Survey) study also showed a correlation between indicators of high body iron levels and cancer incidence (*136*). Of 8556 subjects whose serum iron status was measured in 1971–1975 and who remained cancer-free for the next 4 years, 719 developed some type of cancer during 13–17 years of followup. Those in the 4th and 5th quintiles of transferrin saturation (50–60% and >60%) had elevated risks for cancer of 1.38 and 1.81, respectively, compared to those in the lowest quintile (0–30%).

However, the NHANES I data do not indicate a positive relationship between body iron stores and cardiovascular disease. Analyses of data on 4518 persons demonstrated that transferrin saturation was not related to incidence of coronary heart disease or to myocardial infarction in either men or women (*137*). In fact, a significant inverse association was observed between transferrin saturation and overall mortality and mortality from cardiovascular causes. Another analysis of data on 4237 NHANES participants also found that transferrin saturation and TIBC were not related to myocardial infarction and that serum iron and transferrin saturation were inversely associated with coronary heart disease (*138*). Dietary iron intake based on 24-hour recall was also not associated with coronary heart disease.

Another large epidemiological study involving 44,933 men (Health Professionals Follow-up Study) registered 844 cases of coronary disease in 4 years of follow-up but no relationship was observed between total iron uptake assessed at baseline and the risk of fatal coronary disease and of nonfatal myocardial infarction (*139*). However, the incidence of coronary disease was higher among men in the highest quintile of heme iron consumption as compared to those in the lowest quintile. Heme iron intake, but not total iron intake, was positively correlated with serum ferritin levels in a subgroup of the cohort.

Results from the Nutrition Canada Survey conducted in 1970–1972 also indicated no significant associations between dietary iron and iron supplement use and risk of fatal acute myocardial infarction among 9920 participants (*140*). However, those in the highest category of serum iron (≥175 µg/dL) had an increased risk of fatal acute myocardial infarction.

Since one recent study in Finland indicated that both increased serum ferritin and dietary iron intake were positively associated with acute myocardial infarction, Rabinoff considered the possible mechanism for this effect (*141*). It may be that increased body iron stores enhance infections with certain microbes and these infections damage the heart muscle or blood vessels.

## STABILIZERS AND CONDITIONERS

TOSOM is an efficient emulsifier and anti-spattering agent which is made up of "thermally oxidized soybean oil interacted with mono- and diglycerides of food fatty acids." It is added to frying margarine at a concentration of 0.3%. To test for possible carcinogenic effects of this additive, rats were fed diets containing 3, 6, or 12% TOSOM for 2.5 years (*142*). No treatment-related adverse effects were observed in appearance, weight gain, clinical chemistry and hematology, or histopathology of internal organs. As the rats aged, they developed various lesions, some of which were neoplastic, but no significant differences were seen between the control and experimental groups.

Although potassium bromate has been widely used as an oxidant in bread making, it has been reported to induce renal tumors when rats consumed it in drinking water (but not when it was in bread). An increase in cell proliferation occurred in the proximal tubules of male rats given drinking water containing potassium or sodium bromate (but not potassium bromide) (*143*). Hyaline droplets accumulated in the kidneys of bromate-treated rats and these droplets contained the male-specific urinary protein, $\alpha_{2u}$-globulin. These results suggest that bromate induces an $\alpha_{2u}$-globulin nephropathy which causes cell proliferation and neoplastic changes.

Brominated vegetable oils, used in the manufacture of some citrus-flavored beverages, were fed to rats to test their effects on hepatic secretions and plasma lipoproteins (*144*). After consuming diets with 0.5% brominated vegetable oils for 105 days, a decrease was observed in the hepatic secretion of very-low-density lipoprotein triglycerides and of plasma triglyceride levels. This suggests that these oils adversely affect the synthesis and/or secretion of very-low-density lipoprotein triglycerides.

Piperonyl butoxide, a food additive approved for use in raw cereals in Japan at a maximum level of 24 ppm, was tested for chronic toxicity and carcino-genicity in rats (*145*). Test animals consumed diets containing 0.6, 1.2, or 2.4% of this compound for nearly two years. Piperonyl butoxide was found to induce dose–dependent increases in hepatocellular carcinoma and essential thrombocythemia. Other toxic effects included hemorrhages in the stomach and cecum, anemia, degenerative lesions of the alveoli, and nephrotoxicity. Although these rats were certainly exposed to excessive amounts of this additive (approximately 35,000 times the acceptable daily intake for humans), it may be well to reevaluate its safety as a food additive.

A procedure has been developed for the determination of chlorinated fatty acid bleaching adducts in flour and flour-containing foods (*146*). The bleaching adducts were extracted with supercritical carbon dioxide, purified with acid hydrolysis–methylation and a Florisil column, and determined using gas chromatography with electrolytic conductivity detection. Highest levels of the two most common adducts in cookies and cakes were 40 ppm each and in flour were 300 ppm.

## ENZYMES

In two recent articles the governmental regulatory requirements in the USA (*147*) and the UK (*148*) related to the use of enzymes as food processing aids were summarized. Safety evaluation procedures in the USA for these enzymes, often produced by genetically engineered microbes in culture, were outlined in general and also discussed for several enzymes specifically. Draft guidelines for the safety assessment of microbial enzymes were published by the UK Committee on the Toxicity of Chemicals in Food, Consumer Products, and the Environment in 1992. It is expected that an increasing number of enzymes and other potential food additives produced by recombinant DNA technology will be developed and safety evaluation procedures may have to be further refined.

A report on a safety evaluation of esperase, a proteolytic enzyme used for cleaning meat from bones, was presented by Hjortkjaer et al. (*149*). Meat obtained by this process may contain 0.1% enzyme and the meat may then be used to form a maximum of 10% of meat mixtures and sausages. General toxicity assays in rats revealed that the enzyme caused minor adverse effects which were attributed to its proteolytic activity. However, since heating will inactivate the enzyme, this should be of no concern to consumers of processed foods. No teratogenic or genotoxic effects were observed in other assays. These data, along with information on the production organism (*Bacillus lentus*) and the chemistry and microbiology of the enzyme preparation, indicate that this enzyme is safe for use in food processing.

A lipase enzyme produced by a recombinant *Aspergillus oryzae* strain containing a gene from *Rhizomucor miehei*, can be used in the production of specialty fats, such as those with improved nutritional or functional properties. In an assessment of its safety, it was found to be nongenotoxic (Ames test, mouse lymphoma assay, human lymphocyte assay) and to have no adverse effects on rats fed diets containing up to 1600 ppm lipase for 13 weeks (*150*). At higher concentrations, the enzyme depressed food intake, caused minor changes in kidney weight and urine, and exacerbated the onset of normally occurring chronic myocarditis in male rats.

Acetolactate decarboxylase, used in the fermentation of beer, was found to be nongenotoxic in standard tests and also had no toxic effects on rats (including pregnant females and their offspring) fed for 13 weeks with up to 10,000 ppm of the enzyme (*151*). A concentration of 10,000 ppm is approximately 120,000 times the estimated human intake.

# FAT SUBSTITUTES

A recent issue of the *Journal of Agricultural and Food Chemistry* contained a number of articles related to the chemical characterization (*152*), determination in foods (*153*), safety assessment studies (*154–159*), and clinical evaluations (*160,161*) of SALATRIM, a family of low-calorie fats. SALATRIM is a family of triacylglycerols containing a mixture of long-chain, saturated fatty acids and short-chain fatty acids. These fat substitutes have the physical properties of fats but only about half the calories of an ordinary edible oil and may be used in a variety of foods. Studies reported here indicated that SALATRIM had no mutagenic effects, did not induce chromosomal abnormalities, and, in 13-week feeding studies, had no adverse effects on rats and their cecal flora or on minipigs. In clinical trials with human volunteers, slight and transient increases in serum alanine aminotransferase and serum aspartate aminotransferase were observed. Neither these increases in enzyme activity nor some reported gastrointestinal discomfort were considered clinically significant. SALATRIM appears to be a safe and versatile fat substitute.

Caprenin, a randomized triglyceride containing caprylic (C8:0), capric (C10:0), and behenic (C22:0) acids has functional and organoleptic properties similar to cocoa butter and thus can be used as a confectionery

fat. It provides fewer usable fat calories than ordinary fats because behenic acid is not completely absorbed. Also the short-chain fatty acids have a thermogenic effect. A 91-day feeding study revealed that this fat substitute had no observable adverse effects at a dietary concentration of 15% (*162*). Analyses of fat from fat depot sites in the rats demonstrated that the animals did not store behenic acid.

A series of chromatographic techniques have been described for the isolation and characterization of sucrose polyesters formed by reacting sucrose with methyl esters from olive oil (*163*). Octa-, hepta-, and hexaesters were separated and quantitated by TLC, flame ionization detection, and HPLC.

## LITERATURE CITED

1. Taylor, S.L., and J.A. Nordlee. Chemical additives in seafood products. *Clin. Rev. Aller.* 11:261–291 (1993).

2. Zeiger, E. Mutagenicity of chemicals added to foods. *Mutat. Res.* 290:53–61 (1993).

3. Bamforth, K.J., A.L. Jones, R.C. Roberts, and M.W.H. Coughtrie. Common food additives are potent inhibitors of human liver $17\alpha$-ethinyloestradiol and dopamine sulphotransferases. *Biochem. Pharmacol.* 46:1713–1720 (1993).

4. Fuglsang, G., C. Madsen, S. Halken, et al. Adverse reactions to food additives in children with atopic symptoms. *Allergy* 49:31–37 (1994).

5. Armentia-Alvarez, A., C. Garcia-Moreno, and M.J. Peña-Egido. Residual levels of sulfite in raw and boiled frozen shrimp: variability, distribution and losses. *J. Food Protect.* 57:66–69 (1994).

6. Tsuji, S., K. Fujiwara, M. Kakiuchi, et al. Naturally occurring sulfites in raw and processed foods. *J. Food Hyg. Soc. Japan* 34:303–313 (1993).

7. Rosselló, C., J. Cañellas, I. Santiesteban, and A. Mulet. Simulation of the absorption process of sulphur dioxide in apricots. *Lebensm. Wiss. Technol.* 26:322–328 (1993).

8. Ruiz, E., M.I. Santillana, M. de Alba, et al. High performance ion chromatography determination of total sulfites in foodstuffs. *J. Liq. Chromatogr.* 17:447–456 (1994).

9. Cardwell, T.J., R.W. Cattrall, G.N. Chen, et al. Determination of sulfur dioxide in wines and beverages by flow injection analysis with reductive amperometric detection and electrolytic cleanup. *J. AOAC Int.* 76:1389–1393 (1993).

10. Akasaka, K., H. Ohrui, H. Meguro, et al. Fluorometric determination of total and bound sulfite in wine by *N*-(9-acridinyl)maleimide. *J. AOAC Int.* 76:1385–1388 (1993).

11. Leubolt, R., and H. Klein. Determination of sulphite and ascorbic acid by high-performance liquid chromatography with electrochemical detection. *J. Chromatogr.* 640:271–277 (1993).

12. Fujitani, T. Short-term effect of sodium benzoate in F344 rats and B6C3F1 mice. *Toxicol. Lett.* 69:171–179 (1993).

13. Khan, S.H., M.P. Murawski, and J. Sherma. Quantitative high performance thin layer chromatographic determination of organic acid preservatives in beverages. *J. Liq. Chromatogr.* 17:855–865 (1994).

14. Bruning-Fann, C.S., and J.B. Kaneene. The effects of nitrate, nitrite and N-nitroso compounds on human health: a review. *Vet. Human Toxicol.* 35:521–538 (1993).

15. Laitinen, S., S.M. Virtanen, L. Räsänen, and P.-L. Penttilä. Calculated dietary intakes of nitrate and nitrite by young Finns. *Food Addit. Contam.* 10:469–477 (1993).

16. Dusdieker, L.B., J.P. Getchell, T.M. Liarakos, et al. Nitrate in baby foods. Adding to the nitrate mosaic. *Arch. Pediatr. Adolesc. Med.* 148:490–494 (1994).

17. Lyons, D.J., G.E. Rayment, P.E. Nobbs, and L.E. McCallum. Nitrate and nitrite in fresh vegetables from Queensland. *J. Sci. Food Agric.* 64:279–281 (1994).

18. Tsuji, S., M. Kohsaka, Y. Morita, et al. Naturally occurring of nitrite and nitrate existing in various raw and processed foods. *J. Food Hyg. Soc. Japan* 34:294–302 (1993).

19. Sjöberg, A.-M., and T.A. Alanko. Spectrophotometric determination of nitrate in baby foods: collaborative study. *J. AOAC Int.* 77:425–430 (1994).

20. Jie, N., J. Yang, and J. Li. Fluorimetric determination of nitrite using a new reagent system. *Anal. Lett.* 27:1001–1008 (1994).

21. Misko, T.P., R.J. Schilling, D. Salvemini, et al. A fluorometric assay for the measurement of nitrite in biological samples. *Anal. Biochem.* 214:11–16 (1993).

22. Ensafi, A.A., and M. Keyvanfard. Selective kinetic spectrophotometric determination of nitrite in food and water. *Anal. Lett.* 27:169–182 (1994).

23. Bradberry, S.M., B. Gazzard, and J.A. Vale. Methemoglobinemia caused by the accidental contamination of drinking water with sodium nitrite. *Clin. Toxicol.* 32:173–178 (1994).

24. Phillips, B.J., A.C. Tee, P.A. Carroll, et al. Toxicity to Chinese hamster ovary (CHO) cells of the products of reaction of butylated hydroxyanisole with nitrite at low pH. *Toxicol. in Vitro* 8:117–123 (1994).

25. Kawabe, M., K. Takaba, Y. Yoshida, and M. Hirose. Effects of combined treatment with phenolic compounds and sodium nitrite on two-stage carcinogenesis and cell proliferation in the rat stomach. *Jpn. J. Cancer Res.* 85:17–25 (1994).

26. Xu, G.P., and P.I. Reed. N-Nitroso compounds in fresh gastric juice and their relation to intragastric pH and nitrite employing an improved analytical method. *Carcinogenesis* 14:2547–2551 (1993).

27. Mende, P., D. Ziebarth, R. Preussmann, and B. Spiegelhalder. Occurrence of the nitrosamide precursor pyrrolidin-(2)-one in food and tobacco. *Carcinogenesis* 15:733–737 (1994).

28. Kato, T., S. Takahashi, and K. Kikugawa. Formation of direct-acting mutagens in coffee by treatment with nitrite. *Jpn. J. Toxicol. Environ. Health* 39:189–195 (1993).

29. Erdinger, L., P. Schmezer, R. Razdan, et al. Caffeine-derived N-nitroso compounds. III: Mutagenicity in *S. typhimurium* and in vitro induction of DNA single-strand breaks in rat hepatocytes by mononitrosocaffeidine and dinitrosocaffeidine. *Mutat. Res.* 292:41–49 (1993).

30. Laires, A., J. Gaspar, H. Borba, et al. Genotoxicity of nitrosated red wine and of the nitrosatable phenolic compounds present in wine: tyramine, quercetin and malvidine-3-glucoside. *Food Chem. Toxicol.* 31:989–994 (1993).

31. Mirvish, S.S. Experimental evidence for inhibition of N-nitroso compound formation as a factor in the negative correlation between vitamin C consumption and the incidence of certain cancers. *Cancer Res.* 54(Suppl.):1948s–1951s (1994).

32. Helser, M.A., and J.H. Hotchkiss. Comparison of tomato phenolic and ascorbate fractions on the inhibition of N-nitroso compound formation. *J. Agric. Food Chem.* 42:129–132 (1994).

33. Sen, N.P., P.A. Baddoo, and S.W. Seaman. Studies on the occurrence and formation of 2-(hydroxymethyl)-N-nitrosothiazolidine-4-carboxylic acid (HMNTCA) and 2-(hydroxymethyl)-N-nitrosothiazolidine (HMNTHZ) in various cured smoked meats, fish and cheese. *J. Sci. Food Agric.* 61:353–356 (1993).

34. Fiddler, W., J.W. Pensabene, R.A. Gates, et al. Atlantic menhaden (*Brevoortia tyrannus*) mince and surimi as partial meat substitutes in frankfurters: effect on N-nitrosamine formation. *J. Agric. Food Chem.* 41:2238–2241 (1993).

35. Shahidi, F., R.B. Pegg, and N.P. Sen. Absence of volatile N-nitrosamines in cooked nitrite-free cured muscle foods. *Meat Sci.* 37:327–336 (1994).

36. Sen, N.P., P.A. Baddoo, and S.W. Seaman. Nitrosamines in cured pork products packaged in elastic rubber nettings: an update. *Food Chem.* 47:387–390 (1993).

37. Maxwell, R.J., J.W. Pensabene, and W. Fiddler. Multiresidue recovery at PPB levels of 10 nitrosamines from frankfurters by supercritical fluid extraction. *J. Chromatogr. Sci.* 31:212–215 (1993).

38. Atawodi, S.E., E.N. Maduagwu, R. Preussmann, and B. Spiegelhalder. Preformed volatile nitrosamines in some Nigerian foodstuffs. *Food Chem. Toxicol.* 31:853–855 (1993).

39. Wu,, Y., J. Chen, H. Ohshima, et al. Geographic association between urinary excretion of N-nitroso compounds and oesophageal cancer mortality in China. *Int. J. Cancer* 54:713–719 (1993).

40. Pignatelli, B., C. Malaveille, A. Rogatko, et al. Mutagens, N-nitroso compounds and their precursors in gastric juice from patients with and without precancerous lesions of the stomach. *Eur. J. Cancer* 29A:2031–2039 (1993).

41. Camus, A.-M., O. Geneste, P. Honkakoshi, et al. High variability of nitrosamine metabolism among individuals: role of cytochromes P450 2A6 and 2E1 in the dealkylation of N-nitrosodimethylamine and N-nitrosodiethylamine in mice and humans. *Molec. Carcinogen.* 7:268–275 (1993).

42. Tsutsumi, M., Y. Murakami, S. Kondoh, et al. Comparison of K-*ras* oncogene activation in pancreatic duct

carcinomas and cholangiocarcinomas induced in hamsters by N-nitrosobis(2-hydroxypropyl)amine. *Jpn. J. Cancer Res.* 84:956–960 (1993).

43. Lozano, J.-C., H. Nakazawa, M.P. Cros, et al. G→A mutations in *p53* and Ha-*ras* genes in esophageal papillomas induced by *N*-nitrosomethylbenzylamine in two strains of rats. *Molec. Carcinogen.* 9:33–39 (1994).

44. Takada, N., T. Matsuda, T. Otoshi, et al. Enhancement by organosulfur compounds from garlic and onions of diethylnitrosamine-induced glutathione *S*-transferase positive foci in the rat liver. *Cancer Res.* 54:2895–2899 (1994).

45. Tanaka, T., T. Kojima, T. Kawamori, et al. Chemoprevention of diethylnitrosamine-induced hepatocarcinogenesis by a simple phenolic acid protocatechuic acid in rats. *Cancer Res.* 53:2775–2779 (1993).

46. Elias, P.S. Food irradiation. In *Nutritional Toxicology*. F.N. Kotsonis et al. (eds.). New York, Raven Press. *Target Organ Toxicology Ser.* Pp. 149–180 (1994).

47. Loaharanu, P. Status and prospects of food irradiation. *Food Technol.* 48(5):124–131 (1994).

48. Thayer, D.W. Wholesomeness of irradiated foods. *Food Technol.* 48(5):132–135 (1994).

49. Joseph, A., and M. Dikshit. Effect of irradiation on the proteinase inhibitor activity and digestibility (*in vitro*) of safflower oilcake. *J. Am. Oil Chem. Soc.* 70:935–937 (1993).

50. Maier, P., I. Wenk-Siefert, H.P. Schawalder, et al. Cell-cycle and ploidy analysis in bone marrow and liver cells of rats after long-term consumption of irradiated wheat. *Food Chem. Toxicol.* 31:395–405 (1993).

51. Kilcast, D. Effect of irradiation on vitamins. *Food Chem.* 49:157–164 (1994).

52. Lee, C.J., B.A. Rasco, and F.M. Dong. Effects of sterilizing doses of gamma irradiation on levels of vitamin A, amino acids, and fatty acids in selected dairy products. *J. Food Process. Preserv.* 17:421–436 (1993).

53. Lakritz, L., and D.W. Thayer. Effect of gamma radiation on total tocopherols in fresh chicken breast muscle. *Meat Sci.* 37:439–448 (1994).

54. Fox, J.B., Jr., L. Lakritz, and D.W. Thayer. Effect of reductant level in skeletal muscle and liver on the rate of loss of thiamin due to γ-radiation. *Int. J. Radiat. Biol.* 64:305–309 (1993).

55. Buchalla, R., C. Schüttler, and K.W. Bögl. Effects of ionizing radiation on plastic food packaging materials: a review. Part 1. Chemical and physical changes. *J. Food Protect.* 56:991–997 (1993).

56. Buchalla, R., C. Schüttler, and K.W. Bögl. Effects of ionizing radiation on plastic food packaging materials: a review. Part 2. Global migration, sensory changes and the fate of additives. *J. Food Protect.* 56:998–1005 (1993).

57. Glidewell, S.M., N. Deighton, B.A. Goodman, and J.R. Hillman. Detection of irradiated food: a review. *J. Sci. Food Agric.* 61:281–300 (1993).

58. Stevenson, M.H. Identification of irradiated foods. *Food Technol.* 48(5):141–144 (1994).

59. Helle, N., G. Schulzki, B. Linke, et al. Identifizierung bestrahlter pasteurisierter Eiprodukte: Ein kombiniertes Verfahren zum Einsatz in der Routinekontrolle. *Z. Lebensm. Unters. Forsch.* 197:321–331 (1993).

60. Helle, N., C. Knopfe, J. Mischke, et al. ESR- und HPLC-Untersuchungen zum Nachweis der γ-Bestrahlung bei Eiern. *Z. Lebensm. Unters. Forsch.* 197:440–443 (1993).

61. Crone, A.V.J., M.V. Hand, J.T.G. Hamilton, et al. Synthesis, characterisation and use of 2-tetradecylcyclobutanone together with other cyclobutanones as markers for irradiated liquid whole egg. *J. Sci. Food Agric.* 62:361–367 (1993).

62. Kume, T., T. Ishii, and T.Matsuda. Immunochemical identification of irradiated chicken eggs. *J. Sci. Food Agric.* 65:1–4 (1994).

63. Desrosiers, M.F., F.G. Le, P.M. Harewood, et al. Estimation of the absorbed dose in radiation-processed foods. 4. EPR measurements on eggshell. *J. Agric. Food Chem.* 41:1471–1475 (1993).

64. Hwang, K.T., and G. Maerker. Determination of 6-ketocholestanol in unirradiated and irradiated chicken meats. *J. Am. Oil Chem. Soc.* 70:789–792 (1993).

65. Goodman, B.A., N. Deighton, and S.M. Glidewell. Optimization of experimental parameters for the EPR detection of the 'cellulosic' radical in irradiated foodstuffs. *Int. J. Food Sci. Technol.* 29:23–28 (1994).

66. Uchiyama, S., A. Sugiki, Y. Kawamura, et al. Radical unique to γ-irradiated allspice and cinnamon and its utility for detection of irradiated foods. *J. Food Hyg. Soc. Japan* 34:128–135 (1993).

67. Hayashi, T., S. Todoriki, and K. Kohyama. Applicability of viscosity measuring method to the detection of irradiated spices. *Nippon Shokuhin Kogyo Gakkaishi* 40:456–460 (1993).

68. Hitchcock, C.H.S. Determination of hydrogen using a novel hydrogen-specific electronic sensor: a potential method for detecting irradiated food. *J. Sci. Food Agric.* 62:301–305 (1993).

69. Hayashi, T., S. Todoriki, K. Otobe, and J. Sugiyama. Applicability of impedance measuring method to the detection of irradiation treatment of potatoes. *Nippon Shokuhin Kogyo Gakkaishi* 40:378–384 (1993).

70. Copin, M.P., D. Jehanno, and C.M. Bourgeois. Detection of irradiated deep-frozen foodstuffs by comparison of DEFT and APC counts. *J. Appl. Bacteriol.* 75:254–258 (1993).

71. Hirose, M., H. Yada, K. Hakoi, et al. Modification of carcinogenesis by α-tocopherol, t-butylhydroquinone, propyl gallate and butylated hydroxytoluene in a rat multi-organ carcinogenesis model. *Carcinogenesis* 14:2359–2364 (1993).

72. Page, B.D. Liquid chromatographic method for the determination of nine phenolic antioxidants in butter oil: collaborative study. *J. AOAC Int.* 76:765–779 (1993).

73. Würtzen, G. Scientific evaluation of the safety factor for the acceptable daily intake (ADI). Case study: butylated hydroxyanisole (BHA). *Food Addit. Contam.* 10:307–314 (1993).

74. Whysner, J., C.X. Wang, E. Zang, et al. Dose response of promotion by butylated hydroxyanisole in chemically initiated tumours of the rat forestomach. *Food Chem. Toxicol.* 32:215–222 (1994).

75. Tamano, S., E. Asakawa, P. Boomyaphiphat, et al. Lack of promotion of N-butyl-N-(4-hydroxybutyl)nitrosamine-initiated urinary bladder carcinogenesis in mice by rat cancer promoters. *Teratogen. Carcinogen. Mutagen.* 13:89–96 (1993).

76. Eaton, D.L., and D.M. Hamel. Increase in γ-glutamylcysteine synthetase activity as a mechanism for butylated hydroxyanisole-mediated elevation of hepatic glutathione. *Toxicol. Appl. Pharmacol.* 126:145–149 (1994).

77. Nagai, F., K. Ushiyama, and I. Kano. DNA cleavage by metabolites of butylated hydroxytoluene. *Arch. Toxicol.* 67:552–557 (1993).

78. Schilderman, P.A.E.L., J.M.S. van Maanen, F.J. ten Vaarwerk, et al. The role of prostaglandin H synthase-mediated metabolism in the induction of oxidative DNA damage by BHA metabolites. *Carcinogenesis* 14:1297–1302 (1993).

79. Walton, R.G., R. Hudak, and R.J. Green-Waite. Adverse reactions to aspartame: double-blind challenge in patients from a vulnerable population. *Biol. Psychiatry* 34:13–17 (1993).

80. Eshel, Y., and I. Sarova-Pinhas. Aspartame and seizures. (Letter.) *Neurology* 43:2154–2155 (1993).

81. Shaywitz, B.A., G.M. Anderson, E.J. Novotny, et al. Aspartame has no effect on seizures or epileptiform discharges in epileptic children. *Ann. Neurol.* 35:98–103 (1994).

82. Geha, R., C.E. Buckley, P. Greenberger, et al. Aspartame is no more likely than placebo to cause urticaria/angioedema: results of a multicenter, randomized, double-blind, placebo-controlled, crossover study. *J. Aller. Clin. Immunol.* 82:513–520 (1993).

83. Stokes, A.F., A. Belger, M.T. Banich, and E. Bernadine. Effects of alcohol and chronic aspartame ingestion upon performance in aviation relevant cognitive tasks. *Aviat. Space Environ. Med.* 65:7–15 (1994).

84. Shaywitz, B.A., C.M. Sullivan, G.M. Anderson, et al. Aspartame, behavior, and cognitive function in children with attention deficit disorder. *Pediatrics* 93:70–75 (1994).

85. Curtius, H.C., W. Endres, and N. Blau. Effect of high-protein meal plus aspartame ingestion on plasma phenylalanine concentrations in obligate heterozygotes for phenylketonuria. *Metabolism* 43:413–416 (1994).

86. Shephard, S.E., K. Wakabayashi, and M. Nagao. Mutagenic activity of peptides and the artificial sweetener aspartame after nitrosation. *Food Chem. Toxicol.* 31:323–329 (1993).

87. Hooper, N.M., R.J. Hesp, and S. Tieku. Metabolism of aspartame by human and pig intestinal microvillar peptidases. *Biochem. J.* 298:635–639 (1994).

88. Bell, L.N., and T.P. Labuza. Aspartame stability in commercially sterilized flavored dairy beverages. *J. Dairy Sci.* 77:34–38 (1994).

89. Dinçkaya, M. Çağin, and A. Telefoncu. Enzymatic method for the spectrophotometric determination of aspartame. *Food Chem.* 50:95–97 (1994).

90. Renwick, A.G. A data-derived safety (uncertainty) factor for the intense sweetener, saccharin. *Food Addit. Contam.* 10:337–350 (1993).

91. West, R.W., W.G. Sheldon, D.W. Gaylor, et al. Study of sodium saccharin co-carcinogenicity in the rat. *Food Chem. Toxicol.* 32:207–213 (1994).

92. Suttajit, M., U. Vinitketkaumnuen, U. Meevatee, and D. Buddhasukh. Mutagenicity and human chromosomal effect of stevioside, a sweetener from *Stevia rebaudiana* Bertoni. *Environ. Health Perspect.* 101(Suppl. 3):53–56 (1993).

93. Toskulkao, C., W. Deechakawan, P. Temcharoen, et al. Nephrotoxic effects of stevioside and steviol in rat renal cortical slices. *J. Clin. Biochem. Nutr.* 16:123–131 (1994).

94. Nguyen, N.U., G. Dumoulin, M.-T. Henriet, et al. Carbohydrate metabolism and urinary excretion of calcium and oxalate after ingestion of polyol sweeteners. *J. Clin. Endocrinol. Metab.* 77:388–392 (1993).

95. Beutler, H.O., and M. Dresselhaus-Schroebler. Ringversuche zur Bestimmung von D-sorbit in diätetischen Backwaren. *Dtsch. Lebensm.-Rundsch.* 89:349–351 (1993).

96. Wallis, K.J. Sucralose: features and benefits. *Food Aust.* 45:578–580 (1993).

97. Emerson, J.L., and C.J. Stone. Safety evaluation of flavoring substances. In *Flavor Measurement.* C.-T. Ho and C.H. Manley (eds.). New York, Marcel Dekker, Inc. Pp. 359–372 (1993).

98. Kažimírová, A., and A. Jabloniká. Evaluation of potential mutagenic effect of the liquid smoke preparation UTP in vivo: cytogenetic analysis of mouse bone marrow. *Mutat. Res.* 323:89–92 (1994).

99. Velíšek, J., K. Ledahudcová, B. Kassahun, et al. Chlorine-containing compounds derived from saccharides in protein hydrolysates. II. Levulinic acid esters in soybean meal hydrolysates. *Lebensm. Wiss. Technol.* 26:430–433 (1993).

100. Cruickshank, D., and L.N. Sansom. Inhibition of rat liver aryl sulphotransferase by the food additive vanillin. *Eur. J. Pharmaceut. Sci.* 1:41–47 (1993).

101. Belay, M.T., and C.F. Poole. Determination of vanillin and related flavor compounds in natural vanilla extracts and vanilla-flavored foods by thin layer chromatography and automated multiple development. *Chromatographia* 37:365–373 (1993).

102. Gupta, K.P., K.L. van Golen, K.L. Putman, and K. Randerath. Formation and persistence of safrole–DNA adducts over a 10 000-fold dose range in mouse liver. *Carcinogenesis* 14:1517–1521 (1993).

103. Randerath, K., K.P. Gupta, and K.L. van Golen. Altered fidelity of a nucleic acid modifying enzyme, T4 polynucleotide kinase, by safrole-induced DNA damage. *Carcinogenesis* 14:1523–1529 (1993).

104. Ellahueñe, M.F., L.P. Pérez-Alzola, M. Orellana-Valdebenito, et al. Genotoxic evaluation of eugenol using the bone marrow micronucleus assay. *Mutat. Res.* 320:175–180 (1994).

105. Hasheminejad, G., and J. Caldwell. Genotoxicity of the alkenylbenzenes α- and β-asarone, myristicin and elemicin as determined by the UDS assay in cultured rat hepatocytes. *Food Chem. Toxicol.* 32:223–231 (1994).

106. Delgado, I.F., A.C.M.deA. Nogueira, C.A.M. Souza, et al. Peri- and postnatal developmental toxicity of β-myrcene in the rat. *Food Chem. Toxicol.* 31:623–628 (1993).

107. Miyake, T., and T. Shibamoto. Quantitative analysis of acetaldehyde in foods and beverages. *J. Agric. Food Chem.* 41:1968–1970 (1993).

108. Tarasoff, L., and M.F. Kelly. Monosodium L-glutamate: a double-blind study and review. *Food Chem. Toxicol.* 31:1019–1035 (1993).

109. Spiegel, J.E., R. Rose, P. Karabell, et al. Safety and benefits of fructooligosaccharides as food ingredients. *Food Technol.* 48(1):85–89 (1994).

110. Durán-Merás, I., F. Salinas, A.M. de la Peña, and M.L. Rosas. Simultaneous determination of flavor enhancers inosine 5'-monophosphate and guanosine 5'-monophosphate in food preparations by derivative spectrophotometry. *J. AOAC Int.* 76:754–759 (1993).

111. Durán-Merás, I., A.M. de la Peña, A. Espinosa-Mansilla, and F. Salinas. Multicomponent determination of flavour enhancers in food preparations by partial least squares and principal component regression modelling of spectrophotometric data. *Analyst* 118:807–813 (1993).

112. Poulsen, E. Case study: erythrosine. *Food Addit. Contam.* 10:315–323 (1993).

113. Collins, T.F.X., T.N. Black, and D.I. Ruggles. Teratogenic potential of FD&C Red No. 3 when given by gavage. *Toxicol. Indust. Health* 9:605–616 (1993).

114. Takeda, Y., Y. Goda, H. Noguchi, et al. Spectroscopic characterization of SC-NTR: a subsidiary dye of Allura Red AC dye (FD&C Red No. 40). *Food Addit. Contam.* 11:97–104 (1994).

115. Takeda, Y., T. Yamada, and M. Takeda. Determination of unsulfonated primary aromatic amines in Food Red No. 40 by high performance liquid chromatography. *J. Food Hyg. Soc. Japan* 34:420–425 (1993).

116. Tanaka, T. Reproductive and neurobehavioral effects of amaranth administered to mice in drinking water. *Toxicol. Indust. Health* 9:1027–1035 (1993).

117. Prival, M.J., M.D. Peiperl, and S.J. Bell. Determination of combined benzidine in FD & C Yellow No. 5 (tartrazine), using a highly sensitive analytical method. *Food Chem. Toxicol.* 31:751–758 (1993).

118. Berzas Nevado, J.J., J. Rodríguez Flores, M.J. Villaseñor Llerena. Simultaneous determination of Quinoline Yellow and Sunset Yellow by derivative spectrophotometry and ratio spectra derivative. *Anal. Lett.* 27:1009–1029 (1994).

119. Thuvander, A., and A. Oskarsson. Effects of subchronic exposure to Caramel Colour III on the immune system in mice. *Food Chem. Toxicol.* 32:7–13 (1994).

120. Tanaka, T. Reproductive and neurobehavioural effects of phloxine administered to mice. *Food Chem. Toxicol.* 31:1013–1018 (1993).

121. Hugener, M., A.P. Tinke, W.M.A. Niessen, et al. Pseudo-electrochromatography–negative-ion electrospray mass spectrometry of aromatic glucuronides and food colours. *J. Chromatogr.* 647:375–385 (1993).

122. Uematsu, Y., M. Hirokado, K. Hirata, et al. Determination of residual organic solvents in natural color preparations by standard addition head-space gas chromatography. *J. Food Hyg. Soc. Japan* 34:232–238 (1993).

123. Pikkarainen, S.A., and M.T. Parviainen. Vitamin A levels in bovine and pork liver. *Int. J. Vit. Nutr. Res.* 63:86–88 (1993).

124. Buss, N.E., E.A. Tembe, B.D. Prendergast, et al. The teratogenic metabolites of vitamin A in women following supplements and liver. *Human Exp. Toxicol.* 13:33–43 (1994).

125. Nako, Y., N. Fukushima, T. Tomomasa, K. Nagashima. Hypervitaminosis D after prolonged feeding with a premature formula. *Pediatrics* 92:862–863 (1993).

126. Whittaker, P., J.E. Vanderveen, M.J. Dinovi, et al. Toxicological profile, current use, and regulatory issues on EDTA compounds for assessing use of sodium iron EDTA for food fortification. *Regul. Toxicol. Pharmacol.* 18:419–427 (1993).

127. Hurrell, R.F., S. Ribas, and L. Davidsson. $NaFe^{3+}$ EDTA as a food fortificant: influence on zinc, calcium and copper metabolism in the rat. *Br. J. Nutr.* 71:85–93 (1994).

128. Hamano, T., Y. Mitsuhashi, N. Kojima, et al. Sensitive spectrophotometric method for the determination of ethylenediaminetetraacetic acid in foods. *Analyst* 118:909–912 (1993).

129. Fontecave, M., J.L. Pierre. Iron: metabolism, toxicity and therapy. *Biochimie* 75:767–773 (1993).

130. McCord, J.M. Free radicals and prooxidants in health and nutrition. *Food Technol.* 48(5):106–111 (1994).

131. Herbert, V., S. Shaw, E. Jayatilleke, and T. Stopler-Kasdan. Most free-radical injury is iron-related: it is promoted by iron, hemin, holoferritin and vitamin C, and inhibited by desferoxamine and apoferritin. *Stem Cells* 12:289–303 (1994).

132. Idjradinata, P., W.E. Watkins, and E. Pollitt. Adverse effect of iron supplementation on weight gain of iron-replete young children. *Lancet* 343:1252–1254 (1994).

133. Weinberg, E.D. Association of iron with colorectal cancer. *BioMetals* 7:211–216 (1994).

134. Nelson, R.L., F.G. Davis, E. Sutter, et al. Body iron stores and risk of colonic neoplasia. *J. Natl. Cancer Inst.* 86:455–460 (1994).

135. Knekt, P., A. Reunanen, H. Takkunen, et al. Body iron stores and risk of cancer. *Int. J. Cancer* 56:379–382 (1994).

136. Stevens, R.G., B.I. Graubard, M.S. Micozzi, et al. Moderate elevation of body iron level and increased risk of cancer occurrence and death. *Int. J. Cancer* 56:364–369 (1994).

137. Sempos, C.T., A.C. Looker, R.F. Gillum, and D.M. Markuc. Body iron stores and the risk of coronary heart disease. *New Engl. J. Med.* 330:1119–1124 (1994).

138. Liao, Y., R.S. Cooper, and D.L. McGee. Iron status and coronary heart disease: negative findings from the NHANES I epidemiologic follow-up study. *Am. J. Epidemiol.* 139:704–712 (1994).

139. Ascherio, A., W.C. Willett, E.B. Rimm, et al. Dietary iron intake and risk of coronary disease among men. *Circulation* 89:969–974 (1994).

140. Morrison, H.I., R.M. Semenciw, Y. Mao, and D.T. Wigle. Serum iron and risk of fatal acute myocardial infarction. *Epidemiology* 5:243–246 (1994).

141. Rabinoff, M. Iron, infection and acute myocardial infarction. *Med. Hypoth.* 42:131–132 (1994).

142. Meyer, O., E. Kristiansen, J. Gry, et al. Carcinogenicity study of the emulsifier TOSOM and the release agent TOS in Wistar rats. *Food Chem. Toxicol.* 31:825–833 (1993).

143. Umemura, T., K. Sai, A. Takagi, et al. A possible role for cell proliferation in potassium bromate ($KBrO_3$) carcinogenesis. *J. Cancer Res. Clin. Oncol.* 119:463–469 (1993).

144. Mocchiutti, N.O., C.A. Bernal, and Y.B. Lombardo. Ingeta crónica de aceites vegetales bromados: su acción sobre la secreción hepática y catabolismo de lipoproteínas plasmáticas. *Arch. Latinoamericanos Nutr.* 42:403–408 (1992).

145. Takahashi, O., S. Oishi, T. Fujitani, et al. Chronic toxicity studies of piperonyl butoxide in F344 rats: induction of hepatocellular carcinoma. *Fund. Appl. Toxicol.* 22:293–303 (1994).

146. Heikes, D.L. Procedure for supercritical fluid extraction and gas chromatographic determination of chlorinated fatty acid bleaching adducts in flour and flour-containing food items utilizing acid hydrolysis–methylation and Florisil column cleanup techniques. *J. Agric. Food Chem.* 41:2034–2037 (1993).

147. Zeman, N.W., and W.M. Teague. Safety evaluation of food enzymes from genetically engineered organisms. In *Molecular Approaches to Improving Food Quality and Safety*. D. Bhatnagar and T. E. Cleveland (eds.). New York: Van Nostrand Reinhold. Pp. 83–98 (1992).

148. Battershill, J.M. Guidelines for the safety assessment of microbial enzymes used in food. *Food Addit. Contam.* 10:479–488 (1993).

149. Hjortkjaer, R.K., M. Stavnsbjerg, P.B. Pedersen, et al. Safety evaluation of esperase. *Food Chem. Toxicol.* 31:999–1011 (1993).

150. Broadmeadow, A., C. Clare, and A.S. de Boer. An overview of the safety evaluation of the *Rhizomucor miehei* lipase enzyme. *Food Addit. Contam.* 11:105–119 (1994).

151. de Boer, A.S., R. Marshall, A. Broadmeadow, and K. Hazelden. Toxicological evaluation of acetolactate decarboxylase. *J. Food Protect.* 56:510–517 (1993).

152. Softly, B.J., A.S. Huang, J.W. Finley, et al. Composition of representative SALATRIM fat preparations. *J. Agric. Food Chem.* 42:461–467 (1994).

153. Huang, A.S., L.R. Robinson, L.G. Gursky, et al. Identification and quantification of SALATRIM 23CA in foods by the combination of supercritical fluid extraction, particle beam LC–mass spectrometry, and HPLC with light-scattering detector. *J. Agric. Food Chem.* 42:468–473 (1994).

154. Hayes, J.R., and E.S. Riccio. Genetic toxicology studies of SALATRIM structured triacylglycerols. 1. Lack of mutagenicity in the *Salmonella*/microsome reverse mutation assay. *J. Agric. Food Chem.* 42:515–520 (1994).

155. Hayes, J.R., C.J. Rudd, J.C. Mirsalis, et al. Genetic toxicology studies of SALATRIM structured triacylglycerols. 2. Lack of genetic damage in *in vitro* mammalian cell assays and the *in vivo* micronucleus assay. *J. Agric. Food Chem.* 42:521–527 (1994).

156. Hayes, J.R., N.H. Wilson, D.H. Pence, and K.D. Williams. Subchronic toxicity studies of SALATRIM structured triacylglycerols in rats. 1. Triacylglycerols composed of stearate and butyrate. *J. Agric. Food Chem.* 42:528–438 (1994).

157. Hayes, J.R., N.H. Wilson, D.H. Pence, and K.D. Williams. Subchronic toxicity studies of SALATRIM structured triacylglycerols in rats. 2. Triacylglycerols composed of stearate, acetate, and propionate. *J. Agric. Food Chem.* 42:539–551 (1994).

158. Hayes, J.R., N.H. Wilson, D.H. Pence, and K.D. Williams. Subchronic toxicity studies of SALATRIM structured triacylglycerols in rats. 3. Triacylglycerols composed of stearate, acetate, propionate, and butyrate. *J. Agric. Food Chem.* 42:552–562 (1994).

159. Hayes, J.R., N.H. Wilson, M.C. Roblin, et al. 28-Day continuous dosing study in minipigs with SALATRIM structured triacylglycerol composed of stearate, acetate, and propionate. *J. Agric. Food Chem.* 42:563–571 (1994).

160. Finley, J.W., G.A. Leveille, R.M. Dixon, et al. Clinical assessment of SALATRIM, a reduced-calorie triacylglycerol. *J. Agric. Food Chem.* 42:581–596 (1994).

161. Finley, J.W., C.G. Walchak, J.C. Sourby, and G.A. Leveille. Clinical study of the effects of exposure of various SALATRIM preparations to subjects in a free-living environment. *J. Agric. Food Chem.* 42:597–604 (1994).

162. Webb, D.R., F.E. Wood, T.A. Bertram, and N.E. Fortier. A 91-day feeding study in rats with caprenin. *Food Chem. Toxicol.* 31:935–946 (1993).

163. Rios, J.J., M.C. Pérez-Camino, G. Márquez-Ruiz, and M.C. Dobarganes. Isolation and characterization of sucrose polyesters. *J. Am. Oil Chem. Soc.* 71:385–390 (1994).

# 8

# Indirect Additives, Residues, and Contaminants

Health risks to consumers of fishery products contaminated with inorganic or organic chemicals were discussed and evaluated by Ahmed et al. (*1,2*). Although only a small proportion of fishery products contain appreciable amounts of potentially hazardous contaminants, shellfish and finfish can accumulate chemicals, such as heavy metals, polychlorinated biphenyls, dioxins, chlorinated hydrocarbon insecticides, processing-related contaminants, and aquaculture-related chemicals from their environment. Each of these potential toxicants was considered, with information on how seafoods acquire these chemicals and their known toxic effects along with a realistic evaluation of human health risks and practical recommendations on ways to reduce or prevent contamination.

A recent volume on chemical contaminants in drinking water, edited by Wang (*3*), considered various aspects of exposure assessment, toxicology, and risk assessment for a number of well-studied chemicals. Different chapters discussed sources of contamination, reactions of contaminants with chlorinated water purification compounds, pharmacokinetic studies to estimate internal exposures and to determine interactions of different contaminants, and problems with specific chemicals, including radon, chloroform, trichloroethylene, selenium, aldicarb, and nickel.

## ANTIMICROBIAL DRUGS

Use of antibiotics in farm animals and in seafood farming operations has the potential to adversely affect human health. As many as 10–15% of individuals in a population may exhibit allergic-type reactions to antimicrobial agents, most commonly penicillins and sulfonamides. Residues of antibiotics in meat or fish could, if present in high enough concentrations, trigger allergic reactions in such sensitive individuals. Although such cases may occur, Dayan (*4*) contends that most reports of such reactions are not well substantiated. In addition, the fact that residue levels in foods are much smaller than doses which a patient would receive to treat an infection and the fact that exposure to antibiotics by the oral route is much less likely to induce allergic symptoms than exposure by other routes makes it unlikely that residues in foods would normally provoke serious symptoms. However, in order to minimize any such reactions, withholding periods should be observed by farmers, injection sites should be discarded at slaughterhouses, and residue levels should be monitored by regulatory agencies.

Another issue concerning antibiotics is that their widespread use could select for antibiotic-resistant, pathogenic strains of bacteria. Shah et al. (*5*) pointed out that resistance to antibiotics has become more common in some species since the introduction of some drugs in veterinary medicine. Resistance to quinolines in *Campylobacter* spp. and to chloramphenicol in *Yersinia* appears to have increased since the use of these antibiotics became more common in treatment of poultry and swine. However, resistance to tetracycline and ampicillin in *Salmonella typhimurium* has apparently decreased in recent years. Although the potential does exist for creating multi-drug-resistant human pathogens, with our current levels of veterinary drug usage, this has not happened as yet. The authors caution, however, that we should not be complacent. Wiedemann (*6*), in a discussion of the development of antibiotic resistance in microbes and the origin of resistant strains in humans, concurs that veterinary use of antibiotics probably has had very little to do with the problem of antibiotic treatment of human infections in hospitals.

Methods to assess the effects of antimicrobial residues on human gut flora were evaluated by Corpet (*7*). Experimental procedures discussed included methods to investigate effects on aerobes vs. anaerobes, the use of plate counts and minimal inhibitory concentrations, statistical analyses, human trials, and experiments with gnotobiotic mice inoculated with human flora. It appears that most drug-resistant enterobacteria in untreated humans originate from resistant bacteria in raw foods rather than from selection of resistant bacteria by drug residues in foods.

Recent developments in the liquid chromatographic analyses of residues of antibiotics (aminoglycosides, chloramphenicol, tetracyclines, sulfonamides, β-lactams, macrolides, etc.) in food products of animal origin were reviewed by Shaikh and Moats (*8*). Cleanup procedures, such as ultrafiltration, liquid–liquid partition, solid-phase extraction, immunoaffinity, and matrix–solid phase dispersion were also discussed. Many of these procedures can be automated for rapid analysis and some may be used for direct screening of residues in meat and milk.

An HPLC procedure with a photodiode array detector has been devised for the simultaneous determination of 21 synthetic antibacterial compounds in fish and meat products (*9*). Recoveries of most of the antibiotics from spiked samples were >70% and detection limits for each compound were 0.05–0.1 µg/g except for thiamphenicol (0.25 µg/g). Simple bacteriological and thin-layer chromatographic methods were described for the determination of drug residues in meat when the animals had been treated with penicillin G and an amino-glycoside antibiotic (*10*).

## Sulfonamides

In treating mastitis, antibiotics are often infused directly into the mammary gland and this may result in high levels of antibiotic residues in milk. In an investigation into the elimination of sulfonamide residues from milk, cows were treated with sulfadimidine (SDM) or sulfa-methoxypyridazine (SMP) at the recommended doses, and milk samples were collected and analyzed until residues were no longer detected (*11*). When all 4 quarters were treated, residues of SDM and SMP were detectable up to 57 and 24 hours, respectively, after the last dose. When only one quarter was treated, very low, but detectable, residues were present in milk from the other quarters during the first day after the last treatment. It was recommended that 4 milkings after the last dose would be an adequate withdrawal period for these sulfonamides.

Pharmacokinetics of sulfamonomethoxine (SMM) and sulfadimethoxine (SDM) in rainbow trout at 15°C were studied after oral administration (gavage) of these drugs (*12*). Elimination half-lives of SMM and SDM were, respectively, 32.6 and 24.5 hours. $N^4$-acetyl metabolites of both compounds were also detected in the tissues, and these had a longer half-life of elimination. The currently stipulated withdrawal period of 30 days appears to be adequate for SMM and SDM but metabolites of these drugs may persist for longer periods of time.

Determination of residues of sulfonamides in animal tissue first requires an efficient means of extracting the antibiotics from the matrix. Shearan et al. (*13*) compared matrix solid-phase dispersion (MSPD) with a standard solvent extraction method for the extraction of sulfamethazine in pork muscle. Residue concentrations determined using both methods compared favorably. The MSPD method saved time and manipulative steps and was suitable for application to other detection systems. When HPLC was used for detection, the limit of detection was 0.025 µg/g. A solid-phase extraction column of Cyclobond-I was found to effectively remove contaminating substances from milk and allow determination of 9 sulfonamides by reversed-phase HPLC with a diode array detector (*14*). In experiments with dry milk powder, supercritical fluid extraction was determined to be another effective means of extracting sulfamethazine residues (*15*).

Other analytical methods described for the determination of sulfonamide residues included: (a) a collaborative study of a liquid chromatographic method for determination of sulfamethazine residues in milk (*16*) (this method was found to be capable of detecting residues at levels of ≥10 ppb and was adopted first action by AOAC International); (b) liquid chromatographic method with post-column derivatization with *p*-dimethylamino-benzaldehyde for the determination of 6 sulfonamides in liver and kidney tissue (*17*); (c) a continuous column separation method for use in simultaneous determination of 9 sulfonamides (*18*); (d) a fully automated determination of sulfamethazine in ovine plasma using a solid-phase extraction column and liquid chromatography (*19*); (e) an HPLC method for determination of residues of sulfisomidine and $N^4$-acetylsulfisomidine in swine muscle, kidney, liver, and plasma (*20*); and (f) a confirmatory method for sulfonamide residues in animal tissues utilizing gas chromatography and pulsed positive ion-negative ion chemical ionization mass spectrometry (*21*).

## Tetracyclines

Plasma pharmacokinetics and elimination of oxytetracycline in veal calves has been investigated by Meijer et al. (*22,23*). Healthy male calves were given 5 daily intramuscular injections of oxytetracycline. At 2, 7, 10, and 12 days after the last dose, the animals were slaughtered, and kidney, liver, and muscle tissues were analyzed for antibiotic residues. Antibiotic concentrations were highest in the kidney at all sampling times, with 2.2–3.6 µg/g detected on day 2 and 0.35–0.66 µg/g detected on day 12. Corresponding values for muscle tissue were 0.6–1.3 µg/g and 0.03–0.075 µg/g, respectively. Elimination rates of this drug in tissues correlated highly with plasma elimination rates, and it was possible to estimate tissue residues from plasma elimination rates. Following both intravenous and intramuscular injections, oxytetracycline is eliminated fairly rapidly during the first 2 days and then is eliminated slowly, with a $t_{1/2}$ of 93–98.5 hours. Therefore, long withdrawal periods may be required following use of this antibiotic.

The Delvotest P assay, originally designed to test for penicillin residues in milk, has been evaluated for its use in detecting oxytetracycline residues in chicken tissues (*24*). Chickens were gavaged with two daily doses of this antibiotic for 4 days and then were decapitated at intervals of 0.5 to 8 hours after the final dose. Analyses of kidney, liver, and breast muscle using the standard plate assay with *Bacillus cereus* as the test organism revealed that residue levels peaked at 1 hour and then declined so that at 8 hours antibiotic levels in serum, kidney, and liver were undetectable, 0.78, and 0.2 µg/g, respectively. The Delvotest P performed in a fashion similar to the plate test and could be performed more rapidly. At concentrations ≥0.62 μg/g all Delvotest P assays were positive while at concentrations between 0.2 and 0.41 μg/g, responses were mixed (positive, doubtful, and negative) and at concentrations ≤0.1 μg/g, all responses were negative.

A comparative study of HPLC methods for the determination of tetracycline antibiotics was conducted by White et al. (*25*). A review of a number of parameters (mobile phases, buffers, use of EDTA, and column composition) indicated that polymeric columns with a pH 2 buffer containing acetonitrile provided the best results with mixtures of tetracycline, oxytetracycline, and chlortetracycline.

Other analytical methods developed for the determination of this family of antibiotics include: (a) an HPLC method with photodiode array detection for analysis of 6 tetracyclines in kidney tissue (*26*); (b) a liquid chromatographic method with a programmable fluorimetric detector for the determination of oxytetracycline and chlortetracycline residues in animal tissues (*27*); (c) a continuous HPLC separation method for residues of 5 tetracyclines in foods which uses a bioassay with *Bacillus subtilis* for detection of the antibiotics (*28*); (d) a microtiter bioassay method utilizing *B. cereus* and triphenyltetrazolium chloride as an indicator for the detection of tetracyclines in milk (*29*); and (e) an automated continuous flow chemiluminometric method for determination of tetracyclines in honey (*30*). This method is based on the chemiluminescence produced by reaction of tetracyclines with *N*-bromosuccinamide in alkaline solutions. Bergner-Lang and Mikisch (*31*) point out that a complete analysis of residues of tetracyclines in foods should also quantitate levels of their 4-epimers. These epimers may already exist in the test samples and may also be generated during sample preparation methods.

## β-Lactams (Penicillin Derivatives)

Elimination of procaine penicillin G by feedlot steers was monitored after groups of animals were injected intramuscularly (im) daily for 5 days with 24,000 or 66,000 U/kg or were given a single intramuscular or subcutaneous injection of 66,000 U/kg (*32,33*). Plasma samples were collected at intervals over the next 12 days and analyzed for antibiotic residues. The subcutaneous injections produced a lower mean maximum concentration but had a longer elimination half-life than the im injections. The single im injection produced the highest mean maximum concentration but had the shortest elimination half-life. Analyses of the data indicate that withdrawal periods of 10 and 21 days, respectively, are required for the lower

and higher doses administered for 5 days. For some applications the benzathine salt of penicillin G is used because it is absorbed from the injection site more slowly and therefore lasts for a longer time. In experiments comparing the depletion of penicillin G residues from tissues of steers treated with procaine or benzathine penicillins, Korsrud et al. (*34*) confirmed that residues of penicillin G in the injection site of benzathine-treated animals were 30–60 times higher than the regulatory maximum residue limit even after the recommended withdrawal periods. Therefore, when this form of penicillin is used in food-producing animals, residue levels must be closely monitored.

In an evaluation of 5 milk antibiotic screening assays, samples of milk from 172 cows with mild to moderate clinical mastitis were tested (*35*). One hundred cows had been treated with intramammary doses of amoxicillin or cephapirin and the other 72 had received no antibiotics but only doses of oxytocin. A high percentage of false positive results were obtained with most of the tests: CITE®probe (β-lactam) (43.6%), Delvotest-P® (37.7%), Charm Farm® (81.7%), LacTek® (2.6%), and *Bacillus stearothermophilus* var. *calidolactis* disk assay (18.8%). The most reliable assay, LacTek, is based on a liquid-phase competitive ELISA. The low specificity of CITEprobe, which uses a binding protein on a membrane matrix, is apparently due to the presence of serum or plasma proteins which interfere with the binding of β-lactams. The other 3 assays are based on the antibiotic's inhibition of growth of some indicator organism. Apparently milk from mastitic cows has other inhibitory substances which interfere with the performance of these assays.

Chromatographic methods developed for the determination of β-lactam antibiotics in milk include: an automated liquid chromatographic cleanup method followed by liquid chromatographic analysis for determination of amoxicillin and ampicillin (*36*); a reversed-phase HPLC method using pulsed amperometric detection for determination of several penicillins (*37*); and an HPLC–mass spectrometric method for confirming residues of penicillin G, ampicillin, amoxicillin, cloxacillin, and cephapirin in milk (*38*).

## Chloramphenicol and Its Derivatives

Following oral administration of chloramphenicol (CAP) (30 or 50 mg/kg body weight) to chickens, this drug was absorbed rapidly (maximal plasma concentrations within 0.72 h) but incompletely (bioavailability of 29–38%) (*39*). Antibiotic levels in the plasma also decreased rapidly, with a half-life of about 7 h, with some of the CAP eliminated from the body and the rest distributed widely to the tissues and metabolized. After 6 days of withdrawal, CAP concentrations in muscle, liver, and kidney were 0.43, 0.026, and 0.043 µg/g, respectively. After 12 days of withdrawal, CAP residues were below the limit of detection in all tissues, but two CAP metabolites, nitroso-chloramphenicol and nitrophenyl-aminopropanedione, were still present at concentrations of 0.26–3.04 µg/g in these tissues.

An HPLC method for detection of CAP residues in eggs has been developed and used to monitor residues in eggs of hens treated with medicated feed containing 800 mg CAP/kg (40). CAP was detectable in albumen and yolk of eggs laid for up to 3 and 8 days, respectively, after dosing. Maximum antibiotic level detected in albumen was 0.25 ppm (day 1 after dosing) and in yolk was 0.56 ppm on day 3. An HPLC procedure with UV diode array detection has also been found to be a sensitive method for detection of CAP in chicken muscle tissue (41). None of 50 chicken samples obtained from Spanish slaughterhouses were found to contain detectable levels of CAP.

Two rapid ELISAs utilizing polyclonal antibodies in dipstick and immunofiltration formats have been developed for the detection of CAP residues in raw milk (42). Since the milk can be analyzed directly with a sensitivity of 1 ng CAP/mL, these assays would be suitable as field tests. Confirmation of CAP residues in milk can be achieved by a GC–MS method (43).

Pharmacokinetics of a thiamphenicol dose of 25 mg/kg body weight was investigated in lactating cows injected intravenously (iv) or intramuscularly (im) with the antibiotic (44). Following the iv dose, thiamphenicol appeared in the milk with a penetration half-life of 36.9 min, was eliminated from the milk with a half-life of 3.6 h, and reached a peak concentration in the milk of 23.1 µg/mL at 2.5 h. The corresponding values following an im dose were 50.6 min, 5.9 h, and 17.4 µg/mL at 3.4 h.

Thiamphenicol residues in meat have been determined at concentrations as low as 10 ppb by reversed-phase HPLC following a relatively simple extraction procedure utilizing ethyl acetate (45). HPLC has also been effectively used to determine residues of florfenicol and its metabolite florfenicol amine in fish muscle and liver (46). Detection limits were 20 ng/g in muscle and 50 ng/g in liver.

## Quinoline Antibiotics

Absorption, distribution, and elimination of radiolabeled danofloxacin were monitored in tissues of broiler chickens dosed with 25 µg/mL of the antibiotic in drinking water for 5 days (47). Danofloxacin itself was the major residue in all tissues. Residue concentrations at 6 h after withdrawal were highest in the liver (0.612 µg/g), followed by kidney and muscle (0.406 and 0.099 µg/g, respectively). Residues were eliminated rapidly, with concentrations of 0.056, 0.02, and 0.003 µg/g detected in these 3 tissues, respectively, at 48 h of withdrawal.

A reliable HPLC method with fluorescence detection has been developed for the simultaneous determination of danofloxacin, benofloxacin, enrofloxacin, and ofloxacin in chicken tissues (48). A confirmatory method utilizing HPLC–electrospray ionization tandem mass spectrometry was developed by Schneider et al. (49) for identification of danofloxacin residues in chicken and cattle liver.

Absorption and elimination of flumequine in rainbow trout, dosed orally or intraarterially with 5 mg/kg of this antibiotic, were found to be temperature-dependent processes (50). Following oral administration, maximum plasma concentrations were about twice as high in fish maintained at 13°C than in those at 3°C. Elimination half-life was also much longer at the colder (736 h) than at the warmer temperature (285 h). Metabolic processes in fish are slower at lower ambient temperatures and this fact must be considered in calculating appropriate withdrawal periods.

Several methods have been described for the determination of quinoline antibiotics in seafood, including the following: a microbiological assay using *Vibrio anguillarum* for the detection of sarafloxacin and oxolinic acid in plasma of Atlantic salmon (51); a reversed-phase HPLC method for the determination of oxolinic acid in oysters and sea water (52); and an HPLC method with fluorescence detection for the determination of oxolinic acid and flumequine in fish tissues (53). Oxolinic acid can also be used as an antibacterial agent to control diseases in crops such as rice. An HPLC method was also found to be effective in analyzing residues of oxolinic acid in crops (54).

## Macrolide Antibiotics

Tilmicosin is one drug prescribed for treatment of bovine respiratory disease but there is some concern about residue levels in milk. In an assessment of the persistence of such residues, 6 lactating cows were injected subcutaneously with 10 mg tilmicosin/kg body weight and milk samples were monitored for the next 4½ weeks (55). Antibiotic residues were highest in the first two days after the injection, with maximum concentrations in different cows ranging from 9.65 to 16.91 µg/mL. Persistence of the drug in the animals also varied, with residues undetectable in one cow after 19 days while another had detectable residues for 31 days. Because of the extended and unpredictable amounts of drug present in milk of treated cows, this drug is not recommended for treatment of dairy cows. A reversed-phase HPLC method with UV detection has been developed for the simultaneous determination of tilmicosin and tylosin in animal tissues such as muscle and kidney (56).

Another drug used to treat bovine respiratory disease, spiramycin, has been examined for its pharmacokinetics and tissue residues in calves (57). Eighteen year-old calves were given 2 intramuscular injections of 100,000 IU spiramycin/kg at 48-h intervals and residues were monitored in plasma, liver, kidney, and the injection site. Elimination half-lives of spiramycin were 67, 64, and 145 h for injection sites, kidney, and liver, respectively. Neospiramycin, a degradation product, was also detected in these tissues. Based on the data obtained in this study, a withdrawal time of 35 days was recommended.

Two methods have been developed for the determination of erythromycin in foods: a liquid chromatographic method with electrochemical detection for analysis of salmon tissue (58) and an HPLC method with fluorimetric determination for analysis of eggs and liver (59).

## Nitrofuran Antibiotics

A new and rapid HPLC method for the determination of nitrofurantoin, furazolidone, and furaltadone in feed and milk has been described (60). Simultaneous determination of nitrofurazone and furazolidone by liquid chromatography with UV detection has been accomplished by Rupp et al. for samples of shrimp muscle (61) and for channel catfish muscle (62).

## Other Antibiotics

Since nearly half of the drug formulations available in France for treatment of mastitis by the intramammary route contain aminoglycoside antibiotics, experiments were conducted with lactating cows to determine the rate of elimination of these antibiotics (63). Eight commercial drug formulations containing neomycin, dihydrostreptomycin, kanamycin, or gentamicin mixed with some other antibiotics (penicillin, bacitracin, cephalexin, colistin, or tetracycline) were infused into the four quarters of the cows' udders. Aminoglycoside antibiotics were detectable in milk during at least 5 milkings after treatment and in some cases were present for 15 milkings. Based on this data, withdrawal periods should be from

3–8 days for the different antibiotic formulations. Use of an on-line sample enrichment technique, liquid chromatographic separation with postcolumn derivatization and fluorescence detection has been found to effectively determine residues as low as 10 ppb streptomycin and 20 ppb dihydrostreptomycin in porcine and bovine muscle and kidney (64).

Other HPLC methods developed for detection of antibiotic residues in foods include procedures for determination of spectinomycin in swine, calf, and chicken plasma (65) and bicozamycin and its benzoyl ester derivative in blood, muscle, liver, and kidney of yellowtail (66).

# OTHER VETERINARY DRUGS

## Antiprotozoal Drugs

An HPLC method has been devised for the detection of salinomycin, monesin, lasalocid, and narasin in feed and animal tissues (67).

ELISAs utilizing monoclonal antibodies have been developed for the detection of residues of the coccidiostats salinomycin (68), halofuginone (69), and dimetridazole and other nitroimidazoles (70) in poultry tissues. These assays do not require extensive sample preparation and are capable of detecting the drugs in the low ppb range.

## Anthelminthics

Ivermectin has been proposed as an effective drug to control salmon lice (crustacean parasites) in salmon farms but more information is needed on withdrawal times if this drug is to be used. Experiments with salmon grown in water from the coast of Scotland demonstrated that depuration of an oral dose of this antiparasitic agent was a function of both time and temperature since metabolic activity of the fish is directly related to temperature (71). One day after the last medicated feeding, ivermectin residues in skin and muscle were, respectively, 83.3 and 116.8 μg/kg. Withdrawal periods of 750 and 1000°D (degree days) were required to reduce drug residues to undetectable levels in the muscle and skin. Such long withdrawal periods, corresponding to 200 days at 5°C or 67 days at 15°C, would not be practical since salmon would likely become reinfected during the withdrawal period and suffer significant parasitic damage.

An HPLC method with fluorescence detection revealed that ivermectin residues in salmon were about 10 times higher in the liver than in the muscle and the skin and confirmed that excretion of this drug is relatively slow in these fish as compared to cattle (*72*).

Recently described, modified methods for the determination of ivermectin residues in animal tissues include: a liquid chromatographic method with fluorescence detection with a detection limit of 2 ppb (*73*); an HPLC method with fluorescence detection and a quantitation limit of 5 ppb (*74*); and liquid chromatography with laser-induced fluorescence detection and automated derivatization (*75*).

Other methods designed to determine residues of anthelminthic drugs in animals include: HPLC determination of albendazole in bovine milk with fluorometric detection (*76*); liquid chromatography/mass spectrometry for determination of moxidectin residues in bovine tissues (*77*); and a monoclonal antibody–based ELISA for hygromycin B in swine kidney (*78*).

## Tranquilizers

The tranquilizer and growth promoter diazepam and its metabolites are used for the fattening of several species and have been found to accumulate in the liver. In an experiment to determine the effects of cooking on diazepam residues, liver samples were taken from bulls treated 12–24 hours previously with an oral dose of diazepam and were then boiled for 1 hour (*79*). Cooking was found to degrade only 11–30% of this drug and two of its metabolites (temazepam and dimethyldiazepam) although nearly 50% of another metabolite (oxazepam) was destroyed. These compounds, with the exception of oxazepam, were even more heat stable when heated in a standard solution.

A liquid chromatographic method has been developed for the simultaneous determination of the tranquilizer xylazine and its major metabolite 2,6-dimethylaniline in swine and bovine kidney (*80*). Recoveries of 76–84% were achieved with spiked samples, and concentrations as low as 25–100 ppb could be detected.

## Hormones and Hormone-Like Drugs

Although the use of β-adrenergic agonists such as clenbuterol has been banned by the European Community, these drugs are still sometimes used to promote the growth of farm animals. Residue concentrations of clenbuterol were measured in the liver and retinal tissues of 20 cattle dosed for 30 days with the drug followed by 140 days of withdrawal (*81*). Detectable levels of clenbuterol were present in the liver through 56 days of withdrawal and remained well above detectable concentrations in the retina during the entire withdrawal period. Treat-

ment of lactating cows for 3 weeks with clenbuterol resulted in maximal residue levels of 22.5 ng/mL in milk (*82*). Concentrations of the drug in milk were rapidly depleted during withdrawal (with a half-life of 16 h) and reached concentrations of <0.05 ng/mL at day 5.

Confirmatory analysis of clenbuterol by GC–MS has been achieved by simultaneous analysis of two different derivatives of this compound (*83*). These two derivatives, trimethylsilyl and *tert*-butyldimethylsilyl, provide four high intensity diagnostic ions for analysis and therefore meet the requirements of the European Community for confirmatory analysis.

Other procedures have been developed for the determination of β-agonist and hormone residues in animals, including the following: (a) capillary gas chromatography to detect clenbuterol and salbutamol in calf urine (*84*); (b) HPLC–multidimensional gas chromatography to detect stilbene hormones (diethylstilbestrol, hexestrol, and dienestrol) in corned beef (*85,86*); (c) use of a commercially available ELISA (designed for the detection of progesterone in milk) for the detection of progesterone in beef (*87*); (d) GC–MS with selected ion monitoring for detection of the anabolic steroid 19-nortestosterone in bovine serum (*88*); (e) liquid chromatography–thermospray mass spectrometry for detection of trenbolone in bovine bile and feces (*89*); and (f) an ELISA for the detection of carazolol in tissues and urine of pigs (*90*).

# PESTICIDES

## Overviews and Multi-Residue Methods

Current recommendations for a healthy diet pose a dilemma for some people: On the one hand, we are being encouraged to eat more fruits and vegetables while, on the other hand, concerns have been raised about the health effects of pesticide residues in these crops. A survey of nearly 1800 people in Washington state elicited information on their attitudes and behaviors related to this problem (*91*). Analyses of results from the questionnaires indicated that persons with health concerns about pesticides had higher scores for residue-reducing behaviors, general environmental concerns, and perceived susceptibility to cancer. Those with less concern about pesticides generally saw greater benefits from pesticide use and had greater trust in regulations and monitoring programs to control residue levels. Fear of pesticide residues did not appear to decrease consumption of fruits and vegetables but did affect types of foods purchased ("organic" or "commercial") and other residue-reducing behaviors.

In an investigation into possible causes of increasing rates of mortality due to some types of cancer in industrialized countries, data from WHO were used to calculate age-specific rates of cancer mortality for a number of sites during 1968 to 1986 and these were compared with patterns of cancer in farmers in 8 countries as reported in 20 studies (92). Cancer at many sites appears to be increasing in the general populations in industrialized countries and also in farmers. Among these are Hodgkin's disease, multiple myeloma, leukemia, skin melanomas, and cancers of the lip, stomach, and prostate. These excesses in farmers occur against a background of substantial deficits in total mortality, heart disease, and many other specific diseases. The reasons for this excess mortality from some kinds of cancer are unknown but possible risk factors, such as exposure to pesticides, solvents, engine exhausts, and animal viruses, should be further studied since the general population is increasingly exposed to some of these agents as well.

Two studies of European agricultural workers with a relatively high exposure to pesticides demonstrated a greater incidence of genotoxic lesions in their lymphocytes than was observed in controls from the general population. Sister chromatid exchanges in lymphocytes of 70 Spanish workers employed in flower and/or fruit cultivation were found to be significantly higher (after controlling for age and tobacco use) than in 69 controls without occupational exposure to pesticides (93). These effects appeared to be additive, increasing with length of exposure. A significant increase in micronucleated peripheral lymphocytes was observed in 71 Italian floriculturists compared to that observed in 75 healthy blood donors living in the same area (94). A dose–response relationship was also observed between duration of exposure and micronucleus frequency.

While the general population is not usually exposed to high concentrations of a particular pesticide, residues of numerous pesticides can be detected in foods, albeit at very low levels. To assess the genotoxicity of such a complex mixture, data were obtained on residues of 100 pesticides in common Italian foods and on the frequency of consumption of these foods (95). Average exposure of an adult was estimated to be 716 µg pesticides/day, ranging from 148 µg of dithiocarbamates to 1 µg of pirimiphos-ethyl. A mixture containing the 15 most common pesticides in the proportions found in foods was made and tested for genotoxic effects. The mixture caused no significant increase in mutations in the Ames test or in micronuclei in rats dosed with 1, 10,

or 100 µg/kg. A small but significant increase was observed in sister chromatid exchanges in human lymphocytes exposed to this pesticide mixture in vitro.

Another potential dietary source of pesticides is contaminated groundwater which may contain low levels of several pesticides and/or fertilizers. Two mixtures, representative of groundwater contamination in California and in Iowa, were prepared and given to rats and mice as drinking water to determine possible reproductive and developmental effects (96). Both mixtures contained ammonium nitrate and atrazine in addition to 5 (California) or 4 (Iowa) other pesticides. Drinking water in these experiments contained pesticides at concentrations similar to means detected in groundwater surveys conducted in these states. Other groups of rodents consumed water containing 10 or 100 times these mean concentrations of pesticides. None of the study animals appeared to suffer any adverse effects in clinical signs of toxicity, in fertility or reproductive performance, in embryo/fetal toxicity, or in the incidence of fetal malformations.

A survey of data from the literature and from toxicity information submitted to the EPA's Office of Pesticide Programs on the mutagenicity of 10 pesticides was presented (97). It is intended that this be the first in a series of such publications published in the Genetic Activity Profile format. This will provide a more complete database on genotoxic assessments of pesticides and allow comparisons between information submitted to the EPA and other publicly available information. Results from different genotoxicity assays may not be consistent, and this compilation of data should aid in making risk assessment decisions.

Although regulatory agencies from different countries have access to basically the same toxicological information on pesticides, they often make widely divergent regulatory decisions. In order to obtain some insight into the main concerns among and between nations with regard to pesticide management, Nilsson et al. (98) analyzed information from 11 countries on procedures for registering, restricting, or banning registration for certain selected pesticides. Regulatory agencies must somehow balance political interests, commercial considerations, and scientific integrity in formulating policies to protect human health and environment. In some countries, nonscientific considerations strongly influence decisions about pesticide management and these are not always based on rational considerations. One of the main differences between countries is in the interpretation of carcinogenicity studies in animals: what is the significance to humans of rodent carcinogenicity studies, of methods for dose–response extrapolations, of the use of high challenge doses, of different methods of exposure assessment? The authors point out that there is a tremendous duplication of effort in different countries that could be substantially reduced by more effective international cooperation.

Application of the Delaney Clause to pesticide residues in foods presents a paradox (*99,100*). This Clause has the laudable purpose of prohibiting chemicals "shown to induce cancer" from being used as food additives. The EPA, as directed by the Federal Food, Drug, and Cosmetic Act (FFDCA), determines appropriate tolerances for pesticide residues in or on raw agricultural commodities (Section 408 of FFDCA) and sets tolerances for pesticide residues in processed foods (Section 409). In the case of processed foods, the residues are treated as food additives because they are added directly or indirectly to the foods or they have become concentrated during processing. In setting 408 tolerances, the EPA may consider both benefits and risks of the use of a pesticide, but in setting 409 tolerances, it may only consider toxic or carcinogenic risks (Delaney Clause). Recent court decisions have pointed out that any risk for carcinogenicity precludes approval of the chemical even if the risk is "negligible." Therefore, it has become extremely difficult to obtain approval for any new pesticides even though they may be manifestly less toxic or less carcinogenic than pesticides currently in use. Possible solutions to this problem are discussed in these articles.

Two broad classes of pesticides are recognized: conventional chemical pesticides and biological pesticides. The latter class includes microbial agents (viruses, bacteria, and fungi) and biochemical pesticides (pheromones, hormones, repellents, and natural insect and plant growth regulators). A recent review by McClintock et al. (*101*) discussed fundamental information and data necessary for evaluation of biochemical pesticides and the criteria for classifying a pesticide as "biochemical" rather than as a conventional chemical pesticide. Biochemical pesticides are considered to be a category of pesticide which requires less experimental data to demonstrate no significant adverse effect to humans.

During a 32-month period ending in December 1991, a total of 13,230 samples of domestic and imported agricultural food commodities in Canada were analyzed for residues of >200 pesticides (*102*). Of these, 224 samples contained violative residues (often resulting from the presence of a pesticide on a food for which it was not approved) and another 2501 samples contained detectable but nonviolative residues. A much greater percentage of imported than Canadian foods contained pesticide residues. Captan, endosulfan, dimethoate,

phosalone, and diazinon were the most frequently detected pesticides on domestic foods. Among Canadian foods, carrots, beans, and apples were most frequently contaminated, with 3.3, 0.93, and 0.7% of samples, respectively, with detectable residues. Among imported foods, strawberries, spinach, grapes, carrots, beans, and oranges were most often contaminated (14.5, 7.2, 6.0, 5.6, 4.4, and 4.2% of samples, respectively).

Highlights of a 1991 study of pesticide residues in foods in the UK presented information on foods with high or frequent levels of contamination (*103*). Nearly all of the 42 samples of carrots tested contained residues of triazophos and some also contained violative residues of other compounds. Detectable levels of ethylene thiourea were found in 20 of 27 samples of potato crisps. Three of 256 potato samples, 6 of 108 rice samples, and 6 of 81 lettuce samples contained violative residues of some pesticides. Most of the New Zealand lamb samples contained detectable $p,p'$-DDE and some Chinese meat and meat products contained excessive levels of organochlorine pesticides. However, it was estimated that overall, with the exception of chlorpropham in potatoes, the intakes of organochlorine pesticides declined or remained at very low levels since the last such survey in 1984–1985.

A recent volume on safeguarding food quality contains a number of chapters which describe procedures and approaches for the detection of various residues and contaminants in foods (*104*). Residues in crop plants, meat, and milk were considered along with discussions of the influence of feeds on residues and contaminants in animal products.

A multiresidue method utilizing solid-phase extraction columns and gas–liquid chromatography with electron capture and nitrogen phosphorus detectors has been devised for the determination of 74 pesticide residues in wine (*105*). Detection limits for each compound were 0.01–0.02 mg/L and recoveries from spiked samples averaged 70–110% for most of the pesticides. Only very polar pesticides were not recovered very well.

Experimental conditions for the extraction of organochlorine, organophosphorus, and organonitrogen pesticides from grains by supercritical carbon dioxide extraction were investigated and optimized (*106*). In most cases >80% of residues were recovered using this technique. An improved LC analytical method was also developed for the detection of carbofuran in grains.

Other papers on multiresidue methods for analysis of pesticide residues included: a review of thin-layer chromatographic methods for analyses of various environmental samples (*107*); a rapid GC method for the screening of fruits and vegetables for organochlorine and organophosphate residues (*108*); simultaneous analysis for 25 pesticides in crops using GC and their identification by GC–MS (*109*); and capillary GC with atomic emission detection for the analysis of pesticides in plants with complex matrices such as onions and radishes (*110*). The use of enzyme sensors to detect various families of pesticides was also reviewed and discussed by Marty et al. (*111*).

## Fumigants

Australian fruit packaged for export must be certified free of certain insect pests (fruit flies and coddling moths) and this can be accomplished by fumigation with methyl bromide. Residues of methyl bromide were determined in apples (*112*) and on several cultivars of sweet cherry, apple, nashi, plum, and red and green capsicums (*113*) after fumigation with 40–45 g methyl bromide/m$^3$ for 2 hours at 17°C followed by 2 hours of ventilation and up to 3 weeks' storage at 1°C. Methyl bromide concentrations in the apples, cherries, plums, nashi, and capsicums after 1 day of storage averaged 3.8–6.0, 4.6–11.0, 3.8, 6.8–12.1, and 24.2–28.3 ppm, respectively. Residue levels decreased steadily during storage to undetectable levels. This required 12 or more days for most fruits, but plums and cherries took only 5–6 days.

In an assessment of the reproductive toxicity of methyl bromide, rats were fed fumigated diets containing 200 or 500 ppm total bromine for two successive generations, for a total of 36 weeks (*114*). Food consumption was significantly lower among the higher dose rats and body weights of the pups exposed to the higher dose were lower. But no other adverse effects were observed in reproductive parameters or in gross and histopathological examinations of the exposed animals of both groups. Therefore, the minimum toxic level was designated 500 ppm in feed and the no observed adverse effect level was 200 ppm.

A headspace method, used previously for detection of methyl bromide in nuts, has been successfully used to analyze 63 off-the-shelf spices and seasonings, 83 grain-based, dried, or highly seasoned table-ready items, 30 dried fruits and trail mixes, and 38 oil-based items (*115*). No detectable methyl bromide was present in any of these samples. Methyl bromide was detected in fortified samples of these various foods, with recoveries ranging from 56% for spices and seasonings to a low of 30% for oil-based foods.

Phosphine, another fumigant gas, was applied to samples of coffee beans, rice, wheat and wheat flour, and several types of dried legumes. After a week of fumigation, the cereals (rice and wheat) had higher amounts of free phosphine in the void spaces of their containers than

the coffees and the legumes (*116*). This indicated that the legumes and coffee absorbed more of the phosphine than the other foods. In fact, lower grades of robusta coffee with dark, rough-surfaced husks had higher phosphine residue levels than higher grades of coffee (*117*). The lower-grade coffees also desorbed phosphine faster during storage than the higher-grade coffees.

## Fungicides

Hexachlorobenzene (HCB), a persistent and widespread organochlorine contaminant, is used as a fungicide and is also a by-product of industrial chlorination processes. Relatively high levels of HCB have been detected during surveys of breast milk from Spanish women from 1984–1991 (*118*). Samples were collected from women in rural and in industrialized areas. A great deal of variation was noted in contaminant levels, with mean levels in different populations ranging from 0.87 to 4.99 ppm. It appears that a great number of milk samples exceed the highest acceptable level of 0.5 ppm. Populations with the highest HCB levels came from both agricultural and industrial areas.

Total serum thyroxine levels in rats, orally dosed with 2.6 or 3.5 mmol HCB/kg for 2 or 4 weeks, were significantly decreased as compared to controls (*119*). Free thyroxin levels also decreased and thyroid-stimulating hormone levels increased. The major metabolite of HCB, pentachlorophenol, also induced hypothyroidism in these animals, although apparently by a different mechanism.

In a recent review, Dearfield (*120*) summarized and discussed data on the genotoxicity of ethylene thiourea (ETU) accumulated from numerous assays. Although this compound induces mutations and other genotoxic effects in some assays, it is not very potent. Results from some in vivo assays, in particular, are not very clear and such experiments should be repeated to better ascertain the risk from exposure to this compound.

Potato samples were obtained from 9 commercial stores in the UK at 2-month intervals from November to June to test for residues of tecnazene, a fungicide and sprout suppressant (*121*). None of the samples had residue levels which exceeded the UK maximum advisory limit of 5 mg/kg. Two tecnazene metabolites were detected in all treated potatoes but at much lower levels than the parent compound.

A majority of the 74 samples of bananas purchased at supermarkets in Germany were found to have thiabendazole residues of <0.7 µg/g in the whole fruit and <0.1 µg/g in the edible portion (*122*). Very small amounts of the fungicide were transferred from the fruit to hands during consumption and no residue transfer occurred if the bananas were first washed with warm water.

Effects of home processing of oranges into marmalade on residues of the fungicides imazalil, 2-phenylphenol, and thiabendazole were investigated by Friar and Reynolds (*123*). Heating of the orange pulp with sugar and water on a stove for 4 hours was more effective in reducing residues of thiabendazole (22% decrease) and 2-phenylphenol (48% decrease) than was heating in a microwave oven for 1 hour (no decrease in thiabendazole, 13% decrease in 2-phenylphenol). Both heating procedures actually increased detectable residues of imazalil by about 50%. Apparently imazalil residues were more easily extracted from processed fruit than from raw fruit.

Residues of the systemic fungicide fosetyl-aluminum were measured in orange and tangerine fruits during 4 weeks after a fall application (*124*). Residue levels of phosphonic acid (a metabolite of the fungicide) increased in both fruits during this time to reach a maximum of 4.3 mg/kg in pulp of the oranges and of 10.6 in the tangerines. The increasing residue concentrations were probably a result of translocation of the fungicide from the leaves to the fruit.

Numerous procedures have been described for the determination of fungicide residues in fruits and vegetables. Among these are: (a) solid-phase partition cartridges containing macroporous diatomaceous earth for the extraction of 14 fungicides from lettuce, peppers, peaches, apples and strawberries (*125*); (b) a collaborative study of a gas chromatographic procedure with nitrogen–phosphorus detection for the determination of ethylene urea in finished drinking water (*126*) (adopted first action by AOAC International); (c) a spectrophotometric method for the determination of maneb and zineb and their decomposition products in cucumbers and tomatoes (*127*); (d) a review of chromatographic methods for the determination of benomyl in crops (*128*) and a magnetic particle-based ELISA for determination of benomyl in fruit juices (*129*); (e) analyses of dithiocarbamate fungicides by second derivative UV spectroscopy (*130,131*); (f) an HPLC method for determination of carbendazim residues in crops, grains, and wines with fluorescence detection (*132*) and in wine by a competitive inhibition enzyme immunoassay (*133*); (g) a simple method for the preparation of citrus fruit peel for GC analysis of biphenyl residues (*134*); (h) a GC method for determination of pentachlorophenol residues in wine (*135*); (i) a monoclonal antibody–based ELISA for detection of thiabendazole in potatoes and apples (*136*); (j) determination of captan in water, peaches, and apple juice by magnetic particle-based immuno-

assay (*137*); and (k) a comparative study of an ELISA and a GC–MS method for determination of captan and its degradation product, tetrahydrophthalimide, in baby foods (*138*). The ELISA was found to give higher values than GC–MS and also gave some false-positive results.

Malachite green and some other triphenylmethane dyes are used in fish farming to control fungal diseases and ectoparasites. An HPLC method has been developed for the determination of residues of malachite green, crystal violet, and brilliant green in muscle tissue of trout (*139*). Compounds were identified by UV/visible light spectra, with detection limits of 1.8–3.9 µg/kg.

## Herbicides and Growth Regulators

Adverse effects on human health associated with exposure to phenoxy herbicides have been reported by some authors and disputed by others. Hardell et al. (*140*) examined data from 105 cases of histopathologically confirmed non-Hodgkin's lymphoma (NHL) and from 335 controls from a previous case–control study of malignant lymphoma. Analyses indicated that no specific occupation was associated with NHL but that exposure to phenoxyacetic acids, chlorophenols, and organic solvents yielded odds ratios of 5.5, 4.8, and 2.4, respectively, for contracting this disease. Exposures to DDT, asbestos, and tobacco products were not associated with risk for NHL. In a recent letter, Hadju (*141*) criticized a recent review article which pointed out an association between phenoxy herbicides and NHL and soft-tissue sarcomas. Although some epidemiological studies have noted such an association, many others have not confirmed it. Further studies with more accurate assessments of actual exposures are needed.

Since atrazine is the second most widely used herbicide in the USA, its possible toxicity is of relevance to human health. Brusick (*142*) reviewed and evaluated numerous investigations into the genotoxicity of this compound. Use of an expert judgment approach resulted in an equivocal conclusion as to atrazine's genotoxicity while a weight of evidence method led to the conclusion that atrazine does not pose a mutagenic hazard.

When the phenoxy herbicide 2,4-D is applied to wheat fields in spring to control weeds, the mature seeds do not contain significant levels of residues. To determine whether this herbicide could be safely applied later in the growing season, some Canadian fields were sprayed when the wheat was in the soft-dough stage (about 3 weeks before maturity) (*143*). Analyses of the mature wheat seeds from fields treated with 526 and 1052 g 2,4-D/ha revealed herbicide levels of 0.03–0.10 mg/kg and 0.08–0.26 mg/kg, respectively. Since such herbicide residue levels are close to or exceed the Canadian tolerance limit of 0.1 mg/kg, such a late application of the herbicide is not recommended.

Concentrations of the herbicide thifensulfuron applied postemergence at rates of 8 and 16 g/ha (2–4 times the recommended level) to greenhouse-grown soybeans were found to decline in the foliage, with half-lives ranging from 5 to 20 days (*144*). Radiolabelled residues in mature soybean seeds were extremely low (0.4–1.6 ppb).

Methods have been described for the determination of: (a) seven classes of herbicide residues in crops, food, and environmental samples by chromatographic methods (*145*); alachlor in milk, eggs, and liver by commercial immunoassays (*146*); (c) paraquat and diquat in potatoes by high-performance capillary electrophoresis with UV detection (*147*) and liquid chromatography (*148*) and in low-moisture foods using silica column cleanup and liquid chromatography with UV detection (*149*); (d) atrazine in foods by enzyme immunoassay (*150*) and by immunoassay in microtiter plates and in a dipstick format (*151,152*); (e) phenylurea herbicides in milk by reversed-phase HPLC (*153*); (f) the phenylurea diuron by immunoassay (*154*); (g) arylurea herbicides by ELISA (*155*); and (h) sulfonylurea herbicides by gas–liquid chromatography and mass spectrometry (*156*).

## Acaricides

Residues of formic acid, used to control tracheal mites in bees, were found to be present in higher levels in honey from hives treated in the summer than those treated in the spring (*157*). Experiments were carried out in Alberta, Canada, where some mite-infested hives were treated with 88% formic acid on May 28 and June 7, others were treated with 65% formic acid on June 29, July 6, and July 13, and others remained untreated. Honey from hives treated in the spring and their controls contained 1.7–1.8 $\mu$mol formic acid/g honey (no significant difference). However, honey from those treated in the summer contained an average of 7.9 $\mu$mol/g compared to 2.5 $\mu$mol/g in their controls. Naturally occurring levels of formic acid in 25 samples of honey from various parts of Canada ranged from 1.0 to 3.3 $\mu$mol/g. This natural variation reflects the different flower sources used for making the honey.

Methods have been developed for the determination of: fluvalinate residues recovered from honey by supercritical fluid extraction and determined by HPLC (*158*); amitraz, bromopropylate, coumaphos, cymiazole,

and fluvalinate residues in honey by GC–MS (*159*); and formetanate hydrochloride in pome, citrus, and stone fruits by coupled-column cation exchange liquid chromatography (*160*). A limited survey of 15 fruits from retail stores and farmers' markets revealed that only 2, an apple and an imported Asian pear, had detectable levels of this acaricide, of 0.03 and 0.07 ppm, respectively.

## Insecticides

Carbamate and organophosphate pesticides can depress cholinesterase activity in blood and therefore this is a potentially useful indicator of pesticide exposure. However, plasma cholinesterase activity is also lowered during some stages of pregnancy and this can complicate interpretation of these tests. Recent analyses of cholinesterase activity in 203 pregnant women revealed a high correlation between activity of this enzyme and self-reported pesticide exposure (*161*). Once enzyme activities were referenced, by trimester, to a larger sample of 1050 plasma cholinesterase values from 535 pregnant women, the effects of pesticide exposure could be discerned.

Some previous investigations have noted an association between agricultural pesticide use and non-Hodgkin's lymphoma in men, but not in women. In a recent, population-based, case–control study of women (184 cases, 707 controls) in eastern Nebraska, no increased risk for this disease was observed in women who had ever worked or lived on a farm (*162*). However, relatively few of these women actually handled pesticides. Among women who reported personally using organophosphate pesticides and using chlorinated hydrocarbons with dairy cattle, significant 4.5- and 3.0-fold increases in risk, respectively, were noted. Pesticide-related risks were also greater among women with a family history of cancer, suggesting that both genetic and environmental factors may be involved in carcinogenesis.

A survey of 348 "organically" and conventionally grown fruits and vegetables obtained in retail outlets in Australia revealed that 12% of the "organic" and 30% of the conventional produce contained detectable levels of one or more pesticides (*163*). Chlorpyrifos, endosulfan, and dieldrin were most frequently encountered, accounting for about 70% of the positive assays. Eleven other pesticides were detected much less frequently. Of 18 samples containing residues above the maximum residue limits, 3, which contained excess chlorpyrifos, were "organically" grown. While these organic farmers may not have used pesticides themselves, there may have been some carryover of pesticides in soil from previous farmers or there may have been problems of pesticides drifting in from neighboring fields.

Of 806 composite milk samples tested by the FDA for pesticide residues in 1990–1991, 398 contained one or more pesticides for a total of 455 positive tests (*164*). Together, dieldrin and *p,p'*-DDE accounted for 84.4% of these positive tests. Other compounds detected in >3 samples included chlorpyrifos, heptachlor epoxide, heptachlor, and hexachlorobenzene. None of the composite milks contained levels of residues which approached regulatory limits. Occurrence of pesticides varied nationally, with no residues detected in milk from 7 metropolitan areas while all the samples from 4 other areas contained residues of *p,p'*-DDE.

Spraying of eggplants at the recommended rates with endosulfan, fenvalerate, and decamethrin resulted in residues of only decamethrin above the tolerance level (*165*). A little more than 4 days were required for this pesticide to dissipate to levels below the regulatory limits. When these pesticides were applied at twice the recommended rate, waiting periods of 2.57, 6.5, and 0.14 days were required for endosulfan, decamethrin, and fenvalerate, respectively, to reach acceptable levels.

In an investigation of carryover of pesticides in soybeans during processing into tofu, soybeans were spiked with captan (2.87 ppm), chlorpyrifos (11.2 ppm), malathion (7.9 ppm), and dichlorvos (5.01 ppm) and the pesticide residues were monitored at different steps during tofu production (*166*). Concentrations of all these compounds decreased sharply during the first stage—making of soybean milk—and were further eliminated during subsequent stages, so that the final tofu contained 0.014, 0.82, 0.72, and 0.06 ppm, respectively of the 4 pesticides.

A small-scale, multiresidue method involving gas chromatographic analysis has been developed for the determination of organochlorine and pyrethroid residues in ethanol extracts of vegetables (*167*). When this method was used to screen 15 vegetable samples from the Singapore market, five were found to contain detectable levels of organochlorine pesticides.

**ORGANOCHLORINES.** The publication, last year, of research demonstrating that the women in a cohort who were diagnosed with breast cancer within 6 months of an initial examination had significantly higher levels of serum DDE than matched controls who did not develop this type of cancer has generated much discussion. Acquavella et al. (*168*) stated that DDT is not considered to be a mammary carcinogen in animals and that other epidemiological studies correlating DDT and mortality from cancer have not yielded positive results. Moreover, they pointed out that the cases in this study most likely already had cancer when serum samples were analyzed and that the developing breast cancer may have altered metabolism, thereby giving an inaccurate estimate of actual body burdens of the pesticide. The authors of the 1993 research, Wolff et al. (*169*), replied that IARC has concluded that there is sufficient evidence that DDT is an animal carcinogen and that it is a possible human carcinogen. The negative epidemiological studies mentioned presented either nonspecific data (cancer in general, not specifically breast cancer) or conclusions based on mortality data. However, the 5-year survival rate for breast cancer patients is now >75% and therefore incidence, rather than mortality, is a more appropriate measure. The authors concede that all of their cases would have had a small, as yet undetected, cancer at time of the initial screening and that this tumor may have already affected metabolic processes. Further analyses of members of this cohort who developed cancer within 9 years of sampling are underway.

Analyses of tissue from 44 breast cancer patients in Finland indicated that DDE concentrations in adipose tissue were positively correlated with the amount of estrogen receptors in the cancer tissue (*170*). It may be that DDE exerts an indirect carcinogenic effect by increasing estrogen receptors. In another group of 9 patients with estrogen-receptor-positive mammary adenocarcinoma, mean adipose tissue concentrations of DDE were substantially higher (2132 μg/kg) than in 17 noncancerous controls (765 μg/kg) and in 9 estrogen-receptor negative breast cancer patients (609 μg/kg) (*171*). Although the number of cases analyzed is small, these data support the hypothesis that DDE enhances formation of hormone-responsive cancers.

From a cohort of >57,000 women in the San Francisco area originally examined in the late 1960s, 2097 cases of primary breast cancer (occurring >6 months after the examination) were identified up to 1990. Analyses of blood samples obtained from 150 of these breast cancer patients (50 each of white, black, and Asian women) and from 150 matched controls revealed no significant differences in serum DDE levels between cases (43.3 ppb) and controls (43.1 ppb) either considered as a whole or for each separate racial group (*172*). Organochlorine levels were significantly higher among black and Asian women than among white women. Data on the estrogen receptor status of the tumors were available for only 45% of the cases and no difference in serum DDE levels was observed between these cases and their controls.

Analyses of adipose tissue samples from 25 fatal accident cases in El Paso, Texas revealed the presence of DDT, DDE, lindane, and heptachlor in 72, 100, 96, and 44%, respectively (*173*). Mean concentrations of the 4 compounds were, respectively, 1.5, 4.96, 0.2, and 0.12 ppm. These data indicate that the residents were widely exposed in the past to DDT or were more recently exposed through water and foods from areas of past DDT application, were exposed to a dispersed source of lindane (water and/or food), and were recently exposed to heptachlor. These pesticide levels are considered moderate and comparable to those observed in other areas in the USA.

Of 51 milk samples from women in an agricultural area of Turkey analyzed for organochlorine pesticide residues, all contained DDE (mean of 2389 ppb) and hexachlorocyclohexane isomers (mean of 774 ppb) and 88% contained aldrin (mean of 47 ppb) (*174*). Although these levels are moderately high, they are somewhat lower than residue levels in human milk samples obtained 4–6 years earlier from other areas in Turkey. The average concentration of total DDT derivatives was above the limits recommended by WHO.

To determine whether fish advisories posted on the basis of the percentage of fish sampled which contain >100 ppb chlordane really protect fish eaters from excess exposure to this pesticide, serum chlordane levels were compared among non-fish-eaters and persons consuming at least 1 pound of fish/week from rivers in Missouri with different advisories (*175*). Analyses of the data revealed no significant differences between the groups in serum chlordane levels even when data were controlled for other possible exposures such as use of pesticides in work or around the home or living in a home which had been treated with chlordane. Therefore, the fish advisories do not appear to protect people from chlordane exposure. Serum chlordane levels were <1.5 ppb for 90% of the participants, and the highest concentration measured was 13 ppb. All these values are well below levels known to cause adverse effects in humans.

Analyses of daily total diet samples from 20 vegetarians living in a metropolitan area of India revealed average DDT and benzene hexachloride (hexachlorocyclohexane) levels of 19.24 µg and 77.15 µg, respectively (*176*). The concentrations of these pesticides in fatty foods were much higher than in nonfatty foods but these two categories contributed nearly equally to total intake of the pesticides. Milk, in particular, contained high concentrations of both chemicals: 5.19 mg total BHC/kg and 0.63 mg total DDT/kg. Blood levels of these compounds reflected intake.

Reports from a 1993 workshop on the analytical and environmental chemistry of toxaphene have been published in a recent issue of *Chemosphere* (*177*). Toxaphene is a potent rodent carcinogen and therefore its presence in edible fish may pose a hazard for humans. Various research papers presented at the conference discussed procedures for the determination of toxaphene and related compounds and results from testing of human milk samples from Nicaragua, of Great Lakes fish, and of fish and marine mammals from the northeastern Atlantic. Contamination of fish and marine mammals with this compound is of particular significance to humans in the northern latitudes who depend heavily on these animals for food. Toxaphene concentrations reported in these species were: Great Lakes trout, >900 ppb; Arctic salmon, nearly 3000 ppb; Baltic salmon, nearly 2000 ppb; northern North Sea cod liver, 580 ppb; hake liver from off the coast of Ireland, 1300 ppb; harbor porpoise blubber, 6800 ppb; and white-beaked dolphin, 19,000 ppb.

A total of 229 samples of Spanish meat and meat products were analyzed for residues of organochlorine pesticides (*178*). All samples contained detectable levels of hexachlorobenzene (HCB) and hexachlorocyclohexane (HCH) and 7% contained dieldrin. Lamb appeared to be more heavily contaminated than other meats, with average levels of 49 ppb HCB and 112 ppb HCH. DDT and/or DDE were detected in 83% of the lamb samples (mean of 25 ppb). Only 4 meat samples (all pork) contained pesticide levels above the maximum residue limits. Further analyses of 30 samples of pork from Spanish pigs revealed that male pigs had higher levels of HCB (15 vs. 11 ppb), and lindane (γ-HCH, 57 vs. 21 ppb) (*179*). Mean lindane concentrations were highest in the medium-weight pigs (58 ppb) while HCB levels were slightly higher in the heaviest pig legs compared to other weights. Average total DDT residues in muscle from pigs from two abattoirs in Kenya were 0.53 ppm and 1.23 ppm (*180*). Other organochlorine pesticides (heptachlor, aldrin, and dieldrin) were detected in the fat from a small number of pigs from one abattoir. Different feeding practices appear to account for the different residue levels.

An investigation was conducted on the effects of different cooking processes on residues of DDT (*181*) and on isomers of HCH (*182*) in lamb. Grilling, roasting, and pressure cooking effectively reduced DDT residues by about 75% in the meat and reduced lindane levels by 17–39%. However, other HCH isomers were decreased by only 0–36 %.

Residue levels of chlorinated pesticides which were detected in 90% of 208 samples of sterilized Spanish milk from retail outlets were generally observed to have declined since previous surveys (*183*). However, 32% of the samples were contaminated with chlordane at levels which exceeded the recommended maximum residue limits. Based on an average consumption of 343 mL milk/day in Spain, it appears that this sterilized milk does not pose a health risk.

Most of 150 samples of Argentinian butter analyzed for organochlorine pesticides were found to contain detectable levels of lindane (0.002–0.188 ppm) and heptachlor (0.0005–3.41 ppm) (*184*). Over half the samples contained aldrin and α-HCH and about 30% contained dieldrin and DDT/DDE. Relatively few samples exceeded tolerance levels: 17 for heptachlor epoxide, 10 for dieldrin, 4 for lindane and 2 for DDT.

Organochlorine pesticides detected in 16 species of marine fish caught near a sewage outfall on the coast of Australia were found to be present primarily in the liver (*185*). HCB, chlordane, dieldrin and DDT/DDE were present in the highest concentration. Muscle tissue from these fish contained very low levels of these pesticides, often at or near the limits of detection of the assay.

Of 83 potato and 25 carrot samples from Greece which were analyzed for residues of lindane, 40% of the potatoes tested positive (not detected–250 ppb) and 56% of the carrots were positive (not detected–90 ppb) (*186*). Only 3 potato samples and none of the carrots exceeded maximum residue limits.

Of 19 processed food products imported into Hawaii from western Pacific Rim countries which were analyzed for organochlorine pesticides, 9 contained detectable residues (*187*). DDT was the most commonly found chemical, being detected in black bean sauce, pepper leaves, sesame seeds, and udon noodles. Lindane and chlorpyrifos were detected in 3 foods each, chlordane in 2 foods, and heptachlor and dieldrin in one each. Very low levels of these pesticides were detected, with the highest being chlorpyrifos at 10.95 ppb in roasted peas.

Accurate determination of organochlorine residues in foods requires an efficient means of extraction of food matrices. Several recent papers describe new or modified procedures for extraction. Among these are a reversed-phase solid-phase extraction with octyldecyl-silica for analyses of milk (*188*); supercritical fluid extraction of poultry tissues (*189*); gel permeation chromatography, sweep codistillation, and Florisil column adsorption chromatography for cleanup of samples of animal fats (*190*); matrix solid-phase dispersion extraction of fish muscle (*191*); a sandwich-type extraction column with on-line sulfuric acid treatment for analyses of vegetable oils and oil seeds (*192*); and a redesigned simultaneous steam distillation-solvent extraction apparatus for analyses of biological samples (*193*).

**ORGANOPHOSPHATES.** Exposure to organophosphate pesticides was found to significantly decrease activity of serum cholinesterase in agricultural workers at the end of the work day as compared to the beginning of the day (*194*). These greenhouse workers also had significantly lower serum cholinesterase levels than residents living in the same city in Mexico. Although no obvious signs of organophosphate intoxication were evident among the workers, it is apparent that they are experiencing a subclinical intoxication and primary prevention programs should be instituted to minimize contact with pesticides.

Sixty samples of green coffee beans imported into the USA from 21 countries were analyzed for residues of organochlorine, organophosphate, and carbamate pesticides (*195*). Positive results were obtained with only 4 samples: 3 contained chlorpyrifos (0.01, 0.02, and 0.04 ppm) and one contained 0.01 ppm pirimiphos-methyl. Although there are no U.S. EPA tolerances for these pesticides in green coffee beans, the concentrations detected here were so low that regulatory action was not warranted.

An investigation of the fate of chlorpyrifos-methyl on wheat during storage for 28 months at 20°C revealed that about 70% of the applied insecticide remained in the wheat as bound residues (*196*). When this wheat was fed to rats, the residues were released, metabolized and eliminated, primarily through the urine. Pesticide metabolites were also detected in feces but not in tissues. None of the rats showed signs of clinical toxicity during the 13-day feeding trial.

Fate of four organophosphates (dichlorvos, chlorpirifos-methyl, malathion, and fenitrothion) and of methyl bromide applied to unhulled and brown rice was investigated during a storage period of about three months and during cooking (*197*). Pesticide residues decreased to about one-third the initial levels during storage but bromide concentrations persisted longer. Washing of the rice and cooking by steaming removed nearly all the pesticides but bromide levels remained at about 41% of the initial concentrations. Grinding the rice to make noodles followed by cooking of the noodles removed all of the organophosphates and left only about 5% of the bromide. Similar experiments with buckwheat (treated with the same pesticides and methyl bromide) revealed that the half-lives of the pesticides during storage were ≥90 days (*198*). Bromide residues decreased rapidly at first and then increased. After processing the buckwheat into noodles, no dichlorvos was detected but 40–61% of the other pesticides and 21% of the methyl bromide remained.

Residues of three organophosphates (acephate, methamidophos, and pirimiphos-methyl), which are widely used to control insect pests in crops, were monitored in tomatoes grown in a greenhouse (199). The pesticides were applied at recommended rates and then ripe fruits were collected for analyses at 1 hour after spraying and at intervals during the next 56 days. Depletion of the residues to maximum residue limits recommended by FAO/WHO would require waiting periods of 3–4 days after application of acephate, 1–3 days for methamidophos, and 7–16 days for pirimiphos-methyl, depending on the rate of application of the pesticide. Because tomatoes are perishable and must be harvested frequently, insecticides with long post-application waiting periods would not be very useful.

Fenthion residues in olives and olive products were monitored following two field experiments in which the olive plants were treated 3 or 5 times (200). Degradation of this pesticide on olives was slow, with a half-life of about 38 days, and 5 metabolites, in addition to the parent compound, were detected. When the olives were processed into oil, fenthion residues were concentrated about 3 times. Degradation of fenthion residues in olive oil stored for up to a year at room temperature or in the freezer also proceeded slowly (201). Although concentrations of the parent compound decreased during storage, concentrations of the toxic metabolite, fenthion sulfoxide, increased so that total fenthion residues remained unchanged after a year of storage.

In an investigation of the thermal stability of 6 organophosphate insecticides, these compounds were added to water and to lean ground beef and heated at 70 or 80°C for 1–2 hours (202). All of the pesticides were degraded to some extent by heat but >50% of many of the residues remained after heating for 1 hour at 70°C (an approximation of normal cooking). Generally, the compounds were more stable when heated in water than when added to meat and cooked. Nevertheless, cooking cannot be considered an effective means of eliminating residues of these pesticides from foods.

Fifteen chicken samples obtained from supermarkets in Portugal were analyzed for residues of chlorpyrifos, fenitrothion, ethion, and methidathion (203). Neither of the first two compounds was detected in these samples although the gas chromatographic procedure used was capable of detecting 3.2–5.6 μg fenitrothion/kg and 2.2–2.5 μg chlorpyrifos/kg in fortified samples. Ethion was detected in 4 samples of muscle tissue and its associated skin, with a range of 31.3 to 51.4 μg/kg in muscle and of 381.3 to 1796.8 μg/kg in skin. Methida-

thion was present in concentrations of 3.25–4.41 μg/kg in muscle and of 199.04–1205.0 μg/kg in skin. Residues of both pesticides in muscle were below the maximum residue limits established by FAO/WHO while residues in skin were well above these limits.

Rapid antibody-based field tests have been devised and evaluated for the detection of residues of fenitrothion and pirimiphos-methyl in stored grains (204). Methanol extracts of grains and an enzyme-labeled component were added to tubes, allowed to incubate and then reacted with a chromogen. Results can be read by eye or a portable field photometer with a limit of detection of 0.1 ppm for fenitrothion and of 0.03 ppm for pirimiphos-methyl in grain. Data obtained using these field tests correlated well with that obtained using more precise laboratory methods.

Use of a wide-bore capillary columns for the gas chromatographic determination of 23 organophosphate pesticides in 5 fortified food extracts was found, by a collaborative study, to be equal or superior to the packed columns specified in the official AOAC method (205). Other modifications which have been devised for the gas chromatographic determination of organophosphorus insecticides include a splitless injection of samples of oils to be tested into the gas chromatograph (206) and extraction of pesticides from rice using supercritical fluid extraction and quantitation using an atomic emission detector (207).

CARBAMATES. An unusual and severe case of aldicarb poisoning was reported in a 43-year-old man in Arizona (208). About 15–20 minutes after eating dinner, the victim suddenly developed severe nausea, vomiting, and diarrhea. He was very weak, brachycardic, had slurred speech and abundant secretions in the throat. His red blood cell cholinesterase and plasma pseudocholinesterase activities were depressed and he required intubation for 5 days. Aldicarb and its metabolites were detected in blood samples. The patient had no known exposure to aldicarb but the onset of symptoms so soon after eating suggested that he consumed some contaminated food. The source of the aldicarb was never identified.

A large-scale poisoning of grazing sheep which occurred in Washington state in 1989 was traced to aldicarb residues in the fields. Of 318 sheep in one group, 288 died suddenly, most of the deaths occurring within minutes of each other. The other 30 sheep died later or were euthanized when they became very ill. Although the approximately 1300 sheep grazing in nearby fields were not acutely affected by the pesticide, followup over the next 3 years revealed that they suffered an unusually high number of deaths and also exhibited low fertility and poor health (*209*). Lambs born to these sheep had an increased number of limb and gastrointestinal malformations. All 6 men present in the field about the time of the sheep deaths reported symptoms such as headaches, shortness of breath, burning sensation in the mouth, muscle aches, dizziness, and fatigue. Three years after the incident, 5 of the men were still seeking medical attention or reporting symptoms they felt were related to the poisoning incident. Such chronic health effects have not been previously reported.

The decline in residues of oxamyl on tomatoes during cool storage (15°C) was found to be more rapid under modified atmospheres consisting of 1.5% oxygen + 98.5% nitrogen or 1.5% oxygen + 4% carbon dioxide + 94.5% nitrogen than in air (*210*). Fruit ripened more quickly in air than it did in either modified atmosphere.

A recent review by McGarvey (*211*) described HPLC methods for analysis of 31 *N*-methylcarbamate pesticides and 46 of their metabolites. Techniques for extraction of the pesticides from plants, water and soil, for cleanup of extracts, for chromatographic separation, and for detection by UV absorbance, fluorescence, electrochemical methods and mass spectrometry were discussed.

Two sampling protocols were used to investigate optimal conditions for sample collection, storage, and analysis to ensure the validity of an LC method for determination of carbamate residues in beef, chicken, and duck liver (*212*). Residue depletion during storage at –5°C varied with the species, with greater depletion in duck than in beef liver. Certain carbamate compounds were also more stable than others. These studies emphasized the need for cold temperatures to prevent degradation of carbamate residues during analysis.

Numerous improved and modified methods have been developed for the determination of carbamate pesticide residues in foods. These include: (a) an HPLC method for carbofuran residues in tomatoes grown in hydroponics (*213*); (b) a mixed, selective adsorbent for cleanup during supercritical fluid extraction of 3 carbamate pesticides from chicken muscle (*214*); (c) supercritical fluid extraction and HPLC for detection of thiocarbamate pesticides in apples (*215*); (d) automatic GC analysis with electron capture detection for determination of *N*-methylcarbamates in milk (*216*); (e) simple gas–liquid chromatography with nitrogen–phosphorus detection for determination of aldicarb and its metabolites in oranges (*217*); (f) an LC method for *N*-methylcarbamate pesticides in bovine, swine and poultry liver (*218*); and (g) detection of aldicarb sulfone and carbofuran in fortified meat and liver using a commercial ELISA (*219*).

**PYRETHROIDS.** Deltamethrin, a synthetic pyrethroid, can be used to control insect infestations in saskatoon shrubs. In a recent study the persistence of deltamethrin residues in saskatoon berries was monitored after 4 applications of the pesticide during a one-month period (*220*). Berries collected one day after the last spraying contained an average of 0.22 ppm deltamethrin. After 7 and 39 days, residue levels had declined to 0.08 and 0.01 ppm, respectively. A 21-day waiting period after the last deltamethrin application should be sufficient to dissipate residues of this pesticide.

Carryover of deltamethrin into tissues of animals was measured in pigs fed for 4–5 months on wheat treated postharvest with deltamethrin at the maximum recommended rate (*221*). Residue levels in flour made from the wheat averaged 0.95 mg/kg. At slaughter deltamethrin concentrations in liver and kidney were undetectable while concentrations in muscle and fat averaged 0.002–0.003 and 0.015–0.03 mg/kg, respectively. Under these conditions, deltamethrin residues in pigs did not reach a level of toxicological significance.

Methods developed for determination of pyrethroid residues in foods included: (a) determination of natural pyrethrins and 12 synthetic pyrethroids in vegetables, fruits, grains, beans, and green tea leaves by gas chromatography with electron capture detection (*222*) (different extraction methods were used for preparation of samples of the different crop plants); (b) determination of multiple pyrethroid residues in fruits and vegetables by capillary gas chromatography (*223*); and (c) quantitation of the synthetic pyrethroid bioresmethrin in grains by enzyme immunoassay (*224*).

# POLYHALOGENATED AROMATIC HYDROCARBONS

## Multiple Polyhalogenated Compounds

**TOXICOLOGICAL STUDIES.** While some organochlorine compounds are certainly quite toxic and their presence in foods and water is a matter of serious concern, other organochlorines apparently do not pose a health risk to humans. Willes et al. (*225*) discussed several important principles related to the evaluation of chlorinated organics for their potential toxicity. Chemical structures of these compounds and their resulting physical and chemical properties determine their metabolism and biological activities in mammals. As we now know, not even all chemicals of a particular class, for example polychlorinated biphenyls (PCBs), are equivalent. Non-

*ortho* coplanar PCBs (congeners 77, 126, 169) are associated with more toxic effects than mono-*ortho*-chlorine substituted PCBs (congeners 105, 118, 156), which in turn are more toxic than di-*ortho*-substituted PCBs (congeners 138, 153, 180). Therefore, concentrations of these PCB congeners are often converted to toxic equivalents (TEQ), an expression of the amount of 2,3,7,8-tetrachloro-dibenzo-*p*-dioxin (TCDD) which would induce the same toxicity as the amounts of the PCBs in the sample. Most experiments demonstrate that there are threshold concentrations, below which adverse effects do not occur. It appears that many of the anthropogenic chlorinated organic compounds of concern are also produced in nature in small amounts. Therefore, there may already be biological mechanisms for dealing with low concentrations of some of these contaminants.

Sampling and design considerations relevant to epidemiological investigations of the health effects of organochlorine molecules were discussed by Woodruff et al. (*226*). Biomarkers of exposure, conversions of organochlorine levels to TEQs, etiologic and toxicokinetic considerations, quality control and quality assurance, and statistical sampling were considered. Because such small concentrations of contaminants are involved in these studies, it is essential that the epidemiologists and the statisticians utilize a carefully worked out methodology and describe it completely so that data from different sources can be compared and so that toxic or carcinogenic effects, if they exist, can be discerned.

Some studies have demonstrated immunotoxic or hepatotoxic effects of organochlorine contaminants in laboratory animals. Since salmon and herring from the Baltic Sea contain relatively high levels of PCBs, polychlorinated dibenzo-*p*-dioxins (PCDDs) and dibenzofurans (PCDFs), a study was conducted to compare immunologic parameters in 23 Swedish males who consumed high levels of these fish (average of 606 g/week) and in another group of 20 other males with virtually no fish consumption (*227*). The fish eaters had approximately 2.5–3.0 times the concentration of PCBs (9.4 pg/g for 5 congeners measured) and PCDD/Fs (64 pg TEQ/g fat) in their blood and 6.7 times the level of DDT (0.4 ng/g) in blood as the nonconsumers. Fish eaters also had significantly higher levels of organic mercury in erythrocytes than non-fish-eaters. White blood cell concentrations and major lymphocyte subsets were similar in the two groups but numbers and proportions of natural killer cells were significantly lower among the fish consumers. Numbers of natural killer cells were significantly and negatively correlated with blood levels of DDT and PCB congeners 126 and 118 but were not significantly correlated with organic mercury levels.

Because the Inuit of northern Quebec consume large quantities of fish and sea mammals, they are exposed to high levels of some bioaccumulating organochlorines. Breast milk from women in this population has also been found to contain high levels of PCBs (1052 ng/g fat), DDE (1212 ng/g), and hexachlorobenzene (HCB, 136 ng/g) (*228*). These PCB concentrations were about 7-fold higher and the pesticide levels were about 4 times higher than those recorded for milk from women in southern Quebec. Statistically significant negative associations were observed between the height of male infants born to these Inuit women and concentrations of PCBs, PCDD/Fs, HCB, and mirex in breast milk (*229*). However, significant associations were not noted between organochlorine exposure and birth weight, head circumference, or blood TSH (thyroglobulin) level. Height of female infants was positively correlated with PCBs/PCDD/Fs in mother's milk.

Numerous other studies have reported measurements of organochlorine contaminants in breast milk, including the following: (a) analyses of 412 samples from Canadian women from across the country (*230*); (b) analyses of milk from 2 Yusho patients and from 9 Japanese controls (*231*) [as expected, TEQ of PCBs, PCDDs, and PCDFs in milk from Yusho women were much higher (55.1, 417.3, and 23.8 pg/g fat) than in controls (21.8, 8.1, and 4.8 pg/g)]; (c) analyses of milk from Swedish women from 1967 to 1989 (*232,233*); (d) analyses of 115 Welsh breast milk samples collected in 1990–1991 (*234*); (e) analyses of up to 1400 milk samples from German women, collected since 1984 (*235*); and (f) analyses of milk from 38 New Zealand women in 1987–1988 (*236*). Studies containing milk samples which spanned a number of years often reported a decline in concentrations of some organochlorines, such as pesticides, while concentrations of others, like PCBs, were more stable. Declines in contaminant levels were also noted as women nursed their second or third child as compared to the first.

Adipose tissue samples from various human populations have also been analyzed to determine levels of chlorinated contaminants and their increasing or decreasing trends. Screening of such tissue from 75 individuals in Wales in 1990–1991 revealed the presence of 0.2–1.8 µg total PCBs/g adipose tissue, with 29 PCB congeners identified (*237*). Congeners 138, 153, and 180 were the most abundant. Concentrations of DDT/DDE ranged from 0.11–5.6 µg/g. Older subjects had higher levels of both classes of contaminants and also had a greater proportion of the more persistent and higher chlorinated PCBs. Despite reductions in the use of these compounds in the past 20 years, there appears to be little change in concentrations in human adipose tissue in this area during the past 10 years.

A total of 68 formalin-preserved adipose tissue samples collected between 1928 and 1985 by major research centers in Japan were analyzed for organochlorine residues (*238*). PCB residues were first detected in samples from the 1940s, soon after their use started in Japan, and concentrations increased until about 1980 and then remained steady. DDT residues were detectable at very low levels in the oldest samples and started to rise in the mid 1940s and peaked in the early 1960s. Hexachlorocyclohexane (HCH) residues were first recorded in samples from the late 1940s and peaked in the mid 1960s. Chlordane residues were first detected in the late 1950s and have been on the increase since. These temporal trends in residue concentrations to some extent reflect usage of these chemicals but these contaminants are very persistent and residue levels decline slowly.

Organochlorine contaminants in 277 adipose tissue samples collected in Poland in 1989–1992 included *p,p'*-DDE (mean of 5.745 mg/kg fat), total HCH (0.318 mg/kg), and PCBs (0.856 mg/kg) (*239*). Residue levels appeared to increase with increasing age up to about age 55 and then declines were observed in most types of residues (but not in DDE concentrations).

Of 3 non-*ortho* coplanar PCBs assayed in 28 adipose tissue samples from Atlanta, Georgia, PCB 169 was found in the highest concentration (mean of 69 ppt); lowest in concentration was PCB 77 (11.7 ppt) (*240*). However, PCB congener concentrations varied greatly from one individual to another. Concentrations of TCDD averaged 10.4 ppt and were more similar among individuals. When expressed as toxic equivalents, 4 of the PCB congeners made a larger contribution to toxicity than did the TCDD residues.

Serum TCDD levels in six Michigan Vietnam veterans were found to be elevated (20.4–131 ppt) while 44 other veterans had serum TCDD concentrations <8.5 ppt (*241*). For comparison, pooled blood samples from residents of different areas in Vietnam contained 3.4–28 ppt TCDD. Total PCDD/F congeners in these veterans averaged 1068 ppt. In contrast, mean concentrations of non-*ortho* coplanar, mono-*ortho*-substituted and di-*ortho*-substituted PCBs in the veterans' sera were 227, 50,500, and 117,000 ppt, respectively. These PCB levels (which are not related to service in Vietnam) account for 67% of the toxic equivalents measured in the serum.

**OCCURRENCE IN FOODS.** A comprehensive survey of foods in the Netherlands for residues of 2,3,7,8-chlorine substituted dioxins, furans, and planar PCBs was combined with information on average daily intake of foods from different categories in order to estimate the contribution of different food groups to intake of these chlorinated compounds (*242*). The main sources of these compounds in the diet were found to be fats and oils used in baked and processed foods, margarine, and cooking oils (contributing 27% to toxic equivalent uptake), dairy products (20%), and cheese (15%). Most of the remainder of these chlorinated compounds was consumed in meat, fish, butter, and eggs. This information was then used to determine whether elevated levels of contaminants in milk from cows grazing near municipal incinerators would increase average daily intakes of these organochlorines. Examination of sheep grazing near these incinerators demonstrated that their flesh also contained elevated levels of dioxins and PCBs. While most Dutch people do not consume much mutton, a subgroup of the population, the Dutch Turks, do. A food frequency survey was conducted within this population to determine their potential exposure to toxic organochlorines (*243*). In contrast to the rest of the Dutch population, the main routes of exposure of the Dutch Turks were butter (21%), mutton (19%), beef (17%), and cheese (10%). Analyses of the information obtained in both these studies indicated that the Turks had a slightly higher intake of dioxins and PCBs than the general Dutch population but that the median exposure of both groups was within acceptable limits. The data also demonstrated that small increases in contaminant levels in different food groups would affect the two populations differently. Fortunately, efforts to reduce these contaminants in cow's milk will most likely also reduce levels in mutton.

Analyses of 30 cow's milk samples collected in Madrid, Spain, in 1990–1991 revealed that all contained detectable levels of PCBs and most also were contaminated with lindane, heptachlor epoxide, and *p,p'*-DDE (*244*). Residues of chlorinated compounds exceeded EEC maximum residue levels in 16.6% of the milk samples. All 129 samples of meat from Madrid also contained PCBs and a high percentage also had residues of *p,p'*-DDE and one or more isomers of HCH. Residues of α- and β-HCH exceeded regulatory limits in 2.7–5.4% of lamb and in 3.3–10% of chicken samples.

Fish are another prominent source of dietary organochlorine pesticides, PCBs, and dioxins among some human populations. Fillets of 11 species of commercial fish from the Great Lakes were analyzed for residues of 39 PCB congeners and 24 other organochlorine compounds (*245*). Highest PCB and organochlorine concentrations were found in eel (753 and 607 ppb wet weight, respectively) and trout (633 and 1404 ppb, respectively). Toxaphene was the most abundant pesticide in trout and p,p'-DDE was the major component in eels. Perch and carp contained the lowest residue levels. Average concentrations of these contaminants in fish from most sites were below international guideline levels but some individual fish and fish caught near known point sources of pollution exceeded these limits. In addition, analyses indicated that total organochlorine concentrations in these fish were 5–72 times higher than the sum of the total PCBs and organochlorine pesticides measured (246). This unknown chlorinated material migrates with the high-molecular-weight lipid fraction in gel permeation chromatography but has, so far, not been identified.

Assays of 431 Lake Michigan trout and salmon caught by sport fishermen in 1985 and of 86 of the same species from 1990 revealed that the predominant organochlorine compounds were PCBs in both years (247). Other contaminants, in order of importance, were DDT and its metabolites, chlordane and its metabolites, and dieldrin. Highest concentrations of all these compounds were detected in lake trout (2.44, 1.83, 0.32, and 0.13 µg/g, respectively) in 1990. Concentrations of these contaminants in chinook salmon (the next most contaminated fish) in 1990 were 1.05, 0.48, 0.14, and 0.08 µg/g, respectively. At the mean sizes taken by anglers, some fish species, particularly rainbow trout and coho salmon, have much lower concentrations of organochlorine contaminants. Therefore, stocking lakes with these species may aid in reducing the exposure of sport fishermen to these contaminants.

Analyses of cod caught in the Northwest Atlantic revealed that levels of PCBs and other organochlorine contaminants were highest in liver tissue and were generally near or below the limit of detection (2 ng/g) in muscle tissue (248). One exception was hexachlorobenzene (HCB), which was detected at very low levels in all muscle tissue samples. Mean liver concentrations of different organochlorines ranged from <10 ng/g for β- and γ-HCH, mirex, heptachlor epoxide, and endrin to >70 ng/g for Aroclors 1254 and 1260 and p,p'-DDE. Liver tissue from cod caught off the Scottish coast varied in DDE concentrations (68.5–266.7 ng/g) and in PCB levels (73.1–633.4 ng/g for one congener) according to the location where they were caught (249). Analyses of muscle tissue of herring caught in the same locations revealed contaminant levels that were about 20-fold lower. The Scottish fish were caught close to shore and were therefore exposed to higher concentrations of pollutants.

Highest concentrations of toxic PCB and PCDD/F congeners (expressed as toxic equivalents, TEQ) in

freshwater and marine Dutch fish were found in cod liver, with 504 ng TEQ/kg in samples from 1991 (250). Liver from pike and perch was contaminated with 79 ng TEQ/kg but muscle tissue from the various fish had much lower levels.

Wild eels from some German rivers and lakes are highly contaminated with PCBs and organochlorine pesticides and therefore >99% of the eels sold in Germany are imported. In a survey of 54 imported eel samples, mean levels of different organochlorine contaminants were only 1–5% of the German regulatory limits and no samples exceeded these limits (251). Wild eels (as compared to farmed eels) had somewhat higher residue levels but these were well within the limits.

Pike, perch, and lake bream caught in a Finnish river near the effluent from a pulp mill and downstream from the mill were analyzed for chlorinated contaminants (252). A variety of chlorinated compounds were detected. Most fish contained 2,3,7,8-TCDF (<2–12 pg/g fresh weight) as the primary PCDD/F congener as well as traces of hexachlorinated naphthalenes and detectable levels of polychlorinated diphenyl ethers. Two coplanar PCBs were detected, with PCB 77 present in the greatest concentrations (8–73 pg/g).

METHODS FOR DETECTION. As with many organic contaminants, separation of polyhalogenated aromatic hydrocarbons from food matrices presents a major challenge to accurate determination of residues. Norén and Sjövall (253) reviewed data on the use of Lipidex (a lipophilic gel) to analyze samples of human milk, cod liver oil, bile, urine, and water for organochlorine contaminants. Structures, properties, and mechanisms of action of these gels were described along with filtration and batch extraction procedures for use with different foods and biological matrices. Schenk et al. (254) developed a rapid, multiresidue solid-phase extraction technique to be used in conjunction with gas chromatography for determination of organochlorine pesticides and polychlorinated biphenyls (PCBs) in nonfatty fish, crabmeat, shrimp, and scallops. This extraction procedure reduced organic solvent consumption by 95% and hazardous waste by 85% compared to the AOAC method, and 10 food samples could be processed through extraction and cleanup in <2 hours. Another extraction technique, solid-phase microextraction with poly(dimethylsiloxane)-coated silica fibers suspended and equilibrated in the headspace, has been applied by Page and Lacroix (255) to the analyses of foods for volatile halogenated contaminants. This procedure responds well to less volatile analytes and thereby can complement headspace GC with gas sampling. However, increasing lipid materials in the foods decreased headspace extraction.

An inexpensive, efficient, and reliable method utilizing a column containing activated carbon and Celite 545 has been adapted for use by Kočan et al. (*256*) for the separation of different PCBs and PCDD/Fs from biological samples such as human adipose tissue, butter, eggs, and fish. This method may be used with both mass spectrometric and electron-capture detection.

An automated HPLC system consisting of an amino column and a porous graphitic column, which can be eluted in both directions individually and in combination, has been developed by Zebühr et al. (*257*) for the separation of PCBs, PCDD/Fs, and polycyclic aromatic hydrocarbons (PAHs) from complex standard mixtures and from biological samples such as fish. The method separates the contaminants into 5 structurally related groups which are then ready for injection into GC/MS apparatus.

Rahman et al. (*258*) developed a procedure for the determination of a variety of PCBs and organochlorine pesticides using two parallel capillary GC columns of different polarity. Of a number of commercially available columns tested, two, which afforded the highest number of separated compounds, were chosen and found to be very stable and to provide reproducible results in analyses of fish.

Non-*ortho* coplanar PCBs have been effectively detected in milk at low ppt levels by use of the Carbosphere activated carbon methodology which was developed for analysis of toxic PCDD/F congeners (*259*). Samples of milk from women in the Netherlands were found to contain an average planar PCB level of 9.2 pg TEQ/g fat. Milk from cows grazing near municipal incinerators and a metal reclamation plant contained 1.1–6.1 pg TEQ of planar PCBs/g fat and 1.3–12.9 pg TEQ of PCDD/Fs/g.

## Polychlorinated Biphenyls (PCBs)

TOXICOLOGICAL STUDIES. Data from major studies and monitoring programs on temporal trends of PCB levels in the environment were summarized and reviewed by Fensterheim (*260*). Adequate data were available to discuss changes in PCB concentrations in foods for human consumption, in adipose tissue and serum samples from humans, and in various fish and shellfish species. Dramatic declines have occurred in contaminant levels in many environmental compartments since regulations were instituted for control of PCBs in the USA 15 years ago. The FDA's Total Diet Study reported that PCB intake in 1971 was 6.9 μg/day and had declined to 0.05 μg/day for the years 1987–1990. In 1972, 62% of

adipose tissue samples tested by the EPA contained >1 ppm PCBs; by 1984, this percentage had decreased to 2%. Studies by the National Oceanic and Atmospheric Administration and other groups documented 2- to 10-fold declines in the levels of PCBs in fish and shellfish from the early 1970s to the late 1980s. These decreases in contaminants are expected to continue but probably at a lower rate because the more highly chlorinated congeners will take longer to degrade.

Ahlborg et al. (*261*) reported on a 1993 consultation meeting sponsored by the WHO-European Centre for Environment and Health and the International Programme on Chemical Safety. A project has been initiated to create a database containing information relevant to setting Toxic Equivalency Factors (TEFs) for PCDD/Fs and dioxin-like PCBs. Available data on the relative toxicities of these PCBs were collected, evaluated, and discussed to derive TEFs for dioxin-like PCBs. The Consultation recommended TEFs for 3 non-*ortho* coplanar PCBs of 0.0005 (congener 77), 0.1 (congener 126), and 0.01 (congener 169). For 8 mono-*ortho*-substituted PCBs, TEFs ranged from 0.00001 to 0.0005 and for 2 di-*ortho* substituted PCBs, TEFs were 0.0001 and 0.00001. For some congeners, these TEF values are similar to toxic equivalents (TEQs) previously proposed by Safe. But for 3 of the congeners, the TEFs differ by an order of magnitude or more. It was recommended that this evaluation process be extended to include PCDDs, PCDFs, and other dioxin-like halogenated pollutants.

Environmental and health impacts of PCBs were reviewed by Safe (*262,263*). Some congeners elicit a variety of toxic responses in humans and laboratory animals and many of these effects, like the toxic effects of 2,3,7,8-tetrachlorodibenzo-*p*-dioxin (TCDD), are mediated through the aryl hydrocarbon (Ah) receptor. Structure–activity investigations have identified two major classes of congeners which elicit TCDD-like responses—the coplanar PCBs and their mono-*ortho* coplanar derivatives. Short-term effects of PCBs in occupationally exposed people appear to be reversible and no consistent carcinogenic effects have been reported. Research on reproductive and developmental effects of PCBs continues in studies with laboratory animals and with exposed populations of humans.

Analysis of human tissues for PCB residues, as it has evolved over the years in response to poisoning incidents and as part of large surveys, was reviewed by Schecter et al. (*264*). Among the episodes discussed were the 1968 Yusho rice oil poisoning in Japan, a 1987 transformer incident in Guam, a 1981 transformer fire in New York, and a 1984 capacitor explosion in the USA.

The large surveys measured PCBs and some other organochlorine residues in mothers' milk from various geographic regions and in blood samples from veterans of the Vietnam War. Several analytical approaches have been used in these studies because, as yet, there is no consensus as to how to best analyze blood for PCBs. Not many laboratories are equipped or experienced enough to analyze tissue samples for these contaminants and testing can be very expensive. Therefore, substantial work remains before PCB analyses in human tissues becomes routine.

Recent surveys in Spain (*265*), Canada (*266*), and Germany (*267*) documented PCB levels in breast milk samples. A total of 408 Spanish milk samples were analyzed. Mothers living in cereal-producing provinces had the lowest levels (0.59–0.68 ppm on a fat basis) and those living in coastal fishing areas had the highest levels of total PCBs (1.28 ppm). Analyses of 109 milk samples from Inuit women in Arctic Quebec for 8 non-*ortho*, mono-*ortho*, and di-*ortho* coplanar PCB congeners revealed that, on the average, they had approximately 863 ppb of these congeners, with a TEQ value of 108.2 ppt. In contrast, milk from women in southern Quebec contained an average of approximately 107 ppb of these congeners, with a TEQ of 29.3. Coplanar PCB levels in plasma of 10 highly exposed Canadian fishermen were determined to be 900 ppt while plasma TEQ levels in controls were only 36 ppt. Comparison of milk samples obtained in an area of Germany in 1984–1985 with others from the same area tested in 1990–1991 revealed that concentrations of some low-chlorinated congeners (28, 49, and 52) increased during this time while concentrations of some more highly chlorinated congeners (138 and 153) decreased significantly.

PCB residues in serum of 23 residents of New Bedford, Massachusetts, were compared with PCB concentrations found in locally caught bluefish and lobster (*268*). The serum samples used in this study were selected from a larger, previously analyzed group because they contained high PCB levels and could therefore be more easily analyzed for specific congeners. Total PCB concentrations in serum ranged from 23 to 214 ppb and in the fish and in lobster were about 424–1328 ppb (wet weight) and 3725 ppb, respectively. The pattern of PCB congeners detected in human serum was found to be more closely related to that observed in the lobster than that in the bluefish. The residents appeared to have been exposed to PCBs from the seafood they ate and also occupationally since many of them had worked in a capacitor plant.

During 1978–1979, more than 2000 people in Taiwan were exposed to high levels of PCBs contaminat-

ing their cooking oil. The resulting health effects were called Yu-Cheng (oil disease). Followup studies continue of the persons originally exposed to the contaminated oil and of the children born to exposed women. An examination of 55 such Yu-Cheng children (aged 6–12 years) and a matched group of 55 controls in 1991 revealed that the Yu-Cheng children were smaller and had less total lean mass and soft tissue than controls (*269*). Other parameters measured, including serum parathyroid hormone, vitamin D, calcium, and alkaline phosphatase levels and joint laxity were similar in exposed children and controls.

In another study, 27 Yu-Cheng children and 27 controls were given a battery of neurophysiological and neuropsychological tests at 7–12 years of age (*270*). Compared to controls, the Yu-Cheng children had lower scores on the full scale IQ tests of the WISC-R and had longer latency and reduced amplitude scores on tests of auditory event–related potentials (P300). No significant differences were noted between the groups in results on tests of somatosensory evoked potentials and pattern visual evoked potentials. It appeared that prenatal exposure to PCBs affected high cortical function rather than the sensory pathway in the developing brain.

Behavioral activity and measurements were made for 115 Yu-Cheng children and their controls during 6 years of followup. Yu-Cheng children had mean activity scores 5–44% higher than their controls and behavior scores on the Rutter scale 7–43% higher than controls (*271*). It appeared that in utero exposure to heat-degraded PCBs caused mildly disordered behavior and increased activity levels in children and these effects persisted for several years.

Another mass exposure to PCBs in cooking oil occurred in Japan in 1968, the Yusho incident. In a 1988 followup of 259 Yusho patients, blood PCB levels were determined to average 3.84 ppb and serum triglyceride levels were 114.3 mg/dL (*272*). A weak but statistically significant correlation was noted between these two variables when the data were analyzed by multiple regression analysis. Triglyceride levels for those in the 4th quartile of serum PCB concentration (>6.1 ppb) averaged 127.65 mg/dL compared to those in the 1st quartile (<2.7 ppb) with an average of 98.36 mg/dL.

During a 2-year study, a group of 80 female monkeys (*Macaca mulatta*) consuming daily doses of 0, 5, 20, 40, or 80 μg Aroclor 1254/kg body weight were monitored for effects on health (*273,274*). Some statistically significant, dose-related treatment effects were noted including inflammation and/or prominence of the tarsal glands, eye exudate, and various finger- and toenail changes. Among clinical and analytical laboratory findings, treated monkeys exhibited decreases in erythrocyte and reticulocyte counts, hematocrit, mean platelet volume, serum cholesterol, and antibody production to sheep red blood cells and also alterations in the percentage of T-helper and T-suppressor cells. Many of the effects observed in these studies occurred at doses lower than those previously reported for nonhuman primates. Analytical and quality control procedures for the determination of PCB levels in tissues of these monkeys were described (275). PCB concentrations in fat, blood, and milk rose with increasing dosage. Elevated PCB levels in infants exposed in utero and through their mothers' milk decreased after weaning (to uncontaminated foods). But it was approximately 100 weeks after weaning before PCB concentrations in their adipose tissue reached background levels similar to controls.

Effects of a 20-week exposure to 3.2 mg Aroclor 1016 or Aroclor 1260/kg/day, followed by a withdrawal period of 24 or 44 weeks, on regional brain concentrations of biogenic amines were investigated in the pig-tailed macaque (*Macaca nemestrina*) (276). During the 24- and 44-week withdrawal periods, brain concentrations of PCBs declined about 60–66% for the Aroclor 1016-treated monkeys and about 75% for the Aroclor 1260-treated monkeys from the levels measured immediately after the exposure period. However, in spite of decreasing PCB concentrations in the brain, the significant decrease in brain dopamine levels, observed in monkeys sacrificed immediately after the dosing period, did not change during the withdrawal periods. Therefore, this subchronic exposure to PCBs resulted in persistent changes in brain dopamine levels.

Subchronic toxicity of the non-*ortho* coplanar PCB 126 was investigated in a 13-week study with rats (277). Rats were fed diets containing 0.1, 1.0, 10, or 100 ppb congener 126 and were monitored for general health effects during this time. No adverse effects were observed in rats fed the lowest dose but at the 1 ppb level, mild histopathological changes were observed in the thymus, thyroid, bone marrow, and liver. A multitude of other toxic effects were noted in rats fed 10 and 100 ppb, including decreased growth, biochemical and hematological changes, and histopathological abnormalities.

Immunosuppressive effects of 3 nona-chlorinated and 1 deca-chlorinated biphenyls and diphenyl ethers were studied in two strains of mice (278). The biphenyls suppressed the splenic plaque-forming cell response to sheep red blood cells but demonstrated only a minimal induction of hepatic microsomal ethoxyresorufin *O*-deethylase (EROD) activity (an Ah-receptor mediated activity). Therefore, it appears that this immunosuppressive action is unrelated to Ah induction. Some of the highly chlorinated diphenyl ethers inhibited the antigenic response to trinitrophenyl-lipopolysaccharide and some, at high concentrations, suppressed the splenic plaque-forming cell response.

Kafafi et al. (279,280) described a new thermodynamic model for calculating dissociation constants of complexes formed between PCBs and Ah receptors. Binding of PCBs (and also of PCDD/Fs) to these receptors depends on the physicochemical properties (lipophilicity, electron affinity, entropy, and electronic energy gap) of the individual congeners. This model can qualitatively explain and quantify the Ah receptor and aryl hydrocarbon hydroxylase (AHH)- and EROD-inducing activities of all 209 PCBs and PCDD/Fs. These activities also correlate well with TEQ factors and in vivo toxic effects of these congeners.

Some congeners are known to bioaccumulate while others are more readily metabolized or degraded. In an investigation of the properties of these different congeners, Borlakoglu and Wilkins (281) found a significant correlation between the extent of halosubstitution in PCB congeners and their rate of hydroxylation by hepatic microsomes. Poly-*ortho* substitutions had no relationship to rate of metabolism but PCBs with adjacent unsubstituted carbons (*meta-para* positions) were more easily metabolized by cytochrome P450 enzymes. These structural features of the molecules help to explain why some are more persistent than others.

Mechanisms by which PCBs may interfere with endocrine functions were discussed by McKinney and Waller (282). Some simple molecular recognition models were offered which explain how different structural features of PCBs allow them to mimic natural hormones, such as thyroid hormone and some steroid hormones. The non-*ortho*-substituted congeners may be able to interact more readily with receptors while *ortho*-substituted molecules have less dioxin-like activity and therefore may be less toxic or have different mechanisms of toxicity.

**OCCURRENCE IN FOODS.** Concentrations one mono-*ortho* (congener 105) and of 3 non-*ortho* coplanar (congeners 77, 126, and 169) PCBs were determined in retail samples of fish, beef, pork, poultry, eggs, and fish liver oil in Finland (283). The predominant congener in all samples was 105, ranging from a low average concentration of 22 pg/g fresh weight in beef to a high of 30,000 pg/g in fish liver oil. Of the non-*ortho* coplanar congeners, highest levels were found for congener 77 (3.2–100 pg/g). However, because of differences in relative toxicity of these congeners, congener 105 was the major contributor to TEQ only in Baltic herring and salmon while congener 77 was the major contributor in other fish. For the rest of the food samples, congener 126 was mainly responsible for toxicity. Total TEQ ranged from 0.27 pg/g for poultry, through 19 pg/g for salmon, to 126 pg/g for fish liver oil. It was estimated that, on the average, Finns would consume 170 pg TEQ/day, with about 70% of the total coming from fish, 25% from meat, and 5% from eggs.

Analyses of 5 samples of Baltic cod liver oil collected between 1971 and 1989 were analyzed for total PCBs and for the presence of 15 PCB congeners (*284*). During this time period, total PCB levels were fairly constant (6.7–9.5 μg/g) except for 1980, when there was a peak of 17 μg/g. Relative amounts of the different congeners were similar but not identical from year to year. In 1989, the non-*ortho* coplanar congeners constituted 0.3% of the total amount of all the congeners determined but accounted for 16.4% of the TEQ. In the same year, mono-*ortho* PCBs constituted 44% of the measured PCB congeners and accounted for 81% of the TEQ. A dose of 5 or 15 g of cod liver oil would supply an average of 6.6 or 20 ng TEQ and 49 or 150 μg total PCBs.

Trout from remote mountain lakes in Spain were found to have much lower mean concentrations of 28 PCB congeners (4.87 ng/g) than mullet collected from the Mediterranean coast (38.4 ng/g) (*285*). Relative proportions of tri- to pentachlorobiphenyls were higher in the trout while the hexachlorobiphenyl congeners predominated in the mullet. These data reflect the fact that the primary source of contaminants for the trout is atmospheric deposition while the mullet live near point source inputs of these contaminants.

Winter flounder who live off the southern New England coast spend the summer as one mixed population but in the winter they return to one of 3 discrete spawning grounds to reproduce. These spawning areas have different degrees and sources of PCB contamination and this was found to be reflected in PCB concentrations detected in the different populations of flounder (*286*). Liver samples from fish caught in the New Bedford area had 85–100-fold higher levels of total PCBs than fish from the two Rhode Island locations and both liver and flesh from those fish had PCB concentrations exceeding tolerance limits. The non-*ortho* congeners contributed more to the TEQ of these fish than other congeners.

Crabs collected at several sites in a fjord area of southern Norway, which has been contaminated with organochlorine compounds from a magnesium production plant, were found to contain 0.6–2.05 μg of 12 PCB congeners/g fat in the hepatopancreas (*287*). These PCB concentrations have declined about 30% between 1990 and 1992. Non-*ortho* coplanar congeners accounted for 2–7% of the total PCBs, with congener 126 contributing most to the toxic potential. Consumption of crabs from this area would probably add enough TEQ to the diet to exceed acceptable weekly intakes.

Recent data on PCB concentrations in blood plasma and muscle tissue of cattle suspected of being contaminated with PCBs revealed a good correlation between the two measurements (*288*). When plasma levels of PCB congeners 138, 153, and 180 exceed 1.03, 1.36, and 1.12 μg/kg, respectively, then muscle tissue PCB concentrations will most likely exceed established maximum residue limits. This information can be used to monitor cattle in farms suspected of being contaminated.

Questions have been raised about the potential health risks of using PCB-contaminated sewage sludge to fertilize farm fields. Will crop plants take up PCBs from soil and thereby become unsafe to eat? During a 5-year period, the Madison [Wisconsin] Metropolitan Sewerage District has conducted field experiments, including analyses of >1400 soil and crop tissue samples, to determine the fate of PCBs in sludge applied as fertilizer (*289*). Eight different sludge treatments (using different concentrations and loading rates) were tested and concentrations of 79 PCB congeners were monitored in surface soil, corn stover, and corn grain. Most of the 2-, 3-, 4- and 5-chlorinated PCB congeners (about 85% of the total PCBs in sludge) disappeared from the soil with half-lives of 4–58 months while more highly chlorinated congeners persisted longer. No evidence was observed for translocation of any PCB congeners from the soil into grain or stover of the corn plants.

METHODS FOR DETECTION. An interlaboratory study involving 17 laboratories in Sweden examined the accuracy of current methods for the analysis of coplanar and mono-*ortho*-chlorinated biphenyls (*290*). Laboratories were provided with herring oil samples spiked with high or low levels of 3 coplanar PCBs (congeners 77, 126, and 169) and two mono-*ortho* PCBs (congeners 105 and 118). For extraction, most laboratories used column chromatography or gel permeation chromatography in combination with some type of carbon column fractionation or HPLC fractionation. Quantitation was achieved with GC with electron capture detection (mono-*ortho* PCBs) and GC/MS (coplanar PCBs). Results from different laboratories varied somewhat, with some laboratories consistently reporting values which were too high or too low while others obtained results very close to the calculated values.

Several detection techniques have been evaluated for determination of PCBs in fatty tissues (*291*). GC conditions were optimized to separate interfering contaminants such as phthalates and/or chlorinated pesticides from PCBs. Advantages and drawbacks of GC with an electron capture detector, GC/MS, and GC with an atomic emission detector were discussed and various approaches for calculating PCB concentrations were compared.

Supercritical fluid extraction (SFE) has been used in different procedures for PCB analyses. Johansen et al. (*292*) described on-line coupled SFE and GC for the determination of PCBs and other organochlorine contaminants in human milk and blood serum. A combination of SFE with supercritical fluid chromatography was used by Mills and Jeffries (*293*) to rapidly extract and isolate PCBs from milk.

Since non-*ortho* coplanar PCBs are considered to be the most toxic congeners, methods have been devised to selectively isolate and detect these congeners. Ford et al. (*294*) utilized a semi-automated carbon/glass fiber column with a programmable pumping and valving system for the separation of coplanar PCBs which were then quantitated by GC/MS. Use of this technique for analyses of fats from narwhal, beluga, and ringed seal revealed the presence of these congeners in all species at ppt levels. Stalling et al. (*295*) used polystyrene divinylbenzene beads covalently bonded to $C_{60}$ and $C_{70}$ fullerenes as an electron donor–acceptor adsorbent to fractionate and enrich coplanar PCBs from other PCB congeners. Following this enrichment step, specific PCB isomers can be quantitated by GC/MS.

Improvements in GC methods for determination of PCB congeners have been described. Galceran et al. (*296*) found that DB-17 columns used in combination with a DB-5 or a CP-Sil8CB column allowed separation and identification of some related PCB isomers: 118–149, 138–163, and 153–105–132. This method was used in the analysis of spiked samples of powdered milk and performed well when used by several different laboratories. König et al. (*297*) utilized selectively *o*-substituted cyclodextrins as chiral stationary phases for the separation of some tetra-, penta-, and hexachlorobiphenyls with 3 chlorine substituents in the 4 *ortho* positions by enantioselective gas chromatography.

A new method based on enhanced photoactivated luminescence (EPL) was developed by Vo-Dinh et al. (*298*) for the rapid detection of PCBs. This method combines photoactivation by UV irradiation, excitation of the photoproduct complex, and fluorescence detection of the product. EPL can be used as a spot test under field conditions and can detect PCBs in the ppb range.

## Polychlorinated Dibenzo-*p*-dioxins (PCDDs) and Polychlorinated Dibenzofurans (PCDFs)

RISK ASSESSMENT AND TOXICOLOGICAL STUDIES. Published data on the toxicity and mechanisms of action of PCDDs and PCDFs have been reviewed by Heuvel and Lucier (*299*). Sources and environmental fate of these compounds were detailed and results of toxicity and carcinogenicity assays in laboratory animals were summarized. The importance of the Ah (arylhydrocarbon) receptor in mediating the physiological effects of these organochlorines and procedures for calculating toxic equivalency factors were described. Finally, the questions surrounding the appropriateness of extrapolating from animal data to assess human health risks and the use of dose–response relationships was discussed.

Interim results from a major reassessment of the human health risks resulting from exposure to dioxin, which was initiated by EPA, were reported by Birnbaum (*300*). Recently reported studies have presented much new information on the sensitivity of various toxic endpoints, the shapes of dose–response curves, and the relative potencies of dioxin-like PCBs. It appears that not all Ah-mediated responses are non-linear and that the shapes of dose–response curves for different effects are not the same. This implies the existence of multiple mechanisms of action following ligand-binding to Ah receptors. The toxicity of dioxin-like PCBs appears to be less than that previously reported. Further investigations are in progress, which should shed more light on the risks to humans of exposure to PCDD/Fs.

Feeley and Grant (*301*) described the approach to risk assessment of PCDD/Fs in Canada. Since these compounds are nongenotoxic, it can be assumed that a toxicity threshold exists. Therefore, based on a no observed adverse effect level of 1 ng/kg body weight/day (obtained from a complete database review of animal studies), incorporation of a 100-fold safety factor to compensate for inter- and intraspecies variability, and calculation of TEQ factors for 17 PCDD/F congeners found in foods, an average lifetime tolerable intake of 600 pg TEQ/day was estimated for a 60-kg person. The current estimated average Canadian intake of PCDD/Fs is 2.0–4.2 pg TEQ/kg/day, well within the suggested tolerable intake.

Tysklind et al. (*302*) constructed a toxic equivalency scale for 20 PCDFs based on the induction of EROD activity in rat hepatoma cells. $ED_{50}$ values for EROD induction potency varied over nearly 7 orders of magnitude. Relative toxicities of the individual compounds were calibrated against the assay results for

2,3,7,8-tetrachlorodibenzo-*p*-dioxin (TCDD) to generate toxic equivalency factors. A total of 87 PCDFs were characterized using 37 physicochemical parameters, and an analysis of quantitative structure–activity relationships was performed. Predictions from this model indicate that a large number of PCDF congeners will be potent EROD inducers.

Toxicity equivalents (TEQs) of individual PCDD/Fs in a food are an expression of the toxicity of an equivalent amount of TCDD, the reference compound. Although this concept is quite useful in estimating the toxic potential of a contaminated food, McLachlan (*303*) points out that these compounds are only toxic if they actually reach their target tissue. In other words, even though a particular compound may be very toxic to liver cells in culture, if it is poorly absorbed from the gut, its real toxic potential to an animal ingesting it may be quite low. A better expression of toxicity, exposure toxicity equivalents (ETE), has been proposed to account for this factor of bioavailability: congener-specific transfer rates would be calculated for different steps in the transfer pathway (feed→milk; milk→human) and these would be incorporated into an equation to yield an ETE factor. More research is necessary to determine approximate transfer rates for different processes.

Two studies on a total of 4 nursing infants indicated that their absorption of PCDD/Fs and PCBs from their mothers' milk was >90% (*304,305*). Concentrations of these compounds were measured in samples of breast milk and in the feces of the infants and the amount absorbed was calculated by subtracting output from input. Analyses of individual congeners indicated that all were easily absorbed.

Available data on the toxicokinetics and metabolism of PCDDs and PCDFs were reviewed by Van den Berg et al. (*306*). Absorption, body distribution, and metabolism of these compounds vary greatly among different species and therefore caution must be exercised in extrapolating results from laboratory animals to humans. In humans, most of the body burden of PCDD/Fs is concentrated in adipose tissue (unlike that of most laboratory animals) and elimination of these compounds is dramatically slower than in any other mammalian species studied. Compounds with chlorine substitutions at the 2,3,7, and 8 positions have the greatest biological activity and toxicity. In addition, complex mixtures containing a variety of PCDD/F congeners, as well as PCBs and organochlorine pesticides, may be present in foods, and the interactions among these compounds will affect the toxic potential of the mixture.

Role of the Ah receptor in mediating the biological effects, toxicity, and carcinogenicity of PCDD/Fs has been reviewed by Okey et al. (*307*) and by Nebert et al. (*308*). Most, if not all, toxic effects of these compounds involve interactions with the Ah receptor but the exact mechanism by which this causes toxicity is unknown. The Ah receptor is known to enhance transcription of genes encoding cytochrome P450 enzymes in the CYP1A subfamily and may also mediate expression of other genes regulating cell growth and differentiation. Recently genes for two subunits, the DNA-binding and ligand-binding moieties, of the Ah receptor have been cloned and experiments with these should aid in elucidating specific mechanisms and pathways leading to toxic effects. Three types of DNA response elements which control genes in the Ah gene battery were also described.

In 1976, an accidental explosion in Seveso, Italy, exposed thousands of people to TCDD. Results of monitoring for cancer incidence among persons in three zones of decreasing TCDD contamination during the years 1977–1986 have been published (*309*). For the most highly exposed population, 14 cancer cases were identified in 4568 person-years of follow-up. Among the moderately exposed (zone B) and least-exposed populations (zone R), 112 (in 31,384 person-years) and 765 (in 209,941 person-years) total malignancies, respectively, were diagnosed. Among those in zone B who had lived in the area for >5 years, increased incidences were observed for hepatobiliary cancer (relative risk = 2.8) for all subjects, for multiple myeloma (RR = 5.3) and myeloid leukemia (RR = 3.7) in women, and for lympho-reticulosarcoma in men (RR = 5.7). In zone R, the incidences of soft-tissue tumors, and non-Hodgkin's lymphoma were increased. These populations will be monitored for further evidence on cancer incidence related to dioxin exposure.

Three rare conditions, angiosarcoma, porphyria cutanea tarda, and skin lesions characteristic of chloracne, occurred in a worker who had been exposed to waste oil contaminated with TCDD (*310*). The man was employed at a truck terminal when it was sprayed with waste oil to control dust; he had extensive dermal exposure to the oil and undoubtedly inhaled contaminated dust. This case supports the etiological connection between exposure to TCDD and subsequent development of soft-tissue sarcoma and porphyria cutanea tarda.

A review of data on concentrations of PCDD/Fs in human tissues from general population surveys in many geographical locations (Vietnam, former USSR, Cambodia, Thailand, Germany, USA, South Africa, Japan, China) was presented by Schecter et al. (*311*). In some cases the data have been converted to TEQs and in others, the percentage contribution of particular congeners has been calculated. Generally, between fourteen and sixteen 2,3,7,8-chlorine-substituted congeners can be detected in human tissues. In some less industrialized areas low levels of total PCDD/Fs are the norm (100–160 ppt on a lipid basis in blood or adipose tissue) while higher levels are noted in industrialized areas (886 and 1591 ppt in Germany and the USA). However, results from other areas were unexpectedly high (1890 ppt in Guam) or low (161 ppt in St. Petersburg, Russia).

Other general population surveys reported the following levels of contaminants in human tissues: an average TCDD concentration of 5.38 ppt in adipose tissue samples obtained from 865 cadavers in the coterminous 48 states of the USA (*312*); average TCDD and TEQ levels of 4.0 and 15.6 ppt in 100 breast milk samples collected from all the provinces in Canada (*313*); and an average of 3.28 ppt TCDD and of 1811.7 ppt of total PCDD/Fs in 17 samples of adipose tissue from Spain (*314*).

Other recent studies have compared residue levels of PCDD/Fs in human tissues with dietary exposure to these compounds. From surveys done in Germany, it was estimated that average intakes of TCDD and of total TEQs were approximately 25 and 164 pg/person/day (*315*). As a percentage of total TEQs consumed, fish and fish products, milk and milk products, and meat and meat products contributed 37%, 33.6%, and 22%, respectively. A strong, positive correlation was observed between TCDD levels in breast milk of 41 women in the Netherlands and the consumption of animal but not vegetable fats and proteins (*316*).

Concentrations of chlorinated and brominated dioxins and dibenzofurans in tissues of persons after known occupational or accidental exposures to these compounds were summarized and discussed by Schecter et al. (*317*). Data were presented for each of the following populations: workers in the USA exposed to a PCB transformer fire, German chemical workers exposed to dioxin while cleaning up after an explosion, workers at a municipal incinerator in New York, a chemist exposed to brominated and chlorinated dioxins, U.S. veterans and Vietnamese civilians exposed to Agent Orange, and Japanese Yusho victims who consumed contaminated rice oil. Longitudinal data from the same population demonstrated that some PCDF congeners are eliminated from humans more rapidly than TCDD. In fact, elevated levels of TCDD were observed in some German workers up to 36 years after exposure, indicating that some congeners are remarkably persistent (*318*).

At relatively high doses, TCDD causes immunotoxic effects in rodents along with other signs of general toxicity. However, in experiments reviewed by Neubert

et al. (*319*) lower TCDD doses, more relevant to human exposures, were found to exert immunotoxic effects in rats and marmosets (*Callithrix jacchus*). Following low doses of TCDD, decreases were observed in helper-inducer T cells and in the numbers and percentages of certain B cell types. Lymphocytes from a group of workers moderately exposed to PCDD/Fs during decontamination work in a chemical plant in Germany were examined by flow cytometry and monoclonal antibodies raised against several cell surface receptors to see whether any similar changes in lymphocytes occurred in humans (*320*). Only slight effects were observed in some of the 14 receptor combinations tested and none appeared to be of medical relevance. Lymphocytes from adult humans appear to be less sensitive than those of marmosets to the effects of TCDD.

Lymphocyte cultures from healthy volunteers were treated in vitro with $10^{-7}$–$10^{-14}$ M TCDD in the presence or absence of stimulation by pokeweed mitogen (*321*). All stimulated lymphocyte cultures showed dose-dependent significant increases of cytochrome P450 (CYP1A1) enzyme activity at concentrations of $10^{-7}$–$10^{-9}$ M TCDD but not at lower concentrations of TCDD. However, there was no effect on lymphocyte surface marker distributions nor any suppression of lymphocyte proliferation in mitogen-stimulated cells at any TCDD concentration. These data indicate that induction of CYP1A1 activity was not correlated with direct immunotoxic effects in human lymphocytes in vitro.

In contrast to results from the previous experiments, TCDD was shown to affect human tonsillar lymphocytes in in vitro experiments (*322*). While high-density human B cells were not affected by TCDD, mitogen-induced proliferation of low-density B cells and antibody secretion were both suppressed by TCDD. Further research is needed to clarify immunotoxic effects of TCDD in humans.

It is well known that TCDD is a potent animal carcinogen but its carcinogenic effects in humans remain controversial. Lucier et al. (*323*) reviewed data from many types of animal studies and discussed aspects of the metabolism of TCDD and its carcinogenic effects which may be relevant to human disease. These investigations included animal bioassays for cancer, studies of possible mechanisms of carcinogenicity, initiation–promotion studies, and biochemical responses to TCDD exposure. Since TCDD does not interact directly with DNA and is not genotoxic, it acts as a promotor of tumor growth. Interaction with the Ah receptor appears to be a necessary early step in this process, and TCDD may act by altering a number of receptor and hormone systems involved in cell growth and differentiation. Animal studies have demonstrated that there are different dose–response curves for different effects of TCDD. This, along with variations in the sensitivity of different species and of different individual animals and humans, makes it difficult to predict human risks from exposure to low background levels of TCDD.

Two recent rodent studies illustrate the difficulties in estimating carcinogenicity of PCDD/F congeners from their biochemical or physiological effects in short-term assays. Schrenk et al. (*324*) compared tumor-promoting effects of 1,2,3,4,6,7,8-heptachlorodibenzo-*p*-dioxin (HpCDD) and of a defined mixture of 49 PCDDs with TCDD toxic equivalents (TE) calculated from data on induction of CYP1A activity in primary cultures of hepatocytes and with international TCDD equivalents (ITE, calculated from both induction and toxicity data). Following induction with *N*-nitrosomorpholine, rats were treated for 13 weeks with HpCDD or the PCDD mixture. Although analysis of the data on promotion was complicated by variability in results among individuals of all groups, it was concluded that at low doses the promoting potency of the two treatments was overestimated by the TEs and ITEs of the PCDDs present in the liver of treated rats. Another series of experiments, with rats induced with diethylnitrosamine and then treated for 30 weeks with TCDD, demonstrated that the dose–response effects of TCDD on cell proliferation of altered hepatic foci (a marker for developing tumors) were different from previously reported dose–response relationships for induction of CYP1A enzyme activity (*325*). Both of these studies demonstrate that different physiological effects of PCDDs may have different dose–response curves even though they may both be mediated by Ah receptors.

Uptake and metabolism of TCDD and 2,3,7,8-TCDF were compared in experiments with rat and human hepatic microsomes and in rat hepatocytes and liver slices (*326*). TCDD pretreatment (≥1 μM) significantly enhanced the hepatic uptake and metabolism of TCDD in in vitro assay systems. TCDF metabolism was also induced by TCDD. However, at lower doses (0.01 and 0.1 μM), metabolism of TCDD was not induced and, therefore, it might be expected that exposure to very low doses of TCDD would result in the persistence of TCDD/F in the body for much longer periods. Quantitatively, metabolism of TCDF in human microsomes was quite low.

A review of data on developmental and reproductive toxicity of dioxins and related compounds in several species was presented by Peterson et al. (*327*). Reported symptoms of developmental toxicity in mammals include prenatal mortality, decreased growth, structural malformations, and functional alterations. At relatively low doses, functional effects are the most sensitive signs of toxicity, with effects on the male reproductive system and behavior noted in rats and neurobehavioral effects observed in monkeys. Human infants exposed during the Yu-Cheng and Yusho episodes developed an ectodermal dysplasia syndrome which was manifested as toxic effects in the skin, teeth, and the central nervous system. The relationship of some of these effects to dioxin interactions with the Ah receptor was discussed.

As noted in studies of the carcinogenic effects of different PCDD/Fs, ITE factors are not always good predictors of complex in vivo physiological processes. In studies of the teratogenic potency of 2,3,4,7,8-penta-CDF and of 3 PCDD/F mixtures in mice, dose–response data were calculated for induction of cleft palate (*328*). However, comparison of these results to calculated ITE values revealed that the ITE factor for the penta-CDF overestimated its teratogenic potency by about 2.5 times. ITE for the mixtures more closely predicted their teratogenicity but the research indicates that the predictability of these ITE factors will depend on the specific composition of congeners in a mixture.

Since animal studies have demonstrated that dioxins influence plasma thyroid hormone levels, effects of PCDD/Fs in breast milk on these hormone levels in 38 healthy breast-fed Dutch infants was investigated (*329*). For comparison, infants were divided into low-exposure (mean of 18.6 ng TEQ/kg milk fat, range of 8.7–28.0 ng/kg) and high-exposure (mean of 37.5 ng/kg, range of 29.2–62.7 ng/kg) groups. Blood samples from the high exposure infants, at 1 and 11 weeks, had significantly higher concentrations of total thyroxine (tT$_4$) and of thyroxine/thyroxine-binding globulin ratios as compared to low-exposure infants. At 11 weeks, mean plasma concentrations of thyrotropin were also significantly higher in the high-exposure infants. It appears that these elevated levels of PCDD/Fs in milk affected the thyroid hormone regulatory system in infants.

OCCURRENCE IN FOODS. In a recent review, Rappe (*330*) discussed the sources, environmental concentration, and human exposure assessment to PCDD/Fs. Primary sources of these compounds are chemical reactions occurring during the synthesis of some pesticides and the chlorinated bleaching of pulp; heating of chlorinated organic and inorganic compounds (as in incinerators); photochemical processes acting on emissions in the atmosphere; and enzymatic reactions which might occur in sewage sludge. Almost all of the PCDD/Fs found to accumulate in biological systems are the 2,3,7,8-substituted tetra-, penta-, and hexachlorinated congeners because other congeners are usually metabolized and excreted fairly rapidly. Background levels of these compounds in biota and in human tissues were briefly summarized. Estimates of dioxin balance in humans indicate that excretion and deposition in tissues exceed intake from food and this discrepancy is not understood.

A mathematical model has been developed to describe the transfer of 17 PCDD/Fs in emissions from a source, such as an incinerator, to cow's milk (*331*). The model considers processes occurring in the atmosphere as well as pharmacokinetics of these compounds in the cow. The values of 3 parameters, bioavailability of dioxins in the cow and wash-off of dry and wet deposition by rain, were unknown but were estimated by calibrating the model to a set of 70 analyzed milk samples originating from cows grazing near municipal waste incinerators.

A German survey of 39 samples of commercial baby food, including powder products based on milk, soya, and grain as well as ready-to-serve meals, was conducted to determine residue levels of PCDD/Fs in these foods (*332*). Babies were estimated to ingest a daily average of 3.05, 0.11, 10.7, and 4.54 pg ITE/kg body weight from milk-based powders, soya-based powders, cereals prepared with whole milk, and ready-to-eat foods, respectively. For comparison, mean daily intake of these contaminants from human milk was estimated to be 161 pg ITE/kg in Germany.

Samples of milk from 160 individual Bavarian farms in rural areas remote from sources of pollution ($n = 17$) and from farms located near waste incinerators or other potential sources of PCDD/F emissions ($n = 143$) were analyzed for these contaminants (*333*). Total TE for the 17 congeners detected ranged from 0.48 to 5.62 pg/g on a fat basis and averaged 1.0 pg/g for milk from the rural farms and 1.85 pg/g for milk from farms near sources of pollution. In concentration, octa-substituted PCDD exceeded all the other congeners but in terms of toxicity, 3 congeners, TCDD, 2,3,4,7,8-penta-CDF, and 1,2,3,7,8-penta-CDD, accounted for nearly 80% of the TE. In some cases, characteristic patterns of congeners were detected on nearby farms, which presumably resulted from some local point source of pollution. Data from another study in Germany indicated that PCDD/F levels in soil (even up to a concentration of 30 pg ITE/g dry matter) had no effect on PCDD/F levels in milk of cows grazing in that area (*334*). Increasing contaminant levels on grass were associated with increasing levels in milk. Moreover, the carryover of specific congeners from grass to milk differed considerably, with TCDD having the highest carryover factor.

Sewage sludge is potentially a very useful fertilizer but it may contain a variety of organic and inorganic residues which could present problems if they are incorporated into the human food chain. Wild et al. (*335*) reviewed information on background levels of 17 PCDD/Fs in soils in the UK and in milk. Implications for the transfer of PCDD/Fs from contaminated sludge to cows by soil ingestion, plant ingestion, and from air and water were calculated for different sludge application rates. It appears that livestock would be primarily exposed to increased PCDD/F levels by ingestion of sludge adhering to vegetation. Therefore, application of sludge by injection rather than by spraying could minimize this exposure.

Residues from chemical manufacturing processes used as landfill material in 1900–1921 in a city in Germany have resulted in high levels of PCDD/F contamination in the soil (up to 14,530 ng ITE/kg dry soil). Fruits from apple and pear trees grown on soil with different levels of contamination were analyzed for PCDD/Fs to estimate uptake from soil (*336*). Even though peels account for <20% of the fresh weight of the fruits, they contained >50% of the ITE. These contaminants were not removed from the peel by washing but could be removed from the fruit by peeling. No correlation was found between soil and fruit concentrations of PCDD/Fs and it appeared that the fruits acquired these contaminants from airborne emissions.

During a 4-year Canadian National Dioxin Sampling Program, fish and shellfish were collected at marine and freshwater sites near 46 pulp and paper mills using the chlorine bleaching process (*337*). Analyses of >1000 samples for 2,3,7,8-substituted PCDD/Fs resulted in recommendations for closure of commercial fisheries at 8 sites and recommendations to limit consumption of fish from 11 other sites. Marine species found with excessive levels of contaminants included oysters, clams, dungeness crabs, prawns and shrimp. Contaminated freshwater species included sucker, whitefish, chub, Dolly Varden char, burbot, walleye, and bullhead. The most prominent congeners detected were TCDD and TCDF and highest levels were invariably in liver of fish and digestive organs and hepatopancreas of crabs and lobsters. The most contaminated fish samples came from the Great Lakes, where whole-body concentrations of TCDD in lipid-rich lake trout were often >100 pg/g and total $T_4CDD$ congeners were >1200 pg/g. Highest concentrations of $T_4CDD$ and $T_4CDF$ detected during the survey were >500 pg/g and >14,500 pg/g, respectively, in crab hepatopancreas. Other studies on fish from rivers in Alberta (*338*) and British Columbia (*339*), Canada, which receive effluents from a bleached-kraft mill revealed that whitefish had PCDD/F residues at least an order of magnitude higher than suckers and some species of predatory fish (*338*). This is apparently due to the fact that whitefish preferably consume filter-feeding insects which accumulate contaminants from the sediment.

Cod caught in the northwest Atlantic off the coast of Labrador have been analyzed to determine concentrations of PCDD/Fs (*340*). Neither muscle nor ovary tissue had detectable concentrations of these contaminants. Total PCDD/F levels in liver ranged from 2.1 to 21.9 ppt, with an average of 7.1 ppt. TCDF was the predominant congener, accounting for about 70% of the total PCDD/Fs.

Soft-shell clams, blue crabs, and American lobsters were collected from the Newark/Raritan Bay estuary and analyzed for PCDD/F congeners (*341,342*). TCDD concentrations in clams, crabs, and lobsters from the most polluted area were 11–20, 71.5, and 34.4 ppt, respectively, while TCDF levels in the same animals from these areas were 3.5–5.0, 67.1, and 40.8 ppt, respectively. TCDD concentrations in clams from the most polluted areas approach the advisory limit of 25 ppt for no consumption. Clams transplanted from the polluted site to a relatively less polluted site eliminated PCDD/Fs to achieve concentrations similar to the native populations in this area (0.1–0.6 ppt) in 4 months. Average contaminant levels in crabs from the polluted site exceeded the "no consumption advisory for crabs" of 50 ppt while average concentrations in lobsters exceeded the "limited consumption" (25 ppt) advisory. The source of the dioxin contamination in this area is believed to be contaminated soil at a former pesticide manufacturing plant along a river feeding into the bay.

Since trace levels of PCDD/Fs have been reported in some cellulose-containing consumer products, six such products (tea bags, milk cartons, writing paper, disposable diapers, and packaging paper for fatty and non-fatty foodstuffs) were analyzed for TCDD (*343*). With a detection limit of 2 ppt for the method used, only the packaging for non-fatty foods (bread bags) contained detectable TCDD (6.8 ppt).

METHODS FOR DETECTION. Analytical methods and sampling procedures for determining concentrations of PCDD/Fs in foods and environmental samples near municipal waste incinerators in the Netherlands were detailed by de Jong et al. (*344*). Strategies for sampling different materials, pretreatment, extraction, and cleanup of samples and protocols for high resolution GC–high resolution MS were described. These methods were capable of accurately measuring ultra-

trace levels of these contaminants in most of the biological samples.

Rapid screening of fish tissues for PCDD/Fs has been accomplished by King et al. (*345*) using a saponification step, followed by extraction into hexane, cleanup using gel permeation chromatography and measurement by capillary GC–low resolution MS with selected ion monitoring. Another method for the determination of PCDD/Fs in fish, developed by Sherry et al. (*346*), used a dichloromethane extraction followed by cleanup by size exclusion chromatography, mini acid/base silica columns and HPLC on basic alumina and activated carbon and quantification by GC with mass selective detection.

Cleanup of samples prior to identification and quantitation of PCDD/Fs continues to present a challenge, particularly for some biological samples. Recent research reports described several alternative methods for clean up: a powdered charcoal–silica gel column (*347*); a pyreneylethylsilica gel column (*348*); and solid-phase extraction with a bonded benzene sulfonic acid cartridge in series with a silica cartridge (*349*).

## Other Polyhalogenated Compounds

A population-based, case–control study was conducted in several Massachusetts towns whose residents had been exposed to tetrachloroethylene (PCE)-contaminated drinking water (from the lining in drinking-water pipes) for up to 10 years (1968–1979) (*350*). A total of 2366 controls and 61 cases of bladder cancer, 35 of kidney cancer, and 34 of leukemia were investigated to determine their exposure to PCE and any other factors which might influence cancer development. A computer model, developed to estimate PCE exposure, assigned a relative cumulative exposure score to each resident based on the geometry, size, age, and water flow through pipes supplying the household and the person's length of residence in that household (*351*). An elevated risk was determined for leukemia (odds ratio of about 2) whether or not latency was considered. For subjects above the 90th percentile of exposure, the odds ratio of developing leukemia was 5.84 and for bladder cancer was 4.03. No increased risk was observed for kidney cancer.

Drinking water contaminated with trichloroethylene (TCE) is also viewed as hazardous. Rodents exposed to high doses of TCE develop cancer but Steinberg and DeSesso (*352*) argue that these studies have been used inappropriately to assess human risks. Malignancy in these rodents appears to arise from repeated cycles of cell necrosis and regeneration caused by very high doses of this chemical. However, human epidemiological studies have not demonstrated a toxic or carcinogenic effect of TCE in workers with a substantial exposure. The authors argue that the current EPA limit of 5 µg/L is about 10-fold too stringent.

Cancer risks to populations exposed to tri- and tetrachloroethylene were investigated by Vartiainen et al. (*353*) in two Finnish villages whose drinking water supplies were contaminated with these compounds. TCE levels in the water measured as high as 212 µg/L. Although analyses of urine samples (24-hour) from 95 residents of one village and from 21 in the other town revealed that they excreted averages of 19 and 7.9 µg TCE/day (compared to averages of 2–4 µg/day in residents of control villages), no increased incidences of total cancer, liver cancer, non-Hodgkin's lymphoma, Hodgkin's disease, multiple myeloma, or leukemia were observed among residents of the two affected villages as compared to cancer data from all of Finland. However, because there may be a long latent period for cancer development, cancer incidence in these populations will be monitored in the future.

Polychlorinated terphenyls (PCTs) have properties and characteristics similar to PCBs and are used industrially for many of the same applications (hydraulic fluids, electrical equipment, sealants, plasticizers, paints, etc.). In a survey to detect PCT levels in shellfish, clams, and mussels from the coast of Spain near the mouth of the Ebro river, samples were analyzed by high-resolution GC with electron capture detection and mass spectrometric detection on the selected ion monitoring mode (*354*). PCT concentrations ranged from 3 to 790 ng/g dry mass while total PCBs in the same shellfish ranged from 128 to 2950 ng/g. The toxicological significance of PCT contamination is not yet understood, but contaminant levels should be monitored.

A total of 34 salmon from 3 water courses in Finland were analyzed for the presence of polychlorinated diphenyl ethers (PCDEs) (*355*). Concentrations of the PCDE congeners ranged from 0.02–2.4 ng/g fresh weight. Analyses of PCDEs present in fly ash and in a wood preservative revealed that many of the congeners found in fish were also present in the preservative. Salmon from some areas contained higher concentrations of PCDEs than others but their potential toxicity is not known at present.

A review of the literature and a health assessment of polybrominated dibenzo-*p*-dioxins (PBDDs) and dibenzofurans (PBDFs) was presented by Mennear and Lee (*356*). These compounds may be produced in trace amounts in the production of brominated flame retardants and may also be produced in incinerators and other places where organic compounds are heated in the pres-

ence of bromine. Biological effects of these compounds are similar to those of PCDD/Fs, including interactions with the Ah receptor and carcinogenic, immunotoxic, and reproductive/developmental effects in laboratory animals. They should be considered potential human toxicants and carcinogens.

# POLYCYCLIC AROMATIC HYDROCARBONS (PAHs)

## Toxicological Investigations

PAHs are a potent class of environmental carcinogens produced by pyrolysis of a variety of organic materials, such as petroleum fuels, tobacco, wood, and some foods. In a recent review, Jernström and Gräslund (*357*) discussed bioactivation of these compounds to form bay-region diol epoxides of benzo[a]pyrene (BP), structures of the DNA adducts formed by these activated compounds, and mutations occurring as a result of these DNA interactions. Studies with mammalian systems clearly show that the predominant result of the formation of BP–DNA adducts is the formation of transversion mutations involving GC base pairs flanked by purines and, in some cases, by AT base pairs. Recent research has provided a great deal of information on the biochemical and molecular events involved in PAH-induced mutagenesis and subsequent carcinogenesis.

Most studies of the toxicological effects of PAHs in humans have involved workers with a high occupational exposure to these compounds, usually in the atmosphere of their factories. Principal methods which have been developed recently to detect exposure to PAHs by examining white blood cell DNA and blood proteins for PAH adducts have been reviewed by dell'Omo and Lauwerys (*358*). These methods include immunoassays, $^{32}$P-postlabeling assays, and synchronous fluorescence spectrophotometry. Applications of these procedures for epidemiological studies of numerous workers in different environments were summarized and discussed. Van Hummelen et al. (*359*) reported data on cytogenetic aberrations in workers with 3 different levels of exposure to PAHs. Workers with the middle level of exposure were found to have statistically significant increases in sister chromatid exchanges in lymphocytes and positive correlations between cytogenetic markers and measures of exposure (airborne PAH levels and urinary hydroxypyrene concentrations). Incidence of micronuclei in exposed workers was not a sensitive biomarker of PAH exposure.

Humoral immunity was assessed in male workers in a Polish foundry who were exposed to high levels of PAHs in ambient air (360). Compared to workers with 3–5-magnitude lower exposure, the high-exposure workers were found to have a marked depression in mean serum IgG and IgA levels. In these same workers IgM levels tended to decrease while IgE levels tended to increase but these trends were not significant. The immunosuppression described here may be related to the frequent development of lung cancer reported in such workers.

In an investigation of the effects of transplacental exposure to carcinogens, pregnant patas monkeys (*Erythrocebus patas*) were orally dosed with 5–50 mg BP/kg on days 50, 100, or 150 of gestation (361). BP induced high, dose-dependent levels of DNA adducts in all fetal organs, with higher levels produced during mid-gestation. During early gestation and at lower BP doses, adduct levels were higher and similar in fetal lung and liver and in maternal liver and placenta. While adduct levels decreased relatively rapidly during the first 10–15 days after BP treatment, 10% of adducts persisted for as long as 50 days. It appeared that mid-gestation was the time of maximal sensitivity to transplacental DNA damage.

Dihydrodiol dehydrogenase(s) (DD) catalyzes reactions which are thought to detoxify the ultimate and proximate carcinogenic metabolites of PAHs. However, as Penning (362) points out in a recent review, the products of these detoxification reactions may not be innocuous. The immediate products of DD reactions are transient catechols which then auto-oxidize to PAH-*o*-quinones. Superoxide anions, hydrogen peroxide, and semiquinone radicals are also generated by these reactions. In addition to the toxic effects of these oxidizing agents, some PAH-*o*-quinones also exert cytotoxic and genotoxic effects. Therefore, it appears that these DD reactions are, in fact, another pathway of PAH activation.

Rodents are widely used as convenient mammalian species for toxicological and carcinogenic investigations, but some differences in physiology between rodents and humans mean that these animals are not always good predictors of adverse effects in humans. Lesca et al. (363) compared three major xenobiotic-binding proteins in humans and pigs: the Ah receptor which binds to dioxins and related compounds and the 4S and 8S proteins which bind to BP and other PAHs. All three porcine proteins appear to have binding characteristics similar to those of the corresponding human proteins and this indicates that the pig should be a good model for pharmacological and toxicological investigations of PAHs

and chlorinated compounds interacting with the Ah receptor.

**OCCURRENCE IN FOODS.** Despite the fact that Chinese women smoke less than men, they have a higher rate of lung cancer, suggesting that they may be more exposed to some other environmental pollutant. In an investigation of one such source of contaminants, Li et al. (364) analyzed samples of fumes from 3 cooking oils commercially available in China for PAHs. Concentrations of BP and dibenzo(a,h)anthracene (DBahA) in fumes from the 3 oils heated to 265°C ranged from 0.305 to 0.463 μg BP/g and from 3.725 to 5.736 μg DBahA/g. Highest concentrations of both compounds were detected in a refined vegetable oil, with lower levels in soybean and another vegetable oil. Concentrations of these two PAHs were about the same or a little lower in fume samples from the kitchen of a restaurant and were 2–3 times as high in fumes from oil used in a shop to deep-fry youtiao (a twisted, fried bread). Air samples from the youtiao shop, the restaurant kitchen, and the kitchen using the refined vegetable oil contained 4.18, 0.49, and 7.62 μg BP/100 m³, respectively. China has no established maximum allowable concentration (MAC) for BP but a comparison of these values to the Russian MAC for BP in air (0.1 μg/100 m³) indicates a serious air quality problem, which may be related to the high lung cancer incidence.

Following the huge 1989 oil spill into Prince William Sound, Alaska, a program was instituted to test fish caught by commercial fishermen for oil residues as manifested by the presence of PAHs (365). Following an initial organoleptic examination during which obviously contaminated fish were rejected, samples were sent to a laboratory for analysis of edible tissues for 25 PAHs. Naphthalene and 2-methylnaphthalene were the most frequent contaminants. Of a total of 221 fish samples tested in 1989, 14% had no detectable PAHs, 85% contained trace levels, and 1% contained 5–12 μg PAH/kg edible flesh. For 47 fish tested in 1990, 87% had trace levels of PAHs and 13% had 5–12 μg/kg. Whether this apparent increasing trend in residue levels is real will have to be determined.

Following a massive oil spill in the Arabian Gulf during the 1991 war, concentrations of PAHs were measured in edible parts of fish collected in April 1992 at 4 locations on the western side of the Gulf (366). Average total PAH levels were 105.3 μg/kg dry weight (21.06 μg/kg wet weight), with a maximum concentration of 112.72 μg/kg wet weight. Pyrene and phenanthrene were the most frequently detected contaminants. Although consumption of these fish would certainly increase exposure to PAHs, the major contaminants in these fish are among the least toxic PAHs and therefore are probably not a major health hazard.

Muscle, liver, and ovaries of 10 cod caught in the northwest Atlantic at a location removed from any coastal point source of pollution were analyzed for 27 PAHs (*367*). None of the muscle tissue contained any PAHs while 2 of the ovaries and all of the liver had detectable levels of a few PAHs. Of the parental PAHs detected, only fluorene (72 ng/g dry weight) was detected in the ovaries and acenaphthene (18 ng/g), fluorene (28 ng/g), and chrysene (22 ng/g) were present in liver. Some alkylated PAHs were detected at higher levels.

During a 5-year period, a total of 870 composite oyster samples from coastal and estuarine areas of the Gulf of Mexico were analyzed for PAH contamination (*368*). Oysters from some sites had relatively high PAH concentrations (>1000 ng/g dry weight) in some years but there was a large variability from year to year. This suggested that the source of contamination was episodic, related to occasional small oil spills or discharges from some point source. Changes in the mean concentrations of some populations also displayed a cyclic pattern which probably reflects large-scale climatic factors which influence precipitation and therefore atmospheric deposition and storm-water runoff.

More commonly, food is contaminated with PAHs during cooking or smoking. For example, during grilling of lamb over a charcoal fire, concentrations of 7 PAHs increased from 1.1 ppb in the raw meat to a maximum of 197.2 ppb after 3 min (*369*). Pyrene (49 ppb), chrysene (40.9 ppb), fluoranthene (36.4 ppb), and 9-methylanthracene (28 ppb) were the major PAHs formed. Continued cooking after 3 min caused a decline in PAH levels, perhaps because the fat, containing the PAHs, melted off the meat and dripped into the fire. Broiling of some vegetables, such as sweet potato, pumpkin, pimiento, and sweet pepper, also significantly increased PAH concentrations (*370*). Highest levels were detected in pimiento after 10 min cooking at 300°C (5.26 ppb) and after 30 min at 200°C (11.36 ppb).

Since smoked meat products sometimes contain excessive levels of PAHs, 735 samples of smoked meat from 124 meat-processing firms in the former East Germany were analyzed for their BP content (*371*). Many of these plants were using out-of-date smoking technologies. However, only 25 of the samples analyzed contained >1 ppb and only 3 samples had >2 ppb. It appears that these plants continue to produce safe foods even with their old equipment.

PAH concentrations have also been measured in a variety of smoked foods and liquid smoke preparations.

Total PAHs ranged from 6.3–43.7 ppb and carcinogenic PAHs ranged from 0.3 to 10.2 ppb in 18 liquid smoke preparations and seasonings obtained in Michigan (*372*) while BP concentrations ranged from 0.1 to 336.6 ppb in 11 liquid smoke preparations obtained in Brazil (*373*). Three of the Brazilian samples and none of the Michigan samples of liquid smoke had BP levels >10 ppb (maximum recommended by FAO/WHO). Only 23 of 44 Brazilian smoked food samples contained detectable levels of BP (0.1–5.9 ppb). For the Michigan smoked foods, the ranges of total and carcinogenic PAHs, respectively, of five foods were: 22 poultry samples, 2.8–22.4 and non-detectable–5.5 ppb; 22 pork and beef samples, 2.6–29.8 and non-detectable–7.4 ppb; 18 fish and shrimp samples, 9.3–86.6 and 0.2–16.1 ppb. Meats processed with natural wood smoke had higher levels of total and carcinogenic PAHs than those processed with liquid smoke preparations.

PAH concentrations were monitored in a liquid smoke flavor spiked with a mixture of 6 PAHs to a final concentration of 91.1 ppb during 164 hours' storage in a low-density polyethylene bottle (*374*). PAH concentrations in the flavor decreased rapidly to 21.9 ppb at 27 min and to undetectable levels by the end of the experiment. PAHs were adsorbed to the walls of the container and then diffused into the packaging material.

Sewage sludge is a rich source of nutrients for plants and so may be applied to fields as a fertilizer. However, some sludges may contain significant levels of PAHs. In a discussion of the importance of soil-to-plant transfer of PAHs, Wild and Jones (*375*) considered PAH concentrations of sludges in the UK and uptake of PAHs from the soil by plants and compared this data to other PAH sources such as waste disposal and atmospheric deposition. PAHs are strongly associated with the organic matter in soil and so are not readily absorbed by plant roots. In fact, even with root crops like carrots, PAHs from the soil are primarily associated with the outside peel of the carrot and little penetrates to the inside. Data on atmospheric deposition of PAHs in the UK indicate that this source currently contributes about 16 times as much PAHs to the soil as does sludge. Some of these volatilized PAHs, of course, are deposited on the above-ground parts of plants.

METHODS FOR DETECTION. Because of the ubiquity and toxicity of PAHs, numerous recent papers have detailed methods for their determination. (Not all of these could be included here and interested persons should more thoroughly search the literature.) Furton et al. (*376*) highlighted advances in the past 3 years in chromatographic and related methods for analyses of PAHs. Procedures reviewed included sample preparation, supercritical fluid extraction, GC, LC, supercritical fluid chromatography, and composite methods (LC–LC, LC–GC, etc.). Another review by Wise et al. (*377*) considered various aspects of PAH determination by reversed-phase LC using fluorescence detection. Experience acquired by the National Institute of Standards and Technology in the LC analysis of PAHs was summarized, including criteria for selection of appropriate columns, approaches to analyzing complex PAH mixtures, and accurate quantitation of PAHs in environmental samples.

Capillary electrophoresis with UV-laser-excited native fluorescence has been utilized by Nie et al. (*378*) for the ultrasensitive determination of several PAHs. Achieved mass detection limits were in the range of $3$–$15 \times 10^{-20}$ mol, with a linear response spanning 4 orders of magnitude. This level of sensitivity should be sufficient for analyzing chemical contaminants and their metabolites in individual mammalian cells.

Two cleanup methodologies were compared for the preparation of seafood samples for GC/MS determination of nanogram/gram levels of PAHs (*379*). Both methods, the modified FDA method (involving a liquid–liquid partition and elution through 3 different solid-phase extraction cartridges) and the National Marine Fisheries Service method (involving purification through a deactivated silica gel/alumina column and gel permeation HPLC) quantitated 18 PAHs at concentrations ranging from 1–5 ppb. The NMFS method produced cleaner extracts with fewer interfering matrix components.

## PACKAGING MATERIALS

A reference collection of monomers and other starting substances required as standards for enforcement of European Community legislation on food contact materials has been established by Gilbert et al. (*380*). The substances have been characterized by mass spectrometry and appropriate chromatographic methods to identify any impurities. This collection has been supplemented by a database containing infra-red and mass spectra and a handbook collating various information to assist enforcement laboratories in the selection and interpretation of analytical methods for the identification of different plastics.

As more used plastics are collected for recycling, much concern has been voiced as to whether recycled plastics can be safely used for food packaging. If the plastics were originally used to contain detergents, pesticides, or motor oil, residues of these substances may not be easily removed from the containers. Begley and Hollifield (*381*) discussed migration from different designs of recycled packaging and approaches to realistically measuring the migration of toxic materials into foods. A two-layer, laminated packaging design may provide an effective barrier to migration. Franz et al. (*382*) evaluated a 3-layered polypropylene design for a cup, with a buried layer of recycled polypropylene in the middle. This design minimizes migration from the recycled materials. A general approach to evaluating the use of recycled plastics in food packaging material was presented.

Proceedings from the "Sixth International Symposium on Migration in Food Packaging Plastics" have recently been published (*383*). Various presentations included: several discussions of regulations controlling food packaging in the European Community (EC), the Nordic countries, and the USA; reports on the evaluation of plastics for food contact materials, of polymeric coatings on metals and paper substrates, and of packaging materials designed to be heated; and the impact of recycling and environmental legislation on packaging plastics.

Another issue of *Food Additives and Contaminants* was devoted to reports from another international conference, "High Temperature Testing of Packaging Materials." EC regulations for high temperature testing of food contact materials were discussed by Rossi (*384*). Background debate regarding appropriate testing procedures for microwave susceptors and other packaging was described along with the proposed framework of temperatures and times required for testing. The most stringent testing will require 2 hours at 175°C with olive oil as the food simulant.

Piringer et al. (*385*) discussed the use of various high-temperature-resistant sorbents as simulants for testing. A correct evaluation of food contact materials used in high-temperature applications requires distinguishing between volatile and non-volatile migrants, between additives and decomposition products, and between overall and specific migration. No universally applicable solvent has been found which can evaluate all these parameters for all packaging materials.

Current EC and Dutch regulations on testing overall migration from packaging materials into olive oil in a microwave oven were compared by Rijk and De Kruijf (*386*). Conventional heating can be used to heat the oil before adding it to the package, but handling oil at temperatures of 150–175°C is hazardous. Prototypes of migration cells which can be used for high temperature migration tests (while starting the tests at room temperature) were described.

Jickells and Castle (*387*) described a testing scheme whereby a microwave susceptor is heated in an enclosed system and potential volatile migrants are detected by GC/MS or GC with flame ionization detection. This approach was used to test 15 model substances, with boiling points ranging from 77 to 440°C, which were incorporated into susceptors. Migration into microwaved foods and into test simulants was measured and the relationship between boiling points and migration levels was calculated. Migration to both simulants was much higher than to foods, indicating that these simulants are suitable for screening for volatiles and results would err on the side of safety.

Risch (*388*) discussed the current regulatory status of packaging materials intended for high temperature use in the USA. A great deal of recent research has focused on volatile compounds which may be liberated from microwave susceptors, and research methods used in these studies were described. Further investigations continue to improve testing methods for non-volatile compounds.

High temperatures (>302°F) caused the release of numerous volatile compounds from 11 microwave susceptor products tested using a newly developed protocol (*389*). The analytical procedure used headspace concentration capillary gas chromatography and mass spectrometry to identify the volatile chemicals. More than 140 unique chromatographic peaks were tabulated but only 44 chemicals were identified, including benzene (in 3 samples at ≤0.22 μg/in.$^2$), 1,1,1-trichloroethane (4 samples at 75–122 μg/in.$^2$), and 2-(2-butoxyethoxy)ethanol. These compounds probably originate primarily from the paper and adhesive components of the susceptor.

Benzene, at concentrations of 2–50 μg/dm$^2$, was detected in 7 of 26 samples of the poly(tetrafluoroethylene) coatings of non-stick cookware analyzed by GC/MS (*390*). Benzene was also present in some samples of non-stick frying pans with various polymer coatings at concentrations of 6–30 μg/dm$^2$. However, none of the foods (puddings, cakes, and roast potatoes) cooked in these pans had detectable levels of benzene. Although some microwave susceptors were also found to contain benzene, no benzene was detected in foods microwaved with these susceptors, even when the foods were cooked longer or at higher microwave powers than recommended.

## Styrene

Migration of styrene from thermoset polyester cookware into foods under normal cooking conditions was found to range from <5 to 5 μg/kg and 5–30 μg/kg, depending on the residual styrene monomer content (9 or 380 mg/kg) in the polyester (*391*). Styrene migration into olive oil was significantly greater than into other foods when samples were was heated to 175°C for 2 h. Migration of styrene was less from used pans as compared to new ones. Migration into olive oil was measured by addition of cyclohexane to the oil and coevaporating the styrene with the solvent (*392*). The condensed vapors were then injected into a GC/MS apparatus in the SIM mode.

"Vapor phase" migration of styrene was measured from general purpose and high impact polystyrene into cooking oil (*393*). Pieces of the polymer were placed in a closed container but not in direct contact with the oil. Then the apparatus was heated to the test temperature (120–180°C) and oil samples were analyzed after 10 days to determine how much of the vaporized styrene they had absorbed. The amount of styrene absorbed was proportional to the square root of the time of exposure, and diffusion coefficients calculated for vapor phase migration were found to be similar to those previously calculated for liquid phase migration of styrene.

## Phthalates

A scientific evaluation of data-derived safety factors for the tolerable daily intake (TDI) of diethylhexylphthalate (DEHP) was presented by Morgenroth (*394*). Using data on peroxisome proliferation and assuming that this is related to hepatocarcinogenicity, a TDI of 8 mg/kg body weight is obtained when a data-derived safety factor of 6.25 is used. Using data from teratogenicity studies, a TDI of 0.04 mg/kg was calculated.

DEHP, a known rodent hepatocarcinogen, also induces proliferation of hepatic peroxisomes and it is thought that the two effects are related. (Peroxisomes function in the degradation of long-chain fatty acids.) Bentley et al. (*395*) reviewed the processes associated with hepatic peroxisome proliferation in rodents and discussed its significance for humans. Rats and mice are extremely sensitive to DEHP while monkeys and humans are relatively insensitive or non-responsive at DEHP concentrations which induce significant proliferation in rodents. Evidence from primary hepatocyte cultures from rodents and monkeys indicates that this differential response is not due to different metabolic capabilities of the peroxisomes of the different species (*396*). It may be that differences in sensitivity to peroxisome proliferators are related to differences in receptor molecules or to differences in partitioning of fatty acids into alternate metabolic pathways.

Phthalates were found to be the major plasticizers present in printing inks on the outside of 33 samples of oriented polypropylene food packaging obtained in England and Spain (*397*). Other new plasticizers, *N*-ethyl-toluenesulfonamide and tris(2-ethylhexyl)trimellitate, were also detected in many samples. Analyses of foods packaged in these materials revealed that only phthalates and di(2-ethylhexyl) adipate were present in detectable concentrations. In some cases migration into foods was significant, with 0.79 mg detected in a 100-g chocolate bar. This is >15% of the tolerable daily intake of this plasticizer for a 20-kg child.

Effects of several cooking methods (roasting, boiling, frying, and freeze-drying) on DEHP residues in eggs, liver, and breast meat of hens were investigated (*398*). The hens had been fed diets containing 1% DEHP for 4 weeks before samples were collected. Before cooking, DEHP residues in eggs, liver, and meat were in the following ranges: 12.3–44.15 ppm, 2.8–16.5 ppm, and 1.27–3.54 ppm, respectively. While cooking did reduce DEHP concentrations in the poultry products, results were quite variable for all cooking methods, with a range of 47–94% of the original DEHP remaining in the samples after cooking.

An analytical procedure for the determination of 2-ethyl-1-hexanol (2-EH), a hydrolytic product of DEHP, in drinking water has been described (*399*). Following complaints about an unpleasant taste and smell in some Italian bottled water, samples were analyzed for DEHP and 2-EH and were found to contain both in concentrations of 2–30 and 2–10 µg/L, respectively. Examination of the packaging material indicated that cap gaskets contained 2-EH as an impurity in the plastic used to manufacture them.

## Adipates

Polyvinyl chloride cling films may contain the plasticizer di-2-(ethylhexyl) adipate (DEHA), which has been shown to migrate into certain foods. Metabolism and pharmacokinetics of deuterium labeled DEHA was investigated in 6 male volunteers (*400*). Following an oral dose of 46 mg, no DEHA was detected in plasma but a metabolite, 2-ethylhexanoic acid (EHA), was present. Approximately 8.6% of the administered dose was excreted in the urine as an EHA conjugate and another 3.5% was excreted as other oxidized metabolites in the urine. Urinary EHA concentrations were used as a screening tool to estimate daily intakes of DEHA in 112 individuals in the UK (*401*). The median intake was estimated to be 2.7 mg/day, with a range of 1–11 mg/day.

The polymeric plasticizers poly(butylene adipate) and poly(propylene adipate) are commonly used as partial replacements for DEHA in flexible films and tubing because of lower rates of migration into foods. When these polymers were exposed in vitro to simulated gastric and intestinal hydrolysis, a partial hydrolysis of the polymers was observed (*402*). Very little of the monomer was detected. Rather, the plasticizers were degraded to smaller oligomer units because the ester linkages in the molecules were more resistant to hydrolysis, thereby preventing a complete breakdown of the polymers.

## Mineral Hydrocarbons

Migration of mineral hydrocarbons from waxed paper packaging into retail samples of breads, cereals, biscuits, and candies and into foods during microwave heating was measured by Castle et al. (*403*). Wax hydrocarbons were detected in the outer surface of bread (up to 50 mg/kg), in crackers (up to 185 mg/kg), in soft chews and toffee candies (110–1300 mg/kg), and into foods microwaved in waxed bags (210–1650 mg/kg). Distribution of the hydrocarbons (primarily *n*-alkanes) in the foods was similar to that in the wax coating on the papers, indicating that transfer occurred largely by adhesion to foods rather than by migration (which would favor lower molecular weight compounds). During microwaving, about 60% of the wax on the paper was transferred to the foods. The bread samples also contained up to 550 mg mineral oil/kg dispersed through the loaf. The source of this oil was probably the food processing machinery.

Jute and sisal fibers are commonly treated with a raw mineral oil (batching oil) before being spun and used to make sacks. This batching oil has been detected in samples of hazelnuts, cocoa beans, and other nuts and seeds stored in these bags. Samples of hazelnuts which were in contact with the bags had 115 mg oil/kg while those from the middle of the bags had 40 mg oil/kg (*404*). The nut meats contained 5 mg/kg. Highest concentrations of oil in cocoa beans were in the shells of the beans in contact with the sack (420 mg/kg), with lower levels in beans from the middle (40 mg/kg). Inside kernels from these two bean samples contained 17 and 8 mg oil/kg, respectively. Carryover of these residues was observed in samples of cocoa butter (28–48 mg oil/kg).

## Other Packaging Components

Oligomers extracted by boiling water from two nylon films used in boil-in-bag packaging were identified and quantified by UV spectrophotometry, HPLC, and LC coupled to mass spectrometry (*405*). Up to 1.5% of the original weight of the bag was lost to the water as caprolactam and cyclic oligomers up to the nonamer. Thickness and type of film used and boiling time were the most important factors affecting migration. Since food being boiled in the bag is separated from the nylon by a polyolefin and adhesive barrier, results of these migration studies would be relevant if the water used for boiling food in the bag was then used to prepare some other parts of a meal or drink.

Overall and specific migration of bisphenol A diglycidyl ether (BADGE) monomer and *m*-xylenediamine (XDA) hardener from an epoxy resin (which may be used to coat the inside of food storage containers) were tested by exposure of a resin sample to 3 water-based food simulants for 10 days at 40°C (*406*). Overall migration from the resin was below the maximum permitted level of 10 mg/dm², with the greatest migration observed in acetic acid (4 mg/dm²). Migration of XDA was well below the maximum limit of 8.3 mg/dm² in all the simulants as was the migration of BADGE into distilled water and into 15% ethanol. However, excessive amounts of BADGE and its hydrolysis products migrated into the acetic acid (7.4 compared to the limit of 3.3 mg/dm²).

Effects of electron beam irradiation on the behavior of antioxidant additives present in polypropylene food packaging material were investigated (*407*). Pouches containing one of 3 food simulants (distilled water, 3% acetic acid, 15% ethanol) were irradiated with doses of 2, 5, or 10 kGy and the held for 10 days at 40°C. Neither of the parent antioxidants, Irganox 1010 or Irgafos 168, were detected in the food simulants although their concentrations decreased in the polypropylene bags during testing. Concentrations of three degradation products of these antioxidants increased in all the food simulants as a function of irradiation dose. After 2 kGy irradiation, concentrations of two of these products in the three simulants were similar while after 10 kGy, concentrations were about twice as high in ethanol as in the other two simulants.

# OTHER ORGANIC RESIDUES

## Toxic Oil Syndrome

In 1981, an epidemic of a previously unrecognized illness affecting >20,000 people and causing 457 deaths occurred in Spain. Since it was associated with consumption of aniline-denatured cooking oil, it was called toxic oil syndrome (TOS) even though the specific toxin(s) was never definitively identified. A 7-year follow-up of a systematically chosen 5% sample of the 20,643 people officially recognized as affected by TOS was conducted by Abaitua Borda et al. (*408*) to determine mortality rates in the ensuing years. Nearly all persons (or their relatives) in the sample were contacted, and standardized mortality rates were calculated and compared to mortality in the general population. A clear-cut excess in mortality occurred in 1981 and a significant mortality excess occurred among people <65 years old during 1982–1983. Beyond this time, through March 1988, no excess mortality was observed in this cohort.

An 8-year follow-up of 332 affected persons by Alonso-Ruiz et al. (*409*) investigated the long-term evolution of TOS without the selection bias of inpatient management. The course of the disease was usually severe and disabling during the first 2 years, with an acute phase (2 months) characterized by pulmonary edema, rash, eosinophilia, and myalgia, followed by an intermediate phase (second to fourth months) with severe myalgia, altered liver function, and pulmonary hypertension, and finally an early chronic phase with scleroderma, polyneuropathy, joint contractures and functional limitations. After 2 years there was more variability in the chronic manifestations of the disease with symptoms such as muscle cramps, chronic musculoskeletal pain, and chronic lung disease as the most prominent symptoms. At the end of 8 years' follow-up, there were 10 TOS-related deaths, 16% of patients had some TOS-related physical symptoms, and 47% had some health-related complaints, although these were subtle in most cases.

A review by Yoshida et al. (*410*) considered the immunotoxicological manifestations of TOS. Data gathered from TOS patients revealed a number of adverse effects on the immune system, including high levels of circulating eosinophils and non-antigen specific IgE, deficiencies in circulating basophils and CD3$^+$ and CD8$^+$ T cells, reduced B and T lymphocyte responses to mitogens, and production of autoantibodies. These and other immunopathologic symptoms were discussed in relation to pathogenic mechanisms involved in the disease, with an emphasis on oxidative stress as a central feature of anilide-induced injury.

Eosinophilia-myalgia syndrome (EMS), first reported in 1990 and related to ingestion of L-tryptophan supplements, has many pathological features (including inflammatory lesions of coronary arteries) in common with TOS. An immunohistochemical analysis of lesions in the hearts of 4 TOS victims was compared to that of 3 victims of EMS (*411*). Evidence indicated that cellular immune mechanisms with substantial T cell infiltration were involved in cardioneuropathy in both diseases. Cytotoxic/suppressor T cells were more prominent around nerves, ganglia, and some arteries in EMS cases while B cells were more prominent around arteries in TOS where some humoral immune response may be involved.

Skin lesions are another common symptom in both TOS and EMS. Immunohistochemical studies utilizing antibodies to detect 6 different growth factors in 7 EMS and in 6 TOS skin biopsy specimens revealed the presence of all the growth factors in specimens from both syndromes (*412*). However, two factors, transforming growth factor-β and platelet-derived growth factor$_{AA}$, were more prevalent in EMS than in TOS samples, indicating that pathogenic mechanisms in the 2 diseases differ.

Examination of fibrotic skin and nerve tissues from TOS patients with cDNA probes for types I, III, and IV collagens revealed the presence of high levels of types I and III in fibrotic skin areas while type IV collagen mRNA was abundant in the fibrotic areas around nerves (*413*). Cultured fat-storing cells derived from a cirrhotic rat liver, when challenged with cooking oil associated with TOS, increased their synthesis of type I collagen mRNA and this resulted in increased collagen synthesis (*414*). It appears that the toxin(s) in toxic oil stimulates collagen synthesis by increasing transcription of collagen genes.

Since the toxin(s) in oil associated with TOS has never been identified, 6 control and 8 case samples were analyzed by GC/MS for residues of PCDDs and PCDFs (*415*). Results demonstrated no differences between case and control samples, with all having very low levels of these chlorinated contaminants (<1 ng/g in most cases).

## Benzene

Several reports in the past few years have documented detectable benzene levels in a variety of foods. In some cases, the source of the benzene was apparently the reaction between two food additives (benzoate and ascorbic acid) while, in other cases, the source was apparently some component used to prepare the food. McNeal et al. (*416*) analyzed over 50 foods for benzene, including some previously reported to contain naturally occurring benzene and some containing the two preservatives implicated in benzene formation. Highest benzene levels were detected in two samples of liquid smoke (121 and 21 ng/g), imitation strawberry preserves (38 ng/g), two brands of taco sauce (9 and 22 ng/g), duck sauce (7 ng/g),

imitation grape jelly (5 ng/g), and barbecue sauce (5 ng/g). All other foods tested, including fruits and fruit juices, sodas, eggs, smoked fish, coffee, and other jams, contained ≤2 ng/g. Aqueous solutions of 0.04% sodium or potassium benzoate and 0.025% ascorbic acid (concentrations typically used in soft drinks) were found to contain about 300 ng benzene/g after 20 hours of exposure to strong UV light or to 45°C in an oven. Benzene formation was much slower when these solutions were kept in the dark at room temperature, but concentrations of 266 ng/g were reached after 8 days under these conditions.

## Acrylamide Monomers

Cultivated mushrooms are generally grown in a composting substrate with a capping or casing soil which may contain polyacrylamide because of its water-holding capacity. Although polyacrylamide itself is inert, agricultural grade polymers may contain 200–500 mg of water-soluble monomers/kg. Analyses of mushrooms (*Agaricus bisporus*) grown in such a medium, using a method with a detection limit of 0.5 μg/kg, did not detect any acrylamide monomers (*417*). It appears that these monomers do not bioaccumulate, perhaps because of their high water solubility or their degradation in the composting mix or in the mushrooms.

## Formaldehyde

Formaldehyde may be present in foods either as a result of natural metabolic processes or from some processing technique or packaging. A method has been developed for the quantitative determination of formaldehyde in milk by liquid chromatography (*418*). Average formaldehyde levels detected in fresh milk and in commercial 2% milk from cows fed a typical North American dairy diet were 0.027 and 0.164 mg/kg, respectively.

## Propylene and Ethylene Glycols

Bait fish, which contain added antifreeze compounds (propylene and ethylene glycols), are not considered acceptable for human consumption but they are occasionally illegally diverted to human food use. A GC–tandem MS method has been developed for confirmation of the identity of these glycols in fish (*419*). The method does not require derivatization or preliminary cleanup. Analyses, using this procedure, of suspected anchovy lots embargoed by California in 1991 confirmed the identities of these two compounds in the fish.

# HEAVY METALS — MULTIRESIDUE STUDIES

Exposure of young mammals, including human children, to heavy metals has been associated with learning deficits and neurobehavioral defects. In a recent investigation of prolonged behavioral effects of lead and mercury, squirrel monkeys (*Saimiri sciureus*) were exposed in utero to these metals and then were evaluated at 5–6 years of age with a series of behavioral tests (*420*). Monkeys were trained to press levers under concurrent schedules of reinforcement in which separate, random interval reinforcement schedules operated independently on the two levers. Those monkeys exposed to methyl mercury (0.7–0.9 ppm in maternal blood) and those exposed to >40 µg lead/dL maternal blood were less sensitive to reinforcement rates than control monkeys and when reinforcement schedules changed, the exposed monkeys were slower to adapt to the new pattern. These results suggest that learning deficits associated with heavy metal exposure may be caused by an insensitivity to changing reinforcement contingencies.

## Occurrence in Foods

A survey of over 500 samples of a variety of foods from retail markets in Greece was conducted to determine concentrations of lead and cadmium in the foods (*421*) and to estimate exposure to heavy metals in the nearby population (*422*). Highest concentrations of both Cd (474–477 ppb) and Pb (113–178 ppb) were present in beef and lamb liver. High levels of Pb were also detected in tomatoes and dark wine (both 210 ppb) and in fish (194 ppb), while vegetables (74 ppb) and pastes (63 ppb) contained relatively high levels of Cd. However, in terms of consumption, fruit and tomatoes contributed the most Pb and white bread and leafy vegetables the most Cd to average daily intakes. Data from food frequency questionnaires indicated that the people in this area of northern Greece had an average daily consumption of 179 µg Pb and of 44.5 µg Cd.

Data collected around 1980 in Japan revealed that the general Japanese population had an average daily intake (from food) of 30–40 µg Cd and of 33–38 µg Pb. Ten years later, analyses of duplicate diets from 274 Japanese farmers in 5 prefectures demonstrated that dietary intakes of both metals had decreased significantly to 17–25 µg Cd and 10.8–12.2 µg Pb per day (*423*). Some geographic variations in heavy metal intake were observed and men tended to have a higher Cd intake than women. Reductions in general atmospheric lead levels during the past decade may be partially responsible for decreased levels in food items. Decreased intake of rice (formerly a major source of dietary Cd in Japan) is partly responsible for the reduction of this metal in dietary samples.

Analyses of fresh and canned specimens of two species of bivalve mussels collected at several places along the Chilean coast demonstrated that all had heavy metal (Cd, Pb, Cu, Hg) concentrations below the permitted levels of 1 ppm for Cd and Hg, 5 ppm for Pb, and 20 ppm for Cu (*424*). Heavy metal concentrations were not correlated with the size of the mussels nor were they increased by the canning process. Significantly higher metal concentrations were detected in visceral and mantle tissue, and removal of these tissues before canning was recommended. Two species of bivalve mollusks cultured along the coast of Malaysia and purchased at markets in the capital city were found to contain elevated levels of arsenic and cadmium (*425*). Average As concentrations in samples obtained from different markets ranged from 3.84–5.3 µg/kg (permissible limit, 1 µg/g) and average Cd levels ranged from 0.25–1.42 µg/g (legislative limit, 1 µg/g). Concentrations of lead and copper in these mollusks were below regulatory limits.

Sources of elevated levels of some heavy metals in brined, canned Jordanian cheese preserved in glass jars or tin cans was investigated (*426*). Heavy metal concentrations in fresh sheep's milk and in fresh cheese were generally low but concentrations of some metals (Pb, Fe, Sn, Cu) increased during brining (presumably from impurities in the salt used) and cheese in tin containers had even higher levels of some metals (Cd, Ni, Pb, Sn, Cu, As), perhaps as a result of leaching from the containers. The authors recommend the use of a purified salt and glass jars for preservation of this cheese.

A total of 1582 samples of muscle, liver, and kidney samples from cattle and pigs slaughtered in central Moravia were analyzed, during a monitoring program, for Cd, Hg, and Pb (*427*). Metal concentrations which exceeded regulatory limits were recorded for Cd in 13.1% of cow kidneys, for lead in 1.9% of bull liver samples, and for Hg in 0.5% of cow muscle, 5.5% of bull kidney, and 0.8% of swine kidneys.

Inuit people living in coastal areas of northern Canada consume several marine mammals in relatively large amounts. A survey of muscle, liver, and kidney tissue from walrus living in this area revealed that the muscle contained low levels of mercury compared to other marine mammals (*428*). None of the muscle and only some of the liver samples exceeded Canadian regulatory guidelines for Hg in fish. Concentrations of lead in liver and of cadmium in kidney were higher relative to other marine mammals and may be of concern to local people consuming large amounts of walrus.

Several important food crops in Pakistan have been surveyed to detect potentially harmful levels of heavy metals. Wheat and wheat products were found to have very low levels of As and Hg (*429*), but concentrations of Pb and Cd were high enough that the average daily intake of wheat would contribute 41% and 93%, respectively, to the established weekly tolerance levels for these metals. Analyses of vegetable oils, sugars, and teas obtained from wholesale agencies in Pakistan revealed that they vary greatly in their heavy metal contents (*430*). Cd was not detected in any sugar. Unrefined beet sugar had higher mean Pb (0.33 ppm) and Cu (5.45 ppm) levels than cane sugar. Highest concentrations of Cd, Cu, and Pb in oils were 0.033, 0.263, and 0.154 ppm, respectively. Tea leaves contained up to 0.9 ppm Cd, 9.2 ppm Cu, and 5.2 ppm Pb. Generally these metal concentrations would not be considered a health problem.

Crop plants grown near or on polluted land may accumulate elevated levels of some toxic metals. This was illustrated by studies in Nigeria near an old lead–zinc mine (*431*); in Poland in industrialized as compared to rural areas (*432*); and in India in fields receiving industrial waste effluents (*433*). Lead, copper, and cadmium were the metals accumulated to potentially dangerous levels, with some plants and parts of plants being more efficient at absorbing these metals from soil than others.

Since mushrooms are known to bioaccumulate some heavy metals, Vetter (*434*) examined 88 specimens of a variety of common Hungarian mushrooms for concentrations of arsenic and cadmium. Most of the samples had undetectable levels of As, with the exception of some species of *Agaricus* and its relatives (3.47–26.5 ppm, dry weight). In contrast, all the mushrooms contained detectable Cd, with an average concentration of 4.9 ppm. Highest concentration was 86 ppm in an *Agaricus* and most members of this genus contained significantly more Cd than other genera.

Analyses of 3 Spanish red wines (young, crianza, and reserva) for heavy metals revealed concentrations of 106–186 µg Cu/L, 77–124 µg Pb/L, and 1.3–2.2 µg Cd/L (*435*). Highest levels of Cd were in the young wine; the reserva wine (aged 12 months in an oak barrel and 14 months in a bottle) had the highest concentrations of the other two metals.

Of 52 samples of Spanish bottled vinegars analyzed for heavy metals, only 3 had concentrations of Pb + As + Hg which exceeded the legal limit of 1 ppm (*436*). Mean Cd, Pb, and Ni concentrations (0.035, 0.67, and 0.105 ppm, respectively) were highest in the wine vinegar and lowest in the alcohol or apple vinegars.

## Analytical Methods

Numerous methods have been described for the determination of multiple metals in foods. Among these are procedures for the detection of cadmium and lead in raw milk by graphite furnace atomic absorption spectrophotometry (AAS) (*437*); (b) cadmium, zinc, copper, and silver in lobster digestive gland by gel chromatography followed by AAS and polarography (*438*); (c) trace elements in edible oils and margarines by instrumental neutron activation analysis (*439*) and by AAS (*440*); (d) aluminum, strontium, and titanium in diet test samples using inductively coupled plasma atomic emission spectrometry (*441*); and (e) and cadmium, copper, lead, iron, chromium, nickel, and zinc in liver paste, applesauce, minced fish, wheat bran, milk powder, and two composite diets by AAS after dry ashing (*442*). This last report summarizes an interlaboratory study which concluded that the method gave acceptable results for all the metals.

## ALUMINUM

### Occurrence and Detection in Foods

A total of 64 kinds of foods obtained in shops, warehouses, and factories in Tianjin, China, were analyzed for aluminum (*443*). Aluminum concentrations varied greatly, generally being higher in foods of plant origin, but most foods contained <10 ppm. Daily intake of Al from an average diet in Tianjin was estimated to be 3.79 mg/person.

Using inductively coupled plasma atomic emission spectrometry, a total of 34 infant formulas (29 cow's milk–based and 5 soy-based) available in Italy were analyzed for Al (*444*). Generally, higher Al levels were present in the soy milk formulas (0.39–1.01 mg/L) than in the cow's milk formulas (0.03–0.85 mg/L). Although all these Al concentrations would provide an infant with less than the provisional tolerable weekly intake, most of the soy formulas contained considerably more Al than most of the cow's milk formulas.

Cultivated winged beans (*Psophocarpus tetragonolobus*) are being promoted as an important new protein source in tropical areas. Because Al is abundant in tropical soils, part of an assessment of the plant's nutritional quality included analyses of Al levels in all the edible plant parts (*445*). All parts of the plant accumulated Al to very high levels, especially in the young or immature stages: leaves (1620 ppm); pods (1000 ppm); seeds (150 ppm); and tubers (25,000 ppm). Whether such high Al levels would pose a health risk is unknown.

Concern has been raised that foods packaged in aluminum containers or cooked in aluminum pans might acquire excessive amounts of aluminum. Changes in Al concentrations in 7 varieties of soft drinks packaged in aluminum cans were monitored over a 12-month period of storage at room temperature (*446*). Aluminum concentrations in all the sodas increased from a low of 0.039–0.055 ppm at time 0 to highs of 0.188–0.849 ppm after 12 months. More acidic sodas had higher aluminum concentrations. However, possible daily intakes of Al in these drinks would be almost negligible compared to total daily dietary intakes.

Migration of Al from packaging materials and cookware into foods and beverages was also monitored during cooking or storage (*447*). Very low levels of Al were detected in cola after storage for 5–6 months in internally lacquered cans (<0.25 ppm). However, an acidic drink stored in an uncoated aluminum bottle for 5 days acquired 7 mg Al/L. Large amounts of Al also migrated into acidic foods from cooking pans: mashed tomatoes boiled in an uncoated aluminum pan for 60 min contained 10–15 mg Al/kg. However, since most pans are now made with stainless steel or teflon-coated aluminum, this is probably not a major source of aluminum intake.

Other investigations into leaching of aluminum from cookware confirmed that more acidic liquids dissolved more aluminum during cooking (*448,449*). Foods or liquids with a high pH (>10) also chemically corroded the pots during boiling. When foods or liquids are in contact with aluminumware during prolonged storage at room temperature, Al is dissolved by an electrochemical corrosion which is enhanced by the presence of complexing agents and electrolytes (such as NaCl).

A simple method for direct, routine determination of aluminum in wines by graphite furnace atomic absorption spectrometry has been developed (*450*). A survey of 98 red wines from southern France detected a mean aluminum content of 0.763 mg/L (range, 0.25–2.55 mg/L). Wines stored in bottles with aluminum caps can dissolve Al from the caps, as demonstrated by the higher Al concentration in wine near corks covered with an aluminum cap as compared to a lead–tin cap.

## Biological and Toxicological Effects

One of the most well-known and controversial toxic effects attributed to aluminum is its role in Alzheimer's disease (AD). A recent review by Copestake (*451*) summarized the debate in recent years and discussed a number of epidemiological studies investigating the association between aluminum in drinking water and the incidence of AD. Results from several such studies support a role for aluminum in the development of this disease, but as yet the evidence is far from conclusive. Heredity and advancing age are the only established etiological factors so far.

Tau protein and amyloid β (Aβ) protein are two of the major proteins found in the neuritic senile plaques characteristic of AD. To determine whether aluminum exposure influences the expression of these proteins, the frontal cortices of the brains of 5 AD patients, of 6 controls, and of 15 dialysis patients (who are often exposed to high levels of Al) were examined immunochemically to detect Aβ protein and tau protein (*452*). AD-like changes in tau protein processing were observed in the brains of dialysis patients following prolonged exposure to aluminum.

In a recent review, Greger (*453*) discussed various aspects of aluminum metabolism in humans and laboratory animals. Possible dietary sources of aluminum include water, food additives, and contamination from aluminum utensils and containers. Various studies have estimated that the average dietary intake ranges from 2 to 33.3 mg Al/day. Some individuals consume much higher levels in pharmaceutical products such as antacids. Generally ingested aluminum is not absorbed efficiently but absorption may be enhanced by the presence of other compounds in foods. Distribution and excretion of aluminum were also considered along with a brief description of the toxic effects of aluminum.

While some epidemiological studies indicate that Al in drinking water is positively correlated with AD, others have provided negative or marginal correlations. Experiments by Edwardson et al. (*454*), in which volunteers consumed an Al-containing orange drink with or without sodium silicate, demonstrated that dissolved silicon reduced peak plasma levels of Al to about 15% of the levels detected after consuming the drink without Si. Therefore, studies investigating a link between Al in drinking water and some toxic effect must also consider Si levels in the water.

Tea leaves are known to contain high levels of aluminum but the bioavailability of this Al has been questioned. In some in vitro experiments, Powell et al. (*455*) attempted to ascertain the gastrointestinal bioavailability of Al in tea. In the presence of human gastric juices (pH 2.3), >90% of the Al in the tea infusion was associated with small-molecular-weight components (< 3000 Da). However, when foods and drinks pass into the small intestine, the pH rises to nearly neutral and, at this pH, only 5% of the Al is in the small-molecular-weight fraction. Most of the Al in the small bowel appears to be associated with high-molecular-weight polyphenols and is therefore not very bioavailable.

Following the ingestion of Al-containing antacids by 6 patients with duodenal ulcer and by 2 healthy volunteers, peak serum Al levels (54.5 µg/L) were reached within 30 min (*456*). Serum levels then returned to the initial levels of 6.8 µg/L by 3 hours after dosing. The ingested Al was rapidly excreted in the urine and eliminated in the feces. Therefore, provided renal function is normal, high Al intakes from antacids should not present a problem.

To determine whether increased plasma Al levels following ingestion of Al-containing antacids affected indices of bone formation, serum samples from healthy volunteers and from persons regularly consuming antacids were analyzed for Al, osteocalcin, and procollagen I C-terminal peptide (*457*). Chronic consumption of Al-containing antacids resulted in higher serum Al concentrations: 9.0 and 11.8 µg/L in men and women, respectively, as compared to 4.0 and 5.4 µg/L, respectively, in controls. However, the increased serum Al levels were not associated with significant changes in most indices of bone formation.

In vitro effects of 10–50 µM Al on primary cultures of marrow cells and calvarial osteoblasts isolated from rats demonstrated that in younger, sub-confluent cultures Al suppressed proliferation of both cell types (*458*). This may be related to the bone formation defect associated with Al toxicity in growing rats. In confluent cultures, however, Al selectively stimulated collagen production and periosteal fibroblast and osteoblast DNA synthesis. This effect is consistent with the development of osteomalacia in humans and animals receiving toxic doses of Al.

After 5–7 weeks of consuming diets containing 3.5% sodium citrate and 1000 µg Al/g, young mice had significantly higher levels of Al in liver, bone, spinal cord, and brain nuclear fraction as compared to tissues of mice consuming diets with the citrate and 3 µg Al/g (*459*). Neurotoxicity, as measured with the NIEHS Neurobehavioral Test Battery, revealed that the high-dose mice had a lower grip strength and greater startle responsiveness. No evidence was detected for Al-induced brain lipid and protein oxidative damage.

Hematological effects of excess aluminum in living organisms were reviewed by Zaman et al. (*460*). Among the effects on red blood cells, Al has been reported to reduce the deformability of erythrocytes and to produce peroxidative changes in erythrocyte membranes. Al inhibits heme synthesis in vitro but this effect is not well investigated in vivo. Changes in white blood cells have also been reported but these also require further investigation.

## ARSENIC

### Occurrence and Detection in Foods

Analyses of 21 samples of different types of Spanish milk obtained from retail stores revealed that they contained 0.14 to 0.77 ng As/g (*461*). The lowest concentration was in pasteurized whole milk while the highest concentrations were in full-fat powdered milk, evaporated milk, and semi-skimmed UHT milk. At these low concentrations, milk consumption would not appreciably contribute to the FAO/WHO permitted daily intake of 2 µg As/kg body weight.

Organic arsenicals are fed to meat-type poultry to promote growth but are not currently approved for egg-producing poultry. To determine whether these compounds would cause the deposition of excess arsenic in eggs, hens were fed diets containing 14–112 ppm As (arsanilic acid or roxarsone) or control diets for 10 weeks followed by a 2-week withdrawal period (*462*). Within 1 week of treatment, As levels in eggs increased from barely detectable levels to approximately 750 and 2000 ppb in yolks and 37 and 96 ppb in albumen of eggs from hens fed 56 and 112 ppm arsanilic acid and to >800 ppb As in yolks and 32 ppb in albumen from hens fed 56 ppm roxarsone. Meat-type poultry are usually fed 14 ppm roxarsone or 35 ppm arsanilic acid. If egg-laying hens were fed the same concentrations their eggs would contain approximately 80–150 ppb arsenic, which is below the tolerance limit of 500 ppb.

Using electroanalytical techniques involving differential-pulse cathodic-stripping voltammetry, 2 brands and types of canned tuna fish were analyzed for traces of arsenic (*463*). Both varieties, a brand of chunk light tuna (1.62 µg As/g) and another brand of albacore solid white tuna (2.41 µg As/g), contained concentrations of arsenic below the maximum allowable limit set by the FDA (2.6 ppm).

Total arsenic measured in muscle tissue from 10 male and 10 female Norway lobsters caught in the

Adriatic Sea averaged 14.2 and 13.26 ppm, respectively (*464*). Assuming that 3% of the total arsenic is in the more toxic inorganic form, it may be fairly easy to exceed the maximum intake recommended by WHO of 2 µg/kg body weight/day by consuming these lobsters.

A method has been developed for the determination of arsenic in ground plant tissues using graphite furnace atomic absorption spectrophotometry (*465*). The method eliminates the time and labor of the plant digestion step and was successfully used in analyses of spinach and corn.

## Toxicological Effects

Blackfoot disease, a peripheral vascular disorder resulting in gangrene in the lower extremities, is endemic in some villages in Taiwan where the well water contains high levels of arsenic. While arsenic levels in well water from an unaffected area in Taiwan were measured at <0.7 µg/L, groundwater in the endemic area contained 671 µg dissolved As/L (*466*). The predominant arsenic species in this water are $As^{+3}$ and $As^{+5}$, with an $As^{+3}/As^{+5}$ ratio of 2.6. Methyl arsenicals were below the detection limit. A comparison of other trace elements in well water from the endemic and non-endemic areas revealed that the former also had a Pb level about 4-fold higher, a chromium level about 7-fold higher, and a sodium level about 8.6-fold higher than the latter. Zinc concentrations were about the same.

Arsenic has been shown to give negative effects in the Ames mutagenicity test. However, an ethyl acetate extract of well water from the blackfoot disease area in Taiwan was shown to induce mutations in *Salmonella typhimurium* whether or not an S9 was used (*467*). The nature of these mutagens is being investigated.

Assessments have been made of trace element levels in the urine (*468*), blood (*469*), and hair (*470*) of blackfoot disease patients. Urinary Zn, Cd, Pb, and Cu levels in the patients were 0.9, 1.5, 1.7, and 3.1 times the levels in urine of controls. Patients had an average of about 50% more As in blood and hair compared to controls, but concentrations of Cu and Zn were similar to controls. Selenium concentrations were about 25% lower in blood and 15% lower in hair of patients than in controls. Whether variations in these other trace elements are etiologically related to the disease or are a consequence of the disease process is unknown.

Age- and sex-adjusted prevalence of diabetes mellitus was assessed in 891 adults living in the region of high exposure to arsenic in Taiwan and found to be 2-fold higher than that of residents in other areas in Taiwan (*471*). A dose–response relationship was ob-

served between cumulative arsenic exposure and prevalence of diabetes and this remained significant after adjustment for age, sex, body mass index, and activity level at work. For those with a cumulative As exposure >15 ppm-yr, the multivariate odds ratio for this disease was 10.05.

Lymphocytes from 282 Argentinian individuals who had been drinking water containing >0.13 ppm As for at least 20 years contained a significantly higher frequency of sister chromatid exchanges (SCEs) than lymphocytes from 155 control individuals who drank water containing a mean of 0.02 ppm As (*472*). Other factors, such as occupational exposure to pesticides or to other chemicals in manufacturing plants, did not appear to be relevant. Other adverse health effects noted in this exposed population included hyperkeratosis, melanosis, and basal cell carcinoma. In vitro studies with phytohemagglutinin-stimulated lymphocytes from healthy volunteers demonstrated that very low concentrations of both tri- and pentavalent arsenic enhanced DNA synthesis (*473*).

Although seafoods contain fairly high concentrations of arsenic, the arsenic is primarily in the form of organoarsenicals which are believed to be less toxic than inorganic As. Consumption of crab or shrimp containing arsenobetaine by 6 volunteers was followed by rapid excretion of this compound, unchanged, in the urine, with approximately 70% of the ingested dose excreted within 37 hours (*474*). On the other hand, consumption of nori, a seaweed which contains arsenic primarily as a single arsenosugar compound, resulted in the excretion of as many as 6 metabolites in urine of volunteers. A wide variation was observed among the volunteers in urinary arsenic excretion patterns. Overall retention of the organoarsenic compounds from nori was longer than for the As compounds in crab.

## CADMIUM

## Occurrence and Detection in Foods

Total flow of cadmium in the Swedish environment during the past 50 years was discussed by Bergbäck et al. (*475*). Industrial sources of emissions have been metal industries, zinc and copper mines, and producers of phosphorus fertilizers, and these accounted for a majority of emissions in 1970. In 1990, consumption emissions from the use of cadmium in various products, particularly rechargeable nickel–cadmium batteries, accounted for more than 70% of emissions. Significant amounts of cadmium have been added to arable land from the use of phosphorus fertilizers and this becomes mobilized in acidic soils such that plant uptake and leaching into groundwater is facilitated. This has resulted in higher cadmium levels in wheat and oats. Since human exposure to cadmium is currently close to levels that cause detrimental effects, efforts should be made to decrease emissions, to decrease soil acidity by liming, and to monitor foods with the potential to accumulate heavy metal residues.

In an assessment of current cadmium intake in the new German provinces (formerly East Germany), data were collected from 950 women and 866 men on their 24-hour dietary consumption of 60 food items (*476*). Daily Cd intake from all sources was estimated as 9.7–10.9 µg for women and 11.5–14.0 µg for men. The contributions of various food groups to this total were: bread and pastries (36–37%), potatoes (18–19%), meat (11–14%), vegetables (9–12%), and other (22%). These daily intakes are <20% of the WHO recommended levels.

Examination of tissues from wild game has demonstrated that Cd tends to accumulate in liver and kidneys rather than in muscle, and that older animals carry a greater body burden than younger ones. Liver from 59 deer killed in Connecticut contained an average of 1.71 mg Cd/kg dry weight, with 6 samples exceeding the proposed action level of 4.8 mg/kg (*477*). Where data were available, it was observed that kidney levels of Cd were usually at least 10 times higher than liver concentrations. Liver concentrations of Cd in caribou of different ages from northern Canada killed in the spring and the autumn ranged from 4.62 to 9.17 mg/kg dry weight and from 1.38 to 6.96 mg/kg, respectively (*478*). Kidney Cd concentrations were about 10 times higher than those in liver. Muskoxen living in the same area had about 10-fold lower levels than caribou. Regular weekly consumption of kidney from caribou or older muskoxen would probably result in a Cd intake in excess of the WHO provisional weekly tolerable intake. Most of the kidney samples from deer and wild boar in a nature reserve in Germany were also found to have excessive Cd levels and, in some cases, liver Cd levels were above the recommended limits (*479*).

Analyses of saucer scallops (*480*) and oysters (*481*) collected along the Australian coast disclosed contamination with 0.41–1.44 ppm Cd (wet weight) and 0.17–9.2 ppm, respectively, in the edible parts. Cd concentrations in oysters exceeded recommended limits at 5 of the 10 sites sampled. Cd levels in scallops were below the maximum permitted concentration of 2 mg/kg. However, the digestive gland of the scallops contained about a 100-fold higher concentration of Cd. When scallops were frozen whole, some of this Cd in the digestive gland migrated out to muscle tissue and may cause that tissue to exceed regulatory limits. An improved procedure, involving treatment of tissues in a microwave acid digestion bomb followed by electrothermal atomic absorption spectrometry has been developed for the determination of Cd in seafood (*482*). Analyses of seafoods frequently consumed along the Mediterranean coast of Spain revealed that highest concentrations (up to 45.75 ng/g fresh weight) occurred in squid, shrimp, and related species.

Comparison of Cd concentrations in 24-hour duplicate food samples from Japanese farmers and forestry workers in 1990 with a similar set of samples from 1980 revealed that Cd intake from the diet had decreased by 37% in males and 14% in females during this period (*483*). This was accompanied by decreases of 49–53% in blood Cd levels. The principal factors responsible for reduced dietary Cd intake were the absolute decrease in rice consumption and probably lower Cd levels in Japanese rice in 1990. In 1980, rice accounted for about 72% of the daily intake of Cd while in 1990, it supplied only 33–36% of dietary Cd in this population.

Cadmium levels were investigated in oats, carrots, and spinach as a function of soil acidity and addition of a phosphorus fertilizer containing Cd (*484*). In most cases, Cd levels in plants increased with increasing fertilizer application and with increasing acidity. In comparable soils, with similar fertilizer application, highest Cd levels were detected in spinach and lowest levels were in oats. Of the total Cd accumulated in carrot plants, only 18% was present in the roots.

Uptake of Cd from polluted soils by lettuce was found to vary for different cultivars (*485*). In addition, fertilization of the polluted soils with cow manure increased plant growth and decreased Cd concentrations from an average of 102 ppm to an average of 28 ppm. Ten lettuce cultivars grown in non-polluted soils accumulated only 0.6–1.2 ppm Cd in the leaves.

Greenhouse experiments measured uptake of Cd by swiss chard from soils fertilized with composted materials containing sewage sludge (*486*). Plants grown on composts containing 5.41–6.91 ppm Cd had Cd concentrations of 1.39–1.75 ppm. If such composted materials are used to start young plants which will then be transplanted to fields or gardens outside, there is probably little risk in producing edible plants with excessive levels of Cd.

Recently, U.S. EPA regulations concerning land application of sewage sludge have been published in an effort to control human exposures to Cd from crops grown in sludge-amended soils. However, uptake of Cd by plants is a complex process depending on soil types and acidity as well as the cultivars of plants grown. Stern (*487*) presented a re-analysis of this model of Cd uptake using Monte Carlo probabilistic analysis of exposure variables with Cd uptake slopes restricted to soils with pH ≤6.5. This approach appears to give a more realistic assessment of Cd uptake.

## Biological and Toxicological Effects

Outside of occupational exposures, the main route of human exposure to Cd is through food. Bioavailability of Cd in foods, however, is not well understood. Most toxicological studies test the effects of inorganic Cd added to the diet but in real food Cd is complexed with organic molecules. Groten and van Bladeren (*488*) reviewed available data on Cd speciation in foods, metallothionein, absorption and metabolism of Cd from food, and other dietary factors affecting Cd uptake. For animal foods where Cd is bound to metallothionein, its availability is apparently similar to that of Cd salts. However, little is known of speciation of Cd, and therefore its bioavailability, in plant foods.

Although exposed to foods with similar Cd levels, different individuals in a population may exhibit different degrees of toxicity. Slob and Krajnic (*489*) presented a methodological framework for modelling the relation between external and internal dose which takes into account interindividual variabilities in intake and toxicokinetics. Such a model can be used for risk analyses of different subgroups in a population and can predict the effects of increased (or decreased) Cd concentrations in foods.

Residents in several areas in Japan have been exposed to elevated levels of Cd, particularly in rice, as a result of pollution from mining and other industrial activities. Many of these people suffer symptoms of renal dysfunction and osteomalacia characteristic of itai-itai disease. A follow-up study of 3178 residents living in the Kakehashi River basin from 1981 to 1991 compared mortality rates and urinary levels of protein and $\beta_2$-microglobulin ($\beta$2-MG) (*490,491*). Analyses of data, adjusting for age, revealed that elevated urinary protein and $\beta$2-MG in women and urinary protein in men were the factors most associated with increased mortality rates in these Cd-exposed persons. Urinary Cd levels of approximately 4 μg/g creatinine appeared to be the threshold for development of β-microglobulinuria ($\beta$-MG-uria) in Cd-exposed persons (*492*). Significance of slightly increased urinary $\beta$-MG is not presently understood, but $\beta$-MG levels >1000 μg/L in urine were irreversible, even when Cd intake was significantly decreased, and led to increased mortality (*493*). In a study of 1850 residents in a Cd-polluted area, total Cd intake was significantly associated with $\beta$-MG-uria and a dose–response relationship was observed (*494*).

In vitro tests with cultures of renal proximal tubule cells from 11 individuals without a known exposure to excess Cd were used to investigate toxic responses to ionic Cd over a 16-day period (*495*). Nearly a 3-fold variation in sensitivity to Cd was observed for the different cultures, with $TD_{50}$ (dose producing 50% lethality) values ranging from 1.7 to 4.9 μg/mL. These differences were not related to race, sex, or age of the persons the cells were cultured from nor were they related to culture age or passage number of the cell culture. It appears that there is a heterogeneous response to Cd in the human population.

During a long-term chronic toxicity assay, rhesus monkeys were fed diets containing 0, 3, 10, 30, or 100 ppm cadmium chloride and monitored for toxic effects on general health (*496*). Monkeys consuming ≥10 ppm Cd had reduced body weights and heights compared to controls and low-dose monkeys. At the 2 lowest doses, no effects were observed on renal function. Monkeys consuming 100 ppm Cd developed some signs of renal dysfunction (glucose and protein in urine) but none suffered aggravated renal function or renal failure during the 9 years of the study.

Hospital admissions records for an area in the Netherlands which has been exposed to Cd and Zn pollution from zinc-producing factories for over 100 years were compared with those from a noncontaminated area and with national averages (*497*). Frequencies of several diseases associated with Cd (renal insufficiency, nephrolithiasis, hypertension, cancer, immaturity of the newborn) did not differ in the different areas. However, there was a higher rate of admissions for atherosclerosis in the polluted area, particularly among men >40 years old. Possible influence of Cd exposure on the development of atherosclerosis requires more research.

Effects of Cd ingestion on bones were investigated in female mice with $^{45}$Ca prelabelled skeletons who were fed Ca-deficient diets containing 0, 5, or 25 ppm Cd for 32 days (*498*). While the 0 ppm controls exhibited an immediate decrease in fecal Ca excretion in response to the Ca-deficient diet, mice consuming Cd increased their fecal Ca excretion. This indicates that Cd, in conjunction with a Ca-deficient diet, had an early, direct effect on bone. Analyses of the skeletons of the mice revealed that the high Cd dose significantly decreased skeletal weight. This may be similar to the effects of itai-itai disease in postmenopausal Japanese women exposed to Cd.

# HALOGENS

## Bromine

Data on the natural occurrence of bromine in the environment and its toxicity have been summarized and discussed by Flury and Papritz (*499*). Bromine occurs naturally in foods, with concentrations as high as 72 mg/kg being reported in celery. However, most foods contain ≤10 mg Br/kg fresh weight, and average daily intakes have been estimated to range from 7.6 to 16.6 mg/person. Mammalian toxicity of Br appears to be low. Nevertheless, to avoid the risk of chronic toxicity, it has been recommended that drinking water Br levels not exceed 1 mg/L. A method utilizing unsuppressed ion chromatography with UV detection has been developed for the detection of bromide ions in foods which have been microwave digested in a sealed vessel (*500*).

## Chlorine

A case–control study involving 327 cases of bladder cancer and 261 other-cancer controls (matched for age and sex) was conducted in Colorado to investigate the association between bladder cancer and drinking water disinfection methods (*501*). (Colorectal and lung cancer patients were excluded from the controls because of previously reported associations with chlorinated surface waters.) After adjustment of the data for cigarette smoking, tap water and coffee consumption, and medical factors, years of exposure to chlorinated surface water were significantly associated with risk for bladder cancer. An odds ratio of 1.8 was calculated for those with >30 years' exposure as compared to those with 0 exposure.

In order to obtain a more accurate assessment of the association between chlorinated compounds in drinking water and carcinogenicity, a method must be devised for determining the mutagenicity and/or carcinogenicity of the water. Koivusalo et al. (*502*) discussed various approaches to this problem and evaluated their use in analyses of drinking water in Finland. Although concentrations of chloroform and other trihalomethanes have been used to estimate mutagenic potential, only about 10% of the chlorinated organic compounds in water are volatile and some of the non-volatile compounds are potent mutagens. Furthermore, all chlorinated waters are not equivalent in mutagenicity: Finnish surface waters, for example, contain high levels of humic substances and therefore higher levels of chlorinated, mutagenic substances than drinking water in some other

areas. Therefore, drinking water mutagenicity, rather than simply the use of chlorine dininfectants, may be a more appropriate measure to compare with incidence of cancer.

Formation of mutagens by chlorination of fractions of humic water has been investigated (*503*). The humic acid fraction produced slightly more mutagenicity than the fulvic acid fractions. But, because there are more fulvic acids than humic acids in natural waters, chlorinated fulvic acids contribute more to mutagenicity than the humic acids. One of the most potent mutagenic compounds detected in chlorinated water is called MX [3-chloro-4-dichloromethyl-5-hydroxy-2(5H)-franone]. Ogawa et al. (*504*) described a GC method with electron capture detection for determination of this compound in water samples.

Chlorine is also a widely used disinfectant in food-processing plants. To determine its uptake by chicken frankfurters from a chlorinated recycling brine used for chilling, frankfurters with and without a processing casing were immersed in water containing 1.1–11.3 mM hypochlorite for 1, 4, or 24 hours (*505*). Chlorine was quickly taken up by the frankfurters, increasing with increasing hypochlorite concentrations and with time. Casing retarded the uptake of chlorine at higher concentrations but was not an effective chlorine barrier. This method can be used to determine chlorine uptake during actual processing conditions in order to ascertain whether any health risk is involved.

## Fluorine

An incident of mass fluoride poisoning occurred in a small Eskimo settlement in Alaska in 1992 when a malfunction occurred in the fluoridation equipment for the drinking water supply (*506,507*). At least 296 people were poisoned, reporting symptoms of nausea, vomiting, diarrhea, abdominal pain, and paresthesias. One death occurred—a 41-year-old male who consumed an estimated 17.9 mg fluoride/kg—and one person with severe symptoms was evacuated to a regional hospital. It was estimated that at the peak of contamination the water supply contained 150 ppm fluoride (compared to the recommended range of fluoridation of 0.7–1.2 ppm) and the minimum dose causing symptoms was 0.3 mg/kg (not including fluoride in water consumed in prepared foods). Although the estimated serum half-life of fluoride (from the hospitalized patient) was 3.5 h, symptoms of disordered mineral homeostasis and cellular damage, including abnormalities in serum magnesium, phosphorus, and lactate dehydrogenase concentrations, persisted for at least 19 days in some victims.

A recent review by Spittle (*508*) discussed available data on allergy and hypersensitivity to fluoride. Although some other recent articles concluded that the evidence of allergic reactions to fluorides was unconvincing, this paper described cases of urticaria, contact dermatitis, and stomatitis occurring in response to fluoride and recurring with appropriate challenges. Therefore, it appears that there are some individuals who are hypersensitive to fluoride.

Other reports from populations exposed to fluoridated water or to water with somewhat elevated levels of fluoride indicate that fluoride ingestion may have other adverse effects. A higher prevalence in diffuse opacities (29% compared to 14%) in the enamel of teeth of 4- to 5-year-olds was found in English children living in a community with fluoridated water (1 ppm F) than in children residing in a community without fluoridated water (<0.2 ppm F) (*509*). None of the defects observed were of cosmetic significance.

Ten of 25 young Indian adults who had been drinking water containing 2–13 ppm fluoride since birth and had evidence of dental and skeletal fluorosis, were also found to have impaired glucose tolerance (*510*). Compared to controls consuming water containing <1 ppm F and to the 15 subjects with normal glucose tolerance, the 10 subjects had significantly higher fasting serum fluoride levels, higher fasting serum immunoreactive insulin, and lower fasting glucose. Six months after being provided with drinking water containing <1 ppm F, serum fluoride levels fell significantly and these abnormalities in glucose tolerance were reversed.

Because elevated fluoride consumption decreases fertility in most animal species studied, an epidemiological study was initiated to compare fertility in white women living in areas with high fluoride levels in drinking water (≥3 ppm F) with that of women living in nearby areas with lower fluoride exposure (*511*). Analysis of data over an 18-year period, with corrections for socio-demographic variables, demonstrated a decrease in annual total fertility rate with increasing fluoride levels. Although this study attempted to eliminate or minimize sources of error such as inaccurate data, selection bias, and improper analytical methods, caution should be used in interpreting results because they are based on population data rather than on data for individual women.

Tea is one of the few foods which is a good source of fluoride. In an investigation of the effects of methods for preparation of tea infusions and of the type of tea leaves on fluoride levels in tea, concentrations of fluoride in tea were found to vary from 1.55–3.21 mg/L (*512*). Leaching of fluoride was found to reach a maximum at 6 minutes of brewing and was greatest when leaf particle sizes were smallest (leaf powder). Addition of milk after brewing of tea (English style) did not affect fluoride concentrations but addition of milk and subsequent boiling (Indian style) did reduce fluoride levels. It was estimated that a person consuming 2–6 cups of tea/day would ingest 0.3–1.9 mg fluoride.

## Iodine

Prevalence of thyroid dysfunction was assessed in 1061 adults in 5 coastal areas of Japan that produce iodine-rich seaweed (*513*). Among those testing negative for thyroid autoantibody, hypothyroidism was more prevalent in subjects with elevated iodide concentrations in morning urine (≥75 µmol/L). These subjects had higher serum levels of thyroglobulin and TSH and lower levels of free thyroxin but no visible evidence of goiter. In 2 subjects who restricted their kelp ingestion for 2–2.5 months, urinary iodide levels decreased to about 2–3% of the initial value along with marked reductions in TSH, thyroglobulin, and thyroid volume, and an increase in free thyroxin. These results demonstrate that excessive intakes of iodine can cause development of hypothyroidism.

Consumption of excessive amounts of iodine by a population may also result in an increased incidence of thyrotoxicosis as was observed in Vigo, a coastal, urban area in northwestern Spain (*514*). Because this part of Spain is considered iodine-deficient, the use of iodized salt was made mandatory in 1985. However, previous studies had shown that residents of Vigo consumed sufficient amounts of iodine prior to supplementation. During the 5 years after supplementation was started, residents in this city had an average incidence rate of thyrotoxicosis of 7.68/100,000 as compared to a rate of 3.1/100,000 in the 5 years before supplementation. Both nodular and diffuse goiters were observed in the cases of thyrotoxicosis.

Iodination of cheese during cheese-making was investigated in the manufacture of Edam cheese (*515*). Iodate in salt baths did not diffuse to a large extent into cheese during ripening, apparently because the iodate was reduced and bound to proteins. On the other hand, iodide added to the culture did homogeneously iodinate the cheese, with about 10% of the iodide added being found in the cheese. Little of this iodide subsequently leached out in the salt bath.

A survey of retail whole and 2% milk samples collected across Canada revealed that mean iodine levels were 302 (range of 128–1304 µg/L) and 292 µg/L (range of 87–888 µg/L), respectively (*516*). These values are not significantly different from those measured several years earlier, prior to the ban on the use of ethylenediamine dihydroiodide (EDDI) to prevent foot rot in cattle. Apparently this ban has had little effect on iodine levels in milk. Iodine intakes of up to 1 mg/day are considered safe for most individuals and so most people would probably not exceed this limit by consuming milk. However, those drinking a lot of milk and also consuming significant amounts of seafood may approach or exceed this recommended intake.

Nine laboratories participating in an AOAC International/International Dairy Federation collaborative study on a liquid chromatographic method for the determination of iodine in milk concluded that the method performed well; the method was adopted first action by AOAC International (517). Milk samples were first filtered and then the filtrate was subjected to reversed phase ion-pair LC with electrochemical detection. Effects of solvent type on determination of total iodine in milk powder by inductively coupled plasma mass spectrometry were investigated and the use of an ammonia solution rather than nitric acid was found to give superior results (518). Three different neutron activation analysis methods were developed for the detection of ppb levels of iodine in foods (519). One of these methods, involving bismuth sulfide coprecipitation followed by radiochemical purification, provided the best detection limit and the highest precision.

# LEAD

## Occurrence and Detection in Foods

Concentrations of lead were monitored in Manchego cheese during various steps in the cheese-making process (520). An average of 210 µg Pb/kg dry weight was detected in the raw milk (a mixture of cow's and goat's milks), with a similar concentration in the finished cheese. At some steps in the process, Pb concentrations increased somewhat, perhaps due to outside contamination. However, average consumption of 5.3 g of this cheese/day (as estimated in Spain) would contribute only 0.57 µg Pb/day.

Chickens living in a polluted environment (near industrial sites or roads) may acquire a significant body burden of lead and this may in turn be passed on to consumers of chicken. Because garlic has been reported to antagonize lead toxicity in animals, an experiment was designed to determine whether feeding garlic to chickens would prevent lead deposition in their tissues or remove lead already consumed (521). Five groups of chickens were orally dosed as follows: (A) 5 mg Pb/kg body weight/day; (B) 5 mg Pb/kg/day together with 2 g homogenized garlic/kg/day; (C) same lead and garlic doses as group B but lead was administered during the first week and garlic during the second week; (D) distilled water; and (E) garlic only. Pb concentrations of 10 and 23.35 mg/kg fresh weight were accumulated by the chickens in group A in muscle and liver tissue, respectively. Garlic reduced these levels by 40% and 63%, respectively, in group B birds and by 61% and 78.5%, respectively, in group C birds. It appears that garlic feeding is a potentially useful way of reducing lead contamination in chickens. No information was given on the organoleptic properties of these treated chickens.

A survey of 55 samples of different species of dried fish from markets in Nigeria revealed relatively high levels of lead contamination (522). In comparison with the WHO limit of 8 ppm and the British standard of 5 ppm, the averages of 8.99 ppm in whole fish and 6.7 ppm in muscle tissue in the Nigerian fish were certainly too high. These concentrations were also much higher than Pb contamination in fish reported from other African countries. These high lead levels are apparently the result of unregulated waste disposal, particularly from some industrial sites.

Three *Spirulina* and 5 eukaryotic algal food products obtained in Spain have been analyzed for nutrient composition and for heavy metal content (523). Although lead concentrations were relatively high in some samples, these seaweed products are usually consumed as supplements, and therefore a normal dose would not contain an excessive amount of lead. However some lots of these products did approach or exceed the proposed maximum permissible lead concentration (2 ppm), including *Chlorella*, 8.1 ppm; *Spirulina*, 1.3–6.7 ppm; dulce (*Palmaria palmata*), 28 ppm; and *Fucus*, 0.5–163 ppm. Continued monitoring of these products is recommended.

A method utilizing atomic absorption spectrometry with electrothermal atomization with palladium–magnesium nitrate as a modifier has been developed for the determination of lead in mussels (524).

Determination of ultratrace levels of lead in infant formula has been accomplished by isotope dilution inductively coupled plasma mass spectrometry (525). Detection limit was estimated to be 0.1 ng/g infant formula. The method produced results in good agreement with certified values in standard reference milk powder.

Two papers (526,527) reviewed recent data on lead in wines with attention to sources of lead—in vineyard soils, uptake of lead by plants, deposition on grapes from industrial sources or emissions from cars, and leaching from brass fittings on winery equipment, from lead capsules used to cover the wine bottles, and from leaded crystal decanters. Lead levels in wines have been steadily declining as we have come to realize the significant adverse effects caused by lead exposure and have taken steps to reduce sources of lead in the environment. Organolead compounds in wines have been identified by capillary GC/microwave-induced plasma atomic emission spectrometry (*528*). Analyses of 14 wines from southern France revealed that all contained trimethyllead at concentrations of 8.1–112 ng/L. Ethyllead was generally found in older wines and in wines made from grapes grown near industrial areas.

Moonshine whiskey produced in illegal stills, often automobile radiators with lead-soldered parts, continues to cause lead poisoning in some people in rural Southern communities. Nine such patients with elevated blood lead levels were identified in a hospital in Alabama (*529*). All case patients had been evaluated at a hospital for alcohol-related conditions and all reported a history of moonshine ingestion of 0.2–1.4 L/day. Blood lead levels ranged from 16 to 259 µg/dL. Analysis of 3 moonshine samples revealed lead concentrations of 7000, 76,000, and 97,000 µg/dL compared to <0.1 µg/dL in municipal water from the county where the hospital is located. The two most contaminated samples had been distilled in automobile radiators.

Seventy calcium supplements available in Canada and the USA were analyzed for lead contamination (*530*). The supplements were categorized into bonemeal, dolomite, chelated calcium (lactate, gluconate, etc.), natural-source calcium carbonate (limestone derived from fossilized oyster shells), and refined calcium carbonate (produced in a laboratory). Mean lead concentrations, normalized to 800 mg Ca, for the different categories were, respectively, 11.33, 4.17, 1.64, 6.05, and 0.92 µg. For comparison, lead levels in milk have been reported to average 0.71 µg/800 mg Ca. Little inter-lot variability was noted in lead levels in most types of supplements, but this was not true for bonemeal, with a range of 2.85–42.74 µg Pb/800 mg Ca. Bonemeal, dolomite, and oyster shell calcium, if used as the primary calcium source, could easily supply excess lead, especially in the diets of children.

Two types of "natural" folk remedies, hai ge fen (*531*) and azarcon (*532*) contain high levels of lead and have been associated with lead poisoning incidents. Hai ge fen (clamshell powder), part of a Chinese herbal preparation, was found to contain 225 ppm Pb and 600 ppm arsenic. Tea made from the herbal preparation contained 301 mg Pb/L and 64 µg As/L. After consuming a daily cup of this tea for several weeks, a patient had a blood Pb level of 76 µg/dL. Azarcon is a lead tetroxide salt, containing 96% lead, used by Mexicans and Mexican–Americans for treatment of digestive problems. In toxicological studies with rats, pure lead tetroxide and azarcon caused somewhat different effects, although both were quite toxic.

The source of elevated lead levels in household drinking water is often traced to the pipes carrying the water. Several recent cases of lead poisoning detected in children in Arizona and southern California occurred in households using bulk-stored water (*533*). Water drawn from the bulk storage tanks at the homes was found to contain 450–1050 ppb Pb (EPA drinking water standard, 15 ppb). Testing of the water as delivered in trucks by the supplier revealed no excess lead; the problem was finally traced to brass fittings on the storage tanks at the homes.

Release of lead from crystal decanters containing 24% lead oxide was investigated using new and used decanters and a dry sherry (pH 3.55) as the test liquid (*534*). During storage for 2 months, 50, 163, and 1410 µg Pb/L was leached from decanters used for 20 years, for 10 years, or unused, respectively. When the new decanter was used in 3 successive two-month testing periods, significantly less lead was leached during each period: 1410, 330, and 150 µg/L. It appears that after sufficient aging, leaded crystal may be safe for adults to use.

Studies in two isolated rural Mexican communities demonstrated that blood lead levels in women in the villages were significantly related to storage of food and cooking in lead-glazed ceramics and to meat and cheese consumption (*535*). The correlation with meat and cheese may be due to the fact that these foods were prepared or cooked in lead-glazed pots. Blood lead levels were increased by 71–72% in women who used lead-glazed ceramics as compared to those who did not. A quick color test has been evaluated as a screening tool for determining leachable lead from ceramicware (*536*). This test has a sensitivity of 1–5 µg Pb/mL when used for testing undecorated wares. Of 197 pieces tested, 95% had leachable lead at ≥2 µg/mL.

## Toxicological Effects

Papers from a 1991 international neurotoxicology conference on "New Dimensions of Lead Neurotoxicity" have been published in an issue of *NeuroToxicology* (*537*). Recent advances in molecular, biochemical, cellular, neurophysiological, and neuropharmacological mechanisms of lead toxicity were discussed. Other participants summarized research on developmental, cognitive, neurobehavioral, and sensory effects of low levels of lead in children and in laboratory animals. Approaches to the assessment of toxic effects in exposed children, cellular targets of lead, and trends in the management of lead poisoning were other important topics considered.

Numerous other recent reviews summarized and discussed available data on various aspects of lead toxicity. Carrington et al. (*538*) presented a hazard assessment for lead based on neurobehavioral, cognitive, and electrophysiological deficits observed in children with blood lead levels as low as 10 μg/dL. Elevated blood pressure and other adverse effects in adults have been observed at blood lead levels of 30 μg/dL. Lead ingestion rates producing these blood lead levels were estimated to be 60 (for children of ages ≤6 years), 150 (children >6 years old), 250 (pregnant women), and 750 (other adults) μg/day. Provisional tolerable daily intakes for lead were calculated for these age groups, respectively, as 0.67, 1.67, 2.77, and 8.33 μg Pb.

Lockitch (*539*) reviewed environmental sources of lead (dust, water, paint chips, folk remedies, food supplements, food preparation utensils) and various toxic effects of lead. With severe or chronic exposure, lead causes hematological, gastrointestinal, and neurological dysfunction and may also lead to chronic nephropathy, hypertension, and reproductive impairment. Less severe exposures are associated with poor pregnancy outcome, impaired neurobehavioral development, reduced stature in children, and high blood pressure in adults.

Leggett (*540*) presented an age-specific kinetic model for lead metabolism in humans. The model was originally developed for the International Commission on Radiological Protection for calculating exposures to radionuclides in the environment (including isotopes of lead). Additional features were added to the model to take into account the chemical effects of lead and to include physiological and environmental data on its reactions. In addition, the model has a modular design so that specific parameters or model components can be modified to incorporate new information or address specific problems. Transport of lead between compartments is assumed to follow linear, first-order kinetics. The model has been shown to be consistent with human data from persons exposed to Pb under a variety of experimental and natural conditions.

Evidence relating elevated blood lead levels and high blood pressure in recent epidemiological studies of the general population and of occupational cohorts was explored by Hertz-Picciotto and Croft (*541*). Data from different studies were not pooled because of numerous differences in protocols and information gathered by the various researchers. Rather, evidence was evaluated and

methodology critiqued and recommendations were made for future studies to highlight critical areas where more information is needed and to suggest more in-depth approaches which might lead to more definitive results. Considered overall, the data suggest that increased body burdens of lead have a small but significant effect on blood pressure and that decreasing exposure to lead should reduce cardiovascular disease.

In a recent review considering the mechanism of lead toxicosis, Donaldson and Knowles (*542*) summarized data from several studies demonstrating that a number of biological effects of lead involve peroxidative changes in tissues. Arachidonate appears to be the principal source of these tissue peroxides while glutathione acts as a protectant. Pb-induced alterations in arachidonate metabolism may also cause changes in structure and function of cell membranes, thereby adversely affecting physiological processes.

In a delightfully literary and comprehensive discussion of cell culture models for lead toxicity, Tiffany-Castiglioni (*543*) described the history of the use of neuronal and glial cells and tumor derived cell lines in toxicity investigations. In the early exploratory phase, cells were challenged with massive amounts of lead (50–500 μM) and lead uptake and general toxicity to different cell types were studied. Then, during the expansion phase, subcellular targets (such as membranes, enzymes, Ca-mediated processes) of lead were examined and more biologically relevant doses were used. Now, in the intensification phase of cell culture studies, molecular targets of Pb toxicity are being scrutinized to elucidate the effects of Pb on neuritogenesis and/or synaptogenesis. Some cells, such as astroglia, adapt to and tolerate the presence of intracellular lead. The mechanism for this tolerance to Pb should be another area of intensive research.

In order to assess the strength of reported negative associations between cognitive functions in children and exposure to low levels of lead, Schwartz (*544*) used meta-analytical techniques to examine data from four cross-sectional studies and from three longitudinal studies relating blood lead levels to full-scale IQ. A highly significant correlation was observed between IQ and lead exposure, with an increase from 10 to 20 μg Pb/dL blood associated with a decrease of 2.6 IQ points. There was no evidence that this effect was limited to disadvantaged children and no evidence of a threshold down to blood concentrations of 1 μg/dL. Experiments with primates have also demonstrated an adverse effect of lead at concentrations of 10 μg/dL on cognitive functions.

A cross-sectional study of 139 children (7–9 years old) in Mexico City investigated the relationship between blood lead levels and neurobehavioral development (*545*). Mean blood lead was 19.4 µg/dL, with individual values ranging from about 7 to 40 µg/dL. A significant negative trend was noted between blood lead concentrations and full-scale IQ. Moreover, children with higher lead levels performed more poorly on psychometric tests and had poorer educational attainment than those with lower lead levels.

In another study of cognitive effects of lead, word recognition abilities were assessed in 636 New Zealand children (8–12 years old) and compared to their blood lead levels (*546*). After the data were adjusted for confounding covariates, children with blood lead levels ≥8 ppm had mean test scores which were 3 points lower than the mean scores of children with blood lead levels of 0–3 ppm. This is equivalent to about a 4–6 months' delay in word recognition ability in those with moderately elevated blood lead concentrations.

Lead also appeared to have an adverse effects on some aspects of attention measured with a neuropsychological test battery (*547*). Performance of 79 subjects (aged 19 and 20 years) on two of four attention factors (focus-execute and shift) was inversely related to dentin lead levels in deciduous teeth. Mean dentin lead concentration was 13.7 µg/g, with a range of 2.9–51.8 µg/g. This exposure to lead impaired the ability of these adolescents to select and respond to critical information and to shift focus adaptively. (These children grew up when the use of lead additives in gasoline was at its peak. Dentin lead levels in children who grew up a decade later averaged 3 µg/g.)

Some evidence indicates that the adverse effects of early exposure to high lead levels can be reversed. Of a group of 141 Danish children who had shown lead-related deficits in verbal intelligence and visuomotor coordination at age 8, in most cases no lead-related effects were observed when the children were retested at age 15 (*548*). However, children with a history of neonatal jaundice and relatively high lead exposure (dentin lead >18.7 µg/g) did exhibit mild neurobehavioral deficits in verbal IQ and visuomotor coordination when retested. These children may have an increased sensitivity to lead.

Twenty-eight children attending a kindergarten near a lead battery recycling factory in Taiwan were found to have elevated blood lead levels (average of 15.6 µg/dL) and IQ scores 7 points lower than those of a control group with 8 µg Pb/dL in blood (*549*). Two years after the factory closed the two groups were reexamined. Blood lead levels in the exposed and control groups declined to 8.5 and 7 µg/dL, respectively, and average IQ scores of the two groups were within 2.5 points.

These children were not iron deficient nor were they socioeconomically disadvantaged.

Relatively high lead exposures have also been associated with adverse effects on growth. Data on blood lead levels, growth, and socioeconomic factors were recorded for 111 Mexican children at 6 months and for 73 children at 18 months of age (*550*). Maternal blood lead (1–33 µg/dL) at 36 weeks' pregnancy was inversely related to head circumference of children at 6 and 18 months. Significant and negative relationships were also found between blood lead levels (means of 7.008 and 8.539 µg/dL in females and males) and height in 133 12- and 13-year-olds in Italy (*551*). Serum concentrations of gonadotropins and sex steroid hormones were not related to blood lead in females but were decreased in males with blood lead >9.9 µg/dL.

Data collected from 645 male participants (aged 43–90 years) during a longitudinal study on aging, when subjected to multivariate analysis, revealed a statistically significant and positive association between blood lead levels (range 4–26 µg/dL) and 24-hour urinary excretion of epinephrine (*552*). Non-significant negative associations were observed between 24-hour dopamine and 2-hour serotonin excretion and a nonsignificant positive association between blood lead and 24-hour excretion of norepinephrine was also observed. It appears that low levels of lead can affect epinephrine metabolism.

A comparison was made of the incidence of proteinuria in 900 women in a Yugoslavian town with low levels of lead contamination (blood lead averaged 5.1 µg/dL) with that in 602 women in a town with a lead smelter, refinery, and battery plant about 25 miles away (blood lead averaged 17.1 µg/dL) (*553*). An increased incidence of proteinuria was observed in women from the smelter town, with women in the upper tenth percentile of blood lead having an odds ratio of 4.5 for proteinuria ≥1+. This suggests that chronic exposure to lead may lead to renal dysfunction.

Numerous studies of workers occupationally exposed to lead have documented adverse neurobehavioral effects. One recent study found that the most highly exposed workers averaged scores 5–22% lower than reference groups on tests for manual dexterity and verbal memory/learning (*554*). Significant negative correlations were found between blood lead levels in exposed workers and motor and sensory nerve conduction velocity of the radial nerve (*555*). Examination of the nerve conduction velocities in large myelinated nerve fibers of two lead-exposed workers (blood lead levels averaged 74 and 93 µg/dL) demonstrated that the faster nerve fibers were more sensitive to lead than the slower fibers (*556*).

Chronic lead exposure in cynomolgus monkeys was found to induce ultrastructural alterations in the testis (*557*). Sixteen monkeys were assigned to a control group or to an exposure group (1500 µg lead acetate/kg body weight/day) with lead exposure occurring only during infancy, only during post-infancy, or during the whole lifetime of 9 years. Compared to the controls, the seminiferous epithelium of all treated animals was decreased in height and Sertoli cells contained elevated numbers of lysosomes and lipid droplets. Effects of these changes on fertility have not been determined.

# MERCURY

## Occurrence and Detection in Foods

A new source of mercury pollution in South America is the multitude of gold-miners who use tons of mercury to recover gold from low-grade ores and sediments. Some of this mercury is vaporized during heating of the mercury–gold amalgamate and other mercury is lost directly to the ground or water during each stage of the process. Miners are exposed directly to the mercury vapors as well as metallic mercury and residents in the mining areas and for many miles downstream are exposed to mercury-contaminated fish. Nico and Taphorn (*558*) analyzed fish from remote gold-mining regions in the Upper Cuyuní River system in Venezuela. In this preliminary report, data are presented on 9 species of fish indicating that they have accumulated low to moderate levels of mercury. These results may be conservative, however, because most of the fish analyzed were small and mercury concentrations in fish generally increase with increasing age and body size. Highest Hg concentration in muscle tissue (0.86 µg/g) was detected in a large aimara, a locally important food fish.

Fish in lakes in Canada and the northern USA in areas remote from point sources of pollution also have elevated levels of mercury. Driscoll et al. (*559*) investigated this problem in lakes in the Adirondack area of New York State. Mercury levels in yellow perch generally increased with age and size as has been reported from other lakes. However, compared to fish of the same species and age from lakes in Michigan, the New York fish had greater body burdens of mercury. A mercury level of 1.2 µg/g was detected in a 12-year-old fish. Generally, lakes with lower pHs and higher dissolved aluminum levels were associated with higher mercury levels in fish. Another characteristic of lakes which apparently influences fish contamination is the size of the lake. Bodaly et al. (*560*) found that methylation of mercury occurred faster in warmer water and, since smaller lakes reach higher temperatures than larger ones during the summer in Canada, they produce more bioavailable methyl mercury.

Seafood may also contain fairly high levels of mercury. A recent survey of 449 fish from the Canary Islands found that mercury ranged from 0.014 to 0.97 ppm in fresh fish and from 0.043 to 0.172 ppm in salted fish (*561*). An evaluation of different methods for digestion of fish prior to analysis indicated that treatment with a 1:1 mixture of nitric and sulfuric acids for 15 h at 45°C gave the best results. Sand flathead fish from Port Phillip Bay, Australia, were recently found to contain less than half the mercury of specimens of these fish collected about 15 years previously (0.23 vs. 0.5 ppm) (*562*).

Brown shrimp transferred from an uncontaminated area to a cage in a mercury-contaminated estuary, Lavaca Bay, Texas, were found to bioaccumulate mercury at the rate of 22 ppb/day (*563*). From an average baseline of 347 ppb, concentrations increased to 1170 ppb in 36 days. These levels were higher than those of the natural population of shrimp in this bay, indicating that the natural population is probably quite mobile.

About 65% of the world's cinnabar deposits are located in the Mt. Amiata area of Italy. Although mining activities in the area ceased in 1980, the surrounding area still probably contains elevated levels of mercury. In an analysis of vegetables grown in gardens near the old mines, Barghigiani and Ristori (*564*) found that only a few varieties contained appreciable contamination. These included lettuce and beets, both with large leaf areas to absorb airborne mercury, and rosemary and sage, both of which are evergreens and would be exposed for longer periods than plants with deciduous leaves. Consumption of vegetables from the most contaminated gardens could provide 290 µg Hg/week to an adult. However, the most long-lived people in Tuscany, and perhaps of Italy, live in the Mt. Amiata region.

Although most problems of mercury-contaminated foods or water can be traced to some type of mining or industrial activity, there appear to be some situations where the mercury finds its way naturally into groundwater. Some residential well water in a pristine, granitic Maine coastal area has been found to contain mercury in excess of the EPA's drinking water guideline of 2 µg/L (*565*). Mercury levels ranging from 0.04 to 6.2 µg/L were recorded in 26 well water samples. The mercury is apparently a natural part of the underlying rock and its presence in some wells depends on the well's construction, its depth, and the types of intersected fracture zones in the vicinity of the well.

Several recent papers detailed analytical methods for the determination of mercury in: fish and other biological specimens using cold vapor atomic absorption spectrophotometry (566,567); biological samples by cold vapor generation for inductively coupled argon plasma/atomic emission spectrometric analysis (568); and biological samples using dithiocarbamate extraction and gold (Au III) back extraction for concentration of mercury prior to determination by anodic stripping voltammetry (569).

## Toxicological Effects

Epidemiological and clinical features of minamata disease, caused by ingestion of fish contaminated with methyl mercury, were reviewed by Igata (570). Over 2000 people living near Minamata Bay in Japan were poisoned by mercury discharged into the bay from a chemical factory. Diagnosis of the disease is usually easy in those with more severe symptoms of peripheral neuropathy, but it is more difficult to correctly identify less severely affected persons. Following a survey to elicit all symptoms definitely associated with the disease, a multivariate analysis was performed to help distinguish mildly poisoned persons from those with many similar symptoms which were due to other conditions such as aging. Characteristics of this disease were compared to cases of methyl mercury poisoning occurring elsewhere in the world.

All forms of mercury are known to have nephrotoxic effects even though their primary effects may be on the nervous system. Recent advances in understanding the renal transport and toxicity of mercury were reviewed by Zalups and Lash (571). Four primary areas of research were discussed: renal tubular transport, accumulation and handling of mercury, mechanisms and target site specificity of mercury-induced renal injury, and the factors influencing the susceptibility to mercury-induced renal injury.

Data from the literature regarding the genotoxicity of 29 mercury-containing compounds were reviewed by De Flora et al. (572). Overall, mercury compounds generally fail to induce point mutations in bacterial assays but often exert clastogenic effects in eukaryotic cells. Inorganic mercury compounds also induce the generation of reactive oxygen species and glutathione depletion in mammalian cells. Methyl mercury and other ionizable organomercury compounds were often more potent in short-term genotoxicity tests than inorganic compounds. In most cases, however, cytogenetic studies monitoring the peripheral lymphocytes of persons exposed to mercury accidentally or occupationally do not demonstrate genotoxic effects. In vitro studies by Yamada et al. (573) provided evidence that methyl and ethyl mercury can act to potentiate the effects of known clastogens. It appears that these compounds interfere with repair of DNA lesions caused by the clastogens.

Monkeys (*Macaca fascicularis*) orally dosed with methyl mercury (50 µg Hg/kg body weight) for 6, 12, or 18 months were found to attain a steady-state of total mercury in blood of 1.1 µg/g in about 4 months (574). Elimination $T_{1/2}$ of mercury from blood and brain were 26 and 35 days, respectively. However, mercury persisted for much longer in some regions of the brain.

Exposure of adult female monkeys to 0, 50, 70, or 90 µg methyl mercury/kg/day prior to and during pregnancy resulted in a range of blood mercury levels in the infants of 1.04 to 2.46 ppm. When these offspring reached 7–9 years of age they were trained and tested on a spatial delayed alternation task (575). Performance of all treated monkeys was similar and so combined data for treated monkeys was compared to data from control (unexposed) monkeys. No significant differences were noted between control and treated monkeys in initial button training, number of sessions required to reach criterion on 0.1 sec delay, or in performance on the variable delay schedule. It appears that in utero exposure to methyl mercury did not adversely affect the spatial memory of adult monkeys.

# TIN

## Occurrence and Detection in Foods

A method utilizing inductively coupled plasma atomic emission spectrometry has been developed for the determination of tin in canned foods with a quantitation limit of 0.5 µg/g (576). Samples of canned fruits, vegetables, meat, and salmon were sequentially digested with nitric and hydrochloric acids and then analyzed for tin. For foods packed in tin plate cans, tin concentrations ranged from 19.8 (mushrooms) to 87.7 (apricots) µg/g. Asparagus in a high tin fillet can contained 81.2 µg/g and evaporated milk in a tin plate can with lacquered ends had 19.3 µg Sn/g. None of the foods packed in cans lacquered inside contained detectable tin except for a can of clams. In this case, examination of the can revealed some corrosion at the side seam.

Tributyltin antifouling paints have been widely used for boats and other apparatus in marine environments. Now, it is apparent that some shellfish and finfish are accumulating this compound. A survey of oysters from 53 Gulf of Mexico coastal sites was conducted to determine the extent of butyltin contamination in shell-fish (*577*). The geometric mean concentrations for 1989, 1990, and 1991 were 85, 30, and 43 ng Sn/g tissue, respectively. Generally during these three years, butyltin levels decreased in the less polluted areas but did not change substantially in the more polluted areas.

Surveys of shellfish collected along the Danish coast revealed that clams and mussels concentrated tributyltin, with the extent of organotin contamination related to proximity of marinas and commercial ship-ping activities (*578*). Organotin concentrations in *Mya arenaria* ranged from 0.65–11.85 μg/g and in *Littorina littorea* ranged from 0.6–2.2 μg/g. Seasonal variations were noted, with decreases related to removal of pleasure craft in the winter.

A method for the simultaneous determination of 4 organotin compounds in fish and shellfish by use of gas chromatography with a flame photometric detector has been developed by Tsunoda (*579*). Analyses of 8 species of seafood revealed the presence of dibutyltin (up to 0.674 μg/g), tributyltin (up to 0.669 μg/g), and triphenyltin (up to 0.186 μg/g). Some species were more frequently contaminated than others and some speci-mens contained more than one organotin compound.

Several other procedures have been described for the determination of total tin and tributyltin in biological tissues using graphite furnace atomic absorption spec-trometry (*580*); inorganic and organotin compounds in biological samples by liquid chromatography with in-ductively coupled plasma mass spectrometric detection (*581*); organotin compounds in biological samples using gas chromatography/helium atmospheric pressure microwave-induced plasma/atomic emission detection (*582*); and tin in biological materials by atomic absorp-tion spectrometry and neutron activation analysis (*583*).

## Toxicological Effects

Data-derived safety factors for bis(tri-*n*-butyltin)oxide (TBTO) were evaluated by Penninks (*504*). Lymphoid organs and lymphoid function in laboratory animals appear to be the most sensitive to the effects of TBTO toxicity. Therefore, estimated tolerable daily intakes (TDI) have been derived from results of these assays and the inclusion of a safety factor of 100 to allow for differences in metabolism and toxicity in humans. If a reduction in thymus weight is taken as the toxic effect, then the TDI would be 5 mg/kg/body weight and if impaired lymphoid function is the measure of toxicity, the TDI would be 0.25 mg/kg. Since TBTO is metabolized to dibutyltin compounds in the environment and in fish, it may be

more appropriate to calculate a combined TDI for both tri- and dibutyltin compounds.

In vitro experiments have demonstrated that tri-*n*-butyltin chloride is an effective promoter of morphologi-cal transformation and induces the expression of proliferin in C3H10T1/2 cells (*585*). Some other butyltin com-pounds, but not inorganic tin (stannic chloride), were also inducers of proliferin. These results suggest that butyltin compounds may act as tumor promoters.

Experiments with rats fed diets containing 1, 10, 50, 100, or 200 mg tin/kg (added as stannous chloride) for 28 days indicated that high dietary levels of this metal affected the iron, copper, and zinc status of the animals (*586*). Concentrations of these other metals were de-pressed in plasma and tibia and, in many cases, in the kidney and spleen as well. If effects of tin were similar in humans and if these results were extrapolated to humans, high dietary tin (75 mg/kg) could decrease plasma and tissue concentrations of iron, copper, and zinc up to 15%.

## OTHER MINERALS

### Asbestos

An epidemiological study involving 690 male Norwe-gian lighthouse keepers, exposed to asbestos in drinking water, investigated the incidence of cancer during a follow-up period from 1960 to 1991 (*587*). Drinking water was collected in cisterns from off asbestos–cement roofs, and large amounts of asbestos fibers (1760 to 71,350 million fibers/L) were detected in water samples. Analysis of incident cases of cancer in the whole cohort revealed no statistically significant excess risk for any type of cancer. But, among men exposed ≥20 years previously, 11 cases of stomach cancer occurred when only 4.57 were expected. No cases of malignant meso-thelioma were recorded. This study is limited by the fact that the rate of weathering of the asbestos tiles is unknown and therefore it is hard to accurately determine exposure. If weathering and fiber concentrations did not become significant until 1970, then further follow-up may be needed to detect carcinogenic effects of this exposure to asbestos.

### Chromium

Wastes generated during tanning are included in some commercially available organic fertilizers. How-ever, chromium, an important ingredient in the tanning process, may be present at very high concentrations in tannery meal. In a experiment to determine whether this chromium is taken up by plants, swiss chard was grown in soil amended with 5, 10, or 15% of a tannery waste fertilizer containing 5900 ppm Cr (*588*). Compared to control plants, those grown in 10 and 15% tannery waste fertilizer contained significantly higher Cr concentrations: averages of 4.9 and 6.9 ppm, respectively. At these high fertilizer application rates, swiss chard growth was also inhibited.

## Copper

Oysters collected in the Erhjin Chi estuary in Taiwan in 1989 were green in color due to high concentrations of copper (*589*). Copper levels in the surrounding water and sediment were elevated by large discharges from plants acid-cleaning scrap metal. Oysters bioaccumulated nearly 100 times as much copper as clams and mussels living in the same area. The highest copper concentration recorded was 4.401 mg Cu/g oyster tissue, with an average of 2.194 mg/g found for 85 samples analyzed. Oysters from other estuaries in Taiwan were found to have average copper levels ranging from 67.8–682 µg/g. For an average Taiwanese, consuming about 4 g oysters daily, ingestion of these contaminated oysters would result in a copper intake of about 12.6 mg/day, about 14 times the safe dietary levels suggested by FAO/WHO.

A rapid method using a fast-program slurry electrothermal atomic absorption procedure has been developed for the determination of copper in biscuits, bread, and cereals (*590*). Copper levels found in 16 such samples ranged from 1.05 to 2.96 µg/g.

## Magnesium

One of the high-incidence foci of motor neuron disease (amyotrophic lateral sclerosis) in the western Pacific is the Kii Peninsula in Japan. The etiology of this disease is believed to involve environmental factors, for example mineral deficiencies or excesses in local water and food supplies. Consequently, drinking water samples from several regions on the Kii Peninsula were analyzed for concentrations of eight metals (*591*). Some variation was observed in levels of all the metals but the only significant difference was observed with magnesium. The region of high incidence, Hohara, had significantly lower Mg concentrations (averages of 0.93–1.67 mg/L) than nearby regions (1.6–4.33 mg/L) with few or no cases of motor neuron disease. Of all the individual samples tested in Hohara, 84% had Mg levels <1.7 mg/L while this was true for only 7.5% of individual samples from

other regions. Low levels of Mg in drinking water are also found in regions of New Guinea with motor neuron disease but not in Guam, another high-incidence focus of the disease.

## Nickel

A puzzling case of chronic urticaria was observed in a 39-year-old woman who had a history of allergic rhinitis and contact dermatitis (*592*). Eight attacks of angioedema occurred within 3 months and the patient was not symptom-free for more than 2 days. A preference for nuts, lettuce, and licorice was noted in the patient's diet. Since the patient reacted strongly to skin tests with nickel sulfate, she was admitted to the hospital and put on an elimination diet. Urticaria resolved with this diet but reappeared with an oral challenge with nickel. Thereafter, the patient followed a nickel-restricted diet and has been free of skin lesions for more than a year.

An open, prospective trial, involving 90 patients with known contact sensitivity to nickel, tested the effects of a low nickel diet in reducing persistent episodes of dermatitis not triggered by cutaneous contact with nickel (*593*). Patients were advised to avoid foods with a high nickel content, such as bran, oats, soy, dried legumes, chocolate, nuts, and licorice. After 1–2 months on the diet, 58 subjects improved, 17 did not, and the remainder reported some possible benefit. Of 55 patients responding to a questionnaire after an average of 1.8 years' follow-up, 40 stated that their dermatitis definitely improved when they followed the diet. The evidence indicates that at least some nickel-sensitive people can benefit from a nickel-restricted diet.

A method utilizing differential pulse cathodic stripping voltammetry was developed for the determination of nickel in infant formulas (*594*). This method was rapid, inexpensive, and free of interferences often encountered in atomic absorption spectrometry analyses.

## Selenium

A commercial sewage-sludge plus cement-kiln dust product recommended for liming and fertilizing agricultural land was found to have a selenium content of 4.7 ppm. In an experiment to determine whether plants grown in soil containing this product would absorb excessive amounts of selenium, swiss chard was grown in pots containing 0, 5, or 10% of this sludge–cement dust mixture (*595*). (These application rates are probably well above what would normally be added to acidic agricultural soils.) Analyses of leaves from plants grown with 0, 5, or 10%

of the additive showed that they contained 0.03, 0.11, and 0.15 ppm Se, respectively.

Kashin–Beck disease is a degenerative osteoarticular disorder endemic to some selenium-deficient areas, particularly in China. Recently, an animal model of this disease has been developed by feeding mice a selenium-deficient diet along with fulvic acid supplemented drinking water (596). This dietary regime induced degeneration of the articular cartilage in the knees of mice. This model can be used to test the hypothesis that the production of superoxide radicals from fulvic acid and an inability of the body to remove these radicals because of Se deficiency is responsible for disease symptoms. In China, dietary Se supplementation and better drinking water have drastically reduced the number of cases of Kashin–Beck disease.

However, the margin of safety for selenium supplementation is small because high levels of dietary selenium also induce an increase in superoxide radicals. In vitro cultures of rat hepatocytes had decreased intracellular levels of reduced glutathione and increased oxygen consumption in the presence of added selenite (597). The superoxide ion and its reactive metabolites appeared to be involved in the cytotoxic effects of Se. Young rats fed diets containing 0.05, 0.4 (control level), 2.05, or 4.05 mg Se were found to be adversely affected by both high and low Se levels (598). Deficient animals had lower glutathione peroxidase levels while those given excess Se had decreased hepatic concentrations of retinol and retinyl palmitate (vitamin A) and decreased enzymatic antioxidant defenses.

## Thallium

Thallium is one of the most toxic of the heavy metals, probably because it has the same charge and an ionic radius similar to potassium, which has many critical functions in the body. It is not very often found in food or drinking water but its use as a rodenticide and in some technological applications allows for occasional serious incidents of contamination. Mulkey and Oehme (599) reviewed the chemistry of thallium, its occurrence and distribution, production and uses, and absorption, distribution, and excretion in the body. Clinical toxicology, diagnosis, and treatment of thallium poisoning were also discussed. Various mechanisms proposed to account for thallium's toxicity were evaluated.

## Vanadium

In a recent review, Dafnis and Sabatini (600) discussed the biochemistry and pathophysiology of vanadium. Vanadium is a widely distributed metal but is rarely present in high concentrations in living organisms, with one exception being a marine tunicate that can accumulate vanadium from sea water to an internal concentration of 1 M. From experience with miners, it has become evident that vanadium has a low toxicity when ingested but a high toxicity when inhaled. A variety of toxic effects have been described in humans, including dermatitis, respiratory symptoms, and effects on the cardiovascular and central nervous systems. On a cellular level, vanadate inhibits Na-K ATPase activity. Its effects on the kidney were also described along with a discussion of whether vanadium is involved in the pathogenesis of various renal diseases.

Léonard and Gerber (601) reviewed the available data on the mutagenicity, carcinogenicity, and teratogenicity of vanadium compounds. From various assays, it appears that vanadium is not clastogenic and is only weakly mutagenic. It does have marked mitogenic activity which may cause aneuploidy. Data are inadequate to assess the carcinogenicity of vanadium and its direct effects on development of the embryo or fetus. However, since it can interfere with mitosis, these effects are also a possibility.

Four vanadium compounds tested in human lymphocyte cultures in vitro did not induce structural chromosomal aberrations but did increase numerical aberrations and micronuclei (602). Examination of the micronuclei of affected cells with fluorescence in situ hybridization indicated that vanadium, indeed, has aneuploidogenic potential.

# RADIONUCLIDES IN FOODS

## Occurrence and Detection in Foods

During a 6-year period (1987–1992) foods from a hospital kitchen in northeastern Poland were monitored for plutonium (603). Most of the foods were purchased from local shops and came from the local area except for some spices, beverages, and citrus fruits. Estimated annual intake of $^{239,240}$Pu was highest in the first year (774 mBq) after the Chernobyl accident and declined to a low of about 90 mBq in the last year of the study. During the first two years, large daily fluctuations in plutonium levels were observed which may reflect variable levels of external contamination. Assuming that only $10^{-5}$ of the Pu present as an external contaminant is absorbed and that $10^{-3}$ of Pu in root crops is absorbed after ingestion, approximately 0.02–2.0 mBq

Pu would have been assimilated from food during this period. However, only a very small fraction of human exposure occurs through food; most Pu is inhaled from the air.

A survey of 16 types of foods from different provinces in China revealed that plutonium and neptunium concentrations were highest in tea and spinach (*604*). Concentrations of these radioactive elements in the various foods ranged from 0.0001–0.001 Bq/kg. While radioactivity in the same types of foods from different regions of the country differed, not enough samples were analyzed to distinguish a pattern.

Field measurements to determine the environmental behavior of radionuclides deposited in southern Bavaria after the Chernobyl accident were summarized by Jacob et al. (*605*). Studies on the fate of radioactive ruthenium, iodine, and barium were continued for several weeks after the explosion while studies on cesium were continued for a longer period because of its longer half-life. Natural deposition on plants was measured and experiments were conducted to determine the effects of deposition at different times in the plants' life cycles to estimate carryover into edible parts of the foods. Transfer of radio-iodine and cesium into milk was also investigated.

Effectiveness of sprinkling in removing the $^{134}$Cs applied to wheat plants by foliar aspersion was investigated in a series of experiments in Italy (*606*). In general, the shorter the time between contamination and sprinkling, the more radioactivity was removed: sprinkling within 8 hours of contamination removed >70% of the radiocesium applied. Strawberry plants were found to rapidly absorb a foliar application of radiocesium, with >90% of the isotope incorporated into the plant (and 44% into the berries) within 8 weeks (*607*). On the other hand, only 44% of the radioactive strontium applied to the strawberry plants was absorbed into the plant and none was detected in the fruit. It appears that radioactive cesium liberated from a nuclear accident is much more likely than strontium to be taken up and translocated to edible parts of the plant.

Transfer coefficients of $^{137}$Cs from feed into chicken meat and eggs were determined by Voigt et al. (*608*). In different experiments, laying hens were provided with feed containing 1880 Bq/kg from contaminated grass pellets or with feed containing 1100 Bq/kg from contaminated wheat produced after the Chernobyl accident. Transfer factors from grass to eggs, to leg meat, and to breast meat were calculated as 0.2, 1.2, and 1.6 day/kg, respectively. Transfer factors from contaminated wheat were about twice as high. Addition of 0.66 g ammonium-ferro-cyano-ferrate/kg of feed reduced the

transfer from grass by a factor 3 to 4 and the transfer from wheat by a factor of 8 to 14.

Radiocesium levels in muscle tissue of roe deer in Germany were measured during 1986–1990 (*609*). Highest $^{137}$Cs concentrations were detected in 1987 at 700 Bq/kg muscle, but by 1989–1990 radioactivity had decreased to levels observed before the Chernobyl accident. $^{134}$Cs levels also peaked in 1987 but at lower levels because of the shorter half-life of this isotope. Radiocesium levels in the deer varied according to the season, probably reflecting the types of plants and mushrooms the deer were consuming.

Following the Chernobyl accident, there has been a great deal of concern about the transfer of radionuclides from soil or air to vegetation, to cows, and finally to milk. Several recent research projects have provided data on this process. Radiocesium concentrations in soil in different areas of Belarus were compared with radioactivity in milk from cows grazing on fields in small family farms in these areas (*610*). Transfer factors, the ratios of $^{137}$Cs in milk (Bq/L) to that in soil (kBq/m²) were calculated for soils with 37 to >1480 kBq/m². The soil–milk transfer factors were found to decrease with increasing soil contamination. This may reflect a non-linear uptake of $^{137}$Cs by plants.

Transfer of $^{137}$Cs from feed to cow's milk was investigated by assaying contamination in grass and other fodder components from 10 farms in northeastern Italy and comparing it to milk from cows on these farms (*611*). At the time of this study, 2 years after the Chernobyl accident, natural pasture grass from one field still contained 2285 Bq/kg dry matter of radioactivity. Transfer factors, ratios of radioactivity in milk to radioactivity consumed in feed each day, ranged from 0.0028 to 0.0512 d/L. The farm with the highest transfer factor supplemented the usual grass and hay feed with about 30% maize silage. It may be that radioactivity in maize silage is more bioavailable to cows.

Another experiment in Italy measured the transfer of $^{90}$Sr, $^{134}$Cs, and $^{137}$Cs from feed into milk of a cow fed for 14.5 weeks with alfalfa hay contaminated by the Chernobyl accident (*612*). Transfer coefficients calculated for the 3 isotopes, respectively, were 0.0008, 0.0029, and 0.0031 d/L. Radioactivity was transferred from feed to milk in a two-phase process with a fast biological half-life of about 1–2 days followed by a longer half-life of 8–37 days. Biological elimination could be described by a two-compartment model for radiocesium and by a one-compartment model for strontium.

More than 150 data sets from 11 countries giving time-dependent concentrations of $^{131}$I and $^{137}$Cs in feed and milk of cows after the Chernobyl accident were evaluated by Kirchner (*613*) using a minimal compartmental modelling approach. Transfer of cesium was adequately described by a three-compartment model while for iodine, a two-compartment model was adequate for most of the data. Weathering half-lives for iodine and cesium on plants appeared to be 9.1 and 11.1 days, respectively, and equilibrium feed-to-milk transfer factors were calculated as 0.0034 and 0.0054 d/L, respectively. These transfer coefficients were compared with pre-Chernobyl estimates and environmental and dairy-related factors known to influence transfer factors were discussed.

Abbott and Rood (*614*) developed a dynamic food chain model and computer code, COMIDA, to estimate radionuclide concentrations in agricultural products after an acute fallout event. This program was used to estimate yearly harvest concentrations for 5 human crop types and integrated concentrations for 4 animal products. The model includes seasonal transport processes, discrete soil and vegetation compartments, and estimates for assimilation into animals. Results obtained with this computer model were compared with other models. This model will be used by the Department of Energy to evaluate accidental releases from nuclear power plants.

Because measurement of $^{90}$Sr contamination of foods is so time consuming, Yu (*615*) recommended that imported foods be examined for $^{131}$I and that these levels be used to estimate radiostrontium contaminations. Possible accident scenarios were proposed which may release different relative amounts of these isotopes. Then, by using a dynamic food chain model, relative activities of the two isotopes in specific foods can be calculated and estimates can be made of $^{90}$Sr concentrations from the measured levels of $^{131}$I. Stella et al. (*616*) proposed the use of two inorganic exchangers, consisting of partially reduced tin dioxide and normal copper chromate, for the radiochemical isolation and purification of $^{90}$Sr from milk. The use of both of these exchangers is effective in removing radiobarium interference.

Aside from accidents, $^{90}$Sr may be released to the environment from liquid effluent releases from nuclear power–generating facilities. Numerous nuclear reactors are situated along the shores of the Great Lakes and these along with 5 uranium mines, and a number of uranium mills, nuclear fuel fabrication and conversion facilities, and radioactive waste management facilities are undoubtedly a source of radioactive contamination. Since all the Great Lakes eventually flow into Lake Ontario, specimens of brown trout were collected in Lake Ontario and $^{90}$Sr levels in their skeletons were compared to those from fish in another New York lake with no nearby nuclear facilities (*617*). Average $^{90}$Sr levels in the bones of fish from the two lakes, respectively, averaged 10.755 and 2.81×10$^{-7}$. These results were discussed relative to the different radioactive inputs into the lakes.

$^{63}$Nickel is also produced in nuclear reactors by activation of nickel in structural steel. Cod, herring, and sprat from the Baltic Sea were analyzed for radionickel (*618*) in a study to determine whether this radionuclide accumulates in fish. Contrary to the uniform distribution of stable nickel ($^{62}$Ni) throughout the fish, the radio-isotope was concentrated in the fillet with skin and scale. It appears that radionickel was adsorbed to the surface of the fish and remained there in the mucus. Specific activity of the nickel (radioactive/stable forms) in cod was particularly high, suggesting that the fish spend a lot of time in the vicinity of nuclear power plant discharges.

One of the products of the radioactive decay of uranium is $^{210}$Pb. Therefore in a study of radioactive contamination of foods, radioactive lead levels were measured in 13 vegetables grown in gardens about 1 km and 5 km from a uranium mine in Brazil and in a garden at some distance away (control) (*619*). Levels of radioactivity in garden vegetables grown 5 km from the mine were nearly the same as those grown in the control garden. However, radioactive lead levels were about 8-fold higher in turnips and 2–3-fold higher in many of the other vegetables grown near the mine. Interestingly, no differences were observed in radioactivity in carrots or manioc grown at the three sites. Weisshaar (*620*) described a procedure for the determination of $^{210}$Pb in a variety of foods by measuring the beta-emission of the daughter nuclide $^{210}$Bi. In a survey of foods from German markets, the samples most highly contaminated with this isotope were tea, lettuce, spinach, and kale. Average daily intake of radioactive lead from a hospital diet was 0.07 Bq.

## Biological and Toxicological Effects

Previous reports have indicated an increase in thyroid cancer in some areas of Belarus which received heavy fallout from the Chernobyl nuclear accident in 1986. An examination of the recorded incidence of childhood leukemia in this area revealed no significant differences between the pre-Chernobyl era (1979–1985) and the post-Chernobyl period (1986–1991) (*621*). Differences were still not significant when data for males and females were examined separately. However, it is known that some cancers have a long latency period and monitoring of this population will be continued.

Diet samples collected as duplicate portions and in a market basket survey in Japan were analyzed for $^{226}$Ra and for four stable alkaline earth metals (622). Estimated daily intakes of radium ranged from 32 mBq in Kyushu in the southwest to 20–21 mBq in Chubu and Kita-Nippon in the northeast. This may reflect geological differences in the different regions. In terms of food sources of radium, bean, animal, and fish products supplied 37%, grains, oils, and other foods, 30%, fruits and vegetables, 24%, and eggs, milk, and milk products, 9% of dietary radium.

Marmosets gavaged with mixtures of neptunium and plutonium citrates were found to absorb 0.001–0.002 of the administered dose (623). Gastrointestinal absorption of plutonium and americium in potatoes (bound to phytate or citrate) was 0.003 and 0.0006 of the dose, respectively. Where comparable studies were available, humans appear to absorb less of these compounds than laboratory animals. But data are not available on human absorption of these elements from vegetable foods.

## LITERATURE CITED

1. Ahmed, F.E., D. Hattis, R.E. Wolke, and D. Steinman. Risk assessment and management of chemical contaminants in fishery products consumed in the USA. *J. Appl. Toxicol.* 13:395–410 (1993).

2. Ahmed, F.E., D. Hattis, R.E. Wolke, and D. Steinman. Human health risks due to consumption of chemically contaminated fishery products. *Environ. Health Perspect.* 101(Suppl. 3):297–302 (1993).

3. Wang, R.G.M. (ed.). *Water Contamination and Health. Integration of Exposure Assessment, Toxicology, and Risk Assessment.* New York, Marcel Dekker (1994).

4. Dayan, A.D. Allergy to antimicrobial residues in food: assessment of the risk to man. *Vet. Microbiol.* 35:213–226 (1993).

5. Shah, P.M., V. Schäfer, and H. Knothe. Medical and veterinary use of antimicrobial agents: implications for public health. A clinician's view on antimicrobial resistance. *Vet. Microbiol.* 35:269–274 (1993).

6. Wiedemann, B. Monitoring of resistant organisms in man and identification of their origin. *Vet. Microbiol.* 35:275–284 (1993).

7. Corpet, D.E. An evaluation of methods to assess the effect of antimicrobial residues on the human gut flora. *Vet. Microbiol.* 35:199–212 (1993).

8. Shaikh, B., and W.A. Moats. Liquid chromatographic analysis of antibacterial drug residues in food products of animal origin. *J. Chromatogr.* 643:369–378 (1993).

9. Ishii, R., M. Horie, Y. Hoshino, et al. Simultaneous determination of residual synthetic antibacterials in fish and meat products by high performance liquid chromatography with photodiode array detector. *J. Food Hyg. Soc. Japan* 35:173–179 (1994).

10. Lin, S.-Y., and F. Kondo. Simple bacteriological and thin-layer chromatographic methods for determination of individual drug concentrations treated with penicillin-G in combination with one of the aminoglycosides. *Microbios* 77:223–229 (1994).

11. Roudaut, B., and M. Garnier. Sulphonamide and dapsone residues in bovine milk following intramammary infusion. *Food Addit. Contam.* 10:461–468 (1993).

12. Uno, K., T. Aoki, and R. Ueno. Pharmacokinetics of sulphamonomethoxine and sulphadimethoxine following oral administration to cultured rainbow trout (*Oncorhynchus mykiss*). *Aquaculture* 115:209–219 (1993).

13. Shearan, P., M. O'Keeffe, and M.R. Smyth. Comparison of matrix solid phase dispersion (MSPD) with a standard solvent extraction method for sulphamethazine in pork muscle using high performance liquid and thin layer chromatography. *Food Addit. Contam.* 11:7–15 (1994).

14. Agarwal, V.K. Application of solid phase extraction for the analysis of sulfonamides in milk by high performance liquid chromatography. *J. Liq. Chromatogr.* 16:3793–3799 (1993).

15. Malik, S., S.E. Duncan, J.R. Bishop, and L.T. Taylor. Extraction and detection of sulfamethazine in spray-dried milk. *J. Dairy Sci.* 77:418–425 (1994).

16. Weber, J.D., and M.D. Smedley. Liquid chromatographic method for determination of sulfamethazine residues in milk: collaborative study. *J. AOAC Int.* 76:725–729 (1993).

17. Bui, L.V. Liquid chromatographic determination of six sulfonamide residues in animal tissues using postcolumn derivatization. *J. AOAC Int.* 76:966–976 (1993).

18. Tsai, C.-E., and F. Kondo. Simple continuous and simultaneous determination of multiple sulfonamide residues. *J. Food Protect.* 56:1067–1072 (1993).

19. Hubert, Ph., P. Chiap, B. Evrard, et al. Fully automated determination of sulfamethazine in ovine plasma using solid-phase extraction on disposable cartridges and liquid chromatography. *J. Chromatogr.* 622:53–60 (1993).

20. Nishikawa, M., Y. Takahashi, and Y. Ishihara. High performance liquid chromatographic determination of sulfisomidine and N4-acetylsulfisomidine in swine tissues. *J. Liq. Chromatogr.* 16:4031–4047 (1993).

21. Mooser, A., and H. Koch. Confirmatory method for sulfonamide residues in animal tissues by gas chromatography and pulsed positive ion–negative ion–chemical ionization mass spectrometry. *J. AOAC Int.* 76:976–982 (1993).

22. Meijer, L.A., K.G.F. Ceyssens, W.T. de Jong, and B.I.J.A.C. de Grève. Correlation between tissue and plasma concentrations of oxytetracycline in veal calves. *J. Toxicol. Environ. Health* 40:35–45 (1993).

23. Meijer, L.A., K.G.F. Ceyssens, W.T. de Jong, and B.I.J.A.C. de Grève. Three phase elimination of oxytetracycline in veal calves; the presence of an extended terminal elimination phase. *J. Vet. Pharmacol. Therap.* 16:214–222 (1993).

24. Bugyei, K., W. Black, S. McEwen, and A.H. Meek. Detecting oxytetracyline residues in chicken tissues using the Delvotest® P system. *J. Food Protect.* 57:141–145 (1994).

25. White, C.R., W.A. Moats, and K.L. Kotula. Comparative study of high performance liquid chromatographic methods for the determination of tetracycline antibiotics. *J. Liq. Chromatogr.* 16:2873–2890 (1993).

26. DeGroot, J.M., B. Wyhowski de Bukanski, and S. Srebrnik. Multiresidue analysis of tetracyclines in kidney by HPLC and photodiode array detection. *J. Liq. Chromatogr.* 16:3515–3529 (1993).

27. Horii, S. Liquid chromatographic determination of oxytetracycline and chlortetracycline residues in animal tissues. *J. Liq. Chromatogr.* 17:213–221 (1994).

28. Tsai, C.-E., and F. Kondo. Simple continuous and simultaneous determination of tetracycline residues. *Res. Vet. Sci.* 56:277–283 (1994).

29. Suhren, G., and W. Heeschen. Detection of tetracyclines in milk by a *Bacillus cereus* microtitre test with indicator. *Milchwissenschaft* 48:259–263 (1993).

30. Halvatzis, S.A., M.M. Timotheou-Potamia, and A.C. Calokerinos. Continuous flow chemiluminometric determination of tetracyclines in pharmaceutical preparations and honey by oxidation with *N*-bromosuccinimide. *Analyst* 118:633–637 (1993).

31. Bergner-Lang, B., and E. Mikisch. Zur Bedeutung der 4-Epimeren von Oxytetracyclin-, Tetracyclin- und Chlortetracyclin-Rückständen bei der HPLC-Bestimmung in Lebensmitteln tierischer Herkunft. *Dtsch. Lebensm.-Rundsch.* 90:39–41 (1994).

32. Papich, M.G., G.O. Korsrud, J.O. Boison, et al. A study of the disposition of procaine penicillin G in feedlot steers following intramuscular and subcutaneous injection. *J. Vet. Pharmacol. Therap.* 16:317–327 (1993).

33. Korsrud, G.O., J.O. Boison, M.G. Papich, et al. Depletion of intramuscularly and subcutaneously injected procaine penicillin G from tissues of plasma of yearling beef steers. *Can. J. Vet. Res.* 57:223–230 (1993).

34. Korsrud, G.O., J.O. Boison, M.G. Papich, et al. Depletion of penicillin G residues in tissues and injection sites of yearling beef steers dosed with benzathine penicillin G alone or in combination with procaine penicillin G. *Food Addit. Contam.* 11:1–6 (1994).

35. van Eenennaam, A.L., J.S. Cullor, L. Perani, et al. Evaluation of milk antibiotic residue screening tests in cattle with naturally occurring clinical mastitis. *J. Dairy Sci.* 76:3041–3053 (1993).

36. Moats, W.A. Determination of ampicillin and amoxicillin in milk with an automated liquid chromatographic cleanup. *J. AOAC Int.* 77:41–45 (1994).

37. Kirchmann, E., R.L. Earley, and L.E. Welch. The electrochemical detection of penicillins in milk. *J. Liq. Chromatogr.* 17:1755–1772 (1994).

38. Straub, R.F., and R.D. Voyksner. Determination of penicillin G, ampicillin, amoxicillin, cloxacillin and cephapirin by high-performance liquid chromatography–electrospray mass spectrometry. *J. Chromatogr.* 647:167–181 (1993).

39. Anadón, A., P. Bringas, M.R. Martinez-Larrañaga, and M.J. Diaz. Bioavailability, pharmacokinetics and residues of chloramphenicol in the chicken. *J. Vet. Pharmacol. Therap.* 17:52–58 (1994).

40. Samouris, G., B. Nathanael, H. Tsoukali-Papadopoulou, and N. Papadimitriou. Determination of chloramphenicol residues in eggs by high performance liquid chromatography (HPLC). *Vet. Human Toxicol.* 35:406–409 (1993).

41. Ramos, M., Th. Reuvers, A. Aranda, and J. Gómez. Determination of chloramphenicol in chicken muscle by high performance liquid chromatography and UV-diode array detection. *J. Liq. Chromatogr.* 17:385–401 (1994).

42. Schneider, E., E. Märtlbauer, R. Dietrich, et al. Zwei immunchemische Schnelltests zum Nachweis von Chloramphenicol in Rohmilch. *Arch. Lebensmittelhyg.* 45:43–45 (1994).

43. Kijak, P.J. Confirmation of chloramphenicol residues in bovine milk by gas chromatography/mass spectrometry. *J. AOAC Int.* 77:34–40 (1994).

44. Mestorino, N., M.F. Landoni, M. Alt, and J.O. Errecalde. The pharmacokinetics of thiamphenicol in lactating cows. *Vet. Res. Commun.* 17:295–303 (1993).

45. Psomas, J.E., and E.G. Iosifidoy. High performance liquid chromatographic analysis of residues of thiampenicol [*sic*] in beef muscle. *J. Liq. Chromatogr.* 16:2653–2660 (1993).

46. Hormazabal, V., I. Steffenak, and M. Yndestad. Simultaneous determination of residues of florfenicol and the metabolite florfenicol amine in fish tissues by high-performance liquid chromatography. *J. Chromatogr. Biomed. Appl.* 616:161–165 (1993).

47. Lynch, M.J., J.R. Rice, J.F. Ericson, et al. Residue depletion studies on danofloxacin in the chicken. *J. Agric. Food Chem.* 42:289–294 (1994).

48. Horie, M., K. Saito, N. Nose, and H. Nakazawa. Simultaneous determination of benofloxacin, danofloxacin, enrofloxacin and ofloxacin in chicken tissues by high-performance liquid chromatography. *J. Chromatogr. B* 653:69–76 (1994).

49. Schneider, R.P., J.F. Ericson, M.J. Lynch, and H.G. Fouda. Confirmation of danofloxacin residues in chicken and cattle liver by microbore high-performance liquid chromatography electrospray ionization tandem mass spectrometry. *Biol. Mass Spectrom.* 22:595–599 (1993).

50. Sohlberg, S., A. Aulie, and N.E. Søli. Temperature-dependent absorption and elimination of flumequine in rainbow trout (*Oncorhynchus mykiss* Walbaum) in fresh water. *Aquaculture* 119:1–10 (1994).

51. Giles, J.S., H. Hariharan, and S.B. Heaney. A microbiological assay for determining sarafloxacin and oxolinic acid concentrations in Atlantic salmon plasma. *Microbiologica* 17:155–158 (1994).

52. Pouliquen, H., L. Pinault, and H. Le Bris. Determination of oxolinic acid in seawater, marine sediment, and Japanese oyster (*Crassostrea gigas*) by high-performance liquid chromatography. *J. Liq. Chromatogr.* 17:929–945 (1994).

53. DeGroot, J.M., B. Wyhowski de Bukanski, and S. Srebrnik. Oxolinic acid and flumequine in fish tissues: validation of an HPLC method; analysis of medicated fish and commercial fish samples. *J. Liq. Chromatogr.* 17:1785–1794 (1994).

54. Shiga, N., and O. Matano. High-performance liquid chromatographic method for the determination of oxolinic acid residues in crops. *J. Chromatogr.* 643:311–315 (1993).

55. Helton-Groce, S.L., T.D. Thomson, and R.S. Readnour. A study of tilmicosin residues in milk following subcutaneous administration to lactating dairy cows. *Can. Vet. J.* 34:619–621 (1993).

56. Chan, W., G.C. Gerhardt, and C.D.C. Salisbury. Determination of tylosin and tilmicosin residues in animal tissues by reversed-phase liquid chromatography. *J. AOAC Int.* 77:331–333 (1994).

57. Sanders, P., P. Guillot, M. Dagorn, et al. Pharmacokinetics and tissue residues of spiramycin in cattle after intramuscular administration of multiple doses. *Am. J. Vet. Res.* 55:358–362 (1994).

58. Janeček, M., and M.A. Quilliam. Determination of erythromycin A by liquid chromatography and electrochemical detection, with application to salmon tissue. *J. Chromatogr. Biomed. Appl.* 619:63–69 (1993).

59. Zierfels, G., and M. Petz. Fluorimetrische Bestimmung von Erythromycin-Rückständen in Lebensmitteln tierischer Herkunft nach Derivatisierung mit FMOC und HPLC-Trennung. *Z. Lebensm. Unters. Forsch.* 198:307–312 (1994).

60. Galeano Díaz, T., L. Lopez Martínez, M. Martínez Galera, and F. Salinas. Rapid determination of nitrofurantoin, furazolidone and furaltadone in formulations, feed and milk by high performance liquid chromatography. *J. Liq. Chromatogr.* 17:457–475 (1994).

61. Rupp, H.S., R.K. Munns, and A.R. Long. Simultaneous determination of nitrofurazone and furazolidone in shrimp (*Penaeus vannamei*) muscle tissue by liquid chromatography with UV detection. *J. AOAC Int.* 76:1235–1239 (1993).

62. Rupp, H.S., R.K. Munns, A.R. Long, and S.M. Plakas. Simultaneous determination of nitrofurazone, nitrofurantoin, and furazolidone in channel catfish (*Ictalurus punctatus*) muscle tissue by liquid chromatography. *J. AOAC Int.* 77:344–350 (1994).

63. Moretain, J.P., and J. Boisseau. Elimination of aminoglycoside antibiotics in milk following intramammary administration. *Vet. Q.* 14:109–112 (1993).

64. Gerhardt, G.C., C.D.C. Salisbury, and J.D. MacNeil. Determination of streptomycin and dihydrostreptomycin in animal tissue by on-line sample enrichment liquid chromatography. *J. AOAC Int.* 77:334–337 (1994).

65. Haagsma, N., J.R. Keegstra, and P. Scherpenisse. High-performance liquid chromatographic determination of spectinomycin in swine, calf and chicken plasma. *J. Chromatogr. Biomed. Appl.* 615:289–295 (1993).

66. Ise, N., H. Shibatani, M. Oshita, et al. Determination of bicozamycin and its benzoylester derivative in yellowtail tissues by high performance liquid chromatography. *J. Liq. Chromatogr.* 16:2399–2414 (1993).

67. Asukabe, H., H. Murata, K.-I. Harada, et al. Improvement of chemical analysis of antibiotics. XX. Basic study on high-performance liquid chromatographic determination of four polyether antibiotics pre-derivatized with 1-bromoacetylpyrene. *J. Chromatogr. A* 657:349–356 (1993).

68. Elissalde, M.H., R.C. Beier, L.D. Rowe, and L.H. Stanker. Development of a monoclonal-based enzyme-linked immunosorbent assay for the coccidiostat salinomycin. *J. Agric. Food Chem.* 41:2167–2171 (1993).

69. Rowe, L.D., R.C. Beier, M.H. Elissalde, and L.H. Stanker. Production and characterization of monoclonal antibodies against the poultry coccidiostat halofuginone. *J. Agric. Food Chem.* 42:1132–1137 (1994).

70. Stanker, L.H., C. McKeown, B.E. Watkins, et al. Detection of dimetridazole and other nitroimidazole residues in turkey using an immunoassay. *J. Agric. Food Chem.* 41:1332–1336 (1993).

71. Roth, M., G. Rae, A.S. McGill, and K.W. Young. Ivermectin depuration in Atlantic salmon (*Salmo salar*). *J. Agric. Food Chem.* 41:2434–2436 (1993).

72. Kennedy, D.G., A. Cannavan, S.A. Hewitt, et al. Determination of ivermectin residues in the tissues of Atlantic salmon (*Salmo salar*) using HPLC with fluorescence detection. *Food Addit. Contam.* 10:579–584 (1993).

73. Salisbury, C.D.C. Modified method for the determination of ivermectin residues in animal tissues. *J. AOAC Int.* 76:1149–1151 (1993).

74. DeGroot, J.M., B. Wyhowski de Bukanski, and S. Srebrnik. Determination of ivermectin residues in meat and liver by HPLC and fluorometric detection. *J. Liq. Chromatogr.* 17:1419–1426 (1994).

75. Rabel, S.R., J.F. Stobaugh, R. Heinig, and J.M. Bostick. Improvements in detection sensitivity for the determination of ivermectin in plasma using chromatographic techniques and laser-induced fluorescence detection with automated derivatization. *J. Chromatogr. Biomed. Appl.* 617:79–86 (1993).

76. Chu, P.-S., R.Y. Wang, T.A. Brandt, and C.A. Weerasinghe. Determination of albendazole-2-aminosulfone in bovine milk using high-performance liquid chromatography with fluorometric detection. *J. Chromatogr. Biomed. Appl.* 620:129–135 (1993).

77. Khunachak, A., A.R. Dacunha, and S.J. Stout. Liquid chromatographic determination of moxidectin residues in cattle tissues and confirmation in cattle fat by liquid chromatography/mass spectrometry. *J. AOAC Int.* 76:1230–1235 (1993).

78. Kamps-Holtzapple, C., L.H. Stanker, and J.R. DeLoach. Development of a monoclonal antibody-based ELISA for the anthelmintic hygromycin B. *J. Agric. Food Chem.* 42:822–827 (1994).

79. Bastos, M.deL., and M.E. Soares. Effect of cooking on diazepam and its metabolites in liver of bulls. *J. Agric. Food Chem.* 41:965–967 (1993).

80. Holland, D.C., R.K. Munns, J.E. Roybal, et al. Simultaneous determination of xylazine and its major metabolite, 2,6-dimethylaniline, in bovine and swine kidney by liquid chromatography. *J. AOAC Int.* 76:720–724 (1993).

81. Elliott, C.T., S.R.H. Crooks, J.G.D. McEvoy, et al. Observations on the effects of long-term withdrawal on carcass composition and residue concentrations in clenbuterol-medicated cattle. *Vet. Res. Commun.* 17:459–468 (1993).

82. Stoffel, B., and H.H.D. Meyer. Effects of the β-adrenergic agonist clenbuterol in cows: lipid metabolism, milk production, pharmacokinetics, and residues. *J. Anim. Sci.* 71:1875–1881 (1993).

83. van Rhijn, J.A., W.A. Traag, and H.H. Heskamp. Confirmatory analysis of clenbuterol using two different derivatives simultaneously. *J. Chromatogr. Biomed. Appl.* 619:243–249 (1993).

84. García Regueiro, J.A., B. Pérez, and G. Casademont. Determination of clenbuterol and salbutamol in urine by capillary gas chromatography with capillary columns of 100 μm. *J. Chromatogr. A* 655:73–76 (1993).

85. Chappell, C.G., C.S. Creaser, and M.J. Shepherd. On-line high performance liquid chromatography—multidimensional gas chromatography and its application to the determination of stilbene hormones in corned beef. *J. High Res. Chromatogr.* 16:479–482 (1993).

86. Medina, M., J.M. Grases, P. Rodriguez, and J. Bosch. Method for the determination of DES, hexestrol and dienestrol residues in bovine urine using GC-MSD. *Anal. Lett.* 26:2361–2370 (1993).

87. Hashimoto, T., T. Miyazaki, T. Itoh, et al. Measurement of progesterone in beef by enzyme immunoassay (EIA). *J. Food Hyg. Soc. Japan* 34:211–215 (1993).

88. Perona, M., and I. Pavan. Determination of anabolic steroid 19-nor-testosterone in bovine serum by GC-SIM–MS. *J. Chromatogr. Sci.* 31:429–432 (1993).

89. Hewitt, S.A., W.J. Blanchflower, W.J. McCaughey, et al. Liquid chromatography–thermospray mass spectrometric assay for trenbolone in bovine bile and faeces. *J. Chromatogr.* 639:185–191 (1993).

90. Rattenberger, E., and O. Herr. Entwicklung eines Enzymimmuno-Tests zum Nachweis des Beta-Blockers Carazolol. *Arch. Lebensmittelhyg.* 44:135–137 (1993).

91. Dittus, K.L., V.N. Hillers, and K.A. Beerman. Attitudes and behaviors about pesticide residues, susceptibility to cancer, and consumption of fruits and vegetables. *J. Nutr. Education* 25:245–250 (1993).

92. Davis, D.L., A. Blair, and D.G. Hoel. Agricultural exposures and cancer trends in developed countries. *Environ. Health Perspect.* 100:39–44 (1992).

93. Carbonell, E., N. Xamena, A. Creus, and R. Marcos. Cytogenetic biomonitoring in a Spanish group of agricultural workers exposed to pesticides. *Mutagenesis* 8:511–517 (1993).

94. Bolognesi, C., M. Parrini, F. Merlo, and S. Bonassi. Frequency of micronuclei in lymphocytes from a group of floriculturists exposed to pesticides. *J. Toxicol. Environ. Health* 40:405–411 (1993).

95. Dolara, P., A. Vezzani, G. Caderni, et al. Genetic toxicity of a mixture of fifteen pesticides commonly found in the Italian diet. *Cell Biol. Toxicol.* 9:333–343 (1993).

96. Heindel, J.J., R.E. Chapin, D.K. Gulati, et al. Assessment of the reproductive and developmental toxicity of pesti-

cide/fertilizer mixtures based on confirmed pesticide contamination in California and Iowa groundwater. *Fund. Appl. Toxicol.* 22:605–621 (1994).

97. Dearfield, K.L., H.F. Stack, J.A. Quest, et al. A survey of EPA/OPP and open literature data on selected pesticide chemicals tested for mutagenicity. I. Introduction and first ten chemicals. *Mutat. Res.* 297:197–233 (1993).

98. Nilsson, R., M. Tasheva, and B. Jaeger. Why different regulatory decisions when the scientific information base is similar?—human risk assessment. *Regul. Toxicol. Pharmacol.* 17:292–322 (1993).

99. Winter, C.K. Pesticide residues and the Delaney Clause. *Food Technol.* 47(7):81–86 (1993).

100. Dunkelberger, E., and R.A. Merrill. The Delaney paradox reexamined: regulating pesticides in processed foods. *Food Drug Law J.* 48:411–439 (1993).

101. McClintock, J.T., J.L. Kough, and R. D. Sjoblad. Regulatory oversight of biochemical pesticides by the U.S. Environmental Protection Agency: health effects considerations. *Regul. Toxicol. Pharmacol.* 19:115–124 (1994).

102. Neidert, E., R.B. Trotman, and P.W. Saschenbrecker. Levels and incidences of pesticide residues in selected agricultural food commodities available in Canada. *J. AOAC Int.* 77:18–24 (1994).

103. Anonymous. Pesticide residues in 1991. *Food Chem. Toxicol.* 31:389–390 (1993).

104. Sommer, H., B. Petersen, and P. von Wittke (eds.). *Safeguarding Food Quality.* New York, Springer-Verlag (1993).

105. Holland, P.T., D.E. McNaughton, and C.P. Malcolm. Multiresidue analysis of pesticides in wines by solid-phase extraction. *J. AOAC Int.* 77:79–86 (1994).

106. King, J.W., M.L. Hopper, R.G. Luchtefeld, et al. Optimization of experimental conditions for the supercritical carbon dioxide extraction of pesticide residues from grains. *J. AOAC Int.* 76:857–864 (1993).

107. Rathore, H.S., and T. Begum. Thin-layer chromatographic methods for use in pesticide residue analysis. *J. Chromatogr.* 643:271–290 (1993).

108. Pylypiw, H.M., Jr. Rapid gas chromatographic method for the multiresidue screening of fruits and vegetables for organochlorine and organophosphate pesticides. *J. AOAC Int.* 76:1369–1373 (1993).

109. Hong, J., Y. Eo, J. Rhee, et al. Simultaneous analysis of 25 pesticides in crops using gas chromatography and their identification by gas chromatography–mass spectrometry. *J. Chromatogr.* 639:261–271 (1993).

110. Stan, H.-J., and M. Linkerhägner. Capillary gas chromatography—atomic emission detection: a useful instrumental method in pesticide residue analysis of plant foodstuffs. *J. High Res. Chromatogr.* 16:539–548 (1993).

111. Marty, J.-L., N. Mionetto, T. Noguer, et al. Enzyme sensors for the detection of pesticides. *Biosens. Bioelectron.* 8:273–280 (1993).

112. Jessup, A.J., and R. Sloggett. Residues in apples and their packaging following fumigation with methyl bromide. *Aust. J. Exp. Agric.* 33:499–502 (1993).

113. Jessup, A.J., R.F. Sloggett, and N.M. Quinn. Residues of methyl bromide and inorganic bromide in fumigated produce. *J. Agric. Food Chem.* 42:108–111 (1994).

114. Kaneda, M., N. Hatakenaka, S. Teramoto, and K. Maita. A two-generation reproduction study in rats with methyl bromide-fumigated diets. *Food Chem. Toxicol.* 31:533–542 (1993).

115. Daft, J.L. Methyl bromide determination in selected foods by headspace technique. *J. AOAC Int.* 76:1083–1091 (1993).

116. Rangaswamy, J.R., and N. Gunasekaran. Free phosphine in the void space of food commodities during phosphine fumigation. *Lebensm. Wiss. Technol.* 26:447–449 (1993).

117. Rangaswamy, J.R. Effect of physical attributes of robusta coffee on phosphine residue. *Lebensm. Wiss. Technol.* 26:210–214 (1993).

118. Conde, C., C. Maluenda, and C. Arrabal. Hexachlorobenzene (HCB) in human milk in Spain from 1984 to 1991. *Bull. Environ. Contam. Toxicol.* 51:827–831 (1993).

119. van Raaij, J.A.G.M., C.M.G. Frijters, and K.J. van den Berg. Hexachlorobenzene-induced hypothyroidism. Involvement of different mechanisms by parent compound and metabolite. *Biochem. Pharmacol.* 46:1385–1391 (1993).

120. Dearfield, K.L. Ethylene thiourea (ETU). A review of the genetic toxicity studies. *Mutat. Res.* 317:111–132 (1994).

121. Buckley, D.C., A.R.C. Hill, V.L. Sivyer, and J.P.G. Wilkins. Residues of tecnazene and its metabolites in potatoes in commercial stores. *Crop Protect.* 13:87–92 (1994).

122. Königer, M., and P.R. Wallnöfer. Untersuchungen über das Verhalten von Thiabendazol bei Bananen. *Dtsch. Lebensm.-Rundsch.* 89:384–385 (1993).

123. Friar, P.M.K., and S.L. Reynolds. The effect of home processing on postharvest fungicide residues in citrus fruit: residues of imazalil, 2-phenylphenol and thiabendazole in 'home-made' marmalade, prepared from Late Valencia oranges. *Food Addit. Contam.* 11:57–70 (1994).

124. Pelegrí, R., M. Gamón, R. Coscollá, et al. The metabolism of fosetyl-aluminium and the evolution of residue levels in oranges and tangerines. *Pestic. Sci.* 39:319–323 (1993).

125. Di Muccio, A., R. Dommarco, D.A. Barbini, et al. Application of solid-phase partition cartridges in the determination of fungicide residues in vegetable samples. *J. Chromatogr.* 643:363–368 (1993).

126. Longbottom, J.E., K.W. Edgell, E.J. Erb, and V. Lopez-Avila. Gas chromatographic/nitrogen-phosphorus detection method for determination of ethylene thiourea in finished drinking waters: collaborative study. *J. AOAC Int.* 76:1113–1120 (1993).

127. Walash, M.I., F. Belal, M.E. Metwally, and M.M. Hefnawy. Spectrophotometric determination of maneb, zineb and their decomposition products in some vegetables and its application to kinetic studies after greenhouse treatment. *Food Chem.* 47:411–416 (1993).

128. Singh, R.P., and M. Chiba. Determination of benomyl and its degradation products by chromatographic methods in water, wettable powder formulations, and crops. *J. Chromatogr.* 643:249–260 (1993).

129. Itak, J.A., M.Y. Selisker, S.W. Jourdan, et al. Determination of benomyl (as carbendazim) and carbendazim in water, soil, and fruit juice by a magnetic particle-based immunoassay. *J. Agric. Food Chem.* 41:2329–2332 (1993).

130. Schwack, W., and S. Nyanzi. Analysis of dithiocarbamate fungicides. Second-derivative UV-spectroscopic determination of $CS_2$, COS, and thiram (TMTD). *Z. Lebensm. Unters. Forsch.* 198:3–7 (1994).

131. Schwack, W., and S. Nyanzi. Analysis of dithiocarbamate fungicides. Reaction products of the thiuram disulphide fungicide thiram (TMTD) during acid hydrolysis. *Z. Lebensm. Unters. Forsch.* 198:8–10 (1994).

132. Regis-Rolle, S.D., and G. M. Bauville. High-performance liquid chromatographic method for the determination of carbendazim residues in crops, grains, and wines with fluorescent detection. *Pestic. Sci.* 37:273–282 (1993).

133. Bushway, R.J., L.R. Paradis, L.B. Perkins, et al. Determination of methyl 2-benzimidazolecarbamate in wine by competitive inhibition enzyme immunoassay. *J. AOAC Int.* 76:851–856 (1993).

134. Anklam, E., and A. Müller. A simple method of sample preparation for analysis of biphenyl residues in citrus fruit peels by gas chromatography. *Z. Lebensm. Unters. Forsch.* 198:329–330 (1994).

135. Cooper, J.F., J. Tourte, and P. Gros. Determination of pentachlorophenol residues in wine and corks by solvent extraction methodology and specific gas chromatography detection. *Chromatographia* 38:147–150 (1994).

136. Brandon, D.L., R.G. Binder, R.E. Wilson, and W.C. Montague, Jr. Analysis of thiabendazole in potatoes and apples by ELISA using monoclonal antibodies. *J. Agric. Food Chem.* 41:996–999 (1993).

137. Itak, J.A., M.Y. Selisker, D.P. Herzog, et al. Determination of captan in water, peaches, and apple juice by a magnetic particle-based immunoassay. *J. AOAC Int.* 77:86–91 (1994).

138. Yeung, J.M., and W.H. Newsome. Survey of total tetrahydrophthalidimide in baby foods using both enzyme-linked immunosorbent assay and gas chromatography/mass spectrometry: a comparative study. *J. AOAC Int.* 76:1225–1229 (1993).

139. Fink, W., and J. Auch. Nachweis von Malachitgrün-, Kristallviolett- und Brillantgrün-Rückständen in Speisefischen mittels HPLC. *Dtsch. Lebensm.-Rundsch.* 89:246–251 (1993).

140. Hardell, L., M. Eriksson, and A. Degerman. Exposure to phenoxyacetic acids, chlorophenols, or organic solvents in relation to histopathology, stage, and anatomical localization of non-Hodgkin's lymphoma. *Cancer Res.* 54:2386–2389 (1994).

141. Hajdu, S.I. The health effects of agrichemicals: herbicides and soft tissue sarcomas. (Letter.) *Human Pathol.* 24:1383–1384 (1993).

142. Brusick, D.J. An assessment of the genetic toxicity of atrazine: relevance to human health and environmental effects. *Mutat. Res.* 317:133–144 (1994).

143. Cessna, A.J., and F.A. Holm. Residues of 2,4-D in wheat following application after heading. *Can. J. Plant Sci.* 74:199–203 (1994).

144. Brown, H.M., L.B. Brattsten, D.E. Lilly, and P.J. Hanna. Metabolic pathways and residue levels of thifensulfuron methyl in soybeans. *J. Agric. Food Chem.* 41:1724–1730 (1993).

145. Lehotay, S.J., and R.W. Miller. Evaluation of commercial immunoassays for the detection of alachlor in milk, eggs and liver. *J. Environ. Sci. Health* B29:395–414 (1994).

147. Wigfield, Y.Y., K.A. McCormack, and R. Grant. Simultaneous determination of residues of paraquat and diquat in potatoes using high-performance capillary electrophoresis with ultraviolet detection. *J. Agric. Food Chem.* 41:2315–2318 (1993).

148. Worobey, B.L. Liquid chromatographic method for determination of diquat and paraquat herbicides in potatoes: collaborative study. *J. AOAC Int.* 76:881–887 (1993).

149. Chichila, T.M.P., and D.M. Gilvydis. Determination of paraquat and diquat in low-moisture food crops using silica column cleanup and liquid chromatography with UV detection. *J. AOAC Int.* 76:1323–1328 (1993).

150. Wittmann, C., and B. Hock. Analysis of atrazine residues in food by an enzyme immunoassay. *J. Agric. Food Chem.* 41:1421–1425 (1993).

151. Giersch, T. A new monoclonal antibody for the sensitive detection of atrazine with immunoassay in microtiter plate and dipstick format. *J. Agric. Food Chem.* 41:1006–1011 (1993).

152. Wigfield, Y.Y., and R. Grant. Analysis for atrazine in fortified cornmeal and corns using a commercially available enzyme immunoassay microtiter plate. *Bull. Environ. Contam. Toxicol.* 51:171–177 (1993).

153. Laganà, A., G. Fago, A. Marino, and B. Pardo-Martinez. Rapid method for determination of phenylurea herbicides in milk. *Chromatographia* 38:88–92 (1994).

154. Karu, A.E., M.H. Goodrow, D.J. Schmidt, et al. Synthesis of haptens and derivation of monoclonal antibodies for immunoassay of the phenylurea herbicide diuron. *J. Agric. Food Chem.* 42:301–309 (1994).

155. Schneider, P., M.H. Goodrow, S.J. Gee, and B.D. Hammock. A highly sensitive and rapid ELISA for the arylurea herbicides diuron, monuron, and linuron. *J. Agric. Food Chem.* 42:413–422 (1994).

156. Klaffenbach, P., and P.T. Holland. Analysis of sulfonylurea herbicides by gas–liquid chromatography III— Mass spectrometry and multiresidue determination. *Biol. Mass Spectrom.* 22:565–578 (1993).

157. Liu, T.P., L.T.Y. Chu, and P. Sporns. Formic acid residues in honey in relation to application rate and timing of formic acid for control of tracheal mites, *Acarapis woodi* (Rennie). *Am. Bee J.* 133:719–721 (1993).

158. Atienza, J., J.J. Jiménez, J.L. Bernal, and M.T. Martín. Supercritical fluid extraction of fluvalinate residues in honey. Determination by high-performance liquid chromatography. *J. Chromatogr. A* 655:95–99 (1993).

159. Fernández Muíño, M.A., and J.S. Lozano. Gas chromatographic–mass spectrometric method for the simultaneous determination of amitraz, bromopropylate, coumaphos, cymiazole and fluvalinate residues in honey. *Analyst* 118:1519–1522 (1993).

160. Niemann, R.A. Determination of formetanate hydrochloride in selected fruits by coupled-column cation exchange liquid chromatography. *J. AOAC Int.* 76:1362–1368 (1993).

161. de Peyster, A., W.O. Willis, C.A. Molgaard, et al. Cholinesterase and self-reported pesticide exposure among pregnant women. *Arch. Environ. Health* 48:348–352 (1993).

162. Zahm, S.H., D.D. Weisenburger, R.C. Saal, et al. The role of agricultural pesticide use in the development of non-Hodgkin's lymphoma in women. *Arch. Environ. Health* 48:353–358 (1993).

163. Collins, M., and W. Nassif. Pesticide residues in organically and conventionally grown fruit and vegetables in New South Wales, 1990–91. *Food Aust.* 45:429–431 (1993).

164. Trotter, W.J., and R. Dickerson. Pesticide residues in composited milk collected through the U.S. Pasteurized Milk Network. *J. AOAC Int.* 76:1220–1225 (1993).

165. Raha, P., H. Banerjee, A.K. Das, and N. Adityachaudhury. Persistence kinetics of endosulfan, fenvalerate, and decamethrin in and on eggplant (*Solanum melongena* L.). *J. Agric. Food Chem.* 41:923–928 (1993).

166. Miyahara, M., and Y. Saito. Effects of the processing steps in tofu production on pesticide residues. *J. Agric. Food Chem.* 42:369–373 (1994).

167. Wan, H.B., M.K. Wong, P.Y. Lim, and C.Y. Mok. Small-scale multi-residue method for the determination of organochlorine and pyrethroid pesticides in vegetables. *J. Chromatogr. A* 662:147–152 (1994).

168. Acquavella, J.F., B.K. Ireland, and J.M. Ramlow. Organochlorines and breast cancer. (Letter.) *J. Natl. Cancer Inst.* 85:1872–1873 (1993).

169. Wolff, M.S., N. Dubin, and P.G. Toniolo. Organochlorines and breast cancer. (Reply.) *J. Natl. Cancer Inst.* 85:1873–1875 (1993).

170. Mussalo-Rauhamaa, H., and P. Pantzar. Selenium and DDE in breast fat of breast cancer patients: their relationship to hormone receptors in breast tissue. (Letter.) *J. Natl. Cancer Inst.* 85:1964–1965 (1993).

171. Dewailly, É., S. Dodin, R. Verreault, et al. High organochlorine body burden in women with estrogen receptor-positive breast cancer. *J. Natl. Cancer Inst.* 86:232–234 (1994).

172. Krieger, N., M.S. Wolff, R.A. Hiatt, et al. Breast cancer and serum organochlorines: a prospective study among white, black, and Asian women. *J. Natl. Cancer Inst.* 86:589–599 (1994).

173. Redetzke, K.A., and H.G. Applegate. Organochlorine pesticides in adipose tissue of persons from El Paso, Texas. *J. Environ. Health* 56(3):25–27 (1993).

174. Üstünbas, H.B., M.A. Öztürk, E. Hasanoğlu, and M. Doğan. Organochlorine pesticide residues in human milk in Kayseri. *Human Exp. Toxicol.* 13:299–302 (1994).

175. Evans, R.G., D.W. Roberts, A.M. Murgueytio, et al. Relationship between fish consumption and serum chlordane levels. *J. Environ. Health* 56(10):17–22 (1994).

176. Kashyap, R., L.R. Iyer, and M.M. Singh. Evaluation of daily dietary intake of dichloro-diphenyl-trichloroethane (DDT) and benzene hexachloride (BHC) in India. *Arch. Environ. Health* 49:63–66 (1994).

177. Bidleman, T.F., and D.C.G. Muir (eds.). *Analytical and Environmental Chemistry of Toxaphene.* Proceedings of a workshop held at Burlington, Ontario, Canada, 4–6 February 1993. *Chemosphere* 27(10) (1993).

178. Herrera, A., A.A. Ariño, M.P. Conchello, et al. Organochlorine pesticide residues in Spanish meat products and meat of different species. *J. Food Protect.* 57:441–444 (1994).

179. Ariño, A., A. Herrera, P. Conchello, and R. Lazaro. Hexachlorobenzene and hexachlorocyclohexane residues in pork as affected by weight and sex. *Bull. Environ. Contam. Toxicol.* 51:647–650 (1993).

180. Kotonya, R., G.M. Mutungi, and L.W. Kanja. Organochlorine pesticides in swine tissues form abattoir material collected in Nairobi, Kenya. *Bull. Environ. Contam. Toxicol.* 53:39–45 (1994).

181. Bayarri, S., P. Conchello, A. Ariño, et al. DDT, DDT metabolites, and other organochlorines as affected by thermal processing in three commercial cuts of lamb. *Bull. Environ. Contam. Toxicol.* 52:554–559 (1994).

182. Conchello, M.P., A. Herrera, A. Ariño, et al. Effect of several kitchen treatments on hexachlorocyclohexane residues in ovine meat.*Bull. Environ. Contam. Toxicol.* 51:612–618 (1993).

183. Garrido, M.D., M. Jodral, and R. Pozo. Organochlorine pesticides in Spanish sterilized milk and associated health risks. *J. Food Protect.* 57:249–252 (1994).

184. Lenardón, A., M.I. Maitre de Hevia, and S. Enrique de Carbone. Organochlorine pesticides in Argentinian butter. *Sci. Total Environ.* 144:273–277 (1994).

185. Miskiewicz, A.G., and P.J. Gibbs. Organochlorine pesticides and hexachlorobenzene in tissues of fish and invertebrates caught near a sewage outfall. *Environ. Pollut.* 84:269–277 (1994).

186. Aplada-Sarlis, P., K.S. Liapis, and G.E. Miliadis. Contamination of potato tubers and carrots in Greece with lindane residues. *Bull. Environ. Contam. Toxicol.* 52:135–140 (1994).

187. Gans, D.A., W.W. Kilgore, and J. Ito. Residues of chlorinated pesticides in processed foods imported into Hawaii from western Pacific Rim countries. *Bull. Environ. Contam. Toxicol.* 52:560–567 (1994).

188. Mañes, J., G. Font, and Y. Picó. Evaluation of a solid-phase extraction system for determining pesticide residues in milk. *J. Chromatogr.* 642:195–204 (1993).

189. Snyder, J.M., J.W. King, L.D. Rowe, and J.A. Woerner. Supercritical fluid extraction of poultry tissues containing incurred pesticide residues. *J. AOAC Int.* 76:888–892 (1993).

190. Armishaw, P., and R.G. Millar. Comparison of gel permeation chromatography, sweep codistillation, and Florisil column adsorption chromatography as sample cleanup techniques for the determination of organochlorine pesticide residues in animal fats. *J. AOAC Int.* 76:1317–1322 (1993).

191. Lott, H.M., and S.A. Barker. Comparison of a matrix solid phase dispersion and a classical extraction method for the determination of chlorinated pesticides in fish muscle.*Environ. Monitoring Assessment* 28:109–116 (1993).

192. Seidel, V., I. Tschernuter-Meixner, and W. Lindner. Sandwich-type extraction column with on-line sulphuric acid treatment for the determination of organochlorine compounds in vegetable oil or oil seeds by gas chromatography with electron-capture detection. *J. Chromatogr.* 642:253–262 (1993).

193. Seidel, V., and W. Lindner. Universal sample enrichment technique for organochlorine pesticides in environmental and biological samples using a redesigned simultaneous steam distillation–solvent extraction apparatus. *Anal. Chem.* 65:3677–3683 (1993).

194. López-Carillo, L., and M. López-Cervantes. Effect of exposure to organophosphate pesticides on serum cholinesterase levels. *Arch. Environ. Health* 48:359–363 (1993).

195. Jacobs, R.M., and N.J. Yess. Survey of imported green coffee beans for pesticide residues. *Food Addit. Contam.* 10:575–577 (1993).

196. Singh, K., S.U. Khan, M.H. Akhtar, et al. Nature and bioavailability of nonextractable (bound) residues in stored wheat treated with chlorpyrifos-methyl. *J. Agric. Food Chem.* 41:2421–2425 (1993).

197. Nakamura, Y., Y. Sekiguchi, S. Hasegawa, et al. Reductions in postharvest-applied dichlorvos, chlorpyrifos-methyl, malathion, fenitrothion, and bromide in rice during storage and cooking processes. *J. Agric. Food Chem.* 41:1910–1915 (1993).

198. Tsumura, Y., S. Hasegawa, Y. Sekiguchi, et al. Residues of post-harvest application pesticides in buckwheat after storage and processing into noodles. *J. Food Hyg. Soc. Japan* 35:1–7 (1994).

199. Antonious, G.F., and J.C. Snyder. Residues and half-lives of acephate, methamidophos, and primiphos-methyl in leaves and fruit of greenhouse-grown tomatoes. *Bull. Environ. Contam. Toxicol.* 52:141–148 (1994).

200. Cabras, P., V.L. Garau, M. Melis, et al. Persistence and fate of fenthion in olives and olive products.*J. Agric. Food Chem.* 41:2431–2433 (1993).

201. Lentza-Rizos, C., E.J. Avramides, and R.A. Roberts. Persistence of fenthion residues in olive oil.*Pestic. Sci.* 40:63–69 (1994).

202. Coulibaly, K., and J.S. Smith. Thermostability of organophosphate pesticides and some of their major metabolites in water and beef muscle. *J. Agric. Food Chem.* 41:1719–1723 (1993).

203. Lino, C.M., M.I. Noronha da Silveira. Chlorpyrifos, ethion, fenitrothion, and methidathion residues in chickens. *Bull. Environ. Contam. Toxicol.* 52:425–431 (1994).

204. Beasley, H.L., J.H. Skerritt, A.S. Hill, and J.M. Desmarchelier. Rapid field tests for the organophosphorus pesticides, fenitrothion and pirimiphos-methyl—reliable

estimates of residues in stored grain. *J. Stored Prod. Res.* 29:357–369 (1993).

205. Parfitt, C.H. Wide-bore capillary gas chromatographic determination of organophosphorus pesticide resides in foods: interlaboratory trial. *J. AOAC Int.* 77:92–101 (1993).

206. Grob, K., M. Biedermann, and A.M. Giuffré. Determination of organophosphorus insecticides in edible oils and fats by splitless injection of the oil into a gas chromatograph (injector-internal headspace analysis). *Z. Lebensm. Unters. Forsch.* 198:325–328 (1994).

207. Skopec, Z.V., R. Clark, P.M.A. Harvey, and R.J. Wells. Analysis of organophosphorus pesticides in rice by supercritical fluid extraction and quantitation using an atomic emission detector. *J. Chromatogr. Sci.* 31:445–449 (1993).

208. Burgess, J.L., J.N. Bernstein, and K. Hurlbut. Aldicarb poisoning. A case report with prolonged cholinesterase inhibition and improvement after pralidoxime therapy. *Arch. Intern. Med.* 154:221–224 (1994).

209. Grendon, J., F. Frost, and L. Baum. Chronic health effects among sheep and humans surviving an aldicarb poisoning incident. *Vet. Human Toxicol.* 36:218–223 (1994).

210. McGarvey, B.D., A.A. Reyes, and M. Chiba. Decline of oxamyl residues in tomatoes in cool, modified-atmosphere storage. *HortScience* 29:297–298 (1994).

211. McGarvey, B.D. High-performance liquid chromatographic methods for the determination of N-methylcarbamate pesticides in water, soil, plants and air. *J. Chromatogr.* 642:89–105 (1993).

212. Ali, M.S., J.D. White, R.S. Bakowski, et al. Analyte stability study of *N*-methylcarbamate pesticides in beef and poultry liver tissues by liquid chromatography. *J. AOAC Int.* 76:1309–1316 (1993).

213. Ling, C.F., G.P. Melian, F. Jiminez-Conde, and E. Revilla. High-performance liquid chromatographic analysis of carbofuran residues in tomatoes grown in hydroponics. *J. Chromatogr.* 643:351–355 (1993).

214. Murugaverl, B., A. Gharaibeh, and K.J. Voorhees. Mixed adsorbent for cleanup during supercritical fluid extraction of three carbamate pesticides in tissues. *J. Chromatogr. A* 657:223–226 (1993).

215. Howard, A.L., C. Braue, and L.T. Taylor. Feasibility of thiocarbamate pesticide analysis in apples by supercritical fluid extraction and high-performance liquid chromatography. *J. Chromatogr. Sci.* 31:323–329 (1993).

216. Ballesteros, E., M. Gallego, and M. Valcárcel. Automatic gas chromatographic determination of *N*-methylcarbamates in milk with electron capture detection. *Anal. Chem.* 65:1773–1778 (1993).

217. Albelda, C., Y. Picó, G. Font, and J. Mañes. Determination of aldicarb, aldicarb sulfoxide, and aldicarb sulfone in oranges by simple gas–liquid chromatography with nitrogen–phosphorus detection. *J. AOAC Int.* 77:74–78 (1994).

218. Ali, M.S., J.D. White, R.S. Bakowski, et al. Extension of a liquid chromatographic method for *N*-methylcarbamate pesticides in cattle, swine, and poultry liver. *J. AOAC Int.* 76:907–910 (1993).

219. Lehotay, S.J., and R.J. Argauer. Detection of aldicarb sulfone and carbofuran in fortified meat and liver with commercial ELISA kits after rapid extraction. *J. Agric. Food Chem.* 41:2006–2010 (1993).

220. Westcott, N.D., and R.A. Reichle. Deltamethrin residues on Saskatoon berries. *J. Agric. Food Chem.* 41:2153–2155 (1993).

221. Marti-Mestres, G.N., J.-F.M. Cooper, J.-P.M. Mestres, et al. Effects of a supplemented deltamethrin and piperonyl butoxide diet on residues in products of animal origin. 1. Feeding study in pigs. *J. Agric. Food Chem.* 41:2416–2420 (1993).

222. Nakamura, Y., Y. Tonogai, Y. Tsumura, and Y. Ito. Determination of pyrethroid residues in vegetables, fruits, grains, beans, and green tea leaves: applications to pyrethroid residue monitoring studies. *J. AOAC Int.* 76:1348–1361 (1993).

223. Pang, G.-F., C.-L. Fan, Y.-Z. Chao, and T.-S. Zhao. Rapid method for the determination of multiple pyrethroid residues in fruit and vegetables by capillary column gas chromatography. *J. Chromatogr. A* 667:348–353 (1994).

224. Hill, A.S., D.P. McAdam, S.L. Edward, and J.H. Skerritt. Quantitation of bioresmethrin, a synthetic pyrethroid grain protectant, by enzyme immunoassay. *J. Agric. Food Chem.* 41:2011–2018 (1993).

225. Willes, R.F., E.R. Nestmann, P.A. Miller, et al. Scientific principles for evaluating the potential for adverse effects from chlorinated organic chemicals in the environment. *Regul. Toxicol. Pharmacol.* 18:313–356 (1993).

226. Woodruff, T., M.S. Wolff, D.L. Davis, and D. Hayward. Organochlorine exposure estimation in the study of cancer etiology. *Environ. Res.* 65:132–144 (1994).

227. Svensson, B.-G., T. Hallberg, A. Nilsson, et al. Parameters of immunological competence in subjects with high consumption of fish contaminated with persistent organochlorine compounds. *Int. Arch. Occup. Environ. Health* 65:351–358 (1994).

228. Dewailly, É., P. Ayotte, S. Bruneau, et al. Inuit exposure to organochlorines through the aquatic food chain in Arctic Québec. *Environ. Health Perspect.* 101:618–620 (1993).

229. Dewailly, E., S. Bruneau, P. Ayotte, et al. Health status at birth of Inuit newborn prenatally exposed to organochlorines. *Chemosphere* 27:359–366 (1993).

230. Mes, J., D.J. Davies, J. Doucet, et al. Levels of chlorinated hydrocarbon residues in Canadian human breast milk and their relationship to some characteristics of the donors. *Food Addit. Contam.* 10:429–441 (1993).

231. Matsueda, T., T. Iida, H. Hirakawa, et al. Toxic evaluation of PCDDs, PCDFs and coplanar PCBs in breast-fed babies of yusho and healthy mothers. *Chemosphere* 27:187–194 (1993).

232. Vaz, R., S.A. Slorach, and Y. Hofvander. Organochlorine contaminants in Swedish human milk: studies conducted at the National Food Administration 1981–1990. *Food Addit. Contam.* 10:407–418 (1993).

233. Norén, K. Contemporary and retrospective investigations of human milk in the trend studies of organochlorine

contaminants in Sweden. *Sci. Total Environ.* 139/140:347–355 (1993).

234. Duarte-Davidson, R., S.C. Wilson, and K.C. Jones. PCBs and other organochlorines in human tissue samples from the Welsh population: II—milk. *Environ. Pollut.* 84:79–87 (1994).

235. Fürst, P., C. Fürst, and K. Wilmers. Human milk as a bioindicator for body burden of PCDDs, PCDFs, organochlorine pesticides, and PCBs. *Environ. Health Perspect.* 102(Suppl. 1):187–193 (1994).

236. Bates, M.N., D.J. Hannah, S.J. Buckland, et al. Chlorinated organic contaminants in breast milk of New Zealand women. *Environ. Health Perspect.* 102(Suppl. 1):211–217 (1994).

237. Duarte-Davidson, R., S.C. Wilson, and K.C. Jones. PCBs and other organochlorines in human tissue samples from the Welsh population: I—adipose. *Environ. Pollut.* 84:69–77 (1994).

238. Loganathan, B.G., S. Tanabe, Y. Hidaka, et al. Temporal trends of persistent organochlorine residues in human adipose tissue from Japan, 1928–1985. *Environ. Pollut.* 81:31–39 (1993).

239. Ludwicki, J.K., and K. Góralczyk. Organochlorine pesticides and PCBs in human adipose tissues in Poland. *Bull. Environ. Contam. Toxicol.* 52:400–403 (1994).

240. Patterson, D.G., Jr., G.D. Todd, W.E. Turner, et al. Levels of non-*ortho*-substituted (coplanar), mono- and di-*ortho*-substituted polychlorinated biphenyls, dibenzo-*p*-dioxins, and dibenzofurans in human serum and adipose tissue. *Environ. Health Perspect.* 102(Suppl. 1):195–204 (1994).

241. Schecter, A., H. McGee, J. Stanley, and K. Boggess. Chlorinated dioxin, dibenzofuran, coplanar, mono-ortho, and di-ortho substituted PCB congener levels in blood and semen of Michigan Vietnam veterans compared with levels in Vietnamese exposed to Agent Orange. *Chemosphere* 27:241–252 (1993).

242. Theelen, R.M.C., A.K.D. Liem, W. Slob, and J.H. van Wijnen. Intake of 2,3,7,8 chlorine substituted dioxins, furans, and planar PCBs from food in the Netherlands: median and distribution. *Chemosphere* 27:1625–1635 (1993).

243. Theelen, R.M.C., and A.K.D. Liem. Exposure to 2,3,7,8-chlorine substituted dioxins, furans and planar PCBs from food by Dutch Turks: relevance of mutton. *Chemosphere* 28:675–682 (1994).

244. Hernández, L.M., M.A. Fernández, B. Jiménez, et al. Organochlorine pollutants in meats and cow's milk from Madrid (Spain). *Bull. Environ. Contam. Toxicol.* 52:246–253 (1994).

245. Newsome, W.H., and P. Andrews. Organochlorine pesticides and polychlorinated biphenyl congeners in commercial fish from the Great Lakes. *J. AOAC Int.* 76:707–710 (1993).

246. Newsome, W.H., P. Andrews, H.B.S. Conacher, et al. Total organochlorine content of fish from the Great Lakes. *J. AOAC Int.* 76:703–706 (1993).

247. Miller, M.A., N.M. Kassulke, and M.D. Walkowski. Organochlorine concentrations in Laurentian Great Lakes

Salmonines: implications for fisheries management. *Arch. Environ. Contam. Toxicol.* 25:212–219 (1993).

248. Hellou, J., W.G. Warren, and J.F. Payne. Organochlorines including polychlorinated biphenyls in muscle, liver, and ovaries of cod, *Gadus morhua. Arch. Environ. Contam. Toxicol.* 25:497–505 (1993).

249. Kelly, A.G., and L.A. Campbell. Organochlorine contaminants in liver of cod (*Gadus morhua*) and muscle of herring (*Clupea harengus*) from Scottish waters. *Marine Pollut. Bull.* 28:103–108 (1994).

250. de Boer, J., C.J.N. Stronck, W.A. Traag, and J. van der Meer. Non-ortho and mono-ortho substituted chlorobiphenyls and chlorinated dibenzo-p-dioxins and dibenzofurans in marine and freshwater fish and shellfish from the Netherlands. *Chemosphere* 26:1823–1842 (1993).

251. Karl, H., and I. Lehmann. Organochlorine residues in the edible part of eels of different origins. *Z. Lebensm. Unters. Forsch.* 197:385–388 (1993).

252. Koistinen, J., J. Paasivirta, and M. Lahtiperä. Bioaccumulation of dioxins, coplanar PCBs, PCDEs, HxCNs, R-PCNs, R-PCPHs and R-PCBBs in fish from a pulp-mill recipient watercourse. *Chemosphere* 27:149–156 (1993).

253. Norén, K., and J. Sjövall. Liquid–gel partitioning and enrichment in the analysis of organochlorine contaminants. *J. Chromatogr.* 642:243–251 (1993).

254. Schenck, F.J., R. Wagner, M.K. Hennessy, and J.L. Okrasinski, Jr. Screening of organochlorine pesticide and polychlorinated biphenyl residues in nonfatty seafood products by tandem solid-phase extraction cleanup. *J. AOAC Int.* 77:102–104 (1994).

255. Page, B.D., and G. Lacroix. Application of solid-phase microextraction to the headspace gas chromatographic analysis of halogenated volatiles in selected foods. *J. Chromatogr.* 648:199–211 (1993).

256. Kočan, A., J. Petrík, J. Chovancová, and B. Drobná. Method for the group separation of non-*ortho*-, mono-*ortho*- and multi-*ortho*-substituted polychlorinated biphenyls and polychlorinated dibenzo-*p*-dioxins/polychlorinated dibenzofurans using activated carbon chromatography. *J. Chromatogr. A* 665:139–153 (1994).

257. Zebühr, Y., C. Näf, C. Bandh, et al. An automated HPLC separation method with two coupled columns for the analysis of PCDD/Fs, PCBs and PACs. *Chemosphere* 27:1211–1219 (1993).

258. Rahman, M.S., S. Bøwadt, and B. Larsen. Dual-column GC analysis of Mediterranean fish for ten organochlorine pesticides and sixty two chlorobiphenyls. *J. High Res. Chromatogr.* 16:731–735 (1993).

259. van der Velde, E.G., J.A. Marsman, A.P.J.M. de Jong, et al. Analysis and occurrence of toxic planar PCBs, PCDDs and PCDFs in milk by use of carbosphere activated carbon. *Chemosphere* 28:693–702 (1994).

260. Fensterheim, R.J. Documenting temporal trends of polychlorinated biphenyls in the environment. *Regul. Toxicol. Pharmacol.* 18:181–201 (1993).

261. Ahlborg, U.G., G.C. Becking, L.S. Birnbaum, et al. Toxic equivalency factors for dioxin-like PCBs. Report on

a WHO-ECEH and IPCS consultation, December 1993. *Chemosphere* 28:1049–1067 (1994).

262.  Safe, S.H. Polychlorinated biphenyls (PCBs): Environmental impact, biochemical and toxic responses, and implications for risk assessment. *Crit. Rev. Toxicol.* 24:87–149 (1994).

263.  Safe, S. Toxicology, structure–function relationship, and human and environmental health impacts of polychlorinated biphenyls: progress and problems. *Environ. Health Perspect.* 100:259–268 (1992).

264.  Schecter, A., J. Stanley, K. Boggess, et al. Polychlorinated biphenyl levels in the tissues of exposed and nonexposed humans. *Environ. Health Perspect.* 102(Suppl. 1):149–158 (1994).

265.  Conde, C., C. Maluenda, and C. Arrabal. Organochlorine residues in human milk in Spain. Polychlorinated biphenyls (PCBs) from 1988 to 1991. *Bull. Environ. Contam. Toxicol.* 51:832–837 (1993).

266.  Dewailly, É., J.J. Ryan, C. Laliberté, et al. Exposure of remote maritime populations to coplanar PCBs. *Environ. Health Perspect.* 102(Suppl. 1):205–209 (1994).

267.  Georgii, S., Gh. Bachour, I. Elmadfa, and H. Brunn. PCB-Kongenere in Frauenmilch aus Mittelhessen. Vergleichende Untersuchungen für die Jahre 1984/95 und 1991/92. *Dtsch. Lebensm.-Rundsch.* 89:239–245 (1993).

268.  Burse, V.W., D.F. Groce, S.P. Caudill, et al. Determination of polychlorinated biphenyl levels in the serum of residents and in the homogenates of seafood from the New Bedford, Massachusetts, area: A comparison of exposure sources through pattern recognition techniques. *Sci. Total Environ.* 144:153–177 (1994).

269.  Guo, Y.L., C.J. Lin, W.J. Yao, et al. Musculoskeletal changes in children prenatally exposed to polychlorinated biphenyls and related compounds (Yu-Cheng children). *J. Toxicol. Environ. Health* 41:83–93 (1994).

270.  Chen, Y.-J., and C.-C. Hsu. Effects of prenatal exposure to PCBs on the neurological function of children: a neuropsychological and neurophysiological study. *Dev. Med. Child Neurol.* 36:312–320 (1994).

271.  Chen, Y.-C.J., M.-L.M. Yu, W.J. Rogan, et al. A 6-year follow-up of behavior and activity disorders in the Taiwan Yu-Cheng children. *Am. J. Public Health* 84:415–521 (1994).

272.  Hirota, Y., K. Kataoka, S. Tokunaga, et al. Association between blood polychlorinated biphenyl concentration and serum triglyceride level in chronic "Yusho" (polychlorinated biphenyl poisoning) patients. *Int. Arch. Occup. Environ. Health* 65:221–225 (1993).

273.  Arnold, D.L., F. Bryce, R. Stapley, et al. Toxicological consequences of Aroclor 1254 ingestion by female rhesus (*Macaca mulatta*) monkeys. Part 1A. Prebreeding phase: clinical health findings. *Food Chem. Toxicol.* 31:799–810 (1993).

274.  Arnold, D.L., F. Bryce, K. Karpinski, et al. Toxicological consequences of Aroclor 1254 ingestion by female rhesus (*Macaca mulatta*) monkeys. Part 1B. Prebreeding phase: clinical and analytical laboratory findings. *Food Chem. Toxicol.* 31:811–824 (1993).

275.  Mes, J., D.L. Arnold, and F. Bryce. Determination of polychlorinated biphenyls in postpartum blood, adipose tissue, and milk from female rhesus monkeys and their offspring after prolonged dosing with Aroclor® 1254. *J. Anal. Toxicol.* 18:29–35 (1994).

276.  Seegal, R.F., B. Bush, K.O. Brosch. Decreases in dopamine concentrations in adult, non-human primate brain persist following removal from polychlorinated biphenyls. *Toxicology* 86:71–87 (1994).

277.  Chu, I., D.C. Velleneuve, A. Yagminas, et al. Subchronic toxicity of 3,3',4,4',5-pentachlorobiphenyl in the rat. I. Clinical, biochemical, hematological, and histopathological changes. *Fund. Appl. Toxicol.* 22:457–468 (1994).

278.  Harper, N., L. Howie, K. Connor, et al. Immunosuppressive effects of highly chlorinated biphenyls and diphenyl ethers on T-cell dependent and independent antigens in mice. *Toxicology* 86:123–135 (1993).

279.  Kafafi, S.A., H.Y. Afeefy, A.H. Ali, et al. Binding of polychlorinated biphenyls to the aryl hydrocarbon receptor. *Environ. Health Perspect.* 101:422–428 (1993).

280.  Kafafi, S.A., H.Y. Afeefy, A.H. Ali, et al. Affinities for the aryl hydrocarbon receptor, potencies as aryl hydrocarbon hydroxylase inducers and relative toxicities of polychlorinated biphenyls. A congener specific approach. *Carcinogenesis* 14:2063–2071 (1993).

281.  Borlakoglu, J.T., and J.P.G. Wilkins. Correlations between the molecular structures of polyhalogenated biphenyls and their metabolism by hepatic microsomal monooxygenases. *Comp. Biochem. Physiol.* 105C:113–117 (1993).

282.  McKinney, J.D., and C.L. Waller. Polychlorinated biphenyls as hormonally active structural analogues. *Environ. Health Perspect.* 102:290–297 (1994).

283.  Himberg, K.K. Coplanar polychlorinated biphenyls in some Finnish food commodities. *Chemosphere* 27:1235–1243 (1993).

284.  Falandysz, J., S. Tanabe, and R. Tatsukawa. Most toxic and highly bioaccumulative PCB congeners in cod-liver oil of Baltic origin processed in Poland during the 1970s and 1980s, their TEQ-values and possible intake. *Sci. Total Environ.* 145:207–212 (1994).

285.  Sánchez, J., M. Solé, and J. Albaigés. A comparison of distributions of PCB congeners and other chlorinated compounds in fishes from coastal areas and remote lakes. *Int. J. Environ. Anal. Chem.* 50:269–284 (1993).

286.  Elskus, A.A., J.J. Stegeman, J.W. Gooch, et al. Polychlorinated biphenyl congener distributions in winter flounder as related to gender, spawning site, and congener metabolism. *Environ. Sci. Technol.* 28:401–407 (1994).

287.  Johansen, H.R., O.J. Rossland, and G. Becher. Congener specific determinations of PCBs in crabs from a polluted fjord region. *Chemosphere* 27:1245–1252 (1993).

288.  Hädrich, J., and F. Baum. Beurteilung der PCB-Belastungssituation landwirtschaftlicher Nutztiere durch Bestimmung des PCB-Gehaltes im Blutplasma. 2. Mitteilung: Validierung, Erweiterung und praktische Anwendung des Beurteilungsverfahrens. *Arch. Lebensmittelhyg.* 44:69–73 (1993).

289. Gan, D.R., and P.M. Berthouex. Disappearance and crop uptake of PCBs from sludge-amended farmland. *Water Environ. Res.* 66:54–69 (1994).

290. de Voogt, P., P. Haglund, L.B. Reutergårdh, et al. Fishing for quality in environmental analysis. Interlaboratory study on non- and mono-ortho chlorinated biphenyls. *Anal. Chem.* 66:305A–311A (1994).

291. Hajšlova, J., K. Holadova, V. Kocourek, et al. Determination of PCBs in fatty tissues by means of several detection techniques. *Z. Lebensm. Unters. Forsch.* 197:562–569 (1993).

292. Johansen, H.R., C. Thorstensen, T. Greibrokk, and G. Becher. On-line SFE-GC for determination of PCBs in human milk and blood serum. *J. High Res. Chromatogr.* 16:148–152 (1993).

293. Mills, A.G., and T.M. Jefferies. Rapid isolation of polychlorinated biphenyls from milk by a combination of supercritical-fluid extraction and supercritical-fluid chromatography. *J. Chromatogr.* 643:409–418 (1993).

294. Ford, C.A., D.C.G. Muir, R.J. Norstrom, et al. Development of a semi-automated method for non-ortho PCBs: application to Canadian Arctic marine mammal tissues. *Chemosphere* 26:1981–1991 (1993).

295. Stalling, D.L., C.Y. Guo, and S. Saim. Surface-linked $C_{60/70}$-polystyrene divinylbenzene beads as a new chromatographic material for enrichment of coplanar PCBs. *J. Chromatogr. Sci.* 31:265–278 (1993).

296. Galceran, M.T., F.J. Santos, D. Barceló, and J. Sanchez. Improvements in the separation of polychlorinated biphenyl congeners by high-resolution gas chromatography. Application to the analysis of two mineral oils and powdered milk. *J. Chromatogr. A* 655:275–284 (1993).

297. König, W.A., B. Gehrcke, T. Runge, and C. Wolf. Gas chromatographic separation of atropisomeric alkylated and polychlorinated biphenyls using modified cyclodextrins. *J. High Res. Chromatogr.* 16:376–378 (1993).

298. Vo-Dinh, T., A. Pal, and T. Pal. Photoactivated luminescence method for rapid screening of polychlorinated biphenyls. *Anal. Chem.* 66:1264–1268 (1994).

299. Vanden Heuvel, J.P., and G. Lucier. Environmental toxicology of polychlorinated dibenzo-*p*-dioxins and polychlorinated dibenzofurans. *Environ. Health Perspect.* 100:189–200 (1993).

300. Birnbaum, L.S. EPA's reassessment of dioxin risk: directed health research. *Chemosphere* 27:469–475 (1993).

301. Feeley, M.M., and D.L. Grant. Approach to risk assessment of PCDDs and PCDFs in Canada. *Regul. Toxicol. Pharmacol.* 18:428–437 (1993).

302. Tysklind, M., D. Tillitt, L. Eriksson, et al. A toxic equivalency factor scale for polychlorinated dibenzofurans. *Fund. Appl. Toxicol.* 22:277–285 (1994).

303. McLachlan, M.S. Exposure toxicity equivalents (ETEs): a plea for more environmental chemistry in dioxin risk assessment. *Chemosphere* 27:483–490 (1993).

304. McLachlan, M.S. Digestive tract absorption of polychlorinated dibenzo-*p*-dioxins, dibenzofurans, and biphenyls in a nursing infant. *Toxicol. Appl. Pharmacol.* 123:68–72 (1993).

305. Pluim, H.J., J. Wever, J.G. Koppe, et al. Intake and faecal excretion of chlorinated dioxins and dibenzofurans in breast-fed infants at different ages. *Chemosphere* 26:1947–1952 (1993).

306. Van den Berg, M., J. De Jongh, H. Poiger, and J.R. Olson. The toxicokinetics and metabolism of polychlorinated dibenzo-*p*-dioxins (PCDDs) and dibenzofurans (PCDFs) and their relevance for toxicity. *Crit. Rev. Toxicol.* 24:1–74 (1994).

307. Okey, A.B., D.S. Riddick, and P.A. Harper. The Ah receptor: mediator of the toxicity of 2,3,7,8-tetrachlorodibenzo-*p*-dioxin (TCDD) and related compounds. *Toxicol. Lett.* 70:1–22 (1994).

308. Nebert, D.W., A. Puga, and V. Vasiliou. Role of the Ah receptor and the dioxin-inducible [*Ah*] gene battery in toxicity, cancer, and signal transduction. *Ann. N.Y. Acad. Sci.* 685:624–640 (1993).

309. Bertazzi, P.A., A.C. Pesatori, D. Consonni, et al. Cancer incidence in a population accidentally exposed to 2,3,7,8-tetrachlorodibenzo-*para*-dioxin. *Epidemiology* 4:398–406 (1993).

310. McConnell, R., K. Anderson, W. Russell, et al. Angiosarcoma, porphyria cutanea tarda, and probable chloracne in a worker exposed to waste oil contaminated with 2,3,7,8-tetrachlorodibenzo-p-dioxin. *Br. J. Indust. Med.* 50:699–703 (1993).

311. Schecter, A., P. Fürst, C. Fürst, et al. Chlorinated dioxins and dibenzofurans in human tissue from general populations: a selective review. *Environ. Health Perspect.* 102(Suppl. 1):159–171 (1994).

312. Orban, J.E., J.S. Stanley, J.G. Schwemberger, and J.C. Remmers. Dioxins and dibenzofurans in adipose tissue of the general US population and selected subpopulations. *Am. J. Public Health* 84:439–445 (1994).

313. Ryan, J.J., R. Lizotte, L.G. Panopio, et al. Polychlorinated dibenzo-*p*-dioxins (PCDDs) and polychlorinated dibenzofurans (PCDFs) in human milk samples collected across Canada in 1986–87. *Food Addit. Contam.* 10:419–428 (1993).

314. González, M.J., B. Jiménez, L.M. Hernández, et al. Levels of PCDDs and PCDFs in adipose tissue from Spanish people. *Chemosphere* 27:97–104 (1993).

315. Beck, H., A. Dross, and W. Mathar. PCDD and PCDF exposure and levels in humans in Germany. *Environ. Health Perspect.* 102(Suppl. 1):173–185 (1994).

316. Pluim, H.J., I. Kramer, J.W. van der Slikke, et al. Levels of PCDDs and PCDFs in human milk: dependence on several parameters and dietary habits. *Chemosphere* 26:1889–1895 (1993).

317. Scheter, A., J.J. Ryan, Y. Masuda, et al. Chlorinated and brominated dioxins and dibenzofurans in human tissue following exposure. *Environ. Health Perspect.* 102(Suppl. 1):135–147 (1994).

318. Zober, A., and O. Päpke. Concentrations of PCDDs and PCDFs in human tissue 36 years after accidental dioxin exposure. *Chemosphere* 27:413–418 (1993).

319. Neubert, R., R. Stahlmann, M. Korte, et al. Effects of small doses of dioxins on the immune system of marmosets and rats. *Ann. N.Y. Acad. Sci.* 685:662–686 (1993).

320. Neubert, R., L. Maskow, J. Webb, et al. Chlorinated dibenzo-p-dioxins and dibenzofurans and the human immune system. 1. Blood cell receptors in volunteers with moderately increased body burdens. *Life Sci.* 53:1995–2006 (1993).

321. Lang, D.S., S. Becker, G.C. Clark, et al. Lack of direct immunosuppressive effects of 2,3,7,8-tetrachlorodibenzo-p-dioxin (TCDD) on human peripheral blood lymphocyte subsets in vitro. *Arch. Toxicol.* 68:296–302 (1994).

322. Wood, S.C., H.G. Jeong, D.L. Morris, and M.P. Holsapple. Direct effects of 2,3,7,8-tetrachlorodibenzo-p-dioxin (TCDD) on human tonsillar lymphocytes. *Toxicology* 81:131–143 (1993).

323. Lucier, G., G. Clark, C. Hiermath, et al. Carcinogenicity of TCDD in laboratory animals: implications for risk assessment. *Toxicol. Indust. Health* 9:631–668 (1993).

324. Schrenk, D., A. Buchmann, K. Dietz, et al. Promotion of preneoplastic foci in rat liver with 2,3,7,8-tetrachlorodibenzo-p-dioxin, 1,2,3,4,6,7,8-heptachlorodibenzo-p-dioxin and a defined mixture of 49 polychlorinated dibenzo-p-dioxins. *Carcinogenesis* 15:509–515 (1994).

325. Maronpot, R.R., J.F. Foley, K. Takahashi, et al. Dose response for TCDD promotion of hepatocarcinogenesis in rats initiated with DEN: histologic, biochemical, and cell proliferation endpoints. *Environ. Health Perspect.* 101:634–642 (1993).

326. Olson, J.R., B.P. McGarrigle, P.J. Gigliotti, et al. Hepatic uptake and metabolism of 2,3,7,8-tetrachlorodibenzo-p-dioxin and 2,3,7,8-tetrachlorodibenzofuran. *Fund. Appl. Toxicol.* 22:631–640 (1994).

327. Peterson, R.E., H.M. Theobald, and G.L. Kimmel. Developmental and reproductive toxicity of dioxins and related compounds: cross-species comparisons. *Crit. Rev. Toxicol.* 23:283–335 (1993).

328. Nagao, T., G. Golor, H. Hagenmaier, and D. Neubert. Teratogenic potency of 2,3,4,7,8-pentachlorodibenzofuran and of three mixtures of polychlorinated dibenzo-p-dioxins and dibenzofurans in mice. Problems with risk assessment using TCDD toxic-equivalency factors. *Arch. Toxicol.* 67:591–597 (1993).

329. Pluim, H.J., J.J.M. de Vijlder, D. Olie, et al. Effect of pre- and postnatal exposure to chlorinated dioxins and furans on human neonatal thyroid hormone concentrations. *Environ. Health Perspect.* 101:504–508 (1993).

330. Rappe, C. Sources of exposure, environmental concentrations and exposure assessment of PCDDs and PCDFs. *Chemosphere* 27:211–225 (1993).

331. Slob, W., and J.A. Van Jaarsveld. A chain model for dioxins: from emission to cow's milk. *Chemosphere* 27:509–516 (1993).

332. Frommberger, R. Belastung des Säuglings mit Dioxinen und Furanen durch Säuglingsnahrung des Handels im Vergleich zur Belastung durch Humanmilch. *Dtsch. Lebensm.-Rundsch.* 89:137–142 (1993).

333. Lassek, E., D. Jahr, and R. Mayer. Polychlorinated dibenzo-p-dioxins and dibenzofurans in cows milk from Bavaria, FRG. *Chemosphere* 27:519–534 (1993).

334. Fürst, P., G.H.M. Krause, D. Hein, et al. PCDD/PCDF in cow's milk in relation to their levels in grass and soil. *Chemosphere* 27:1349–1357 (1993).

335. Wild, S.R., S.J. Harrad, and K.C. Jones. The influence of sewage sludge applications to agricultural land on human exposure to polychlorinated dibenzo-p-dioxins (PCDDs) and -furans (PCDFs). *Environ. Pollut.* 83:357–369 (1994).

336. Müller, J.F., A. Hülster, O. Päpke, et al. Transfer pathways of PCDD/PCDF to fruits. *Chemosphere* 27:195–201 (1993).

337. Whittle, D.M., C. Mageau, R.K. Duncan, et al. Canadian national dioxin sampling program: dioxins and furans in biota near 46 pulp and paper mills using the chlorine bleaching process. *Chemosphere* 27:279–286 (1993).

338. Owens, J.W., S.M. Swanson, and D.A. Birkholz. Bioaccumulation of 2,3,7,8-tetrachlorodibenzo-p-dioxin, 2,3,7,8-tetrachlorodibenzofuran and extractable organic chlorine at a bleached-kraft mill site in a northern Canadian river system. *Environ. Toxicol. Chem.* 13:343–354 (1994).

339. Law, F.C.P., and J.A. Gudaitis. A preliminary assessment of human health risks due to consumption of fish contaminated by dioxins and furans in the Fraser and Thompson Rivers. *Chemosphere* 28:1079–1086 (1994).

340. Hellou, J., and J.F. Payne. Polychlorinated dibenzo-p-dioxins and dibenzofurans in cod (*Gadus morhua*) from the Northwest Atlantic. *Marine Environ. Res.* 36:117–128 (1993).

341. Brown, R.P., K.R. Cooper, A. Cristini, et al. Polychlorinated dibenzo-p-dioxins and dibenzofurans in *Mya arenaria* in the Newark/Raritan Bay estuary. *Environ. Toxicol. Chem.* 13:523–528 (1994).

342. Hauge, P.M., T.J. Belton, B.E. Ruppel, et al. 2,3,7,8-TCDD and 2,3,7,8-TCDF in blue crabs and American lobsters from the Hudson-Raritan estuary and the New York Bight. *Bull. Environ. Contam. Toxicol.* 52:734–741 (1994).

343. Garattini, S., G. Mariani, E. Benfenati, and R. Fanelli. Preliminary survey on 2,3,7,8-TCDD in cellulose-containing consumer products on the Italian market. *Chemosphere* 27:1561–1564 (1993).

344. de Jong, A.P.J.M., A.K.D. Liem, and R. Hoogerbrugge. Study of polychlorinated dibenzodioxins and furans from municipal waste incinerator emissions in the Netherlands: analytical methods and levels in the environment and human food chain. *J. Chromatogr.* 643:91–106 (1993).

345. King, T.L., J.F. Uthe, and C.J. Musial. Rapid screening of fish tissue for polychlorinated dibenzo-p-dioxins and dibenzofurans. *Analyst* 118:1269–1275 (1993).

346. Sherry, J.P., J. Carron, D. Leger, et al. An MSD-based method for the detection of chlorinated dibenzo-p-dioxins and chlorinated dibenzofurans in fish. *Chemosphere* 27:651–664 (1993).

347. Tsuda, S., M. Kawano, T. Wakimoto, and R. Tatsukawa. Application of charcoal/silica-gel column for analysis of polychlorinated dibenzo-p-dioxins (PCDDs) and polychlorinated dibenzofurans (PCDFs). *Chemosphere* 27:2117–2122 (1993).

348. Pyell, U., and P. Garrigues. Clean-up by high-performance liquid chromatography of polychlorodibenzo-p-dioxins

and polychlorodibenzofurans on a pyrenylethylsilica gel column. *J. Chromatogr. A* 660:223–229 (1994).

349.    Chang, R.R., W.M. Jarman, and J.A. Hennings. Sample cleanup by solid-phase extraction for the ultratrace determination of polychlorinated dibenzo-*p*-dioxins and dibenzofurans in biological samples. *Anal. Chem.* 65:2420–2427 (1993).

350.    Aschengrau, A., D. Ozonoff, C. Paulu, et al. Cancer risk and tetrachloroethylene-contaminated drinking water in Massachusetts. *Arch. Environ. Health* 48:284–292 (1993).

351.    Webler, T., and H.S. Brown. Exposure to tetrachloroethylene via contaminated drinking water pipes in Massachusetts: a predictive model. *Arch. Environ. Health* 48:293–297 (1993).

352.    Steinberg, A.D., and J.M. DeSesso. Have animal data been used inappropriately to estimate risks to humans from environmental trichloroethylene? *Regul. Toxicol. Pharmacol.* 18:137–153 (1993).

353.    Vartiainen, T., E. Pukkala, T. Rienoja, et al. Population exposure to tri- and tetrachloroethene and cancer risk: two cases of drinking water pollution. *Chemosphere* 27:1171–1181 (1993).

354.    Galceran, M.T., F.J. Santos, J. Caixach, et al. Environmental analysis of polychlorinated terphenyls: distribution in shellfish from the Ebro Delta (Mediterranean). *J. Chromatogr.* 643:399–408 (1993).

355.    Koistinen, J., P.J. Vuorinen, and J. Paasivirta. Contents and origin of polychlorinated diphenyl ethers (PCDE) in salmon from the Baltic Sea, Lake Saimaa and the Tenojoki River in Finland. *Chemosphere* 27:2365–2380 (1993).

356.    Mennear, J.H., and C.-C. Lee. Polybrominated dibenzo-*p*-dioxins and dibenzofurans: literature review and health assessment. *Environ. Health Perspect.* 102(Suppl. 1):265–274 (1994).

357.    Jernström, B., and A. Gräslund. Covalent binding of benzo[a]pyrene 7,8-dihydrodiol 9,10-epoxides to DNA: molecular structures, induced mutations and biological consequences. *Biophys. Chem.* 49:185–199 (1994).

358.    dell'Omo, M., and R.R. Lauwerys. Adducts to macromolecules in the biological monitoring of workers exposed to polycyclic aromatic hydrocarbons. *Crit. Rev. Toxicol.* 23:111–126 (1993).

359.    Van Hummelen, P., J.P. Gennart, J.P. Buchet, et al. Biological markers in PAH exposed workers and controls. *Mutat. Res.* 300:231–239 (1993).

360.    Szczeklik, A., J. Szczeklik, Z. Galuszka, et al. Humoral immunosuppression in men exposed to polycyclic aromatic hydrocarbons and related carcinogens in polluted environments. *Environ. Health Perspect.* 102:302–304 (1994).

361.    Lu, L.-J.W., L.M. Anderson, A.B. Jones, et al. Persistence, gestation, stage-dependent formation and interrelationships of benzo[a]pyrene-induced DNA adducts in mothers, placentae and fetuses of *Erythrocebus patas* monkeys. *Carcinogenesis* 14:1805–1813 (1993).

362.    Penning, T.M. Dihydrodiol dehydrogenase and its role in polycyclic aromatic hydrocarbon metabolism. *Chem.-Biol. Interact.* 89:1–34 (1993).

363.    Lesca, P., R. Witkamp, P. Maurel, and P. Galtier. The pig as a model for studying Ah receptor and other PAH-binding proteins in man. *Biochem. Biophys. Res. Commun.* 200:475–481 (1994).

364.    Shuguang, L., P. Dinhua, and W. Guoxiong. Analysis of polycyclic aromatic hydrocarbons in cooking oil fumes. *Arch. Environ. Health* 49:119–122 (1994).

365.    Saxton, W.L., R.T. Newton, J. Rorberg, et al. Polycyclic aromatic hydrocarbons in seafood from the Gulf of Alaska following a major crude oil spill. *Bull. Environ. Contam. Toxicol.* 51:515–522 (1993).

366.    Al-Yakoob, S., T. Safeed, and H. Al-Hashash. Polycyclic aromatic hydrocarbons in edible tissue of fish from the Gulf after the 1991 oil spill. *Marine Pollut. Bull.* 27:297–301 (1993).

367.    Hellou, J., J.F. Payne, and C. Hamilton. Polycyclic aromatic compounds in Northwest Atlantic cod (*Gadus morhua*). *Environ. Pollut.* 84:197–202 (1994).

368.    Jackson, T.J., T.L. Wade, T.J. McDonald, et al. Polynuclear aromatic hydrocarbon contaminants in oysters from the Gulf of Mexico (1986–1990). *Environ. Pollut.* 83:291–298 (1994).

369.    Nakano, M., and M. Fukushima. Formation of polycyclic aromatic hydrocarbons (PAHs) in lamb during roasting. *J. Food Hyg. Soc. Japan* 35:41–45 (1994).

370.    Tateno, T., and S. Suenaga. Polycyclic aromatic hydrocarbons produced by grill of vegetables—effects of various grilled temperature and time. *J. Food Hyg. Soc. Japan* 35:206–209 (1994).

371.    Westphal, K., K. Potthast, and G. Übermuth. Benzo-a-pyrengehalte in geräucherten Fleischerzeugnissen aus traditionellen Räucheranlagen ehemaliger DDR-Betriebe. *Fleischwirtschaft* 74:543–546 (1994).

372.    Gomaa, E.A., J.I. Gray, S. Rabie, et al. Polycyclic aromatic hydrocarbons in smoked food products and commercial liquid smoke flavourings. *Food Addit. Contam.* 10:503–521 (1993).

373.    Yabiku, H.Y., M.S. Martins, and M.Y. Takahashi. Levels of benzo[*a*]pyrene and other polycyclic aromatic hydrocarbons in liquid smoke flavour and some smoked foods. *Food Addit. Contam.* 10:399–405 (1993).

374.    Šimko, P., P. Šimon, V. Khunová, et al. Kinetics of polycyclic aromatic hydrocarbon sorption from liquid smoke flavour into low density polyethylene packaging. *Food Chem.* 50:65–68 (1994).

375.    Wild, S.R., and K.C. Jones. The significance of polynuclear aromatic hydrocarbons applied to agricultural soils in sewage sludges in the U.K. *Waste Management Res.* 12:49–59 (1994).

376.    Furton, K.G., E. Jolly, and G. Pentzke. Recent advance in the analysis of polycyclic aromatic hydrocarbons and fullerenes. *J. Chromatogr.* 642:33–45 (1993).

377.    Wise, S.A., L.C. Sander, and W.E. May. Determination of polycyclic aromatic hydrocarbons by liquid chromatography. *J. Chromatogr.* 642:329–349 (1993).

378.    Nie, S., R. Dadoo, and R.N. Zare. Ultrasensitive fluorescence detection of polycyclic aromatic hydrocarbons

in capillary electrophoresis. *Anal. Chem.* 65:3571–3575 (1993).

379. Nyman, P.J., G.A. Perfetti, F.L. Joe, Jr., and G.W. Diachenko. Comparison of two clean-up methodologies for the gas chromatographic/mass spectrometric determination of low nanogram/gram levels of polynuclear aromatic hydrocarbons in seafood. *Food Addit. Contam.* 10:489–501 (1993).

380. Gilbert, J., J. Bush, A. Lopez de Sa, et al. Establishment of a reference collection of substances and an analytical handbook of reference data to support enforcement of EC regulations on food contact materials. *Food Addit. Contam.* 11:71–77 (1994).

381. Begley, T.H., and H.C. Hollifield. Recycled polymers in food packaging: migration considerations. *Food Technol.* 47(11):109–112 (1993).

382. Franz, R., M. Huber, and O.-G. Piringer. Verfahren zur Prüfung und Bewertung von Recyclingkunststoffen für deren Einsatz in der Lebensmittelverpackung unter dem Aspekt der Migration durch eine funktionelle Barriere. *Dtsch. Lebensm.-Rundsch.* 89:317–324 (1993).

383. Ashby, R., and P. Tice (eds.). *Sixth International Symposium on Migration in Food Packaging Plastics. Food Addit. Contam.* 11(2) (1994).

384. Rossi, L. European Community controls for high temperature testing of food contact materials. *Food Addit. Contam.* 10:615–620 (1993).

385. Piringer, O., E. Wolff, and K. Pfaff. Use of high temperature-resistant sorbents as simulants for testing. *Food Addit. Contam.* 10:621–629 (1993).

386. Rijk, R., and N. de Kruijf. Migration testing with olive oil in a microwave oven. *Food Addit. Contam.* 10:631–645 (1993).

387. Jickels, S.M., and L. Castle. Combined compositional analysis and threshold of regulation as a possible control measure for microwave susceptors. *Food Addit. Contam.* 10:647–653 (1993).

388. Risch, S. Safety assessment of microwave susceptors and other high temperature packaging materials. *Food Addit. Contam.* 10:655–661 (1993).

389. McNeal, T.P., and H.C. Hollifield. Determination of volatile chemicals released from microwave-heat-susceptor food packaging. *J. AOAC Int.* 76:1268–1275 (1994).

390. Jickells, S.M., M.R. Philo, J. Gilbert, and L. Castle. Gas chromatographic/mass spectrometric determination of benzene in nonstick cookware and microwave susceptors and its migration into foods on cooking. *J. AOAC Int.* 76:760–764 (1993).

391. Jickells, S.M., P. Gancedo, C. Nerin, et al. Migration of styrene monomer from thermoset polyester cookware into foods during high temperature applications. *Food Addit. Contam.* 10:567–573 (1993).

392. Nerin, C., P. Gancedo, and J. Cacho. Determination of styrene in olive oil by coevaporation, cold trap, and GC/MS/SIM. *J. Agric. Food Chem.* 41:2003–2005 (1993).

393. Lehr, K.M., G.C. Welsh, C.D. Bell, and T.D. Lickly. The 'vapour-phase' migration of styrene from general purpose

polystyrene and high impact polystyrene into cooking oil. *Food Chem. Toxicol.* 31:793–798 (1993).

394. Morgenroth, V., III. Scientific evaluation of the data-derived safety factors for the acceptable daily intake. Case study: diethylhexylphthalate. *Food Addit. Contam.* 10:363–373 (1993).

395. Bentley, P., I. Calder, C. Elcombe, et al. Hepatic peroxisome proliferation in rodents and its significance for humans. *Food Chem. Toxicol.* 31:857–907 (1993).

396. Dirven, H.A.A.M., P.H.H. van den Broek, M.C.E. Peeters, et al. Effects of the peroxisome proliferator mono(2-ethylhexyl)phthalate in primary hepatocyte cultures derived from rat, guinea pig, rabbit and monkey. *Biochem. Pharmacol.* 45:2425–2434 (1993).

397. Nerín, C., J. Cacho, and P. Gancedo. Plasticizers from printing inks in a selection of food packagings and their migration to food. *Food Addit. Contam.* 10:453–460 (1993).

398. Ishida, M. Reduction of phthalate in chicken eggs, liver and meat by several cooking methods. *J. Food Hyg. Soc. Japan* 34:529–531 (1993).

399. Vitali, M., V. Leoni, S. Chiavarini, and C. Cremisini. Determination of 2-ethyl-1-hexanol as contaminant in drinking water. *J. AOAC Int.* 76:1133–1137 (1993).

400. Loftus, N.J., W.J.D. Laird, G.T. Steel, et al. Metabolism and pharmacokinetics of deuterium-labelled di-2-(ethylhexyl) adipate (DEHA) in humans. *Food Chem. Toxicol.* 31:609–614 (1993).

401. Loftus, N.J., B.H. Woollen, G.T. Steel, et al. An assessment of the dietary uptake of di-2-(ethylhexyl) adipate (DEHA) in a limited population study. *Food Chem. Toxicol.* 32:1–5 (1994).

402. Castle, L., J. Nichol, and J. Gilbert. Migration from plasticized films into foods. 6. Hydrolysis of polymeric plasticizers under simulated gastric and intestinal conditions. *Food Addit. Contam.* 10:523–529 (1993).

403. Castle, L., J. Nichol, and J. Gilbert. Migration of mineral hydrocarbons into foods. 4. Waxed paper for packaging dry goods including bread, confectionery and for domestic use including microwave cooking. *Food Addit. Contam.* 11:79–89 (1994).

404. Grob, K., A. Artho, M. Biedermann, and H. Mikle. Verunreinigung von Haselnüssen und Schokolade durch Mineralöl aus Jute- und Sisalsäcken. *Z. Lebensm. Unters. Forsch.* 197:370–374 (1993).

405. Darkby, C.T., and O. Lawson. Analysis of migrants from nylon 6 packaging films into boiling water. *Food Addit. Contam.* 10:541–553 (1993).

406. Simal Gándara, J., P. López Mahía, P. Paseiro Losada, et al. Overall migration and specific migration of bisphenol A diglycidyl ether monomer and *m*-xylylenediamine hardener from an optimized epoxy-amine formulation into water-based food simulants. *Food Addit. Contam.* 10:555–565 (1993).

407. Bourges, F., G. Bureau, and B. Pascat. Effects of electron beam irradiation on the migration of antioxidants and their degradation products from commercial polypropylene into food simulating liquids. *Food Addit. Contam.* 10:443–452 (1993).

408. Abaitua Borda, I., E.M. Kilbourne, M. Posada de la Paz, et al. Mortality among people affected by toxic oil syndrome. *Int. J. Epidemiol.* 22:1077–1084 (1993).

409. Alonso-Ruiz, A., M. Calabozo, F. Perez-Ruiz, and L. Mancebo. Toxic oil syndrome. A long-term follow-up of a cohort of 332 patients. *Medicine* 72:285–295 (1993).

410. Yoshida, S.H., J.B. German, M.P. Fletcher, and M.E. Gershwin. The toxic oil syndrome: a perspective on immunotoxicological mechanisms. *Regul. Toxicol. Pharmacol.* 19:60-79 (1994).

411. Hayashi, T., and T.N. James. Immunohistochemical analysis of lymphocytes in postmortem study of the heart from fatal cases of the eosinophilia myalgia syndrome and of the toxic oil syndrome. *Am. Heart J.* 127:1298–1308 (1994).

412. Kaufman, L.D., B.L. Gruber, J.J. Gomez-Reino, and F. Miller. Fibrogenic growth factors in the eosinophilia-myalgia syndrome and the toxic oil syndrome. *Arch. Dermatol.* 130:41–47 (1994).

413. Gomez-Reino, J.J., M. Sandberg, P.E. Carreira, and E. Vuorio. Expression of types I, III and IV collagen genes in fibrotic skin and nerve lesions of toxic oil syndrome patients. *Clin. Exp. Immunol.* 93:103–107 (1993).

414. Hernández-Muñoz, I., M. Paz de la Torre, M.A. Pedraza, et al. Toxic oil stimulates collagen synthesis acting at a pretranslational level in cultured fat-storing cells. *Gastroenterology* 106:691–701 (1994).

415. Guitart, R., L. Nørgaard, G. Mariani, et al. Analysis of polychlorinated dioxins and furans in samples of the toxic oil syndrome. *Human Exp. Toxicol.* 12:273–278 (1993).

416. McNeal, T.P., P.J. Nyman, G.W. Diachenko, and H.C. Hollifield. Survey of benzene in foods by using headspace concentration techniques and capillary gas chromatography. *J. AOAC Int.* 76:1213–1219 (1993).

417. Castle, L. Determination of acrylamide monomer in mushrooms grown on polyacrylamide gel. *J. Agric. Food Chem.* 41:1261–1263 (1993).

418. Kaminski, J., A.S. Atwal, and S. Mahadevan. Determination of formaldehyde in fresh and retial milk by liquid column chromatography. *J. AOAC Int.* 76:1010–1013 (1993).

419. Matusik, J.E., P.P. Eilers, E.M. Waldron, et al. Confirmation of identities of propylene and ethylene glycols in anchovies by tandem mass spectrometry. *J. AOAC Int.* 76:1344–1347 (1993).

420. Newland, M.C., S. Yezhou, B. Lögdberg, and M. Berlin. Prolonged behavioral effects of *in utero* exposure to lead or methyl mercury: reduced sensitivity to changes in reinforcement contingencies during behavioral transitions and in steady state. *Toxicol. Appl. Pharmacol.* 126:6–15 (1994).

421. Tsoumbaris, P., and H. Tsoukali-Papadopoulou. Heavy metals in common foodstuff: quantitative analysis. *Bull. Environ. Contam. Toxicol.* 53:61–66 (1994).

422. Tsoumbaris, P., and H. Tsoukali-Papadopoulou. Heavy metals in common foodstuff: daily intake. *Bull. Environ. Contam. Toxicol.* 53:67–70 (1994).

423. Watanabe, T., S. Shimbo, M. Yasumoto, et al. Reduction to one half in dietary intake of cadmium and lead among Japanese populations. *Bull. Environ. Contam. Toxicol.* 52:196–202 (1994).

424. De Gregori, I., D. Delgado, H. Pinochet, et al. Cadmium, lead, copper and mercury levels in fresh and canned bivalve mussels *Tagelus dombeii* (Navajuela) and *Semelle sólida* (Almeja) from the Chilean coast. *Sci. Total Environ.* 148:1–10 (1994).

425. Mat, I. Arsenic and trace metals in commercially important bivalves, *Andara granosa* and *Paphia undulata*. *Bull. Environ. Contam. Toxicol.* 52:833–839 (1994).

426. Ereifej, K.I., and S.H. Gharaibeh. The levels of cadmium, nickel, manganese, lead, zinc, iron, tin, copper and arsenic in the brined canned Jordanian cheese. *Z. Lebensm. Unters. Forsch.* 197:123–126 (1993).

427. Simakova, A., J. Kamenik, R. Brazdil, and J. Bardon. Blei-, Cadmium- und Quecksilbergenan in Rind- und Schweinefleisch in Mittelmähren. *Fleischwirtschaft* 73:1187–1188 (1993).

428. Wagemann, R., and R.E.A. Stewart. Concentrations of heavy metals and selenium in tissues and some foods of walrus (*Odobenus rosmarus rosmarus*) from the Eastern Canadian Arctic and sub-Arctic, and associations between metals, age, and gender. *Can. J. Fish. Aquat. Sci.* 51:426–436 (1994).

429. Ahmad, S., S. Waheed, A. Mannan, et al. Evaluation of trace elements in wheat and wheat by-products. *J. AOAC Int.* 77:11–17 (1994).

430. Sattar, A., N. Ahmad, and L.A. Khan. Potentiometric stripping analysis of selected heavy metals in biological materials. *Nahrung* 37:220–225 (1993).

431. Chukwuma, C., Sr. Comparison of the accumulation of cadmium, lead and zinc in cultivated and wild plant species in the derelict Enyigba lead-zinc mine. *Toxicol. Environ. Chem.* 38:167–173 (1993).

432. Kretowska-Kutas, M. Determination of the level of certain trace elements in vegetables in differently contaminated regions. *Nahrung* 37:456–462 (1993).

433. Barman, S.C., and M.M. Lal. Accumulation of heavy metals (Zn, Cu, Cd & Pb) in soil and cultivated vegetables and weeds grown in industrially polluted fields. *J. Environ. Biol.* 15:107–115 (1994).

434. Vetter, J. Data on arsenic and cadmium contents of some common mushrooms. *Toxicon* 32:11–15 (1994).

435. Arcos, M.T., M.C. Ancín, J.C. Echeverría, et al. Study of lability of heavy metals in wines with different degrees of aging through differential pulse anodic stripping voltammetry. *J. Agric. Food Chem.* 41:2333–2339 (1993).

436. Acosta, A., C. Díaz, A. Hardisson, and D. González. Levels of Cd, Pb, and Ni in different types of vinegars. *Bull. Environ. Contam. Toxicol.* 51:852–856 (1993).

437. Jeng, S.L., S.J. Lee, and S.Y. Lin. Determination of cadmium and lead in raw milk by graphite furnace atomic absorption spectrophotometer. *J. Dairy Sci.* 77:945–949 (1994).

438. Chou, C.L., J.F. Uthe, and R.D. Guy. Determination of free and bound Cd, Zn, Cu, and Ag ions in lobster (*Homarus americanus*) digestive gland extracts by gel chromatography

followed by atomic absorption spectrophotometry and polarography. *J. AOAC Int.* 76:794–798 (1993).

439.  Iskander, F.Y. Determination of seventeen elements in edible oils and margarine by instrumental neutron activation analysis. *J. Am. Oil Chem. Soc.* 70:803–805 (1993).

440.  Martín-Polvillo, M., T. Albi, and A. Guinda. Determination of trace elements in edible vegetable oils by atomic absorption spectrophotometry. *J. Am. Oil Chem. Soc.* 71:347–353 (1994).

441.  Krushevska, A., and R.M. Barnes. Inductively coupled plasma atomic emission spectrometric determination of aluminium, barium, silicon, strontium and titanium in food after sample fusion. *Analyst* 119:131–134 (1994).

442.  Jorhem, L. Determination of metals in foodstuffs by atomic absorption spectrophotometry after dry ashing: NMKL interlaboratory study of lead, cadmium, zinc, copper, iron, chromium, and nickel. *J. AOAC Int.* 76:798–813 (1993).

443.  Xu, G.-S., R.-P. Jin, Z.-W. Zhang, et al. Preliminary study on aluminum content of foods and aluminum intake of residents in Tianjin. *Biomed. Environ. Sci.* 6:319–325 (1993).

444.  Coni, E., G. Bellomonte, and S. Caroli. Aluminium content of infant formulas. *J. Trace Elem. Electrolytes Health Dis.* 7:83–86 (1993).

445.  Harder, D.K. Aluminum contents of the edible portions of the winged bean, *Psophocarpus tetragonolobus* (L.) DC. (Fabaceae): field study and caveat. *Plant Foods Human Nutr.* 45:127–137 (1994).

446.  Šeruga, M., J. Grgić, and M. Mandić. Aluminium content of soft drinks from aluminium cans. *Z. Lebensm. Unters. Forsch.* 198:313–316 (1994).

447.  Müller, J.P., A. Steinegger, and C. Schlatter. Contribution of aluminium from packaging materials and cooking utensils to the daily aluminium intake. *Z. Lebensm. Unters. Forsch.* 197:332–341 (1993).

448.  Mei, L., and T. Yao. Aluminum contamination of food from using aluminumware. *Int. J. Environ. Anal. Chem.* 50:1–8 (1993).

449.  Nagy, E., and K. Jobst. Aluminium dissolved from kitchen utensils. *Bull. Environ. Contam. Toxicol.* 52:396–399 (1994).

450.  Larroque, M., J.C. Cabanis, and L. Vian. Determination of aluminum in wines by direct graphite furnace atomic absorption spectrometry. *J. AOAC Int.* 77:463–466 (1994).

451.  Copestake, P. Aluminium and Alzheimer's disease—an update. *Food Chem. Toxicol.* 31:679–685 (1993).

452.  Harrington, C.R., C.M. Wischik, F.K. McArthur, et al. Alzheimer's disease-like changes in tau protein processing: association with aluminium accumulation in brains of renal dialysis patients. *Lancet* 343:993–997 (1994).

453.  Greger, J.L. Aluminum metabolism. *Annu. Rev. Nutr.* 13:43–63 (1993).

454.  Edwardson, J.A., P.B. Moore, I.N. Ferrier, et al. Effect of silicon on gastrointestinal absorption of aluminium. *Lancet* 342:211–212 (1993).

455.  Powell, J.J., S.M. Greenfield, H.G. Parkes, et al. Gastro-intestinal availability of aluminium from tea. *Food Chem. Toxicol.* 31:449–454 (1993).

456.  Nagy, E., and K. Jobst. The kinetics of aluminium-containing antacid absorption in man. *Eur. J. Clin. Chem. Clin. Biochem.* 32:119–121 (1994).

457.  Sharp, C.A., J. Perks, M. Worsfold, et al. Plasma aluminium in a reference population: the effects of antacid consumption and its influence on biochemical indices of bone formation. *Eur. J. Clin. Invest.* 23:554–560 (1993).

458.  Kidder, L.S., G.L. Klein, C.M. Gundberg, et al. Effects of aluminum on rat bone cell populations. *Calcif. Tissue Int.* 53:357–361 (1993).

459.  Oteiza, P.I., C.L. Keen, B. Han, and M.S. Golub. Aluminum accumulation and neurotoxicity in Swiss-Webster mice after long-term dietary exposure to aluminum and citrate. *Metabolism* 42:1296–1300 (1993).

460.  Zaman, K., A. Zaman, and J. Batcabe. Hematological effects of aluminum on living organisms. *Comp. Biochem. Physiol.* 106C:295–293 (1993).

461.  Cervera, M.L., J.C. Lopez, and R. Montoro. Arsenic content of Spanish cows' milk determined by dry ashing hydride generation atomic absorption spectrometry. *J. Dairy Res.* 61:83–89 (1994).

462.  Donoghue, D.J., H. Hairston, C.V. Cope, et al. Incurred arsenic residues in chicken eggs. *J. Food Protect.* 57:218–223 (1994).

463.  Higham, A.M., and R.P.T. Tomkins. Determination of trace quantities of selenium and arsenic in canned tuna fish by using electroanalytical techniques. *Food Chem.* 48:85–93 (1993).

464.  Sekulić, B., J. Sapunar, and D. Bažulić. Arsenic in Norway lobster (*Nephrophs norvegicus* L.) from Kvarnerić Bay—Northeastern Adriatic. *Bull. Environ. Contam. Toxicol.* 51:460–463 (1993).

465.  Kukier, U., M.E. Sumner, and W.P. Miller. Determination of arsenic in plant tissue using a slurry sampling graphite furnace. *Commun. Soil Sci. Plant Anal.* 25:1149–1159 (1994).

466.  Chen, S.-L., S.R. Dzeng, M.-H. Yang, et al. Arsenic species in groundwaters of the Blackfoot disease area, Taiwan. *Environ. Sci. Technol.* 28:877–881 (1994).

467.  Lu, F.-J., C.-L. Hong, M.-F. Lu, and H. Shimizu. Mutagenicity of drinking well water. *Bull. Environ. Contam. Toxicol.* 51:545–550 (1993).

468.  Pan, T.C., C.J. Horng, S.R. Lin, et al. Simultaneous determination of Zn, Cd, Pb, and Cu in urine of patients with blackfoot disease using anodic stripping voltammetry. *Biol. Trace Elem. Res.* 38:233–241 (1993).

469.  Wang, C.T., C.W. Huang, S.S. Chou, et al. Studies on the concentration of arsenic, selenium, copper, zinc and iron in the blood of blackfoot disease patients in different clinical stages. *Eur. J. Clin. Chem. Clin. Biochem.* 31:759–763 (1993).

470.  Wang, C.T., W.T. Chang, C.W. Huang, et al. Studies on the concentrations of arsenic, selenium, copper, zinc and iron in the hair of blackfoot disease patients in different clinical stages. *Eur. J. Clin. Chem. Clin. Biochem.* 32:107–111 (1994).

471.  Lai, M.-S., Y.-M. Hsueh, C.-J. Chen, et al. Ingested inorganic arsenic and prevalence of diabetes mellitus. *Am. J. Epidemiol.* 139:484–492 (1994).

472. Lerda, D. Sister-chromatid exchange (SCE) among individuals chronically exposed to arsenic in drinking water. *Mutat. Res.* 312:111–120 (1994).

473. Meng, Z. Effects of arsenic on DNA synthesis in human lymphocytes. *Arch. Environ. Contam. Toxicol.* 25:525–528 (1993).

474. Le, X.-C., W.R. Cullen, and K.J. Reimer. Human urinary arsenic excretion after one-time ingestion of seaweed, crab, and shrimp. *Clin. Chem.* 40:617–624 (1994).

475. Bergbäck, B., S. Anderberg, and U. Lohm. Accumulated environmental impact: the case of cadmium in Sweden. *Sci. Total Environ.* 145:13–28 (1994).

476. Müller, M., M. Anke, C. Thiel, et al. Zur Cadmiumaufnahme Erwachsener in den neuen Bundesländern. *Ernährungs-Umschau* 40:240–243 (1993).

477. Musante, C.L., M.R. Ellingwood, and D.E. Stilwell. Cadmium contamination of deer livers in Connecticut. *Bull. Environ. Contam. Toxicol.* 51:838–843 (1993).

478. Gamberg, M., and A.M. Scheuhammer. Cadmium in caribou and muskoxen from the Canadian Yukon and Northwest Territories. *Sci. Total Environ.* 143:221–234 (1994).

479. Lusky, K., A. Lippert, M. Stoyke, et al. Untersuchungen auf Umweltkontaminanten in Reh-, Rot-, Dam-, Muffel- und Schwarzwild. *Fleischwirtschaft* 74:189–191 (1994).

480. Francesconi, K.A., E.J. Moore, and L.M. Joll. Cadmium in the saucer scallop, *Amusium balloti*, from Western Australian waters: concentrations in adductor muscle and redistribution following frozen storage. *Aust. J. Mar. Freshwater Res.* 44:787–797 (1993).

481. Peerzada, N., A. Padovan, and M. Guinea. Concentrations of heavy metals in oysters from the coastline of Northern Territory, Australia. *Environ. Monitoring Assessment* 28:101–107 (1993).

482. Cabrera, C., M.L. Lorenzo, C. Gallego, et al. Cadmium contamination levels in seafood determined by electrothermal atomic absorption spectrometry after microwave dissolution. *J. Agric. Food Chem.* 42:126–128 (1994).

483. Watanabe, T., O. Iwani, S. Shimbo, and M. Ikeda. Reduction in cadmium in blood and dietary intake among general populations in Japan. *Int. Arch. Occup. Environ. Health* 65:S205–S208 (1993).

484. He, Q.B., and B.R. Singh. Crop uptake of cadmium from phosphorus fertilizers: I. Yield and cadmium content. *Water Air Soil Pollut.* 74:251–265 (1994).

485. Kuo, T.-c., and Y.-t. Huang. Cadmium uptake by lettuce cultivars grown on cadmium-polluted soil. *J. Agric. Assoc. China* 161:27–32 (1993).

486. Rutzke, M., W.H. Gutenmann, S.D. Williams, and D.J. Lisk. Cadmium and selenium absorption by swiss chard grown in potted composted materials. *Bull. Environ. Contam. Toxicol.* 51:416–420 (1993).

487. Stern, A.H. Monte Carlo analysis of the U.S. EPA model of human exposure to cadmium in sewage sludge through consumption of garden crops. *J. Exp. Anal. Environ. Epidemiol.* 3:449–469 (1993).

488. Groten, J.P., and P.J. van Bladeren. Cadmium bioavailability and health risk in food. *Trends Food Sci. Technol.* 5:50–55 (1994).

489. Slob, W., and E.I. Krajnc. Interindividual variability in modeling exposure and toxicokinetics: a case study on cadmium. *Environ. Health Perspect.* 102:78–81 (1994).

490. Nishijo, M., H. Nakagawa, Y. Morikawa, et al. Prognostic factors of renal dysfunction induced by environmental cadmium pollution. *Environ. Res.* 64:112–121 (1994).

491. Nakagawa, H., M. Nishijo, Y. Morikawa, et al. Urinary $\beta_2$-microglobulin concentration and mortality in a cadmium-polluted area. *Arch. Environ. Health* 48:428–435 (1993).

492. Nogawa, K., and T. Kido. Biological monitoring of cadmium exposure in itai-itai disease epidemiology. *Int. Arch. Occup. Environ. Health* 65:S43–S46 (1993).

493. Iwata, K., H. Saito, M. Moriyama, and A. Nakano. Renal tubular function after reduction of environmental cadmium exposure: a ten-year follow-up. *Arch. Environ. Health* 48:157–163 (1993).

494. Kido, T., and K. Nogawa. Dose–response relationship between total cadmium intake and $\beta_2$-microglobulinuria using logistic regression analysis. *Toxicol. Lett.* 69:113–120 (1993).

495. Sens, M.A., D.J. Hazen-Martin, J.E. Bylander, and D.A. Sens. Heterogeneity in the amount of ionic cadmium necessary to elicit cell death in independent cultures of human proximal tubule cells. *Toxicol. Lett.* 70:185–191 (1994).

496. Masaoka, T., F. Akahori, S. Arai, et al. A nine-year chronic toxicity study of cadmium ingestion in monkeys. I. Effects of dietary cadmium on the general health of monkeys. *Vet. Human Toxicol.* 36:189–194 (1994).

497. Houtman, J.P.W. Prolonged low-level cadmium intake and atherosclerosis. *Sci. Total Environ.* 138:31–36 (1993).

498. Wang, C., and M.H. Bhattacharyya. Effect of cadmium on bone calcium and $^{45}Ca$ in nonpregnant mice on a calcium-deficient diet: evidence of direct effect of cadmium on bone. *Toxicol. Appl. Pharmacol.* 120:228–239 (1993).

499. Flury, M., and A. Papritz. Bromide in the natural environment: occurrence and toxicity. *J. Environ. Qual.* 22:747–758 (1993).

500. Miyahara, M., and Y. Saito. Determination of bromide ions in food by unsuppressed ion chromatography with ultraviolet detection after microwave digestion in a sealed PTFE vessel. *J. Agric. Food Chem.* 42:1126–1131 (1994).

501. McGeehin, M.A., J.S. Reif, J.C. Becher, and E.J. Mangione. Case–control study of bladder cancer and water disinfection methods in Colorado. *Am. J. Epidemiol.* 138:492–501 (1993).

502. Koivusalo, M.T., J.J.K. Jaakkola, and T. Vartiainen. Drinking water mutagenicity in past exposure assessment of the studies on drinking water and cancer: application and evaluation in Finland. *Environ. Res.* 64:90–101 (1994).

503. Långvik, V.-A., and B. Holmbom. Formation of mutagenic organic by-products and AOX by chlorination of fractions of humic water. *Water Res.* 28:553–557 (1994).

504. Ogawa, S., H. Kita, Y. Hanasaki, et al. Determination of the potent mutagen 3-chloro-4-dichloromethyl-5-hydroxy-2(5*H*)-franone (MX) in water by gas chromatography with electron-capture detection. *J. Chromatogr.* 643:221–226 (1993).

505. Tsai, L.-S., V.G. Randall, and J.E. Schade. Chlorine uptake by chicken frankfurters immersed in chlorinated water. *J. Food Sci.* 58:987–990 (1993).

506. Gessner, B.D., M. Beller, J.P. Middaugh, and G.M. Whitford. Acute fluoride poisoning from a public water system. *New Engl. J. Med.* 330:95–99 (1994).

507. Foulkes, R.G. Case report: mass fluoride poisoning, Hooper Bay, Alaska. *Fluoride* 27:32–36 (1994).

508. Spittle, B. Allergy and hypersensitivity to fluoride. *Fluoride* 26:267–273 (1993).

509. Weeks, K.J., K.M. Milsom, and M.A. Lennon. Enamel defects in 4- to 5-year-old children in fluoridated and non-fluoridated parts of Cheshire, UK. *Caries Res.* 27:317–320 (1993).

510. Trivedi, N., A. Mithal, S.K. Gupta, et al. Reversible impairment of glucose tolerance in patients with endemic fluorosis. *Diabetologia* 36:826–828 (1993).

511. Freni, S.C. Exposure to high fluoride concentrations in drinking water is associated with decreased birth rates. *J. Toxicol. Environ. Health* 42:109–121 (1994).

512. Gulati, P., V. Singh, M.K. Gupta, et al. Studies on the leaching of fluoride in tea infusions. *Sci. Total Environ.* 138:213–222 (1993).

513. Konno, N., H. Makita, K. Yuri, et al. Association between dietary iodine intake and prevalence of subclinical hypothyroidism in the coastal regions of Japan. *J. Clin. Endocrinol. Metab.* 78:393–397 (1994).

514. Galofré, J.C., L. Fernández-Calvet, M. Ríos, and R.V.G. García-Mayor. Increased incidence of thyrotoxicosis after iodine supplementation in an iodine sufficient area. *J. Endocrinol. Invest.* 17:23–27 (1994).

515. Wiechen, A., and W. Hoffmann. Untersuchungen zur Jodierung von Käse beim Herstellungsprozeß. *Milchwissenschaft* 49:74–78 (1994).

516. Fischer, P.W.F., and A. Giroux. Iodine content of Canadian retail milk samples. II. After the ethylenediamine dihydroiodide ban. *Food Res. Int.* 26:277–281 (1993).

517. Sertl, D., and W. Malone. Liquid chromatographic method for determination of iodine in milk: collaborative study. *J. AOAC Int.* 76:711–719 (1993).

518. Vanhoe, H., F. Van Allemeersch, J. Versieck, and R. Dams. Effect of solvent type on the determination of total iodine in milk powder and human serum by inductively coupled plasma mass spectrometry. *Analyst* 118:1015–1019 (1993).

519. Rao, R.R., and A. Chatt. Determination of nanogram amounts of iodine in foods by radiochemical neutron activation analysis. *Analyst* 118:1247–1251 (1993).

520. Zurera-Cosano, G., R. Moreno-Rojas, and M.A. Amaro-Lopez. Effects of processing on the concentration of lead in Manchego-type cheese. *Food Addit. Contam.* 11:91–96 (1994).

521. Hanafy, M.S.M., S.M. Shalaby, M.A.A. El-Fouly, et al. Effect of garlic on lead contents in chicken tissues. *Dtsch. Tierärztl. Wschr.* 101:157–158 (1994).

522. Okoye, C.O.B. Lead and other metals in dried fish form Nigerian markets. *Bull. Environ. Contam. Toxicol.* 52:825–832 (1994).

523. Ortega-Calvo, J.J., C. Mazuelos, B. Hermosin, and C. Saiz-Jimenez. Chemical composition of *Spirulina* and eukaryotic algae food products marketed in Spain. *J. Appl. Phycol.* 5:425–435 (1993).

524. Bermejo-Barrera, P., M. Aboal-Somoza, R.M. Soto-Ferreiro, and R. Domínguez-González. Palladium–magnesium nitrate as a chemical modifier for the determination of lead in mussel slurries by electrothermal atomic absorption spectrometry. *Analyst* 118:665–668 (1993).

525. Thompson, J.J. Determination of ultratrace levels of lead in infant formula by isotope dilution inductively coupled plasma mass spectrometry. *J. AOAC Int.* 76:1378–1384 (1993).

526. Henick-Kling, T., and G.S. Stoewsand. Lead in wine. *Am. J. Enol. Vitic.* 44:459–463 (1993).

527. Ough, C.S. Lead in wines—a review of recent reports. *Am. J. Enol. Vitic.* 44:464–467 (1993).

528. Lobinski, R., J. Szpunar-Lobinska, F.C. Adams, et al. Speciation analysis of organolead compounds in wine by capillary gas chromatography/microwave-induced-plasma atomic emission spectrometry. *J. AOAC Int.* 76:1262–1267 (1993).

529. Pegues, D.A., B.J. Hughes, and C.H. Woernle. Elevated blood lead levels associated with illegally distilled alcohol. *Arch. Intern. Med.* 153:1501–1504 (1993).

530. Bourgoin, B.P., D.R. Evans, J.R. Cornett, et al. Lead content in 70 brands of dietary calcium supplements. *Am. J. Public Health* 83:1155–1160 (1993).

531. Markowitz, S.B., C.M. Nunez, S. Klitzman, et al. Lead poisoning due to *hai ge fen*. The prophyrin content of individual erythrocytes. *JAMA* 271:932–934 (1994).

532. Yáñez, L., L. Batres, L. Carrizales, et al. Toxicological assessment of azarcon, a lead salt used as a folk remedy in Mexico. I. Oral toxicity in rats. *J. Ethnopharmacol.* 41:91–97 (1994).

533. Centers for Disease Control. Lead-contaminated drinking water in bulk-water storage tanks—Arizona and California, 1993. *Morbid. Mortal. Weekly Rep.* 43:751,757–758 (1994).

534. Barbee, S.J., and L.A. Constantine. Release of lead from crystal decanters under conditions of normal use. *Food Chem. Toxicol.* 32:285–288 (1994).

535. Rojas-López, M., C. Santos-Burgoa, C. Ríos, et al. Use of lead-glazed ceramics is the main factor associated to high lead in blood levels in two Mexican rural communities. *J. Toxicol. Environ. Health* 42:45–52 (1994).

536. Dolan, S.P., S.G. Capar, R.M. Jacobs, et al. Sensitivity of the quick color test for indicating lead release from ceramicware. *J. AOAC Int.* 77:454–457 (1994).

537. Multiple authors. *New Dimensions of Lead Neurotoxicity: Redefining Mechanisms and Effects.* Proceedings of the Ninth International Neurotoxicology Conference,

Little Rock, Arkansas, October 28–31, 1991.*NeuroToxicology* 14(2–3) (1993).

538. Carrington, C.D., D.M. Sheehan, and P.M. Bolger. Hazard assessment of lead. *Food Addit. Contam.* 10:325–335 (1993).

539. Lockitch, G. Perspectives on lead toxicity. *Clin. Biochem.* 26:371–381 (1993).

540. Leggett, R.W. An age-specific kinetic model of lead metabolism in humans.*Environ. Health Perspect.* 101:598–616 (1993).

541. Hertz-Picciotto, I., and J. Croft. Review of the relation between blood lead and blood pressure. *Epidemiol. Rev.* 15:352–373 (1993).

542. Donaldson, W.E., and S.O. Knowles. Is lead toxicosis a reflection of altered fatty acid composition of membranes? *Comp. Biochem. Physiol.* 104C:377–379 (1993).

543. Tiffany-Castiglioni, E. Cell culture models for lead toxicity in neuronal and glial cells. *NeuroToxicology* 14:513–536 (1993).

544. Schwartz, J. Low-level lead exposure and children's IQ: a meta-analysis and search for a threshold. *Environ. Res.* 65:42–55 (1994).

545. Muñoz, H., I. Romieu, E. Palazuelos, et al. Blood lead level and neurobehavioral development among children living in Mexico City. *Arch. Environ. Health* 48:132–139 (1993).

546. Fergusson, D.M., and L.J. Horwood. The effects of lead levels on the growth of word recognition in middle childhood. *Int. J. Epidemiol.* 22:891–897 (1993).

547. Bellinger, D., H. Hu, L. Titlebaum, and H.L. Needleman. Attentional correlates of dentin and bone lead levels in adolescents. *Arch. Environ. Health* 49:98–105 (1994).

548. Damm, D., P. Grandjean, T. Lyngbye, et al. Early lead exposure and neonatal jaundice: relation to neurobehavioral performance at 15 years of age. *Neurotoxicol. Teratol.* 15:173–181 (1993).

549. Rabinowitz, M. Declining blood lead levels and cognitive change in children. (Letter.) *JAMA* 270:827 (1993).

550. Rothenberg, S.J., L. Schnaas-Arrieta, I.A. Pérez-Guerrero, et al. Prenatal and postnatal blood lead level and head circumference in children to three years: preliminary results from the Mexico City Prospective Lead Study.*J. Exposure Anal. Environ. Epidemiol.* 3(Suppl. 1):1–8 (1993).

551. Vivoli, G., G. Fantuzzi, M. Bergomi, et al. Relationship between low lead exposure and somatic growth in adolescents. *J. Exposure Anal. Environ. Epidemiol.* 3(Suppl. 1):201–209 (1993).

552. Payton, M., H. Hu, D. Sparrow, et al. Relation between blood lead and urinary biogenic amines in community-exposed men. *Am. J. Epidemiol.* 138:815–825 (1993).

553. Factor-Litvak, P., Z. Stein, and J. Graziano. Increased risk of proteinuria among a cohort of lead-exposed pregnant women. *Environ. Health Perspect.* 101:418–421 (1993).

554. Schwartz, B.S., K.I. Bolla, W. Stewart, et al. Decrements in neurobehavioral performance associated with mixed exposure to organic and inorganic lead. *Am. J. Epidemiol.* 137:1006–1021 (1993).

555. Hirata, M., and H. Kosaka. Effects of lead exposure on neurophysiological parameters. *Environ. Res.* 63:60–69 (1993).

556. Sata, F., S. Araki, K. Murata, et al. Are faster or slower large myelinated nerve fibers more sensitive to chronic lead exposure? A study of the distribution of conduction velocities. *Environ. Res.* 62:333–338 (1993).

557. Singh, A., C. Cullen, A. Dykeman, et al. Chronic lead exposure induces ultrastructural alterations in the monkey testis. *J. Submicrosc. Cytol. Pathol.* 25:479–486 (1993).

558. Nico, L.G., and D.C. Taphorn. Mercury in fish from gold-mining regions in the upper Cuyuni River system, Venezuela. *Fresenius Environ. Bull.* 3:287–292 (1994).

559. Driscoll, C.T., C. Yan, C.L. Schofield, et al. The mercury cycle and fish in the Adirondack Lakes. *Environ. Sci. Technol.* 28:136A–143A (1994).

560. Bodaly, R.A., J.W.M. Rudd, and R.J.P. Fudge, and C.A. Kelly. Mercury concentrations in fish related to size of remote Canadian Shield lakes. *Can. J. Fish. Aquat. Sci.* 50:980–987 (1993).

561. Diaz, C., A. González Padrón, I. Frías, et al. Concentrations of mercury in fresh and salted marine fish from the Canary Islands. *J. Food Protect.* 57:246–248 (1994).

562. Fabris, G.J., C. Monahan, G. Nicholson, and T.I. Walker. Total mercury concentrations in sand flathead, *Platycephalus bassensis* Cuvier & Valenciennes, from Port Phillip Bay, Victoria. *Aust. J. Mar. Freshwater Res.* 43:1393–1402 (1992).

563. Palmer, S.J., and B.J. Presley. Mercury bioaccumulation by shrimp (*Penaeus aztecus*) transplanted to Lavaca Bay, Texas. *Marine Pollut. Bull.* 26:564–566 (1993).

564. Barghigiani, C., and T. Ristori. Mercury levels in agricultural products of Mt. Amiata (Tuscany, Italy). *Arch. Environ. Contam. Toxicol.* 26:329–334 (1994).

565. Sidle, W.C. Naturally occurring mercury contamination in a pristine environment?*Environ. Geol.* 21:42–50 (1993).

566. Gutierrez, J., H. Travieso, and M.A. Pubillones. Rapid determination of inorganic and methyl mercury in fish. *Water Air Soil Pollut.* 68:315–323 (1993).

567. Winfield, S.A., N.D. Boyd, M.J. Vimy, and F.L. Lorscheider. Measurement of total mercury in biological specimens by cold vapor atomic fluorescence spectrometry. *Clin. Chem.* 40:206–210 (1994).

568. Anderson, K.A., B. Isaacs, M. Tracy, and G. Möller. Cold-vapor generation for inductively coupled argon plasma/atomic emission spectrometry analysis. Part 3. Mercury. *J. AOAC Int.* 77:473–480 (1994).

569. Lo, J.-M., and J.-D. Lee. Dithiocarbamate extraction and Au(III) back extraction for determination of mercury in water and biological samples by anodic stripping voltammetry. *Anal. Chem.* 66:1242–1248 (1994).

570. Igata, A. Epidemiological and clinical features of Minamata disease. *Environ. Res.* 63:157–169 (1993).

571. Zalups, R.K., and L.H. Lash. Advances in understanding the renal transport and toxicity of mercury. *J. Toxicol. Environ. Health* 42:1–44 (1994).

572. De Flora, S., C. Bennicelli, and M. Bagnasco. Genotoxicity of mercury compounds. A review. *Mutat. Res.* 317:57–79 (1994).

573. Yamada, H., T. Miyahara, H. Kozuka, et al. Potentiating effects of organomercuries on clastogen-induced chromosome aberrations in cultured Chinese hamster cells. *Mutat. Res.* 290:281–291 (1993).

574. Vahter, M., N.K. Mottet, L. Friberg, et al. Speciation of mercury in the primate blood and brain following long-term exposure to methyl mercury. *Toxicol. Appl. Pharmacol.* 124:221–229 (1994).

575. Gilbert, S.G., T.M. Burbacher, and D.C. Rice. Effects of *in utero* methylmercury exposure on a spatial delayed alternation task in monkeys. *Toxicol. Appl. Pharmacol.* 123:130–136 (1993).

576. Sumitani, H., S. Suekane, A. Nakatani, and K. Tatsuka. Inductively coupled plasma atomic emission spectrometric determination of tin in canned food. *J. AOAC Int.* 76:1374–1377 (1993).

577. Garcia-Romero, B., T.L. Wade, G.G. Salata, and J.M. Brooks. Butyltin concentrations in oysters from the Gulf of Mexico from 1989 to 1991. *Environ. Pollut.* 81:103–111 (1993).

578. Kure, L.K., and M.H. Depledge. Accumulation of organotin in *Littorina littorea* and *Mya arenaria* from Danish coastal waters. *Environ. Pollut.* 84:149–157 (1994).

579. Tsunoda, M. Simultaneous determination of organotin compounds in fish and shellfish by gas chromatography with a flame photometric detector. *Tohoku J. Exp. Med.* 169:167–178 (1993).

580. Pang, F.Y., Y.L. Ng, S.M. Phang, and S.L. Tong. Determination of total tin and tributyltin in biological tissues. *Int. J. Environ. Anal. Chem.* 53:53–61 (1993).

581. Kumar, U.T., J.G. Dorsey, J.A. Caruso, and E.H. Evans. Speciation of inorganic and organotin compounds in biological samples by liquid chromatography with inductively coupled plasma mass spectrometric detection. *J. Chromatogr. A* 654:261–268 (1993).

582. Suzuki, T., R. Matsuda, Y. Saito, and H. Yamada. Application of helium microwave-induced plasma emission detection system to analysis of organotin compounds in biological samples. *J. Agric. Food Chem.* 42:216–220 (1994).

583. Chiba, M., V. Iyengar, R.R. Greenberg, and T. Gills. Determination of tin in biological materials by atomic absorption spectrophotometry and neutron activation analysis. *Sci. Total Environ.* 148:39–44 (1994).

584. Penninks, A.H. The evaluation of data-derived safety factors for bis(tri-*n*-butyltin)oxide. *Food Addit. Contam.* 10:351–361 (1993).

585. Parfett, C.L.J., and R. Pilon. Tri-*n*-butyltin chloride promotes morphological transformation and induces proliferin expression in C3H10T1/2 cells. *Cancer Lett.* 71:167–176 (1993).

586. Pekelharing, H.L.M., A.G. Lemmens, and A.C. Beynen. Iron, copper and zinc status in rats fed on diets containing various concentrations of tin. *Br. J. Nutr.* 71:103–109 (1994).

587. Anderson, A., E. Glattre, and B.V. Johansen. Incidence of cancer among lighthouse keepers exposed to asbestos in drinking water. *Am. J. Epidemiol.* 138:682–687 (1993).

588. Grubinger, V.P., W.H. Butenmann, G.J. Doss, et al. Chromium in swiss chard grown on soil amended with tannery meal fertilizer. *Chemosphere* 28:717–720 (1994).

589. Han, B.-C., W.-L. Jeng, T.-C. Hung, and M.-S. Jeng. Copper intake and health threat by consuming seafood from copper-contaminated coastal environments in Taiwan. *Environ. Toxicol. Chem.* 13:775–780 (1994).

590. Viñas, P., N. Campillo, I.L. García, and M.H. Córdoba. Analysis of copper in biscuits and bread using a fast-program slurry electrothermal atomic absorption procedure. *J. Agric. Food Chem.* 41:2024–2027 (1993).

591. Iwami, I., C.-S. Moon, T. Watanabe, and M. Ikeda. Association of metal concentrations in drinking water with the incidence of motor neuron disease in a focus on the Kii Peninsula of Japan. *Bull. Environ. Contam. Toxicol.* 52:109–116 (1994).

592. Abeck, D., I. Traenckner, V. Steinkraus, et al. Chronic urticaria due to nickel intake. *Acta Dermatol. Venereol. (Stockh.)* 73:438–439 (1993).

593. Veien, N.K., T. Hattel, and G. Laurberg. Low nickel diet: an open, prospective trial. *J. Am. Acad. Dermatol.* 29:1002–1007 (1993).

594. Barbera, R., M.J. Esteve, R. Farre, and J.C. Lopez. A DPCSV method for the determination of nickel in infant formulas. *Food Chem.* 49:427–430 (1994).

595. Gutenmann, W.H., G.J. Doss, and D.J. Lisk. Selenium in swiss chard grown on sewage sludge–cement kiln dust amended soil. *Chemosphere* 27:1461–1463 (1993).

596. Yang, C., E. Wolf, K. Röser, et al. Selenium deficiency and fulvic acid supplementation induces fibrosis of cartilage and disturbs subchondral ossification in knee joints of mice: an animal model study of Kashin-Beck disease. *Virch. Archiv A* 423:483–491 (1993).

597. Kitahara, J., Y. Seko, and N. Imura. Possible involvement of active oxygen species in selenite toxicity in isolated rat hepatocytes. *Arch. Toxicol.* 67:497–501 (1993).

598. Albrecht, R., M.A. Pélissier, and M. Boisset. Excessive dietary selenium decreases the vitamin A storage and the enzymatic antioxidant defense in the liver of rats. *Toxicol. Lett.* 70:291–297 (1994).

599. Mulkey, J.P., and F.W. Oehme. A review of thallium toxicity. *Vet. Human Toxicol.* 35:445–453 (1993).

600. Dafnis, E., and S. Sabatini. Biochemistry and pathophysiology of vanadium. *Nephron* 67:133–143 (1994).

601. Léonard, A., and G.B. Gerber. Mutagenicity, carcinogenicity and teratogenicity of vanadium compounds. *Mutat. Res.* 317:81–88 (1994).

602. Migliore, L., R. Bocciardi, C. Macrì, and F. Lo Iacono. Cytogenetic damage induced in human lymphocyte by four vanadium compounds and micronucleus analysis by

fluorescence in situ hybridization with a centromeric probe. *Mutat. Res.* 319:205–213 (1993).

603. Pietrzak-Flis, Z., and G. Orzechowska. Plutonium in daily diet in Poland after the Chernobyl accident. *Health Phys.* 65:489–492 (1993).

604. Shouling, H., M. Junjie, Z. Qingchang, et al. Survey of $^{237}$Np and plutonium isotopes in principal foodstuffs in China. *Appl. Radiat. Isot.* 44:1490 (1993).

605. Jacob, P., H. Müller, G. Pröhl, et al. Environmental behaviour of radionuclides deposited after the reactor accident of Chernobyl and related exposures. *Radiat. Environ. Biophys.* 32:193–207 (1993).

606. Anguissola Scotti, I. Cs-134 levels in wheat related to time elapsed between contamination and sprinkling. *Environ. Exp. Botany* 34:213–216 (1994).

607. Zehnder, H.J., P. Kopp, J.J. Oertli, and U. Feller. Uptake and transport of radioactive cesium and strontium into strawberries after leaf contamination. *Gartenbauwissenschaft* 58:209–213 (1993).

608. Voigt, G., H. Müller, H.G. Paretzke, et al. $^{137}$Cs transfer after Chernobyl from fodder into chicken meat and eggs. *Health Phys.* 65:141–146 (1993).

609. Brunn, H., S. Georgii, and U. Eskens. $^{137}$Cesium and $^{134}$cesium in roe deer from North and Middle Hesse (Germany) subsequent to the reactor accident in Chernobyl. *Bull. Environ. Contam. Toxicol.* 51:633–639 (1993).

610. Knatko, V.A., V.V. Gurkov, V.D. Asimova, et al. Soil–milk transfer of $^{137}$Cs in an area of Byelorussia after the Chernobyl accident. *J. Environ. Radioactivity* 22:269–278 (1994).

611. Belli, M., U. Sansone, E. Piasentier, et al. $^{137}$Cs transfer coefficients from fodder to cow milk. *J. Environ. Radioactivity* 21:1–8 (1993).

612. Fabbri, S., G. Piva, R. Sogni, et al. Transfer kinetics and coefficients of $^{90}$Sr, $^{134}$Cs, and $^{137}$Cs from forage contami-nated by Chernobyl fallout to milk of cows. *Health Phys.* 66:375–379 (1994).

613. Kirchner, G. Transport of iodine and cesium via the grass–cow–milk pathway after the Chernobyl accident. *Health Phys.* 66:653–665 (1994).

614. Abbott, M.L., and A.S. Rood. COMIDA: a radio-nuclide food chain model for acute fallout deposition. *Health Phys.* 66:17–29 (1994).

615. Yu, K.N. Monitoring $^{90}$Sr contamination in terms of $^{131}$I contamination in imported food. *Health Phys.* 65:318–321 (1993).

616. Stella, R., M.T. Ganzerli Valentini, and L. Maggi. Determination of $^{90}$Sr in milk by using two inorganic exchang-ers. *Appl. Radiat. Isot.* 44:1093–1096 (1993).

617. Manos, C.G., Jr., R.. Kinney, and D.J. Lisk. Analysis of strontium-90 in the bones of brown trout (*Salmo trutta*) from Lake Ontario. *Chemosphere* 26:2031–2037 (1993).

618. Skwarzec, B., E. Holm, P. Roos, and J. Pempkowiak. Nickel-63 in Baltic fish and sediments. *Appl. Radiat. Isot.* 45:609–611 (1994).

619. Santos, P.L., R.C. Gouvea, and I.R. Dutra. Lead-210 in vegetables and soils form an area of high natural radio-activity in Brazil. *Sci. Total Environ.* 138:37–46 (1993).

620. Weisshaar, R. Blei-210 in Lebensmitteln. *Dtsch. Lebensm.-Rundsch.* 89:205–208 (1993).

621. Ivanov, E.P., G. Tolochko, V.S. Lazarev, and L. Shuvaeva. Child leukaemia after Chernobyl. (Letter.) *Nature* 365:702 (1993).

622. Shiraishi, K., M. Yamamoto, K. Yoshimizu, et al. Daily intakes of alkaline earth metals in Japanese males. *Health Phys.* 66:30–35 (1994).

623. Ham, G.J., J.D. Harrison, D.S. Popplewell, et al. The gastrointestinal absorption of neptunium, plutonium and americium in a primate (*C. jacchus*). *Sci. Total Environ.* 145:1–6 (1994).

# 9

# Naturally Occurring Toxicants and Food Constituents of Toxicological Interest

# SEAFOOD TOXINS

In a recent review on seafood toxins, Saavedra-Delgado and Metcalfe (*1*) compared the clinical presentations of the more common seafood poisonings (ciguatera, scombrotoxicosis, and shellfish poisonings), of bacterial and viral infections, and of a number of rare seafood poisonings. Differential diagnosis of these toxicoses and methods for distinguishing them from seafood allergy were presented along with a description of the marine organisms most commonly implicated and their general geographic distributions.

Surveillance programs on foodborne disease in England and Wales reported that 16 general outbreaks, 1 family outbreak, and 20 sporadic cases of scombroid poisoning, 78 incidents of suspected scombroid poisoning, 1 family outbreak of ciguatera, and 1 family outbreak of red whelk poisoning occurred during 1989–1991 (*2*). Most of the cases of scombrotoxicosis followed consumption of scombroid fish such as mackerel and tuna, although pilchards and sardines were implicated in one outbreak each. The ciguatera cases had eaten red snapper imported from Oman.

A semi-automated assay based upon mitochondrial dehydrogenase activity in the presence of veratridine and ouabain has been developed for the detection of sodium channel–specific marine toxins, such as saxitoxins, brevetoxins, and ciguatoxins (*3*). This assay can be completed in 4–6 hours and requires substantially less sample than the mouse bioassay.

## Ciguatera

The ecological, clinical and socioeconomic aspects of ciguatera fish poisoning were reviewed by Lewis and Ruff (*4*). Ciguatera is circumtropical in origin, with toxic fish concentrating toxins produced by coral reef dinoflagellates. Although people living on Pacific atolls are most commonly affected, world travel and worldwide distribution of fish cause the appearance of ciguatera in unexpected places and probably contribute to >25,000 cases annually. Another review, by Lewis and Holmes (*5*), focused on the origin and transfer of toxins involved in ciguatera. Ciguatoxins, which are potent activators of voltage-dependent sodium channels in a variety of tissues, originate as gambiertoxins in the dinoflagellate *Gambierdiscus toxicus*. Certain environmental conditions (sometimes related to human activities) favor the growth of these dinoflagellates and toxin production. The toxins are then concentrated up the food chain and may result in ciguatera outbreaks.

The history of ciguatera research at the University of Hawaii was recounted by Scheuer (*6*). Much of the research revolved around attempts to define the molecular structure of ciguatoxin(s) and led to the discovery of some other marine toxins.

A severe case of ciguatera poisoning was reported from a non-endemic area, Rhode Island (USA) (*7*). The victim had consumed a large portion of a fish soup made from an unidentified fish (which he had been told was cod) and arrived at an emergency room with severe gastrointestinal distress and paresthesias. Shortly thereafter he developed respiratory distress and lapsed into a coma. Following intensive treatment, the patient recovered and was discharged after 9 days. Cod has never been reported as a source of ciguatoxin and since these fish inhabit temperate waters they would not be expected to be toxic. The authors suspect that the soup, which tested positive for ciguatoxin, was made with an imported fish. The victim had been drinking heavily the night before this incident and had consumed two bottles of beer just before lunch. This may have contributed to the severity of his symptoms.

Development of polymyositis following an episode of ciguatera poisoning has previously been reported in two cases. Another incidence of polymyositis occurred in a businessman who had contracted ciguatera in the Bahamas (*8*). Six months following the initial symptoms, the patient had erythematous skin and diffuse muscle wasting and sensitivity. No other cause for these symptoms was determined, but the symptoms did resolve after administration of methylprednisolone.

A family outbreak of ciguatera on Reunion Island was traced to consumption of shark, which is rarely associated with this disease (*9*). Besides the usual gastrointestinal symptoms and paresthesias, the victims experienced severe cardiac symptoms, brachycardia which persisted for a month, and muscular aches which lasted for 3 months.

An epidemiological study of a confirmed outbreak of ciguatera involving 15 people of different ages on Kauai revealed that increasing age and body weight were associated with increasing severity and duration of symptoms (*10*). Since previous exposure to ciguatera is known to exacerbate symptoms in subsequent poisoning episodes, the correlation with age is believed to be related to prior subclinical toxin exposure. Severity of brachycardia was also associated with the amount of fish eaten, which is consistent with an increased dose of ciguatoxin.

In an investigation of the paradoxical reversal of temperature perception commonly experienced by ciguatera patients, five subjects with acute ciguatera poisoning were tested to determine whether they could distinguish a range of temperatures of water baths and to assess the severity of the paradoxical symptoms associated with cold water baths (*11*). All subjects could detect differences in temperature and correctly differentiate warmer and colder water baths. However, all reported intense burning pain and tingling when their hands were immersed in cold (0, 10, or 20°C) water. This intense nerve discomfort most likely results from an exaggerated and intense nerve depolarization occurring in peripheral small A-delta myelinated, and in particular, in C-polymodal nociceptor fibers.

Effects of ciguatoxin extracted from poisonous moray eels on sodium and calcium channels in cells have been investigated in cultured mouse NG108-15 neuroblastoma × glioma hybrid cells (*12*) and in *Torpedo* synaptosomes (*13*). Intracellular calcium ion levels increased in the hybrid cells in response to 5–25 nM ciguatoxin, and this increase was prevented by tetrodotoxin (which blocks voltage-gated sodium channels). Ciguatoxin did not cause an increase in acetylcholine (ACh) release from synaptosomes incubated in a calcium ion–free medium. However, subsequent addition of calcium ions to the medium caused a large ACh release from these cells. This release was also inhibited by tetrodotoxin, suggesting that ciguatoxin activates the reversed operation of the $Na^+/Ca^{2+}$-exchange system allowing the entry of $Ca^{2+}$ in exchange for $Na^+$.

Spatial distribution of ciguateric dinoflagellates was investigated in the waters and corals around Mayotte Island (Indian Ocean) (*14*). The greatest abundance of all species of dinoflagellates, particularly *G. toxicus*, occurred on dead corals on the inner slope of the barrier reef. Some macroalgae appeared to be stimulatory and some inhibitory to growth of *G. toxicus*.

Toxin analysis of three strains of *G. toxicus* revealed the presence of 3 distinct maitotoxins which are structurally related to ciguatoxins (*15*). Two of the toxins were relatively large (molecular weights >3000) and the third was small (molecular weight of 1060). However, when tested with guinea pig atria, vas deferens, and ilea, all three exerted a similar direct contractile effect which required calcium influx through voltage-sensitive calcium channels.

Six specimens of narrow-barred Spanish mackerel (*Scomberomorus commersoni*) captured off the Australian coast and associated with cases of ciguatera were analyzed for water-soluble and lipid-soluble toxins (*16*). Ciguatoxin-like and scaritoxin-like toxins (lipid soluble) were detected in all specimens, as were significant amounts of water-soluble toxins. The most important water-soluble compound was unidentified but was present in a fraction which tested positive for alkaloids. Cooking of the fish removed large amounts of the water-soluble toxins into the cooking water but they were not destroyed and would still constitute a hazard if the cooking water was consumed as in a soup.

The water-soluble toxins from *S. commersoni* were found to be chromatographically indistinguishable from toxins detected in extracts from a cyanobacterium, *Trichodesmium erythraeum*, which frequently forms blooms in Australian coastal waters (*17*). Partial purification of the toxic extract revealed the presence of a peptide and an alkaloid. Lipid-soluble toxins similar to those detected in the mackerel were also present in lipid extracts of the cyanobacterium. This suggests that the cyanobacteria are the source of the major toxins in the Australian ciguateric mackerel.

Extracts of herbivorous and carnivorous ciguateric fish, when tested in a mouse bioassay, produced different results, indicating that there was some difference in the toxins present (*18*). Herbivorous species were more toxic and appeared to contain an unidentified toxin which caused hind leg paralysis (HLP) in the mice. In mice with HLP, 93% died while of those with no symptoms of HLP, only 51% died.

An extraction method selective for ciguatoxin in fish has been developed and its efficiency assessed by use of a mouse bioassay (*19*). Approximately 63% of spiked ciguatoxin was recovered using ether–water partitioning and the method appeared to be reliable enough to quantify ciguatoxin in the flesh of fish.

Three cytotoxicity assays—neutral red uptake assay, observation of morphological alterations in baby hamster kidney cells, and the measurement of $Ca^{2+}$ concentrations in human lymphocytes—were evaluated for their ability to detect maitotoxin-like activity from *G. toxicus* (*20*). As compared to results from the mouse bioassay, all of the cytotoxicity assays detected the toxins. The neutral red assay proved to be particularly sensitive, and since it can be automated it has potential as a screening method. An ionspray mass spectrometry procedure has been optimized to identify a number of polyether toxins, including ciguatoxin and maitotoxin (*21*).

## Tetrodotoxin

Tetrodotoxin (TTX), a potent neurotoxin which affects neuromuscular function, has also been observed to have direct effects on the central nervous system. Following consumption of a reticulated blowfish (*Arothron reticularis*), a Thai man presented at an emergency room with nausea but soon thereafter stopped breathing and lost consciousness (*22*). He remained in a deep coma for 36 hours and then rapidly recovered so that he was nearly normal by 50 hours. These severe symptoms resembled cranial diabetes insipidus and indicated that TTX crossed the blood–brain barrier to suppress cerebral, hypophysial, and brainstem functions. The effects were apparently reversible.

Although tetrodotoxin can be synthesized by several species of marine microbes, only a few varieties of fish accumulate TTX and are associated with human exposures to this toxin. Analysis of liver from a toxic pufferfish (*Takifugu vermicularis snyderi*) revealed that TTX was bound to high-molecular-weight substances which appeared to be protein in nature (*23*). These complexes could be hydrolyzed by a protease but not by a ribonuclease or a deoxyribonuclease. It may be that pufferfish and other toxic species owe their toxicity to such high-molecular-weight substances which accumulate and concentrate TTX from organisms lower on the food chain.

A high-molecular-weight, TTX-binding substance from the body fluids of shore crabs was bound to CNBr-activated Sepharose to produce an affinity gel column which was useful in purifying TTX (*24*). The gel was very specific for TTX and was particularly useful in detecting TTX in samples with low toxin concentrations.

Recent studies of freshwater lakes in Japan indicate that TTX and TTX-producing bacteria are present in sediments in these lakes (*25*). A total of 17 TTX-producing bacteria belonging to 5 genera (*Bacillus*, *Micrococcus*, *Alcaligenes*, *Caulobacter*, and *Flavobacterium*) were isolated and identified. Studies with a marine bacterium, *Alteromonas tetraodonis*, demonstrated that TTX was produced during stationary phase growth and that at least 100-fold more TTX was produced when phosphate was limited than when it was sufficient (*26*).

## Paralytic Shellfish Poisoning (PSP)

Alaska experienced a record-breaking incidence of PSP in the spring of 1994, with 7 outbreaks involving at least 16 people reported from the Kodiak Island area (*27*). Analyses of mussels from the affected beaches revealed PSP toxin concentrations as high as 19,000 μg/100 g shellfish. One fatality occurred: a 61-year-old woman, who had been ill after eating mussels 3 days earlier, insisted on eating them again and died about 6 hours after consuming 6 contaminated mussels. Despite widespread warnings, some people continued to harvest shellfish for personal use because they believed that a lifetime of consuming local shellfish would make them immune to the toxins.

Several major blooms of dinoflagellates occurred in southern Tasmania in 1993 and these resulted in a number of PSP cases. Recently it was discovered that an Australian species of freshwater cyanobacteria, *Anabaena circinalis*, can also produce PSP toxins (*28*). Although there have been no reported human poisonings from this organism, it is also known to produce extensive blooms, including one which contaminated 1000 km of the Darling River in 1991. Toxins from *A. circinalis* could accumulate in freshwater mussels, causing inland outbreaks of PSP in Australia.

PSP-associated dinoflagellates (*Gymnodinium catenatum*) from Japan, Tasmania, and Spain were cultured under similar conditions and then examined to determine similarities and differences in toxin production (*29*). Variations in salinity, temperature, and concentrations of nitrate and phosphate did not affect toxin profiles. The primary toxins produced by all the strains were those of the *N*-sulfocarbamoyl group (C1–C5, gonyautoxins 5 and 6), but the relative amounts of each varied with the geographical origins of the strains. Only the Australian isolates produced the newly found 13-deoxydecarbamoyl toxins. Toxin profiles of different Japanese populations of the dinoflagellates, *Alexandrium tamarense* and *A. catenella* were also found to vary by geographical location (*30*). Furthermore, the total amount of toxins produced by some strains was nearly twice that produced by others.

In a recent review, Cembella et al. (*31*) discussed recent data on PSP toxin accumulation and biotransformation in commercially important natural populations of sea scallops and surfclams from the Gulf of Maine. Comparative data on anatomical distribution and spatio-temporal variations in toxin composition in the bivalve mollusks were considered and the dinoflagellates responsible for toxin production in this area were described.

The geographic distribution and the frequency of shellfish poisoning incidents appear to be increasing worldwide. Since the mid 1970s, PSP has spread from the open coast of Washington throughout much of Puget Sound. Since the still unaffected areas in the Sound include some of the most important sport and commercial shellfish beds, a study has been made of physical and chemical factors controlling PSP distribution (*32*). PSP originally entered the area when a major coastal bloom of *A. catenella* was moved south and into the Sound by an unusually large riverine discharge. The current distribution of PSP in shellfish and dinoflagellates in this area was found to be related to concentrations of dissolved nitrogen and the extent of vertical mixing of the water column. The author expresses concern that increased nitrogen discharge to the Sound from rapid urbanization and other, non-point sources could spread PSP to important shellfish-harvesting areas.

Investigations of factors affecting the distribution of PSP have also been carried out in the waters around Newfoundland (*33*). PSP intoxication of mussels in this area occurs not only during blooms of *Alexandrium fundyense* during the summer but also, in some locations, during the winter. Results of this study indicated that toxic, cultured mussels ingested resuspended cysts of *A. fundyense* during the winter and that areas where strong winds stirred up the muddy bottom were more likely to harbor toxic mussels.

Analyses of short-necked clams collected in Mikawa Bay, Japan, during a red tide in 1991 revealed the presence of high concentrations of PSP toxins (*34*). Approximately 90% of the total toxicity was identified by HPLC as the *N*-sulfocarbamoyl toxins, C1 and C2. Boiling of the clams for 10 min at pH 1 caused a 4–5-fold increase in toxicity in the mouse bioassay. Shellfish toxicity reached a maximum in mid-April shortly after a peak in the numbers of *A. tamarense*.

Boiling or steaming of lobsters contaminated with PSP decreased total toxicity in the hepatopancreas by about 65%, with decreases of 90–100% in gonyautoxins 2 and 3 and of 60% in saxitoxin (*35*). Hepatopancreas from the raw lobsters contained 85–127 µg PSP toxins/ 100 g (guideline level 80 µg/100 g). Toxin levels in claw and tail meat increased slightly after cooking but were still much lower (0.9–2.7 µg/100 g) than those detected in raw hepatopancreas. Although very little PSP toxin could be detected in the cooking water or steam condensate after cooking of the lobsters, it appeared that the toxins were leached out during cooking but were greatly diluted in the cooking water.

Two new PSP toxins, with a toxicity (by mouse bioassay) between that of saxitoxin and some of the gonyautoxins, were detected in a crab (*Zosimus aeneus*) from Okinawa (*36*). Analyses utilizing HPLC, electrophoresis, electrospray ionization mass spectrometry, and NMR indicated that their structures were carbamoyl-*N*-hydroxysaxitoxin and carbamoyl-*N*-neosaxitoxin.

An interlaboratory comparison, involving 18 European laboratories, has been made of methods for the detection of saxitoxin in liquid samples and in shellfish extracts (*37*). Each laboratory used a method of choice, with 4 HPLC methods and 1 ELISA being evaluated. All methods proved adequate for analysis of the saxitoxin solution, but interfering substances in the shellfish extract caused inaccurate results. A 3-year project, involving 15–20 European laboratories, has been initiated with the aims of improving the accuracy of PSP analyses

and of preparing reference materials for analyses. Procedures have been described for the detection of saxitoxin-induced protein in crabs by ELISA (*38*) and the detection of PSP toxins by reversed-phase HPLC (*39,40*).

## Domoic Acid (Amnesic Shellfish Poisoning)

During a two-year period following a California epidemic of domoic acid poisoning affecting hundreds of pelicans, a total of 1182 bivalve shellfish samples were analyzed for this toxin (*41*). Of these, 4.5% contained detectable levels of domoic acid, with maximum concentrations of 47, 1.9, and 29 ppm in mussels, oysters, and razor clams, respectively. Domoic acid was also detected in anchovies and crabs. Results of this monitoring indicate that low levels of domoic acid may be present in a number of marine species along the California coast. However, data collected from offshore fisheries (crabs and anchovies) were not always a reliable indicator of toxicity in nearshore bivalves and vice versa.

Elevated levels of domoic acid were detected in Pacific razor clams collected along the coast of Washington in the autumn of 1991 (*42,43*). Most of the toxin was present in the edible portion of the animals (36.4 vs 13.7 µg/g edible and inedible tissue). Contaminated clams, containing 10 or 48 µg toxin/g, maintained for 3 months under controlled conditions lost very little of the toxin.

A recent review compared the geographical distributions, seasonal patterns, growth requirements and histories of occurrences of two domoic-acid producing diatoms, *Pseudonitzschia pungens* and *P. australis* (*44*). Another two papers (*45,46*) also reported information on the occurrence of these two species along the west coast of the USA and their potential for toxin production. Monitoring of populations of these diatoms and an understanding of factors inducing them to bloom should aid in preventing future outbreaks of domoic acid poisoning.

Two recent papers presented procedures for the determination of domoic acid levels in biological samples by HPLC (*47,48*). Polyclonal antibodies developed against cell surface antigens of toxigenic and non-toxigenic strains of *P. pungens* have been used to produce an immunofluorescence assay which successfully differentiated between 31 toxic and 17 nontoxic isolates (*49*). This assay has great potential for use in monitoring programs.

## Diarrhetic Shellfish Poisoning (DSP)

Cases of DSP have been reported for the first time from the UK (*50,51*) and from South Africa (*52*). About 1–2 hours following consumption of imported mussels, which had been purchased in Yorkshire in the spring of 1994, two persons developed typical DSP symptoms (chills, nausea, abdominal pain, vomiting, and diarrhea). These symptoms persisted for 36 h. Uneaten mussels from the same batch were found, by bioassay, to contain DSP toxins and, by HPLC, to contain okadaic acid. Investigation of a number of South African cases of shellfish poisoning with DSP-like symptoms, occurring in the autumns of 1991 and 1992, revealed that the illness coincided with red tides along the west and south coasts. Analyses of extracts of mussels from the affected areas demonstrated the presence of DSP toxins, and one of the prominent red tide organisms, *Dinophysis acuminata*, appeared to be the source of the toxin.

A DSP red tide also occurred along the eastern coast of Canada in late July of 1990 and was associated with a subsurface population of *Dinophysis norvegica* (*53*). Although no human cases of DSP were described, okadaic acid levels in *D. norvegica* were as high as 32.6 pg/cell; in scallops exposed to red tide water, levels reached a maximum of 469 ng/g tissue. Such a bloom certainly has the potential to cause DSP if it occurs in areas where shellfish are harvested for consumption.

Okadaic acid is known to be a potent tumor promoter, to increase phosphorylation of several proteins, and to modulate a variety of cellular functions. Recent experiments with cultured cerebellar neurons provided further evidence for the neurotoxic effects of this toxin (*54*). These effects do not appear to affect excitatory amino acid receptors or voltage-sensitive calcium channels in cell membranes.

A method utilizing capillary electrophoresis coupled with a liquid chromatography-linked protein phosphatase bioassay has been developed for the sensitive detection of DSP toxins and hepatotoxic microcystins in marine and freshwater samples (*55*). Improved procedures for derivatization reactions and HPLC were devised in research designed to optimize DSP detection and determination (*56*). Because of its sensitivity to okadaic acid, *Daphnia magna* has been used in a bioassay to detect this toxin (*57*). This organism can detect okadaic acid at concentrations 10 times lower than the threshold of the mouse bioassay.

## Other Toxins

Snake mackerel, also known as escolar or the castor oil fish, has been responsible for recent outbreaks of diarrhea in North Carolina, Alabama, Georgia, and Texas (*58*). This fish is renowned for its purgative effects and is sometimes purposely consumed for that function. How-

ever, in these cases, the victims became ill after consuming the fish at restaurants. In the North Carolina incident, the fish were also contaminated with histamine, thereby also causing symptoms of scombroid poisoning. Although the diarrhea caused by this fish is not, in itself, serious, it is debilitating and could pose a threat to those in precarious health.

Introduction of a green alga, *Caulerpa taxifolia*, from tropical regions into the Mediterranean has raised concerns about the toxins it produces, apparently as a defense against herbivorous fish. There have been several reports of human poisonings following consumption of fish which had eaten *Caulerpa*. Aqueous and methanolic extracts of this alga and 4 purified toxins were evaluated for toxicity in mice, mammalian cells in culture, and in sea urchin eggs (*59*). Of the compounds tested, caulerpenyne, the major metabolite of this alga, was the most active against sea urchin eggs and is probably of greatest concern. An HPLC method has been described for the determination of caulerpenyne in algae (*60*).

Following a serious outbreak of poisoning due to consumption of a normally edible red alga on Guam in 1991, extracts of the toxic algae were tested for palytoxin using a recently developed ELISA. Results were inconclusive due to matrix interference. Therefore, a more sensitive palytoxin selective assay utilizing a hemolysis neutralization assay (which is based on the in vitro hemolytic activity of palytoxin) was devised (*61*). Hemolytic destruction of red cells could be observed in cultures containing as little as 10 pg palytoxin/mL, and this destruction was inhibited by anti-palytoxin monoclonal antibodies. Extracts of the toxic algae also exerted hemolytic activity but this was not inhibited by anti-palytoxin antibodies. The algal toxicity has recently been found to be due to polycavernosides A and B, new glycoside macrolides (*62*). The reason for the sudden and transient appearance of these toxins in these red algae remains unexplained.

The poisonous coral reef crab, *Lophozozymus pictor*, has been responsible for several fatalities among persons in Singapore and the Philippines. Analyses of different parts of poisonous specimens revealed that the gut and hepatopancreas contained the highest concentrations of toxins (*63*). Crabs which were kept in tanks and fed non-poisonous fish were found to lose nearly all their toxicity within 24 days. These data indicate that the toxin has an exogenous origin. Toxic fractions from these crabs exerted effects similar to palytoxin when given to mice or added to cultures of rat erythrocytes or HeLa cells (*64*). However, unlike palytoxin, this new toxin gives an intense blue fluorescence under UV light and migrates differently when analyzed by high performance capillary electrophoresis and reverse-phase HPLC.

Three species of carnivorous gastropods commonly consumed in Japan have been found to contain toxins in their salivary glands (*65*). The major toxin present in *Neptunea lyrata* has been identified as tetramine, while those present in the other species have not yet been isolated and characterized. One of the other species, *Charonia sauliae*, has been reported to also contain tetrodotoxin in its digestive gland.

Proteinaceous toxins have been isolated from the skin mucus of two species of eels: the common European eel (*Anguilla anguilla*) and the pike eel (*Muraenesox cinereus*) (*66*). Both toxins were similar to one previously isolated from Japanese eels and were unstable acidic proteins. These toxins are very sensitive to heat and, as such, are not considered a threat to humans consuming the eels. However, they could enter wounds in the hands of persons handling these fish.

# BIOGENIC AMINES

Formation of biogenic amines in foods and their adverse effects were reviewed by Halász et al. (*67*) with particular reference to amines produced by food-associated microbes. The presence of these compounds in fish, meat, cheese, and alcoholic beverages has received much attention but relatively little information is available on biogenic amines in vegetables and in prepacked convenience foods.

Although foods rich in histamines may cause allergy-like symptoms such as sneezing, skin flushing and itching, diarrhea, and shortness of breath, these reactions are not IgE-mediated and therefore do not represent a true food allergy. In a study of 45 persons with a history of chronic headache or intolerance to wine or foods, 33 showed some improvement in symptoms after 4 weeks on a histamine-free diet (no fish, cheese, hard-cured sausages, pickled cabbage, or alcoholic beverages) (*68*). Later challenges with histamine-rich foods caused symptoms to reappear. It is believed that these histamine-sensitive patients are deficient in the enzyme diamine oxidase.

Inoculation of various ground meats with *Proteus morganii* and subsequent incubation at 5–7°C until spoilage resulted in histamine levels as high as 10.58, 22.49, 18.14, 61.73, and 981.3 μg/g in beef, pork, mutton, poultry, and mackerel, respectively (*69*). Maximum histamine levels in the various meats occurred 1–2 days prior to the organoleptic changes associated with spoilage. Although histamine concentrations increased during the period of bacterial growth, they also continued after the bacterial population stabilized.

A survey of 209 microbial strains associated with food revealed that 16 of 16 *Enterococcus*, 7 of 14 *Lactococcus*, 2 of 3 *Proteus*, and 3 of 10 *Pseudomonas aeruginosa* strains had the ability to produce tyramine in a tyrosine-containing broth (*70*). A number of other bacterial strains, including species of *Acinetobacter*, *Bacillus*, *Escherichia*, *Salmonella*, *Shigella*, and *Yersinia* tested negative as did most yeast strains.

A method utilizing silica gel TLC and spectrofluorometry has been devised for the separation, identification, and estimation of 8 biogenic amines (histamine, cadaverine, putrescine, phenylethylamine, tyramine, tryptamine, spermidine, and spermine) (*71*). Application of this method for the analysis of dry sausage and fish samples obtained in Egyptian markets indicated that all 8 amines were present in the sausage and that all except tyramine, tryptamine, and phenylethylamine were present in fish.

## Seafood

Two outbreaks of scombrotoxic fish poisoning involving 7 people were reported in England and Wales in June, 1994 (*72*). Both were traced to consumption of canned tuna containing high levels of histamine.

An examination of 80 strains of lactic acid bacteria isolated from vacuum-packed, sugar-salted fish from Denmark revealed that none produced histamine while 52 were capable of producing tyramine (*73*). All except 3 of these isolates were identified as *Carnobacterium* spp. Tyramine production peaked during exponential growth and was reduced by lowering storage temperatures from 9 to 4°C.

A new procedure for the HPLC determination of biogenic amines utilizing precolumn derivatization with ortho-phthaldehyde and fluorometric detection was used in an investigation of the incidence of amine contamination in canned sardines (*74*). Of 7 biogenic amines detected in 41 batches of sardines, spermidine, histamine, and agmatine were present at the highest levels, with average concentrations of 4.24, 2.09, and 1.58 mg/kg, respectively. Approximately 96% of the 369 cans analyzed contained <100 mg histamine/kg and about 86% had <10 mg/kg. Only 4 contained >200 mg/kg.

An enzymatic method for detection of histamine in fish was developed and found to reliably detect this amine at concentrations of 3–30 mg/kg (*75*). Fish samples were extracted with perchloric acid, then neutralized and reacted with diamine oxidase to form hydrogen peroxide. Addition of peroxidase and a chromogen in reduced form allowed detection of this reaction by use of a spectrophotometer set at 596 nm. The diamine oxidase used was very specific and interference from other amines was generally not a problem.

Determination of histamine, cadaverine, putrescine, and spermidine in fish products can also be achieved by ion exchange chromatography with integrated pulsed amperometric detection (76). Estimated detection limits varied from 5 ng (putrescine) to 25 ng (spermidine).

## Meat

Fifty samples of dry sausage obtained from markets in Cairo, Egypt, were analyzed for the presence of 8 biogenic amines (77). Putrescine and cadaverine were detected most commonly (in 94–96% of samples) and at the highest mean concentrations—38.6 and 19.2 mg/kg, respectively. Phenylethylamine was least common, present in only 18% of samples, while spermine concentrations were the lowest—an average of 1.75 mg/kg.

Vacuum packaging of beef can greatly extend its shelf life but the potential remains for the accumulation of biogenic amines since proteolytic and decarboxylating bacteria can grow in an anaerobic environment. In experiments to monitor biogenic amine formation, beef carcasses were sprayed with water, 200 ppm chlorine, or 3% lactic acid, fabricated, vacuum-packaged and stored at 1°C for up to 120 days (78). Significant levels of tyramine were detected at day 20 in all treatments and controls, and they increased to 50 ppm at 60 days and 180 ppm at 120 days. Although the beef samples were still organoleptically acceptable at 60 days, they could present a hazard to individuals sensitive to biogenic amines.

A preliminary survey of lactic acid bacteria, including 13 pure cultures used as starter cultures, 4 strains isolated from commercial starter preparations, and 10 isolates from dry sausages, revealed that only 1 culture, *Lactobacillus brevis* (traditionally used for bakery products), was capable of producing histamine and tyramine in MRS broth (79). However, later investigations of 42 lactic acid bacteria isolated from Finnish dry sausages during ripening demonstrated that 4 of them could produce both tyramine (577–1087 ppm) and histamine (725–1083 ppm) in broth while another 6 produced only tyramine (402–900 ppm) (80). These amine-positive strains are apparently contaminants.

Efforts to control these amine-producing contaminants include decreasing pH of the media by the addition of lactic acid or glucono-delta-lactone (GDL) (81,82). During manufacture of dry sausages with different starter cultures, GDL effectively suppressed histamine production. GDL also inhibited growth and histamine and tyramine production by an amine-positive *Lactobacillus* strain in broth cultures.

An optimized perchloric acid extraction process coupled with reversed-phase HPLC analysis with fluorescence detection has been developed for the determination of putrescine, cadaverine, histamine, tyramine and 2-phenylethylamine in meat products, especially fermented sausages (83). Detection limit was 0.5 mg/kg.

## Alcoholic Beverages

Following a case of hypertensive crisis after consumption of beer on tap by a patient using an irreversible monoamine oxidase inhibitor (MAOI), a total of 98 beer samples (49 on tap and 49 bottled or canned) were analyzed for tyramine (84). Tyramine levels in all the bottled beers were <3.5 mg/L and therefore safe for those using MAOI. However, 4 of the tap beers had potentially dangerous tyramine concentrations (>10 mg/L) ranging from 26.34 to 112.91 mg/L. These were lager beers which were brewed by a secondary fermentation process.

Two liquid chromatographic methods for the determination of biogenic amines were described: ion-pair LC with postcolumn derivatization for the detection of amines in beers and their raw materials (85); HPLC with electrochemical coulometric detection after precolumn derivatization for the detection of amines in wines (86).

## Other Foods

A survey of a variety of vegetables revealed that most had very low biogenic amine concentrations (87). Spermidine and diaminobutane were the main compounds detected. Significant levels of histamine and tyramine were also present in sauerkraut. Since amines from raw vegetables were partially extracted into water during cooking, the amine content of cooked and canned vegetables could be decreased considerably by simply discarding the cooking water.

Total biogenic amine concentrations in soybeans were found to increase from <280 ppm to about 1800 ppm during fermentation to form tempe (88). Addition of *Lactobacillus plantarum* to the soybeans during fermentation by the mold *Rhizopus oligosporus* partially inhibited biogenic amine formation (to about 1000 ppm). Home cooking by stewing had little effect on amine concentrations but frying in oil resulted in significant losses of both tyramine and putrescine.

An automated ion exchange chromatographic method has been devised for the determination of biogenic amines in leafy vegetables (*89*). Total concentration of these amines was found to range from 14 to 20 μg/g fresh weight, with spermidine as the principal component.

## MUTAGENS AND CARCINOGENS IN HEATED AND PROCESSED FOODS

### Heterocyclic Amines

A recent review by Eisenbrand and Tang (*90*) summarized information in the literature on the chemistry and formation of heterocyclic amines and their biological effects, including their metabolism, mutagenicity, DNA adduct formation, and carcinogenicity. Estimates of human dietary exposure to these compounds were presented and potential health risks were discussed. Another review by Skog (*91*) discussed the precursors and reaction conditions important for mutagen formation during normal domestic cooking. Structures of the mutagens were described, as were results of studies on their formation in cooked meats and in model systems. It is expected that an understanding of these processes will suggest potential inhibitors of mutagen formation and procedures which would significantly decrease mutagens in cooked foods.

BIOLOGICAL EFFECTS. Since 2-amino-3-methylimidazo[4,5-*f*]quinoline (IQ) is carcinogenic when administered to rodents, it has recently been tested in macaques (38 cynomolgus and 2 rhesus monkeys) to assess its potential for inducing tumors in primates (*92*). Monkeys were gavaged 5 times per week with 10 or 20 mg IQ/kg body weight for up to 91 months. Hepatocellular carcinomas were induced in 55% of the low-dose and in 95% of the high-dose animals, but were not observed in any of the controls treated with vehicle only. Average latent periods at the high- and low-dose levels were 43 and 60 months, respectively. Although these IQ doses are much higher than would be encountered in a normal grilled hamburger, the high percentage of treated animals developing cancer in a relatively short time (about one seventh of their life span) and the presence of other carcinogenic heterocyclic amines in cooked meats indicates that we should be concerned about harmful effects in humans.

In an assessment of the carcinogenicity of 3-amino-1-methyl-5H-pyrido[4,3-*b*]indole acetate (Trp-P-2), male and female rats were maintained on diets containing 0, 30, or 100 ppm Trp-P-2 for 112 weeks (*93*). In the highest dose groups, incidences of the following tumors were significantly increased: hepatocellular adenomas, transitional cell tumors in the urinary bladder, and fibroadenomas/fibromas of the mammary gland in males; mammary tumors, malignant lymphomas, and adenomas and adenocarcinomas of the clitoral gland in females.

Dose-dependency of tumor induction by 2-amino-1-methyl-6-phenylimidazo[4,5-*b*]pyridine (PhIP) has been investigated in experiments with rats fed diets containing 25 or 100 ppm PhIP for up to 104 weeks (*94*). Incidences of mammary adenocarcinomas in females were 7% and 47% in the low- and high-dose groups and of colon adenocarcinomas were 43% for males and 13% for females fed 100 ppm PhIP. No colon tumors were observed in the low-dose group. However, another 8-week experiment with rats fed 25, 100, or 400 ppm PhIP revealed a clear dose-dependence in the induction of aberrant crypt foci (preneoplastic lesions) in the colons of treated animals.

High doses of heterocyclic amines are known to be carcinogenic to rodents, but whether lower levels of these compounds, more typical of the usual human exposure, are also carcinogenic remains to be determined. In one such experiment, male rats fed a choline-deficient diet (to induce a high level of hepatocyte proliferation) for 20 or 40 weeks, also consumed 0.4 or 4 ppm dietary 2-amino-3,8-dimethylimidazo[4,5-*f*]quinoxaline (MeIQx) (*95*). At the higher dose, MeIQx approximately doubles the number and the area of glutathione-S-transferase (GST)-positive foci (preneoplastic changes) in the liver at both 20 and 40 weeks. No significant effects were observed in livers of rats fed a choline-sufficient diet supplemented with MeIQx or the choline-deficient diet with 0.4 ppm MeIQx.

To assess the promoting ability of some heterocyclic amines, rats were initiated with diethylnitrosamine, subjected to partial hepatectomy and then gavaged over a period of 10 days with MeIQx or IQ (*96*). After one month their livers were examined for GST-positive foci but no differences were observed between control and experimental animals. At least in this system, these compounds do not act as promoters of carcinogenicity.

Some carcinogens act by activating oncogenes, such as the *ras* family of genes or by inactivating the tumor suppressor gene, *p*53. In some tissues, heterocyclic amines appear not to induce such mutations: none of 11 colon tumors induced by IQ and of 9 induced by PhIP, and only 1 of 7 induced by 2-amino-6-methyldipyrido[1,2-*a*:3',2'-*d*]imidazole (Glu-P-1) in rats contained a mutation in the Ki-*ras* oncogene (*97*). Female rats fed 100 or 400 ppm PhIP developed mammary carcinomas but only 2 of 10 induced at the low dose and 1 of 7 at the high dose were found to contain mutations in the Ha-*ras* oncogene (*98*). None of the animals in these two studies had mutations in other *ras* genes.

On the other hand, IQ appeared to activate the *ras* gene in liver tumors and possibly in lung tumors in mice (*99*). Mice were given 4 ip injections of IQ during the first 3 weeks of life and then sacrificed at 22 months for tumor analyses. None of 15 liver tumors from control mice but 7 of 34 liver tumors in IQ-treated mice contained mutant Ha-*ras* genes. As regards lung tumors, 20 of 26 from control mice and 49 of 54 from treated mice contained mutant Ki-*ras* genes. IQ also activated Ha-*ras* and Ki-*ras* genes in rat Zymbal's gland tumors (*100*). All nine tumors induced by dietary IQ (0.015% for 55 weeks) had mutations in one or the other of these *ras* oncogenes.

Analysis of mutations induced by 9 heterocyclic amines in the *lacZ* gene of *E.coli* revealed that 99.5% of them were frameshift mutations (*101*). A small number of transversions (GC→TA) were caused by MeIQx, PhIP, and several other of the amines. Since transversions rather than frameshifts are reported to be important in activating oncogenes, these results may indicate why heterocyclic amines are relatively modest carcinogens despite their strong mutagenicity in the Ames assay. In another in vitro system, 75% of the mutations induced by PhIP in the dihydrofolate reductase gene of Chinese hamster ovary cells were found to be transversions with only a few frameshifts and deletions (*102*).

Further research with PhIP has confirmed its mutagenicity in rodents. Analyses by DNA fingerprinting of mouse tumor cell lines exposed to PhIP indicated that PhIP induced recombinational mutations which would result in chromosomal instability, a characteristic of many tumor cells (*103*). PhIP also induced mutations in epithelial stem cells in the base of crypts in the small intestine of orally exposed mice (*104*). Although the intestinal cells do not effectively activate PhIP, hepatic microsomes readily convert PhIP to a proximate mutagen (*N*-hydroxy-PhIP) and this relatively stable compound can reach the small intestine via the systemic circulation. Therefore, it appears that metabolic activation does not necessarily occur in the target tissue.

IQ has been reported to cause chromosomal aberrations in both Chinese hamster lung fibroblasts in vitro (*105*) and in hepatocytes of rats gavaged with 12.5, 25, or 50 mg IQ per kg body weight per day for 1 to 28 days (*106*). Metabolic activation with an S9 mix was required for the genotoxic effects to occur in vitro. The in vivo assay was very sensitive, not requiring partial hepatectomy or mitogen treatment.

Following a single oral dose of radiolabelled IQ, MeIQx, or PhIP to lactating rats with 5-day-old pups, radioactivity in the dams was highest in liver and kidney; mammary gland showed the next highest concentration (*107*). Levels of DNA–heterocyclic amines in the mammary gland ranged from 0.2 to 2.2 adducts/$10^7$ nucleotides. IQ–DNA adduct levels were about 11 times higher in the liver than in mammary gland while PhIP adducts were about 4 times lower in liver. Radioactivity was also detected in nursing pups; amine–DNA adducts in their livers ranged from 0.25 to 0.46 adducts/$10^8$ nucleotides. Thus, breast milk is a potential route of exposure to these carcinogenic heterocyclic amines.

Comparison of IQ–DNA adduct levels in rat hepatic nuclear and mitochondrial DNA revealed that after a single dose of IQ, adduct levels were about 2 times higher in nuclear DNA, while after a series of IQ doses, adduct levels were similar in the two types of DNA (*108*). In contrast, a single dose of PhIP produced similar adduct levels in nuclear and mitochondrial DNA while multiple doses resulted in significantly higher levels in mitochondrial DNA. The C8–guanine adduct accounted for 72 and 40% of the nuclear and mitochondrial adducts of IQ, respectively, and for 48 and 15% of the PhIP adducts in these DNAs.

Several analyses of DNA adducts formed by heterocyclic amines have shown the C8–guanine adduct to be predominant. These included: (a) in vitro experiments with polynucleotides and in vivo experiments with cynomolgus monkeys dosed with IQ, MeIQx, and PhIP (*109*); (b) analyses of DNA from rats dosed with PhIP (*110*); and rats dosed with MeIQx (*111*). Other experiments on in vivo adduct formation in mice demonstrated that consumption of a high-fat diet (25% beef fat, hydrogenated vegetable oil or non-hydrogenated vegetable oil) compared to a diet containing 1% fat increased the binding of MeIQx to hepatic DNA although only the hydrogenated oil caused a statistically significant increase (*112*). Hepatic microsomes isolated from mice fed high-fat diets also had a greater capacity to activate MeIQx compared to microsomes from mice on a low-fat diet.

In addition to being mutagenic on their own, at least some heterocyclic amines [3-amino-1,4-dimethyl-5*H*-pyrido[4,3-*b*]indole (Trp-P-1) and Trp-P-2] have been shown to enhance the damage caused by other mutagens. UV irradiation of *Escherichia coli* causes formation of cyclobutane dimers and (6–4)photoproducts. However, within 30 min, healthy cells can repair about 60% of the former and 90% of the latter photoproducts. Incubation of irradiated cells with 0.02 to 20 µg/mL Trp-P-1 (concentrations too low to be mutagenic or carcinogenic) was found to inhibit repair of both types of photolesions in a dose-dependent manner (*113*).

Trp-P-2 is also cytotoxic to cultured rat hepatocytes by causing leakage of DNase and cell death (*114*). This effect requires metabolic activation and is also correlated with DNA strand breaks in these cells.

Although Trp-P-1 is readily absorbed from the rat intestine, freeze-dried gastrointestinal microbes, lactic acid bacteria and yeast were found to significantly reduce this absorption (*115*). In vitro freeze-dried cells bound 51–87% of Trp-P-1 and, in vivo, coadministration of freeze-dried cells with Trp-P-1 reduced uptake of this compound by 40–65%. However, the significance of this binding in the normal intestine is uncertain because large populations of intestinal bacteria inhabit the large, not the small, intestine and heterocyclic amines may not directly reach the large intestine.

Myocyte degeneration and mitochondrial changes have been observed in hearts of 10 monkeys (rhesus and cynomolgus) gavaged with 10 or 20 mg IQ for 5 days per week for 48–80 months (*116*). All the monkeys had developed hepatocellular carcinomas, but their hearts appeared normal upon gross inspection. However, light microscopic examination disclosed numerous abnormalities (necrosis, atrophy, and hypertrophy) of myocytes, and the electron microscope revealed mitochondrial swelling, myofibrillar loss and disorganization of the sarcomeres. Fetal rat myocytes exposed to the activated forms of IQ and PhIP also exhibited swollen and irregular mitochondria (*117*). In addition, leakage of enzymes from the cells was observed (more so in IQ-treated cells) and DNA adducts were produced (more in PhIP-treated cells). Hearts of rats orally dosed with IQ or PhIP were also found to contain foci of chronic inflammation with myocyte necrosis and myofibrillar dissolution and disarray. Other studies with rats injected ip with PhIP demonstrated that this compound significantly decreased the activity of complex I in the mitochondrial electron transport chain in the heart, diaphragm, and psoas major but not in the liver (*118*). All these experiments indicate that IQ and PhIP exert cardiotoxic as well as carcinogenic effects.

Radiolabelled Trp-P-1 injected into β-naphthoflavone (BNF)-treated mice was found to selectively bind to endothelial cells of heart and kidney (*119*) and to endothelial cells in the vena cava and in the pulmonary and the hepatic portal vascular systems (*120*). Since BNF induces P450 enzymes, it appeared that Trp-P-1 was converted to an active form by cytochrome P450 and may then play a role in cardiovascular disease. No

such localized binding to endothelial cells was observed in mice pretreated with corn oil instead of BNF. Thus, Trp-P-1, PhIP, and other food mutagens may play a role in cardiac degeneration and decline of mitochondrial function.

**OCCURRENCE AND DETECTION IN FOODS.** Commercial heat-processed Finnish foods were assayed for mutagenicity (Ames test) and for their content of the heterocyclic amines MeIQx, PhIP, and DiMeIQx (sum of 2-amino-3,4,8-trimethylimidazo[4,5-*f*]quinoxaline and 2-amino-3,7,8-trimethylimidazo[4,5-*f*]quinoxaline) (*121*). Of all the foods tested, flame-broiled fish had the highest mutagenic activity, followed by grilled pork and grilled chicken. Commercially produced meat patties were not mutagenic. PhIP was present in the highest concentration (0.5–3.8 ng/g cooked food); MeIQx and DiMeIQx were present in lower concentrations (0.04–0.4 ng/g and 0.03–0.2 ng/g) in the mutagenic samples. Considerable differences in mutagenicity and heterocyclic amine content were observed between equivalent products from different manufacturers, indicating that processing techniques have a marked effect on mutagen formation.

PhIP and MeIQx were also reported to be the predominant heterocyclic amines present in grilled bacon (<0.1–52 ppb and 0.9–18 ppb, respectively) and in grilled beef (0.8–3.2 ppb) (*122*). However, in this study no heterocyclic amines were detected in grilled fish. Significantly higher concentrations of PhIP and MeIQx were present in bacon fat drippings and pan scrapings than in the cooked meats. Combined grilled fish and meat scrapings contained 144 ppb PhIP, 29 ppb MeIQx, and 77 ppb 2-aminoαcarboline.

Meat from 16 different animal species was fried under standard conditions and then assayed for mutagenicity in the Ames test (*123*). A sample of beef was fried with each of the other meats and then mutagenicity was expressed relative to that in beef. Fried beef consistently induced more mutations, followed by goat and pheasant. Fried hare, rabbit, and minced elk contained only about 40% the mutagenicity of the fried beef. Mutagenicity was not correlated with creatinine, protein, carbohydrate, or fat contents of the different meats.

Microwave cooking of beefburgers, with and without the use of a flavoring, was found to produce burgers with much lower levels of mutagens (*124*). For example, in one series of experiments, the numbers of revertants induced in TA98 by uncooked beef and beef that was fried and unflavored, fried and flavored, microwaved and unflavored, or microwaved and flavored were, respectively, 15, 134, 226, 31, and 48. A flavor testing panel rated the microwaved, flavored burgers equally acceptable to traditionally fried burgers.

Analysis of a bacteriological-grade beef extract revealed the presence of two new mutagenic compounds (*125*). Structure of one of these compounds was determined to be 2-amino-4-hydroxymethyl-3,8-dimethyl-imidazo[4,5-*f*]quinoxaline by UV and mass spectral analyses and ¹H-NMR. Concentration of this compound in the beef extract was estimated to be 6 ng/g.

Only 10 of 24 commercial beef flavors tested were found to be mutagenic in the Ames test (50–3200 revertants induced/g) (*126*). MeIQx was detected in two of the mutagenic flavors and MeIQx and DiMeIQx were present in one mutagenic sample tested. In another study, all except one of 22 beef and chicken bouillon samples tested contained mutagens active in the Ames assay (*127*). Beef bouillon samples, on the average, induced more revertants/g (346) than chicken and turkey samples (135).

Determination of MeIQx, DiMeIQx, and PhIP in foods by gas chromatography–negative ion mass spectrometry has been described (*128*). In addition, an HPLC method with electrochemical detection has been developed for the determination of ten heterocyclic amines in foods (*129*).

**BIOACTIVATION OF HETEROCYCLIC AMINES.** To ascertain the contribution of CYP1A2 to the metabolism of PhIP and MeIQx in humans, 6 male volunteers were dosed with a placebo or furafylline, a selective inhibitor of CYP1A2, prior to consuming a test meal containing a known amount of amines (*130*). Urine was monitored for the next 28 hours for the presence of unchanged PhIP and MeIQx. Without furafylline, subjects excreted only an average of 2.6% of the ingested dose of MeIQx and 1.2% of PhIP as the parent compound. Inhibition of CYP1A2 activity resulted in an average of 31% of the MeIQx and 4.2% of the PhIP doses being excreted unchanged. Calculations based on the efficiency of inhibition of CYP1A2 and the percentage of these amines normally eliminated in urine indicated that, in humans, CYP1A2-catalyzed metabolism accounts for 91% of the elimination of ingested MeIQx and 70% of ingested PhIP, most likely via *N*-hydroxylation.

In cynomolgus monkeys, PhIP is extensively metabolized, with only about 1% of an administered dose being excreted in the urine unchanged. Four PhIP metabolites were detected in urine, bile, and plasma, with the most prominent one in all tissues being PhIP-4'-sulfate (*131*). Clearance of PhIP and its metabolites from plasma was rapid. PhIP did form DNA adducts in white blood cells, and these were still detectable a week after dosing. This suggests that PhIP is activated by *N*-hydroxylation and detoxified by 4'-hydroxylation in cynomolgus monkeys.

Hepatic microsomes from humans, cynomolgus monkeys, and rats were incubated with 8 different heterocyclic amines to determine their relative abilities to activate these compounds (*132*). Compared to rats and humans, monkeys had almost no ability to activate the quinoxaline-type amines (IQx and MeIQx) but could activate the other compounds. For most of the compounds, the human microsomes were the most efficient at transforming the heterocyclic amines into mutagens.

Phase II activation of *N*-hydroxy-IQ, *N*-hydroxy-PhIP, and *N*-hydroxy-MeIQx was studied in vitro using cytosolic preparations from liver, kidney, colon, and heart of cynomolgus monkeys and of rats (*133*). All four phase II enzymes were capable of activating these amines but the extent of activation varied with the species and the tissues. These differences may be related to the differential toxic effects observed in various organs and species.

In vitro studies using hepatic microsomes from PCB-treated rats demonstrated that they metabolized DiMeIQx to form two major and three minor metabolites (*134*). It appeared that DiMeIQx was first hydroxylated at the 2-amino or the 8-methyl group and these compounds were further metabolized to produce proximate mutagens.

Normal intestinal bacteria are capable of converting IQ to 7-hydroxy-IQ, a direct-acting mutagen. To test whether this compound exerts carcinogenic effects on the rat colon, male rats were infused intrarectally three times per week with pure, synthetic 7-OH-IQ during a 21-month period (*135*). Although colon cancer developed in most rats of a positive control group dosed with *N*-nitrosomethylurea, 7-OH-IQ did not induce colon cancer in the rats.

## Cholesterol Oxides

A large number of cholesterol oxidation products (COPS) have been identified and some appear to exert cytotoxic, mutagenic, or carcinogenic effects. In experiments with rat hepatocytes in culture, three COPS were found to inhibit gap junctional communication between cells (*136*). Addition of cholesterol to the cultures did not abolish this effect, suggesting that this inhibitory effect was not directly related to suppression of cholesterol synthesis. Inhibition of intercellular communication may be an early sign of the cytotoxicity or tumor-promoting effects of these COPS.

A survey of Australian foods revealed that spray-dried egg powders contained the highest COPS levels (31–113 mg/100 g powder), with lower concentrations detected in spray-dried full cream milk powders (2.1–3.4 mg/100 g), sweet biscuits (2.1–7.8 mg/100 g), cake mixes (1.6–3.1 mg/100 g), mayonnaise (6.8 mg/100 g) and baby foods containing egg (0.2–0.5 mg/100 g) (*137*). COPS were undetectable in fresh eggs and eggs stored at 4°C for 6 weeks.

In an attempt to control lipid oxidation in dried egg powders, the diets of laying hens were supplemented with 25–200 mg vitamin E/kg feed (*138*). This resulted in dose-dependent increases of this antioxidant vitamin in the dried egg powders and decreases in oxysterols and other oxidized lipids formed during prolonged storage at ambient temperatures.

Research with both eggs and milk demonstrated that appropriate packaging and storage conditions can also minimize COPS formation. Formation of COPS in spray-dried egg powder was found to be very slow in a freezer at –20°C but was significantly increased by exposure to diffuse daylight and to heat (*139*). The β-epoxide of cholesterol was the main derivative obtained after prolonged exposure to light, while the 7-oxidized compounds were more prominent in heated samples.

COPS levels in whole milk powders dried by 3 different processes were found to be uniformly low immediately after processing, but those samples processed by direct-fired heaters in the presence of high levels of oxides of nitrogen ($NO_x$) accumulated the highest levels of COPS during storage under suboptimal conditions (*140*). The use of oxygen-impermeable packaging systems and oxygen absorbers in the packages effectively suppressed COPS formation in dried milk during 6 months of storage, regardless of drying method.

Small sun-dried fish from retail stores in Taiwan were found to contain 4.82–65.7 ppm total COPS, with 7α-hydroxycholesterol as the main derivative (*141*). These fish are traditionally dried in the sun for 1–2 days and are then stored for several months exposed to the air and without packaging. Total COPS in Japanese samples of canned and boiled squid, dried squid, and dried sardines were measured as 11, 14.6, and 28.7 mg/100 g, respectively (*142*). Other Japanese samples of boiled, dried fish contained 6.9–18.8 mg total COPS/100 g while salted, dried fish contained 0.96–13.8 mg COPS/100 g (*143*).

When cholesterol is heated by itself, very little oxidation occurs. However, recent studies of the oxidation process demonstrated that cholesterol is unstable when heated with fats, particularly unsaturated fats (*144*). Vitamin E supplementation of veal calves enhanced the stability of cholesterol in their membranes as evidenced by a 60% suppression of cholesterol oxidation in cooked meat from supplemented, compared to control, calves.

Procedures for the determination of cholesterol and phospholipid hydroperoxides by HPLC with mercury drop electrochemical detection (*145*) and cholesterol oxides in heated lard by TLC and HPLC (*146*) have been described. Several extraction, separation, and detection methods for the analysis of COPS from heated lard were devised and evaluated by use of liquid chromatography (*147*).

## Other Lipid Oxidation Products

BIOLOGICAL EFFECTS. In a recent review, Aubourg (*148*) discussed the special characteristics and reactivity of malondialdehyde, one of the most significant products of lipid degradation. Reaction of this compound with free amino groups may have carcinogenic and mutagenic implications and it may interact with important constituents of foods during and after processing.

Dietary oxidized lipids constituting 10% of the diet for 8 weeks caused the accumulation of high levels of fluorescent peroxidation products in the red blood cell membranes of rats and significantly decreased membrane fluidity (*149*). An increase in the activity of membrane-bound acetylcholinesterase and $(Na^+K^+)ATPase$ and a decrease in the content of membrane polyunsaturated fatty acids also occurred. These changes point out the potential for adverse effects of dietary oxidized lipids.

Diabetic humans and animals are known to have higher levels of oxidized serum lipoproteins. Both normal and diabetic rats fed a fat-free diet had very low levels of oxidized lipids in their serum proteins. However, when oxidized corn oil was added to the diets, the quantity of oxidized serum lipoproteins increased about 5-fold in normal rats and about 16-fold in diabetic rats (*150*). A high intake of oxidized lipids in fried foods could, especially in diabetics, contribute to atherosclerosis.

OCCURRENCE AND CONTROL IN FOODS. High molecular weight autoxidation products formed in commercially available rapeseed, soybean, and sunflower oils at 60°C in the dark have been identified using high-performance size-exclusion chromatography (HPSEC) (*151*). During 13 days' storage under these conditions, triacylglycerol dimers increased about 2.5- to 10-fold and polar triacylglycerols increased approximately 5.5- to 35-fold in the different oils, with the greatest changes observed in the sunflower oil. No higher oligomeric compounds were detected. During 4 steps in the refining process for these oils little change was observed in the diacylglycerol and polar triacylglycerol concentrations in the oils (*152*). However, an increase in triacylglycerol dimers was detected by HPSEC following the bleaching and deodorization steps.

Production of oxo- and hydroxy-fatty acids during heating to 180°C for 4 days was monitored in safflower oil, olive oil, and a fast-food fat (mostly tallow) (*153*). Safflower oil accumulated the greatest amounts of mono- and polyhydroxy-fatty acids while the fast-food fat formed the highest levels of oxo-fatty acids. At least half of the maximal concentration of these compounds was formed during hours 16–24 of heating of each oil.

Total polar compounds were monitored in sunflower oil used for 75 repeated deep-fat fryings of potatoes (*154*). Fresh oil was added every 4–5 fryings to replenish the amount absorbed by the potatoes. Total polar components increased rapidly during the first 20 fryings, from 5.09 to 15.99 mg/100 mg oil, and continued to increase slowly to 17.99 mg/100 mg until the 30th frying. Triglyceride dimers also increased until the 30th frying while triglyceride polymers increased throughout the experiment. The data indicate that with frequent turnover of fresh oil, the critical level of 25% polar material is rarely reached.

Transfer of lipids between a frying medium (canola oil) and mackerel steaks containing 12% fat was measured following deep-fat frying for 7 min at 180°C (*155*). Analyses of fatty acids in the oil, in fish skin, and in fish meat before and after frying demonstrated that extensive lipid exchanges had occurred during frying. Longer chain *n*-3 fatty acids of the mackerel were not affected by the frying, and only small quantities of polar compounds, polymers, and geometrical fatty acid isomers of the long-chain polyunsaturated fatty acids were formed during frying.

In an investigation of the potential for lipid oxidation during sun-drying of fish, initial rate of oxygen uptake has been measured in a model system consisting of highly polyunsaturated fish oil exposed to different temperatures and light conditions (*156*). An increase of temperature from 30 to 40°C increased oxygen consumption by 82% in the dark and by about 200% in the light. Oxygen consumption in the light as compared to the dark increased by 53% at 30°C and by about 157% at 40°C. Thus both environmental factors contribute significantly to lipid oxidation.

Exposure of cod liver oil to UV light for up to 12 hours resulted in the formation of several toxic aldehydes and of acrolein and malonaldehyde (*157*). Concentrations of propanal and malonaldehyde peaked after

2 hours of treatment while acrolein levels peaked at 6 hours and formaldehyde and acetaldehyde concentrations reached a maximum after 12 hours of exposure.

**ANALYTICAL METHODS.** Numerous improvements in analytical procedures for the determination of lipid oxides in foods have been described. These involve: solid phase extraction methods (*158*); use of Fourier transform infrared spectroscopy (*159*); iron-based spectrophotometry (*160*); reversed-phase HPLC with UV and evaporative light-scattering detectors (*161*); thermoluminescence measurements (*162*); an organic phase enzyme electrode (*163*); and an automated system based on flow injection (*164*). In addition, methods were described for the determination of cyclic fatty acid monomers in heated fats (*165*) and for determination of lipid oxidation volatiles in meat (*166*) and in frying oils (*167*).

## OTHER COMPOUNDS IN HEATED AND PROCESSED FOODS

### Urethane (Ethyl Carbamate)

Results from a survey of urethane concentrations in beverages and foods in Denmark indicated that the estimated daily intake of this carcinogen was about 2 µg per person, although those with the highest level of alcohol consumption may be exposed to 7 µg per day (*168*). Average urethane concentrations in spirits, fortified wines, wine, beer, bread, and yogurts and other acidified milk products were, respectively, 534, 30, 7, 3, 3.5, and 0.2 µg per L or kg.

Concentrations of methyl and ethyl carbamates (MC and EC) were determined in 48 alcoholic beverages, 12 samples of bread and toast, 10 of soy sauce, and 14 of yogurt and buttermilk obtained in Canada by a newly developed method utilizing GC with a thermal energy analyzer for detection and GC-high resolution mass spectrometry for confirmation (*169*). MC levels were much lower than EC concentrations in most samples, the exception being yogurt and buttermilk, where MC concentrations ranged up to 4.3 µg/kg and EC up to 0.4 µg/kg. Two soy sauce samples originating in the USA had high levels of EC (57–59 µg/kg) and MC (0.6 µg/kg), while those originating in Canada and Asia had much lower EC (up to 6.5 µg/kg) concentrations. MC and EC measured in toast averaged 2.7 and 15.7 µg/kg (dark toast) and 2.2 and 4.3 µg/kg (light). Most alcoholic beverages contained only traces of MC, although one sample of a fruit brandy had 28 µg MC/kg along with 2344 µg EC/kg.

Two recent 2-year storage studies examined some factors related to urethane formation in wines. Both confirmed the importance of storage temperature and of urea concentrations in the newly made wine. In addition, one study demonstrated that citrulline levels and probably some other compounds affected urethane production (*170*). Urease-treated wines, with no detectable urea at the beginning of the experiment, still accumulated urethane during storage for 6 months but to significantly lower concentrations than the untreated wines (*171*). It was recommended that urea concentrations in wine should be reduced to <2 mg/L in order to keep urethane concentrations within acceptable limits.

Solid-phase extraction with Extrelut followed by analysis using gas chromatography–selected ion monitoring–mass spectrometry was used to determine urethane concentrations in 18 soy sauces (*172*). Although the number of samples of different soy sauces was small, the fermented soy sauces tended to have higher urethane concentrations than the non-fermented sauces.

Following a collaborative study, a capillary gas chromatography procedure using a thermal energy analyzer system was adopted first action by AOAC International for the determination of urethane in alcoholic beverages (*173*).

## Cross-linked Amino Acids and Sugar–Lysine Compounds

Analyses of acid hydrolysates of heated skim milk revealed the presence of an unknown ninhydrin-positive compound (*174*). This compound was identified by $^1$H-NMR spectroscopy as two isomeric forms of histidinoalanine, a cross-linked amino acid not previously known to be present in foods. Concentrations of this amino acid ranged between 50 and 1800 mg/kg protein in some heated milk products, which is comparable to concentrations of another cross-linked amino acid, lysinoalanine. The formation of these cross-linked amino acids can reduce digestibility of food proteins and lower the availability of some essential amino acids.

Heat treatment of soy protein with glucose and in alkali was found to reduce available lysine by 78–85% and by 7–24%, respectively (*175*). In the first case, lysine reacts to form fructose-lysine while under alkaline conditions, lysinoalanine is formed. Both reactions could lower the nutritional value of the heated soy protein. In addition, glucose-lysine Maillard reaction products are mutagenic in the Ames test and clastogenic to Chinese hamster ovary cells in systems without metabolic activation (*176*). These Maillard reaction products were also found to reduce AHH activities in the small intestine (but

not in liver, kidney, or lungs), and thus they may affect the metabolism of dietary xenobiotics (*177*).

## Hydroxymethylfurfural

5-(Hydroxymethyl)furfural (HMF), a decomposition product of glucose and fructose present in a variety of foods, has been shown to be mutagenic and to cause breaks in DNA strands. In an investigation of the possible mechanisms for this genotoxicity, HMF was subjected to allylic sulfonation and chlorination and then tested for mutagenicity and cytotoxicity (*178*). Both derivatives were directly mutagenic (without metabolic activation) to *S. typhimurium* and to human lymphoblast cells in culture.

Analytical procedures have been described for the determination of HMF in breakfast cereals by reversed-phase liquid chromatography (*179*) and in diversely colored and turbid food samples using a stopped-flow injection technique and spectrophotometric analysis (*180*).

## Aromatic Amines

Mutagen formation in breads, cookies, flour, and meat-substitute patties during cooking has been assayed using the Ames/Salmonella test with and without metabolic activation (*181*). Heating of all these foods increased their mutagenicity; evidence from the type of mutations induced, the requirement for metabolic activation, and behavior during extraction suggests that these mutagens are amines. Although the authors suspected that these compounds were heterocyclic amines, they could not be identified as any of the known heterocyclic amines.

Certain amino acids when heated alone or in combination with other amino acids form new aromatic amine mutagens which appear to differ from the known heterocyclic amine mutagens found in cooked meats (*182*). Only cysteine produced mutagens when heated alone, but arginine when heated with any one of five other amino acids formed mutagens.

## β-Carbolines

Conditions influencing the formation of 1-methyl-1,2,3,4-tetrahydro-β-3-carboxylic acid (MTCA), a precursor of mutagenic *N*-nitroso compounds, were studied in model systems and during the fermentation of grape juice (*183*). MTCA was produced by a reaction between tryptophan and acetaldehyde released by yeast during growth and alcoholic fermentation. Low pH and high temperature accelerated this reaction while sulfur dioxide inhibited it. Another β-carboline, THCA, was also formed at high storage temperatures by a reaction between formaldehyde and tryptophan.

# COFFEE AND CAFFEINE

Summaries of salient presentations at the Seventh International Caffeine Workshop held in 1993 in Greece have been recently published (*184*). Major workshop topics included caffeine intake studies and effects of caffeine on calcium metabolism, the heart, behavior, mental performance, and exercise, and possible carcinogenic effects of caffeine and coffee.

## Metabolism of Caffeine

Human hepatic microsomal preparations from adults were found to produce significantly higher levels of dimethylxanthines when incubated with caffeine than liver microsomes isolated from human fetuses, neonates, and infants (*185*). Formation of dimethylxanthines increased significantly with age in the neonate-infant group (0–300 days of age) and was correlated with CYP1A2 microsomal concentrations. In contrast, total dimethylxanthines decreased significantly with increasing gestational age in fetal samples. Neither CYP1A1 nor CYP1A2 were present in fetal microsomes, suggesting that metabolism of caffeine in these samples depended on CYP3A.

A series of V79 Chinese hamster cells genetically engineered to stably express single forms of rat cytochromes P450IA1, P450IA2, P450IIB1, or human P450IA2 and rat liver epithelial cells expressing murine P450IA2 were used to investigate which P450 forms were responsible for different pathways of methylxanthine metabolism (*186*). Four primary demethylated and hydroxylated metabolites were produced from caffeine by cells containing human, rat, and murine P450IA2, but there were differences in the relative amounts of the metabolites. Cells containing the human and mouse cytochromes predominantly catalyzed the 3-demethylation of caffeine, while the rat cytochrome mediated about equal amounts of 3- and 1-demethylation. Theophylline was primarily metabolized by 8-hydroxylation and all cell lines were able to carry out this reaction.

## Genotoxicity and Carcinogenicity

A review of published data on the genotoxic, mutagenic, and antimutagenic effects of coffee by Nehlig and Debry (*187*) concluded that moderate to normal consumption

of coffee and caffeine by humans is extremely unlikely to induce mutagenic effects. While coffee and caffeine are mutagenic to bacteria and, at high concentrations, are genotoxic to cultured mammalian cells, these effects are abolished by the presence of liver extracts containing detoxifying enzymes. Mutagenicity of coffee is most likely due to reactive compounds such as methylglyoxal and other aliphatic dicarbonyls, in combination with hydrogen peroxide, and to heterocyclic amines generated during roasting.

The presence of a possibly new mutagen with DNA-breaking activity has been detected in extracts of brewed and instant coffee (*188*). The active gel fraction was mutagenic in the Ames test without metabolic activation and was inhibited by high concentrations of inorganic salts. DNA breakage was not caused by chemiluminescent materials or active oxygen radicals. The nature of the mutagenic compound(s) remains to be determined.

Several epidemiological studies presented evidence that coffee and caffeine intake do not have carcinogenic effects. A Danish study of 49 colorectal cancer patients, 171 subjects with adenomas, 171 persons testing positive for occult blood but without cancer or adenomas, and 362 age- and sex-matched controls found that coffee consumption was unrelated to cancer incidence but was actually protective against the development of adenomas (*189*). A Greek hospital-based case–control study of 189 women with ovarian cancer and 200 controls found no consistent association between coffee intake and cancer incidence (*190*). Caffeine intake was also not related to development of breast cancer in a cohort of 34,388 Iowa women (aged 55–69 years) followed for 5 years (*191*). During this period there were 580 incident cases of breast cancer, but even when the data were adjusted for other known risk factors, coffee consumption appeared to be unrelated to cancer.

Freshly brewed drip coffee fed to rats for 2 or 6 weeks did not appear to stimulate cell proliferation in rat urinary bladder epithelium (*192*). Rats were provided with undiluted coffee or coffee diluted 10 times as their only source of drinking water, and then bladder tissue was examined histopathologically at the end of the experiment. Although uracil, a known cell proliferating agent, induced hyperplasia in bladder epithelium of rats used as positive controls, coffee had no hyperplastic effect.

## Effects on Reproduction and Development

Numerous studies have indicated that high intakes of caffeine have detrimental effects on various aspects of reproduction and development but the effects of low or moderate doses remain controversial. Data from a study of 1909 married women in the USA demonstrated that increased intakes of caffeine (as assessed during early pregnancy) were associated with some delay in conception (*193*). Odds ratios for delayed conception were 1.39, 1.88, and 2.24 for caffeine intakes of 1–150, 151–300, and >300 mg/day, respectively, compared to women who ingested no caffeine. These ratios were calculated after controlling for smoking, parity, and last method of birth control used. Average time to conception in the no-caffeine group was 4.5 menstrual cycles while women in the highest consumption group conceived after an average of 5.5 cycles.

Caffeine use among 1050 women with primary infertility as compared to that of 3833 fertile women was found to be somewhat higher in the groups whose infertility was related to tubal disease or to endometriosis (*194*). After controlling for age, cigarette and alcohol consumption, number of sexual partners, contraception, body mass index, and exercise, relative risks for infertility due to tubal disease were 1.2, 0.9, and 1.5 for caffeine intakes of 3.1–5, 5.1–7, and >7 g/month, respectively, The risks associated with endometriosis at these levels of caffeine intake were 1.1, 1.9, and 1.6, respectively.

A study of 7025 Canadian mothers indicated that caffeine intake during pregnancy (as determined by telephone interview a few weeks after delivery) was associated with intrauterine growth retardation (birth weight <10th percentile for sex and gestational age) but not to low birth weight (birth weight <2.5 kg) or to preterm delivery (*195*). Adjusted odds ratios for delivering an infant with intrauterine growth retardation were 1.0, 1.28, 1.42, and 1.57 for women with average daily caffeine intakes of 0–10, 11–150, 151–300, and >300 mg, respectively.

However, among 628 French women interviewed during their first visit to a maternity clinic, caffeine intake was not significantly related (when the data were controlled for effects of smoking) to birth weight in their infants delivered several months later (*196*). In the data analyses, caffeine consumption groups were: ≤400 (*n* = 356), 401–800 (*n* = 69), and >800 (*n* = 15) mg/day. A significant effect of alcohol consumption on birth weight was noted.

A recent review by Sivak (*197*) on coteratogenic effects of caffeine pointed out that most studies in human populations have demonstrated that caffeine does not negatively affect birth outcome and does not appear to enhance the adverse effects of alcohol or smoking. Coteratogenicity studies in rodents given a single large dose of caffeine show that this compound can enhance the teratogenicity of nicotine, alcohol, ionizing radiation, and some chemical carcinogens. But the relevance of these studies to humans is questionable because humans are not typically exposed to caffeine in this way.

Data on caffeine intake by 331 Canadian women with miscarriages and by 993 controls with a normal pregnancy at the same gestational period when the cases experienced fetal loss indicated that there was strong association between caffeine intake during pregnancy and fetal loss (*198*). Adjusted odds ratios for fetal loss (compared to a caffeine intake of <48 mg/day) of daily intakes of 48–162, 163–321, and >321 mg/day were 1.15, 1.95, and 2.62. A moderate association was also noted between miscarriage and caffeine intake in the month prior to pregnancy.

A review of experimental and epidemiological data on the effects of maternal caffeine consumption on newborns concluded that moderate caffeine consumption (≤300 mg/day) during gestation and lactation had no significant effects on the fetus and newborn infant (*199*). Large doses of caffeine, not usually encountered by humans, have been shown to cause malformations in rodent pups and decrease birth weights. Maternal caffeine consumption may also affect hematologic parameters, sleep, and some behavioral measures in rodents. Particularly since caffeine has a prolonged half-life in mothers during the third trimester and in the fetus, pregnant women should be advised to consume caffeine in moderation.

Infant monkeys exposed to caffeine in utero were tested on a variable ratio schedule at 30 days of age to determine any residual effects of this exposure (*200*). Pregnant females in the high- and low-dose groups were given caffeine-containing drinking water to provide daily intakes of 10–15 or 24–30 mg caffeine/kg body weight/day. (Pregnant women consuming 300 mg caffeine/day would have a daily intake of about 6 mg/kg.) On the variable ratio schedule, the low-dose infant monkeys did not differ significantly from controls while the high-dose infants had consistently longer pause times and longer interresponse times than the controls. Thus, high levels of caffeine exposure in utero can affect behavior of infant monkeys.

Administration of 30 or 60 mg caffeine/kg/day to pregnant rats was found to increase the incidence of apnea in their offspring in a dose-dependent manner (*201*). Caffeine-exposed pups also grew more slowly in utero and after birth. Although these levels of caffeine exposure are much higher than normal human consumption, they suggest that caffeine abuse by pregnant women may affect respiratory function of their infants and may be related to sudden infant death syndrome.

## Effects on the Cardiovascular System

Data from 9740 subjects (aged 40–59 years) in the Scottish Heart Health Survey demonstrated a slight negative correlation between coffee consumption (primarily instant coffee) and the incidence of coronary heart disease (202). This relationship was observed after adjustment of the data for various other risk factors. However, the authors caution that these results should not be construed to mean that coffee has a protective effect, only that they do not support an etiological role for coffee for cardiovascular disease.

Among a group of 5115 healthy young adults, approximately balanced according to age (18–24 and 25–30 years), sex, race (black and white), and educational level (high school graduate or less and beyond high school), no consistent correlation was observed between consumption of caffeine and caffeinated beverages and either blood pressure or serum cholesterol, triglyceride, or lipoprotein levels (203). Analyses were controlled for a number of possible confounding variables, including age, sex, race, alcohol and cigarette consumption, body mass index, and physical activity. A similar inconsistent relationship was observed between levels of various blood lipid fractions and consumption of caffeine-containing beverages in 1035 white women aged 65–90 years (204).

However, data from a health and nutrition survey of 1879 German adults indicated that those with a higher coffee intake (>400 mL/day) had higher levels of total cholesterol and LDL-cholesterol and lower levels of triglycerides in serum than those with lower intakes (<200 mL/day) of coffee (205). Linear regression analyses demonstrated increases of 1.66 and 1.58 mg LDL-cholesterol/dL per cup of coffee consumed each day.

An unidentified compound(s) in the lipid fraction of boiled coffee has previously been shown to raise serum cholesterol levels. When 15 volunteers were fed various coffee oil fractions for 4 weeks, the non-triglyceride fraction was found to significantly elevate mean cholesterol levels while other coffee oil fractions had no significant effect (206). Further studies demonstrated that two compounds in the non-triglyceride fraction, cafestol and kahweol, increased cholesterol levels by 66 mg/dL during a 6-week period. Oil from Robusta coffee beans, which contains cafestol but negligible kahweol, also raised serum cholesterol and triglycerides and depressed serum γ-glutamyl transferase (GGT) activity. Norwegians who habitually consume 5–9 cups of boiled coffee/day were also found to have elevated serum cholesterol and depressed GGT levels compared to controls. Thus it appears that cafestol, and possibly also kahweol, are responsible for the elevation of serum cholesterol and also affect liver function enzymes. Further evidence for the role of these diterpene alcohols in raising some serum lipoproteins came from a German study (207). Both cafestol and kahweol were extracted from a lipid fraction of Arabica coffee beans; when these compounds were fed to volunteers for 30 days, mean concentrations of total cholesterol, LDL-cholesterol, and triglycerides were elevated.

Although caffeine is known to have a pressor effect, chronic caffeine use abolishes this effect. To investigate this phenomenon in the elderly, an acute oral dose of caffeine (250 mg) was given after 48 hours of caffeine abstention to 8 normotensive subjects (aged 67–82 years) who were regular caffeine users (208). This dose was found to elevate both supine and standing systolic and diastolic blood pressure but did not affect pulse rate. However, when this acute dose was given following 6 days of normal caffeine intake (mean 490 mg/day) supplemented with an additional 250 mg caffeine/day and then 12 hours of abstention from any caffeine, there were no significant effects on any blood pressure measurement. It appears that acute caffeine ingestion is unlikely to have a significant pressor effect in regular caffeine users since the normal period of caffeine abstinence (overnight) is too short to abolish caffeine tolerance.

In another trial involving 150 male, normotensive, habitual coffee drinkers (mean of 4.5 cups/day), no significant differences were observed in resting blood pressure or heart rate in groups which (a) continued normal caffeine consumption, (b) changed to decaffeinated coffee, or (c) consumed no coffee for 2 months (209). However, a significant reduction in ambulatory systolic and diastolic blood pressures occurred in groups (b) and (c) after the 8 weeks. This suggests that cessation of caffeinated coffee consumption can reduce ambulatory blood pressure in normotensive men.

## Effects on Mineral Metabolism

Data from an epidemiological cohort study of 980 postmenopausal women (aged 50–98 years) indicated that increasing lifetime intakes of caffeinated coffee were associated with decreased bone mineral density (BMD) at both the hip and spine (210). BMD values were 4–5% lower in women in the highest quintile (average of 217 cup-years) of coffee consumption compared to the lowest quintile (26.1 cup-years average). This relationship was independent of measures of age, obesity, parity, and use of alcohol, tobacco, estrogen, and calcium supplements. However, caffeinated coffee consumption was not related to bone mineral density in women who reported drinking at least one glass of milk per day during their adult lives. It appears that adequate dietary calcium intake can prevent the reduction in bone mineral density by caffeinated coffee. A recent review of research related to risks of osteoporosis due to caffeine consumption concluded that younger women with an adequate calcium intake can consume moderate amounts of coffee with no deleterious effects because they can increase the efficiency of calcium absorption from the intestine (*211*). However, older women do not seem to be able to compensate as well by increased intestinal calcium absorption and so find it more difficult to maintain calcium balance.

Caffeine may also interfere with the development of the mineral structure in teeth. The enamel surface of molars of rat pups exposed to caffeine in utero showed a significantly different pattern of etching when exposed to acid as compared to teeth from pups not exposed to caffeine (*212*). The more diffuse lines on teeth of treated pups suggested that the enamel crystallites were smaller in this group. In addition, significantly more calcium and phosphorus was leached from teeth of treated pups than from control pups when the teeth were exposed to an acid solution. These structural changes translated into a higher caries score when pups from mothers fed diets providing 2 mg caffeine/100 g body weight were themselves fed a cariogenic diet (*213*).

## Effects on the Nervous System and Behavior

In a study of the effects of an acute dose of caffeine on mental performance and EEG, 20 female, non-smoking, regular coffee consumers were dosed with 0,1.5, 3, and 6 mg caffeine/kg (*214*). Physiological measurements were taken and subjects were tested with a rapid information processing task (RIP). The dominant frequencies of the $\alpha$ and the $\beta$ bands of the EEGs showed significant dose-dependent increases with increasing caffeine doses. Significant increases in reaction time and processing rate were observed in most subjects at the higher caffeine doses.

Acute effects of caffeine on operant behavior in rhesus monkeys were assessed using an operant test battery of complex food-reinforced tasks which are thought to depend on several relatively specific brain functions (*215*). Injected caffeine doses of 5.6–20 mg/kg given 15 min pretesting, induced significant dose-dependent decreases in accuracy and percent tasks completed in measures of time estimation. No consistent effects were observed on tests of short-term memory and attention and of motivation to work for food while low

caffeine doses increased performance on tasks involving learning and color and position discrimination.

Nerve conduction velocity and synaptic transmission were examined in rats dosed with caffeine in drinking water during a 10-day period (estimated average consumption 597.4 mg caffeine/10 days) (*216*). Nerve conduction velocity in the caudal nerve of the tail was decreased significantly in the caffeine-treated animals while the amplitude of indirectly evoked extracellular muscle action potentials was unaffected.

Using radioligand binding assays, the effects of chronic caffeine ingestion (about 100 mg caffeine/kg body weight/day for 4 days) on a variety of central nervous system receptors and on calcium channels in mice was investigated (*217*). The densities of cortical $A_1$ adenosine, of 5 $HT_1$ and 5 $HT_2$ serotonergic, and of muscarinic and nicotinic receptors increased by 20–50% and increases were also noted in binding sites associated with $GABA_A$ receptors and with calcium channels. Cortical $\beta_1$ and $\beta_2$ adrenergic receptors were reduced by about 25%. These results demonstrate that a wide range of biochemical alterations in the central nervous system occur in response to chronic caffeine ingestion.

## Other Physiological Effects

Two recent epidemiological studies demonstrated that moderate coffee consumption decreases the activity of some liver enzymes. Analyses of blood samples from 2250 elderly (≥65 years) Italian men and women (CASTEL Study) showed that those drinking ≥3 cups brewed Italian coffee/day had serum levels of $\gamma$-glutamyl transferase (GGT), alanine amino transferase, and alkaline phosphatase which were 17%, 10.3%, and 4.7% less than those in persons drinking 0–2 cups of coffee/day (*218*). Multivariate regression analyses taking into account age, smoking, and alcohol consumption confirmed that the reduction in liver enzyme activity with increased coffee intake was significant. Coffee consumption was also found to be inversely related to serum GGT levels in a cohort of 2494 male, Japanese, self-defense officials aged 48–56 years (*219*). Body mass index, alcohol use, and smoking were positively related to serum GGT levels but the effects of coffee were independent of these other variables.

Physiological responses of 8 healthy, male, non-obese volunteers to low blood glucose levels were investigated after they drank caffeine-free cola with or without added caffeine (400 mg) (*220*). A hyperinsulinemic glucose clamp technique was used to maintain plasma glucose levels at 5 mmol/L for 90 min, followed by 60 min at 3.8 mmol/L, and then 2.8 mmol/L for another 60 min. Caffeine caused a rapid decrease in cerebral artery velocity. When glucose levels were lowered to 3.8 mmol/L, only those participants given caffeine had warning symptoms and "felt hypoglycemic." Levels of several hormones (epinephrine, norepinephrine, cortisol, and growth hormone) were higher after the caffeine dose as compared to the placebo. These data suggest that persons ingesting moderate amounts of caffeine may develop hypoglycemic symptoms if plasma glucose levels fall into the low–normal range.

Caffeine and other methylxanthines are known to be competitive antagonists of adenosine receptors and therefore chronic caffeine ingestion leads to up-regulation of these receptors in animals. To determine whether similar effects occur in humans, 19 healthy, male, non-smokers were given 3 oral doses of 250 mg caffeine/day for 7 days (221). Platelets obtained at baseline and at 12 and 60 h after the last dose of caffeine were examined for antiaggregation responses to adenosine and prostacyclin receptors. Caffeine induced an up-regulation of these receptors and this action may be related to caffeine withdrawal symptoms.

## TOXICITY OF MUSHROOMS

During a 2-year survey of wild mushrooms in commercial distribution, a total of 344 samples of 15 varieties of mushrooms were examined by the FDA. Eleven of these, designated as morels or mixed wild mushrooms, were found to contain toxic look-alike species (222). The toxic species were identified as the false morel and the early false morel (*Gyromitra esculenta* and *Verpa bohemica*). All of the contaminated batches were imported from France or India. This report also includes a comprehensive listing and description of toxic mushrooms which are similar in appearance to edible wild varieties.

Two foci of *Lepiota* mushroom poisoning involving 10 people occurred in rural areas of Spain in 1989 (223). In both cases, the mushrooms were picked locally on farmland. Five of the patients recovered completely after suffering intestinal symptoms while the others incurred some liver damage. Three developed fulminant hepatitis and two subsequently died of acute respiratory distress.

Cases of poisoning due to ingestion of toxic mushrooms are rare in Australia and no fatalities have been recorded so far. This is probably due to the reluctance of Australians to collect wild mushrooms and also to the absence, until recently, of the highly toxic death cap (*Amanita phalloides*). Barbato (224) reviewed various

syndromes associated with mushroom poisoning but pointed out that little is known of indigenous, poisonous mushrooms in Australia.

Clinical symptomology and management of mushroom poisoning was reviewed by Köppel (225). Adverse reactions in humans may result from specific toxins in mushrooms, immunologically active mushroom antigens, difficulties in digesting large amounts of mushrooms, and effects of mushrooms on ethanol metabolism. Seven types of mushroom poisoning can be distinguished. Of these, phalloides, orellanus, gyromitra, and paxillus syndromes are the most serious and may have fatal consequences.

Carcinogenic compounds have been detected in *Agaricus bisporus*, the commonly eaten, cultivated mushroom of the Western hemisphere. In an attempt to assess the potential carcinogenicity of these mushrooms, Toth and Gannett (226) reviewed available data on the carcinogenic potency of these compounds (hydrazines and diazonium salts), their concentrations in mushrooms, and results of a long-term carcinogenicity assay in mice. Estimates (based on admittedly inadequate data) suggest that one would need to consume >1 lb. raw mushrooms per day for 50 years to induce cancer.

Extracts of *A. bisporus* have also been reported to be mutagenic. Agaritine, one of the proposed mutagenic compounds, was tested in the Ames assay but its mutagenic profile, both in the presence and in the absence of an activation system, differed from that of mushroom extracts (227). Evidence from other experiments with mushroom extracts, treated with tyrosinase, catalase, and superoxide dismutase, indicated that phenolic and quinoid compounds, by generating reactive oxygen species, may be responsible for at least part of the mutagenicity of mushrooms.

Embryotoxic and teratogenic potential of monomethylhydrazine (MMH), a toxic component of the false morel (*G. esculenta*), was studied in pregnant rats (228). The rats received an intragastric dose of 1 or 5 mg MMH/kg body weight on day 6 of pregnancy or an iv infusion providing 1.2–13.2 mg MMH/kg/day during days 6–13 of pregnancy. Serum concentrations of MMH in the lower dose groups were similar to those observed in human volunteers after consuming a single mushroom meal. A dose-dependent, statistically significant increase in resorptions and a decrease in pregnancy rate was noted in all but the lowest dose groups. However, no evidence of teratogenicity was observed.

People in mountainous areas of Japan believe that toxins in *Amanita muscaria* can be reduced by drying, storing, or cooking. Ibotenic acid (IBO), one of the main physiologically active constituents in this mushroom, can readily be converted to the hallucinogen muscimol (MUS) by decarboxylation. In experiments monitoring the stability of these two compounds, both heating and drying of mushrooms were found to decrease IBO and increase MUS (*229*). Both compounds were stable when mushrooms were stored under dry or salted conditions. Boiling or soaking of mushrooms in water leached most of the active compounds into the water.

Three specimens of *A. phalloides* at two different stages of carpophore development were divided into 6 parts (cap, gills, ring, stipe, volva, and bulb) and analyzed for phallotoxins and amatoxins (*230*). Highest toxin levels were detected in the ring and lowest concentrations in the bulb. Amatoxins were more plentiful in the cap, gills, and ring while phallotoxins were more concentrated in the bulb and volva. An improved HPLC method for the detection of amatoxins and phallotoxins in *Amanita* sp. has been developed (*231*).

## ALKALOIDS

### Pyrrolizidine Alkaloids

Drought and conflict in southern Tadjikistan in 1992 led to a delay in the wheat harvest and contamination of the wheat seeds with those of a heliotrope. After the wheat was ground and used to make bread, cases of liver toxicity began appearing at the local hospital (*232*). As of March 1993, a total of 3906 cases were recorded, with an overall fatality rate of 1.3%. Early symptoms of intoxication included abdominal pain and nausea and these later progressed to hepatomegaly, ascites, and finally to coma and death in the most severely poisoned patients. The contaminating seeds were first reported to be from *Heliotropium lasocarpium*, which contains lasiocarpine as its main pyrrolizidine alkaloid. However, a later report indicated that the dominant alkaloid in the contaminated wheat was heliotrine and the responsible plant was most likely *H. popovii* (*233*). This plant species was responsible for a similar epidemic in Afghanistan in 1976.

A more common dietary source of pyrrolizidine alkaloids in Western countries is the use of comfrey (*Symphytum* sp.) in herbal teas. An improved capillary gas chromatographic procedure was developed to analyze comfrey-containing products purchased at retail health food stores in the Washington, D.C. area (*234*). Of 11 products tested, 9 were found to contain detectable levels of these alkaloids (0.1–400 ppm). The highest concentrations were found in bulk comfrey root (400 ppm of intermedine) followed by bulk comfrey leaf (95 ppm intermedine) while lowest levels were present in products combining comfrey leaf with one or more products. Teas produced from comfrey roots and leaves also contained alkaloids.

Investigation of severe losses of yaks in Bhutan revealed that the animals were consuming at least 5 species of plants (*Senecio* and *Ligularia*) which contained pyrrolizidine alkaloids (*235*). Since the population in this area depends heavily on yaks as a source of milk and cheese, there is concern that the human population may be exposed to dangerous levels of these toxins. The toxic plants appear to be less palatable to yaks than the other plants in the area but they tend to become dominant in overgrazed pastures.

Cytotoxic effects of 8 pyrolizidine alkaloids were measured in cultured bovine kidney epithelial cells and then compared to determine structural features important for toxicity (*236*). A dose-dependent inhibition of colony growth was observed with 4 macrocyclic alkaloids with $\alpha,\beta$-unsaturation while saturated macrocyclic and open diester compounds only slightly inhibited growth and a necine base compound had no effect on growth.

### Glycoalkaloids from *Solanum* sp.

Exposure of potato tubers to light results in greening (an increase in chlorophyll) and an accumulation of the glycoalkaloids $\alpha$-chaconine and $\alpha$-solanine. Exposure of commercial White Rose potatoes to fluorescent light for 20 days increased total glycoalkaloid concentrations from 1.24 to 3.74 mg/100 g fresh potato and more than doubled chlorogenic acid concentrations to 15.8 mg/100 g (*237*). Protease inhibitor concentrations were essentially unchanged by the light exposure. Experiments to delay greening of potatoes by immersion in water indicated that chlorophyll formation and glycoalkaloid synthesis are not physiologically linked.

Comparison of glycoalkaloid formation in 20 potato varieties exposed to light for 48 hours revealed that only a small increase in total glycoalkaloids occurred in some varieties (average 8 mg/100 g freeze-dried matter, FDM) while a much larger increase was seen in other varieties (39 mg/100 g FDM) (*238*). These differences in alkaloid accumulation were still observed when 6 of these varieties were further tested during 7 days' exposure to light (*239*).

Since the toxicity of glycoalkaloids depends on the carbohydrate residues attached to the steroidal secondary 3-OH group, the fate of these groups following ingestion becomes important. Friedman et al. (*240*) investigated the acid-catalyzed hydrolysis of these residues in α-chaconine and α-solanine and found that 8 different compounds could be isolated. By varying the reaction conditions, the amounts of specific compounds formed could be optimized. These results should facilitate characterization of alkaloid metabolites in animals and aid in assessment of their relative toxicities.

Bioavailability and disposition of $^3$H-solanine was compared in rats and hamsters following an oral dose of 170 μg/kg (*241*). Mean bioavailability of total radioactivity was about 29% for rats and 57% for hamsters. About 40% of the dose was excreted by hamsters and 90% by rats within 7 days. Based on these results and toxicological data from the literature, it appears that the hamster is a better model for humans in chronic toxicity assays.

Improved procedures have been described for the determination of solanum glycoalkaloids by thin-layer chromatographic screening (*242*), by reversed-phase HPLC (*243*), and by immunoassay using monoclonal antibodies (*244*). Tomatine, a glycoalkaloid present in species of *Solanum* (potatoes) and *Lycopersicon* (tomatoes) can be effectively detected by liquid chromatography after derivatization (*245*).

## Aconitine

A mini-epidemic of aconitine poisoning has been reported from Hong Kong, with over 25 cases, including 3 fatalities, reported during the past 5 years (*246–248*). The victims, afflicted with a variety of ailments, consumed aconitine in herbal teas and preparations containing the root of *Aconitum* spp. Traditional Chinese methods for preparing these remedies involve a curing process which hydrolyzes much of the aconitine. However, some samples tested were obviously prepared better than others. Symptoms of poisoning included nausea and vomiting, numbness in the mouth and extremities, hypotension, and cardiac arrhythmias.

Several cases of food poisoning in Japan in 1992 were traced to consumption of honey (*249*). Examination of the honey revealed that nearly 70% of the pollen in it belonged to *Aconitum* plants, and HPLC analysis demonstrated the presence of 9.8 ppm aconitine. The implicated honey produced neurotoxic effects when fed to rats.

An HPLC-atmospheric pressure chemical ionization mass spectrometry method has been developed for the determination of alkaloids from *Aconitum* sp. (*250*). Detection limits were approximately 1–5 ng/injection.

## Other Alkaloids

Another Chinese herbal product, marketed as an aid to losing weight, was responsible for at least 70 cases of progressive interstitial fibrosis of the kidney in Belgium (*251*). Thirty of the cases suffered terminal renal failure, and a pathological examination of some of the diseased kidneys revealed lesions very similar to those observed in cases of Balkan endemic nephropathy (BEN) (*252*). Analyses of the herbal mixtures showed that they contained the nephrotoxin aristolochic acid, from the plant *Aristolochia*, instead of the alkaloid tetrandrine from the plant *Stephania*. The Chinese words for these two herbs are similar and it is believed that the toxic herb was accidentally substituted for *Stephania*. Since the renal lesions were similar in these cases and in cases of BEN, it may be that victims of BEN are consuming aristolochic acid from some source.

## PHENOLIC COMPOUNDS

### Flavonoids

Quercetin, a flavonoid widely distributed in edible fruits and vegetables, is a potent in vitro mutagen but is not carcinogenic in long-term feeding studies in rodents. Metabolic studies using porcine liver and hamster kidney demonstrated that quercetin was rapidly O-methylated by these tissues and that the genotoxic potential of the methylated compound was effectively neutralized (*253*). The rate of O-methylation was up to 3 orders of magnitude greater than that of catechol estrogens and catecholamines. In fact this rapid rate of O-methylation of quercetin apparently explains the paradox of tumor promotion by quercetin in estradiol-induced carcinogenesis in hamster kidneys (*254*). In the absence of quercetin, dietary estradiol, activated to catechol estradiol, can be inactivated by O-methylation. However, coadministration of quercetin causes competitive inhibition of the O-methyltransferase and more of the catechol estradiol remains intact to generate potentially mutagenic free radicals and kidney tumors.

Studies on the in vitro binding of quercetin to DNA indicate that the flavonoid does not have any preferred sites for binding (*255*). The binding does not involve electrostatic interactions and may be intercalative in nature. Flavonoid interactions with DNA can induce significant concentration-dependent nuclear DNA degradation along with lipid peroxidation (*256*). In vitro experiments with myricetin and rat liver nuclei demonstrated that these effects were enhanced by iron(III) and copper(II). DNA damage was stimulated by catalase, superoxide dismutase (SOD), mannitol, and sodium azide in the presence of copper(II). Lipid peroxidation was significantly inhibited only by SOD in the presence of copper(II). These results demonstrate that flavonoids, which are generally considered antioxidant and anticarcinogenic compounds, can also exert pro-oxidant effects.

Aqueous extracts of guarana (*Paullinia cupana*), which is a constituent of some soft drinks, tested positive for genotoxicity in experiments with *E. coli* and *Salmonella* (*257*). Addition of an S9 microsomal mix and of catalase inhibited the genotoxicity of these extracts, suggesting that reactive oxygen species are involved. The mutagenic activity was related to the presence of a complex containing caffeine, a flavonoid, and potassium.

## Coumarins and Furocoumarins

An unanticipated consequence of the Gulf War in 1991 was an outbreak of phytophotodermatitis involving 11 workers in the celery harvest in southern Israel (*258*). During Iraqi missile attacks, the workers were confined to their homes. The celery, which remained in the fields for 2–3 weeks after maturity, accumulated high levels of total psoralens—84 µg/g fresh weight. (The following year, celery harvested in this area, at the correct time, contained only 26 µg psoralens/g.) After handling the celery with moist hands and then being exposed to bright sunlight, the patients experienced severe swelling of the hands and intense pain. Symptoms resolved rapidly after the workers were treated with sulfadiazine and prednisone.

Severe phytophotodermatitis in two young boys making limeade prompted the analyses of two varieties of limes for phototoxic coumarins (*259*). Immature Persian limes from the same tree the boys had picked from were found to contain 3.9 µg psoralen and 128.7 µg bergapten/g fresh weight of the rind. In contrast, the rind of mature key limes contained no detectable psoralens and only 20.9 µg bergapten/g. Much lower concentrations or undetectable levels of these compounds were detected in the pulp of both varieties. Bergapten has about 27.5 times the phototoxic activity of psoralens and is probably the primary compound responsible for phytophotodermatitis.

A series of 14 naturally occurring coumarins were investigated for their effects on murine hepatic cytochrome P450s, namely ethoxyresorufin *O*-dealkylase (EROD) and pentoxyresorufin *O*-dealkylase (PROD) activities (*260*). Several of these compounds, which are naturally present in the human diet, were potent inhibitors of EROD and/or PROD. Because these enzymes are known to be active in metabolizing xenobiotic compounds, these natural coumarins, when consumed in the diet, may be capable of modulating carcinogenesis.

## Tannins

Condensed tannins in a variety of foods are known to reduce the nutritional value of those foods, perhaps by interfering with digestion or the absorption of nutrients. To determine whether tannins from faba beans inhibit proteolytic enzymes, pigs fed high- and low-tannin diets (3.5% and <0.1% catechin equivalents) were fitted with cannulas in the duodenum and the ileum to sample the intestinal contents at different times (*261*). Trypsin and chymotrypsin activities in the duodenum and chymotrypsin activities in the ileum were similar in both experimental groups. However, trypsin activity was significantly reduced in ileal digesta of pigs on the high-tannin diet as compared to those on the low-tannin diet.

In rats fed for 28 days with varying amounts of tannins extracted from cowpeas or black tea (up to 0.057%), tannin consumption did not significantly affect growth rate or apparent protein digestibility (*262*). Apparent calcium absorption, but not magnesium absorption, was reduced during days 11–18 in rats fed all levels of tea tannins and >0.0171% cowpea tannin. By week 4, this apparent decrease in calcium absorption disappeared and calcium absorption was similar in all groups. Bone calcium levels did not vary during the 4 weeks.

Dose-dependent increases in the weight of the parotid salivary gland and in the production of proline-rich proteins in saliva were observed in rats fed diets containing 0–1.99% condensed tannins from faba beans (*263*). These proline-rich proteins can effectively bind tannins and thereby reduce their antinutritional effects.

In order to improve the nutritional quality of high-tannin foods, several techniques have been evaluated for removal or degradation of tannins. Soaking of faba bean seeds in distilled water was found to leach out 20–27% of the tannins while soaking in 0.1 M sodium carbonate solution extracted up to 80% of the tannins (*264*). Fermentation of sorghum seeds for 14 h with a traditional Sudanese culture consisting primarily of lactic acid bacteria decreased the tannin content by as much as 92% (*265*).

## Gossypol

A recent review on gossypol considered results from numerous clinical and experimental studies on the possible genotoxic effects of this polyphenol from cotton plants (*266*). Under normal physiological conditions, the evidence indicates that gossypol has weak, if any, genotoxic effects in mammals. However, there is a need for further research to determine the significance of the weak increases in sister chromatid frequencies observed in a number of studies. Also, more definitive, comprehensive data should be collected on tumorigenicity of this compound in animals.

## TOXIC AMINO ACIDS

Two recent reviews discussed the possible role of dietary excitatory amino acids in neurologic disorders. Meldrum (*267*) summarized information on toxicity of high doses of glutamate and aspartate to neonatal rodents as well as data on domoic acid (shellfish toxin), acromelic acid (mushroom toxin), β-ODAP (β-*N*-oxalyl-L-α,β-diaminopropionic acid), a toxic constituent of grass peas, and BMAA (β-methylamino-L-alanine), a toxin in cycad fruits. In vitro and in vivo studies with these toxins to elucidate their mechanisms of action were described. Lipton and Rosenberg (*268*) primarily discussed the toxicity of glutamate.

Four neurological diseases (lathyrism, Western Pacific motor neuron disease, cassavism, and an encephalopathy and tardive dystonia) occurring periodically in developing regions of the world were described by Spencer et al. (*269*). These diseases have been related to consumption of grass pea, cycad, cassava, and mildewed sugar cane, respectively. Typically, outbreaks of these diseases occur during times of famine when the populations are otherwise nutritionally stressed and when the implicated foods are eaten in larger quantities or without adequate preparation to remove toxins.

Although proteins of higher organisms contain almost exclusively the L form of amino acids, D-amino acids are present in varying amounts in different food items. Concentrations of these D-amino acids and their formation in foods were reviewed by Zagon et al. (*270*). Data on the toxicity of these compounds in humans are inadequate, but studies with animals indicate that they may have toxic effects on the liver and kidney.

## Tryptophan Contaminants

The epidemic of eosinophilia-myalgia syndrome (EMS), which began in 1989, has been linked to the intake of supplemental tryptophan. Philen et al. (*271*) analyzed 101 lots of L-tryptophan that were associated with cases of EMS or with asymptomatic consumers of tryptophan supplements for the presence of 6 contaminating compounds. Analyses of data which controlled for time of manufacture of the supplements showed that 1,1'-ethylidenebis[L-tryptophan] (EBT) was present in higher levels in case lots but the association lacked statistical significance. These results do not rule out the possibility that EBT is the etiologic agent for EMS but they suggest that other chemical contaminants may also be involved. Other evidence suggesting that EBT is not totally responsible for symptoms of EMS derives from experiments comparing the effects of case-associated tryptophan with effects of pure tryptophan with added EBT. In such experiments, the case-associated sample inhibited binding of radiolabelled tryptophan to rat hepatic nuclear envelopes differently from the control tryptophan with added EBT (*272*). In in vitro experiments, EBT (or a breakdown product) was found to be incorporated into proteins. If this happens in vivo, EBT may adversely affect the function of the proteins.

Two of the diastereoisomeric breakdown products [(−)-(1*S*,3*S*)- and (−)-(1*R*,3*S*)-1-methyl-1,2,3,4-tetrahydro-β-carboline-3-carboxylic acid] of EBT were tested for cytotoxicity in spinal cord cultures derived from fetal mice (*273*). Addition of the *S*-isomer, but not the *R*-isomer or the parent compound, EBT, caused the death of 30–35% of the neurons in culture. Antisera against the murine interleukin-1 receptor prevented the neuronal death associated with this compound.

Other in vitro experiments to determine the possible mechanisms of action of EBT indicated that this contaminant enhanced the release of eosinophil cationic protein from human peripheral blood normodense eosinophils, up-regulated interleukin 5 receptor levels on these eosinophils, and stimulated human splenic T-cells to produce bioactive and immunoreactive interleukin 5 (*274*). L-Tryptophan without this contaminant had none of these effects. An HPLC method has been developed to determine levels of EBT in L-tryptophan preparations (*275*).

### *Lathyrus* Toxins

A dietary survey was carried out in northern Ethiopia, an endemic area for lathyrism, and various foods prepared from grass peas (*Lathyrus sativus*) were analyzed to determine their content of β-ODAP (*276*). Analyses of field samples of the peas revealed a great variation in β-ODAP concentrations: 128–985 mg/100 g dry seeds. Normally, grass pea is consumed primarily as an ingredient in a traditional Ethiopian gravy and as a snack, either roasted or boiled. The bread form is widely consumed only in times of famine. Preparation of foods in the laboratory using grass peas with a known toxin content and traditional methods of preparation revealed that steeping the seeds in excess water could leach out about 30% of the β-ODAP. However, grass pea bread and roasted seeds contained elevated levels of β-ODAP as compared to the raw seeds they were prepared from. Thus traditional food preparation methods do not effectively reduce the levels of this neurotoxin in foods made with grass peas.

Since grass peas are reported to have an excellent flavor, it would be useful to determine what factors could be controlled to minimize production of the neurotoxin β-ODAP in these plants. In greenhouse experiments with a variety of *L. sativus* selected for low toxin levels, both zinc deficiency and excess iron in the growth medium were found to dramatically increase levels of β-ODAP (*277*). Addition of β-ODAP to the growth medium enhances transport of zinc to the shoots. It appears that β-ODAP acts as a carrier for zinc and, under conditions of zinc deficiency (as in soils leached of micronutrients by flooding monsoon rains), concentrations of β-ODAP in grass pea seeds increase significantly. Ethiopian soils, rich in iron (a biological antagonist of zinc), may also be quite low in available zinc.

In vitro experiments to assess the cytotoxicity of β-ODAP demonstrated that concentrations of 1 pM caused significant leakage of enzymes and ions from sagittal slices of mouse brain (*278*). Furthermore, extensive vacuolation and degeneration of neurons was observed in some areas of the brain. In contrast, nearly a billion-fold higher concentrations of BMAA (the cycad toxin) were required to elicit similar effects in the brain slices.

## Cycad Toxins

Investigations of endemic motor neuron disease occurring in 3 areas of the Western Pacific (Guam, Kii Peninsula of Japan, and West New Guinea) have suggested that toxins in cycad fruits, consumed in traditional medicines or as a food during times of food scarcity, were possible etiological agents. An epidemiological study in the Kii region of Japan sought to determine the present and past medicinal use of cycad in this area (*279*). Surveys were conducted among wholesale dealers of traditional medicines in nearby major Japanese cities,

pharmacies and households in small towns in and near the endemic area, and over 200 older inhabitants of the endemic area. Cycad appeared to be a more popular remedy in the past but its use did not appear to be more prevalent in the endemic area than in other areas of Japan. According to the older residents, cycad nuts were not eaten as a food but were sometimes used as toys and the trees were sometimes grown in gardens. The data presented here do not support the hypothesis that cycad toxins were a causative agent of motor neuron disease in this area.

## CYANOGENIC COMPOUNDS

### Cassava

Nearly 100 samples of two fermented cassava foods (gari and foofoo) purchased at 9 local markets in Freetown, Sierra Leone, were analyzed for cyanide concentrations and other parameters of quality (pH, particle size, microbial contamination and water content) (*280*). Mean concentrations of cyanide (both free cyanide and cyanohydrin) were 8.6 and 28.2 mg/kg dry matter for gari and foofoo, respectively. These levels are higher than the Codex guidelines and indicate that some samples had unacceptably high cyanide levels.

Several steps in the production of gari from a high-cyanide variety of cassava were varied in an attempt to produce gari with low residual levels of cyanide (*281*). Increasing the mash moisture content to 80% (natural moisture level was 65%) and sun-heating the mash for 2 days reduced cyanide levels in the original cassava by 99.3%, to 2.6 mg/kg dry weight. This is a little higher than the 2 ppm permissible by the Nigerian FDA but cyanide levels could presumably be decreased further by using a low-cyanide cassava cultivar.

Fermentation is also known to reduce the levels of cyanogenic compounds in cassava products. A mixed culture obtained from a yogurt coconut toddy fermentation and containing yeast and species of *Lactobacillus, Streptococcus*, and *Corynebacterium* degraded about 75% of the bound cyanide in cassava tubers and 67–85% of that in cassava peels (*282*). Free cyanide was present in higher concentrations in the fermented products but this could easily be eliminated by sun drying. The fermentation process appeared to be more efficient with a low-cyanide cassava strain.

Epidemiological observations from around the globe suggest that the incidence of malnutrition-related diabetes mellitus is related to cassava consumption.

Using dogs as a model, the possible effects of linamarin (the main cyanogenic glucoside in cassava) on blood sugar levels were investigated (*283*). Half an hour after receiving a dose of linamarin, plasma insulin and insulin binding to erythrocytes and to mononuclear leukocytes were significantly lower in malnourished dogs than in normal dogs. This resulted in abnormally high glucose levels in the malnourished dogs. These results suggest that a high cyanide intake from cassava can alter carbohydrate tolerance in poorly fed populations and thereby contribute to the onset of diabetes.

Several improved procedures for the determination of linamarin in cassava and cassava products have been developed (*284–286*).

## Other Plant Foods

The extraction of linseed oil from flax seed leaves a protein-rich meal which could be used as a food or feed ingredient. Several Canadian cultivars of flax grown at different locations were analyzed for the presence of antinutritional factors (*287*). Mean HCN levels in different strains ranged from 8.0 to 9.7 μg HCN/100 g ground seed and were significantly influenced by growth location and season. Laboratory-prepared raw linseed meal also contained 42–51 units of trypsin inhibitor activity (compared to 1650 units detected in soybean meal).

Extraction of linseed meal with a two-phase solvent system consisting of hexanes and methanol with added ammonia and water was found to effectively remove >90% of the cyanogenic glucosides present (*288*). Concentrations of these glucosides, linustatin and neolinustatin, were measured by a column chromatographic method utilizing Sephadex LH-20 (*289*).

Jojoba meal, the residue after extraction of the valuable jojoba oil, also is rich in proteins but has been found to inhibit the growth of laboratory animals. Recently a method has been developed for the isolation and purification of large quantities of simmondsin, a cyanogenic compound, from jojoba meal (*290*). This should be helpful in determining whether this compound or some other is responsible for growth retardation. A new simmondsin compound, simmondsin ferulate, has been isolated from jojoba meal (*291*). Its potential toxicity has not yet been tested.

Several processing techniques, such as soaking, sprouting, cooking, and fermentation were evaluated for their effectiveness in removing antinutrients from pearl millet (*292*). While soaking was found to drastically reduce cyanide levels (by about 84%), sprouting actually increased measurable cyanide (by 6–10 times) by activating enzymes which hydrolyzed cyanogens to produce

HCN. Fermentation also increased detectable cyanide but cooking, by driving off volatile HCN, effectively removed much of the cyanide in the millet.

Soaking of apricot kernels was also found to effectively remove >97% of the HCN, 35% of the tannins, and 21% of the phytate present (*293*). Although soaking also removed small amounts of protein and sugars, the reduction in antinutritional compounds resulted in a nutritionally well-balanced apricot kernel flour which could safely be incorporated into human foods.

Fruits of the plant nai habarala (*Alocasia cucullata*), which grows in Sri Lanka, are not normally eaten. Two recent fatalities in children consuming these fruits demonstrated that the fruits are toxic (*294*). Symptoms of poisoning indicated that the toxic principle(s) include cyanogenic compounds.

# GLUCOSINOLATES

Significant quantities of glucosinolates are present in cruciferous vegetables and these compounds can be converted to isothiocyanates (ITC) by an endogenous enzyme, myrosinase. Although there is no evidence that consumption of large amounts of vegetables is harmful—in fact, the reverse is often observed in epidemiological studies—some isothiocyanates exhibit clastogenic effects in cell cultures (*295*). Benzyl-, phenyl-, and phenethyl-ITCs induced significant chromosomal damage in SV40-transformed Indian muntjac cells in the absence of metabolic activation.

One of the major glucosinolate hydrolysis products found in cruciferous vegetables, 1-isothiocyanato-3-(methylsulphinyl)-propane (IMSP), has been tested for acute toxicity (*296*) and for its effects on xenobiotic metabolizing enzymes (*297*). A dose-dependent increase in multifocal hemorrhages and mucosal damage was observed in the stomachs of rats gavaged with a single dose of 0.3–2.0 mmol IMSP/kg body weight. No significant changes were noted in the liver, kidney, or blood chemistry. IMSP was detected in urine of treated rats, indicating that this compound had been absorbed from the gastrointestinal tract. When rats were gavaged daily for a week with lower concentrations of IMSP approximating those present in the human diet (1–100 μmol IMSP/kg), no histological lesions were observed in the alimentary tract. Neither were any effects observed on the activities of hepatic phase I or phase II xenobiotic metabolizing enzymes. Significant increases in these enzymes in the intestine were only observed in rats given the highest dose.

A survey of 10 different cruciferous vegetables purchased at markets in Taiwan demonstrated that leaf mustard and radish had the highest glucosinolate levels (2815 and 1724 mg/kg fresh weight, respectively) while Chinese cabbage and cauliflower had the lowest levels (89 and 117 mg/kg) (*298*). Myrosinase activity did not directly correlate with glucosinolates, as the highest enzyme activities were present in radish and broccoli (22.6 and 9.9 μmol/min/mg protein) and the lowest activities were in kale and Chinese cabbage (2.02 and 2.45 μmol/min/mg protein).

Total glucosinolate levels in 4 types of Portuguese cabbage and in one hybrid white cabbage were found to vary from 3.3 to 8.1 mmol/kg fresh weight (*299*). Boiling reduced glucosinolate concentrations in the cabbages by >50%, with most of the loss accounted for by glucosinolates detected in the cooking water.

Fertilization of cruciferous plants with nitrogen and sulfur compounds can significantly affect glucosinolate levels. Leaves of thousand-headed kale (*Brassica oleracea* var. *Acephala*) top-dressed with ammonium sulfate contained 33–56% more total glucosinolates than leaves of plants fertilized with calcium ammonium nitrate (*300*). On sulfur-sufficient soils, application of sulfur only marginally increased, and addition of nitrogen significantly increased, glucosinolate levels in seeds of oilseed rape (*301*). However, on sulfur-deficient soils, a sulfur fertilizer dramatically increased seed glucosinolate concentrations and concomitant addition of nitrogen resulted in even higher levels. Analyses of rape seeds from plants grown under these different regimes revealed that supplying large amounts of both N and S resulted in particularly high levels of 2-hydroxy-but-3-enyl, which is a glucosinolate with known goitrogenic effects (*302*).

Assessment of glucosinolate levels in broccoli by 3 different methods revealed that the thymol method gave better results than enzyme immobilization and gas–liquid chromatographic techniques (*303*). Other analytical procedures recently developed for glucosinolate determination include: X-ray fluorescence spectroscopy (*304*); GC–MS and GC–Fourier transform infrared spectroscopy (*305*); micellar electrokinetic capillary chromatography (*306*); and anion exchange chromatography on a silica trialkylammonium exchanger (*307*).

## PROTEASE INHIBITORS

Consumption of raw soybeans or kidney beans results in a rapid enlargement of the pancreas in rodents. To determine whether this was due to the presence of protease inhibitors or lectins in the raw beans, rats were fed raw soybeans (high trypsin inhibitor and moderate lectin contents), cowpeas (high trypsin inhibitor, low in lectins), kidney beans (low trypsin inhibitor content, high in lectins), or lupinseed (low in both antinutrients) for up to 800 days (*308*) The lupinseed diet caused no pancreatic enlargement. Rats fed soybeans and cowpeas experienced an initial rapid growth in the pancreas, followed by a period of normal growth, and then another period of rapid growth after 350 days. Since rats fed kidney beans had only the first period of enhanced pancreatic growth, it appeared that both lectins and trypsin inhibitors may be responsible for the early growth spurt while only the trypsin inhibitors are involved in later growth.

To determine whether protease inhibitors increase fecal loss of nitrogen by interfering with protein digestion or by enhancing the loss of endogenous nitrogen, pigs were fitted with ileal cannulas and fed homoarginine-labelled test meals with different trypsin inhibitor contents (*309*). Results demonstrated that trypsin inhibitors increase fecal nitrogen by both mechanisms but the losses of amino acids through endogenous secreta appear to be more important than losses of dietary amino acids.

Analyses of a number of legumes and other food plants continue to expand our knowledge of the structure of plant protease inhibitors. These include studies on: five trypsin isoinhibitors of Great Northern Beans (*Phaseolus vulgaris*) (*310*), two protease inhibitors from pigeon pea (*Cajanus cajan*) (*311*), a trypsin/chymotrypsin inhibitor from giant taro (*Alocasia macrorrhiza*) (*312*), structures of trypsin inhibitors from giant taro, taro (*Colocasia esculenta*), and giant swamp taro (*Cyrtosperma chamissonis*) (*313*), and a trypsin inhibitor from amaranth (*Amaranthus hypochondriacus*) (*314*). A high-performance capillary electrophoretic method has been adapted for the determination of both Kunitz and Bowman–Birk protease inhibitors (*315*).

Since these protease inhibitors are proteins themselves, they tend to be heat labile and may be destroyed by ordinary cooking. An investigation into the heat inactivation of trypsin inhibitors in soymilk at pH 6.5 demonstrated that for temperatures up to 125°C, the holding times which effectively killed putrefactive anaerobes also inactivated at least 90% of the trypsin inhibitor activity (*316*). However, at higher temperatures, a longer holding time was required to inactivate the inhibitors than to destroy the microbes. Thus, a UHT process which produces commercially sterile soymilk may not satisfactorily abolish trypsin inhibitor activity.

A combination of high storage temperature (40°C) and high humidity (95%) was capable of inactivating

50% of the trypsin inhibitors in cowpeas (*317*). Under drier conditions and at lower temperatures, only 20–30% of the activity was destroyed. Dry heat was also less effective than moist heat in abolishing trypsin and chymotrypsin inhibitor activity in sorghum (*318*). Activities of these inhibitors in sorghum were also reduced during germination and became undetectable after 6 days. Fermentation of ground lentils for 4 days at 30°C reduced trypsin inhibitor activity to 59–82% of the original beans and also destroyed flatulence factors and improved starch digestibility (*319*).

## PHYTATE

Several lines of evidence indicate that phytate (inositol hexakisphosphate) exerts its antinutritional effects by interfering with the intestinal absorption of dietary minerals. Following germination of pearl millet grain for 2–2½ days, phytate levels decreased dramatically and the HCl-extractability (an index of bioavailability) of Ca, Fe, and Zn increased significantly (*320*). Fermentation of high-tannin (brown sorghum and millet) and no-tannin (maize and white sorghum) cereals with a natural lactic culture from Tanzania was also found to decrease phytate concentrations and increase the in vitro solubility of iron (*321*). This process was more effective with the no-tannin cereals. A more physiologically relevant, in vitro method (utilizing a pancreatic digestion mixture and continuous removal of dialyzable components) has been devised to test the bioavailability of Ca, Mg, Fe, Zn, and Cu from breads with different phytate contents (*322*). Results indicated that although phytate decreased the bioavailability of Ca, Fe, and Zn, other components in the mixture and factors such as pH were also important in determining the bioavailability of dietary minerals.

Addition of several inositol phosphates to cultures of CaCo-2 cells (a human colon adenocarcinoma cell line), reduced the uptake of iron by the cells by 30–65% and reduced zinc uptake by 47–70% (*323*). Furthermore, the presence of phytate decreased the transport of these minerals through the cell cultures.

Investigations of the bioavailability of calcium from legumes demonstrated that the presence of tannins and trypsin inhibitors could not explain the lower availability of legume calcium (compared to casein calcium) in rat diets (*324*). Rather, it appears that phytate and/or oxalate was the culprit. Increased mineral availability to rats fed diets in which phytate has been removed, by soaking and phytase treatment, confirmed that this antinutrient significantly affects the absorption of dietary minerals (*325,326*).

Surveys of 12 leafy vegetables from Nigeria (*327*), of rice, legumes and bread from Kuwait (*328*), and of 29 common foods from Sri Lanka (*329*) revealed a range of phytate concentrations. Often, cooking or processing methods significantly reduced phytate levels. Soaking, sprouting, and boiling of some Nigerian legumes all decreased phytate concentrations, with some procedures eliminating more than half the phytate found in raw samples (*330*). Soaking of soybeans also removes phytate, with soaking at higher temperatures being more effective (*331*). However, soaking at higher temperatures has been reported to cause development of an objectionable flavor.

Among 8 wild and 4 cultivated lupine varieties, phytate concentration in seeds was found to vary from 0.4 to 1.2 g/100 g dry weight (*332*). Low phytate:Ca molar ratios in all varieties indicated that lupine may be a better source of calcium than other legumes, and very low phytate:Zn ratios in some cultivars indicated that they would also be a good source for Zn.

An anion exchange HPLC method with post-column detection has been developed for the determination of phytic acid (*333*).

## OTHER ANTINUTRITIONAL COMPOUNDS

Recent reviews considered available data on the content of various antinutritional compounds in foods and their implications for human health. Liener (*334*) focused primarily on antinutrients in soybeans, discussing their biochemical properties, nutritional significance, physiological action, and their stability under different processing conditions. Data on reductions in antinutrient levels in various cereals, legumes, and tubers were summarized and discussed by Reddy and Pierson (*335*).

Experiments to determine the relative effectiveness of roasting and malting in removing antinutritional compounds from cereals and legumes commonly eaten in India were conducted by Gahlawat and Sehgal (*336*). Roasting of raw ingredients removed about 39–51% of phytate, saponins, and tannins in these foods while malting removed about 54–63% of these antinutrients.

### Saponins

Saponins, which are composed of a carbohydrate attached to a triterpenoid or a steroidal aglycone, are common in legumes and many grain crops. They have been reported to cause hemolysis and permeabilization of the intestine, although they may also have beneficial effects on blood lipids. Saponin concentrations in seeds of six species of lupin were found to vary from 0 in *Lupinus albus* (sweet and bitter) to 467 mg/kg in the bitter variety of *L. angustifolius* (*337*). Three types of saponins were detected: soyasaponin 1, and two bidesmosides of soyasapogenol A.

Saponins A and B comprise about 0.9% of the dry weight of the seeds of quinoa (*Chenopodium quinoa*), an ancient indigenous crop of the Andes (*338*). Scrubbing and washing of the seeds removes about 67% of the saponins. While unwashed bitter quinoa caused significant food aversion and poor food conversion efficiency in rats, processed quinoa had an increased palatability and nutritional quality (*339*). Neither tannins nor protease inhibitors were detected in quinoa seeds but significant phytate levels were present. Total saponin content and composition have been effectively determined by an improved TLC method (*340*).

Using a modified HPLC procedure (*341*), the content of avenacosides A and B (saponins) in 16 oat cultivars and 4 fractions of oat kernels was determined (*342*). Saponin levels differed significantly among the strains, with concentrations ranging from 0.02% to 0.05%. Oat kernels with the smallest particle size had the highest saponin levels and these appeared to be derived mainly from the endosperm.

## Lectins

In a toxicological investigation, lectins from toxic red kidney beans and from non-toxic mountaineer half runner beans were purified and tested for their effects on glucose metabolism in rat everted intestinal sacs (*343*). Neither lectin affected glucose metabolism itself. However, absorption and transport of glucose were inhibited 40 and 72%, respectively, by red kidney bean lectin. These processes were inhibited by <10% by the half runner bean lectin. This interference with absorption and transport of nutrients may partially explain the toxicity of some bean varieties.

Germination of white kidney beans for 7 days decreased lectin concentrations by 85% and reduced the binding capacities of functional lectins towards brush border membranes by 91% (*344*). In addition, germination reduced trypsin inhibitor levels by 76%. Thus, germination may be a useful process for improving the quality of flour made from beans.

## Oligosaccharides

Oligosaccharides of the raffinose family, which are found in relatively high concentrations in some legumes, are known to be causes of flatulence. These carbohydrates cannot be digested by the human digestive system and so pass into the colon where they are fermented by the colonic flora, with the production of hydrogen and other gases. Several procedures have been evaluated for reducing the oligosaccharide content of legumes and thereby increasing the acceptability of these foods. Both germination for 3 days and a debittering process, which involved leaching out of bitter compounds, were found to remove >90% of the α-galactosides in several varieties of lupin seeds (*345*). Human subjects consuming test meals made of these processed lupin samples were found to exhale only about half as much hydrogen after consuming the germinated seeds and about one-eighth as much hydrogen after the debittered seeds as compared to unprocessed lupin. Soaking for 16 h and cooking for 50 min were found to remove about 27% and 29–44% of the raffinose and stachyose, respectively, in cowpea flour (*346*). Treatment of the flour with a crude fungal preparation (*Aspergillus niger*) containing α-galactosidase activity decreased the levels of these oligosaccharides by 82–93%. Incubation of pinto bean and field pea flours with different populations of *Lactobacillus plantarum* and *L. fermentum* for 72 h reduced stachyose concentrations by 27 and 43%, respectively (*347*).

A method for the determination of stachyose based on its inhibitory action on sucrose crystallization has been developed (*348*).

## Phytoestrogens

Estrogenic activity in eleven naturally occurring, multiply hydroxylated chalcones, flavanones, and flavones was assessed using in vitro assays to measure an estrogen receptor-dependent transcriptional response and the promotion of growth of estrogen-dependent MCF7 cells (isolated from a human breast tumor) (*349*). Although several of these flavonoids exhibited relatively weak estrogenic effects in one or both assays, some of them are widely distributed in food plants and thus may be physiologically relevant.

Affinity for cytosolic estrogen receptor binding sites was determined for 4 phytoestrogens found in alcoholic beverages: β-sitosterol and biochanin A from bourbon and genistein and daidzein from beer (*350*). All were capable of binding to the receptors, with genistein being the most potent. Administration of the compounds from bourbon to ovariectomized rats, at concentrations comparable to those found in the liquor, revealed that β-sitosterol produced a weak estrogenic effect only at the lowest dose (6.2 μg/dL) but that bourbon concentrate (containing both phytoestrogens) exerted a dose-dependent estrogenic response.

Female rat pups lactationally exposed to the phytoestrogen coumestrol were found to develop a premature anovulatory syndrome (*351*). The mother rats consumed diets containing 0.01% coumestrol on post-natal days 1 to 21. By 19 weeks of age, 83% of the treated females were in a persistent estrous state while 91% of control animals were cycling regularly. Estradiol stimulation of the treated females at 20 weeks failed to elicit the normal rise in luteinizing hormone, indicating the possibility of a neuroendocrine impairment.

## Vicine and Divicine

A case of acute hemolytic anemia has been reported in a young Greek man (17 years of age) who had recently eaten broad beans (*Vicia faba*) for the first time (*352*). His symptoms included jaundice, low hemoglobin levels (9.6 g/dL vs. a normal value of 14–18 g/dL), and elevated levels of lactate dehydrogenase and bilirubins. Analysis of his red blood cells revealed the absence of glucose-6-phosphate dehydrogenase (G6PD) activity, which is characteristic of persons susceptible to favism. Although the exact mechanism of toxicity is unknown, two pyrimidine β-glucosides (vicine and convicine) in faba beans are believed to be responsible for precipitating hemolytic crises in persons deficient in G6PD.

Divicine, a metabolite of vicine, had been considered to be the compound actually exerting the toxic effects. However, recent analyses have demonstrated that the divicine used in many experiments was not pure and therefore its etiological role has been questioned. McMillan et al. (*353*) chemically synthesized and purified divicine and examined its toxicity to rat erythrocytes. Exposure of these erythrocytes to 1.5 mM divicine dramatically reduced their survival while exposure to 5 mM vicine had no such effect. These results confirm that divicine is a direct-acting hemolytic agent and thus is likely to be the cause of favism.

## OTHER FOOD-RELATED TOXINS

### Ferns

Several recent outbreaks of food poisoning related to consumption of raw or lightly cooked ostrich fern fiddle-

heads raised the possibility that these ferns contain some hitherto unknown toxin (*354*). These ferns were regularly eaten as spring vegetables by Native Americans and are considered a delicacy in coastal areas of the USA and Canada. Thirty-one persons in New York and 33 in western Canada suffered from nausea, vomiting, and diarrhea within an average of 3–6 hours after eating the fiddleheads at restaurants. The short incubation period indicated the presence of a preformed toxin, but tests for *Bacillus cereus* and *Staphylococcus aureus* and for nitrogen/phosphorus and organochlorine pesticides were negative. No other food items were associated with illness and no deficiencies in food handling or storage were identified. Although ferns may accumulate some heavy metals, the symptoms reported were not characteristic of heavy metal poisoning. Most patients recovered quickly—within 24 hours.

An Australian freshwater fern, the nardoo fern (*Marsilea drummondii*), contributed to the demise of the 1860–61 Burke–Wills expedition to cross Australia from north to south (*355*). Aboriginal people in Australia prepared the fern sporocarps by grinding them with water to make a flour paste which could then be made into a bread or eaten in a soup. However, when the expedition members ran out of supplies on the return journey and started eating nardoo, they failed to realize the importance of this method for preparation. They ground the flour in the traditional European way and thus failed to leach out or inactivate the high levels of thiaminase in this fern. As expedition members ate more nardoo, they became progressively weaker and developed muscle wasting and hypothermia. These are classic signs of beriberi, a deficiency disease caused by lack of thiamine. Eventually most of the explorers died but their journals provide probably the first and only description of thiaminase poisoning in humans.

A recent review of Japanese plants known to contain carcinogens focused on bracken ferns, which are commonly eaten in the fiddlehead stage (*356*). Ptaquiloside, a component of these ferns, causes ileal and bladder tumors in laboratory rodents and is also the cause of bracken poisoning in cattle and of bright blindness in sheep consuming these ferns. A significantly higher incidence of esophageal cancer has been reported among people who eat large amounts of bracken ferns. This review also discusses possible carcinogenic effects of cycad and plants containing pyrrolizidine alkaloids.

Exposure to ptaquiloside may occur not only directly from the ferns but also from milk from cows which have been eating bracken. Using a newly developed method for preparation of milk samples, ptaquiloside was detected by reverse-phase HPLC in milk from cows fed 6 kg fresh bracken/day (*357*). Although cattle become sick if they eat too much bracken, these cows appeared healthy, indicating that this ptaquiloside dose was below the level of overt toxicity.

Under weakly alkaline conditions ptaquiloside is converted to the genotoxin dienone-2. In vitro studies with this compound demonstrated that it covalently binds to DNA at adenine and guanine residues (*358*). This attachment results in breaks in the DNA strands and may be the mechanism by which ptaquiloside causes tumors.

## Licorice

Excessive consumption of licorice candies caused edema, hypertension, and hypokalemia in a 34-year-old Spanish man (*359*). Analyses of plasma and urine samples revealed that plasma renin, plasma aldosterone, and urinary aldosterone levels were all so low as to be undetectable, while angiotensin I-converting enzyme (ACE) levels were elevated. The man reported eating about 40 g of licorice candies/day for 2–3 years but had increased his intake to >100 g/day the week before symptoms appeared. Ten days after licorice withdrawal, his blood pressure had returned to normal and the edema had disappeared. However, plasma hormone and ACE levels returned to normal only after 48 days of withdrawal.

Data on the effects of licorice ingestion on blood pressure–regulating hormones were summarized and discussed by Schambelan (*360*). Plasma renin, aldosterone, and vasopressin levels decrease in response to licorice ingestion while atrial natriuretic peptide levels increased. Concentrations of other vasoactive substances may also be altered. Licorice was once prescribed as a treatment for gastric ulcers, but because of its toxic effects in many individuals, it was abandoned as a remedy.

A monoclonal antibody-based ELISA has been developed for the determination of glycyrrhetic acid (the active ingredient in licorice) in biological samples (*361*).

## Spices

Capsaicin, the pungent compound in chili peppers, exerts genotoxic effects in vitro and is carcinogenic to some laboratory rodents. In an investigation of its possible carcinogenicity to humans, a population-based, case–control study of gastric cancer was conducted in Mexico (*362*). Analyses of dietary information from 220 cancer cases and 752 controls demonstrated about a 5.5-fold increased risk of gastric cancer for chili consumers compared to nonconsumers. A highly significant trend was observed for increasing risk associated with

self-reported increased consumption (low, medium, or high). But an increased risk was not associated with increased frequency of consumption. Although this data suggests that chili peppers have carcinogenic effects in humans, the relatively low incidence of gastric cancer in Mexico City, an area with heavy chili pepper consumption, indicates that other factors must play a significant role in carcinogenesis.

Another environmental factor possibly associated with carcinogenesis in Mexico City is the particulate organic matter present in the polluted air of the city. Extracts of this organic matter and extracts of chili pepper were both mutagenic in the Ames test (*363*). Coadministration of both extracts resulted in an additive mutagenic effect except at the highest concentration of chili extract used. At that concentration, the chili extract caused a decrease in the number of mutants induced by the air pollutants. This may be an effect of the high concentrations of antimutagenic compounds, such as chlorophyllin and β-carotene, also present in the extracts. Therefore, in fact, high intakes of chili peppers may be protective rather than carcinogenic.

Testing of two extracts of chili peppers in the mouse bone marrow micronucleus assay revealed that one fraction, containing a mixture of 3 long-chain nitrogen-containing compounds but no capsaicin, was clastogenic at the maximum tolerated dose (*364*). It appears that there may be several toxicological compounds in chili peppers.

Mutagenicity testing of extracts of three spices (caraway, coriander, and black pepper) from Thailand using the Ames assay strains TA98 and TA100 demonstrated the absence of mutagens (*365*). However, when the extracts were treated with nitrite, aqueous and methanolic extracts were mutagenic to TA100 without metabolic activation. Extracts of black pepper induced the most mutations.

## Herbal Preparations

Another case of acute hepatitis induced by ingestion of chaparral has been reported, this time from Australia (*366*). This herbal product, derived from leaves of the creosote bush, became a popular remedy after it was reported to have cured a case of head and neck cancer in the 1960s. The patient had been taking 2 capsules of chaparral/day for about 8 weeks prior to onset of symptoms, which included gastrointestinal upset, dark urine, and pruritis. Following withdrawal of chaparral, the patient recovered slowly, with liver function tests returning to normal after 4 months. It is unclear why hepatotoxic effects of chaparral have only recently become a concern when this product has been available for the past 20 years.

A British patient with a 17-year history of drinking poppy tea was referred to a Drug Dependence Unit for treatment to overcome his dependence on the tea (*367*). Poppy tea drinking rarely induces dependence. However, a thorough investigation revealed that this patient used no other illicit drugs. His early use of the tea had been intermittent, but for the two years prior to presentation he had been boiling about 14 poppy heads (obtained from local florists) for tea daily. The patient was treated with methadone, starting with 30 mg/day.

An epidemic of hepatitis due to ingestion of germander occurring in France in 1992 prompted the investigation of the hepatotoxic effects of this herb. Mice were gavaged with germander tea lyophilisate or a tea fraction containing furano neo-clerodane diterpenoids (the probable toxic compounds) and then examined for liver damage 24 hours later (*368*). Both preparations caused midzonal liver cell necrosis. This effect was prevented by pretreatment with a specific inhibitor of cytochromes P450 and was enhanced by pretreatment with inducers of cytochromes P450 3A. Butylated hydroxyanisole, an inducer of microsomal epoxide hydrolase, attenuated the toxic effects of the germander preparations. These results indicate that the germander toxins are activated by cytochrome P450 3A to form hepatotoxic epoxides, which may be partially inactivated by the epoxide hydrolase.

Besides the natural toxins which may be present in various herbs, there is also the possibility that commercially available herbal preparations may contain undeclared drugs. HPLC and TLC methods have been devised for the detection and quantitation of drugs such as anorexics, hypoglycemics, and antidepressants in herbal preparations with purported slimming activity (*369*).

## Other Foods

Foraging for wild foods always entails the danger of collecting toxic specimens which are similar in appearance to the desired food. While this most commonly occurs with mushrooms, other plant species may also be confused. While searching for wild ginseng in the Maine woods, two brothers collected and tasted the root of a plant later identified as water hemlock (*370*). The younger man, who took 3 bites of the root, started vomiting and having convulsions about 30 min later. Although the men were able to walk out of the woods and obtain medical attention within 45 min of onset of the symptoms, the younger man died. The older man, who had

taken only one bite, suffered some seizures and delirium but recovered with treatment. Water hemlock is considered the most toxic indigenous plant in North America and the root of the plant contains the highest concentration of its neurotoxin, cicutoxin.

Overindulgence in a normally innocuous food can also have untoward effects. A 5-year-old boy admitted to the hospital after a day of abdominal pain and vomiting was found to have an intestinal obstruction (*371*). A laparotomy was performed and a jelly-like bezoar was discovered and then fragmented and squeezed out through the ileocecal valve. Questioning of the parents revealed that the child had eaten a large number of common gel candies the day before admission. These candies contained agar as the gelling agent. This polysaccharide is not digested in humans and apparently formed a strong gel in the intestine which eventually obstructed the terminal ileum.

A study of 4 French children with lymphonodular hyperplasia of the colon and bloody diarrhea revealed that the ingestion of specific foods (orange juice, fruit-flavored sweets, kiwi, milk, and chocolate) exacerbated their symptoms (*372*). The patients did not appear to have IgE-mediated allergic reactions to the foods but clinical challenge tests demonstrated that the foods did indeed worsen symptoms.

Hemolytic anemia following ingestion of onions has been reported in a number of animal species (cattle, horses, sheep, dogs, cats) but not so far in humans. Research with rats indicates that this toxic effect is due to dipropyl, di(1-propenyl), and di(2-propenyl) disulfides present in the onions (*373*). As this onion-induced hemolysis is caused by oxidative reactions, individuals with hereditary deficiencies in antioxidant enzymes, for example glucose-6-phosphate dehydrogenase, may be more susceptible to the toxic effects of these compounds. It may be that the quantity of onions normally eaten is too low to induce hemolytic effects in sensitive humans. Current interest in the potential therapeutic effects of *Allium* vegetables and the use of these disulfides as permitted food additives may increase exposure to these potentially toxic compounds.

## FOOD ALLERGY AND FOOD INTOLERANCE

A random sample of 1483 Dutch adults, surveyed to obtain an estimate of the prevalence food allergy and food intolerance, yielded a self-reported food-sensitive subgroup of 198 persons (12.4% of the total group)

(*374*). Of these food-sensitive individuals, 73 completed double-blind, placebo-controlled food challenges. A total of 12 persons were confirmed to have food allergies or food intolerance, with pork, alcoholic drinks, kiwi, menthol, glucose, vanillin, benzoic acid, sorbic acid, tartrazine, MSG, histamine, and trassi (an Indonesian condiment) identified as the offending foods. Assuming that food allergy/food intolerance is equal among participants, nonparticipants and dropouts, an estimated 2.4% of the adult population would be affected.

Approximately 20% of 18,880 persons responding to a survey on food sensitivity in the UK claimed to be sensitive to one or more foods (*375*). Of the 93 subjects who later completed a double-blind, placebo-controlled challenge, 19.4% had a positive reaction. Extrapolation of results from this study suggested that 1.4–1.8% of the total population is truly affected with food allergy/intolerance. Potential test subjects were lost at every step in the study, with some simply not responding or claiming that the testing protocol was inconvenient, while others were excluded because interview results did not indicate a true food sensitivity. Forty-seven subjects reported severe symptoms in response to intake of specific foods (most commonly shellfish and nuts), including 4 who had suffered anaphylactic reactions.

The pattern of food hypersensitivity was investigated in 112 Israeli subjects with a known food allergy which had developed after age 10 (*376*). Fruits and vegetables were the main allergenic foods in these adults, in contrast to studies with children, where milk and eggs are the main causes of food allergy. Although the majority of patients tested positive to multiple food allergens in skin tests, most had a positive response to only one food following oral challenge. About one-third of the subjects had a history of exercise-induced symptoms after meals.

## Case Reports

Although rice is commonly considered to be hypoallergenic, asthma and urticaria occurring in a 27-year-old Spanish woman were traced to her handling of raw rice and exposure to rice dust (*377*). Similar, but less severe, symptoms occurred when she handled flour made from other cereals and, on one occasion, she presented with systemic anaphylaxis after consuming a Spanish dish made with undercooked wheat flour. However, this woman regularly consumed cooked rice, bread and pastries without incident. Hypersensitivity tests confirmed allergic reactions primarily to raw rice and also to rye, corn, and wheat extracts.

However, allergic reactions to breads and pastries are not always caused by antigens in the grains used. A 48-year-old man in Detroit suffered an anaphylactic reaction after consuming some beignets prepared from a commercial mix (*378*). The patient had previously eaten beignets in a New Orleans restaurant without incident and had brought home a beignet mix purchased from the restaurant. Microscopic examination of the mix revealed the presence of actively crawling mites (*Dermatophagoides farinae*). Skin prick tests to the infested mix and to *D. farinae* were positive, while there was no reaction to an uninfested mix or to other ingredients in the mix. The patient declined a challenge with beignets made from an uninfested mix and continues to eat foods with similar ingredients (without mites) with no problem.

An exercise-induced anaphylactic reaction in a 13-year-old Spanish girl was traced to prior consumption of hazelnuts (*379*). The patient had a 3-year history of respiratory difficulty and urticaria after exercise but there was no seasonal pattern as might be expected for pollen allergies. Skin tests were positive for a mixture of grass and weed pollen and nuts and seeds. An exercise challenge test with hazelnuts was also positive. The girl can eat walnuts and hazelnuts without difficulty but experiences adverse reactions if she exercises afterwards.

Three cases of hypersensitivity to pistachio nuts have been described (*380*). The 3 Spanish adults had histories of facial flushing, angioedema, skin rash, and/or respiratory symptoms after eating these nuts. Skin tests were positive for pistachios for all three. In addition, these subjects had positive reactions to other nuts, including cashews, sunflower seeds, and walnuts, but the pattern of positive reactions differed among the three.

Anaphylaxis occurred in a 14-year-old girl in Colorado on two occasions following consumption of chicken prepared in a teriyaki marinade (*381*). Skin tests using chicken and other components of the meal were negative, but the teriyaki sauce produced a significant wheal. Further investigation of the various ingredients of the sauce identified coriander as the allergenic substance. A spice product containing 8 different ingredients appeared to be the cause of orofacial swelling in a 37-year-old woman in Australia (*382*). Another case with similar symptoms appeared to be related to the consumption of aspartame-containing food and drinks, particularly a specific brand of chewing gum.

Five cases of anaphylaxis due to ingestion of royal jelly (a protein-rich food obtained from bees which has been used as a health tonic) have been described from Australia (*383*). All subjects were adults and had histories of mild, atopic asthma. The subjects reacted within 20 min to 2 h after ingestion of the jelly and symptoms were severe. Skin prick tests done on 4 of the subjects were positive for royal jelly and negative for bee venom. Several other cases of adverse reactions to royal jelly, including one fatality in an 11-year-old asthmatic, were subsequently reported from Australia (*384*). All the cases were persons with a known history of asthma.

Numerous allergic reactions resulting from occupational exposure to foods have been reported, including the following: asthma caused by milk proteins in a worker in a delicatessen factory in Italy (*385*); allergic reactions in Japanese workers engaged in picking and packing okra (*386*); three cases of asthma and rhinitis traced to garlic exposure in a cook and 2 workers in a sausage factory in Finland (*387*); asthma in a French worker in a spice factory as a result of exposure to powdered fenugreek (*388*); and allergic reactions in a Swiss woman employed as a frog skinner in a factory processing and canning frogs' legs (*389*). A protein in the frog's skin was found to be the culprit. The patient returned to work in another part of the factory but even a visit to the frog-processing hall triggers symptoms.

## Reviews

An entire issue of *Clinical Reviews in Allergy* was devoted to various aspects of adverse reactions to seafood. Topics covered included important seafood species implicated in allergic reactions (*390*), allergic reactions to fish (*391*), hypersensitivity to crustacea and mollusks (*392*), and occupational reactions in the seafood industry (*393*). Other papers on seafood toxins and chemical additives in seafood products were discussed in their respective sections in this book.

Allergic reactions to and allergens in crustacea were reviewed by Musmand et al. (*394*). Such reactions most often occur in response to eating shrimp but there is significant cross-reactivity among crustacean species. Crustacea also induce allergic skin reactions in fishermen and food processors and handlers and occupational asthma occurs in sensitive individuals exposed to steam from cooking crabs and other crustacea.

Viens et al. (*395*) reviewed the problem of hidden food allergens in complex foods. A variety of foods and extracts may be added to processed foods to improve their nutritional value or to improve their stability or consumer appeal. In terms of their current level of use and their allergic potential, the most important foods which may act as hidden allergens are nuts, peanuts, soy proteins, celery, cow's milk, hen's eggs, and fish. Since severe anaphylactic reactions have occurred in response to some of these ingredients in complex foods, it is important to limit their use unless they are declared on labels or menus.

Matsuda and Nakamura (*396*) reviewed the molecular structure and immunological properties of 15 food allergens which have been isolated and characterized. These include proteins and glycoproteins from milk, eggs, legumes, rice, and seafood. An understanding of the structure of these allergens may aid in understanding their mode of action and may also lead to methods for minimizing their concentrations in foods.

Immune responses in the intestine in response to dietary protein antigens were detailed by Moreau and Coste (*397*). The gut-associated lymphoid tissue protects the body against pathogenic organisms and excessive doses of food antigens and also plays a role in the development of the immune system and food sensitivity.

## Allergies to Specific Foods

MILK AND MILK PRODUCTS. In a prospective epidemiological study, 1158 Dutch infants were studied for 1 year from birth to determine the incidence of cow's milk protein intolerance (*398*). No dietary interventions were required for 914 of the infants (79%), and 33 infants required changes unrelated to milk consumption. Of the remainder, 80 infants improved on a low-lactose formula (lactose-intolerant), 87 did not improve on a cow's milk–free formula, and 26 infants did improve when cow's milk was eliminated and showed a positive reaction to 2 challenges with cow's milk proteins. Therefore, the calculated incidence of cow's milk protein intolerance was 2.8%. What of the 87 who did not improve on the milk-free formula? A Belgian study of 64 infants with an apparent cow's milk allergy revealed that 31 improved dramatically when fed a cow's milk–free formula (*399*). Symptoms in most of the 33 who did not improve with the new formula did resolve when dust-producing items such as carpets, bedclothes and teddy bears were removed from the house or treated with an acaricide to kill house dust mites.

Twenty children with a known allergy to cow's milk protein were given skin tests and double-blind, placebo-controlled challenges with 3 different milk protein hydrolysate formulae (*400*). Two children each had allergic reactions to a casein hydrolysate and to an extensively hydrolyzed whey protein formula. In contrast, 9 children reacted positively to the partially hydrolyzed whey formula. It appears that the partially hydrolyzed formula is not truly hypoallergenic even though the package labels may indicate this.

Even breast-fed infants may not be safe from the allergenic effects of cow's milk proteins if their mothers drink cow's milk. Studies with 55 Finnish mother–infant pairs, in which the infants were apparently suffering allergic reactions, indicated that 46 of the infants were, in fact, allergic to cow's milk when challenged orally (*401*). β-Lactoglobulin, one of the most important allergenic cow's milk proteins, was present at concentrations up to 8.6 μg/L in the milk of 75% of the mothers when tested 1–2 h after consuming 400 mL skim milk. A great deal of interindividual variation was noted in β-lactoglobulin levels in breast milk.

Intestinal permeability tests were performed in 3 infants with known cow's milk allergy to assess the effects of breast milk and some hypoallergenic formulae on the urinary elimination of orally administered lactulose and mannitol (L/M ratio) (*402*). When the mothers drank cow's milk while nursing their infants, the infants' L/M ratio was abnormal, indicating that the breast milk contained some substance which caused intestinal damage. However, intestinal permeability was normal in the infants when they drank breast milk after their mothers started a milk protein elimination diet. These infants also had abnormal ratios when they were fed hypoallergenic, hydrolyzed-protein, milk substitutes and apparently were extremely sensitive to minute amounts of milk protein.

Although children may outgrow their allergy to milk, they may still experience clinically significant allergic reactions under certain circumstances. Two such cases were recently described (*403*). A 12-year-old, who was able to tolerate milk in baked goods but still avoided drinking milk, developed urticaria, abdominal cramps, and respiratory symptoms when he rode his bicycle after consuming a meal containing pancakes made with milk. A 14-year-old was found to tolerate challenges with dried milk but still had allergic symptoms when given liquid milk.

An examination of the serological reactions to milk proteins in 34 adults with IgE-mediated reactions to cow's milk and cheese revealed that, unlike allergic children, the predominant allergen in 29 subjects was casein (*404*). Sensitization to whey proteins was relatively rare (6 subjects) among these adults but is the most common reaction in children. Most of the subjects were female and about a third of them reported that the milk allergy symptoms started during a pregnancy.

LEGUMES. Peanuts are one of the most allergenic foods known and even a small amount of peanut protein present in other foods has triggered anaphylaxis in sensitive persons. Seven peanut oils from different manufacturers were analyzed to determine whether different processing methods removed all the peanut allergens (*405*). No protein or peanut allergenic material was detected in any of 3 oils produced by hot-pressing and in one sample

produced by cold-pressing. Another cold-pressed sample appeared to contain trace amounts of allergens but protein levels were too low to be detected by the method used. Two other cold-pressed samples contained detectable protein (3.3 and 0.2–0.6 μg/mL) and highly significant amounts of peanut allergens. Therefore, peanut-sensitive individuals should avoid cold-pressed peanut oils and foods made with them, although hot-pressed oils are probably safe.

Several groups reported the production of monoclonal antibodies to allergenic peanut proteins. Such antibodies can be used in an ELISA to detect hidden peanut allergens in foods (*406,407*). For example, one ELISA was capable of detecting 40 μg peanut allergens/mL in vanilla ice cream with added defatted peanut protein. Peanut allergens were also detected in other foods such as a cheesecake mix, chocolate candies and even in a trail mix with the peanuts removed by hand. Monoclonal antibodies have also been useful in investigating the antigenic structure of *Ara h* I, the major peanut allergen (*408*). Four different antigenic sites were identified. These antibodies have also been used to prepare an immunoaffinity column for the purification of *Ara h* I.

Soybean allergy is another common childhood food allergy. Several soy-derived products, including soy sprouts, mold- and acid-hydrolyzed soy sauce, tofu, tempeh, miso, and hydrolyzed vegetable protein, all tested positive for allergenicity in 7 sensitive volunteers (*409*). Processing, particularly fermentation, apparently degraded a large percentage of the allergens in some foods (tofu, tempeh, miso, and mold-hydrolyzed soy sauce). It may be possible to develop processing methods which would further destroy soybean allergens.

One of the major soybean allergens, *Gly m* Bd 30K, has been isolated and characterized (*410*). Amino acid sequence of monomers of this allergen revealed that it was identical to that of the soybean seed 34-kDa oil body–associated protein and it has about 30% sequence homology with *Der p* I, a house dust mite allergen. The purified allergen was used to prepare monoclonal antibodies for a sandwich ELISA to detect this allergen in food extracts (*411*).

FRUITS. Apples contain food allergens which mainly cause oropharyngeal symptoms. Analyses of fruits from 16 apple varieties revealed a great variation in the amounts of the 18-kDa apple allergen (*412*). Seven cultivars contained relatively large amounts of the allergen and provoked greater responses in allergic individuals. Five of these strains (Braeburn, Golden Delicious, Granny Smith, Jonagold, and Cox Orange) are very common in

German markets. In contrast, the varieties with the lowest concentrations of the allergenic protein are of minor economic importance. These included Macoun, Jamba, and Ellison's Orange.

Since allergies to fruits have been associated with latex allergy, three German individuals with a known allergy to latex were tested with extracts of banana and avocado (*413*). All had positive skin reactions to these fruits. One person who was diagnosed with allergic asthma also reacted to tomato extracts.

**SHRIMP.** Two allergens have been isolated from different species of shrimp and characterized. A major heat-stable allergen from *Penaeus indicus*, previously designated as Sa-II, has been shown to be a 34-kDa protein containing 300 amino acids (*414*). Several immunological and biochemical assays indicated that this protein is identical to the shrimp muscle protein tropomyosin. The name *Pen i* I is proposed for this allergen, according to the International Convention.

A similar, heat-stable 39-kDa protein has been isolated from a common Taiwanese shrimp (*Parapenaeus fissurus*) and was determined to be the major allergen in these shrimp (*415*). A monoclonal antibody prepared against this compound also reacted with a 39-kDa protein from crabs but did not react with extracts from cuttlefish, oyster, or pomfret. The proposed name for this allergen is *Par f* I.

**OTHER FOODS.** Eleven purified members of the α-amylase/trypsin inhibitor family were tested for allergenicity in 31 subjects who showed allergic sensitization to wheat flour (*416*). The 3 allergens which induced the strongest skin response in prick tests were the glycosylated subunits of tetrameric α-amylase inhibitors from wheat and barley and a barley monomeric α-amylase inhibitor.

Not only α-amylase inhibitors but also the enzyme itself causes allergic reactions in sensitive individuals. Tests with bakers, some of whom were known to have work-related respiratory symptoms, revealed that some were sensitive to the commercially available α-amylase from *Aspergillus oryzae*, which is widely used as a baking additive (*417*). To determine whether this was a reaction to the enzyme or to some other fungal protein, a highly purified α-amylase was used to challenge these bakers. There were no significant differences between the reactions induced by the crude and purified enzymes and therefore it has been proposed that this occupational allergen be designated *Asp o* II.

An investigation of 31 persons who were allergic to birds, eggs, or both attempted to distinguish common allergens (*418*). The subjects allergic only to eggs were primarily sensitive to egg whites and did not react to allergens from bird feathers. Those who were supposed to be allergic only to bird feathers did not react to egg allergens and some also did not react to the feather antigens tested. IgE from the 13 persons sensitive to both eggs and feathers recognized a 70-kDa protein from egg yolks and 70-, 95-, and 200-kDa proteins from feathers. Preincubation of sera from these patients with extracts from egg yolks or from feathers completely blocked IgE reactions to feather and eggs, respectively. It appeared that the egg yolk protein, α-livetin, led to a cross-sensitization and therefore to the bird-egg syndrome.

A major allergen from oriental-mustard (*Brassica juncea*) has been isolated and characterized and given the name *Bra j* IE (*419*). The structure of this allergen is closely related to a previously isolated allergen from yellow mustard (*Sinapis alba*).

## LITERATURE CITED

1. Saavedra-Delgado, A.M., and D.D. Metcalfe. Seafood toxins. *Clin. Rev. Aller.* 11:241–260 (1993).

2. Sockett, P.N., J.M. Cowden, S. Le Baigue, et al. Foodborne disease surveillance in England and Wales: 1989–1991.*Commun. Dis. Rep.* 3(Rev. 12):R159–R173 (1992).

3. Manger, R.L., L.S. Leja, S.Y. Lee, et al. Tetrazolium-based cell bioassay for neurotoxins active on voltage-sensitive sodium channels: semiautomated assay for saxitoxins, brevetoxins, and ciguatoxins. *Anal. Biochem.* 214:190–194 (1993).

4. Lewis, R.J., and T.A. Ruff. Ciguatera: ecological, clinical, and socioeconomic perspectives. *Crit. Rev. Environ. Sci. Technol.* 23:137–156 (1993).

5. Lewis, R.J., and M.J. Holmes. Origin and transfer of toxins involved in ciguatera. *Comp. Biochem. Physiol.* 106C:615–628 (1993).

6. Scheuer, P.J. Ciguatera and its off-shoots—chance encounters en route to a molecular structure. *Tetrahedron* 50:3–18 (1994).

7. DeFusco, D.J., P. O'Dowd, Y. Hokama, and B.R. Ott. Coma due to ciguatera poisoning in Rhode Island. *Am. J. Med.* 95:240–243 (1993).

8. Stommel, E.W., L.R. Jenkyn, and J. Parsonnet. Another case of polymyositis after ciguatera toxin exposure.*Arch. Neurol.* 50:571 (1994).

9. Le Bouquin, V., G. D'Hooghe, J.P. Quod, and C. Marasse. "Ciguatera", une forme particulière à La Réunion. *Presse Méd.* 22:1061 (1993).

10. Katz, A.R., S. Terrell-Perica, and D.M. Sasaki. Ciguatera on Kauai: investigation of factors associated with severity of illness.*Am. J. Trop. Med. Hyg.* 49:448–454 (1993).

11. Cameron, J., and M.F. Capra. The basis of the paradoxical disturbance of temperature perception in ciguatera poisoning. *Clin. Toxicol.* 31:571–579 (1993).

12. Molgó, J., T. Shimahara, and A.M. Legrand. Ciguatoxin, extracted from poisonous morays eels, causes sodium-dependent calcium mobilization in NG108-15 neuroblastoma × glioma hybrid cells. *Neurosci. Lett.* 158:147–150 (1993).

13. Molgó, J., Y.M. Gaudry-Talarmain, A.M. Legrand, and N. Moulian. Ciguatoxin extracted from poisonous moray eels *Gymnothorax javanicus* triggers acetylcholine release from *Torpedo* cholinergic synaptosomes via reversed Na+–Ca2+ exchange. *Neurosci. Lett.* 160:65–68 (1993).

14. Grzebyk, D., B. Berland, A.B. Thomassin, et al. Ecology of ciguateric dinoflagellates in the coral reef complex of Mayotte Island (S.W. Indian Ocean). *J. Exp. Mar. Biol. Ecol.* 178:51–66 (1994).

15. Holmes, M.J., and R.J. Lewis. Purification and characterisation of large and small maitotoxins from cultured *Gambierdiscus toxicus*. *Nat. Toxins* 2:64–72 (1994).

16. Endean, R., J.K. Griffith, J.J. Robins, et al. Variation in the toxins present in ciguateric narrow-barred Spanish mackerel, *Scomberomorus commersoni*. *Toxicon* 31:723–732 (1993).

17. Endean, R., S.A. Monks, J.K. Griffith, and L.E. Llewellyn. Apparent relationships between toxins elaborated by the cyanobacterium *Trichodesmium erythraeum* and those present in the flesh of the narrow-barred Spanish mackerel *Scomberomorus commersoni*. *Toxicon* 31:1155–1165 (1993).

18. Hokama, Y., J.L. Shirai, and M.A. Islam. Evaluation of bioassay for toxicity of ciguateric fish and associated toxins. *J. Clin. Lab. Anal.* 8:63–69 (1994).

19. Lewis, R.J., and M. Sellin. Recovery of ciguatoxin from fish flesh. *Toxicon* 31:1333–1336 (1993).

20. Diogène, G., A. Dubreuil, J.Ph. Breittmayer, and S. Puiseux-Dao. Cytotoxic quantification of maitotoxin-like activity from the dinoflagellate *Gambierdiscus toxicus*. *Toxicol. in Vitro* 8:37–45 (1994).

21. Lewis, R.J., M.J. Holmes, P.F. Alewood, and A. Jones. Ionspray mass spectrometry of ciguatoxin-1, maitotoxin-2 and -3, and related marine polyether toxins. *Nat. Toxins* 2:56–63 (1994).

22. Tambyah, P.A., K.P. Hui, P. Gopalakrishnakone, et al. Central-nervous-system effects of tetrodotoxin poisoning. *Lancet* 343:538–539 (1994).

23. Nagashima, Y., T. Nagai, K. Shiomi, et al. Tetrodotoxin-associated high molecular weight substances from toxic pufferfish liver. *Nippon Suisan Gakkaishi* 59:1177–1182 (1993).

24. Shiomi, K., S. Yamaguchi, K. Shimakura, et al. Affinity chromatographic purification of tetrodotoxin by use of tetrodotoxin-binding high molecular weight substances in the body fluid of shore crab (*Hemigrapsus sanguineus*) as ligands. *Toxicon* 31:1615–1618 (1993).

25. Do, H.K., K. Hamasaki, K. Ohwada, et al. Presence of tetrodotoxin and tetrodotoxin-producing bacteria in freshwater sediments. *Appl. Environ. Microbiol.* 59:3934–3937 (1993).

26. Gallacher, S., and T.H. Birkbeck. Effect of phosphate concentration on production of tetrodotoxin by *Alteromonas tetraodonis*. *Appl. Environ. Microbiol.* 59:3981–3983 (1993).

27. Anonymous. Toxin reaches record levels in Alaskan PSP outbreaks. *Food Protect. Rep.* 10(7–8):1–2 (1994).

28. Humpage, A.R., J. Rositano, P.D. Baker, et al. Paralytic shellfish poisons from freshwater blue-green algae. *Med. J. Aust.* 159:423 (1993).

29. Oshima, Y., S.I. Blackburn, and G.M. Hallegraeff. Comparative study on paralytic shellfish toxin profiles of the dinoflagellate *Gymnodinium catenatum* from three different countries. *Marine Biol.* 116:471–476 (1993).

30. Kim, C.-H., Y. Sako, and Y. Ishida. Comparison of toxin composition between populations of *Alexandrium* spp. from geographically distant areas. *Nippon Suisan Gakkaishi* 59:641–646 (1993).

31. Cembella, A.D., S.E. Shumway, and N.I. Lewis. Anatomical distribution and spatio-temporal variation in paralytic shellfish toxin composition in two bivalve species from the Gulf of Maine. *J. Shellfish Res.* 12:389–403 (1993).

32. Rensel, J. Factors controlling paralytic shellfish poisoning (PSP) in Puget Sound, Washington. *J. Shellfish Res.* 12:371–376 (1993).

33. Schwinghamer, P., M. Hawryluk, C. Powell, and C.H. MacKenzie. Resuspended hypnozygotes of *Alexandrium fundyense* associated with winter occurrence of PSP in inshore Newfoundland waters. *Aquaculture* 122:171–179 (1994).

34. Okumura, M., S. Yamada, Y. Oshima, and N. Ishikawa. Characteristics of paralytic shellfish poisoning toxins derived from short-necked clams (*Tapes japonica*) in Mikawa Bay. *Nat. Toxins* 2:141–143 (1994).

35. Lawrence, J.F., M. Maher, and W. Watson-Wright. Effect of cooking on the concentration of toxins associated with paralytic shellfish poison in lobster hepatopancreas. *Toxicon* 32:57–64 (1994).

36. Arakawa, O., T. Noguchi, Y. Shida, and Y. Onoue. Occurrence of carbamoyl-*N*-hydroxy derivatives of saxitoxin and neosaxitoxin in a xanthid crab *Zosimus aeneus*. *Toxicon* 32:175–183 (1994).

37. Van Egmond, H.P., H.J. Van den Top, W.E. Paulsch, et al. Paralytic shellfish poison reference materials: an intercomparison of methods for the determination of saxitoxin. *Food Addit. Contam.* 11:39–56 (1994).

38. Smith, D.S., and D.D. Kitts. Development of a monoclonal-based enzyme-linked immunoassay for saxitoxin-induced protein. *Toxicon* 32:317–323 (1994).

39. Franco, J.M., and P. Fernández-Vila. Separation of paralytic shellfish toxins by reversed phase high performance liquid chromatography, with postcolumn reaction and fluorimetric detection. *Chromatographia* 35:613–620 (1993).

40. Janeček, M., M. A. Quilliam, and J.F. Lawrence. Analysis of paralytic shellfish poisoning toxins by automated pre-column oxidation and microcolumn liquid chromatography with fluorescence detection. *J. Chromatogr.* 644:321–331 (1993).

41. Langlois, G.W., K.W. Kizer, K.H. Hansgen, et al. A note on domoic acid in California coastal molluscs and crabs. *J. Shellfish Res.* 12:467–468 (1993).

42. Drum, A.S., T.L. Siebens, E.A. Crecelius, and R.A. Elston. Domoic acid in the Pacific razor clam *Siliqua patula* (Dixon, 1789). *J. Shellfish Res.* 12:443–450 (1993).

43. Horner, R.A., M.B. Kusske, B.P. Moynihan, et al. Retention of domoic acid by Pacific razor clams, *Siliqua patula* (Dixon, 1789): preliminary study. *J. Shellfish Res.* 12:451–456 (1993).

44. Villac, M.C., D.L. Roelke, T.A. Villareal, and G.A. Fryxell. Comparison of two domoic acid-producing diatoms: a review. *Hydrobiologia* 269/270:213–224 (1993).

45. Horner, R.A., and J.P. Postel. Toxic diatoms in western Washington waters (U.S. west coast). *Hydrobiologia* 269/270:197–205 (1993).

46. Villac, M.C., D.L. Roelke, F.P. Chavez, et al. *Pseudonitzschia australis* Frenguelli and related species from the west coast of the U.S.A.: occurrence and domoic acid production. *J. Shellfish Res.* 12:457–465 (1993).

47. Lawrence, J.F., C. Cleroux, and J.F. Truelove. Comparison of high-performance liquid chromatography with radioimmunoassay for the determination of domoic acid in biological samples. *J. Chromatogr. A* 662:173–177 (1994).

48. Lawrence, J.F., B.P.-Y. Lau, C. Cleroux, and D. Lewis. Comparison of UV absorption and electrospray mass spectrometry for the high-performance liquid chromatographic determination of domoic acid in shellfish and biological samples. *J. Chromatogr. A* 659:119–126 (1994).

49. Bates, S.S., C. Léger, B.A. Keafer, and D.M. Anderson. Discrimination between domoic-acid-producing and nontoxic forms of the diatom *Pseudonitzschia pungens* using immunofluorescence. *Marine Ecol. Prog. Ser.* 100:185–195 (1993).

50. PHLS Communicable Disease Surveillance Centre. Diarrhetic shellfish poisoning associated with mussels. *Commun. Dis. Rep.* 4:101 (1994).

51. Anonymous. Diarrhoetic shellfish poisoning (DSP). *Commun. Dis. Environ. Health Scotland Weekly Rep.* 28(15):2 (1994).

52. Pitcher, G.C., D.A. Horstman, D. Calder, et al. The first record of diarrhetic shellfish poisoning on the South African coast. *South African J. Sci.* 89:512–514 (1993).

53. Subba Rao, D.V., Y. Pan, V. Zitko, et al. Diarrhetic shellfish poisoning (DSP) associated with a subsurface bloom of *Dinophysis norvegica* in Bedford Basin, eastern Canada. *Marine Ecol. Prog. Ser.* 97:117–126 (1993).

54. Fernández, M.T., V. Zitko, S. Gascón, et al. Neurotoxic effect of okadaic acid, a seafood-related toxin, on cultured cerebellar neurons. *Ann. N.Y. Acad. Sci.* 679:260–269 (1993).

55. Boland, M.P., M.A. Smillie, D.Z.X. Chen, and C.F.B. Holmes. A unified bioscreen for the detection of diarrhetic shellfish toxins and microcystins in marine and freshwater environments. *Toxicon* 31:1393–1405 (1993).

56. Stockemer, J., and M. Gürke. Optimierung einer HPLC-Methode zur Bestimmung von DSP-Toxinen. *Arch. Lebensmittelhyg.* 44:146–147 (1993).

57. Vernoux, J.P., C. Le Baut, P. Masselin, et al. The use of *Daphnia magna* for detection of okadaic acid in mussel extracts. *Food Addit. Contam.* 10:603–608 (1993).

58. Anonymous. Escolar—The snake mackerel strikes again. *Food Protect. Rep.* 10(9):2–3 (1994).

59. Lemée, R., D. Pesando, M. Durand-Clément, et al. Preliminary survey of toxicity of the green alga *Caulerpa taxifolia* introduced into the Mediterranean. *J. Appl. Phycol.* 5:485–493 (1993).

60. Valls, R., J. Artaud, P. Amade, et al. Determination of caulerpenyne, a toxin from the green alga *Caulerpa taxifolia* (Caulerpaceae). *J. Chromatogr. A* 663:114–118 (1994).

61. Bignami, G.S. A rapid and sensitive hemolysis neutralization assay for palytoxin. *Toxicon* 31:817–820 (1993).

62. Yotsu-Yamashita, M., R.L. Haddock, and T. Tasumoto. Polycavernoside A: a novel glycosidic macrolide from the red alga *Polycavernosa tsudai* (*Gracilaria edulis*). *J. Am. Chem. Soc.* 115:1147–1148 (1993).

63. Chia, D.G.B., C.O. Lau, P.K.L. Ng, and C.H. Tan. Localization of toxins in the poisonous mosaic crab, *Lophozozymus pictor* (Fabricius, 1798) (Brachyura, Xanthidae). *Toxicon* 31:901–904 (1993).

64. Lau, C.O., H.E. Khoo, R. Yuen, et al. Isolation of a novel fluorescent toxin from the coral reef crab, *Lophozozymus pictor*. *Toxicon* 31:1341–1345 (1993).

65. Shiomi, K., M. Mizukami, K. Shimakura, and Y. Nagashima. Toxins in the salivary gland of some marine carnivorous gastropods. *Comp. Biochem. Physiol.* 107B:427–432 (1994).

66. Shiomi, K., K. Utsumi, S. Tsuchiya, et al. Comparison of proteinaceous toxins in the skin mucus from three species of eels. *Comp. Biochem. Physiol.* 107B:389–394 (1994).

67. Halász, A., Á. Baráth, L. Simon-Sarkadi, and W. Holzapfel. Biogenic amines and their production by microorganisms in food. *Trends Food Sci. Technol.* 5:42–49 (1994).

68. Wantke, F., M. Götz, and R. Jarisch. Histamine-free diet: treatment of choice for histamine-induced food intolerance and supporting treatment for chronical headaches. *Clin. Exp. Aller.* 23:982–985 (1993).

69. Teodorović, V., S. Buncic, and D. Smiljanić. A study of factors influencing histamine production in meat. *Fleischwirtschaft* 74:170–172 (1994).

70. Beutling, D. Untersuchungen über die Bildung von Tyramin durch Mikroben mit lebensmittelhygienischer Relevanz. *Arch. Lebensmittelhyg.* 44:83–87 (1993).

71. Shalaby, A.R. Separation, identification and estimation of biogenic amines in foods by thin-layer chromatography. *Food Chem.* 49:305–310 (1994).

72. PHLS Communicable Disease Surveillance Centre. Other food poisoning: June 1994. *Commun. Dis. Rep.* 4:120 (1994).

73. Leisner, J.J., J.C. Millan, H.H. Huss, and L.M. Larsen. Production of histamine and tyramine by lactic acid bacteria isolated from vacuum-packed sugar-salted fish. *J. Appl. Bacteriol.* 76:417–423 (1994).

74. Giorgio, B., C. Tisse, and M. Guerere. A new method for quantitative determination of biogenic amines in canned sardines. *Sci. Aliments* 13:737–750 (1993).

75. López-Sabater, E.I., J.J. Rodríguez-Jerez, A.X. Roig-Sagues, and M.T. Mora-Ventura. Determination of histamine in fish using an enzymic method. *Food Addit. Contam.* 10:593–602 (1993).

76. Draisci, R., S. Cavalli, L. Lucentini, and A. Stacchini. Ion exchange separation and pulsed amperometric detection for determination of biogenic amines in fish products. *Chromatographia* 35:584–590 (1993).

77. Shalaby, A.R. Survey on biogenic amines in Egyptian foods: sausage. *J. Sci. Food Agric.* 62:291–293 (1993).

78. Smith, J.S., P.B. Kenney, C.L. Kastner, and M.M. Moore. Biogenic amine formation in fresh vacuum-packaged beef during storage at 1°C for 120 days. *J. Food Protect.* 56:497–500,532 (1993).

79. Maijala, R.L. Formation of histamine and tyramine by some lactic acid bacteria in MRS-broth and modified decarboxylation agar. *Lett. Appl. Microbiol.* 17:40–43 (1993).

80. Maijala, R., and S. Eerola. Contaminant lactic acid bacteria of dry sausages produce histamine and tyramine. *Meat Sci.* 35:387–395 (1993).

81. Maijala, R., S. Eerola, P. Hill, and E. Nurmi. The influence of some starter cultures and GDL on the formation of biogenic amines in dry sausages. *Agric. Sci. Finl.* 2:403–412 (1993).

82. Maijala, R. Histamine and tyramine production by a *Lactobacillus* strain subjected to external pH decrease. *J. Food Protect.* 57:259–262 (1994).

83. Straub, B., M. Schollenberger, M. Kicherer, et al. Extraction and determination of biogenic amines in fermented sausages and other meat products using reversed-phase-HPLC. *Z. Lebensm. Unters. Forsch.* 197:230–232 (1993).

84. Tailor, S.A.N., K.I. Shulman, S.E. Walker, et al. Hypertensive episode associated with phenelzine and tap beer—a reanalysis of the role of pressor amines in beer. *J. Clin. Psychopharmacol.* 14:5–14 (1994).

85. Izquierdo-Pulido, M.L., M.C. Vidal-Carou, and A. Marine-Font. Determination of biogenic amines in beers and their raw materials by ion-pair liquid chromatography with postcolumn derivatization. *J. AOAC Int.* 76:1027–1032 (1993).

86. Achilli, G., G.P. Cellerino, and G. Melzi d'Eril. Determination of amines in wines by high-performance liquid chromatography with electrochemical coulometric detection after precolumn derivatization. *J. Chromatogr. A* 661:201–205 (1994).

87. Ziegler, W., M. Hahn, and P.R. Wallnöfer. Verhalten biogener Amine bei der Zubereitung ausgewählter pflanzlicher Lebensmittel. *Dtsch. Lebensm.-Rundsch.* 90:108–112 (1994).

88. Nout, M.J.R., M.M.W. Ruikes, H.M. Bouwmeester, and P.R. Beljaars. Effect of processing conditions on the formation of biogenic amines and ethyl carbamate in soybean tempe. *J. Food Safety* 13:293–303 (1993).

89. Simon-Sarkadi, L., and W.H. Holzapfel. Determination of biogenic amines in leafy vegetables by amino acid analyser. *Z. Lebensm. Unters. Forsch.* 198:230–233 (1994).

90. Eisenbrand, G., and W. Tang. Food-borne hetercyclic amines. Chemistry, formation, occurrence and biological activities. A literature review. *Toxicology* 84:1–82 (1993).

91. Skog, K. Cooking procedures and food mutagens: a literature review. *Food Chem. Toxicol.* 31:655–675 (1993).

92. Adamson, R.H., S. Takayama, T. Sugimura, and U.P. Thorgeirsson. Induction of hepatocellular carcinoma in nonhuman primates by the food mutagen 2-amino-3-methylimidazo[4,5-*f*]quinoline. *Environ. Health Perspect.* 102:190–193 (1994).

93. Takahashi, M., K. Toyoda, Y. Aze, et al. The rat urinary bladder as a new target of heterocyclic amine carcinogenicity: tumor induction by 3-amino-1-methyl-5*H*-pyrido[4,3-*b*]indole acetate. *Jpn. J. Cancer Res.* 84:852–858 (1993).

94. Hasegawa, R., M. Sano, S. Tamano, et al. Dose-dependence of 2-amino-1-methyl-6-phenylimidazo[4,5-*b*]pyridine (PhIP) carcinogenicity in rats. *Carcinogenesis* 14:2553–2557 (1993).

95. Sone, H., K. Wakabayashi, H. Kushida, et al. Effects of chronic administration of low doses of 2-amino-3,8-dimethyl-imidazo[4,5-*f*]quinoxaline on glutathione S-transferase placental form-positive foci development in the livers of rats fed a choline-deficient diet. *Jpn. J. Cancer Res.* 84:859–864 (1993).

96. Kleman, M.I., E. Övervik, I. Porsch-Hällström, et al. The heterocyclic amines IQ and MeIQx show no promotive effect in a short-term *in vivo* liver carcinogenesis assay. *Carcinogenesis* 14:2123–2125 (1993).

97. Kakiuchi, H., T. Uhijima, M. Ochiai, et al. Rare frequency of activation of the Ki-*ras* gene in rat colon tumors induced by heterocyclic amines: possible alternative mechanisms of human colon carcinogenesis. *Molec. Carcinogen.* 8:44–48 (1993).

98. Ushijima, T., H. Kakiuchi, H. Makino, et al. Infrequent mutation of Ha-*ras* and *p53* in rat mammary carcinomas induced by 2-amino-1-methyl-6-phenylimidazo[4,5-*b*]pyridine. *Molec. Carcinogen.* 10:38–44 (1994).

99. Herzog, C.R., H.A.J. Schut, R.R. Maronpot, and M. You. *ras* Mutations in 2-amino-3-methylimidazo[4,5-*f*]-quinoline–induced tumors in the CDF$_1$ mouse. *Molec. Carcinogen.* 8:202–207 (1993).

100. Takahashi, M., T. Minamoto, T. Sugimura, and H. Esumi. High frequency and low specificity of *ras* gene mutations in rat Zymbal's gland tumors induced by 2-amino-3-methylimidazo[4,5-*f*]quinoline. *Carcinogenesis* 14:1355–1357 (1993).

101. Watanabe, M., and T. Ohta. Analysis of mutational specificity induced by heterocyclic amines in the *lacZ* gene of *Escherichia coli. Carcinogenesis* 14:1149–1153 (1993).

102. Carothers, A.M., W. Yuan, B.E. Hingerty, et al. Mutation and repair induced by the carcinogen 2-(hydroxy-amino)-1-methyl-6-phenylimidazo[4,5-*b*]pyridine (*N*-OH-PhIP) in the dihydrofolate reductase gene of Chinese hamster ovary cells and conformational modeling of the dG-C8-PhIP adduct in DNA. *Chem. Res. Toxicol.* 7:209–218 (1994).

103. Kitazawa, T., R. Kominami, R. Tanaka, et al. 2-Hydroxyamino-1-methyl-6-phenylimidazo[4,5-*b*]pyridine induction of recombinational mutations in mammalian cell lines as detected by DNA fingerprinting. *Molec. Carcinogen.* 9:67–70 (1994).

104. Brooks, R.A., N.J. Gooderham, K. Zhao, et al. 2-Amino-1-methyl-6-phenylimidazo[4,5-*b*]pyridine is a potent mutagen in the mouse small intestine. *Cancer Res.* 54:1665–1671 (1994).

105. Miura, K.F., M. Hatanaka, C. Otsuka, et al. 2-Amino-3-methylimidazo[4,5-*f*]quinoline (IQ), a carcinogenic pyrolysate, induces chromosomal aberrations in Chinese hamster lung fibroblasts *in vitro*. *Mutagenesis* 8:349–354 (1993).

106. Sawada, S., H. Daimon, S. Asakura, et al. Cumulative effects of chromosome aberrations and sister chromatid exchanges in rat liver induced *in vivo* by heterocyclic amines. *Carcinogenesis* 15:285–290 (1994).

107. Ghoshal, A., and E.G. Snyderwine. Excretion of food-derived heterocyclic amine carcinogens into breast milk of lactating rats and formation of DNA adducts in the newborn. *Carcinogenesis* 14:2199–2203 (1993).

108. Davis, C.D., H.A.J. Schut, and E.G. Snyderwine. Adduction of the heterocyclic amine food mutagens IQ and PhIP to mitochrondrial and nuclear DNA in the liver of Fischer-344 rats. *Carcinogenesis* 15:641–645 (1994).

109. Snyderwine, E.G., C.D. Davis, K. Nouso, et al. $^{32}$P-Postlabeling analysis of IQ, MeIQx and PhIP adducts formed *in vitro* in DNA and polynucleotides and found *in vivo* in hepatic DNA from IQ-, MeIQx- and PhIP-treated monkeys. *Carcinogenesis* 14:1389–1395 (1993).

110. Fukutome, K., M. Ochiai, K. Wakabayashi, et al. Detection of guanine-C8-2-amino-1-methyl-6-phenyl-imidazo[4,5-*b*]pyridine adduct as a single spot on thin-layer chromatography by modification of the $^{32}$P-postlabeling method. *Jpn. J. Cancer Res.* 85:113–117 (1994).

111. Ochiai, M., H. Nagaoka, K. Wakabayashi, et al. Identification of $N^2$-(deoxyguanosin-8-yl)-2-amino-3,8-dimethylimidazo[4,5-*f*]quinoxaline 3',5'-diphosphate, a major DNA adduct, detected by nuclease P1 modification of the $^{32}$P-postlabeling method, in the liver of rat fed MeIQx. *Carcinogenesis* 14:2165–2170 (1993).

112. Alldrick, A.J., T.A. Hô, I.R. Rowland, et al. Influence of dietary fat on DNA binding by 2-amino-3,8-dimethylimidazo[4,5-*f*]quinoxaline (MeIQx) in the mouse liver. *Food Chem. Toxicol.* 31:483–489 (1993).

113. Mori, T., K. Shimoi, Y.F. Sasaki, et al. 3-Amino-1,4-dimethyl-5*H*-pyrido[4,3-*b*]indole (Trp-P-1) inhibits the removal of both cyclobutane dimers and (6–4) photoproducts from the DNA of ultraviolet-irradiated *E. coli. Carcinogenesis* 14:1475–1478 (1993).

114. Segawa, T., H. Ishiga, H. Ueno, et al. Genotoxicity and cytotoxicity of 3-amino-1-methyl-5*H*-pyrido[4,3-*b*]indole (Trp-P-2). *Chemosphere* 28:853–861 (1994).

115. Zhang, X.B., and Y. Ohta. Microorganisms in the gastrointestinal tract of the rat prevent absorption of the mutagen–carcinogen 3-amino-1,4-dimethyl-5*H*-pyrido(4,3-*b*)-indole. *Can. J. Microbiol.* 39:841–845 (1993).

116. Thorgeirsson, U.P., A. Farb, R. Virmani, and R.H. Adamson. Cardiac damage induced by 2-amino-3-methyl-imidazo[4,5-*f*]quinoline in nonhuman primates. *Environ. Health Perspect.* 102:194–199 (1994).

117. Davis, C.D., A. Farb, S.S. Thorgeirsson, et al. Cardiotoxicity of heterocyclic amine food mutagens in cultured myocytes and in rats. *Toxicol. Appl. Pharmacol.* 124:201–211 (1994).

118. Sugiyama, S., M. Takasawa, M. Hayakawa, et al. Detrimental effects of 2-amino-1-methyl-6-phenylimidazo-[4,5-b]pyridine, a mutagenic agent, on mitochondrial respiration among various rat tissues. *Biochem. Molec. Biol. Int.* 30:797–805 (1993).

119. Brittebo, E.B. Metabolic activation of the food mutagen Trp-P-1 in endothelial cells of heart and kidney in cytochrome P450-induced mice. *Carcinogenesis* 15:667–672 (1994).

120. Brittebo, E.B., and I. Brandt. Metabolic activation of the food mutagen 3-amino-1,4-dimethyl-5*H*-pyrido[4,3-*b*]indole (Trp-P-1) in endothelial cells of cytochrome P-450-induced mice. *Cancer Res.* 54:2887–2894 (1994).

121. Tikkanen, L.M., T.M. Sauri, and K.J. Latva-Kala. Screening of heat-processed Finnish foods for the mutagens 2-amino-3,8-dimethylimidazo[4,5-*f*]quinoxaline, 2-amino-3,4,8-trimethylimidazo[4,5-*f*]quinoxaline and 2-amino-1-methyl-6-phenylimidazo[4,5-*b*]pyridine. *Food Chem. Toxicol.* 31:717–721 (1993).

122. Gross, G.A., R.J. Turesky, L.B. Fay, et al. Heterocyclic aromatic amine formation in grilled bacon, beef and fish and in grill scrapings. *Carcinogenesis* 14:2313–2318 (1993).

123. Vikse, R., and P.E. Joner. Mutagenicity, creatine and nutrient contents of pan fried meat from various animal species. *Acta Vet. Scand.* 34:363–370 (1993).

124. Davies, J.E., J.K. Chipman, and M.A. Cooke. Mutagen formation in beefburgers processed by frying or microwave with use of flavoring and browning agents. *J. Food Sci.* 58:1216–1218,1223 (1993).

125. Kim, I.-S., K. Wakabayashi, R. Kurosaka, et al. Isolation and identification of a new mutagen, 2-amino-4-hydroxymethyl-3,8-dimethylimidazo[4,5-*f*]quinoxaline (4-CH$_2$OH-8-MeIQx), from beef extract. *Carcinogenesis* 15:21–26 (1994).

126. Jackson, L.S., W.A. Hargraves, W.H. Stroup, and G.W. Diachenko. Heterocyclic aromatic amine content of selected beef flavors. *Mutat. Res.* 320:113–124 (1994).

127. Stavric, B., T.I. Matula, R. Klassen, and R.H. Downie. Analysis of commercial bouillons for trace levels of mutagens. *Food Chem. Toxicol.* 31:981–987 (1993).

128. Murray, S., A.M. Lynch, M.G. Knize, and N.J. Gooderham. Quantification of the carcinogens 2-amino-3,8-dimethyl- and 2-amino-3,4,8-trimethylimidazo[4,5-*f*]quinoxaline and 2-amino-1-methyl-6-phenylimidazo[4,5-*b*]pyridine in food using a combined assay based on gas chromatography–negative ion mass spectrometry. *J. Chromatogr.* 616:211–219 (1993).

129. Galceran, M.T., P. Pais, and L. Puignou. High-performance liquid chromatographic determination of ten heterocyclic aromatic amines with electrochemical detection. *J. Chromatogr. A* 655:101–110 (1993).

130. Boobis, A.R., A.M. Lynch, S. Murray, et al. CYP1A2-catalyzed conversion of dietary heterocyclic amines to their proximate carcinogens is their major route of metabolism in humans. *Cancer Res.* 54:89–94 (1994).

131. Snyderwine, E.G., M.H. Buonarati, J.S. Felton, and K.W. Turteltaub. Metabolism of the food-derived mutagen/

carcinogen 2-amino-1-methyl-6-phenylimidazo[4,5-*b*]pyridine (PhIP) in nonhuman primates. *Carcinogenesis* 14:2517–2522 (1993).

132. Davis, C.D., R.H. Adamson, and E.G. Snyderwine. Studies on the mutagenic activation of heterocyclic amines by cynomolgus monkey, rat and human microsomes show that cynomolgus monkeys have a low capacity to *N*-oxidize the quinoxaline-type heterocyclic amines. *Cancer Lett.* 73:95–104 (1993).

133. Davis, C.D., H.A.J. Schut, and E.G. Snyderwine. Enzymatic phase II activation of the *N*-hydroxylamine of IQ, MeIQx and PhIP by various organs of monkeys and rats. *Carcinogenesis* 14:2091–2096 (1993).

134. Frandsen, H., P.A. Nielsen, S. Grivas, and J.C. Larsen. Microsomal metabolism of the food mutagen 2-amino-3,4,8-trimethyl-3*H*-imidazo[4,5-*f*]-quinoxaline to mutagenic metabolites. *Mutagenesis* 9:59–65 (1994).

135. Weisburger, J.H., A. Rivenson, J. Reinhardt, et al. Genotoxicity and carcinogenicity in rats and mice of 2-amino-3,6-dihydro-3-methyl-7*H*-imidazolo[4,5-*f*]quinolin-7-one: an intestinal bacterial metabolite of 2-amino-3-methyl-3*H*-imidazo[4,5-*f*]quinoline. *J. Natl. Cancer Inst.* 86:25–30 (1994).

136. Guo, X., Y. Ohno, A. Miyajima, et al. Oxysterols inhibit gap junctional communication between rat hepatocytes in primary culture. *Pharmacol. Toxicol.* 73:10–13 (1993).

137. Sarantinos, J., K. O'Dea, and A.J. Sinclair. Cholesterol oxides in Australian foods. Identification and quantification. *Food Aust.* 45:485–490 (1993).

138. Wahle, K.W.J., P.P. Hoppe, and G. McIntosh. Effects of storage and various intrinsic vitamin E concentrations on lipid oxidation in dried egg powders. *J. Sci. Food Agric.* 61:463–469 (1993).

139. Fontana, A., F. Antoniazzi, M.L. Ciavatta, et al. [1]H-NMR study of cholesterol autooxidation in egg powder and cookies exposed to adverse storage. *J. Food Sci.* 58:1286–1290 (1993).

140. Chan, S.-H., J.I. Gray, E.A. Gomaa, et al. Cholesterol oxidation in whole milk powders as influenced by processing and packaging. *Food Chem.* 47:321–328 (1993).

141. Chen, J.-S., and G.-C. Yen. Cholesterol oxidation products in small sun-dried fish. *Food Chem.* 50:167–170 (1994).

142. Osada, K., T. Kodama, L. Cui, et al. Levels and formation of oxidized cholesterols in processed marine foods. *J. Agric. Food Chem.* 41:1893–1898 (1993).

143. Ohshima, T., N. Li, and C. Koizumi. Oxidative decomposition of cholesterol in fish products. *J. Am. Oil Chem. Soc.* 70:595–600 (1993).

144. Engeseth, N.J., and J.I. Gray. Cholesterol oxidation in muscle tissue. *Meat Sci.* 36:309–320 (1994).

145. Korytowski, W., G.J. Backowski, and A.W. Girotti. Analysis of cholesterol and phospholipid hydroperoxides by high-performance liquid chromatography with mercury drop electrochemical detection. *Anal. Biochem.* 213:111–119 (1993).

146. Chen, Y.C., C.P. Chiu, and B.H. Chen. Determination of cholesterol oxides in heated lard by liquid chromatography. *Food Chem.* 50:53–58 (1994).

147. Chen, B.H., and Y.C. Chen. Evaluation of the analysis of cholesterol oxides by liquid chromatography. *J. Chromatogr. A* 661:127–136 (1994).

148. Aubourg, S.P. Review: Interaction of malondi-aldehyde with biological molecules — new trends about reactivity and significance. *Int. J. Food Sci. Technol.* 28:323–335 (1993).

149. Hayam, I., U. Cogan, and S. Mokady. Dietary oxidized oil enhances the activity of $(Na^+K^+)$ ATPase and acetylcholinesterase and lowers the fluidity of rat erythrocyte membrane. *J. Nutr. Biochem.* 4:563–568 (1993).

150. Stapräns, I., J.H. Rapp, X.-M. Pan, and K.R. Feingold. The effect of oxidized lipids in the diet on serum lipoprotein peroxides in control and diabetic rats. *J. Clin. Invest.* 92:638–643 (1993).

151. Hopia, A. Analysis of high molecular weight autoxidation products using high performance size exclusion chromatography: I. Changes during autoxidation. *Lebensm. Wiss. Technol.* 26:563–567 (1993).

152. Hopia, A. Analysis of high molecular weight autoxidation products using high performance size exclusion chromatography: II. Changes during processing. *Lebensm. Wiss. Technol.* 26:568–571 (1993).

153. Schwartz, D.P., A.H. Rady, and S. Castañeda. The formation of oxo- and hydroxy-fatty acids in heated fats and oils. *J. Am. Oil Chem. Soc.* 71:441–444 (1994).

154. Cuesta, C., F.J. Sánchez-Muniz, C. Garrido-Polonio, et al. Thermoxidative and hydrolytic changes in sunflower oil used in fryings with a fast turnover of fresh oil. *J. Am. Oil Chem. Soc.* 70:1069–1073 (1993).

155. Sebedio, J.L., W.M.N. Ratnayake, R.G. Ackman, and J. Prevost. Stability of polyunsaturated omega-3 fatty acids during deep fat frying of Atlantic mackerel (*Scomber scombrus* L.). *Food Res. Int.* 26:163–172 (1993).

156. Davis, L., L. Goodwin, G. Smith, and M. Hole. Lipid oxidation in salted-dried fish: the effect of temperature and light on the rate of oxidation of a fish oil. *J. Sci. Food Agric.* 62:355–359 (1993).

157. Niyati-Shirkhodaee, F., and T. Shibamoto. Formation of toxic aldehydes in cod liver oil after ultraviolet irradiation. *J. Am. Oil Chem. Soc.* 69:1254–1256 (1992).

158. Raharjo, S., J.N. Sofos, and G.R. Schmidt. Solid-phase acid extraction improves thiobarbituric acid method to determine lipid oxidation. *J. Food Sci.* 58:921–924,932 (1993).

159. van de Voort, F.R., A.A. Ismail, J. Sedman, and G. Emo. Monitoring the oxidation of edible oils by Fourier transform infrared spectroscopy. *J. Am. Oil Chem. Soc.* 71:243–253 (1994).

160. Shantha, N.C., and E.A. Decker. Rapid, sensitive, iron-based spectrophotometric methods for determination of peroxide values of food lipids. *J. AOAC Int.* 77:421–424 (1994).

161. Viinanen, E., and A. Hopia. Reversed-phase high-performance liquid chromatographic analysis of triacylglycerol autoxidation products with ultraviolet and evaporative light-scattering detectors. *J. Am. Oil Chem. Soc.* 71:537–539 (1994).

162. Miyazawa, T., K. Fujimoto, M. Kinoshita, and R. Usuki. Rapid estimation of peroxide content of soybean oil by measuring thermoluminescence. *J. Am. Oil Chem. Soc.* 71:343–345 (1994).

163. Mannino, S., M.S. Cosio, and J. Wang. Determination of peroxide value in vegetable oils by an organic-phase enzyme electrode. *Anal. Lett.* 27:299–308 (1994).

164. Garcia-Mesa, J.A., M.D. Luque de Castro, and M. Valcárcel. Automated determination of peroxides in olive oil by flow injection. *Analyst* 118:891–893 (1993).

165. Sebedio, J.L., J. Prevost, E. Ribot, and A. Grandgirard. Utilization of high-performance liquid chromatography as an enrichment step for the determination of cyclic fatty acid monomers in heated fats and biological samples. *J. Chromatogr. A* 659:101–109 (1994).

166. Mahungu, S.M., S.L. Hansen, and W.E. Artz. Quantitation of volatile compounds in heated triolein by static headspace capillary gas chromatography/infrared spectroscopy–mass spectrometry. *J. Am. Oil Chem. Soc.* 71:453–455 (1994).

167. Ajuyah, A.O., T.W. Fenton, R.T. Hardin, and J.S. Sim. Measuring lipid oxidation volatiles in meats. *J. Food Sci.* 58:270–273,277 (1993).

168. Vahl, M. A survey of ethyl carbamate in beverages, bread and acidified milks sold in Denmark. *Food Addit. Contam.* 10:585–592 (1993).

169. Sen, N.P., S.W. Seaman, M. Boyle, and D. Weber. Methyl carbamate and ethyl carbamate in alcoholic beverages and other fermented foods. *Food Chem.* 48:359–366 (1993).

170. Stevens, D.F., and C.S. Ough. Ethyl carbamate formation: reaction of urea and citrulline with ethanol in wine under low to normal temperature conditions. *Am. J. Enol. Vitic.* 44:309–312 (1993).

171. Kodama, S., T. Suzuki, S. Fujinawa, et al. Urea contribution to ethyl carbamate formation in commercial wines during storage. *Am. J. Enol. Vitic.* 45:17–24 (1994).

172. Fauhl, C., R. Catsburg, and R. Wittkowski. Determination of ethyl carbamate in soy sauces. *Food Chem.* 48:313–316 (1993).

173. Dyer, R.H. Determination of ethyl carbamate (urethane) in alcoholic beverages using capillary gas chromatography with thermal energy analyzer detection: collaborative study. *J. AOAC Int.* 77:64–66 (1994).

174. Henle, T., A.W. Walter, and H. Klostermeyer. Detection and identification of the cross-linking amino acids $N^\tau$- and $N^\pi$-(2'-amino-2'-carboxy-ethyl)-L-histidine ("histidinoalanine", HAL) in heated milk products. *Z. Lebensm. Unters. Forsch.* 197:114–117 (1993).

175. Mao, L.-C., K.-H. Lee, and H.F. Erbersdobler. Effects of heat treatment on lysine in soya protein. *J. Sci. Food Agric.* 62:307–309 (1993).

176. Kitts, D.D., C.H. Wu, H.F. Stich, and W.D. Powrie. Effect of glucose–lysine Maillard reaction products on bacterial and mammalian cell mutagenesis. *J. Agric. Food Chem.* 41:2353–2358 (1993).

177. Kitts, D.D., C.H. Wu, and W.D. Powrie. Effect of glucose–lysine Maillard reaction product fractions on

tissue xenobiotic enzyme systems. *J. Agric. Food Chem.* 41:2359–2363 (1993).

178. Surh, Y.-J., and S.R. Tannenbaum. Activation of the Maillard reaction product 5-(hydroxymethyl)furfural to strong mutagens via allylic sulfonation and chlorination. *Chem. Res. Toxicol.* 7:313–317 (1994).

179. García-Villanova, B., E. Guerra-Hernández, E. Martínez-Gómez, and J. Montilla. Liquid chromatography for the determination of 5-(hydroxymethyl)-2-furaldehyde in breakfast cereals. *J. Agric. Food Chem.* 41:1254–1255 (1993).

180. Espinosa-Mansilla, A., A. Muñoz de la Peña, and F. Salinas. Semiautomatic determination of furanic aldehydes in food and pharmaceutical samples by a stopped-flow injection analysis method. *J. AOAC Int.* 76:1255–1261 (1993).

181. Knize, M.G., P.L. Cunningham, E.A. Griffin, Jr., et al. Characterization of mutagenic activity in cooked-grain-food products. *Food Chem. Toxicol.* 32:15–21 (1994).

182. Knize, M.G., P.L. Cunningham, J.R. Avila, et al. Formation of mutagenic activity from amino acids heated at cooking temperatures. *Food Chem. Toxicol.* 32:55–60 (1994).

183. Herraiz, T., and C.S. Ough. Chemical and technological factors determining tetrahydro-β-carboline-3-carboxylic acid content in fermented alcoholic beverages. *J. Agric. Food Chem.* 41:959–964 (1993).

184. Barone, J.J., and H.C. Grice. Seventh International Caffeine Workshop, Santorini, Greece 13–17 June 1993. *Food Chem. Toxicol.* 32:65–77 (1994).

185. Cazeneuve, C., G. Pons, E. Rey, et al. Biotransformation of caffeine in human liver microsomes from foetuses, neonates, infants and adults. *Br. J. Clin. Pharmacol.* 37:405–412 (1994).

186. Fuhr, U., J. Doehmer, N. Battula, et al. Biotransformation of methylxanthines in mammalian cell lines genetically engineered for expression of single cytochrome P450 isoforms. Allocation of metabolic pathways to isoforms and inhibitory effects of quinolones. *Toxicology* 82:169–189 (1993).

187. Nehlig, A., and G. Debry. Potential genotoxic, mutagenic and antimutagenic effects of coffee: A review. *Mutat. Res.* 317:145–162 (1994).

188. Kato, T., K. Hiramoto, and K. Kikugawa. Possible occurrence of new mutagens with the DNA breaking activity in coffee. *Mutat. Res.* 306:9–17 (1994).

189. Olsen, J., and O. Kronborg. Coffee, tobacco and alcohol as risk factors for cancer and adenoma of the large intestine. *Int. J. Epidemiol.* 22:398–402 (1993).

190. Polychronopoulou, A., A. Tzonou, C.-c. Hsieh, et al. Reproductive variables, tobacco, ethanol, coffee and somatometry as risk factors for ovarian cancer. *Int. J. Cancer* 55:402–407 (1993).

191. Folsom, A.R., D.R. McKenzie, K.M. Bisgard, et al. No association between caffeine intake and postmenopausal breast cancer incidence in the Iowa Women's Health Study. *Am. J. Epidemiol.* 138:380–383 (1993).

192. Lina, B.A.R., A.A.J.J.L. Rutten, and R.A. Woutersen. Effect of coffee drinking on cell proliferation in rat urinary bladder epithelium. *Food Chem. Toxicol.* 31:947–951 (1993).

193. Hatch, E.E., and M.B. Bracken. Association of delayed conception with caffeine consumption. *Am. J. Epidemiol.* 138:1082–1092 (1993).

194. Grodstein, F., M.B. Goldman, L. Ryan, and D.W. Cramer. Relation of female infertility to consumption of caffeinated beverages. *Am. J. Epidemiol.* 137:1353–1360 (1993).

195. Fortier, I., S. Marcoux, and L. Beaulac-Baillargeon. Relation of caffeine intake during pregnancy to intrauterine growth retardation and preterm birth. *Am. J. Epidemiol.* 137:931–940 (1993).

196. Larroque, B., M. Kaminski, N. Lelong, et al. Effects on birth weight of alcohol and caffeine consumption during pregnancy. *Am. J. Epidemiol.* 137:941–950 (1993).

197. Sivak, A. Coteratogenic effects of caffeine. *Regul. Toxicol. Pharmacol.* 19:1–13 (1994).

198. Infant-Rivard, C., A. Fernández, R. Gauthier, et al. Fetal loss associated with caffeine intake before and during pregnancy. *JAMA* 270:2940–2943 (1993).

199. Nehlig, A., and G. Debry. Consequences on the newborn of chronic maternal consumption of coffee during gestation and lactation: a review. *J. Am. Coll. Nutr.* 13:6–21 (1994).

200. Gilbert, S.G., and D.C. Rice. *In utero* caffeine exposure affects feeding pattern and variable ratio performance in infant monkeys. *Fund. Appl. Toxicol.* 22:41–50 (1994).

201. Tye, K., I. Pollard, L. Karlsson, et al. Caffeine exposure in utero increases the incidence of apnea in adult rats. *Reproduct. Toxicol.* 7:449–452 (1993).

202. Brown, C.A., C. Bolton-Smith, M. Woodward, and H. Tunstall-Pedoe. Coffee and tea consumption and the prevalence of coronary heart disease in men and women: results from the Scottish Heart Health Study. *J. Epidemiol. Commun. Health* 47:171–175 (1993).

203. Lewis, C.E., B. Caan, E. Funkhouser, et al. Inconsistent associations of caffeine-containing beverages with blood pressure and with lipoproteins. The CARDIA study. *Am. J. Epidemiol.* 138:502–507 (1993).

204. Carson, C.A., J.A. Cauley, and A.W. Caggiula. Relation of caffeine intake to blood lipids in elderly women. *Am. J. Epidemiol.* 138:94–100 (1993).

205. Berndt, B., G.B.M. Mensink, M. Kohlmeier, et al. Lipoprotein metabolism and coffee intake – who is at risk? *Z. Ernährungswiss.* 32:163–175 (1993).

206. Weusten-Van der Wouw, M.P.M.E., M.B. Katan, R. Viani, et al. Identity of the cholesterol-raising factor from boiled coffee and its effects on liver function enzymes. *J. Lipid Res.* 35:721–733 (1994).

207. Heckers, H., U. Göbel, and U. Kleppel. End of the coffee mystery: diterpene alcohols raise serum low-density lipoprotein cholesterol and triglyceride levels. (Letter.) *J. Intern. Med.* 235:192–193 (1994).

208. Haigh, R.A., G.D. Harper, M. Fotherby, et al. Duration of caffeine abstention influences the acute blood pressure responses to caffeine in elderly normotensives. *Eur. J. Clin. Pharmacol.* 44:549–553 (1993).

209. Superko, H.R., J. Myll, C. DiRicco, et al. Effects of cessation of caffeinated-coffee consumption on ambulatory and resting blood pressure in men. *Am. J. Cardiol.* 73:780–784 (1994).

210. Barrett-Connor, E., J.C. Chang, and S.L. Edelstein. Coffee-associated osteoporosis offset by daily milk consumption. *JAMA* 271:280–283 (1994).

211. Massey, L.K., and S.J. Whiting. Caffeine, urinary calcium, calcium metabolism and bone. *J. Nutr.* 123:1611–1614 (1993).

212. Falster, A.U., S. Yoshino, K. Hashimoto, et al. The effect of prenatal caffeine exposure on the enamel surface of the first molars of newborn rats. *Arch. Oral Biol.* 38:441–447 (1993).

213. Nakamoto, T., S.L. Cheuk, S. Yoshino, et al. Cariogenic effect of caffeine intake during lactation on first molars of newborn rats. *Arch. Oral Biol.* 38:919–922 (1993).

214. Hasenfratz, M., and K. Bättig. Acute dose–effect relationships of caffeine and mental performance, EEG, cardiovascular and subjective parameters. *Psychopharmacology* 114:281–287 (1994).

215. Buffalo, E.A., M.P. Gillam, R.R. Allen, and M.G. Paule. Acute effects of caffeine on several operant behaviors in rhesus monkeys. *Pharmacol. Biochem. Behav.* 46:733–737 (1993).

216. Raya, Á., A.M. Cuervo, F. Macián, et al. Nerve conduction velocity decrease and synaptic transmission alterations in caffeine-treated rats. *Neurotoxicol. Teratol.* 16:11–15 (1994).

217. Shi, D., O. Nikodijević, K.A. Jacobson, and J.W. Daly. Chronic caffeine alters the density of adenosine, adrenergic, cholinergic, GABA, and serotonin receptors and calcium channels in mouse brain. *Cell. Molec. Neurobiol.* 13:247–261 (1993).

218. Casiglia, E., P. Spolaore, G. Ginocchio, and G.B. Ambrosio. Unexpected effects of coffee consumption on liver enzymes. *Eur. J. Epidemiol.* 9:293–297 (1993).

219. Kono, S., K. Shinchi, K. Imanishi, et al. Coffee and serum gamma-glutamyltransferase: a study of self-defence officials in Japan. *Am. J. Epidemiol.* 139:723–727 (1994).

220. Kerr, D., R.S. Sherwin, F. Pavalkis, et al. Effect of caffeine on the recognition of and responses to hypoglycemia in humans. *Ann. Intern. Med.* 119:799–804 (1993).

221. Paul, S., B. Kurunwune, and I. Biaggioni. Caffeine withdrawal: apparent heterologous sensitization to adenosine and prostacyclin actions in human platelets. *J. Pharmacol. Exp. Ther.* 267:838–843 (1993).

222. Gecan, J.S., and S.M. Cichowicz. Toxic mushroom contamination of wild mushrooms in commercial distribution. *J. Food Protect.* 56:730–734 (1993).

223. Ramirez, P., P. Parrilla, F. Sanchez Bueno, et al. Fulminant hepatic failure after *Lepiota* mushroom poisoning. *J. Hepatol.* 19:51–54 (1993).

224. Barbato, M.P. Poisoning from accidental ingestion of mushrooms. *Med. J. Aust.* 158:842–847 (1993).

225. Köppel, C. Clinical symptomatology and management of mushroom poisoning. *Toxicon* 31:1513–1540 (1993).

226. Toth, B., and P. Gannett. *Agaricus Bisporus*: An assessment of its carcinogenic potency. *Mycopathologia* 124:73–77 (1993).

227. Papaparaskeva-Petrides, C., C. Ioannides, and R. Walker. Contribution of phenolic and quinonoid structures in the mutagenicity of the edible mushroom *Agaricus bisporus*. *Food Chem. Toxicol.* 31:561–567 (1993).

228. Slanina, P., E. Cekan, B. Halen, et al. Toxicological studies of the false morel (*Gyromitra esculenta*): embryotoxicity of monomethylhydazine in the rat. *Food Addit. Contam.* 10:391–398 (1993).

229. Tsunoda, K., N. Inoue, Y. Aoyagi, and T. Sugahara. Change in ibotenic acid and muscimol contents in *Amanita muscaria* during drying, storing or cooking. *J. Food Hyg. Soc. Japan* 34:153–160 (1993).

230. Enjalbert, F., C. Gallion, F. Jehl, and H. Monteil. Toxin content, phallotoxin and amatoxin composition of *Amanita phalloides* tissues. *Toxicon* 31:803–807 (1993).

231. Enjalbert, F., C. Gallion, F. Jehl, et al. Amatoxins and phallotoxins in *Amanita* species: high-performance liquid chromatographic determination.*Mycologia* 85:579–584 (1993).

232. Chauvin, P., J.-C. Dillon, A. Moren, et al. Heliotrope poisoning in Tadjikistan. (Letter.) *Lancet* 341:1663 (1993).

233. Mayer, F., and J. Lüthy. Heliotrope poisoning in Tadjikistan. (Letter.) *Lancet* 342:246–247 (1993).

234. Betz, J.M., R.M. Eppley, W.C. Taylor, and D. Andrzejewski. Determination of pyrrolizidine alkaloids in commercial comfrey products (*Symphytum* sp.). *J. Pharm. Sci.* 83:649–653 (1994).

235. Winter, H., A.A. Seawright, H.J. Noltie, et al. Pyrrolizidine alkaloid poisoning of yaks: identification of the plants involved. *Vet. Rec.* 134:135–139 (1994).

236. Kim, H.-Y., F.R. Stermitz, R.J. Molyneux, et al. Structural influences on pyrrolizidine alkaloid-induced cytopathology. *Toxicol. Appl. Pharmacol.* 122:61–69 (1993).

237. Dao, L., and M. Friedman. Chlorophyll, chlorogenic acid, glycoalkaloid, and protease inhibitor content of fresh and green potatoes. *J. Agric. Food Chem.* 42:633–639 (1994).

238. Griffiths, D.W., M.F.B. Dale, and H. Bain. The effect of cultivar, maturity and storage on photo-induced changes in the total glycoalkaloid and chlorophyll contents of potatoes (*Solanum tuberosum*). *Plant Sci.* 98:103–109 (1994).

239. Dale, M.F.B., D.W. Griffiths, H. Bain, and D. Todd. Glycoalkaloid increase in *Solanum tuberosum* on exposure to light. *Ann. Appl. Biol.* 123:411–418 (1993).

240. Friedman, M., G. McDonald, and W.F. Haddon. Kinetics of acid-catalyzed hydrolysis of carbohydrate groups of potato glycoalkaloids α-chaconine and α-solanine. *J. Agric. Food Chem.* 41:1397–1406 (1993).

241. Groen, K., D.P.K.H. Pereboom-de Fauw, P. Besamusca, et al. Bioavailability and disposition of $^3$H-solanine in rat and hamster. *Xenobiotica* 23:995–1005 (1993).

242. Ferreira, F., P. Moyna, S. Soule, and A. Vázquez. Rapid determination of solanum glycoalkaloids by thin-layer chromatographic scanning. *J. Chromatogr. A* 653:380–384 (1993).

243. Houben, R.J., and K. Brunt. Determination of glycoalkaloids in potato tubers by reversed-phase high-performance liquid chromatography.*J. Chromatogr. A* 661:169–174 (1994).

244. Plhak, L., and P. Sporns. Development and production of monoclonal antibodies for the measurement of solanidine potato glycoalkaloids. *Am. Potato J.* 71:297–313 (1994).

245. Takagi, K., M. Toyoda, M. Shimizu, et al. Determination of tomatine in foods by liquid chromatography after derivatization. *J. Chromatogr. A* 659:127–131 (1994).

246. Chan, T.Y.K., B. Tomlinson, and J.A.J.H. Critchley. Aconitine poisoning following the ingestion of Chinese herbal medicines: a report of eight cases.*Aust. N.Z. J. Med.* 23:268–271 (1993).

247. Chan, T.Y.K., and C.S. Cockram. Herb-induced aconitine poisoning presenting as tetraplegia. *Vet. Human Toxicol.* 36:133–134 (1994).

248. But, P.P.-H., Y.-T. Tai, and K. Young. Three fatal cases of herbal aconite poisoning. *Vet. Human Toxicol.* 36:212–215 (1994).

249. Saisho, K., M. Toyoda, K. Takagi, et al. Identification of aconitine in raw honey that caused food poisoning. *J. Food Hyg. Soc. Japan* 35:46–50 (1994).

250. Wada, K., H. Bando, and N. Kawahara. Determination and quantitative analysis of *Aconitum* alkaloids in plants by liquid chromatography—atmospheric pressure chemical ionization mass spectrometry. *J. Chromatogr.* 644:43–48 (1993).

251. Vanhaelen, M., R. Vanhaelen-Fastre, P. But, and J.-L. Vanherweghem. Identification of aristolochic acid in Chinese herbs. (Letter.) *Lancet* 343:174 (1994).

252. Cosyns, J.P., M. Jadoul, J.-P. Squifflet, et al. Chinese herbs nephropathy: A clue to Balkan endemic nephropathy? *Kidney Int.* 45:1680–1688 (1994).

253. Zhu, B.T., E.L. Ezell, and J.G. Liehr. Catechol-*O*-methyltransferase-catalyzed rapid *O*-methylation of mutagenic flavonoids. *J. Biol. Chem.* 269:292–299 (1994).

254. Zhu, B.T., and J.G. Liehr. Quercetin increases the severity of estradiol-induced tumorigenesis in hamster kidney. *Toxicol. Appl. Pharmacol.* 125:149–158 (1994).

255. Ahmed, M.S., V. Ramesh, V. Nagaraja, et al. Mode of binding of quercetin to DNA.*Mutagenesis* 9:193–197 (1994).

256. Sahu, S.C., and G.C. Gray. Interactions of flavonoids, trace metals, and oxygen: nuclear DNA damage and lipid peroxidation induced by myricetin. *Cancer Lett.* 70:73–79 (1993).

257. da Fonseca, C.A.S., J. Leal, S.S. Costa, and A.C. Leitão. Genotoxic and mutagenic effects of guarana (*Paullinia cupana*) in prokaryotic organisms. *Mutat. Res.* 321:165–173 (1994).

258. Afek, U., E. Gross, N. Aharoni, et al. An outbreak of phytophotodermatitis due to celery.*Int. J. Dermatol.* 33:116–118 (1994).

259. Nigg, H.N., H.E. Nordby, R.C. Beier, et al. Phototoxic coumarins in limes. *Food Chem. Toxicol.* 31:331–335 (1993).

260. Cai, Y., D. Bennett, R.V. Nair, et al. Inhibition and inactivation of murine hepatic ethoxy- and pentoxyresorufin

*O*-dealkylase by naturally occurring coumarins. *Chem. Res. Toxicol.* 6:872–879 (1993).

261. Jansman, A.J.M., H. Enting, M.W.A. Verstegen, and J. Huisman. Effect of condensed tannins in hulls of faba beans (*Vicia faba* L.) on the activities of trypsin (*EC* 2.4.21.4) and chymotrypsin (*EC* 2.4.21.1) in digesta collected from the small intestine of pigs. *Br. J. Nutr.* 71:627–641 (1994).

262. Chang, M.-C.J., J.W. Bailey, and J.L. Collins. Dietary tannins from cowpeas and tea transiently alter apparent calcium absorption but not absorption and utilization of protein in rats. *J. Nutr.* 124:283–288 (1994).

263. Jansman, A.J.M., A.A. Frohlich, and R.R. Marquardt. Production of proline-rich proteins by the parotid glands of rats is enhanced by feeding diets containing tannins from faba beans (*Vicia faba* L.). *J. Nutr.* 124:249–258 (1994).

264. Babiker, E.E., and A.H. El Tinay. Effect of reconstitution and Na$_2$CO$_3$ on tannin content and in vitro protein digestibility of faba bean cultivars. *Plant Foods Human Nutr.* 44:119–130 (1993).

265. El Khalifa, A.O., and A.H. El Tinay. Effect of fermentation on protein fractions and tannin content of low- and high-tannin cultivars of sorghum. *Food Chem.* 49:265–269 (1994).

266. de Peyster, A., and Y.Y. Wang. Genetic toxicity studies of gossypol. *Mutat. Res.* 297:293–312 (1993).

267. Meldrum, B. Amino acids as dietary excitotoxins: a contribution to understanding neurodegenerative disorders. *Brain Res. Rev.* 18:293–314 (1993).

268. Lipton, S.A., and P.A. Rosenberg. Excitatory amino acids as a final common pathway for neurologic disorders. *New Engl. J. Med.* 330:613–622 (1994).

269. Spencer, P.S., A.C. Ludolph, and G.E. Kisby. Neurologic diseases associated with use of plant components with toxic potential. *Environ. Res.* 62:106–113 (1993).

270. Zagon, J., L.-I. Dehne, and K.W. Bögl. D-amino acids in organisms and food. *Nutr. Res.* 14:445–463 (1994).

271. Philen, R.M., R.H. Hill, Jr., W.D. Flanders, et al. Tryptophan contaminants associated with eosinophilia-myalgia syndrome. *Am. J. Epidemiol.* 138:154–159 (1993).

272. Sidransky, H., E. Verney, J.W. Cosgrove, et al. Studies with 1,1'-ethylidenebis(tryptophan), a contaminant associated with L-tryptophan implicated in the eosinophilia–myalgia syndrome. *Toxicol. Appl. Pharmacol.* 126:108–113 (1994).

273. Brenneman, D.E., S.W. Page, M. Schultzberg, et al. A decomposition product of a contaminant implicated in L-tryptophan eosinophilia myalgia syndrome affects spinal cord neuronal cell death and survival through stereospecific, maturation and partly interleukin-1-dependent mechanisms. *J. Pharmacol. Exp. Ther.* 266:1029–1035 (1993).

274. Yamaoka, K.A., N. Miyasaka, G. Inui, et al. 1,1'-Ethylidenebis(tryptophan) (peak E) induces functional activation of human eosinophils and interleukin 5 production from T lymphocytes: association of eosinophilia-myalgia syndrome with a L-tryptophan contaminant. *J. Clin. Immunol.* 14:50–60 (1994).

275. Trucksess, M.W., F.S. Thomas, and S.W. Page. High-performance liquid chromatographic determination of 1,1'-ethylidenebis(L-tryptophan) in L-tryptophan preparations. *J. Pharm. Sci.* 83:720–722 (1994).

276. Tekle-Haimanot, R., B.M. Abegaz, E. Wuhib, et al. Pattern of *Lathyrus sativus* (grass pea) consumption and *beta-N*-oxalyl-α-β-diaminoproprionic acid (β-ODAP) content of food samples in the lathyrism endemic region of northwest Ethiopia. *Nutr. Res.* 13:1113–1126 (1993).

277. Lambein, F., R. Haque, J.K. Khan, et al. From soil to brain: zinc deficiency increases the neurotoxicity of *Lathyrus sativus* and may affect the susceptibility for the motorneurone disease neurolathyrism. *Toxicon* 32:461–466 (1994).

278. Pai, K.S., S.K. Shankar, and V. Ravindranath. Billionfold difference in the toxic potencies of two excitatory plant amino acids, L-BOAA and L-BMAA: biochemical and morphological studies using mouse brain slices. *Neurosci. Res.* 17:241–248 (1993).

279. Iwami, O., Y. Niki, T. Watanabe, and M. Ikeda. Motor neuron disease on the Kii Peninsula of Japan: cycad exposure. *Neuroepidemiology* 12:307–312 (1993).

280. Blanshard, A.F.J., M.T. Dahniya, N.H. Poulter, and A.J. Taylor. Quality of cassava foods in Sierra Leone. *J. Sci. Food Agric.* 64:425–432 (1994).

281. Akingbala, J.O., G.B. Oguntimein, and M.K. Bolade. Effect of unit operations of production on the cyanide content and acceptability of gari. *J. Food Process. Preserv.* 17:337–350 (1993).

282. Padmaja, G., M. George, and S.N. Moorthy. Detoxification of cassava during fermentation with a mixed culture inoculum. *J. Sci. Food Agric.* 63:473–481 (1993).

283. Ragoobirsingh, D., H.M. Robinson, and E.Y.St.A. Morrison. Effects of cassava cyanoglucoside, linamarin, on blood sugar levels in the dog. *J. Nutr. Biochem.* 4:625–629 (1993).

284. Essers, S.A.J.A., M. Bosveld, R.M. van der Grift, and A.G.J. Voragen. Studies on the quantification of specific cyanogens in cassava products and introduction of a new chromogen. *J. Sci. Food Agric.* 63:287–296 (1994).

285. Yeoh, H.-H., and C.-K.C. Tan. An enzyme-immobilized microplate for determination of linamarin for large number of samples. *Biotechnol. Tech.* 8:337–338 (1994).

286. Yeoh, H.-H. Nylon-linamarase electrode for rapid determination of linamarin. *Biotechnol. Tech.* 7:761–764 (1993).

287. Bhatty, R.S. Further compositional analyses of flax: mucilage, trypsin inhibitors and hydrocyanic acid. *J. Am. Oil Chem. Soc.* 70:899–904 (1993).

288. Wanasundara, P.K.J.P.D., R. Amarowicz, M.T. Kara, and F. Shahidi. Removal of cyanogenic glycosides of flaxseed meal. *Food Chem.* 48:263–266 (1993).

289. Amarowicz, R., and F. Shahidi. Application of sephadex LH-20 chromatography for the separation of cyanogenic glycosides and hydrophylic phenolic fraction from flaxseed. *J. Liq. Chromatogr.* 17:1291–1299 (1994).

290. Van Boven, M., N. Blaton, M. Cokelaere, and P. Daenens. Isolation, purification, and stereochemistry of simmondsin. *J. Agric. Food Chem.* 41:1605–1607 (1993).

291. Van Boven, M., S. Toppet, M.M. Cokelaere, and P. Daenens. Isolation and structural identification of a new simmondsin ferulate from jojoba meal. *J. Agric. Food Chem.* 42:1118–1121 (1994).

292. Obizoba, I.C., and J.V. Atii. Evaluation of the effect of processing techniques on the nutrient and antinutrient contents of pearl millet (*Pennisetum glaucum*) seeds. *Plant Foods Human Nutr.* 45:23–34 (1994).

293. El-Adawy, T.A., E.H. Rahma, A.A. El-Badawey, et al. Biochemical studies of some non-conventional sources of proteins. Part 7. Effect of detoxification treatments on the nutritional quality of apricot kernels. *Nahrung* 38:12–20 (1994).

294. Goonasekera, C.D.A., V.W.J.K. Vasanthathilake, N. Ratnatunga, and C.A.S. Seneviratne. Is Nai Habarala (*Alocasia cucullata*) a poisonous plant? *Toxicon* 31:813–816 (1993).

295. Musk, S.R.R., and I.T. Johnson. The clastogenic effects of isothiocyanates. *Mutat. Res.* 300:111–117 (1993).

296. Kore, A.M., and M.A. Wallig. Histological and serum biochemical effects of 1-isothiocyanato-3-(methylsulphinyl)-propane in the F344 rat. *Food Chem. Toxicol.* 31:549–559 (1993).

297. Kore, A.M., E.H. Jeffery, and M.A. Wallig. Effects of 1-isothiocyanato-3-(methylsulfinyl)-propane on xenobiotic metabolizing enzymes in rats. *Food Chem. Toxicol.* 31:723–729 (1993).

298. Yen, G.-C., and Q.-K. Wei. Myrosinase activity and total glucosinolate content of cruciferous vegetables, and some properties of cabbage myrosinase in Taiwan. *J. Sci. Food Agric.* 61:471–475 (1993).

299. Rosa, E.A.S., and R.K. Heaney. The effect of cooking and processing on the glucosinolate content: studies on four varieties of Portuguese cabbage and hybrid white cabbage. *J. Sci. Food Agric.* 62:259–265 (1993).

300. Abukutsa, M.O., J.A. Chweya, B.O. Mochoge, and J.C. Onyango. Effect of nitrogen sources and storage on thiocyanate content of kale (*Brassica oleracea* var. *Acephala*) leaves. *Discovery Innovation* 5:367–371 (1993).

301. Zhao, F., E.J. Evans, P.E. Bilsborrow, and J.K. Syers. Influence of sulphur and nitrogen on seed yield and quality of low glucosinolate oilseed rape (*Brassica napus* L). *J. Sci. Food Agric.* 63:29–37 (1993).

302. Zhao, F., E.J. Evans, P.E. Bilsborrow, and J.K. Syers. Influence of nitrogen and sulphur on the glucosinolate profile of rapeseed (*Brassica napus* L). *J. Sci. Food Agric.* 61:295–304 (1994).

303. Alpuche-Solis, A.G,. and O. Paredes-Lopez. Assessment of glucosinolates in broccoli by three different methodologies. *J. Food Biochem.* 16:265–275 (1993).

304. Schnug, E., F. Murray, and S. Haneklaus. Preparation techniques of small sample sizes for sulphur and indirect total glucosinolate analysis in *Brassica* seeds by X-ray fluorescence spectroscopy. *Fat Sci. Technol.* 95:334–337 (1993).

305. Slater, G.P., and J.F. Manville. Analysis of thiocyanates and isothiocyanates by ammonia chemical ionization gas chromatography–mass spectrometry and gas chromatography–Fourier transform infrared spectroscopy. *J. Chromatogr.* 648:433–443 (1993).

306. Feldl, C., P. Møller, J. Otte, and H. Sørensen. Micellar electrokinetic capillary chromatography for determination of indolyl glucosinolates and transformation products thereof. *Anal. Biochem.* 217:62–69 (1994).

307. Elfakir, C., M. Lafosse, and M. Dreux. Retention of some glucosinolates in anion exchange chromatography. Part I: Qualitative study on a silica-trialkylammonium exchanger. *Chromatographia* 37:313–318 (1993).

308. Grant, G., P.M. Dorward, and A. Pusztai. Pancreatic enlargement is evident in rats fed diets containing raw soybeans (*Glycine max*) or cowpeas (*Vigna unguiculata*) for 800 days but not in those fed diets based on kidney beans (*Phaseolus vulgaris*) or lupinseed (*Lupinus angustifolius*). *J. Nutr.* 123:2207–2215 (1993).

309. Barth, C.A., B. Lunding, M. Schmitz, and H. Hagemeister. Soybean trypsin inhibitor(s) reduce absorption of exogenous and increase loss of endogenous protein in miniature pigs. *J. Nutr.* 123:2195–2200 (1993).

310. Bergeron, D., and S.S. Nielsen. Partial characterization of trypsin inhibitors and *N*-terminal sequences of five trypsin isoinhibitors of Great Northern beans (*Phaseolus vulgaris*). *J. Agric. Food Chem.* 41:1544–1549 (1993).

311. Godbole, S.A., T.G. Krishna, and C.R. Bhatia. Purification and characterisation of protease inhibitors from pigeon pea (*Cajanus cajan* (L) Millsp) seeds. *J. Sci. Food Agric.* 64:87–93 (1994).

312. Argall, M.E., J.H. Bradbury, and D.C. Shaw. Aminoacid sequence of a trypsin/chymotrypsin inhibitor from giant taro (*Alocasia macrorrhiza*). *Biochim. Biophys. Acta* 1204:189–194 (1994).

313. Peng, L., J.H. Bradbury, B.C. Hammer, and D.C. Shaw. Comparison of amino acid sequences of the trypsin inhibitors from taro (*Colocasia esculenta*), giant taro (*Alocasia macrorrhiza*) and giant swamp taro (*Cyrtosperma chamissonis*). *Biochem. Molec. Biol. Int.* 31:73–81 (1993).

314. Valdes-Rodriguez, S., M. Segura-Nieto, A. Chagolla-Lopez, et al. Purification, characterization, and complete amino acid sequence of a trypsin inhibitor from amaranth (*Amaranthus hypochondriacus*) seeds. *Plant Physiol.* 103:1407–1412 (1993).

315. Arentoft, A.M., H. Frøkiær, S. Michaelsen, et al. High-performance capillary electrophoresis for the determination of trypsin and chymotrypsin inhibitors and their association with trypsin, chymotrypsin and monoclonal antibodies. *J. Chromatogr. A* 652:189–198 (1993).

316. Kwok, K.C., W.H. Qin, and J.C. Tsang. Heat inactivation of trypsin inhibitors in soymilk at ultra-high temperatures. *J. Food Sci.* 58:859–862 (1993).

317. Piergiovanni, A.R., C. Della Gatta, and P. Perrino. Effects of storage conditions on the trypsin inhibitor content in flour and whole seeds of cowpea (*Vigna unguiculata*). *Lebensm. Wiss. Technol.* 26:426–429 (1993).

318. Mulimani, V.H., and S. Vadiraj. Effects of heat treatment and germination on trypsin and chymotrypsin inhibitory activities in sorghum (*Sorghum bicolor* (L.) Moench) seeds. *Plant Foods Human Nutr.* 44:221–226 (1993).

319. Vidal-Valverde, C., J. Frias, M. Prodanov, et al. Effect of natural fermentation on carbohydrates, riboflavin and

trypsin inhibitor activity of lentils. *Z. Lebensm. Unters. Forsch.* 197:449–452 (1993).

320. Kumar, A., and B.M. Chauhan. Effects of phytic acid on protein digestibility (in vitro) and HCl-extractability of minerals in pearl millet sprouts. *Cereal Chem.* 70:504–506 (1993).

321. Svanberg, U., W. Lorri, and A.-S. Sandberg. Lactic fermentation of non-tannin and high-tannin cereals: effects on *in vitro* estimation of iron availability and phytate hydrolysis. *J. Food Sci.* 58:408–412 (1993).

322. Wolters, M.G.E., H.A.W. Schreuder, G. van den Heuvel, et al. A continuous *in vitro* method for estimation of the bioavailability of minerals and trace elements in foods: application to breads varying in phytic acid content. *Br. J. Nutr.* 69:849–861 (1993).

323. Han, O., M.L. Failla, A.D. Hill, et al. Inositol phosphates inhibit uptake and transport of iron and zinc by a human intestinal cell line. *J. Nutr.* 124:580–587 (1994).

324. Proulx, W.R., C.M. Weaver, and M.A. Bock. Trypsin inhibitor activity and tannin content do not affect calcium bioavailability of three commonly consumed legumes. *J. Food Sci.* 58:382–384 (1993).

325. Larsen, T. Dephytinization of a rat diet. Consequences for mineral and trace element absorption. *Biol. Trace Elem. Res.* 39:55–71 (1993).

326. Rimbach, G., and J. Pallauf. Enhancement of zinc utilization from phytate-rich soy protein isolate by microbial phytase. *Z. Ernährungswiss.* 32:308–315 (1993).

327. Udosen, E.O., and U.M. Ukpanah. The toxicants and phosphorus content of some Nigerian vegetables. *Plant Foods Human Nutr.* 44:285–289 (1993).

328. Mameesh, M.S., and M. Tomar. Phytate content of some popular Kuwaiti foods. *Cereal Chem.* 70:502–503 (1993).

329. Ravindran, V., G. Ravindran, and S. Sivalogan. Total and phytate phosphorus contents of various foods and feedstuffs of plant origin. *Food Chem.* 50:133–136 (1994).

330. Igbedioh, S.O., K.T. Olugbemi, and M.A. Akpapunam. Effects of processing methods on phytic acid level and some constituents in bambara groundnut (*Vigna subterranea*) and pigeon pea (*Cajanus cajan*). *Food Chem.* 50:147–151 (1994).

331. Beleia, A., L.T. Tua Thao, and E.I. Ida. Lowering phytic phosphorus by hydration of soybeans. *J. Food Sci.* 58:375–377,388 (1993).

332. Trugo, L.C., C.M. Donangelo, Y.A. Duarte, and C.L. Tavares. Phytic acid and selected mineral composition of seed from wild species and cultivated varieties of lupin. *Food Chem.* 47:391–394 (1993).

333. Rounds, M.A., and S.S. Nielsen. Anion-exchange high-performance liquid chromatography with post-column detection for the analysis of phytic acid and other inositol phosphates. *J. Chromatogr. A* 653:148–152 (1993).

334. Liener, I.E. Implications of antinutritional components in soybean foods. *Crit. Rev. Food Sci. Nutr.* 34:31–67 (1994).

335. Reddy, N.R., and M.D. Pierson. Reduction in antinutritional and toxic components in plant foods by fermentation. *Food Res. Int.* 27:281–290 (1994).

336. Gahlawat, P., and S. Sehgal. Antinutritional content of developed weaning foods as affected by domestic processing. *Food Chem.* 47:333–336 (1993).

337. Muzquiz, M., C.L. Ridout, K.R. Price, and G.R. Fenwick. The saponin content and composition of sweet and bitter lupin seed. *J. Sci. Food Agric.* 63:47–52 (1993).

338. Ruales, J., and B.M. Nair. Saponins, phytic acid, tannins and protease inhibitors in quinoa (*Chenopodium quinoa*, Willd) seeds. *Food Chem.* 48:137–143 (1993).

339. Gee, J.M., K.R. Price, C.L. Ridout, et al. Saponins of quinoa (*Chenopodium quinoa*): effects of processing on their abundance in quinoa products and their biological effects on intestinal mucosal tissue. *J. Sci. Food Agric.* 63:201–209 (1993).

340. Ng, K.G., K.R. Price, and G.R. Fenwick. A TLC method for the analysis of quinoa (*Chenopodium quinoa*) saponins. *Food Chem.* 49:311–315 (1994).

341. Önning, G., and N.-G. Asp. Analysis of saponins in oat kernels. *Food Chem.* 48:301–305 (1993).

342. Önning, G., N.-G. Asp, and B. Sivik. Saponin content in different oat varieties and in different fractions of oat grain. *Food Chem.* 48:251–254 (1993).

343. Santiago, J.G., A. Levy-Benshimol, and A. Carmona. Effect of *Phaseolus vulgaris* lectins on glucose absorption, transport, and metabolism in rat everted intestinal sacs. *J. Nutr. Biochem.* 4:426–430 (1993).

344. Savelkoul, F.H.M.G., S. Tamminga, P.P.A.M. Leenaars, et al. The degradation of lectins, phaseolin and trypsin inhibitors during germination of white kidney beans, *Phaseolus vulgaris* L. *Plant Foods Human Nutr.* 45:213–222 (1994).

345. Trugo, L.C., A. Farah, and N.M.F. Trugo. Germination and debittering lupin seeds reduce α-galactoside and intestinal carbohydrate fermentation in humans. *J. Food Sci.* 58:627–630 (1993).

346. Somiari, R.I., and E. Balogh. Effect of soaking, cooking and crude α-galactosidase treatment on the oligosaccharide content of cowpea flours. *J. Sci. Food Agric.* 61:339–343 (1993).

347. Duszkiewicz-Reinhard, W., E. Gujska, and K. Khan. Reduction of stachyose in legume flours by lactic acid bacteria. *J. Food Sci.* 59:115–117 (1994).

348. Grases, F., A. Costa-Bauzá, A. García-Raso, and J.G. March. Kinetic-turbidimetric determination of stachyose based on its inhibitory action on sucrose crystallization. *Anal. Lett.* 27:819–829 (1994).

349. Miksicek, R.J. Commonly occurring plant flavonoids have estrogenic activity. *Molec. Pharmacol.* 44:37–43 (1993).

350. Rosenblum, E.R., R.E. Stauber, D.H. Van Thiel, et al. Assessment of the estrogenic activity of phytoestrogens isolated from bourbon and beer. *Alcoholism: Clin. Exp. Res.* 17:1207–1209 (1993).

351. Whitten, P.L., C. Lewis, and F. Naftolin. A phytoestrogen diet induces the premature anovulatory syn-

drome in lactationally exposed female rats. *Biol. Reproduct.* 49:1117–1121 (1993).

352. Riepl, R.L., J. Schreiner, B. Müller, et al. „Dicke Bohnen" als Auslöser einer akuten hämolytischen Anämie. *Dtsch. Med. Wschr.* 118:932–935 (1993).

353. McMillan, D.C., K.L. Schey, G.P. Meier, and D.J. Jollow. Chemical analysis and hemolytic activity of the fava bean aglycon divicine. *Chem. Res. Toxicol.* 6:439–444 (1993).

354. Centers for Disease Control. Ostrich fern poisoning—New York and western Canada, 1994. *Morbid. Mortal. Weekly Rep.* 43:677,683–684 (1994).

355. Earl, J.W., and B.V. McCleary. Mystery of the poisoned expedition. *Nature* 368:683–684 (1994).

356. Hirono, I. Edible plants containing naturally occurring carcinogens in Japan. *Jpn. J. Cancer Res.* 84:997–1006 (1993).

357. Alonso-Amelot, M.E., U. Castillo, and F. De Jongh. Passage of the bracken fern carcinogen ptaquiloside into bovine milk. *Lait* 73:323–332 (1993).

358. Kushida, T., M. Uesugi, Y. Sugiura, et al. DNA damage by ptaquiloside, a potent bracken carcinogen: detection of selective strand breaks and identification of DNA cleavage products. *J. Am. Chem. Soc.* 116:479–486 (1994).

359. Megia, A., L. Herranz, M.A. Martin-Almendra, and I. Martinez. Angiotensin I-converting enzyme levels and renin-aldosterone axis recovery after cessation of chronic licorice ingestion. *Nephron* 65:329–330 (1993).

360. Schambelan, M. Licorice ingestion and blood pressure regulating hormones. *Steroids* 59:127–130 (1994).

361. Mizugaki, M., K. Itoh, M. Hayasaka, et al. Monoclonal antibody-based enzyme-linked immunosorbent assay for glycyrrhizin and its aglicon, glycyrrhetic acid. *J. Immunoassay* 15:21–34 (1994).

362. López-Carrillo, L., M. Hernández Avila, and R. Dubrow. Chili pepper consumption and gastric cancer in Mexico: a case–control study. *Am. J. Epidemiol.* 139:263–271 (1994).

363. Espinosa-Aguirre, J.J., R.E. Reyes, J. Rubio, et al. Mutagenic activity of urban air samples and its modulation by chili extracts. *Mutat. Res.* 303:55–61 (1993).

364. Villaseñor, I.M., and E.J. de Ocampo. Clastogenicity of red pepper (*Capsicum frutescens* L.) extracts. *Mutat. Res.* 312:151–155 (1994).

365. Higashimoto, M., J. Purintrapiban, K. Kataoka, et al. Mutagenicity and antimutagenicity of extracts of three spices and a medicinal plant in Thailand. *Mutat. Res.* 303:135–142 (1993).

366. Smith, B.C., and P.V. Desmond. Acute hepatitis induced by ingestion of the herbal medication chaparral. (Letter.) *Aust. N.Z. J. Med.* 23:526 (1993).

367. Unnithan, S., and J. Strang. Poppy tea dependence. *Br. J. Psychiat.* 163:813–814 (1993).

368. Loeper, J., V. Descatoire, P. Letteron, et al. Hepatotoxicity of germander in mice. *Gastroenterology* 106:464–472 (1994).

369. Parodi, B., G. Caviglioli, A. Bachi, et al. Herbal mixtures with claimed slimming activity: determination

by TLC and HPLC of illegally added drugs. *Pharmazie* 48:678–681 (1993).

370. Centers for Disease Control. Water hemlock poisoning—Maine, 1992. *Morbid. Mortal. Weekly Rep.* 43:229–230 (1994).

371. Yulevich, A., R. Finaly, and A.J. Mares. Candy bezoar: an unusual cause of food bolus bezoar. *J. Pediatr. Gastroenterol. Nutr.* 17:108–110 (1993).

372. Gottrand, F., T. Erkan, D. Turck, et al. Food-induced bleeding from lymphonodular hyperplasia of the colon. *Am. J. Dis. Child.* 147:821–823 (1993).

373. Munday, R., and E. Manns. Comparative toxicity of prop(en)yl disulfides derived from Alliaceae: possible involvement of 1-propenyl disulfides in onion-induced hemolytic anemia. *J. Agric. Food Chem.* 42:959–962 (1994).

374. Jansen, J.J.N., A.F.M. Kardinaal, G. Huijbers, et al. Prevalence of food allergy and intolerance in the adult Dutch population. *J. Aller. Clin. Immunol.* 93:446–456 (1994).

375. Young, E., M.D. Stoneham, A. Petruckevitch, et al. A population study of food intolerance. *Lancet* 343:1127–1130 (1994).

376. Kivity, S., K. Dunner, and Y. Marian. The pattern of food hypersensitivity in patients with onset after 10 years of age. *Clin. Exp. Aller.* 24:19–22 (1994).

377. Lezaun, A., J.M. Igea, S. Quirce, et al. Asthma and contact urticaria caused by rice in a housewife. *Allergy* 49:92–95 (1994).

378. Erben, A.M., J.L. Rodriguez, J. McCullough, and D.R. Ownby. Anaphylaxis after ingestion of beignets contaminated with *Dermatophagoides farinae*. *J. Aller. Clin. Immunol.* 92:846–849 (1993).

379. Martín Muñoz, F., J.M. López Cazaña, F. Villas, et al. Exercise-induced anaphylactic reaction to hazelnut. *Allergy* 49:314–316 (1994).

380. Parra, F.M., M. Cuevas, A. Lezaun, et al. Pistachio nut hypersensitivity: identification of pistachio nut allergens. *Clin. Exp. Aller.* 23:996–1001 (1993).

381. Bock, S.A. Anaphylaxis to coriander: a sleuthing story. *J. Aller. Clin. Immunol.* 91:1232–1233 (1993).

382. Reed, B.E., A.P. Barrett, C. Katelaris, and M. Bilous. Orofacial sensitivity reactions and the role of dietary components. Case reports. *Aust. Dent. J.* 38:287–291 (1993).

383. Thien, F.C.K., R. Leung, R. Plomley, et al. Royal jelly-induced asthma. (Letter.) *Med. J. Aust.* 159:639 (1993).

384. Bullock, R.J., A. Rohan, and J.-A. Straatmans. Fatal royal jelly-induced asthma. *Med. J. Aust.* 160:44 (1994).

385. Rossi, G.L., A. Corsico, and G. Moscato. Occupational asthma caused by milk proteins: report on a case. *J. Aller. Clin. Immunol.* 93:799–801 (1994).

386. Ueda, A., F. Manda, K. Aoyama, et al. Immediate-type allergy related to okra (*Hibiscus esculentus* Linn) picking and packing. *Environ. Res.* 62:189–199 (1993).

387. Seuri, M., A. Taivanen, P. Ruoppi, and H. Tukiainen. Three cases of occupational asthma and rhinitis caused by garlic. *Clin. Exp. Aller.* 23:1011–1014 (1993).

388. Dugue, P., J. Bel, and M. Figueredo. Le fenugrec responsable d'un nouvel asthme professionnel. *Presse Méd.* 22:922 (1993).

389. Holtz, J., E. Fréchelin, B. Noël, and H. Savolainen. A case of frog allergy: antigenic skin protein. *Int. Arch. Aller. Immunol.* 101:299–300 (1993).

390. Moody, M.W., K.J. Roberts, and J.V. Huner. Phylogeny of commercially important seafood and description of the seafood industry. *Clin. Rev. Aller.* 11:159–182 (1993).

391. O'Neil, C., A.A. Helbling, and S.B. Lehrer. Allergic reactions to fish. *Clin. Rev. Aller.* 11:183–200 (1993).

392. Daul, C.B., J.E. Morgan, and S.B. Lehrer. Hypersensitivity reactions to crustacea and mollusks. *Clin. Rev. Aller.* 11:201–222 (1993).

393. Malo, J.-L., and A. Cartier. Occupational reactions in the seafood industry. *Clin. Rev. Aller.* 11:223–239 (1993).

394. Musmand, J.J., C.B. Daul, and S.B. Lehrer. Crustacea allergy. *Clin. Exp. Aller.* 23:722–732 (1993).

395. Vieths, S., K. Fischer, L.I. Dehne, et al. Versteckte Allergene in Lebensmitteln. *Herausgegeben Bundesgesundheitsamt* 37:51–60 (1994).

396. Matsuda, T., and R. Nakamura. Molecular structure and immunological properties of food allergens. *Trends Food Sci. Technol.* 4:289–293 (1993).

397. Moreau, M.C., and M. Coste. Immune responses to dietary protein antigens. In *Intestinal Flora, Immunity, Nutrition and Health.* A.P. Simopoulos et al. (eds.). Basel, Karger. *World Rev. Nutr. Diet.* 74:22–57 (1993).

398. Schrander, J.J.P., J.P.H. van den Bogart, P.P. Forget, et al. Cow's milk protein intolerance in infants under 1 year of age: a prospective epidemiological study. *Eur. J. Pediatr.* 152:640–644 (1993).

399. Casimir, G.J.A., J. Duchateau, B. Gossart, et al. Atopic dermatitis: role of food and house dust mite allergens. *Pediatrics* 92:252–256 (1993).

400. Ragno, V., P.G. Giampietro, G. Bruno, and L. Businco. Allergenicity of milk protein hydrolysate formulae in children with cow's milk allergy. *Eur. J. Pediatr.* 152:760–762 (1993).

401. Sorva, R., S. Mäkinen-Kiljunen, and K. Juntunen-Backman. β-Lactoglobulin secretion in human milk varies widely after cow's milk ingestion in mothers of infants with cow's milk allergy. *J. Aller. Clin. Immunol.* 93:787–792 (1994).

402. Barau, E., and C. Dupont. Allergy to cow's milk proteins in mother's milk or in hydrolyzed cow's milk infant formulas as assessed by intestinal permeability measurements. *Allergy* 49:295–298 (1994).

403. Kaplan, M.S. The importance of appropriate challenges in diagnosing food sensitivity. *Clin. Exp. Aller.* 24:291–293 (1994).

404. Stöger, P., and B. Wüthrich. Type I allergy to cow milk proteins in adults. A retrospective study of 34 adult milk- and cheese-allergic patients. *Int. Arch. Aller. Immunol.* 102:399–407 (1993).

405. Hoffman, D.R., and C. Collins-Williams. Cold-pressed peanut oils may contain peanut allergen. *J. Aller. Clin. Immunol.* 93:801–802 (1994).

406. Uhlemann, L., W.-M. Becker, and M. Schlaak. Nahrungsmittelallergie: identifizierung und Charakterisierung von Erdnußallergenen mit Patientenseren und monoklonalen Antikörpern. *Z. Ernährungswiss.* 32:139–151 (1993).

407. Hefle, S.L., R.K. Bush, J.W. Yunginger, and F.S. Chu. A sandwich enzyme-linked immunosorbent assay (ELISA) for the quantitation of selected peanut proteins in foods. *J. Food Protect.* 57:419–423 (1994).

408. Burks, A.W., G. Cockrell, C. Connaughton, and R.M. Helm. Epitope specificity and immunoaffinity purification of the major peanut allergen, *Ara h I. J. Aller. Clin. Immunol.* 93:743–750 (1994).

409. Herian, A.M., S.L. Taylor, and R.K. Bush. Allergenic reactivity of various soybean products as determined by RAST inhibition. *J. Food Sci.* 58:385–388 (1993).

410. Ogawa, T., H. Tsuji, N. Bando, et al. Identification of the soybean allergenic protein, *Gly m* Bd 30K, with the soybean seed 34-kDa oil-body-associated protein. *Biosci. Biotechnol. Biochem.* 57:1030–1033 (1993).

411. Tsuji, H., N. Bando, M. Kimoto, et al. Preparation and application of monoclonal antibodies for a sandwich enzyme-linked immunosorbent assay of the major soybean allergen, *Gly m* Bd 30K. *J. Nutr. Sci. Vitaminol.* 39:389–397 (1993).

412. Vieths, S., A. Jankiewicz, B. Schöning, and H. Aulepp. Apple allergy: the IgE-binding potency of apple strains is related to the occurrence of the 18-kDa allergen. *Allergy* 49:262–271 (1994).

413. Abeck, D., C. Kuwert, and J. Ring. Koinzidenz von Latex- und Nahrungsmittelallergien. (Letter.) *Dtsch. Med. Wschr.* 118:1585 (1993).

414. Shanti, K.N., B.M. Martin, S. Nagpal, et al. Identification of tropomyosin as the major shrimp allergen and characterization of its IgE-binding epitopes. *J. Immunol.* 151:5354–5363 (1993).

415. Lin, R.-Y., H.-D. Shen, and S.-H. Han. Identification and characterization of a 30 kd major allergen from *Parapenaeus fissurus. J. Aller. Clin. Immunol.* 92:837–845 (1993).

416. Armentia, A., R. Sanchez-Monge, L. Gomez, et al. *In vivo* allergenic activities of eleven purified members of a major allergen family from wheat and barley flour. *Clin. Exp. Aller.* 23:410–415 (1993).

417. Baur, X., Z. Chen, and I. Sander. Isolation and denomination of an important allergen in baking additives: α-amylase from *Aspergillus oryzae* (*Asp o* II). *Clin. Exp. Aller.* 24:465–470 (1994).

418. Szépfalusi, Z., C. Ebner, R. Pandjaitan, et al. Egg yolk α-livetin (chicken serum albumin) is a cross-reactive allergen in the bird-egg syndrome. *J. Aller. Clin. Immunol.* 92:932–942 (1994).

419. Monsalve, R.I., M.A. Gonzalez de la Peña, L. Menendez-Arias, et al. Characterization of a new oriental-mustard (*Brassica juncea*) allergen, *Bra j* IE: detection of an allergenic epitope. *Biochem. J.* 293:625–632 (1993).

# Part III: Foodborne Microbial Illness

# 10

# Mycotoxins

# GENERAL

Three recent papers described current research focus and trends for future research on mycotoxins in Africa (*1*), Spain (*2*), and Hungary (*3*). While research to date has concentrated primarily on aflatoxins, more emphasis is now being placed on other mycotoxins, particularly fumonisins and other *Fusarium* toxins.

Occurrence and significance of mycotoxins in stored products were reviewed by Scudamore (*4*). Surveillance studies of cereals, peanuts, and dried fruits and of human tissues in Europe indicate that contamination with aflatoxins and ochratoxin is relatively low. However, the presence of fumonisins and stable trichothecenes may present more of a challenge and be of more concern toxicologically.

Analyses of 31 corn samples from regions in China with a high incidence of esophageal cancer revealed the presence of high levels of fumonisin $B_1$ (up to 155 ppm), type A trichothecenes (up to 2.03 ppm), and type B trichothecenes (up to 5.83 ppm) and lower levels of aflatoxins (up to 0.038 ppm) (*5*). Highly toxigenic strains of *Fusarium moniliforme* isolated from moldy corn samples were also capable of forming several nitrosamines in the presence of nitrite and precursor amines. The capacity for both nitrosamine and mycotoxin production suggests that these fungi may play an important role in carcinogenesis in humans in this region.

Of a total of 23 strains of *Aspergillus ochraceus* and 11 strains of *Penicillium verrucosum* isolated from beans in Serbia, only 13% of the former and 18% of the latter were capable of producing ochratoxin A when growing on crushed wheat (*6*). All the strains of both species could produce this toxin when growing on one or more types of synthetic media.

Fungal colonization and mycotoxin production were compared in two rice cultivars during two growing seasons in India (*7*). Aflatoxins were detected early in development of the seeds and later declined while T-2 toxin increased steadily during grain development. Ochratoxin A was not detected until harvest.

Of 100 samples of seeds of an Egyptian faba bean cultivar, 7 were found to be naturally contaminated with aflatoxins and 2 contained ochratoxin A (*8*). Mycotoxin levels of 100–200 µg/kg in soil significantly decreased numbers of nodules on bean roots and total nitrogenase activity, thereby adversely affecting nutrition of the bean plants.

A total of 55 species belonging to 23 genera of fungi were isolated from samples of dried fruit (figs, apricots, plums, and raisins) in Egypt (*9*). Analyses for

a variety of mycotoxins demonstrated the presence of ochratoxin A at maximal concentrations of 110–120 mg/kg in apricots and figs and of 280 mg/kg in plums. No mycotoxins were detected in raisins. Of 25 samples of coconut collected from Egyptian markets, 5 contained aflatoxin $B_1$ ($AFB_1$) (15–25 mg/kg) and 3 contained ochratoxin A (50–205 mg/kg) (*10*). A total of 59 fungal species were isolated from the coconut samples, with *Aspergillus* and *Penicillium* being the most common.

At the time of collection of 9 samples of rootstock snack (*Cyperus esculentus*), three were found to be contaminated with trace amounts of aflatoxins (*11*). However, after 120 days of storage at ambient temperatures, all contained $AFB_1$ (95–460 ppb) and three contained ochratoxin A (10–50 ppb). Altogether 12 fungal species were isolated from the samples.

Although a wide range of fungi, including *Aspergillus* spp., were isolated from samples of almonds, cashews, chestnuts, hazelnuts, pistachios, and walnuts collected from markets in Saudi Arabia, only chestnuts contained detectable levels of any of 11 mycotoxins tested (*12*). Aflatoxins $B_1$ and $G_1$ were present at concentrations of 20–60 µg/kg.

In a survey of 329 samples of maize, peanuts, cashews, and copra obtained from farmers and from retail outlets in Thailand, fungal contamination was widespread in maize and peanuts and somewhat lower in the other foods (*13*). Major fungi in peanuts were *Aspergillus flavus* (95%) and *Aspergillus niger* (86%) and in maize were *F. moniliforme* (97%), *A. flavus* (85%), and *Penicillium citrinum* (67%). Mycotoxin analyses on these products were not reported.

To determine whether mycotoxin-contaminated crops left in the field could contaminate groundwater, the binding of aflatoxins $B_1$ and $B_2$ and fumonisin $B_1$ to silty clay loam soils was measured (*14*). Mixtures of 50% silty clay loam soil and moldy corn prevented the leaching of all these mycotoxins. Mixtures containing less soil (20%) permitted the leaching of some $AFB_1$ but not of the other mycotoxins. Therefore the practice of disking contaminated crops into the soil should prevent these mycotoxins from gaining access to groundwater.

In yeast extract cultures, potassium sorbate inhibited growth of *A. ochraceus* and *Penicillium aurantiogriseum* and also inhibited mycotoxin production by these strains (*15*). To determine whether this compound would be useful in preserving high-moisture corn, aerated corn with 28% moisture was treated with 1.5 and 2.5% potassium sorbate and potassium sorbate plus propylene glycol and stored for 193 days (*16*). After storage under these conditions, no molds could be isolated from this corn, although 100% of untreated corn samples with the same initial moisture content were infected with one or more genera of fungi (*Aspergillus*, *Penicillium*, or *Fusarium*).

In experiments with cheese, heat treatment for one hour did not significantly affect mold growth, but liquid smoke applied to the cheese surface completely inhibited growth of *Aspergillus oryzae* and significantly delayed growth of two species of *Penicillium* (*17*). Isoeugenol, one of 8 major phenolic compounds in smoke, was principally responsible for inhibition of mold growth on smoked cheddar cheese. Other phenolic compounds (the antioxidants BHA, propyl paraben, and butyl paraben) effectively inhibited mycelial growth of *Fusarium*, *Penicillium*, and *Aspergillus* in cultures (*18,19*).

Immunotoxic effects of AFB$_1$ and T-2 toxin on granulocyte–macrophage progenitor cells in male mice were investigated in vivo and in vitro (*20*). Myelotoxic effects were observed in in vitro experiments with AFB$_1$ and in mice gavaged for two weeks on alternate days with 0.7 mg AFB$_1$/kg body weight but did not occur in mice treated with T-2 toxin. However, T-2 toxin was clearly cytotoxic to bone marrow cells in vitro.

Neurotoxic effects of 5 mycotoxins (fumonisin B$_1$, slaframine, swainsonine, lolitrems, and paspalitrems) were reviewed by Plumlee and Galey (*21*). These toxins have been detected in animal feeds and have been associated with neurologic diseases. Electrophysiological experiments with several tremorgenic indole alkaloids, including paspalitrems, aflatrem, and penitrem A, demonstrated that these compounds blocked the maxi-K channels of smooth muscle cell membranes (*22*). This inhibition is responsible for some of the toxic effects of these compounds but may not be related to their tremorgenic effects.

Mysterious deaths of archaeologists after opening old tombs and of scholars studying "old books" have been ascribed to curses imposed by long dead pharaohs or priests. However, three recent reports of human illness following exposure to airborne mycotoxins suggest that molds growing in these damp environments, rather than King Tut, may be responsible. After spending 8 hours working with wheat which had been stored in a closed granary for 2 years, a farmer developed acute renal failure (*23*). This illness was apparently caused by inhalation of dust containing ochratoxin, because a toxigenic strain of *A. ochraceus* was isolated from the wheat and laboratory animals breathing dust from the granary also developed renal and hepatic lesions. Another agricultural worker, after exposure to moldy silage, developed neurological symptoms, including dementia and a remarkable tremor (*24*). It appeared that this illness was caused by inhalation of a tremorgenic mycotoxin. Molds

and various mycotoxins, including sterigmatocystin, were found to be present in throat swabs from miners working in deep uranium mines, and it has been suggested (*25*) that such toxins may induce mutations in the *p*53 gene and initiate carcinogenesis.

A variety of chromatographic and ELISA procedures designed to analyze foods and feeds for the presence of mycotoxins was discussed by Richard et al. (*26*). Since mycotoxins constitute a chemically diverse group of compounds, there is no universal method for detection. Current methods are capable of detecting as little as 50 ppb of some mycotoxins. In another review, Panigrahi (*27*) described bioassays, utilizing terrestrial and aquatic plant and animal species, to detect the presence of mycotoxins. A routine screening program would require the use of a battery of such assays to detect all the mycotoxins which might be present.

Of 14 species of microorganisms tested, one (*Bacillus brevis*) was found to be sensitive to 8 common, non-trichothecene mycotoxins but not to 4 trichothecenes. Cells of one yeast strain were sensitive only to the trichothecene mycotoxins. Used in conjunction, these two species could form the basis for a bioassay to detect the presence of several common mycotoxins (*28*).

A procedure for the simultaneous screening of multiple mycotoxins in foods that combines line immunoblot assay and image analysis (a computer-assisted multianalyte assay system) has been developed by Abouzied and Pestka (*29*).

Methods for the detection of fungal contamination in stored grain have been reviewed by Magan (*30*). These include biochemical tests for the presence of specific fungal enzymes or metabolites, including volatiles, electrochemical methods to detect microbial activity, and immunological methods and DNA probes. A new indirect method has been developed for the detection of *Aspergillus* and *Penicillium* by use of an ELISA or the Latex Agglutination Assay sensitive to the almost genus-specific extracellular polysaccharides of these fungi (*31*).

# MYCOTOXINS PRODUCED BY *ASPERGILLUS* SPP.

## Aflatoxins in Humans and Their Biological Effects

Several recent reviews focused on various associations between aflatoxins and human disease. Eaton and Gallagher (*32*) comprehensively summarized data from studies with experimental animals and with humans and discussed its implications for suggested mechanisms of aflatoxin carcinogenesis. The presence of aflatoxins in human breast milk and cord sera, the teratogenic, carcinogenic, and immunotoxic effects of aflatoxins in developing humans, and the possible relationships between aflatoxin exposure and kwashiorkor and Indian childhood cirrhosis were discussed by Raisuddin (*33*). The specific G→T transversion within codon 249 of the tumor suppressor *p*53 gene and its relation to aflatoxin exposure was described by Gerbes and Caselmann (*34*) and evaluated with respect to aflatoxin's purported etiological role in hepatocellular carcinoma (HCC). Development and validation of molecular biomarkers of aflatoxin exposure using experimental and human population studies were described by Groopman et al. (*35*). An extensive research database on the metabolism, macromolecular adduct formation, and general mechanisms of action of aflatoxins has been used to establish such biomarkers.

An improved analytical procedure to increase the overall recovery of aflatoxin–albumin adducts has been developed and validated (*36*). All serum proteins were precipitated with ammonium sulfate and then adducts were determined by radioimmunoassay. Recovery of adducts was increased 8-fold compared to previous methods and the detection limit of this assay was 0.5 pmol $AFB_1$–albumin adducts.

A cross-sectional survey of 250 Taiwanese revealed a significant correlation between urinary aflatoxin metabolites and the background rate of HCC in the subjects' townships of residence (*37*). A 4-fold variation in HCC mortality was observed in the 8 townships. Although hepatitis-B carrier status, alcohol consumption, and cigarette smoking were also related to HCC mortality, the association with aflatoxin exposure remained significant after adjustment for these other factors.

Bioactivation of $AFB_1$ by microsomes from human liver donors was compared with that by microsomes from human lymphoblastoid cell lines expressing transfected CYP1A2 or CYP3A4 (*38*). Results indicated that with normal, relatively low dietary levels of aflatoxins, CYP1A2 is the high affinity P450 enzyme principally responsible for the activation of $AFB_1$ while CYP3A4 is primarily involved with $AFB_1$ detoxification. Tumorous liver tissue from 20 Thai patients with hepatic cancer was found to have a significantly reduced expression of P450 proteins as compared to paired normal tissue (*39*). The tumorous tissue produced a markedly lower level of CYP3A4 and $AFQ_1$ (a detoxification product) as compared to normal tissue in in vitro experiments. Although the expression of two major classes of glutathione S-transferases (GST) was markedly reduced in tumorous, compared to normal,

cytosols, this did not appear to be toxicologically significant. Unlike aflatoxin-resistant species (mouse, hamster) which detoxify $AFB_1$ by conjugation with glutathione, glutathione was not conjugated to $AFB_1$–epoxide by cytosol from either tumorous or normal human tissue.

HCC cells from patients living in areas where food is highly contaminated with aflatoxins often contain a mutation in codon 249 of the *p*53 tumor suppressor gene. In an examination of $AFB_1$ mutagenesis, human HCC (HepG2) cells exposed to $AFB_1$ in vitro were found to preferentially acquire the G to T transversion in the third position of codon 249 (*40*). Two other transversions in adjacent codons were also observed at 2-fold lower frequencies. These results support the proposed etiological role of $AFB_1$ in hepatocarcinogenesis. In contrast, no mutations in the *p*53 gene were detected in cells from HCC induced by injections of $AFB_1$ in 13 rats (*41*). Results from analyses of HCC from 59 Japanese (*42*) and from 21 Hong Kong Chinese (*43*) patients revealed that none of the Japanese and only 2 of the Chinese had the G→T transversion in codon 249. Since the food supplies in these areas are not known to be heavily contaminated with aflatoxins, these results do not negate the proposed etiological role of $AFB_1$ in HCC.

Since primary liver cancer rates have been reported to be relatively high in Nepal, serum samples from 38 Nepalese (15 controls and 23 patients with various liver diseases) were analyzed for the presence of $AFM_1$ (*44*). This mycotoxin was detected in 80% of controls and 52% of the patients, thereby failing to demonstrate a relationship between aflatoxins and liver disease.

Since the small intestine is also exposed to dietary aflatoxins and CYP3A enzymes are present in this organ, explants of rat and human intestinal tissue were used to determine whether $AFB_1$ would form DNA adducts in intestinal cells (*45*). These adducts were detected in both species but only in mature enterocytes containing active CYP3A enzymes. The authors suggest that the lack of adducts in proliferating cells prevents the development of intestinal cancers and further that this $AFB_1$ binding may serve a protective function: The aflatoxin molecules are sequestered in the mature enterocytes which are sloughed off every 5–6 days, thereby eliminating this potential carcinogen from the body.

Since essential oils from some common spices appear to exert a protective effect on human and animal health, several such oils were tested for their ability to suppress the formation of DNA adducts by $AFB_1$ in vitro (*46*). All of the oils tested (cardamom, celery, nutmeg, ginger, xanthoxylum, black pepper, cumin, and coriander) inhibited adduct formation in a dose-dependent manner, with cardamom, celery, and nutmeg being the most potent. The oils also inhibited the formation of activated metabolites of $AFB_1$ and this could be the basis for the reported anticarcinogenic effects of spices.

In an investigation of the possible effects of aflatoxin-contaminated food on kwashiorkor, a retrospective study of hospital records of 36 malnourished South African children with kwashiorkor compared clinical features of the children with detectable aflatoxin in their serum ($n = 21$) with those of children with no detectable aflatoxin (47). Compared to the aflatoxin-negative group, those scored as aflatoxin-positive had significantly lower hemoglobin levels, longer durations of edema and hospital stay, and an increased number of infections. Thus, exposure to dietary aflatoxins appeared to compound the effects of kwashiorkor.

Dietary administration of the antioxidant ethoxyquin is known to exert a protective effect against hepatocarcinogenesis in rats. Ethoxyquin has been shown to induce the synthesis of an aldehyde reductase which detoxifies an activated dialdehydic form of $AFB_1$ (48). The livers of adult rats fed ethoxyquin contain at least 15-fold higher amounts of this enzyme as compared to livers of rats fed control diets. This enzyme appears to be a previously unrecognized protective mechanism for prevention of cytotoxic effects of $AFB_1$–protein adducts.

## Biosynthesis of Aflatoxins

Stereochemical relations during aflatoxin biosynthesis have been investigated recently using chiral HPLC and cell-free extracts of *Aspergillus parasiticus* (49,50). Results indicated that enzymes involved in the steps leading from norsolorinic acid to averufin (norsolorinic acid dehydrogenase) and from versiconal hemiacetal acetate to versicolorin A (a cyclase enzyme) showed strict stereospecificity for their substrates. Some other enzymes did not exhibit strict stereospecificity, and nonenzymatic racemization occurred in versiconal hemiacetal acetate enantiomers.

Another approach to clarification of the details of aflatoxin synthesis involves the cloning of genes coding for biosynthetic enzymes. Production of polyclonal antibodies against sterigmatocystin *O*-methyltransferase (51), one of the key enzymes involved in the latter few synthetic reactions, enabled the screening of a cDNA library from *A. parasiticus* for the gene encoding this enzyme. A clone containing this gene was identified and sequenced and the amino acid sequence of the enzyme was then deduced (52). Another gene, *apa*-2, associated with the

regulation of aflatoxin biosynthesis, has been cloned from *A. parasiticus* and shown to have a high degree of DNA homology with the *A. flavus afl*-2 gene (53).

Analyses of headspace volatiles from cultures of 4 aflatoxigenic and 4 nonaflatoxigenic strains of *A. flavus* grown in submerged cultures for up to 10 days revealed that the aflatoxigenic strains produced a unique series of sesquiterpenes ($C_{15}H_{24}$ compounds) which peaked in 3-day cultures (54). The initiation of aflatoxin synthesis was apparently correlated with the release of these compounds, and the decline of aflatoxin synthesis corresponded to the disappearance of these volatiles.

## Occurrence and Control of Aflatoxins in Foods

Aflatoxin contamination of a variety of foods is common in some countries and during certain seasons. Significant levels of *Aspergillus* spp. contamination were observed in maize (76%), coconut and groundnut (92%), and green gram (44%) from markets in India (55). Of the 1706 isolates of *A. flavus* cultured from these food samples, 48.4% were toxigenic. A survey of Nigerian foods and feeds revealed that groundnut and groundnut-containing products were the most heavily contaminated, with one sample containing 1862 ppb aflatoxins (56). Highest levels of contamination in maize, sunflower meal, and sorghum were 140, 245, and 107 ppb, respectively. None of 10 soybean samples contained detectable aflatoxins.

Recent reviews by Park and Liang (57) and Park (58) described reported human health effects of exposure to aflatoxins and discussed strategies for monitoring contamination levels in human foods and animal feeds and the efficacy of different decontamination procedures. Bhatnagar et al. (59) and Cleveland and Bhatnagar (60) reviewed molecular strategies for control of aflatoxins in food including: (a) control of aflatoxin biosynthesis, (b) environmental factors and biocompetitive microbes which could inhibit growth of *Aspergillus* species and aflatoxin production, and (c) enhancement of host plant resistance to aflatoxin accumulation.

Of four fungicides evaluated for their effects on aflatoxin production in corn and sunflower seeds, Rizolex-T and Vitavax-Captan were effective inhibitors while the other two pesticides were not (61). Preliminary tests with these fungicides in liquid cultures of *A. flavus* did not accurately predict their effectiveness when applied to corn and sunflower seeds.

A series of acidic, alkaline, and neutral food additives was examined for potential use in degradation of aflatoxins in corn and butter beans (62). Treatment of contaminated corn with 0.25% sodium chlorite and with 0.25% ammonium peroxodisulfate for 48 h at 60°C completely degraded $AFB_1$. For the beans, the most effective treatment was boiling for 1 h with 0.5% or 2% sodium sulfite. These results indicate that some food additives may be used to degrade aflatoxins during food processing.

CORN AND OTHER GRAINS. Although Thai maize is highly sought after by egg producers in Japan because of its bright yellow color, problems with aflatoxin contamination have severely restricted exports. An investigation of maize production in Thailand revealed that shelling with a mechanical sheller, which physically damaged kernels, was the most important step in the contamination process (63).

Postharvest resistance to aflatoxin contamination in two maize cultivars was found to be related to activities of the living corn embryo (64). When kernels were wounded through the pericarp, inoculation with *A. flavus* spores resulted in good fungal growth but low aflatoxin concentrations. However, autoclaving or crushing of kernels or otherwise wounding of embryos abolished the resistance to aflatoxin production.

Boiling of aflatoxin-contaminated pastes made from corn and sorghum for 15 min resulted in destruction of nearly half the original amount of $AFB_1$ (312–475 μg/kg) in the grains (65). Boiling for 60 min reduced toxin levels by 80–100%. Fermentation of these contaminated grains to produce ogi, a Nigerian food, destroyed about 71% of $AFB_1$.

PEANUTS AND OTHER LEGUMES. Nearly 77% of 200 isolates of *A. flavus* and *A. parasiticus* cultured from peanuts growing in Israel were capable of producing aflatoxins while 22.5% and 3.5%, respectively, synthesized cyclopiazonic acid and sterigmatocystin (66). Although only one strain produced all 3 mycotoxins, the toxigenic potential of these aspergilli appears to be relatively high and they may pose a threat to human and animal health.

To assess the fate of aflatoxins in naturally contaminated peanuts during processing into peanut protein flour, peanut samples taken from several stages in the process were analyzed for $AFB_1$ (67). Shrivelled peanuts contained significantly more $AFB_1$ (126 ppb) than hand-picked, selected peanuts (9 ppb). Even though the defatted peanut protein flour was made from the hand-picked peanuts, its aflatoxin content (52 ppb) was higher than the permissible level of 30 ppb. The various processing steps appear to concentrate rather than remove $AFB_1$.

A total of 38 groundnut strains from India were screened for resistance to growth of *A. flavus* and aflatoxin production (68). Following inoculation with fungal spores, seeds were incubated at 25°C and 98% humidity for 8 days. Rates of seed colonization for the different cultivars ranged from 14.7% to 73.4% and aflatoxin concentrations ranged from 3900 to 90,000 μg/kg. No relation was observed between sugar content of the seeds and the rate of colonization or the production of aflatoxins.

Gypsum is commonly added to fields during peanut cultivation to increase available calcium and improve peanut quality and germination. To test whether this practice would increase or decrease the susceptibility of these seeds to fungal growth and aflatoxin production, peanuts were grown in fields treated with 550–4400 kg gypsum/ha and then harvested and inoculated with spores of *A. parasiticus* (69). After incubation for 14 d at 25°C, seeds from the treated fields had significantly lower levels of aflatoxins (0.5–1.9 mg/g) compared to those from untreated fields (17.3 mg/g). Peanuts from treated fields also had significantly higher concentrations of calcium (especially the hulls) and significantly lower concentrations of zinc (especially the kernels). Although there was no direct correlation between levels of calcium supplementation during growth and aflatoxin concentrations in peanuts inoculated with different spore loads of *A. parasiticus*, toxin production was lowest in peanuts grown in fields treated with 4400 kg gypsum/ha (70).

Analyses of samples of 100 lots of soybeans following commercial storage in Egypt revealed the presence of numerous species of fungi (71). Approximately 87% of the isolates identified were species of *Aspergillus* and 35% of samples contained detectable levels of aflatoxin (5–35 μg/kg). Although other potentially toxigenic fungi were present, no other mycotoxins were detected.

A soybean phytoalexin, glyceollin, when added to cultures of *A. flavus* at a concentration of 6.25 μg/mL suppressed aflatoxin synthesis by 70% but did not significantly affect fungal growth (72). Glyceollin appears to inhibit $AFB_1$ synthesis since it does not increase $AFB_1$ degradation. Glyceollin is known to accumulate in viable seeds infected with *A. flavus* and this may partially explain why aflatoxin contamination is not a common problem in soybeans.

In experiments to evaluate the potential use of the yeast *Pichia guilliermondii* as a biocontrol agent against *A. flavus* and other fungi on stored soybeans, fungal growth was markedly inhibited when the yeast was coinoculated with *A. flavus* spores on sterilized seeds (73). However, with naturally infected beans, application of the yeast inhibited fungal growth for only a limited period of time and propionic acid proved to be a better fungistatic agent.

**OTHER PLANT PRODUCTS.** Four of seven strains of *A. flavus* isolated from rotting sweet oranges obtained from markets in Nigeria were found to be aflatoxigenic, producing primarily $AFB_1$ (*74*). The optimal temperature for $AFB_1$ production on orange juice medium was 25–30°C.

A sugar content of 65° Brix generally inhibits mold growth on candied fruit. However, recent interest in low-sugar candied fruit has generated interest in other preservatives which might be fungistatic. Chitosan, a deacetylated form of chitin, at a concentration of 3 mg/mL, was found to inhibit growth of *A. parasiticus* by about 62% and $AFB_1$ production by 84% (*75*). Using response surface methodology, a model was derived to predict the number of days to visible mold growth in candied kumquat at various concentrations of chitosan and °Brix.

Inter- and intra-box aflatoxin distribution was determined in 200 12-kg boxes of dried figs in order to devise an effective strategy for sampling large lots of potentially contaminated dried fruit (*76*). About two-thirds of the boxes contained <10μg aflatoxins/kg whereas the most contaminated box contained 227 μg/kg. Of 12 1-kg subsamples analyzed from each of 3 boxes, the highest aflatoxin contamination was 2063 μg/kg. This is consistent with previous observations that individual figs in a lot may be very highly contaminated. Several sampling regimes were evaluated for their probable success in detecting contaminated lots.

Sixteen species of fungi were isolated from watermelon seed samples collected from markets in Nigeria where it is an important food (*77*). Optimal conditions for synthesis of aflatoxins by *A. flavus* and ochratoxin A by *A. ochraceus* were studied in samples of ground, toxin-free melon seeds.

Susceptibility of 21 California almond cultivars to aflatoxigenic *A. flavus* has been investigated (*78*). While seed coat resistance (delay in fungal colonization) was uniformly high for all cultivars, cotyledon resistance (lower rate of disease development) was identified in only 3 cultivars.

Samples of black pepper, cayenne pepper, chili powder, cumin, ground ginger, and paprika from retail outlets in the UK have been analyzed for aflatoxin contamination by a newly developed procedure utilizing an immunoaffinity column for cleanup followed by HPLC with post-column derivatization with pyridinium bromide perbromide (*79*). More than 50% of the samples were contaminated with >1 ppb afla-

toxin. Ginger and chili powder were the most often contaminated, with some samples containing >20 ppb total aflatoxins.

Of 50 different Indian herbal medicines (prescribed for liver disorders) analyzed for aflatoxins, 23 were found to be contaminated at levels of 0.28–2.23 μg/g (*80*). Nearly all of the drug samples were contaminated with one or more species of fungi.

**DAIRY PRODUCTS, MEAT, AND FISH.** It has been reported that when milk contaminated with aflatoxins is made into yogurt, there is a very slight (*81*) or a significant (*82*) decrease in aflatoxin concentrations. In the first study, $AFB_2$, $AFG_1$, and $AFG_2$ levels in milk decreased during yogurt production (4–17%), $AFM_1$ levels increased by 20%, and $AFB_1$ levels remained the same. After 12 days' storage at 4°C, $AFG_1$ and $AFM_1$ levels decreased (13–21%) compared to the starting milk while levels of the other toxins increased by 10–17%. In the second study, recovery of $AFM_1$ (added to milk) in newly made yogurt was 83% while after 13 days of refrigerated storage, the $AFM_1$ concentration in the yogurt had decreased to 41% of the original level.

Exposure of lactating dairy goats to aflatoxin-contaminated feed (200 ppb) for 6 days resulted in $AFM_1$ levels in milk of 1.62 ppb (*83*). Incorporation of 4% HSCAS (hydrated sodium calcium aluminosilicate) into the contaminated diet reduced $AFM_1$ levels in milk to 0.187 ppb. HSCAS added to diets at levels of 1% and 2% also reduced carryover of aflatoxins into milk by 52% and 82%, respectively. Dietary concentrations of 0.5% HSCAS have also been found to reduce the toxic effects of dietary aflatoxins to broiler chicks (*84,85*) and to pigs (*86*).

In a similar type of experiment, rats were fed a diet consisting of 50% peanut butter contaminated with 1500 ppb aflatoxin with or without 0.1 or 1% Volclay, a bentonite clay, for 8 weeks (*87*). Reduced weight gain and liver lesions were observed in the rats without Volclay but these effects were significantly less in those consuming Volclay. The Volclay supplements themselves appeared to have no toxic effects.

Feeding an aflatoxin-contaminated diet (50 or 100 ppb toxin) to walleye fish for 30 days resulted in histopathological changes in the liver and deposition of 5–10 ppb $AFB_1$ in muscle tissue (*88*). After 2 weeks of withdrawal, aflatoxin was no longer detectable in muscles but the liver lesions were still present.

**INHIBITION OF AFLATOXIN PRODUCTION IN SYNTHETIC MEDIA.** Several research labs reported that extracts of spices and herbs were capable of inhibiting growth of

A. *flavus* or A. *parasiticus* and production of aflatoxins in liquid media. These included studies with essential oils of cinnamon, cloves, almond, and cardamom (*89*), cumin, onion, garlic, and cloves (*90*), capsaicin and capsanthin (*91*), extracts of *Amorphophallus campanulatus* (an Indian condiment) (*92*), and extracts of six non-commercial Nigerian herbs and spices (*93*). Potency of the various preparations varied, and at some concentrations certain extracts actually stimulated aflatoxin production. Nevertheless, some of these extracts may be useful in controlling mold growth and mycotoxin production in foods.

Of 6 food preservatives tested, three (sodium acetate, sodium chloride, and benzoic acid) exerted only marginal inhibitory effects on growth of A. *parasiticus* and aflatoxin production (*94*). Both citric and propionic acids at concentrations of 0.5 and 1.0% completely inhibited growth and toxin production both in liquid media and on agar. Sodium metabisulfite was an effective inhibitor only in liquid media.

Nine of twelve surfactants evaluated for their effects on growth and aflatoxin production by A. *flavus* were found to exhibit some inhibitory effects (*95*). Five nonionic compounds (Triton X-100, Tergitol NP-7, Tergitol NP-10, Polyoxyethylene 10 lauryl ether, and Latron AG-98) and one anionic compound (Triton X-301) restricted colony growth on agar and reduced aflatoxin production by 96–99%. Sodium dodecyl sulfate and dodecyltrimethylammonium bromide at concentrations of 1% suppressed conidial germination.

At concentrations of $\geq 5$ µg/g, the fungicide iprodione inhibited growth and toxin production by A. *parasiticus* on agar media (*96*). Another fungicidal compound, iturin A, which is produced by *Bacillus subtilis*, did not consistently reduce growth or aflatoxin production in several strains of A. *flavus* or A. *parasiticus* tested (*97*). In liquid cultures, three organophosphate insecticides (dimethoate, malathion, and selecron) significantly delayed growth of A. *parasiticus* but significantly promoted growth of A. *flavus* (*98*). Treatment of sorghum with these pesticides (5000 mg/kg) suppressed production of aflatoxins by both aspergilli.

Aflatoxins are known to have immunotoxic effects such as the suppression of phagocytosis by rat peritoneal macrophages. Exposure of a solution of $AFB_1$ to ozone, a powerful oxidant, for 6 min apparently destroyed its phagocytosis-suppressing activity (*99*). Whether ozone treatment of aflatoxin-contaminated crops would be a safe and effective control procedure, however, remains to be determined.

Data from a full factorial experimental design testing the effects of inoculum size and various environmental factors demonstrated that inoculum level, water activity, storage temperature, and headspace oxygen all had significant effects on growth of and aflatoxin production by A. *flavus* in synthetic medium under modified atmosphere packaging (*100*). Optimal conditions for growth and toxin production differed slightly but were in the range of 20–25°C, $a_w = 0.95$–0.96, headspace $O_2$ of 10–15%, and an inoculum level of $10^3$–$10^4$ spores/plate. Packaging under almost completely anaerobic conditions inhibited both growth and toxin production irrespective of other factors.

## Detection and Determination of Aflatoxins

Reliable methods for determining the extent of aflatoxin contamination in foods begin with appropriate methods for sampling and toxin extraction. An investigation into the variability of results of aflatoxin analyses of farmers' stock lots of peanuts demonstrated that sampling, sample preparation and analysis accounted for 92.7, 7.2, and 0.1%, respectively, of the total variability (*101*). It was previously thought that fluorescence in dried figs was an indication of the presence of aflatoxins. However, this is no longer considered a dependable means of distinguishing contaminated fruit. Therefore, it is recommended that at least 10 samples of 20 kg each be analyzed from a 20-ton lot in order to determine whether the allowable limit of aflatoxin has been exceeded (*102*).

Grinding of peanut samples in preparation for analysis was investigated as a source of variability by comparison of 4 different mills (*103*). The least variability was observed with a vertical cutter mixer but it took much longer to grind samples than a cheaper type of mill. However, the latter gave more variable results.

A method for the extraction of $AFB_1$ from field-inoculated corn by supercritical fluid extraction has been developed and found to yield 90% analyte recovery when compared to conventional solvent extraction procedures (*104*).

Several reversed-phase HPLC systems with fluorescence detection have been developed for the detection of aflatoxins in corn (*105*), corn and peanuts (*106*), milk powder (*107*), and dried fruit and nuts (*108*). Many of these also include an immunoaffinity column as a cleanup step prior to HPLC. Results of an interlaboratory evaluation of such a method indicated that procedures using immunoaffinity columns have not been sufficiently refined to be recommended as a standard method (*109*).

Rapid and inexpensive methods for detection of the presence of aflatoxins in foods have also been devised. A diphasic dialysis technique was developed and found to quickly and effectively purify a large number of samples of dairy products prior to TLC analysis for aflatoxins (*110*). A minicolumn assay in which AFM$_1$ is adsorbed at an interface of neutral sand and magnesium silicate can demonstrate the presence of ≥0.5 ppb AFM$_1$ in milk as a band of bright blue fluorescence (*111*). A simple, rapid, and reliable aflatoxin detection kit including a UV lamp, a solvent blender for toxin extraction, and adsorbent-coated dip-strips for detecting and quantifying aflatoxin has been assembled for field analyses (*112*).

Methods have also been described for the detection of DNA-damaging mycotoxins using the Drosophila DNA-repair test (*113*) and for the detection of aflatoxigenic molds on coconut cream agar (*114*) and by an ELISA capable of reacting with extracellular and mycelial antigens (*115*).

### Sterigmatocystin

Sterigmatocystin, a hepatocarcinogenic mycotoxin structurally related to aflatoxins, was added to primary cultures of healthy human gastric epithelial cells to investigate its effects on unscheduled DNA synthesis (UDS) (*116*). Following metabolic activation by an S9 mix, sterigmatocystin, at noncytotoxic concentrations ($10^{-6}$–$10^{-4}$ M), induced UDS in the cultured cells. Such a genotoxic effect may be relevant to humans consuming moldy grains and peanuts since this toxin can be produced in human gastric juice.

Biosynthesis of sterigmatocystin by *Aspergillus nidulans* has been elucidated with the isolation and characterization of the gene *verA* (*117*). Disruption of this gene by insertion of extraneous genetic material resulted in the accumulation of versicolorin A but only negligible amounts of sterigmatocystin. This demonstrated that the gene encodes an enzyme necessary for the conversion of versicolorin A to sterigmatocystin.

### Ochratoxin A

Four of 30 stored maize samples and none of 25 dried bean samples tested in Croatia were contaminated with ochratoxin A (OA) at levels of 0.4–400 µg/g (*118*). Approximately 53% of the beans and 26% of the maize samples contained one or more species of *Aspergillus*. Of the 27 isolates of *A. flavus*, 3 produced aflatoxin B$_1$ and 2 produced cyclopiazonic acid when grown on synthetic media. Six of 26 *A. ochraceus* isolates were OA positive on laboratory media.

### Tremorgenic Mycotoxins

Effects of territrem-B, a mycotoxin produced by *Aspergillus terreus* growing on rice culture, were investigated using nerve–muscle preparations from mice (*119*). This toxin induced spontaneous muscle twitching and blocked the potassium current in the nerve terminal but did not affect the sodium, calcium, or calcium-activated potassium currents of the nerve terminal. This blockage of the potassium channel is probably related to its effect on synaptic transmission.

## MYCOTOXINS PRODUCED BY *FUSARIUM* SPP.

A variety of *Fusarium* mycotoxins were detected during a survey of corn and barley produced in South Korea (*120*). Deoxynivalenol (DON), nivalenol (NIV), and zearalenone (ZEA) were the major toxins detected in barley, with average concentrations of 170, 1011, and 287 ng/g, respectively. DON and 15-acetylDON (15-ADON) were the toxins present in greatest amounts on corn, with mean concentrations of 310 and 297 ng/g, respectively. A very high incidence of infection was noted in barley, with ≥90% of samples containing DON and/or NIV and 51% containing ZEA. Levels of contamination were somewhat less in corn, with 65%, 26%, 35%, and 17% containing DON, 15-ADON, NIV, and ZEA, respectively.

A survey of 29 lots of cereals and legumes imported from Australia into Papua New Guinea, revealed that nearly half of the samples, including wheat, soybeans, millet, and rice, were contaminated with *Fusarium* mycotoxins (*121*). DON was present in 13 samples at concentrations ranging from 23–2270 ng/g while NIV was present in 7 of the same samples at 13–1540 ng/g. ZEA at 250–3060 ng/g was detected in 10 samples. None of the barley, mung bean, red bean, or corn samples assayed were contaminated with these toxins.

A high level of contamination with *Fusarium* was also detected in barley samples grown during a wet summer (1987) in Germany (*122*). DON, ZEA, and 3-ADON were detected in 98, 68, and 48% of samples, respectively, at mean concentrations of 399, 39, and 21 µg/kg, respectively. Two or more mycotoxins were present in 77% of samples.

DON and ZEA were also major contaminants of German wheat and wheat bran intended for animal feed, with mean levels, respectively, of 788 and 20 µg/kg in bran and of 204 and 11 µg/kg in wheat (*123*). Incidences of contamination with DON were 100% in bran and 74% in wheat while ZEA was found in 71% of the bran and in 18% of the wheat samples.

Of a total of 174 isolates of *Fusarium* spp. from crop plants and soil in Taiwan, 31% were identified as *F. moniliforme* (*124*). Analyses of 61 strains for mycotoxin production revealed that fusarin C, ZEA, DON, T-2 toxin, or moniliformin were produced by one or more of 18 isolates. Fumonisins $B_1$ and $B_2$ and fusarins A, C, and F have been identified in liquid cultures of 27 *F. moniliforme* strains isolated from maize in Indonesia, the Philippines, and Thailand (*125*). All strains produced detectable levels of both types of mycotoxins but fumonisin:fusarin ratios for different strains varied widely.

Field experiments in Ontario involving inoculation of corn 1–6 weeks after silking with spores of one of three species of *Fusarium* demonstrated that DON and ZEA were the major toxins produced (*126*). Fumonisin and *F. moniliforme* were also detected in all samples whether or not the ears had been inoculated with this strain.

Analyses of 48 samples of swine feeds from Ontario revealed that all except 7 contained detectable levels of fusaric acid (1.4–135.64 µg/g) (*127*). Highest mean concentrations occurred in whole feeds and high moisture corn, with 2–3-fold lower concentrations in wheat, barley, and dry corn. Some of the samples were also contaminated with DON, ZEA, and T-2 toxin, with average concentrations of 3.33, 0.35, and 0.26 µg/g, respectively.

Methods for detection of *Fusarium* toxins by (a) ELISA using monoclonal antibodies directed against T-2 toxin and ZEA (*128*), (b) GC with Fourier transform infrared spectroscopy (*129*), and (c) supercritical fluid chromatography (*130*) have been developed and described. A sensitive GC–MS method has been devised and used to analyze 50 samples of Canadian and imported beer for contamination with DON, NIV, and α-zearalenol (*131*). DON and NIV were detected in 29 and 3 samples, respectively, with the highest levels being 50 and 0.84 ng/mL, respectively.

## Trichothecenes

Trichothecenes are a group of sesquiterpenoid epoxides, some of which have been associated with mycotoxicoses in farm animals and with illness and death in humans who consume moldy grains and other agricultural products. In a recent review, Desjardins et al. (*132*) discussed the chemistry, genetics, and significance of trichothecene biosynthesis. Another review by Yagen and Bialer (*133*) considered the metabolism and pharmacokinetics of T-2 toxin and related trichothecenes.

Examination of 36 isolates (8 species) of *Fusarium*, isolated from corn and wheat grown in Manitoba, demonstrated that *Fusarium graminearum*, *Fusarium poae*, and *Fusarium sporotrichioides* produced the greatest amounts (up to 124.6 µg T-2 toxin/mL) and the greatest number (7 to 8) of trichothecenes (*134*). Isolates of the other species produced 3 to 5 toxins each. Production of DON and fusarenone-X was widespread, with 22 to 23 of the 36 isolates producing each of these toxins.

Addition of 0.11 M sodium bicarbonate to cultures of *Fusarium tricinctum* was found to completely inhibit the synthesis of neosolaniol, acetyl T-2 toxin, and 15-diacetoxyscirpenol (15-DAS) and to inhibit production of DAS and T-2 toxin by 7–51 times (*135*). Incubation of a trichothecene-containing broth with sodium bicarbonate did not cause degradation of the toxins, thereby indicating that the effect of this compound was on the biosynthetic reactions.

Genetic studies utilizing two overlapping cosmid clones carrying a known trichothecene biosynthetic gene isolated from *F. sporotrichioides* provided evidence that several genes involved in trichothecene biosynthesis are closely linked on the chromosome (*136*). Transformation of two T-2 toxin-deficient *F. sporotrichioides* mutants with both of these cosmid clones restored T-2 production to both strains. It is unusual in fungi for genes involved in a specific biosynthetic pathway to be clustered.

Two new modified trichothecenes, 2-deoxy-11-*epi*-3α-hydroxysambucoin and 2-deoxy-11-*epi*-12-acetyl-3α-hydroxysambucoin, have been detected in corn grits infected with a *F. sporotrichioides* strain originally isolated from Ethiopian wheat (*137*). The structures, elucidated using GC–MS, NMR, and X-ray crystallography, contained two 6-membered rings which were *cis*-fused, the first such modified trichothecenes described. Preliminary toxicological studies indicated that these compounds were nontoxic to cultured baby hamster kidney cells.

Sensitive GC methods utilizing electron capture detection have been developed for the detection and quantitation of 13 trichothecenes in corn (*138*) and of 7 trichothecenes in wheat and corn (*139*). Minimum quantifiable limits in corn ranged from 50–200 µg/kg and in wheat ranged from 10–1000 ppb for the different toxins. A disc diffusion type bioassay utilizing yeast has been optimized for the detection of 10 trichothecenes (*140*).

**T-2 TOXIN.** Structural properties and toxicological effects of T-2 toxin were described and structure–function relationships discussed in a recent review by Bergman (*141*). Since trichothecenes penetrate eukaryotic cells and inhibit synthesis of DNA and proteins, these toxins may be potentially useful as antitumor agents.

To determine whether the known immunotoxic effects of T-2 toxin would adversely affect fetuses exposed in utero, pregnant mice were gavaged on gestation days 14–17 with 1.2 or 1.5 mg T-2 toxin/kg body weight (*142*). Significant thymic atrophy was observed in treated fetal mice examined on day 18. Further in vitro experiments demonstrated that T-2 toxin decreased thymocyte proliferation but that this was a result of toxic effects on lymphocyte progenitor cells rather than a direct cytotoxic effect on thymocytes.

Recent studies have shown that T-2 toxin binds to cells in culture, crosses cell membranes, and can inhibit protein synthesis by binding to ribosomes. During a study of T-2 toxin–cell association it was observed that certain steroids (progesterone, estradiol, testosterone, and diethylstilbestrol) increased this association by as much as 500% (*143*). These steroids did not affect the binding of T-2 to isolated ribosomes but the steroids may alter the state of ribosomal aggregation in intact cells such that more toxin can bind to them.

To determine the potential for nonenzymatic degradation of T-2 toxin in aqueous solutions, T-2 was dissolved in deuterated phosphate-buffered saline solutions containing 5% 2-propanol and adjusted to pD 5–12 (*144*). Decomposition, as monitored by NMR, was not observed in solutions of pD 5.0–6.7 even after one year. Above pD 6.7, degradation proceeded via sequential cleavage of ester side chains with an estimated half-life of 4 years at pD 7.4. Therefore, nonenzymatic decomposition of T-2 toxin appears to have negligible toxicological significance.

Previous reports that T-2 toxin was effectively destroyed by treatment with dilute alkaline hypochlorite (0.25% NaOCl + 0.025 M NaOH) for 4 h could not be duplicated in another lab (*145*). Rather, this treatment left a residual of about 3–5% of the T-2 intact and a much longer time (48–72 h) was required to completely destroy all the T-2 toxin.

A monoclonal antibody with a high degree of specificity for T-2 toxin has been isolated and found to effectively neutralize the cytotoxicity of this toxin (*146*). The antibody may be useful in studying mechanisms of toxicity and in treatment of T-2 toxemia.

DEOXYNIVALENOL (VOMITOXIN) AND RELATED COMPOUNDS. Mycological surveys of scabby wheat harvested from 19 fields in Japan demonstrated the presence of 4 species of *Fusarium*: *F. sporotrichioides*, *F. avenaceum*, *F. poae*, and *F. crookwellense* (*147*). The samples also contained 0.03–1.28 μg DON/g and 0.04–1.22 μg NIV/g.

Of 19 strains grown in culture, isolates of *F. poae* and *F. crookwellense* were found to be responsible for the production of NIV and DON.

Analyses of moldy maize samples (most of which had been discarded by farmers) in Nigeria, revealed the presence of NIV (0.8–1.0 mg/kg), DON (4.0–18.8 mg/kg), and 4-acetyl-nivalenol (3.0–15.0 mg/kg) (*148*). Other trichothecenes, including T-2 and HT-2 toxins, had previously been detected in these samples.

No carryover of deoxynivalenol (DON) from contaminated feed to milk was observed in experiments with 18 cows fed for 10 weeks with diets formulated to contain 0, 6, or 12 mg DON/kg of concentrate DM (*149*). DON contamination also did not affect the volume of milk produced.

Some food additives (sodium bisulfite, ammonium phosphate, and L-cysteine) when added to whole wheat flour at typical usage levels were found to reduce DON levels in bread baked from this flour by 38–46% (*150*). The baking process itself (without additives) destroyed about 7% of the DON. Potassium bromate and L-ascorbic acid had no effect on DON concentrations in the baked bread.

Hepatic microsomes from rats fed 6–12 ppm NIV for 2–4 weeks were found to have increased levels of cytochrome P450 activity and, in in vitro systems, increased the formation of aflatoxin–DNA adducts (*151*). NIV also appeared to enhance the activity of cytosolic glutathione S-transferase in hepatic cells and this cytosolic fraction diminished the increased adduct formation. In vivo experiments with rats fed 12 ppm NIV for 2 weeks and then injected with aflatoxin $B_1$ demonstrated that pretreatment with NIV did not increase aflatoxin–DNA adducts in the liver.

To determine whether dietary DON elevates IgE levels as it does IgA levels, mice were fed diets containing 25 ppm DON for up to 24 weeks (*152*). Serum IgE levels measured at weeks 12–24 were 2–5 times higher in treated mice than in controls. When mice were fed DON for 8 weeks and then continued on a toxin-free diet for the next 16 weeks, there was no significant decrease in their IgE levels at weeks 12–24 compared to those of mice fed DON during the whole 24 weeks. These results suggest that DON may function as an etiologic agent in human hypersensitivities as well as in IgA-mediated autoimmune diseases.

An HPLC method for the detection of DON in cow's milk has been developed with a detection limit of 5 ng/mL milk (*153*). In order to develop simpler and more sensitive immunoassays for DON and nivalenol (NIV), three mono- and two dihemisuccinates of NIV have been prepared for use as haptens (*154*). This paper also describes procedures for the bulk production and purification of NIV and 4,15-diacetylnivalenol. Polyclonal antibodies against 15-acetylDON have been used in microtiter plate and membrane-based dipstick ELISAs to detect 15-ADON in wheat, with detection limits of 50–100 ng/g (*155*).

## Fumonisins

Papers from a 1993 symposium on fumonisins have been recently published and include information on and discussion of: fumonisin production in corn by two toxigenic strains (*156*); toxicity of fumonisins and their possible role in human and animal diseases (*157*); mechanisms of fumonisin toxicity (*158*); methods for detection and determination of fumonisins (*159*); and incidence of contamination with toxigenic *Fusarium* and fumonisins in corn and corn-based foods and feeds (*160*).

Recent reviews on fumonisins have been written by Riley et al. (*161*), Nelson et al. (*162*), and Scott (*163*). All consider the chemistry and toxicology of these toxins and analytical methods for their determination.

A new fumonisin, fumonisin $C_1$ ($FC_1$), has been isolated from cultures of *F. moniliforme* (*164*). $FC_1$ is similar in structure to fumonisin $FB_1$ but lacks the amino-end terminal methyl group.

TOXICOLOGICAL EFFECTS. Although fumonisins are known carcinogens, the initiation of liver cancer in rats by $FB_1$ is masked by the hepatotoxic effects of this mycotoxin. In order to study this process in more detail, rats were fed for 21 days with diets containing 250–750 ppm $FB_1$ and then following enhancement of initiated cells by treatment with 2-AAF and partial hepatectomy, liver tissue was examined for the presence of resistant hepatocytes (*165*). The effective dose for cancer initiation was found to be in the range of 14.2–30.8 mg $FB_1$/100 g body weight (equivalent to a daily intake of 0.7–1.5 mg/100 g). At the lowest dose of $FB_1$ tested, this mycotoxin effectively delayed cell proliferation. This may explain why fumonisins are slow cancer initiators. Further studies testing the initiating potential of $FB_2$, $FB_3$, $FA_1$, and their hydrolysis products revealed that only the fumonisin B toxins initiated formation of resistant hepatocytes (*166*). It appears that both a free amino group and an intact fumonisin molecule are important for both the cytotoxic and the carcinogenic effects of these mycotoxins.

Since $FB_1$ is a potent inhibitor of sphingolipid synthesis, it causes the accumulation of the intermediate, sphinganine, in cultured cells. Elevated free sphinganine levels in serum or urine of animals may therefore be indicative of consumption of feed contaminated with fumonisins. Riley et al. (*167*) devised a method for the extraction of free sphingoid bases from serum, urine and various tissues of animals and the LC determination of sphinganine and sphingosine concentrations. An elevated sphinganine:sphingosine ratio in urine of rats fed diets containing 15, 50, or 150 μg $FB_1$/g was closely correlated with histopathological changes observed in their kidneys (*168*).

Disruption of sphingolipid metabolism also results in neurotoxic and mitogenic effects. Mouse cerebellar neurons cultured in the presence of $FB_1$ accumulated free sphinganine and experienced a reduction in total sphingolipids (*169*). Observations on the metabolic fate of some radiolabelled precursors indicated that sphingomyelin synthesis was more sensitive to inhibition by $FB_1$ than was glycolipid formation.

Since it was known that addition of free sphingosine to Swiss 3T3 cells stimulated DNA synthesis, experiments were undertaken to determine whether $FB_1$ had a similar effect (*170*). Indeed, when $FB_1$ was added to these cells, it stimulated the incorporation of thymidine into DNA.

During 3 days following a single oral dose of $^{14}C$-labelled $FB_1$ (8 mg/kg), feces from vervet monkeys were collected and analyzed for radioactive metabolites (*171*). Using an improved, newly described method for extraction of this toxin from feces, radioactivity was found to be concentrated in two spots on TLC. One fraction was identified as $FB_1$ and the other proved to be an equilibrium mixture of two structural isomers of partially hydrolyzed $FB_1$.

$FB_1$ is almost completely hydrolyzed by nixtamalization, a traditional treatment of corn with $Ca(OH)_2$ and heat to produce masa (tortilla flour). However, this process does not completely detoxify this mycotoxin, as shown in some feeding studies with rats (*172*). Compared to controls fed diets with no $FB_1$, rats fed $FB_1$-contaminated corn and nixtamalized, contaminated corn had lower body weights, higher plasma cholesterol levels, and increased incidences of hepatic adenomas and cholangiomas. These effects were not so severe in animals given the nixtamalized feed. Supplementation of the diets with B vitamins and casein increased body weights of the experimental rats but also increased the incidence of neoplastic changes in most groups. Thus, nixtamalization is probably not a useful method for detoxification of $FB_1$-contaminated foods.

BIOSYNTHESIS. Use of radiolabelled methionine (*173*), alanine (*174*), and acetate (*175*) has demonstrated that *F. moniliforme* utilizes all these compounds to synthesize fumonisins. Optimum labelling conditions in the first experiment were the addition of 50 mg unlabelled methionine and 200 μCi of $^{14}$C-labelled methionine to a 30 g corn patty over a period of 9 days. This resulted in [$^{14}$C]FB$_1$ with a specific activity of 36 μCi/mmol. Under static culture conditions, about 5.5% of $^{13}$C-alanine was incorporated intact into FB$_1$. When $^{14}$C-acetate was added to cultures, the label was distributed throughout the fumonisin molecule. Addition of $^{13}$C-labelled amino acids to growing cultures indicated that methionine, glutarate, and serine or alanine are added to the hydrocarbon fumonisin backbone during toxin biosynthesis.

OCCURRENCE AND CONTROL IN FOODS. Surveys of different foods continue to demonstrate that fumonisins most commonly occur in corn and corn-based foods. Analyses of corn from areas in China with high and low incidences of esophageal cancer indicated that 48% of corn from the high incidence area and 25% of that from the low incidence area were contaminated with fumonisins (*176*). Mean concentrations of FB$_1$ in the contaminated samples were 872 and 890 ng/g, respectively, and for FB$_2$ were 448 and 330 ng/g, respectively, in the high- and low-incidence areas.

Seventeen samples of Argentinian corn contaminated with *F. moniliforme* were found to have high levels of total fumonisins (1585–9990 ng/g) (*177*). FB$_1$ was the predominant analogue produced by the *F. moniliforme* strains in culture while one strain of *Fusarium proliferatum*, of three isolated, produced only FB$_2$. FB$_1$ has also been detected in samples of maize from India at levels of 300–366 ppm (*178*). Of 28 samples of the 1991 Georgia corn crop analyzed, 27 tested positive for aflatoxins, 24 were positive for FB$_1$, and 23 contained both mycotoxins (*179*). No correlation was observed between concentrations of the two toxins. However, these results indicate that exposure to both mycotoxins can occur simultaneously.

A total of 58 strains of *Fusarium* isolated in Europe from corn (41), sorghum (4), wheat (6), barley (5), and mixed feeds (2) were grown on corn for 28 days and then analyzed for mycotoxin production (*180*). All strains of *F. moniliforme* and the one tested strain of *F. proliferatum* produced fumonisins, with most strains generating more FB$_1$ than FB$_2$. Highest levels of fumonisins were detected in cultures of isolates from corn. Very little or no fumonisins were present in cultures of *Fusarium subglutinans*. FB$_1$ was also the predominant homolog produced by 33 strains of *F. moniliforme* isolated from Mexican maize (*181*) and by several *F. moniliforme* strains from the culture collection of the Fusarium Research Center (Pennsylvania)

(*182*), although FB$_2$ and FB$_3$ were also present in many cultures.

Control of fumonisin contamination of foods could potentially be achieved at several points. Tests with 15 commercially available corn hybrids grown in 17 locations in the USA demonstrated some variability in susceptibility to fumonisin contamination (5.78–30.53 μg/g) (*183*). Toxin levels were significantly related to June rainfall but not to kernel characteristics such as protein, oil, starch, or total fiber. These results indicate that it should be possible to select for fumonisin-resistant strains, but that weather conditions will still play a major role in determining contamination levels during a given year.

Sieving of 10 fumonisin-contaminated maize samples, taken from bulk shipments, yielded two fractions (whole kernels and fines) with different toxin concentrations (*184*). Ranges of fumonisin levels in fines (<3 mm diameter) and kernels were 12,340–27,460 ng/g and 530–1890 ng/g, respectively. Removal of fines from bulk shipments of maize could remove 26–69% of the contamination and would constitute a preliminary decontamination procedure.

Experiments to determine the thermostability of FB$_1$ in dry contaminated corn disclosed half-lives of 10, 38, 175, and 480 min at 150, 125, 100, and 75°C, respectively (*185,186*). Therefore, under normal drying conditions little FB$_1$ is destroyed.

Following oral or intravenous administration of $^{14}$C-FB$_1$ to laying hens, only trace residues were present in crop, liver, and kidney (*187*). Systemic absorption of oral doses of fumonisin appeared to be poor, with less than 2% of the administered dose being absorbed and no radioactivity detected in muscles or in eggs during the 24-h post-dosing period.

Radioactivity remaining in swine tissues 72 h after a single iv dose with radiolabelled FB$_1$ was approximately 19.8%, while tissue residue levels following intragastric dosing were 10- to 20-fold lower (*188*). Systemic bioavailability of fumonisin following an oral dose was estimated to be 3–6%, with the highest concentration found in liver.

DETECTION AND DETERMINATION. The MTT bioassay which utilizes the tetrazolium salt MTT to measure cell viability and proliferation, has been optimized for the detection of FB$_1$ and FB$_2$ (*189*). Proliferation of turkey lymphocytes was inhibited after 48- and 72-h exposure to these toxins.

Several variations of HPLC procedures for determination of fumonisins in corn, cereal products, laboratory media, and animal excreta have been described (*190–192*).

FB$_1$ labelled on the branch methyl groups with deuterium has been produced by feeding *F. moniliforme* cultures deuterated methionine (*193*). This labelled FB$_1$ was then used as an internal standard in GC–MS and in fast atom bombardment MS procedures for the determination of this toxin in extracts of corn, corn products, and cultures.

Five stable hybridoma cell lines have been constructed to produce monoclonal antibodies against FB$_1$ (*194*). These antibodies were then used in a competitive indirect ELISA. Analyses of food samples with a monoclonal antibody–based competitive ELISA, HPLC, and GC–MS methods revealed that the ELISA gave higher estimates of fumonisin concentrations than HPLC and GC–MS methods (*195*). This may be a result of different methods for sample preparation or of the presence of structurally related compounds which can be detected by the antibodies but not by the other methods.

Effects of heat and different extraction solvents on the recovery of fumonisins added to corn-based foods have been investigated (*196*). Heating of dry or moist corn meal at 190°C for 60 min destroyed 60–80% of the toxins while heating at 220°C for 25 min completely destroyed them. Different solvent systems were more or less effective in extracting the fumonisins depending on the foods examined (corn meal, corn bran flour, corn bran breakfast cereal, mixed cereal for babies). This emphasizes the need for controlled recovery experiments for each type of food analyzed.

## Other Non-Trichothecenes

A sensitive and reliable liquid chromatographic method with fluorescence detection has been developed for the determination of zearalenone and α-zearalenol in barley and Job's tears (used as a health food and herbal remedy in Japan) (*197*). Detection limit was estimated to be 0.2 ng and recoveries averaged 96–103%.

Examination of 25 samples of Peruvian maize from different parts of the country revealed that the most common toxigenic *Fusarium* species were *F. subglutinans* and *F. moniliforme* (*198*). All 8 tested isolates of *F. subglutinans* produced both moniliformin (70–270 mg/kg) and beauvericin (BEA, 50–250 mg/kg) when grown on autoclaved corn kernels. Contamination with *F. subglutinans* and production of BEA and moniliformin were also reported from moldy corn ears collected in Poland (*199*). BEA is known for its insecticidal properties and is also toxic to *Artemia salina*.

A new compound toxic to *Artemia salina* and cytotoxic to 6 of 60 human tumor cell lines has been isolated from cultures of *F. tricinctum* (*200*). This

metabolite, named visoltricin, was examined using UV, IR, MS, and NMR and found to have the structure: 3-[1-methyl-4-(3-methyl-2-butenyl)imidazol-5-yl]-2-propenoic acid.

## MYCOTOXINS PRODUCED BY *PENICILLIUM* SPP.

Examination of 18 samples of wheat, barley, and mixed feed from the UK revealed the presence of several species of *Penicillium* (*201*). *Penicillium verrucosum,* which produced both ochratoxin A (OA) and citrinin, occurred in two samples; subspecies of *P. aurantiogriseum,* most of which produced the naphthoquinone mycotoxins xanthomegnin, viomellein, and vioxanthin were isolated from 11 samples. Thus, there could potentially be 5 nephrotoxic mycotoxins in poorly stored grain.

Of five cultured cell lines used to evaluate the cytotoxicity of OA and citrinin, the most sensitive was the MDCK canine kidney cell line (*202*). The MTT colorimetric assay was a better indicator of toxicity than the measurement of some enzyme activities. LD$_{50}$ values for both mycotoxins were of a similar magnitude as measured in this assay and in rodent assays.

To investigate interactions between OA and citrinin, renal cortical cubes from young adult swine were cultured in vitro in the presence of $10^{-6}$–$10^{-3}$ M citrinin and/or OA (*203*). None of the experiments demonstrated antagonism between the toxins while one showed synergism. However, the synergistic responses were neither strong nor consistent.

### Ochratoxin

Using a newly devised extraction procedure and analysis by ion pair liquid chromatography with fluorescence detection, 36 cows' milk and 40 human milk samples from Sweden were analyzed for OA residues (*204*). Five of the bovine and 23 of the human milk samples contained OA (range of 10–40 ng/L). Analyses of blood samples from the mothers who provided milk demonstrated that all were contaminated with OA, with an average of 167 ng/L (range of 90–940 ng/L).

Carryover of OA from contaminated feed to various tissues and organs of swine and sausages made from them has been investigated in two series of experiments. Feeding pigs a diet containing 0.58 or 0.15 ppm OA for 28 days caused no obvious toxic effects to the animals but did leave residues of 5.2–6.4 µg/kg in liver and 3.0–3.6 µg/kg in kidneys of the high-dose animals (*205*). During another feeding trial of a diet contaminated with 0.1 or 0.4 ppm OA, again no obvious toxicity was noted (206,207). However, in the high-dose pigs, residues of 77, 10.3, 36.9, 50.1, and 43.6 µg OA/kg were detected in blood, muscle, liver, heart, and kidneys, respectively. Of various types of dry sausage made from tissues of this group, fresh salami had the lowest concentration of OA (12 µg/kg) and blood sausage had the highest level (83.3 µg/kg).

Microbial degradation of OA was tested using 27 species of bacteria, 10 yeasts, and 14 molds (208). Only *Acinetobacter calcoaceticus* was capable of degrading this toxin in liquid cultures at 25 or 30°C, with an initial OA concentration of 10 µg/mL. Thin-layer chromatography indicated that the main decomposition product was ochratoxin α (Oα), a much less toxic compound.

OA exerts a number of toxic effects in animals, with the most prominent being nephrotoxicity and urinary tract tumors. Experiments to assess the genotoxicity of OA, its major metabolite in rodents, Oα, and 7 other structurally related compounds revealed that OA and 4 chlorinated compounds induced SOS DNA repair in *E. coli* while ochratoxin B, Oα, citrinin, and one other compound were inactive (209). All except Oα were cytotoxic. Experiments with other tester strains of *E. coli* indicated that an OA-derived free radical was the genotoxic intermediate in bacteria.

OA also forms adducts with DNA in experimental animals. Forty-eight hours following an oral dose of 2.5 mg OA/kg body weight, total DNA adducts in kidney, liver, and spleen of mice were 103, 42, and 2.2 adducts per $10^9$ nucleotides (210). The principal adduct formed in liver differed from that in the kidneys, and adducts persisted in the kidneys for up to 16 days while those in the liver disappeared within 5 days. Both the number and persistence of adducts in the kidney indicate that it is the major site of genotoxic damage.

Nephrotoxic effects of OA have been investigated by Gekle et al. in experiments with Madin-Darby canine kidney (MDCK) cells in vitro and in rats injected ip with 0.5 mg OA/kg/day for 6 days (211–213). Glomerular filtration rates in rats dosed with OA were reduced to 63% that of control rats and excretion of Na+, K+, and Cl⁻ was increased but did not affect excretion of amino acids or phosphate. Total renal vascular resistance also increased. OA blocked the fractional anion conductance of the plasma membrane of the MDCK cells. Since the MDCK cells are considered a model of collecting duct epithelium, it appears that OA acts acutely on the post-proximal parts of the nephron and that its action on the proximal tubules would decrease their capacity to eliminate OA.

Possible adverse effects of OA on rat testes were investigated in animals gavaged every other day for up to 8 weeks with 289 µg OA/kg (214). OA was found to elevate testicular levels of α-amylase, alkaline phosphatase, and γ-glutamyltransferase and these increased enzyme levels may be associated with impairment of spermatogenesis. After about 3 weeks of treatment testicular testosterone levels were approximately double those in control animals.

A sensitive and quantitative ELISA has been developed for the determination of OA in feeds (215). Antibodies for the assay were obtained from the yolk of eggs from immunized hens using an optimized purification procedure.

## Citrinin

Testing of 122 isolates of *Penicillium expansum* from apple packaging plants in Spain revealed that 43% were capable of producing citrinin in laboratory media (216). Most of the citrinin-positive strains originated in decaying apples and most were also able to produce citrinin when grown on apples or apple juice.

Under anhydrous conditions citrinin can be detoxified by heating to 175°C, while under semi-moist conditions only 140°C is required. When heated in the presence of water, citrinin decomposes to form several spots and peaks detectable by TLC and HPLC (217). One of these products, citrinin H1, has been isolated and its structure determined. In standard cytotoxicity assays, citrinin H1 is about 10 times as toxic as citrinin on a unit weight basis. Citrinin H1 was also detected in solutions of citrinin heated to 100°C for 30 min. These results emphasize that the decomposition of a toxin does not always lead to its detoxification.

When citrinin is fed to pregnant rats and mice, it exerts embryotoxic/fetotoxic effects. To determine whether it is also a developmental toxin, cells of *Hydra attenuata* and whole rat embryos in culture were exposed to various citrinin concentrations (218). Neither assay system indicated that citrinin is a primary developmental mycotoxin although it is lethal at high concentrations and may be maternotoxic.

## Patulin

Screening of extracts of 67 different fungi identified 52 patulin-producing strains, including 15 species which were not previously known to produce patulin (219). All of the strains tested were from a culture collection and had been isolated from a variety of substrates.

Both potassium sorbate and cinnamon oil were found to be effective inhibitors of growth of *P. expansum* on laboratory media and of patulin production in apple juice (*220*). Although fungal growth occurred, no patulin was detectable in juice containing 0.1% cinnamon oil or 0.2% sorbate, inoculated with *P. expansum*, and incubated for 7 days. Clove oil and eugenol were less effective inhibitors and benomyl at 2.5 ppm actually stimulated patulin production. Surface application of cinnamon oil and sorbate to apples also decreased spoilage of fruit.

Whole rat embryos in culture exposed for 45 hours to 47 or 55 µM patulin showed a number of developmental defects while those exposed to higher patulin concentrations died (*221*). Anomalies induced included growth retardation, hypoplasia of the mesencephalon and telencephalon, and hyperplasia of the mandibular process.

Two procedures have been described for the HPLC determination of patulin in apple juice (*222,223*). Polyclonal antibodies against patulin hemiglutarate conjugated with bovine serum albumin have been isolated and used in an ELISA to detect patulin (*224*).

## Other Toxins

A very specific monoclonal antibody to cyclopiazonic acid has been raised from a murine hybridoma and has been used in an antibody-immobilized ELISA for the detection of cyclopiazonic acid (*225*). The assay can also be used to detect this mycotoxin in white-mold fermented cheeses.

Luteoskyrin, a hepatotoxic mycotoxin produced by *Penicillium islandicum*, has been shown, by EPR spin-trap techniques, to produce ·OH when mixed with ascorbic acid and ferrous ions (*226*). The EPR signals disappeared in the presence of excess catalase, and the iron-chelator desferoxamine inhibited the formation of these radicals, indicating that they were derived from hydrogen peroxide.

Analyses of molded maize silage in Japan yielded 58 fungal strains capable of producing indole alkaloids (*227*). One isolate, studied in detail, was identified as *Penicillium roqueforti* and was found to produce roquefortine C as the major alkaloid and smaller amounts of roquefortines A, B, and D and festuclavine in cultures. When this isolate was grown on maize, the principal mycotoxins produced were roquefortine A (2.4 mg/kg) and roquefortine C (1.66 mg/kg).

In a study of the biosynthesis of some tremorgenic mycotoxins, [14]C-labelled paxilline and some of its derivatives were fed to submerged cultures of *Penicillium janczewskii* and *Penicillium janthinellum*, which produce penitrem and janthitrem alkaloids, respectively

(*228*). [14]C]Paxilline was incorporated into penitrems and janthitrems at rates of 13.7 and 23.2% and [14]Cβ-paxitriol was incorporated at rates of 10.7 and 34.5%. This indicates that both of these compounds are intermediates in the biosynthesis of these mycotoxins. However, α-paxitriol did not appear to be an intermediate.

## OTHER MYCOTOXINS

### Ergot Alkaloids

A procedure for the semicontinuous and continuous production of pharmaceutically useful ergot alkaloids has been achieved by cultivation of immobilized *Claviceps purpurea* (*229*). A high concentration of $CaCl_2$ (96.9 mM) was found to prolong the productive phase, and restriction of phosphate supplies prevented the problem of a massive increase of outgrowing hyphae.

### Tremorgenic Mycotoxins

Molecular structure of lolitrem B, causative agent of ryegrass staggers in livestock, has been elucidated by the use of NOE NMR (*230*). The configuration of the A/B ring junction was determined and described.

### Sporidesmin

Sporidesmin, another mycotoxin causing illness in grazing ruminants, is a hydrophobic molecule which may affect cell membrane structure and function. To investigate this possibility, sporidesmin molecules in dimyristoyl-sn-3-phosphatidyl choline bilayers were localized in the glycerol-backbone region of the bilayer by examining changes in the phase properties of the bilayers (*231*). Oxidized and reduced forms of sporidesmin apparently perturbed bilayer organization, thereby altering the susceptibility of the bilayer to pancreatic phospholipase $A_2$.

### LITERATURE CITED

1. Anwar, W.A., and C.P. Wild. The Pan African Environmental Mutagen Society, report on inaugural meeting: "Mycotoxins as mutagens and carcinogens: possibilities for disease prevention", Cairo, Egypt, 23–26 January 1993. *Mutat. Res.* 312:61–63 (1994).

2. Sanchis, V., and I. Viñas. Mycotoxin research in Spain. *Rev. Española Cien. Tecnol. Aliment.* 34:134–144 (1994).

3. Rafai, P., Á. Bata, and A. Ványi. Mycotoxin contamination of cereals and feed mixtures in Hungary. *Hung. Agric. Res.* 2(4):12–15 (1993).

4. Scudamore, K.A. Mycotoxins in stored products: myth or menace. *Int. Biodeteriorat. Biodegradat.* 32:191–203 (1993).

5. Chu, F.S., and G.Y. Li. Simultaneous occurrence of fumonisin B$_1$ and other mycotoxins in moldy corn collected from the People's Republic of China in regions with high incidences of esophageal cancer. *Appl. Environ. Microbiol.* 60:847–852 (1994).

6. Škrinjar, M., and G. Dimić. Ochratoxigenicity of *Aspergillus ochraceus* group and *Penicillium verrucosum* var. *cyclopium* strains on various media. *Acta Microbiol. Hung.* 39:257–261 (1992).

7. Usha, C.M., K.L. Patkar, H.S. Shetty, et al. Fungal colonization and mycotoxin contamination of developing rice grain. *Mycol. Res.* 97:795–798 (1993).

8. Mahmoud, A.-L.E., and M.H. Abd-Alla. Natural occurrence of mycotoxins in broad bean (*Vicia faba* L.) seeds and their effect on *Rhizobium*–legume symbiosis. *J. Basic Microbiol.* 34:97–103 (1994).

9. Zohri, A.A., and K.M. Abdel-Gawad. Survey of mycoflora and mycotoxins of some dried fruits in Egypt. *J. Basic Microbiol.* 33:279–288 (1993).

10. Zohri, A.A., and S.M. Saber. Filamentous fungi and mycotoxin detected in coconut. *Zbl. Mikrobiol.* 148:325–332 (1993).

11. Adebajo, L.O. Survey of aflatoxins and ochratoxin A in stored tubers of *Cyperus esculentus* L. *Mycopathologia* 124:41–46 (1993).

12. Abdel-Gawad, K.M., and A.A. Zohri. Fungal flora and mycotoxins of six kinds of nut seeds for human consumption in Saudi Arabia. *Mycopathologia* 124:55–64 (1993).

13. Pitt, J.I., A.D. Hocking, K. Bhudhasamai, et al. The normal mycoflora of commodities from Thailand. 1. Nuts and oilseeds. *Int. J. Food Microbiol.* 20:211–226 (1993).

14. Madden, U.A., and H.M. Stahr. Preliminary determination of mycotoxin binding to soil when leaching through soil with water. *Int. Biodeteriorat. Biodegradat.* 31:265–275 (1993).

15. Garza, S., R. Canela, I. Viñas, and V. Sanchis. Effects of potassium sorbate on growth and penicillic acid production by *Aspergillus ochraceus* and *Penicillium aurantiogriseum. Zbl. Mikrobiol.* 148:343–350 (1993).

16. Yasin, M., M.A. Hanna, and L.B. Bullerman. Potassium sorbate inhibition of mold in high moisture corn. *Trans. Am. Soc. Agric. Eng.* 35:1229–1233 (1992).

17. Wendorff, W.L., W.E. Riha, and E. Muehlenkamp. Growth of molds on cheese treated with heat and liquid smoke. *J. Food Protect.* 56:963–966 (1993).

18. Thompson, D.P., L. Metevia, and T. Vessel. Influence of pH alone and in combination with phenolic antioxidants on growth and germination of mycotoxigenic species of *Fusarium* and *Penicillium. J. Food Protect.* 56:134–138 (1993).

19. Thompson, D.P. Minimum inhibitory concentration of esters of p-hydroxybenzoic acid (paraben) combinations against toxigenic fungi. *J. Food Protect.* 57:133–135 (1994).

20. Dugyala, R.R., Y.-W. Kim, and R.P. Sharma. Effects of aflatoxin B$_1$ and T-2 toxin on the granulocyte-macrophage progenitor cells in mouse bone marrow cultures. *Immunopharmacology* 27:57–65 (1994).

21. Plumlee, K.H., and F.D. Galey. Neurotoxic mycotoxins: a review of fungal toxins that cause neurological disease in large animals. *J. Vet. Intern. Med.* 8:49–54 (1994).

22. Knaus, H.-G., O.B. McManus, S.H. Lee, et al. Tremorgenic indole alkaloids potently inhibit smooth muscle high-conductance calcium-activated potassium channels. *Biochemistry* 33:5819–5828 (1994).

23. Di Paolo, N., A. Guarnieri, F. Loi, et al. Acute renal failure from inhalation of mycotoxins. *Nephron* 64:621–625 (1993).

24. Gordon, K.E., R.E. Masotti, and W.R. Waddell. Tremorgenic encephalopathy: a role of mycotoxins in the production of CNS disease in humans? *Can. J. Neurol. Sci.* 20:237–239 (1993).

25. Venitt, S., and P.J. Biggs. Radon, mycotoxins, p53, and uranium mining. *Lancet* 343:795 (1994).

26. Richard, J.L., G.A. Bennett, P.F. Ross, and P.E. Nelson. Analysis of naturally occurring mycotoxins in feedstuffs and food. *J. Anim. Sci.* 71:2563–2574 (1993).

26. Panigrahi, S. Bioassay of mycotoxins using terrestrial and aquatic, animal and plant species. *Food Chem. Toxicol.* 31:767–790 (1993).

28. Madhyastha, M.S., R. R. Marquardt, A. Masi, et al. Comparison of toxicity of different mycotoxins to several species of bacteria and yeasts: use of *Bacillus brevis* in a disc diffusion assay. *J. Food Protect.* 57:48–53 (1994).

29. Abouzied, M.M., and J.J. Pestka. Simultaneous screening of fumonisin B$_1$, aflatoxin B$_1$, and zearalenone by line immunoblot: a computer-assisted multianalyte assay system. *J. AOAC Int.* 77:495–501 (1994).

30. Magan, N. Early detection of fungi in stored grain. *Int. Biodeteriorat. Biodegradat.* 32:145–160 (1993).

31. Schwabe, M., J. Menke, and J. Krämer. Einsatz des EPS-ELISA zur Bestimmung von Schimmelpilzen der Gattungen *Aspergillus* und *Penicillium* in Lebensmitteln. *Arch. Lebensmittelhyg.* 44:64–66 (1993).

32. Eaton, D.L., and E.P. Gallagher. Mechanisms of aflatoxin carcinogenesis. *Annu. Rev. Pharmacol. Toxicol.* 34:135–172 (1994).

33. Raisuddin, S. Toxic responses to aflatoxins in a developing host. *J. Toxicol.–Toxin Rev.* 12:175–201 (1993).

34. Gerbes, A.L., and W.H. Caselmann. Point mutations of the *P53* gene, human hepatocellular carcinoma and aflatoxins. *J. Hepatol.* 19:312–315 (1993).

35. Groopman, J.D., G.N. Wogan, B.D. Roebuck, and T.W. Kensler. Molecular biomarkers for aflatoxins and their application to human cancer prevention. *Cancer Res.* 54(Suppl.):1907s–1911s (1994).

36. Shebar, F.Z., J.D. Groopman, G.-S. Qian, and G.N. Wogan. Quantitative analysis of aflatoxin–albumin adducts. *Carcinogenesis* 14:1203–1208 (1993).

37. Hatch, M.C., C.-J. Chen, B. Levin, et al. Urinary aflatoxin levels, hepatitis-B virus infection and hepatocellular carcinoma in Taiwan. *Int. J. Cancer* 54:931–934 (1993).

38. Gallagher, E.P., L.C. Wienkers, P.L. Stapleton, et al. Role of human microsomal and human complementary DNA-expressed cytochromes P4501A2 and P4503A4 in the bioactivation of aflatoxin B₁. *Cancer Res.* 54:101–108 (1994).

39. Kirby, G.M., C.R. Wolf, G.E. Neal, et al. *In vitro* metabolism of aflatoxin B₁ by normal and tumorous liver tissue from Thailand. *Carcinogenesis* 14:2613–2620 (1993).

40. Aguilar, F., S. P. Hussain, and P. Cerutti. Aflatoxin B₁ induces the transversion of G → T in codon 249 of the p53 tumor suppressor gene in human hepatocytes. *Proc. Natl. Acad. Sci. USA* 90:8586–8590 (1993).

41. Tokusashi, Y., I. Fukuda, and K. Ogawa. Absence of *p53* mutations and various frequences of ki-*ras* exon 1 mutations in rat hepatic tumors induced by different carcinogens. *Molec. Carcinogen.* 10:45–51 (1994).

42. Hayashi, H., K. Sugio, T. Matsumata, et al. The mutation of codon 249 in the *p53* gene is not specific in Japanese hepatocellular carcinoma. *Liver* 13:279–281 (1993).

43. Ng, I.O.L., L.P. Chung, S.W.Y. Tsang, et al. p53 gene mutation spectrum in hepatocellular carcinomas in Hong Kong Chinese. *Oncogene* 9:985–990 (1994).

44. Okumura, H., O. Kawamura, S. Kishimoto, et al. Aflatoxin M₁ in Nepalese sera, quantified by combination of monoclonal antibody immunoaffinity chromatography and enzyme-linked immunosorbent assay. *Carcinogenesis* 14:1233–1235 (1993).

45. Kolars, J.C., P. Benedict, P. Schmiedlin-Ren, and P.B. Watkins. Aflatoxin B1-adduct formation in rat and human small bowel enterocytes. *Gastroenterology* 106:433–439 (1994).

46. Hashim, S., V.S. Aboobaker, R. Madhubala, et al. Modulatory effects of essential oils from spices on the formation of DNA adduct by aflatoxin B₁ *in vitro*. *Nutr. Cancer* 21:169–175 (1994).

47. Adhikari, M., G. Ramjee, and P. Berjak. Aflatoxin, kwashiorkor, and morbidity. *Nat. Toxins* 2:1–3 (1994).

48. Hayes, J.D., D.J. Judah, and G.E. Neal. Resistance to aflatoxin B₁ is associated with the expression of a novel aldo-keto reductase which has catalytic activity towards a cytotoxic aldehyde-containing metabolite of the toxin. *Cancer Res.* 53:3887–3894 (1993).

49. Yabe, K., Y. Matsuyama, Y. Ando, et al. Stereochemistry during aflatoxin biosynthesis: conversion of norsolorinic acid to averufin. *Appl. Environ. Microbiol.* 59:2486–2492 (1993).

50. Yabe, K., and T. Hamasaki. Stereochemistry during aflatoxin biosynthesis: cyclase reaction in the conversion of versiconal to versicolorin B and racemization of versiconal hemiacetal acetate. *Appl. Environ. Microbiol.* 59:2493–2500 (1993).

51. Liu, B.H., N.P. Keller, D. Bhatnagar, et al. Production and characterization of antibodies against sterigmatocystin O-methyltransferase. *Food Agric. Immunol.* 5:155–164 (1993).

52. Yu, J., J.W. Cary, D. Bhatnagar, et al. Cloning and characterization of a cDNA from *Aspergillus parasiticus* encoding an O-methyltransferase involved in aflatoxin biosynthesis. *Appl. Environ. Microbiol.* 59:3564–3571 (1993).

53. Chang, P.-K., J.W. Cary, D. Bhatnagar, et al. Cloning of the *Aspergillus parasiticus apa-2* gene associated with the regulation of aflatoxin biosynthesis. *Appl. Environ. Microbiol.* 59:3273–3279 (1993).

54. Zeringue, H.J., Jr., D. Bhatnagar, and T.E. Cleveland. $C_{15}H_{24}$ volatile compounds unique to aflatoxigenic strains of *Aspergillus flavus*. *Appl. Environ. Microbiol.* 59:2264–2270 (1993).

55. Bilgrami, K.S., and A.K. Choudhary. Impact of habitats on toxigenic potential of *Aspergillus flavus*. *J. Stored Prod. Res.* 29:351–355 (1993).

56. Atawodi, S.E., A.A. Atiku, and A.G. Lamorde. Aflatoxin contamination of Nigerian foods and feedingstuffs. *Food Chem. Toxicol.* 32:61–63 (1994).

57. Park, D.L., and B. Liang. Perspectives on aflatoxin control for human food and animal feed. *Trends Food Sci. Technol.* 4:334–342 (1993).

58. Park, D.L. Controlling aflatoxin in food and feed. *Food Technol.* 47(10):92–96 (1993).

59. Bhatnagar, D., P.J. Cotty, and T.E. Cleveland. Preharvest aflatoxin contamination. Molecular strategies for its control. In *Food Flavor and Safety. Molecular Analysis and Design*. A.M. Spanier et al. (eds.). *ACS Symp. Ser.* 528:272–292 (1993).

60. Cleveland, T.E., and D. Bhatnagar. Molecular strategies for reducing aflatoxin levels in crops before harvest. In *Molecular Approaches to Improving Food Quality and Safety*. D. Bhatnagar and T. E. Cleveland (eds.). New York: Van Nostrand Reinhold. Pp. 205–228 (1992).

61. El-Kady, I.A., S.S.M. El-Maraghy, A.Y. Abdel-Mallek, and H.A.H. Hasan. Effect of four pesticides on aflatoxin production by *Aspergillus flavus* IMI 89717. *Zbl. Mikrobiol.* 148:549–557 (1993).

62. Tabata, S., H. Kamimura, A. Ibe, et al. Degradation of aflatoxins by food additives. *J. Food Protect.* 57:42–47 (1994).

63. Kawashima, K., P. Siriacha, and S. Kawasugi. Prevention of aflatoxin contamination in Thai maize. 1. Infection of Thai maize with *Aspergillus flavus*. *Japan Agric. Res. Q.* 27:55–60 (1993).

64. Brown, R.L., P.J. Cotty, T.E. Cleveland, and N.W. Widstrom. Living maize embryo influences accumulation of aflatoxin in maize kernels. *J. Food Protect.* 56:967–971 (1993).

65. Adegoke, G.O., E.J. Otumu, and A.O. Akanni. Influence of grain quality, heat, and processing time on the reduction of aflatoxin B₁ levels in 'tuwo' and 'ogi': two cereal-based products. *Plant Foods Human Nutr.* 45:113–117 (1994).

66. Lisker, N., R. Michaeli, and Z.R. Frank. Mycotoxigenic potential of *Aspergillus flavus* strains isolates from

groundnuts growing in Israel. *Mycopathologia* 122:177–183 (1993).

67. Sashidhar, R.B. Fate of aflatoxin B₁ during the industrial production of edible defatted peanut protein flour from raw peanuts. *Food Chem.* 48:349–352 (1993).

68. Ghewande, M.P., G. Nagaraj, S. Desai, and P. Narayan. Screening of groundnut bold-seeded genotypes for resistance to *Aspergillus flavus* seed colonisation and less aflatoxin production. *Seed Sci. Technol.* 21:45–51 (1993).

69. Reding, C.L.C., M.A. Harrison, and C.K. Kvien. *Aspergillus parasiticus* growth and aflatoxin synthesis on Florunner peanuts grown in gypsum-supplemented soil. *J. Food Protect.* 56:593–594,611 (1993).

70. Clavero, M.R.S., M.A. Harrison, and Y.-C. Hung. *Aspergillus parasiticus* NRRL 2667 growth and aflatoxin synthesis as affected by calcium content and initial spore load in single peanuts. *J. Food Protect.* 57:415–418 (1994).

71. El-Kady, I.A., and M.S. Youssef. Survey of mycoflora and mycotoxins in Egyptian soybean seeds. *J. Basic Microbiol.* 33:371–378 (1993).

72. Song, D.K., and A.L. Karr. Soybean phytoalexin, glyceollin, prevents accumulation of aflatoxin B₁ in cultures of *Aspergillus flavus. J. Chem. Ecol.* 19:1183–1194 (1993).

73. Paster, N., S. Droby, E. Chalutz, et al. Evaluation of the potential of the yeast *Pichia guilliermondii* as a biocontrol agent against *Aspergillus flavus* and fungi of stored soya beans. *Mycol. Res.* 97:1201–1206 (1993).

74. Bankole, S.A. Fungi associated with post-harvest rot of sweet orange (*Citrus sinensis*) and aflatoxin B₁ production by isolates of *Aspergillus flavus* on plain and supplemented orange juice. *Nahrung* 37:380–385 (1993).

75. Fang, S.W., C.F. Li, and D.Y.C. Shih. Antifungal activity of chitosan and its preservative effect on low-sugar candied kumquat. *J. Food Protect.* 57:136–140,145 (1994).

76. Sharman, M., S. MacDonald, A.J. Sharkey, and J. Gilbert. Sampling bulk consignments of dried figs for aflatoxin analysis. *Food Addit. Contam.* 11:17–23 (1994).

77. Adebajo, L.O., O.A. Bamgbelu, and R.A. Olowu. Mould contamination and the influence of water activity and temperature on mycotoxin production by two aspergilli in melon seed. *Nahrung* 38:209–217 (1994).

78. Gradziel, T.M., and D. Wang. Susceptibility of California almond cultivars to aflatoxigenic *Aspergillus flavus. HortScience* 29:33–35 (1994).

79. Garner, R.C., M.M. Whattam, P.J.L. Taylor, and M.W. Stow. Analysis of United Kingdom purchased spices for aflatoxins using an immunoaffinity column clean-up procedure followed by high-performance liquid chromatographic analysis and post-column derivatisation with pyridinium bromide perbromide. *J. Chromatogr.* 648:485–490 (1993).

80. Kumar, S., and A.K. Roy. Occurrence of aflatoxin in some liver curative herbal medicines. *Lett. Appl. Microbiol.* 17:112–114 (1993).

81. Blanco, J.L., B.A. Carrion, N. Liria, et al. Behavior of aflatoxins during manufacture and storage of yoghurt. *Milchwissenschaft* 48:385–387 (1993).

82. Hassanin, N.I. Stability of aflatoxin M₁ during manufacture and storage of yoghurt, yoghurt-cheese and acidified milk. *J. Sci. Food Agric.* 65:31–34 (1994).

83. Smith, E.E., T.D. Phillips, J.A. Ellis, et al. Dietary hydrated sodium calcium aluminosilicate reduction of aflatoxin M₁ residue in dairy goat milk and effects on milk production and components. *J. Anim. Sci.* 72:677–682 (1994).

84. Kubena, L.F., R. B. Harvey, W. E. Huff, et al. Efficacy of a hydrated sodium calcium aluminosilicate to reduce the toxicity of aflatoxin and diacetoxyscirpenol. *Poultry Sci.* 72:51–59 (1993).

85. Jindal, N., S.K. Mahipal, and N.K. Mahajan. Effect of hydrated sodium calcium aluminosilicate on prevention of aflatoxicosis in broilers. *Indian J. Anim. Sci.* 63:649–652 (1993).

86. Harvey, R.B., L.F. Kubena, M.H. Elissalde, et al. Comparison of two hydrated sodium calcium aluminosilicate compounds to experimentally protect growing barrows from aflatoxicosis. *J. Vet. Diagn. Invest.* 6:88–92 (1994).

87. Voss, K.A., J.W. Dorner, and R.J. Cole. Amelioration of aflatoxicosis in rats by Volclay NF-BC, microfine bentonite. *J. Food Protect.* 56:595–598 (1993).

88. Hussain, M., M.A. Gabal, T. Wilson, and R.C. Summerfelt. Effect of aflatoxin-contaminated feed on morbidity and residues in walleye fish. *Vet. Human Toxicol.* 35:396–398 (1993).

89. Patkar, K.L., C.M. Usha, H.S. Shetty, et al. Effect of spice essential oils on growth and aflatoxin B₁ production by *Aspergillus flavus. Lett. Appl. Microbiol.* 17:49–51 (1993).

90. Hasan, H.A.H., and A.-L.E. Mahmoud. Inhibitory effect of spice oils on lipase and mycotoxin production. *Zbl. Mikrobiol.* 148:543–548 (1993).

91. Masood, A., J.V.V. Dogra, and A.K. Jha. The influence of colouring and pungent agents of red chilli (*Capsicum annum*) on growth and aflatoxin production by *Aspergillus flavus. Lett. Appl. Microbiol.* 18:184–186 (1994).

92. Prasad, G., S.S. Sahay, and A. Masood. Inhibition in aflatoxin biosynthesis by the extract of *Amorphophallus campanulatus* (OL) and calcium oxalate. *Lett. Appl. Microbiol.* 18:203–205 (1994).

93. Olojede, F., G. Engelhardt, P.R. Wallnofer, and G.O. Adegoke. Decrease of growth and aflatoxin production in *Aspergillus parasiticus* caused by spices. *World J. Microbiol. Biotechnol.* 9:605–606 (1993).

94. Chourasia, H.K. Growth, sclerotia and aflatoxin production by *Aspergillus parasiticus*: influence of food preservatives. *Lett. Appl. Microbiol.* 17:204–207 (1993).

95. Rodriguez, S.B., and N.E. Mahoney. Inhibition of aflatoxin production by surfactants. *Appl. Environ. Microbiol.* 60:106–110 (1994).

96. Arino, A.A., and L.B. Bullerman. Growth and aflatoxin production by *Aspergillus parasiticus* NRRL 2999 as affected by the fungicide iprodione. *J. Food Protect.* 56:718–721 (1993).

97. Klich, M.A., A.R. Lax, J.M. Bland, and L.L. Scharfenstein, Jr. Influence of iturin A on mycelial weight and

aflatoxin production by *Aspergillus flavus* and *Aspergillus parasiticus* in shake culture. *Mycopathologia* 123:35–38 (1993).

98. Hasan, H.A.H., and S.A. Omar. Selective effect of organophosphate insecticides on metabolic activities and aflatoxins biosynthesis by two *Aspergillus* spp. *Cryptogamie Mycol.* 14:185–193 (1993).

99. Chatterjee, D., and S.K. Mukherjee. Destruction of phagocytosis-suppressing activity of aflatoxin $B_1$ by ozone. *Lett. Appl. Microbiol.* 17:52–54 (1993).

100. Ellis, W.O., J.P. Smith, B.K. Simpson, and H. Ramaswamy. Effect of inoculum level on aflatoxin production by *Aspergillus flavus* under modified atmosphere packaging (MAP) conditions. *Food Microbiol.* 10:525–535 (1993).

101. Whitaker, T.B., F.E. Dowell, W.M. Hagler, Jr., et al. Variability associated with sampling, sample preparation, and chemical testing for aflatoxin in farmers' stock peanuts. *J. AOAC Int.* 77:107–116 (1994).

102. Hussain, M., and F. Vojir. Stichprobenplan für die Abnahmeprüfung beim Import getrockneter Feigen. *Dtsch. Lebensm.-Rundsch.* 89:379–383 (1993).

103. Dorner, J.W., and R.J. Cole. Variability among peanut subsamples prepared for aflatoxin analysis with four mills. *J. AOAC Int.* 76:983–987 (1993).

104. Taylor, S.L., J.W. King, J.L. Richard, and J.I. Greer. Analytical-scale supercritical fluid extraction of aflatoxin $B_1$ from field-inoculated corn. *J. Agric. Food Chem.* 41:910–913 (1993).

105. Joshua, H. Determination of aflatoxins by reversed-phase high-performance liquid chromatography with post-column in-line photochemical derivatization and fluorescence detection. *J. Chromatogr. A* 654:247–254 (1993).

106. Urano, T., M.W. Trucksess, and S.W. Page. Automated affinity liquid chromatography system for on-line isolation, separation, and quantitation of aflatoxins in methanol–water extracts of corn or peanuts. *J. Agric. Food Chem.* 41:1982–1985 (1993).

107. Tuinstra, L.G.M.T., A.H. Roos, and J.M.P. van Trijp. Liquid chromatographic determination of aflatoxin $M_1$ in milk powder using immunoaffinity columns for cleanup: interlaboratory study. *J. AOAC Int.* 76:1248–1254 (1993).

108. Niedwetzki, G., G. Lach, and K. Geschwill. Determination of aflatoxins in food by use of an automatic work station. *J. Chromatogr. A* 661:175–180 (1994).

109. Barmark, A.-L., and K. Larsson. Immunoaffinity column cleanup/liquid chromatographic determination of aflatoxins: an interlaboratory study. *J. AOAC Int.* 77:46–52 (1994).

110. Diaz, S., M.A. Moreno, L. Dominguez, et al. Application of a diphasic dialysis technique to the extraction of aflatoxins in dairy products. *J. Dairy Sci.* 76:1845–1849 (1993).

111. Cathey, C.G., Z.G. Huang, A.B. Sarr, et al. Development and evaluation of a minicolumn assay for the detection of aflatoxin $M_1$ in milk. *J. Dairy Sci.* 77:1223–1231 (1994).

112. Sashidhar, R.B. Dip-strip method for monitoring environmental contamination of aflatoxin in food and feed: use of a portable aflatoxin detection kit. *Environ. Health Perspect.* 101(Suppl. 3):43–46 (1993).

113. Obana, H., Y. Kumeda, T. Nishimune, and Y. Usami. Direct detection using the Drosophila DNA-repair test and isolation of a DNA-damaging mycotoxin, 5,6-dihydropenicillic acid, in fungal culture. *Food Chem. Toxicol.* 32:37–43 (1994).

114. Dyer, S.K., and S. McCammon. Detection of toxigenic isolates of *Aspergillus flavus* and related species on coconut cream agar. *J. Appl. Bacteriol.* 76:75–78 (1994).

115. Tsai, G.-J., and M.A. Cousin. Partial purification and characterization of mold antigens commonly found in foods. *Appl. Environ. Microbiol.* 59:2563–2571 (1993).

116. Ji, X.J., T. Ning, Y. Liang, et al. Effects of sterigmatocystin and T-2 toxin on the induction of unscheduled DNA synthesis in primary cultures of human gastric epithelial cells. *Nat. Toxins* 2:115–119 (1994).

117. Keller, N.P., N.J. Kantz, and T.H. Adams. *Aspergillus nidulans verA* is required for production of the mycotoxin sterigmatocystin. *Appl. Environ. Microbiol.* 60:1444–1450 (1994).

118. Cvetnić, Z. Cyclopiazonic acid and aflatoxin production by cultures of Aspergillus flavus isolated from dried beans and maize. *Nahrung* 38:21–25 (1994).

119. Tsai, M.C., W.H. Hsieh, F.T. Peng, et al. Effects of territrem B on motor nerve terminals of mouse skeletal muscle. *Asia Pacific J. Pharmacol.* 8:141–145 (1993).

120. Kim, J.-C., H.-J. Kang, D.-H. Lee, et al. Natural occurrence of *Fusarium* mycotoxins (trichothecenes and zearalenone) in barley and corn in Korea. *Appl. Environ. Microbiol.* 59:3798–3802 (1993).

121. Yuwai, K.E., K.S. Rao, K. Singh, et al. Occurrence of nivalenol, deoxynivalenol, and zearalenone in imported cereals in Papua, New Guinea. *Nat. Toxins* 2:19–21 (1994).

122. Müller, H.-M., and K. Schwadorf. Natural occurrence of *Fusarium* toxins in barley grown in a southwestern area of Germany. *Bull. Environ. Contam. Toxicol.* 51:532–537 (1993).

123. Müller, H.-M., K.-U. Metzger, R. Modi, and J. Reimann. Ergosterin und Fusarientoxine in Weizenkleie und Weizen. *J. Anim. Physiol. Anim. Nutr.* 71:48–55 (1994).

124. Tseng, T.-C. Mycotoxins produced by *Fusarium* spp. of Taiwan. *Bot. Bull. Acad. Sin.* 34:261–269 (1993).

125. Miller, J.D., M.E. Savard, A. Sibilia, et al. Production of fumonisins and fusarins by *Fusarium moniliforme* from Southeast Asia. *Mycologia* 85:385–391 (1993).

126. Schaafsma, A.W., J.D. Miller, M.E. Savard, and R.J. Ewing. Ear rot development and mycotoxin production in corn in relation to inoculation method, corn hybrid, and species of *Fusarium*. *Can. J. Plant Pathol.* 15:185–192 (1993).

127. Smith, T.K., and M.G. Sousadias. Fusaric acid content of swine feedstuffs. *J. Agric. Food Chem.* 41:2296–2298 (1993).

128. Barna-Vetró, I., Á. Gyöngyösi, and L. Solti. Monoclonal antibody-based enzyme-linked immunosorbent assay of *Fusarium* T-2 and zearalenone toxins in cereals. *Appl. Environ. Microbiol.* 60:729–731 (1994).

129. Young, J.C., and D.E. Games. Analysis of *Fusarium* mycotoxins by gas chromatography–Fourier transform infrared spectroscopy. *J. Chromatogr. A* 663:211–218 (1994).

130. Young, J.C., and D.E. Games. Analysis of *Fusarium* mycotoxins by supercritical fluid chromatography with ultra-violet or mass spectrometric detection. *J. Chromatogr. A* 653:374–379 (1993).

131. Scott, P.M., S.R. Kanhere, and D. Weber. Analysis of Canadian and imported beers for *Fusarium* mycotoxins by gas chromatography–mass spectrometry. *Food Addit. Contam.* 10:381–389 (1993).

132. Desjardins, A.E., T.M. Hohn, and S.P. McCormick. Trichothecene biosynthesis in *Fusarium* species: chemistry, genetics, and significance. *Microbiol. Rev.* 57:595–604 (1993).

133. Yagen, B., and M. Bialer. Metabolism and pharmacokinetics of T-2 toxin and related trichothecenes. *Drug Metab. Rev.* 25:281–323 (1993).

134. Abramson, D., R.M. Clear, and D.M. Smith. Trichothecene production by *Fusarium* spp. isolated from Manitoba grain. *Can. J. Plant Pathol.* 15:147–152 (1993).

135. Roinestad, K.S., T.J. Montville, and J.D. Rosen. Inhibition of trichothecene biosynthesis in *Fusarium tricinctum* by sodium bicarbonate. *J. Agric. Food Chem.* 41:2344–2346 (1993).

136. Hohn, T.M., S.P. McCormick, and A.E. Desjardins. Evidence for a gene cluster involving trichothecene-pathway biosynthetic genes in *Fusarium sporotrichioides*. *Curr. Genet.* 24:291–295 (1993).

137. Fort, D.M., C.L. Barnes, M.S. Tempesta, et al. Two new modified trichothecenes from *Fusarium sporotrichioides*. *J. Nat. Prod.* 56:1890–1897 (1993).

138. Croteau, S.M., D.B. Prelusky, and H.L. Trenholm. Analysis of trichothecene mycotoxins by gas chromatography with electron capture detection. *J. Agric. Food Chem.* 42:928–933 (1994).

139. Seidel, V., B. Lang, S. Fraißler, et al. Analysis of trace levels of trichothecene mycotoxins in Austrian cereals by gas chromatography with electron capture detection. *Chromatographia* 37:191–201 (1993).

140. Madhyastha, M.S., R.R. Marquardt, A.A. Frohlich, and J. Borsa. Optimization of yeast bioassay for trichothecene mycotoxins. *J. Food Protect.* 57:490–495 (1994).

141. Bergman, F. Structural properties and pharmacological use of T-2 mycotoxins. *J. Toxicol.–Toxin Rev.* 13:1–10 (1994).

142. Holladay, S.D., B.L. Blaylock, C.E. Comment, et al. Fetal thymic atrophy after exposure to T-2 toxin: selectivity for lymphoid progenitor cells. *Toxicol. Appl. Pharmacol.* 121:8–14 (1993).

143. Middlebrook, J.L., and D.L. Leatherman. Effects of steroids on association of T-2 toxin with mammalian cells. *Toxicon* 32:435–444 (1994).

144. Duffy, M.J., and R.S. Reid. Measurement of the stability of T-2 toxin in aqueous solution. *Chem. Res. Toxicol.* 6:524–529 (1993).

145. Faifer, G.C., V. Velazco, and H.M. Godoy. Adjustment of the conditions required for complete decontamination of T-2 toxin residues with alkaline sodium hypochlorite. *Bull. Environ. Contam. Toxicol.* 52:102–108 (1994).

146. Minervini, F., A. Gyongyosi-Horvath, G. Lucivero, et al. In vitro neutralization of T-2 toxin toxicity by a monoclonal antibody. *Nat. Toxins* 2:111–114 (1994).

147. Sugiura, Y., K. Fukasaku, T. Tanaka, et al. *Fusarium poae* and *Fusarium crookwellense*, fungi responsible for the natural occurrence of nivalenol in Hokkaido. *Appl. Environ. Microbiol.* 59:3334–3338 (1993).

148. Okoye, Z.S.C. *Fusarium* mycotoxins nivalenol and 4-acetyl-nivalenol (fusarenon-X) in mouldy maize harvested from farms in Jos district, Nigeria. *Food Addit. Contam.* 10:375–379 (1993).

149. Charmley, E., H.L. Trenholm, B.K. Thompson, et al. Influence of level of deoxynivalenol in the diet of dairy cows on feed intake, milk production, and its composition. *J. Dairy Sci.* 76:3580–3587 (1993).

150. Boyacioglu, D., N.S. Hettiarachchy, and B.L. D'Appolonia. Additives affect deoxynivalenol (vomitoxin) flour during breadbaking. *J. Food Sci.* 58:416–418 (1993).

151. Yabe, T., H. Hashimoto, M. Sekijima, et al. Effects of nivalenol on hepatic drug-metabolizing activity in rats. *Food Chem. Toxicol.* 31:573–581 (1993).

152. Pestka, J.J., and W. Dong. Progressive serum IgE elevation in the B6C3F1 mouse following withdrawal of dietary vomitoxin (deoxynivalenol). *Fund. Appl. Toxicol.* 22:314–316 (1994).

153. Vudathala, D.K., D.B. Prelusky, and H.L. Trenholm. Analysis of trace levels of deoxynivalenol in cow's milk by high pressure liquid chromatography. *J. Liq. Chromatogr.* 17:673–683 (1994).

154. Lauren, D.R., W.A. Smith, and A.L. Wilkins. Preparation, purification, and NMR spectra of some mono- and dihemisuccinates of the trichothecene mycotoxin nivalenol. *J. Agric. Food Chem.* 42:828–833 (1994).

155. Usleber, E., E. Schneider, E. Märtlbauer, and G. Terplan. Two formats of enzyme immunoassay for 15-acetyldeoxynivalenol applied to wheat. *J. Agric. Food Chem.* 41:2019–2023 (1993).

156. Bacon, C.W., and P.E. Nelson. Fumonisin production in corn by toxigenic strains of *Fusarium moniliforme* and *Fusarium proliferatum*. *J. Food Protect.* 57:514–521 (1994).

157. Norred, W.P., and K.A. Voss. Toxicity and role of fumonisins in animal diseases and human esophageal cancer. *J. Food Protect.* 57:522–527 (1994).

158. Riley, R.T., K.A. Voss, H.-S. Yoo, et al. Mechanism of fumonisin toxicity and carcinogenesis. *J. Food Protect.* 57:638–645 (1994) [corrected version of *J. Food Protect.* 57:528–535 (1994)].

159. Rice, L.G., and P. F. Ross. Methods for detection and quantitation of fumonisins in corn, cereal products and animal excreta. *J. Food Protect.* 57:536–540 (1994).

160. Bullerman, L.B., and W.-Y.J. Tsai. Incidence and levels of *Fusarium moniliforme*, *Fusarium proliferatum* and fumonisins in corn and corn-based foods and feeds. *J. Food Protect.* 57:541–546 (1994).

161. Riley, R.T., W.P. Norred, and C.W. Bacon. Fungal toxins in foods: recent concerns. *Annu. Rev. Nutr.* 13:167–189 (1993).

162. Nelson, P.E., A.E. Desjardins, and R.D. Plattner. Fumonisins, mycotoxins produced by *Fusarium* species: biology, chemistry, and significance. *Annu. Rev. Phytopathol.* 31:233–252 (1993).

163. Scott, P.M. Fumonisins. *Int. J. Food Microbiol.* 18:257–270 (1993).

165. Branham, B.E., and R.D. Plattner. Isolation and characterization of a new fumonisin from liquid cultures of *Fusarium moniliforme. J. Nat. Prod.* 56:1630–1633 (1993).

165. Gelderblom, W.C.A., M.E. Cawood, S.D. Snyman, and W.F.O. Marasas. Fumonisin B$_1$ dosimetry in relation to cancer initiation in rat liver. *Carcinogenesis* 15:209–214,790 (1994).

166. Gelderblom, W.C.A., M.E. Cawood, S.D. Snyman, et al. Structure–activity relationships of fumonisins in short-term carcinogenesis and cytotoxicity assays. *Food Chem. Toxicol.* 31:407–414 (1993).

167. Riley, R.T., E. Wang, and A.H. Merrill, Jr. Liquid chromatographic determination of sphinganine and sphingosine: use of the free sphinganine-to-sphingosine ratio as a biomarker for consumption of fumonisins. *J. AOAC Int.* 77:533–540 (1994).

168. Riley, R.T., D.M. Hinton, W.J. Chamberlain, et al. Dietary fumonisin B$_1$ induces disruption of sphingolipid metabolism in Sprague-Dawley rats: a new mechanism of nephrotoxicity. *J. Nutr.* 124:594–603 (1994).

169. Merrill, A.H., Jr., G. van Echten, E. Wang, and K. Sandhoff. Fumonisin B$_1$ inhibits sphingosine (sphinganine) *N*-acyltransferase and *de novo* sphingolipid biosynthesis in cultured neurons *in situ. J. Biol. Chem.* 268:27299–27306 (1993).

170. Schroeder, J.J., H.M. Crane, J. Xia, et al. Disruption of sphingolipid metabolism and stimulation of DNA synthesis by fumonisin B$_1$: A molecular mechanism for carcinogenesis associated with *Fusarium moniliforme. J. Biol. Chem.* 269:3475–3481 (1994).

171. Shephard, G.S., P.G. Thiel, E.W. Sydenham, et al. Determination of the mycotoxin fumonisin B$_1$ and identification of its partially hydrolysed metabolites in the faeces of non-human primates. *Food Chem. Toxicol.* 32:23–29 (1994).

172. Hendrich, S., K.A. Miller, T.M. Wilson, and P.A. Murphy. Toxicity of *Fusarium proliferatum*-fermented nixtamalized corn-based diets fed to rats: effect of nutritional status. *J. Agric. Food Chem.* 41:1649–1654 (1993).

173. Alberts, J.F., W.C.A. Gelderblom, R. Vleggaar, et al. Production of [$^{14}$C]fumonisin B$_1$ by *Fusarium moniliforme* MRC 826 in corn cultures. *Appl. Environ. Microbiol.* 59:2673–2677 (1993).

174. Branham, B.E., and R.D. Plattner. Alanine is a precursor in the biosynthesis of fumonisin B$_1$ by *Fusarium moniliforme. Mycopathologia* 124:99–104 (1993).

175. Blackwell, B.A., J.D. Miller, and M.E. Savard. Production of carbon 14-labeled fumonisin in liquid culture. *J. AOAC Int.* 77:506–511 (1994).

176. Yoshizawa, T., A. Yamashita, and Y. Luo. Fumonisin occurrence in corn from high- and low-risk areas for human esophageal cancer in China. *Appl. Environ. Microbiol.* 60:1626–1629 (1994).

177. Sydenham, E.W., G.S. Shephard, P.G. Thiel, et al. Fumonisins in Argentinian field-trial corn. *J. Agric. Food Chem.* 41:891–895 (1993).

178. Chatterjee, D., and S.K. Mukherjee. Contamination of Indian maize with fumonisin B$_1$ and its effects on chicken macrophage. *Lett. Appl. Microbiol.* 18:251–253 (1994).

179. Chamberlain, W.J., C.W. Bacon, W.P. Norred, and K.A. Voss. Levels of fumonisin B$_1$ in corn naturally contaminated with aflatoxins. *Food Chem. Toxicol.* 31:995–998 (1993).

180. Visconti, A., and M.B. Doko. Survey of fumonisin production by *Fusarium* isolated from cereals in Europe. *J. AOAC Int.* 77:546–550 (1994).

181. Desjardins, A.E., R.D. Plattner, and P.E. Nelson. Fumonisin production and other traits of *Fusarium moniliforme* strains from maize in northeast Mexico. *Appl. Environ. Microbiol.* 60:1695–1697 (1994).

182. Nelson, P.E., J.H. Juba, P.F. Ross, and L.G. Rice. Fumonisin production by *Fusarium* species on solid substrates. *J. AOAC Int.* 77:522–525 (1994).

183. Shelby, R.A., D.G. White, and E.M. Bauske. Differential fumonisin production in maize hybrids. *Plant Dis.* 78:582–584 (1994).

184. Sydenham, E.W., L. van der Westhuizen, S. Stockenström, et al. Fumonisin-contaminated maise: physical treatment for the partial decontamination of bulk shipments. *Food Addit. Contam.* 11:25–32 (1994).

185. Dupuy, J., P. Le Bars, H. Boudra, and J. Le Bars. Thermostability of fumonisin B$_1$, a mycotoxin from *Fusarium moniliforme*, in corn. *Appl. Environ. Microbiol.* 59:2864–2867 (1993).

186. Le Bars, J., P. Le Bars, J. Dupuy, et al. Biotic and abiotic factors in fumonisin B$_1$ production and stability. *J. AOAC Int.* 77:517–521 (1994).

187. Vudathala, D.K., D.B. Prelusky, M. Ayroud, et al. Pharmacokinetic fate and pathological effects of $^{14}$C-fumonisin B$_1$ in laying hens. *Nat. Toxins* 2:81–88 (1994).

188. Prelusky, D.B., H.L. Trenholm, and M.E. Savard. Pharmacokinetic fate of $^{14}$C-labelled fumonisin B$_1$ in swine. *Nat. Toxins* 2:73–80 (1994).

189. Dombrink-Kurtzman, M.A., G.A. Bennett, and J.L. Richard. An optimized MTT bioassay for determination of cytotoxicity of fumonisins in turkey lymphocytes. *J. AOAC Int.* 77:512–516 (1994).

190. Ware, G.M., O. Francis, S.S. Kuan, et al. Determination of fumonisin B$_1$ in corn by high performance liquid chromatography with fluorescence detection. *Anal. Lett.* 26:1751–1770 (1993).

191. Bennett, G.A., and J.L. Richard. Liquid chromatographic method for analysis of the naphthalene dicarboxaldehyde derivative of fumonisins. *J. AOAC Int.* 77:501–506 (1994).

192. Hopmans, E.C., and P.A. Murphy. Detection of fumonisins B$_1$, B$_2$, and B$_3$ and hydrolyzed fumonisin B$_1$ in corn-containing foods. *J. Agric. Food Chem.* 41:1655–1658 (1993).

193. Plattner, R.D., and B.E. Branham. Labeled fumonisins: production and use of fumonisin $B_1$ containing stable isotopes. *J. AOAC Int.* 77:525–532 (1994).

194. Fukuda, S., A. Nagahara, M. Kikuchi, and S. Kumagai. Preparation and characterization of anti-fumonisin monoclonal antibodies. *Biosci. Biotechnol. Biochem.* 58:765–767 (1994).

195. Pestka, J.J., J.I. Azcona-Olivera, R.D. Plattner, et al. Comparative assessment of fumonisin in grain-based foods by ELISA, GC-MS, and HPLC. *J. Food Protect.* 57:169–172 (1994).

196. Scott, P.M., and G.A. Lawrence. Stability and problems in recovery of fumonisins added to corn-based foods. *J. AOAC Int.* 77:541–545 (1994).

197. Tanaka, T., R. Teshima, H. Ikebuchi, et al. Sensitive determination of zearalenone and α-zearalenol in barley and Job's-tears by liquid chromatography with fluorescence detection. *J. AOAC Int.* 76:1006–1009 (1993).

198. Logrieco, A., A. Moretti, C. Altomare, et al. Occurrence and toxicity of *Fusarium subglutinans* from Peruvian maize. *Mycopathologia* 122:185–190 (1993).

199. Logrieco, A., A. Moretti, A. Ritieni, et al. Natural occurrence of beauvericin in preharvest *Fusarium subglutinans* infected corn ears in Poland. *J. Agric. Food Chem.* 41:2149–2152 (1993).

200. Visconti, A., and M. Solfrizzo. Isolation, characterization, and biological activity of visoltricin, a novel metabolite of *Fusarium tricinctum. J. Agric. Food Chem.* 42:195–199 (1994).

201. Scudamore, K.A., H.J. Clarke, and M.T. Hetmanski. Isolation of *Penicillium* strains producing ochratoxin A, citrinin, xanthomegnin, viomellein and vioxanthin from stored cereal grains. *Lett. Appl. Microbiol.* 17:82–87 (1993).

202. Kitabatake, N., E. Doi, and A.B. Trivedi. Toxicity evaluation of the mycotoxins, citrinin and ochratoxin A, using several animal cell lines. *Comp. Biochem. Physiol.* 105C:429–433 (1993).

203. Braunberg, R.C., C.N. Barton, O.O. Gantt, and L. Friedman. Interaction of citrinin and ochratoxin A. *Nat. Toxins* 2:124–131 (1994).

204. Breitholtz-Emanuelsson, A., M. Olsen, A. Oskarsson, et al. Ochratoxin A in cow's milk and in human milk with corresponding human blood samples. *J. AOAC Int.* 76:842–846 (1993).

205. Tesch, D., and K. Lusky. Untersuchungen zum Einfluß des Mykotoxins Ochratoxin A auf die Tiergesundheit und auf das Rückstandsverhalten beim Schwein. *Arch. Lebensmittelhyg.* 44:77–80 (1993).

206. Lusky, K., D. Tesch, and R. Göbel. Untersuchungen zum Einfluß des Mykotoxins Ochratoxin A auf die Tiergesundheit und auf das Rückstandsverhalten beim Schwein und aus daraus hergestellten Wurstwaren. *Arch. Lebensmittelhyg.* 44:131–134 (1993).

207. Lusky, K., D. Tesch, R. Göbel, and K.-D. Doberschütz. Ochratoxin A. Untersuchungen zum Rückstandsverhalten beim Schwein und in daraus hergestellten Lebensmitteln. *Fleischwirtschaft* 74:558–560 (1994).

208. Hwang, C.-A., and F.A. Draughon. Degradation of ochratoxin A by *Acinetobacter calcoaceticus. J. Food Protect.* 57:410–414 (1994).

209. Malaveille, C., G. Brun, and H. Bartsch. Structure–activity studies in *E. coli* strains on ochratoxin A (OTA) and its analogues implicate a genotoxic free radical and a cytotoxic thiol derivative as reactive metabolites. *Mutat. Res.* 307:141–147 (1994).

210. Pfohl-Leszkowicz, A., Y. Grosse, A. Kane, et al. Differential DNA adduct formation and disappearance in three mouse tissues after treatment with the mycotoxin ochratoxin A. *Mutat. Res.* 289:265–273 (1993).

211. Gekle, M., H. Oberleithner, and S. Silbernagl. Ochratoxin A impairs "postproximal" nephron function in vivo and blocks plasma membrane anion conductance in Madin-Darby canine kidney cells in vitro.*Eur. J. Physiol.* 425:401–408 (1993).

212. Gekle, M., and S. Silbernagl. Mechanism of ochratoxin A-induced reduction of glomerular filtration rate in rats. *J. Pharmacol. Exp. Ther.* 267:316–321 (1993).

213. Gekle, M., and S. Silbernagl. The role of the proximal tubule in ochratoxin A nephrotoxicity in vivo: toxodynamic and toxokinetic aspects. *Renal Physiol. Biochem.* 17:40–49 (1994).

214. Gharbi, A., O. Trillon, A.M. Betbeder, et al. Some effects of ochratoxin A, a mycotoxin contaminating feeds and food, on rat testis. *Toxicology* 83:9–18 (1993).

215. Clarke, J.R., R.R. Marquardt, A. Oosterveld, et al. Development of a quantitative and sensitive enzyme-linked immunosorbent assay for ochratoxin A using antibodies from the yolk of the laying hen.*J. Agric. Food Chem.* 41:1784–1789 (1993).

216. Viñas, I., J. Dadon, and V. Sanchis. Citrinin-producing capacity of *Penicillium expansum* strains from apple packinghouses of Lerida (Spain).*Int. J. Food Microbiol.* 19:153–156 (1993).

217. Trivedi, A.B., M. Hirota, E. Doi, and N. Kitabatake. Formation of a new toxic compound, citrinin H1, from citrinin on mild heating in water. *J. Chem. Soc. Peking Trans. 1* 18:2167–2171 (1993).

218. Yang, Y.G., K. Mayura, C.B. Spainhour, Jr., et al. Evaluation of the developmental toxicity of citrining using *Hydra attenuata* and postimplantation rat whole embryo culture. *Toxicology* 85:179–198 (1993).

219. Okeke, B., F. Seigle-Murandi, R. Steiman, et al. Identification of mycotoxin-producing fungal strains: a step in the isolation of compounds active against rice fungal diseases. *J. Agric. Food Chem.* 41:1731–1735 (1993).

220. Ryu, D., and D.L. Holt. Growth inhibition of *Penicillium expansum* by several commonly used food ingredients. *J. Food Protect.* 56:862–867 (1993).

221. Smith, E.E., E.A. Duffus, and M.H. Small. Effects of patulin on postimplantation rat embryos. *Arch. Environ. Contam. Toxicol.* 25:267–270 (1993).

222. Prieta, J., M.A. Moreno, J. Bayo, et al. Determination of patulin by reversed-phase high-performance liquid

chromatography with extraction by diphasic dialysis. *Analyst* 118:171–173 (1993).

223.   Bartolomé, B., M.L. Bengoechea, F.J. Pérez-Ilzarbe, et al. Determination of patulin in apple juice by high-performance liquid chromatography with diode-array detection. *J. Chromatogr. A* 664:39–43 (1994).

224.   McElroy, L.J., and C.M. Weiss. The production of polyclonal antibodies against the mycotoxin derivative patulin hemiglutarate. *Can. J. Microbiol.* 39:861–863 (1993).

225.   Hahnau, S., and E.W. Weiler. Monoclonal antibodies for the enzyme immunoassay of the mycotoxin cyclopiazonic acid. *J. Agric. Food Chem.* 41:1076–1080 (1993).

226.   Ueno, I., M. Hoshino, T. Maitani, et al. Luteoskyrin, an anthraquinoid hepatotoxin, and ascorbic acid generate hydroxyl radical *in vitro* in the presence of a trace amount of ferrous iron. *Free Rad. Res. Commun.* 19(Suppl.):S95–S100 (1993).

227.   Ohmomo, S., H.K. Kitamoto, and T. Nakajima. Detection of roquefortines in *Penicillium roqueforti* isolated from moulded maize silage. *J. Sci. Food Agric.* 64:211–215 (1994).

228.   Penn, J., and P.G. Mantle. Biosynthetic intermediates of indole-diterpenoid mycotoxins from selected transformations at C-10 of paxilline. *Phytochemistry* 35:921–926 (1994).

229.   Dierkes, W., M. Lohmeyer, and H.-J. Rehm. Long-term production of ergot peptides by immobilized *Claviceps purpurea* in semicontinuous and continuous culture. *Appl. Environ. Microbiol.* 59:2029–2033 (1993).

230.   Ede, R.M., C.O. Miles, L.P. Meagher, et al. Relative stereochemistry of the A/B rings of the tremorgenic mycotoxin lolitrem B. *J. Agric. Food Chem.* 42:231–233 (1994).

231.   Upreti, G.C., and M.K. Jain. Interaction of sporidesmin, a mycotoxin from *Pithomyces chartarum*, with lipid bilayers. *Biosci. Rep.* 13:233–243 (1993).

# 11

# Foodborne Bacterial Intoxications and Infections

# INTRODUCTION

Infectious diseases are emerging or reemerging as major public health problems worldwide. Among the important emerging infections are a number that are either foodborne, or waterborne with the potential to become foodborne. The Centers for Disease Control and its consulting agencies have developed a prevention strategy aimed at these emerging diseases (*1*). Doyle summarized what he believes to be the priorities in reducing foodborne illness (*2*). Areas for emphasis are risk analysis, management, and communications; innovative approaches for producing pathogen-free animal foods; research on implementing HACCP programs; and innovations in educating consumers and those who prepare food. In another paper, Doyle reviewed the identification of *Campylobacter jejuni, Listeria monocytogenes, Vibrio vulnificus,* and *Escherichia coli* O157:H7 as important causes of food-related illness (*3*). These four organisms are uniquely different, yet risks from all of them can be minimized by proper cooking and handling of cooked food. *Campylobacter jejuni* was first known as an obscure veterinary pathogen; now it is recognized as the leading cause of acute bacterial diarrhea in many countries. *Vibrio vulnificus* can produce life-threatening illness in persons with liver dysfunction and a penchant for eating raw or undercooked oysters. *Listeria monocytogenes,* widely distributed in nature and unprocessed foods, is a severe hazard for pregnant women, their fetuses, and immunocompromised persons; certain foods, e.g., low-acid soft cheeses, pose particular risks. *Escherichia coli* O157:H7, of undercooked hamburger fame, is found in many foods but dairy cattle are one of its major reservoirs.

Accelerating ecologic and social change worldwide is at the root of the ascendance of diarrheal disease. Levine and Levine discussed changes in human ecology and behavior that relate to these infections (*4*). In developing countries, crowded and unsanitary living conditions are a major problem. Diminished breast-feeding and large-scale migrations contribute. In industrialized countries, factory agriculture and giant distribution, processing, and retailing networks create an auspicious setting for foodborne pathogens. Other factors are increased foreign travel, importation of food from developing countries, and a growing population of elderly and chronically ill persons. Cholera—both the seventh pandemic due to *Vibrio cholerae* O1 biotype Eltor, and the new epidemic due to *V. cholerae* O139—was cited as an illustration.

Savarino and Bourgeois reviewed some environmental, host, and pathogen-specific factors that shape the epidemiology of infectious diarrhea in developed countries (*5*). They emphasized the ease with which a lapse in water quality, environmental sanitation, agricultural hygiene, or food hygiene can result in large and disseminated outbreaks of illness in an economy based on mass production and distribution. Increasing consumption of natural and unprocessed or minimally processed foods may also pose a public health risk. The authors discussed how techniques from molecular biology assist epidemiologic investigations of diarrheal disease.

Foodborne illness is being attributed to an increasing variety of bacteria, parasites, and viruses. Hedberg et al. discussed the changing epidemiology of foodborne disease nationally and as reflected by surveillance at the Minnesota Department of Health (*6*). Estimates of the number of cases range from 6.5 to 81 million annually in the USA, with from 525 to >7000 associated deaths. The annual cost of this illness may reach $23 billion. Changes in diet and eating habits are reflected in changes in both the type and source of foods eaten. The authors discussed "the other side of Five-A-Day for Better Health," citing large outbreaks of hepatitis A, shigellosis, and salmonellosis caused by unusual serotypes (Chester, Poona, Javiana, and Montevideo), due to widespread distribution of fresh produce. Given the prevailing trends in international trade and national consumption of fresh fruits and vegetables, these outbreaks are likely to occur with increasing frequency. New methods of food production and distribution and the increased consumption of foods in commercial establishments also contribute to the potential for large outbreaks of illness. In addition, some truly new food pathogens have appeared—perhaps most notably, *E. coli* O157:H7. All this has created new challenges for public health surveillance and health education.

Baird-Parker's discussion of the epidemiology and extent of foodborne disease added the dimension of the serious and often chronic sequelae of foodborne illness (*7*). The most publicized of these is hemolytic uremic syndrome (HUS), a dreaded consequence of infection by verotoxin-producing strains of *E. coli* (VTEC). However, foodborne pathogens have also been implicated in other conditions, including ankylosing spondylitis, Reiter's syndrome, nutritional and malabsorption problems, atherosclerosis, and Guillain–Barré syndrome. Foodborne illness is universally underreported, for reasons that were discussed. Changes in agricultural practices and food technology have fostered new problems as well as alleviating a few old ones. Overall, Baird-Parker asserts that foods are becoming "less microbiologically robust, requiring greater care in their production, distribution and storage." Large segments of the population (the very young, the elderly, pregnant women, and immuno-compromised persons) are at particular risk for foodborne illness. Risk assessment, the HACCP system, and the importance of understanding microbial interactions and disease processes were discussed.

Lacey summarized the incidence, types, and clinical features of bacterial food poisoning in the UK (8). Four major pathogens were comprehensively reviewed. Most of the increase in salmonellosis is attributable to *Salmonella enteritidis*, particularly from eggs. The commonest bacterial food pathogen is *Campylobacter*, which causes illness with a seasonal peak in May and June. Although these organisms cause many cases of illness, they are rarely fatal. In contrast, *L. monocytogenes* and *E. coli* O157:H7 rarely produce disease; but when they do, the consequences are often dire. Lacey believes that most foodborne illness could be prevented if society were determined to do so.

Bryan discussed the incidence, causes, and economic impact of foodborne illness in the USA and approaches for its prevention and control (9). A table showed the numbers of outbreaks and cases of foodborne disease of known etiology in the USA, 1973–1987. Places where food mishandling occurs frequently, the changing spectrum of implicated foods, and causative factors in outbreaks were discussed. Surveillance is required not only of foodborne diseases themselves but of foods and food environments at every stage of production and processing. Public education about food safety and training of food-industry and food-service personnel, including both handlers and supervisors, are also part of prevention and control.

Worldwide, growing global markets and free trade have focused the food-safety concerns of nations on risk management and HACCP or HACCP-type approaches (10–12). Adams and Crawford discussed the importance of HACCP and ISO 9000 quality systems in harmonizing free trade in North and South America (10). Rapid social and political changes in Europe have pushed the HACCP concept to the fore there as well. However, van Schothorst pointed out points at which confusion might arise in assigning responsibility and liability for food safety (11). Changing views of food safety are also involved. The author argues that the no-risk policy of the past should be changed to one of risk management. While it is reasonable to insist that all foods be safe when eaten by "normal" people, consumers themselves must assume some responsibility for safety. The zero tolerance policy is unrealistic. The concept of tolerance needs to be

rephrased in terms of limiting the survival, growth, and spread of pathogens and in terms of particular foods and particular groups of consumers. Not all foods need necessarily be safe for everyone. Eyles discussed HACCP and ISO 9000 systems within the framework of Australia's regulatory structure (12). International harmonization and quality assurance of fishery products are of major concern in Pacific Rim countries.

Notermans and Van de Giessen updated the status of foodborne illness in the Netherlands during the 1980s and 1990s (13). Fewer than 20% of cases and outbreaks were of known etiology, but where etiology was known the top three causative agents were *Salmonella, Bacillus cereus,* and *C. perfringens*. Chinese foods accounted for 32% of the outbreaks and 20% of the single cases; meat and meat products, the second leading vehicle, accounted for 12 and 15% of outbreaks and single cases, respectively. Because of lack of information about incidents and causes of foodborne diseases, the National Institute of Public Health and Environmental Protection initiated a sentinel system of reporting in 1987. Participating physicians agreed to report all patients with acute gastroenteritis who had symptoms similar to an established case definition. These patients were requested to complete a questionnaire and send a fecal sample to be analyzed by a regional laboratory. Such sentinel studies and population studies increase the reporting rate of foodborne diseases and the information they provide complements information from case–control and other epidemiologic investigations.

Buchanan and Deroever discussed limits in assessing microbiological food safety (14). Fundamental limitations in the current reporting system constrain its ability to determine the true incidence of foodborne illness. Moreover, traditional detection methods do not permit real-time decisions on the microbiological safety of food products. To compensate for deficiencies in epidemiologic and analytical information, the authors recommend microbiological profiling. Its goals are to specify the pathogens likely to be a problem in a particular food and to identify factors that can be manipulated to control them. In addition to these approaches for assessing microbiological safety—epidemiology, analysis, and risk profiling—an integrated approach to food safety also requires risk assessment and a system for allocating available resources in a cost-efficient manner. In this way, quality and safety can be designed into a product.

Sofos briefly summarized the major techniques in food preservation in the context of current microbiological concerns (15). The techniques discussed were sanitation, low-temperature storage, moisture control and reduction of water activity ($a_w$), pH control, chemical preservatives, fermentation and biopreservation, packaging under modified atmospheres, irradiation, and thermal processing. The concept of hurdles or multiple barriers is based on the observation that control can be achieved through interactions of several factors each of which is at a suboptimal level. Statistical models can predict the contribution of each factor to the total preservation system under a variety of conditions.

Irbe analyzed the microbiologic consequences of replacing the fat in a food with a fat substitute (*16*). Reduced-fat foods differ from full-fat foods in physical and chemical properties and most have not been on the market long enough to establish a record for safety (the presence or absence of pathogens) and stability (the growth of spoilage organisms). After reviewing the limits of $a_w$ and pH that permit growth of specific yeasts, molds, and bacteria and discussing factors that influence microbial growth, Irbe considered the microbiological safety and stability of selected types of foods. The types considered were retorted soups and sauces, bakery and cereal products, fat-type spreads, and cheese. Irbe discussed the effects of processing on the microbiology of these products and predicted the effect of fat substitution.

Many fermented foods are less likely vehicles for foodborne infection or intoxication than fresh foods. This is attributable to the competitive activity and metabolites of typical starter microorganisms. However, certain risks are also associated with fermented foods (*17*). These include mycotoxin contamination of raw materials or mycotoxin production by fungal contaminants, or production of toxic by-products of fermentation. Poorly controlled natural fermentation, suboptimal fermentation starters, and inadequate maturation and storage conditions enhance risk. Risks can be minimized by using only high-quality raw materials, pasteurization, and careful selection of starter cultures. Conventional or recombinant DNA techniques can be used to develop starters with the desired characteristics.

There is a potential for serious outbreaks of foodborne illness at temporary public eating places. Manning and Snider developed a questionnaire on food-safety knowledge and attitudes and a checklist of food-handling practices, and used them to assess the knowledge, attitudes, and practices of 64 workers in 11 temporary establishments at a state fair (*18*). The characteristics of these workers suggest that they are similar to workers at other temporary eating places such as churches. There were notable deficiencies in knowledge and attitudes, particularly in relation to cooling, reheating, and temperature control. In addition, some discrepancies were noted between actual practices, as recorded on the checklist, and

knowledge and attitudes as indicated by the questionnaire. Specifically, knowledge and attitudes about personal hygiene and cross-contamination were not always put into practice. Workers received limited on-the-job training by coworkers or supervisors.

Corthier et al. described the nature and mode of action of *Clostridium botulinum* neurotoxins and the diarrheal enterotoxins produced by foodborne bacteria (*19*). They discussed the ecology of the digestive tract, including interactions among nonpathogenic and potentially pathogenic bacteria. In concluding, they suggested how the disease process could give the pathogen an ecological advantage; and toxin production is the tool by which the pathogen induces disease.

## *STAPHYLOCOCCUS*

### Outbreaks and Epidemiology

In discussing outbreaks of *Staphylococcus aureus* food poisoning in mass-feeding situations, Bergdoll reviewed the enterotoxins involved and clinical features of the illness (*20*). He summarized the types of food involved in outbreaks, sources of contamination, sites of outbreaks, the importance of properly refrigerating vulnerable foods, and the role of infected food handlers in outbreaks. Specific incidents of staphylococcal intoxication illustrated these points. Wieneke et al. reviewed ~350 incidents of staphylococcal food poisoning in the UK, 1969–1990 (*21*). Strains from 79% of incidents produced staphylococcal enterotoxin A (SEA), alone or with another enterotoxin. The number of viable staphylococci in the incriminated foods ranged from none to $1.5 \times 10^{10}$ cfu/g, with a median of $3.0 \times 10^7$. Meat and poultry or their products were the vehicle in 75% of incidents. Seafood accounted for 7% and dairy foods for 8%. Most contamination occurred in the home.

A study in Japan evaluated growth characteristics and toxin production of *S. aureus* strains isolated from healthy subjects, hospitalized patients, toxic food, normal and mastitic milk, and dairy cows (*22*). Strains isolated from toxic food and mastitic milk had a high level of resistance to novobiocin, whereas human strains were sensitive to this antibiotic. Strains from normal and mastitic milk differed according to two biotyping schemes and in their coagulase type.

Gangbar et al. described a case of infective endocarditis, caused by *S. aureus*, in a dairy farmer (*23*). The patient's cows were suspected of having subclinical mastitis. The patient, who had fissures and abrasions on both hands, had previously consulted his physician because of chills, fever, and cellulitis in his hand and arm. He did not wear protective gloves when he attached the cups of the milking machine to the cows' udders, and his hands frequently contacted the milk. Due to lapse of time and the intervening treatment of infected cattle, transmission of the pathogen from mastitic cows or their milk to the farmer could not be proved microbiologically. However, in the absence of any other identifiable source of infection, contact with infected milk was considered the likely cause of the farmer's initial infection and ultimate endocarditis.

## Occurrence and Growth in Foods

Bowen and Henning examined 50 retail samples of natural hard and semihard cheeses for coliform bacteria and *S. aureus* (*24*). A variety of cheeses, including reduced-fat and reduced-cholesterol products and sliced or shredded cheeses, were included. No thermonuclease-positive *S. aureus* or *E. coli* O157:H7 were found. Nine samples had coliform bacteria at levels of $10^1$–$1.1 \times 10^3$ cfu/mL by the violet red–bile agar method; 24 were positive for coliforms when a 25-g sample was used in an enrichment broth. In comparison with results of a Canadian study done in the mid-1970s, these limited results suggest that the microbial quality of natural cheeses on the U.S. retail market in the 1990s is high.

In Pakistan, 48 of 85 *S. aureus* strains isolated from dairy products were enterotoxigenic (*25*). Sixteen strains produced more than one type of enterotoxin. Of the toxigenic strains, 67% produced SEA, 31% produced SEB, 21% produced SED, and 19% produced SEC.

Tamime et al. reported seasonal changes in the microbiologic quality of sheep's milk in Scotland (*26*). Numbers of both total coliforms and *S. aureus* peaked in July, but even these counts were relatively low and the overall quality of bulk sheep's milk was considered very good. Neither *S. aureus* nor coliforms were found after heat treatment. The microbiologic quality of yogurts produced from this milk was high and comparable to that of retail yogurts made from cow's milk.

The survival and growth of *S. aureus* and several other selected microorganisms were monitored during preparation and storage of khoa, a heat-concentrated milk-based product (*27*). Two processing temperatures (63 and 73°C) and milks containing from 3.6 to 6.5% fat were evaluated. *Staphylococcus aureus* was recovered only when milk containing 6.5% fat was heated at the lower temperature. The organism survived during pro-longed storage at 6–7°C. Survival was little influenced by preservative (3000 ppm of potassium sorbate or ascorbic acid) or by reducing the $a_w$ (from .97 to .93).

Mead et al. conducted a microbiologic survey of five poultry-processing plants in the UK (*28*). Neck skin samples were taken from chickens and turkeys after each main stage of processing: bleeding, scalding, defeathering, evisceration, final wash, chilling, and packaging. Although *S. aureus* was readily isolated from the defeathering equipment, mean counts from defeathered carcasses were always $<10^3$ cfu/g. In South Africa, 232 samples of processed meats, ground beef, and broilers were analyzed for total aerobic plate count, *E. coli*, and *S. aureus* (*29*). *Staphylococcus aureus* was found in 23.4% of ground beef, 39.5% of broiler, and 7.1% of processed meat samples. There was no clear relationship between total aerobic plate counts and the occurrence of *E. coli* or *S. aureus*.

A study of the microbial flora of fresh pork after γ-irradiation found no surviving organisms in samples that received an absorbed dose of 1.91 kGy or higher, even after 35 days of refrigerated storage (*30*). In samples that had received 0.57 kGy or no irradiation, *Staphylococcus* was the predominant bacterial organism throughout the first 21 d of storage. However, very few *Staphylococcus* isolates were *S. aureus*.

In Singapore, Ng and Tay tested for enterotoxin production in 111 randomly selected samples of foods and drinks contaminated with coagulase-positive *S. aureus* (*31*). Thirty-six of the strains (32%) were enterotoxigenic by an enzyme-linked immunosorbent assay (ELISA). Of these, 33 were confirmed positive by the reverse passive latex agglutination (RPLA) test. Surprisingly few strains produced SEA. SEB was the most common enterotoxin, produced by 36% of toxigenic strains assayed; 22% produced SEC, 17% produced SED, 11% produced SEA, and 6% produced both SEA and SEC. The "false-positives" by ELISA may have been SEE-producers, which the RPLA kit would fail to detect.

Pasta can become contaminated by *S. aureus* from various sources, and the organism may grow before the pasta is dried. Valik and Görner monitored the survival and growth of *S. aureus* in pasta during drying (*32*). One strain isolated from commercial pasta began to multiply immediately after inoculation, but decreased in numbers when the $a_w$ was reduced to <.93. Another strain apparently continued to grow until the $a_w$ was <.86, although its maximum growth was less than that normally required to produce enterotoxin. The authors concluded that pasta drying procedures are fast enough to prevent enough growth for toxin production.

## Toxins and Virulence Factors

Betley and Harris reviewed the genetics of staphylococcal enterotoxins and relationships between their structure and emetic activity (*33*). There is considerable diversity among the SE genes: *sea* is associated with a family of lysogenic phage; *sed* is located on a plasmid; and *seb* and *sec* appear to be chromosomal. Phages and plasmids bearing SE genes provide a means for horizontal transfer of these genes from enterotoxin producers to enterotoxin nonproducers. Enterotoxin gene expression was discussed in terms of its coordinate regulation and the influence of environmental conditions. Analysis of the effects of staphylococcal enterotoxins on T cells has led to recognition of a class of molecules dubbed "superantigens." The authors discussed the nature of SE's emetic and superantigenic activities and relationships between them.

Daugherty and Low cloned the gene for a phosphatidylinositol-specific phospholipase C (*plc*) from *S. aureus*, expressed it in *E. coli*, and characterized it and its product (*34*). Enzyme activity was abolished by mutagenesis with a tetracycline resistance gene. Oligonucleotide probes detected *plc* in all 15 clinical isolates of *S. aureus* surveyed but not in any of 6 coagulase-negative *Staphylococcus* species. It appears that *plc* is partially under the control of the accessory gene regulator *agr*, which controls transcription of several toxins and virulence factors, but is also regulated in part by *agr*-independent mechanisms. The authors concluded that this phosphatidylinositol-specific phospholipase C is a potential virulence factor.

Further studies of how *agr* regulates synthesis of staphylococcal virulence factors were reported by Novick et al. (*35*). They verified that the RNAIII promoter region encodes the *agr*-specific regulator by cloning it and demonstrating that its induction is sufficient to activate the *agr* response in the absence of any other element of the *agr* system. RNAIII appears to regulate exoprotein production primarily at the level of transcription, but it sometimes also acts at the level of translation. The authors speculate on why the staphylococci evolved an RNA-based global regulator for accessory exoprotein genes, when other organisms depend on regulatory proteins for these functions.

In quantitative studies, Borst and Betley showed that *S. aureus* strain FRI722 produces at least 8 times as much SEA as its parent strain FRI100 (*36*). Sequence analysis of *sea* revealed two mutations in the upstream promoter region of FRI722 at nucleotides −28 and +3 (with the transcriptional initiation site at +1). Both mutations were involved in the increased SEA synthesis.

## Detection and Identification

A collaborative study tested TECRA SET, an ELISA for staphylococcal enterotoxins A–E in foods without identifying the serotype (*37*). Samples of five foods were inoculated with 4–10 ng/g of SE, one serotype per sample. There were also uninoculated control samples of each food. Positive samples turned blue-green. Results were read visually and absorbance was measured using a microtiter plate reader. The method was sensitive and specific, and was adopted first action by AOAC International. Although the collaborative study yielded 100% correct responses, Bergdoll pointed out that this investigation failed to determine the method's sensitivity (*38*). As little as 0.5 ng/g of SE can be detected with some currently available methods, whereas the lowest concentration tested in this trial was 4 ng/g.

German investigators evaluated TECRA SET and three other commercial enzyme immunoassay kits for detecting SE in ground beef and cheddar cheese (*39*). Neither staphylococci nor thermonuclease could be detected in any sample. The SET-EIA yielded two false-positive results for beef samples and two for cheese; RIDASCREEN SET gave one false-positive for ground beef; and TECRA SET gave one false-positive for cheese. When enterotoxigenic *S. aureus* was inoculated into ground beef it grew and the thermonuclease test was positive. Nevertheless, the kits failed to detect enterotoxin in several of the 16 samples tested. VIDAS SET identified 14 positive samples, whereas RIDASCREEN identified only 10. Canadian investigators, however, found that RIDASCREEN could detect SE at levels as low as 0.20–0.30 ng/mL of extract of ham, salami, or mushrooms, 0.30–0.35 ng/mL of cheese extract, and 0.5–0.75 ng/g of foods such as noodles, ham, cheese, salami, and turkey (*40*). The kit simultaneously detects the enterotoxin and identifies its type (A–E). No food component or microbial product except naturally occurring peroxidase gave false-positive results.

Chang and Huang developed a sandwich ELISA for rapid detection of *S. aureus* in processed foods (*41*) Based on detection of protein A, it uses anti-protein A IgG. The authors also formulated a selective enrichment broth to be used in the 24-h incubation preceding the ELISA. The same authors evaluated a latex agglutination kit (AUREUS TEST™) for rapid identification of *S. aureus* (*42*). The latex particles are sensitized with anti–protein A IgG (which binds with protein A) and fibrinogen (which binds with coagulase). Results were obtained within minutes and were comparable to results with the conventional coagulase test, which requires hours.

Tsen et al. reported development of new oligo-nucleotide probes for identification of enterotoxigenic *S. aureus* by colony hybridization (*43*). The probes are complementary to sequences in SEA, SEB, SEC, SED, and SEE. Despite the high degree of homology among the SE genes, each probe allows specific identification with total discrimination from other types of enterotoxin genes. In particular, probes designed for *see* permit discrimination of SEE-producing strains, which are grouped with SEA-producers by RPLA.

Amplification of the *sec⁺* gene for $SEC_1$ by a polymerase chain reaction (PCR) using two nested primer pairs requires as little as 10 fg of total genomic DNA—representing fewer than 10 cells (*44*). However, the presence of bacterial cells or thermonuclease reduces the sensitivity of the PCR.

Matthews and Oliver reported a PCR-based DNA fingerprinting technique suitable for typing *Staphylococcus* species of bovine origin (*45*). The profiles were discrete and reproducible for each species tested.

Wilson et al. used a digoxygenin-labeled total genomic DNA probe to distinguish *S. aureus* from other staphylococci associated with milk and meat (*46*). Its results were comparable to those from conventional methods and were simpler and less costly for large samples. Freney et al. found that Accuprobe®, an acridinium ester–labeled DNA probe, distinguished *S. aureus* from all other *Staphylococcus* species and also detected 26 atypical *S. aureus* strains (*47*). They suggest this as a rapid and specific method for identifying atypical (lacking coagulase, thermonuclease, or fibrinogen affinity factor) *S. aureus* strains.

## Control

Sutherland et al. studied the growth of *S. aureus* in laboratory medium as affected by NaCl concentration (0.5–13.5%, w/v), pH (4.0–7.0), and temperature (10–30°C) (*48*). Growth was modeled using the modified Gompertz equation and the values of the parameters of the curve were derived. From this the growth rate, lag time, and generation time could be calculated. Growth curves could then be generated for any set of conditions within the matrix studied, enabling prediction of growth rate, generation and lag times, and time to 1000-fold increase. With one exception, predictions were fail-safe. The model gave realistic estimates of generation times for shrimp slurry, potato dough, egg noodles, canned ham, and milk. It underestimated the generation time for mayonnaise, cream pastries, and a number of meat-containing foods. Buchanan et al. generated response-surface models for the effects of temperature, pH, NaCl,

and $NaNO_2$ on aerobic and anaerobic growth of *S. aureus* 196E (*49*). Growth kinetics were independent of inoculum size. Quadratic models reasonably predicted the effects of the four variables on growth kinetics and should provide initial estimates of the behavior of *S. aureus* in foods.

Ballesteros et al. found that ethanol has some antibacterial effects against *S. aureus* that are unrelated to reduction of $a_w$ (*50*). Growth occurred in 5 wt% ethanol only after a prolonged lag period. At 6.5 wt% or higher, the number of viable cells of *S. aureus* ATCC 6538P declined during incubation. Growth of strain C-243 was inhibited at concentrations of 7.5 wt%, but this may reflect a greatly extended lag time. Electron microscopy revealed pronounced morphologic changes in walls of cells grown in broth with 5.0–6.5% ethanol.

Although the antimicrobial action of phenolic antioxidants such as BHA and TBHG against *S. aureus* is well established, the antimicrobial action of the widespread naturally occurring phenolic compounds has received less attention. Commercial oleuropein and phenolics extracted from olives inhibited growth and enterotoxin production by *S. aureus* S-6, an SEB producer, in broth and a model food system (*51*). Inhibition was more pronounced when the pH was low and the inoculum size small.

Lee et al. reported a series of studies on the antibacterial effects of food-grade phosphates against *S. aureus* (*52–54*). In synthetic medium, the following MICs were determined against cells in the early exponential phase of growth: 0.1% for sodium ultraphosphate and sodium polyphosphate glassy; 0.5% for sodium acid pyrophosphate, sodium tripolyphosphate, and tetrasodium pyrophosphate (*52*). Thus MICs were lower for phosphates of shorter chain-length. Further tests indicated that cells were lysed in the presence of phosphates. When added before the polyphosphate-containing medium was inoculated, 0.01 M $Ca^{2+}$ or $Mg^{+2}$ prevented growth inhibition by ultraphosphate and sodium polyphosphate glassy (*53*). Moreover, the bactericidal effects of these phosphates were reversed by 0.01 M $Ca^{2+}$ or $Mg^{2+}$ when the metals were added after 1 h of incubation. Growth inhibition by tetrasodium pyrophosphate was prevented when $Fe^{3+}$ was added 1 h before the phosphate; $Ca^{2+}$ and $Mg^{2+}$ were ineffective. Thus the metal content of the environment can substantially alter the antibacterial effects of phosphates. Studies of the antibacterial mechanism indicated that chelation of metal ions is involved (*54*). The authors postulated that the structurally essential metals form cross-bridges between teichoic acid chains in the cell walls of gram-positive bacteria; polyphosphates bind to the cell wall and chelate the metals, disrupting these bridges and causing leakage from the cell.

In screening 37 strains of lactobacilli and leuconostocs for bacteriocin production, Liao et al. found a bacteriocin-like substance in culture filtrate of *Lactobacillus acidophilus* OSU133 (*55*). They named it lacidin A. Lacidin A was strongly bactericidal against *S. aureus* in phosphate buffer; it was bacteriostatic in brain–heart infusion, heat-treated milk, and liquid whole egg. The activity was not due to acid, hydrogen peroxide, or phage and was destroyed by hydrolysis with proteolytic enzymes.

Ballesteros et al. assessed how lowering $a_w$ with NaCl, sucrose, propylene glycol, butylene glycol, or various polyethylene glycols affects *S. aureus* (*56*). The inhibitory effects of NaCl and sucrose were entirely attributable to their lowering of $a_w$. However, the amphipathic solutes also showed specific antibacterial activity that could stem from attack on the cell wall.

Pasteurization of goat's milk at 70°C for 5 min or microfiltration at a 1.4-µm pore size significantly reduces the level of staphylococci and fecal coliforms in the milk and guarantees a low level of contaminant flora in soft cheese (*57*). Development of contaminant flora during acidification of the milk at 22°C was inversely proportional to the initial level of lactic acid bacteria. The rate of acidification was most rapid in raw milk and slowest in microfiltered milk. Pasteurized and microfiltered milks permitted more growth of contaminant bacteria in the drained curds and in 30-d-old ripened cheese than did raw milk. The authors concluded that growth of lactic acid starter during ripening must be optimized, particularly for rennet curd cheese.

# CLOSTRIDIUM

## Clostridium botulinum

*Clostridium botulinum* is of great concern as a human pathogen because its neurotoxins are among the most potent poisons known and it can grow and produce toxin in a variety of foods without causing any signs of "spoilage." Sofos discussed the forms of botulism, characteristics of the causative organism, the nature and activities of *C. botulinum* neurotoxins, methods for detecting the organism and its neurotoxins, and principles of *C. botulinum* control in foods (*58*). He stressed the risks from home-processed foods and product mishandling. The potential for abuse is of particular concern since innovations in food technology have provided large numbers of

partially processed, ready-to-eat, extended shelf-life foods that require refrigeration.

**OCCURRENCE, GROWTH, AND CONTROL IN FOODS.** Gibbs et al. surveyed more than 500 samples of refrigerated packaged foods, purchased from retail markets in the UK, for occurrence of psychrotrophic strains of *C. botulinum* (*59*). None of the samples contained the organism. When samples of carrots, potatoes, lasagna, and smoked trout fillets were inoculated with the organism, no botulinal toxin was detected after incubation at 4 or 10°C for 3 weeks. However, toxin did develop within 1 week in all whole trout that were inoculated.

One likely source of *C. botulinum* spores in honey appears to be dead honey bees and bee pupae. Three strains of type A and one of type F *C. botulinum*, all isolated from contaminated honey, were inoculated at a level of $10^2$–$10^3$ into honey bee workers, larvae, and pupae (*60*). The organisms grew to populations of $10^4$–$10^5$ in dead bees after 10 days of aerobic incubation. Similar growth occurred in pupae, but not in larvae. Coinoculation with *Bacillus alvei* significantly enhanced growth of most *C. botulinum* strains. The authors concluded that the heavy contamination with botulinum spores sometimes encountered in honey could be caused by contamination from dead bees in which the organism had proliferated.

Cheese is rarely implicated as a vehicle of botulism, but a few notable cheese-associated outbreaks have occurred. Malizio et al. pursued earlier clues that arginine supply is related to growth and toxin production by *C. botulinum* (*61*). They measured production of botulinal toxin by a mixture of type A and type B spores in cheddar cheese containing 0, 0.9, or 1.8% NaCl and 1% L-arginine. No toxin was detected in samples without supplemental arginine or in samples with arginine and 1.8% salt. The pH of arginine samples was increased at least 0.5 pH units, to near 6.0, but this alone did not permit growth. The authors discussed the interaction of pH, salts, moisture, temperature, endogenous inhibitors, and inhibitors formed by lactic cultures to prevent growth of *C. botulinum* in cheese and the possible role of arginine metabolism in promoting spore germination and toxin production. Another study showed that polyphosphates delay toxin production in processed pasteurized cheese spreads better than disodium phosphate (*62*). Samples of cheese spread were inoculated with ~$10^4$ spores per gram, held for 3 min at 80°C, then filled into glass containers and incubated at 30°C. At moisture contents of 52–56% no samples were toxic after 20 weeks. However, toxin did form in cheese with 60% moisture. It was first detected at 8 weeks in cheese containing orthophosphate but not until 20 weeks in cheeses containing polyphosphate. Toxin production was thus related to time, moisture, and phosphate type. pH was correlated with toxin production at 8 weeks but not at 20 weeks.

Meng and Genigeorgis used modeling techniques to determine how the lag phase of *C. botulinum* toxigenesis in cooked, vacuum-packaged turkey and chicken breast is affected by temperature, sodium lactate, NaCl, and inoculum size (*63*). The inoculum was a mixture of spores of nonproteolytic *C. botulinum* types B and E. Lag phase was measured as the time from inoculation to detection of the first toxic sample. The resulting regression model explained 94.5% of the variance seen with turkey; results for chicken were similar. The most important factor was temperature ($T^{1/2}$), which accounted for 65% of variance. Lactate concentration explained 21%, and the rest was explained by interactions of inoculum size with $T^{1/2}$ and NaCl concentration. When the lower limit of the 90% confidence interval for the lag phase was used, the predicted lag time was longer than the observed in only 1% of the comparisons. This provides a quantitative demonstration that higher concentrations of lactate and NaCl and lower temperatures significantly delay toxigenesis. A lag-time model for spores of proteolytic *C. botulinum* in broth medium was developed by Whiting and Call (*64*). Variables were temperature (15–37°C), pH (5–7), and NaCl concentration (0–3%). Inoculum size was $10^4$ spores of a 6-strain mixture of types A and B. NaCl had little effect on time to growth, but low pH and temperatures <20°C greatly delayed growth. The regression equations are least-squares fits and are not intended to represent fail-safe times for growth. Nor have they been validated against observational data for growth of *C. botulinum* in foods.

Processing recommendations for home-canned smoked fish to kill *C. botulinum* spores must consider both the moisture content of the fish and the fill of the jar. Heat penetration measurements showed that slow-heating jars are likely to contain drier, more tightly packed fish than faster-heating jars (*65*). Process times were calculated for three levels of moisture loss with dense or loose packing. Based on the worst-case scenario, a process time of 110 min was established as the new recommendation for home-canning smoked fish in pint jars under the conditions specified.

Miller et al. evaluated salts of five organic acids as possible antibotulinal agents (*66*). The product tested was a vacuum-packed formulation of ground turkey breast, artificially inoculated with mixed spores of proteolytic *C. botulinum* and incubated at 28°C. Antibotulinal activity of the monocarboxylic acids (pyruvic,

lactic, acetic, and propionic) was related to the $pK_a$. Possible inhibitory actions of these acids include lowering intracellular pH, altering membrane permeability, and interfering with the electron transport system. Citrate did not fit this pattern, suggesting a different mode of action—perhaps metal chelation. The authors suggested organic acid salts as secondary barriers to control bacterial growth in refrigerated foods. Houtsma et al. showed that the inhibitory effects of sodium lactate on proteolytic strains of *C. botulinum* in culture medium depend on the incubation temperature (*67*). Visible growth was always accompanied by toxin production. Toxigenesis was delayed by 2% sodium lactate (wt/vol) at 15°C and by 2.5% sodium lactate at 20°C. It was completely prevented at 15 and 20°C by 3 and 4% sodium lactate, respectively; however, 4% sodium lactate did not prevent toxin production at 30°C. The inhibition by lactate was not due to lowering of the $a_w$, since NaCl concentrations having the same effect on $a_w$ were not significantly inhibitory. There was no clear synergism between sodium lactate and NaCl.

Nisin is a broad-spectrum bacteriocin produced by *Lactococcus lactis*. Rogers and Montville assessed the influences of food ingredients on nisin's anticlostridial activity in model systems (*68*). A basal yeast extract–peptone–glucose medium was supplemented with three levels of protein, phospholipid, and soluble starch at three pH values, with and without nisin. Samples were inoculated with spores of *C. botulinum* 56A ($10^4$/mL) and incubated at 15, 25, or 35°C. Nisin lost effectiveness as temperature increased. It inhibited *C. botulinum* until its residual level dropped below a threshold, which was 154 IU/mL at 35°C and 12 IU/mL at 15°C. Several significant interactions between nisin and food components were seen. The authors concluded that nisin can provide a secondary barrier to botulinal growth, but only under suboptimal growth conditions.

Some strains of *Pediococcus pentosaceus* produce the bacteriocin pediocin. Crandall et al. investigated the ability of a pediocin-producing strain of *P. pentosaceus* to inhibit botulinal growth and toxin production in minimally processed, vacuum-packaged beef with gravy (*69*). When samples were inoculated with a mixture of type A and B *C. botulinum* spores, toxin was detected by day 31 at 4°C and by day 6 at 10°C. When coinoculated with *C. botulinum*, neither the pediocin producer nor a nonproducer *P. pentosaceus* strain significantly delayed toxigenesis. Thus if spores are present, sous vide beef presents a botulinal hazard even when adequately refrigerated.

Bowles and Miller have tested a variety of compounds for antibotulinal properties in broth cultures

(*70–72*). They reported that a variety of aromatic and aliphatic aldehydes delay germination of mixtures of type A and B spores and are sporicidal at higher concentrations (*70*). Of the 12 compounds tested, 11 either are FDA-approved synthetic flavors or have been granted GRAS status. In nearly all cases, aldehydes containing a benzene ring had lower MICs than aliphatic compounds. Benzaldehyde, the simplest aromatic aldehyde tested, was the most active inhibitor of dipicolinic acid release during germination; pyruvaldehyde, an aliphatic, was least effective. Both types of aldehyde reduced the thermal resistance of *C. botulinum* spores at 80°C. Similar studies with aromatic and aliphatic ketones showed that antibotulinal activity was a function of carbon chain length, location and number of carbonyl groups, and aromaticity (*71*). Like the aldehydes, these compounds are noted for their characteristic flavors and aromas and a number of them have been approved as food additives. Caffeic acid, a hydroxycinnamic acid widely distributed in fruits and vegetables, also showed potential as a food additive to inhibit growth of *C. botulinum* and reduce thermal processing requirements of heat-sensitive foods (*72*). In broth culture it inhibited germination for 6 h at a concentration of 0.78 mM and for 24 h at 3.25 mM; it was sporicidal at concentrations >100 mM. It also had sporostatic activity and delayed toxigenesis when tested in commercial meat broths.

TOXINS. The research group of East and Collins has sequenced several botulinal neurotoxin genes and compared them with other known botulinal toxin sequences, in the context of phylogenetic relationships within the *C. botulinum* species complex (*73–75*). The product of the gene encoding the nonproteolytic *C. botulinum* type B neurotoxin is a protein of 1291 amino acid residues (*73*). The gene showed greatest sequence homology with the gene for proteolytic *C. botulinum* B neurotoxin: 97.7% for the light chain (corresponding to 10 amino acid changes) and 90.2% for the heavy chain (corresponding to 81 amino acid changes). The next highest light-chain sequence identity was 52.1%, with tetanus toxin. Identities with light chains of other botulinum neurotoxins were in the 32–45% range. Most differences were at the carboxy-terminal end, the region important in cell binding. The authors performed a distance-matrix analysis and constructed two dendrograms, one based on relatedness of botulinal neurotoxins and one based on phylogenetic relationships within the *C. botulinum* species complex as derived from 16S rRNA. Major differences between the trees reaffirmed the previously recognized discordance between toxin type and genotypic divisions

within *C. botulinum*. The neurotoxin gene from a *C. botulinum* type A strain associated with infant botulism was sequenced and compared with other clostridial neurotoxins (*74*). The sequence identity between infant and classical type A neurotoxin was 94.9% for the light chain (corresponding to 23 amino acid changes) and 87.1% for the heavy chain (corresponding to 109 amino acid changes). The two neurotoxins, while clearly related, are nonetheless distinct. (The sequence deviation between infant and classical type A toxins is probably substantially greater than the variation within either of the forms.) By comparison, the type E toxins of *C. botulinum* and *C. butyricum* show considerably less divergence, whereas the type F toxins of *C. botulinum* and *C. baratii* show considerably more. The authors concluded that the infant and classical type A neurotoxins are indisputably of common ancestry, but the number of amino acid differences indicates that their divergence was not very recent. The type G neurotoxin gene showed greatest homology (~58%) with the type B neurotoxin of proteolytic and nonproteolytic *C. botulinum* (*75*). Distance matrix dendrograms showed the relationships between light and heavy chains of various clostridial neurotoxins of types A–G.

Be et al. identified functional domains of type A botulinal and tetanus neurotoxins by hydrophobic moment analysis of their amino acid sequences (*76*). Both toxins are water-soluble proteins that form membrane channels as part of their mode of action. Whereas calculations of hydrophobicity suggested only one or two membrane-compatible segments, hydrophobic-moment analysis revealed three such segments in tetanus neurotoxin and five in type A botulinum toxin. Several amphiphilic peptide segments were also identified. There is little sequence homology between these segments—indicating that although high sequence homology is not maintained, functional characteristics are conserved. Other observations suggested that the transmembrane and amphiphilic segments may become exposed upon interaction with the membrane.

IDENTIFICATION. Potter et al. developed an ELISA for detecting botulinal neurotoxins of types A, B, and E in inoculated food samples (*77*). Confirmation by the mouse test indicated that there were no false-negative results and 91 false-positives for ~500 samples tested. The "false-positive" results were thought to be due to inactivated toxin or sublethal levels of toxin.

Doellgast et al. developed a modified ELISA based on detection of sandwich complexes on microtiter plates by a solid-phase enzyme-linked coagulation assay (ELCA) (*78*). With it they were able to measure *C. botulinum* type

A, B, and E neurotoxins, both purified and in crude culture filtrates, at mouse bioassay levels. The assay should be appropriate for feces, blood, and most contaminated foods. In considering alternatives to the sandwich protocol, the authors tested chicken IgG and biotinylated IgG as capture reagents (*79*). This ELISA-ELCA also detected type A, B, and E neurotoxins at mouse-assay levels. A modification of the methods permitted assessment of toxin concentration. Elcatech developed these assays in kit form, and the authors investigated whether the kits could be used to measure polyclonal human and horse antibodies to the toxins (*80*). Specific antibodies to types A, B, and E neurotoxins could be measured, but the sensitivity for indicating the neurotoxin was reduced. The authors suggested that the reduction in sensitivity provides a measure of the specific antibody titer.

Goodnough et al. reported a new enzyme-linked immunoassay for neurotoxins of *C. botulinum* types A, B, and E and toxigenic *C. butyricum* (*81*). Toxin is transferred from agar culture medium to a nitrocellulose support and probed with type-specific antibodies. The toxin types of colonies grown from a mixed inoculum of *C. botulinum* serotypes could be identified.

A number of DNA probes for *C. botulinum* have been reported (*82–85*). McKinney et al. developed a probe specific for group I proteolytic *C. botulinum* (toxin types A, B, and F) (*82*). It did not hybridize to groups II, III, or IV or to any strains of *Clostridium sporogenes*. Campbell et al. developed a PCR method for identifying the botulinal neurotoxin gene, with specific identification of *C. botulinum* toxin types B, E, and F and the type F toxin gene of *C. baratii* (*83*). Szabo et al. used the polymerase chain reaction to develop specific probes for genes for botulinal neurotoxins type A–E (*84*). Type A, B, and E genes could be amplified from crude DNA extracts, vegetative cells, or spore preparations. Fach et al. reported a PCR method for detection of *C. botulinum* type A strains in food samples (*85*).

Dezfulian and Bartlett described their new method for rapid direct identification of type A or B *C. botulinum* colonies (*86*). Based on demonstration of toxigenicity by an enzyme immunoassay and on antimicrobial susceptibility testing, it can be completed in 48 h.

INFANT BOTULISM. The first case of infant botulism in Europe to be linked conclusively to honey was reported (*87*). The patient was a 9-week-old baby girl who had been given pacifiers sweetened with home-canned honey. Strains of *C. botulinum* type B were isolated from the baby's feces and from samples of the honey.

## Clostridium perfringens

Heat-resistant spores of *Clostridium perfringens* are often found in meat and poultry, where they survive the heating process. They undergo rapid vegetative growth in improperly chilled foods, then sporulate and produce enterotoxins in the human intestine. Most *C. perfringens* food poisoning is caused by type A strains. Labbé discussed factors affecting the organism's growth, sporulation, and enterotoxin production (*88*). He described the biochemical properties and mode of action of the enterotoxin and techniques for its purification and assay.

OUTBREAKS AND CLINICAL FEATURES. In 1993, two outbreaks of *C. perfringens* gastroenteritis were caused by contaminated corned beef eaten at St. Patrick's Day dinners (*89*). Both were confirmed by the recovery of ≥10^5 organisms per gram of corned beef. Cultured stool samples from one outbreak also met the alternative criterion of ≥10^6 colonies per gram. The outbreak in Cleveland, Ohio, affected approximately 150 persons, all of whom ate corned beef purchased at the same delicatessen. The meat had been boiled, cooled at room temperature, and refrigerated for several days before reheating and serving. Sandwiches made for catering were held at room temperature for several hours. Meat sold at the delicatessen was held in a warmer at 120°F until it was sliced and served. In Virginia, 86 of 113 persons became ill after attending a traditional St. Patrick's Day dinner. Ten-pound chunks of corned beef were cooked in an oven and refrigerated. About 90 min before serving began, the meat was sliced and placed under heat lamps. The errors in preparing the corned beef associated with these outbreaks are typical of those generally associated with *C. perfringens* food poisoning. Temperature abuse was a contributing factor in virtually all (97%) *C. perfringens* outbreaks reported to CDC from 1973 through 1987.

Common food poisoning is caused by the α toxin of type A *C. perfringens* whereas necrotizing enteritis ("pig-bel") is caused by type C, which produces both α and β toxin. Clarke et al. described a case of enteritis necroticans with midgut necrosis caused by *C. perfringens* (*90*). The patient, a 53-year-old black woman, had eaten chicken stew and sweet potatoes the day before she became ill. Although a complete epidemiologic investigation was not carried out, it is likely that the chicken stew was the vehicle of infection. The authors suggested that concurrent ingestion of sweet potatoes, which contain a trypsin inhibitor, may have contributed to the illness.

To see whether resistance to growth-enhancing antibiotics is increasing in *C. perfringens* isolated from farm animals in Belgium, Devriese et al. determined the MICs of 7 such antibiotics against 95 field isolates of the organism (*91*). Overall, the prevalence of resistance was low and comparable to levels observed in 1979 in the same host species. For 6 of the 7 antibiotics, the $MIC_{90}$'s were well below the permitted feed levels. The exception was flavomycin, which was inactive in vitro but depressed ileal populations of *C. perfringens*.

Results obtained by Mach, Lindsay, and their associates implicate *C. perfringens* type A cytotoxic enterotoxin in the etiology of sudden infant death syndrome (SIDS) (*92,93*). Type A *C. perfringens* vegetative cells and spores were isolated in high numbers from feces of 133 of 164 SIDS infants but from only 1 of 57 infants who died of other causes and 5 of 29 live controls (*92*). Presence of *C. perfringens* type A cytotoxic enterotoxins, determined in fecal samples by an ELISA, was highly correlated with presence of the organism in SIDS cases: 122 SIDS infants tested positive for both enterotoxin and organisms, compared with only 1 of the live controls. Histopathologically, ileal tissue from SIDS infants was strikingly similar to tissue from experimental mice affected by type A cytotoxic enterotoxins. The histopathologic pattern depends on the age of the animal. In mice up to 16 d old, the pathologic change would favor absorption of a high concentration of enterotoxin into the systemic circulation. Developmentally this period corresponds to 6–18 weeks in human infants, when >85% of SIDS cases occur. The authors propose that in immunologically vulnerable infants, systemic distribution of cytotoxic enterotoxin acts parasympathomimetically to trigger a biochemical cascade, altering cardiorespiratory control and possibly causing death. Mach and Lindsay pursued the trigger idea by in vivo and in vitro studies of young rabbits (*93*). Action of the enterotoxin was promoted by an activator in a brush border membrane fraction, which was provisionally identified as interferon-γ. Since viral and bacterial infections induce interferons and immunologically immature infants are predisposed to infection, these observations could explain many cases of SIDS.

**OCCURRENCE AND BEHAVIOR IN FOODS.** To estimate the prevalence of *C. perfringens* in cow's milk, Moustafa and Marth tested samples from 312 quarters of 80 apparently healthy dairy cows (*94*). Twenty-nine samples (9%) yielded *C. perfringens*. Of these, 14 were positive by the pH test and 12 were positive by the California Mastitis Test; however, only 7 samples had a high mastitis test score. Sensitivity of the isolates to 7 anti-

biotics was variable. All strains were resistant to clindamycin and sensitive to tetracycline. Sensitivity to carbenicillin, cephalothin, chloramphenicol, piperacillin, and erythromycin ranged between 31 and 69%. Owing to its prevalence and resistance to antibiotics used therapeutically in humans, *C. perfringens* in milk has the potential to pose a significant public health hazard.

Stolle et al. investigated the microbiologic quality of doner kebabs, a Turkish meat specialty, in the Munich area (*95*). The microflora was composed of aerobic sporeformers, lactic acid bacteria, enterobacteria, pseudomonads, enterococci, and yeasts. No counts of *S. aureus* exceeded the limit, and no salmonellas were found. Eight of 44 samples were positive for *C. perfringens*.

Juneja et al. studied the growth and sporulation potential of *C. perfringens* in cooked ground beef packaged under air or vacuum and stored at various temperatures (*96*). Regardless of packaging, the organisms either declined in number or failed to grow at temperatures of 4, 8, and 12°C. At 15 and 28°C, growth was markedly slower under aerobic conditions than under vacuum. Overall, the data indicated that temperature abuse (28°C) of refrigerated products for up to 6 h will not permit substantial growth of *C. perfringens*, but cyclic abuse and static-temperature abuse for longer periods may permit growth of dangerously high numbers of organisms. Even so, reheating such products to an internal temperature of 65°C before eating would kill vegetative cells and prevent food poisoning. In experiments with precooked 50-g chunks of beef loin, post-packaging pasteurization reduced populations of *C. perfringens* spores and vegetative cells (*97*). Pasteurization in a waterbath to an internal temperature of 60°C for 16 min reduced *C. perfringens* counts by 5 $log_{10}$ in the broth and by 1.5 $log_{10}$ on the surface. This level of control persisted throughout 85 days of refrigerated storage. Growth of indigenous microflora was also suppressed.

The importance of preformed *C. perfringens* enterotoxin in cases of food poisoning is not clear. Mengert et al. reported that stability of the preformed toxin in foods is influenced by time and temperature factors and salt content (*98*).

**TOXINS AND PATHOGENESIS.** Czeczulin et al. reported the cloning, sequencing, and expression of the *C. perfringens* enterotoxin gene (*cpe*) in *E. coli* (*99*). The gene encodes a polypeptide of 319 amino acid residues, with a deduced molecular weight of 35,317. The 5' region had no consensus sequence for a typical signal peptide. CPE from recombinant *E. coli* retained its full cytotoxicity for Vero cells. All or most of its expression in *E. coli* seemed to be driven from a clostridial promoter. The amount of CPE made by recombinant *E. coli* was intermediate between the low level formed by vegetative cultures of *C. perfringens* and the high level formed by sporulating cells. This suggests that sporulation is not essential for *cpe* expression but does enhance it.

Titball et al. expressed the *C*-terminal domain of *C. perfringens* α-toxin in *E. coli* and studied its biochemical and immunologic properties (*100*). Anti-α-toxin serum and antiserum raised against this 124-residue polypeptide (C247–C370) reacted identically when used to map epitopes in the *C*-terminal domain, suggesting that the fragment was structurally and immunologically identical to the corresponding region of the intact α-toxin. The fragment had no sphingomyelinase activity and was not cytotoxic for mouse lymphocytes. Neither the C1–C249 fragment nor the C247–C370 fragment had hemolytic activity when tested individually or sequentially. Together, however, in equimolar amounts, they hemolyzed mouse erythrocytes. The authors concluded that the *C*-terminal region confers hemolytic activity on the *N*-terminal domain, where the phospholipase C activity resides.

The mechanism of action of *C. perfringens* enterotoxin involves multiple steps culminating in cytotoxicity (*101*). First the molecule binds to a protein receptor on mammalian plasma membranes. Once membrane-bound, it becomes progressively more resistant to release by proteases—a phenomenon consistent with insertion into the membrane. The inserted enterotoxin participates in formation of large complexes containing a 70-kDa membrane protein, a 50-kDa membrane protein, and the enterotoxin in a molecular ratio of 1:1:1. When this process is complete, the plasma membrane is freely permeable to ions and small molecules, and disruption of cellular colloidal and osmotic equilibrium causes secondary cellular effects and death.

IDENTIFICATION. A collaborative study compared methods using the iron milk medium and the official AOAC tryptose–sulfite–cycloserine plating medium for detecting and enumerating *C. perfringens* in oysters (*Crassostrea gigas*) (*102*). The selectivity of iron milk medium relies on the rapid growth of *C. perfringens* at 45°C, indicated by the stormy fermentation reaction within 18 h. Compared to the standard method, the iron milk medium method is convenient and rapid and is especially useful in field work. Data analysis revealed no significant differences between estimates from the two methods, and the iron milk method was adopted first action by AOAC International for detection of *C. perfringens* in shellfish.

Attempts to isolate plasmid DNA from *C. perfringens* have been plagued by the presence of a nuclease elaborated by the organism. Results have not been reproducible, and the storage quality of the plasmid DNA has been very poor. Hussain and Purnima developed an improved procedure by combining features of several previously reported procedures (*103*). Steps that help to combat nuclease activity are complete lysis of cells, maintenance of pH between 12.35 and 12.40, incorporation of DEP in the protocol, and incubation on ice until the precipitation stage.

## Other

Galindo et al. developed a PCR hybridization assay for detecting clostridial cells and spores in liquid food samples (*104*). The PCR amplifies a genus-specific portion of the 16S rDNA. The capture oligonucleotide is immobilized on a microtiter plate and positive results are detected by color development. As few as 2–5 cells or spores can be detected in 6 h.

Cigáneková and Kallová tested the anticlostridial activity of a series of alkyl-dimethylamine oxides,

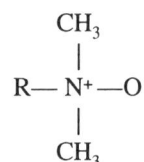

$$R—\overset{\overset{\displaystyle CH_3}{|}}{\underset{\underset{\displaystyle CH_3}{|}}{N^+}}—O$$

where R is a chain of 1–18 carbons (*105*). They also tested (1-methyldodecyl)dimethylamine oxide and Iodaminox. The most effective of the alkyl-dimethylamine oxides was the (1-methyldodecyl)dimethylamine. Its MIC ranged from 7.8 to 78 μmol/L for strains of *C. perfringens* types A, C, D, and E, *C. sporogenes,* and *C. bifermentans.* This same range was seen for the 5 strains of *C. perfringens* type A tested. Iodaminox was about twice as effective (MIC 3.9–31 μmol/L). These two compounds were most active at pH 6 and 40°C.

In addition to *C. botulinum*, strains of *C. butyricum* and *C. baratii* that produce toxins of types E and F, respectively, have been associated with infant botulism. Fujii et al. determined the nucleotide sequence of the gene encoding the nontoxic component of botulinum type E progenitor toxin from *C. butyricum* strain BL6340 and compared it with that from *C. botulinum* type E strain Mashike (*106*). They also compared the deduced amino acid sequences. The two genes differed in only 33 of 3486 bases, corresponding to 17 amino acid residues. Because it appears that the gene encoding certain *C. botulinum* neurotoxin types can be naturally transferred to *C. butyricum* and *C. baratii* and this could have important repercussions in the food industry and infectious microbiology, Zhou et al. investigated the mechanism of transfer of the toxin gene (*107*). A toxin gene probe hybridized with chromosomal DNA from toxigenic *C. botulinum* type E and *C. butyricum* strains but not with their plasmid DNA or with chromosomal DNA from nontoxigenic strains. Phage DNAs of toxigenic strains of the two species were similar or identical, and different from DNAs of phages induced in nontoxigenic strains. However, toxigenic variants could not be obtained by growing nontoxigenic strains in the presence of phage induced from a toxin producer. Interspecies transfer did occur when a recipient strain of nontoxigenic *C. botulinum*, type E–like, was incubated in filter-sterilized growth fluid obtained from culturing a nontoxigenic helper strain of nontoxigenic *C. butyricum* with phage induced from toxigenic *C. butyricum*. The authors postulated that the transfer was a transduction by a defective phage that was made infective by a helper strain. The transfer was strain-specific, perhaps explaining why strains of *C. butyricum* producing a botulinum type E–like toxin are not encountered more often.

*Clostridium sporogenes* PA3679 is frequently used as a model in studies of anaerobic spore-formers. Rodrigo et al. determined the thermal death time curve for PA3679 spores using a computer-controlled thermoresistometer (*108*). Curves were determined in phosphate buffer pH 7 and in mushroom extract acidified to pH 6.65–4.65 with citric acid. The curve for spores in buffer with micropurge was a straight line ($z = 9.5°C$). Without micropurge the curve could be described by two lines, with $z = 10.0°C$ for temperatures of 121 to 132.5°C and $z = 18.3$ for higher temperatures (to 143°C). Spores were less heat resistant in mushroom extract than in buffer. $D_T$ values decreased exponentially as temperature increased. Acidification did not reduce thermal resistance at high temperatures. The same research group evaluated the thermal resistance of PA3679 spores at 110 121°C in phosphate buffer pH 7.0, unacidified mushroom extract (pH 6.7), and mushroom extract acidified to pH 6.22–4.65 with citric acid or glucono–δ-lactone (*109*). Again, spores were less heat resistant in unacidified extract than in buffer. However, acidification had a pH-dependent effect on $D$ values. At 110°C and pH 6.22, $D$ was considerably longer than in unacidified extract. The effect became smaller as pH was further decreased or as temperature was increased. The two acidulants produced comparable results.

Li et al. used an extruded mixture of white corn flour and mechanically deboned turkey to study thermal inactivation and injury of PA3679 spores (*110*). There was a 2-log$_{10}$ reduction in surviving spores at 93.3°C and

a 4- to 5-log$_{10}$ reduction at 115.6°C. Most spores that survived the heat treatments required nutrients not needed by uninjured spores. Moreover, spore counts in the extruded material decreased during 2 weeks of refrigerated storage. The overall quality of the extruded mixture of corn flour and mechanically deboned turkey was excellent.

Welt et al. compared the thermal inactivation rates of microwave-heated and conventionally heated PA3679 spores at steady-state temperatures of 90, 100, and 110°C (*111*). No significant heat-source-related differences were found. To confirm that microwave irradiation had no effect separate from the heating effect, they pumped a spore suspension through the microwave oven, where it received 400 W of microwave power, into a tube outside the oven where it was continuously cooled. No detectable inactivation occurred.

## BACILLUS

The genus *Bacillus* is divided into two subgroups, one of which comprises large-celled gram-positive rods that produce central or terminal ellipsoid or cylindrical spores that do not distend the sporangia. *Bacillus cereus, B. megaterium, B. anthracis, B. thuringiensis*, and *B. cereus* var. *mycoides* are in this group, which includes most clinically important species. Drobniewski reviewed *B. cereus* and related species (*112*). He discussed the isolation and identification of *B. cereus,* the food poisoning and nongastrointestinal disease it causes, and the toxins it produces. Other *Bacillus* species were mentioned briefly. Kramer and Gilbert summarized *B. cereus* gastroenteritis (*113*). They discussed the taxonomy of the genus *Bacillus* and the properties of *B. cereus*, the characteristics and epidemiology of foodborne illness due to *B. cereus*, the exotoxins associated with *B. cereus* food poisoning, and the organism's spore, somatic, and flagellar antigens.

### Outbreaks

An increase in *Bacillus* food poisoning has been noted in Northern Ireland (*114*). Only one incident was identified during the 1980s, but there were 9 in 1991 and 4 in 1992. Only small numbers of persons were affected in these outbreaks, 9 of which involved food from Chinese restaurants. Rice and chicken were the most frequently implicated food sources. In 4 instances, *B. subtilis* was isolated from the implicated food, although two of these foods also contained *B. cereus*. Low numbers of *B.*

*licheniformis* were isolated from one food that allegedly caused illness. *Bacillus cereus* H1 was the most common serotype, but H20 was detected 4 times and H11 once.

In July 1993 a district health department in Virginia received reports of acute gastrointestinal illness in children and staff at two jointly owned child day-care centers after a catered lunch (*115*). Fourteen of 48 persons who ate chicken fried rice became ill, whereas none of the 16 who did not eat this dish became ill. *Bacillus cereus* was isolated from leftover chicken fried rice in numbers exceeding $10^6$/g. The rice had been cooked the evening before the lunch and cooled at room temperature before refrigeration. The next morning it was briefly pan-fried with pieces of cooked chicken and delivered to the day-care centers at about 10:30 a.m., where it was held without refrigeration until served, without reheating, at noon. This outbreak was the emetic type, which is frequently associated with fried rice. *Bacillus cereus* is frequently found in uncooked rice, and heat-resistant spores may survive the initial cooking. If cooked rice is held at room temperature, these spores germinate and vegetative cells multiply rapidly—producing an emetic toxin that can survive brief heating. The food handlers and day-care staff did not realize that cooked rice was a potentially hazardous food.

## Occurrence and Behavior in Foods

Sutherland and Murdoch studied the seasonal occurrence of psychrotrophic *Bacillus* spp. in raw milk in Scotland (*116*). *Bacillus cereus* was the most common psychrotroph. The incidence of psychrotrophs was lowest in winter and highest during the late summer and autumn, whereas the incidence of mesophiles (chiefly *B. subtilis, B. licheniformis,* and *B. pumilus*) peaked during winter. *Bacillus* spores were isolated throughout the milk chain, from farm milk machines to the pasteurized product. The authors found that *B. subtilis* and *B. licheniformis* produce factors antagonistic to growth of *B. cereus* and *B. pumilus* isolates. These factors have not been characterized, and how they affect the incidence and growth of psychrotrophic *Bacillus* spp. in the farm environment or in milk is not known.

Rangasamy et al. examined 91 samples of Australian milk and milk products for contamination by *B. cereus*, using PEMBA medium and the medium of Kim and Goepfert (KG) (*117*). Isolation rates on the two media were comparable. KG and PEMBA yielded, respectively, 6 and 3 positive samples among 24 raw milk samples; 4 and 2 among 12 pasteurized milk samples; 3 and 4 among 15 yogurt samples; 4 and 2 among 10 cheddar cheese samples; 3 and 1 among 10

milk powders; and 4 and 4 among 10 ice cream samples. The organism was not found in 10 UHT milk samples. The contamination level rarely exceeded 500 cfu/mL. The highest contamination level was found in milk powder. The biochemical characteristics of these isolates were summarized.

Growth of psychrotrophic *B. cereus* was modeled by response surface analysis of the individual and interactive effects of $a_w$, pH, temperature, glucose concentration, and starch concentration in BHI broth (*118*). Toxin production was evaluated by an immunologic method and by cytotoxicity for Vero and HEp-2 cells; growth was assessed by optical density measurements and plate counts. These data were used to derive quadratic predictive equations for growth and production of the diarrheagenic toxin. The organism used did not produce the emetic toxin. Temperature and $a_w$ had the greatest influence on both growth and toxin production, and an interaction between temperature and $a_w$ was the only significant interaction found.

Sutherland showed that spores of a toxigenic, psychrotrophic dairy isolate of *B. cereus* did not grow or produce diarrheagenic toxin in creams or dairy desserts at 6°C, whereas at 21°C growth and toxin production were easily demonstrated in creams and some desserts (*119*). In creams, growth was associated with obvious spoilage. However in the flavored desserts, spoilage was not always obvious before significant growth and toxin production occurred. Both the pH and the sugar content of these desserts influenced production of diarrheagenic toxin at 21°C. Sutherland and Limond reported that broth cultures containing high levels of sugars, particularly glucose at >50 g/L, did not support production of diarrheagenic toxin by *B. cereus* even though the organism grew well (*120*). Growth was slower at glucose concentrations of 250–300 g/L, probably because of osmotic effects. Toxin was produced in broths containing lactose at concentrations as high as 150 g/L, although titers decreased with increasing sugar. Broths containing fructose supported toxin production up to the highest level tested, 300 g/L. However, titers were lower and growth was slower at the highest concentrations. Starch at 10 or 50 g/L enhanced toxin production while not affecting growth. These observations could explain the variations in toxin levels previously noted in certain dairy desserts (*119*).

Olm and Scheibner evaluated the influence of pH, temperature, and concentrations on NaCl and nitrite of production of *B. cereus* enterotoxin in BHI broth and several food products (*121*). The plasmid profile of the organisms was determined after every experiment. Both growth and toxin production were strain-dependent under the various conditions. No relationship between enterotoxin production and alterations in the plasmid profile could be demonstrated.

da Silva et al. assessed growth of *B. cereus* naturally present in three types of reconstituted dehydrated foods produced for young children in Brazil, and of *B. cereus* NCTC 2599 spores inoculated into sterilized and unsterilized samples of these foods (*122*). In caramel and chocolate-flavored puddings, indigenous *B. cereus* had mean generation times of 54, 31, and 56 min at 25, 35, and 45°C, respectively. In bean soup with noodles the corresponding generation times were 58, 41, and 31 min. These times were comparable to those for inoculated spores. The indigenous microflora had no influence on generation time. Clearly, *B. cereus* can multiply rapidly in these products and hygienic practices should be observed during their rehydration and storage.

## Toxin Characterization

Papers on *B. cereus* in milk and milk products, presented at a joint seminar of the International Dairy Federation and the Netherlands Institute for Dairy Research in October 1992, were published in *Netherlands Milk and Dairy Journal* (volume 47 No. 2, 1993). This seminar reviewed research on the pathogenicity and toxicology of *B. cereus*. Three papers are summarized here (*123–125*; also *132,133*). Shinagawa reviewed the pathogenicity of *B. cereus* (*123*). Foods most often incriminated in the diarrheal type of food poisoning are meats, soups, puddings, vegetables, and casseroles. Starchy foods, especially boiled rice and fried rice, are the usual vehicles of the emetic type. Epidemiologically, outbreaks with diarrhea resemble *C. perfringens* food poisoning and outbreaks with vomiting resemble staphylococcal food poisoning. The author summarized the biotyping, serotyping, and phage typing of *B. cereus*. In more detail, he considered the purification, properties, and assay of the enterotoxin and emetic toxin. He then discussed the contamination of milk and milk products with *B. cereus* and production of enterotoxin and vacuolation factor in milk. Granum et al. reviewed the production of enterotoxin, hemolysin, and lecithinase (phospholipase C) by *B. cereus* under aerobic and anaerobic conditions (*124*). Because the enterotoxin is inactivated by exposure to pH 3 and is degraded by proteolytic enzymes, ingestion of preformed enterotoxin does not cause the diarrheal syndrome. The organism grows well anaerobically, however, and produces enterotoxin, lecithinase, and hemolysin in the small intestine. Thus the diarrheal syndrome is caused by ingestion of bacterial cells. The infective dose appears to be $10^5$–$10^8$ cells, although

enterotoxin production is difficult to detect in culture until the concentration of cells reaches $10^{10}$/L. The concentration of enterotoxin produced by different strains of *B. cereus* varies by more than two orders of magnitude, and only high-producing strains appear to cause food poisoning. Moreover, psychrotrophic strains that grow poorly at 37°C would not fare well in the small intestine. Of concern to the dairy industry are enterotoxin-producing strains that grow at both 6°C and 37°C. The food industry should be concerned about cell concentrations of $10^8$/L or perhaps as low as $10^6$. Notermans and Tatini investigated the ability of *B. cereus* isolated from foods to grow and produce diarrheal enterotoxin in BHI broth, UHT milk, and rice extract at 10, 15, and 30°C (*125*). Three of the 9 strains evaluated tested negative for enterotoxin with an RPLA test kit (Oxoid), and two of these "negative" strains had been involved in outbreaks of foodborne disease. All strains gave positive results with an ELISA test kit (Tecra), titers ranging from 13 to 5000. However, one outbreak-related strain had a titer of only 35. Two outbreak strains were studied further. They produced enterotoxin in all media at all temperatures that supported growth, but only after cell concentrations reached $10^{10}$/L. Spores of these strains had $D_{90°C}$ values of 6 and 55 min. Spores germinated rapidly in BHI broth at 30°C, but germination in milk was delayed.

Granum and Nissen purified the three components of the *B. cereus* "enterotoxin complex" and determined the sequence of their first 14 or 15 *N*-terminal amino acids (*126*). Proteins of 48, 40, and 34 kDa were obtained. Only one amino acid residue was common to all three; the 48- and 40-kDa proteins had two other homologous amino acids and the 40- and 34-kDa proteins had one other homology. However, the 1–14 sequence of the 34-kDa protein corresponded exactly to the 28–41 sequence of sphingomyelinase, except for a change from glutamic acid to glutamine at position 33. The 34-kDa protein was hemolytic. Only the 40-kDa protein was toxic to Vero cells. The biological activity of the 48-kDa protein is not known.

Hemolysin BL, a hemolytic dermonecrotic vascular permeability factor from *B. cereus*, consists of a binding component (B) and two lytic components ($L_1$ and $L_2$). Beecher and Wong developed a high-yield purification scheme that yielded milligram quantities of highly purified B, $L_1$, and $L_2$, permitting further characterization of the hemolysin (*127*). Combined, the three components had vascular permeability activity at low doses; higher doses caused necrosis. Turbidometric hemolysis assays measuring the activity of B, $L_1$, and $L_2$ combined in various proportions indicated that at high concentrations of one or two components, a small amount of the remaining component(s) confers full hemolytic activity. Erythrocytes were protected from hemolysis by micromolar concentrations of $Zn^{2+}$ but not by $Ca^{2+}$ or $Mg^{2+}$. Heinrichs et al. reported the molecular cloning and characterization of the *hblA* gene, which encodes the B component of hemolysin BL (*128*). The protein, expressed in *E. coli*, produced a ring-shaped zone of hemolysis when combined with purified L components of hemolysin BL. Northern blot analysis of *B. cereus* RNA revealed a 5.1-kilobase transcript that hybridized with a 500-bp probe within the coding sequence for the B component. This suggests that *hblA* is transcribed as part of a polycistronic message that may include the structural genes for the two L components. Further studies of *hblA* should establish whether hemolysin BL is indeed the enterotoxin, as has been proposed.

Rice culture filtrates of an emetic-type *B. cereus* strain contain a toxin that causes formation of cytoplasmic vacuoles in HEp-2 and HeLa cells (*129*). Electron microscopy revealed that these "vacuoles" are actually swollen mitochondria. Rice culture filtrate increased the oxygen consumption of HEp-2 cells and isolated mouse liver mitochondria. The activity was similar to that of 2,4-dinitrophenol, suggesting that the toxin uncouples mitochondrial oxidative phosphorylation. The authors believe the vacuolating and emetic toxins to be identical.

Hansen et al. reported further studies in their ongoing exploration of the active site of phospholipase C from *B. cereus* (*130*). This paper describes the crystal structure of phospholipase C that is inhibited with Tris buffer. The structure of the Tris-inhibited enzyme was determined at 1.9 Å resolution and refined to $R = 20.3\%$. The amine nitrogen in Tris is coordinated to the second of three $Zn^{2+}$ ions in the enzyme's active site, confirming the enzyme's chelating properties and the involvement of the metal ions in catalysis. In crystals of the native enzyme the Zn2 binding site is only partly occupied and thus may have a lower affinity for $Zn^{2+}$ than the other sites. The conclusion that phospholipase C is a 3-zinc metalloenzyme is consistent with biochemical and analytical evidence and with evidence from homologous enzymes.

## Identification

Several selective plating media have been developed for enumeration of *B. cereus*. However, bacterial reference materials are necessary to test laboratory performance or a medium's suitability, and these reference materials must meet a number of requirements. Workers in the Netherlands evaluated the properties of *B. cereus* spores in a reference material prepared from artificially con-

taminated spray-dried milk (*131*). The stability of the reference material was good: the contamination level did not decrease during 1.5 years of storage at –20°C or 4 weeks at 22, 30, or 37°C. Bacteria were distributed evenly enough throughout the material for its homogeneity to be acceptable. Heat treatment and addition of lysozyme to the enumeration medium did not influence the spore count. However, germination of spores at 30 and 38°C depended on how long the spray-dried milk had been stored and on the medium in which it was reconstituted. One month after spray drying, >90% of spores germinated within 30 min. Nine months after spray drying, <10% germinated within this time. The suitability of the reference material was confirmed in a collaborative study, which indicated that the material meets the general requirements for reference materials.

Bennett et al. reported the biological characterization and serological identification of the diarrheal factor from *B. cereus* (*132*). The three antigens selected for investigation had previously been identified in *B. cereus* B4ac and designated as 575, 577, and 580. The *Bacillus* strains studied produced various combinations of these antigens. Antigens were identified serologically and given by mouth to cynomolgus monkeys (*Macaca fascicularis*) in crude or partially purified form. Antigen 577 caused diarrhea; the others did not. However, the activity was lost upon chromatography on DEAE cellulose. The authors prepared a monospecific serum against antigen 577, for identifying the diarrheal toxin in culture fluids and foods.

Christiansson compared several methods for detection of *B. cereus* enterotoxin in milk (*133*). Seven dairy isolates and two reference strains were grown in milk and assayed for enterotoxin. There was no correlation between results with an RPLA kit and an ELISA: the positive-control enterotoxins in neither kit reacted with the antibodies of the other. Agreement between the ELISA and a cytotoxicity test with human embryonic lung cells was qualitatively good. Cytotoxin titers and ELISA titers also agreed well with bacterial counts.

Beecher and Wong have developed two methods that, for the first time, permit detection of a specific well-characterized *B. cereus* toxin (hemolysin BL) in complex samples and on primary culture media (*134*). In one, hemolysin BL's unusual discontinuous hemolysis pattern was produced in sheep- and calf-blood agar around wells filled with crude culture supernatant from hemolysin BL–producing strains. In the other, the pattern was produced around colonies of producing strains grown on nutrient agar medium containing calf serum and sheep or calf blood. These methods detected hemolysin BL production by 41 of 62 previously identified *B.*

*cereus* isolates and by 46 of 136 presumptive *B. cereus* isolates from soil. The nine isolates associated with diarrhea or nongastrointestinal illness all were positive for hemolysin BL.

## *SALMONELLA*

### Epidemiology

TRENDS. Kühn traced the epidemiology of salmonella infections in the two parts of Germany, emphasizing the upsurge of salmonellosis that began around 1985 (*135*). The number of reported cases increased fivefold between 1987 and 1992, quadrupled between 1988 and 1992, and doubled between 1990 and 1992. The largest number of cases (25%) and the highest incidence rate (~950 per 100,000) occur in children 1–4 years old. The proportion of isolates identified as *S. typhimurium* peaked at 60% in 1980, then fell to ~20% 1986 and has changed little since. *Salmonella agona* infections comprised ~20% of the total between 1972 and 1986, but have fallen steadily since then. *Salmonella enteritidis* accounted for <10% of infections in 1985 but for >75% in 1992. In 1991 and 1992, ~80% of the *S. enteritidis* isolates that could be phage-typed were PT 4/6. Krutsch summarized similar information for the city of Nürnberg, which showed roughly the same pattern as the country as a whole (*136*). From 1956 through 1989, 36% of *Salmonella* isolates were *S. typhimurium,* 12% were *S. infantis,* and 11% were *S. enteritidis.* Since 1990 *S. enteritidis* has been the most frequently isolated serotype. Sander discussed the reservoirs of salmonellas and described the clinical features, pathogenesis, and treatment of salmonellosis (*137*).

In Scotland, the number of clinical isolates of *Salmonella* also began to increase in 1985, but the number of veterinary isolates began to decrease slowly (*138*). In 1992, 54% of human isolates were *S. enteritidis* and 81% of these belonged to PT 4. About 22% were *S. typhimurium,* and *S. virchow* and *S. wangata* each accounted for ~5%. During the summer of 1992, *S. wangata,* a previously rare serotype, was responsible for many cases of illness that were part of a wider UK outbreak associated with contaminated poultry from northern England. Ten serotypes accounted for 90% of veterinary isolates. The most common isolate was *S. typhimurium* PT 104; this was followed by *S. mbandaka, S. enteritidis, S. dublin,* and *S. montevideo.* In England and Wales during the second quarter of 1994, salmonella isolates from human feces were distributed as follows: *S.*

*enteritidis* PT 4, 49%; *S. enteritidis* of other phage types, 12%; *S. typhimurium,* 17%; *S. virchow,* 7%; other serotypes, 13%; and *Salmonella* not further identified, 2% (*139*). There were more than 10 reports of 21 serotypes. *Salmonella* infections since 1989 were summarized, but data for years before 1992 are not directly comparable with later data because a new reporting system was implemented in 1992.

ADAPTATION TO HOST SPECIES. Blaha grouped *Salmonella* serovars into three categories (*140*). The distinctions between them may not be clear-cut in some cases. The first category includes serovars that are adapted to and cause epidemics in a specific host. Examples are *S. typhi* and *S. paratyphi* in humans, *S. gallinarum-pullorum* in chickens, *S. abortusequi* in horses, *S. abortusovis* in sheep, *S. choleraesuis* in pigs, and *S. dublin* in cattle. The second category includes sporadically occurring serovars such as *S. agona, S. infantis,* and *S. saintpaul,* which are not species-adapted. These cause occasional infections in humans but are not a primary public health concern. Serovars of the third category are also not adapted to any particular species, but they occur endemically and pose a substantial threat to humans. This group includes *S. typhimurium* and *S. enteritidis.* Salmonellas from all three epidemiologic categories can contaminate a food product; whether they cause human disease depends on their pathogenicity. Salmonellas that can infect a food animal, whether or not they cause disease in that animal, are also passed on to humans via the food chain. The cyclic relationships among contamination, infection, and disease and the role of carriers were illustrated and discussed in terms of reducing risks to human health. Selbitz also discussed the adaptation of salmonella strains to their hosts and its epidemiologic importance for zoonosis (*141*). Because many strains that infect animals can cause illness in humans, Selbitz urged application of modern molecular typing methods to identify and trace infection routes from animals to people.

ANTIBIOTIC RESISTANCE. Veterinary use of antimicrobial agents encourages the emergence of resistant strains. In England and Wales, antimicrobial resistance has been monitored in food-animal isolates of salmonellas since 1970. Wray et al. assessed recent trends by comparing data for 1981, 1989, and 1990 (*142*). Three-quarters of isolates are still sensitive to all 10 agents tested. However, roughly half of *S. typhimurium* isolates were resistant to sulphonamides and tetracyclines. Most of the resistance was seen in bovine isolates of *S. typhimurium.* Multiple resistance was most often encountered in *S. typhimurium* PT DT204C isolated from calves. The percentage of tetracycline-resistant *S. typhimurium* isolates from cattle and pigs increased during the period of the survey. Resistance to chloramphenicol, ampicillin, and trimethoprim also increased in cattle, but neomycin resistance decreased. Many pig isolates were also resistant to ampicillin and trimethoprim, whereas resistance to chloramphenicol and neomycin declined. Although *S. dublin* isolates show a high frequency of multiple resistance in other countries, 98% of *S. dublin* isolates in this survey were sensitive to all agents. Resistance has increased slightly in *S. enteritidis*, but 87% of isolates are still sensitive. Some resistance to apramycin and fluorquinolones has been detected.

Threlfall et al. compared multiple antimicrobial resistance in salmonellas from humans and food animals in England and Wales in 1981, 1988, and 1990 (*143*). In clinical isolates of *S. typhimurium*, the incidence of multiple resistance more than doubled between 1981 and 1988 and increased by a further 7% in the next two years. Resistance and multiple resistance also increased significantly between 1981 and 1990 in *S. virchow*. In poultry isolates of *S. virchow,* multiple resistance was common in a phage type associated with poultry imported from France. Resistance to kanamycin was seen in bovine, porcine, and human isolates of *S. typhimurium* but the rate decreased between 1981 and 1990. Gentamicin resistance emerged in bovine and porcine isolates of *S. typhimurium* during this period. The authors stress that the continuing use of a wide range of antimicrobials in calf husbandry has promoted emergence of multiply resistant strains of *S. typhimurium* in cattle, whereas antimicrobials are used less intensively in poultry and multiple resistance remains rare. In veterinary medicine, prophylactic use of antimicrobial agents with cross-resistance to those used in clinical medicine should be discouraged.

In Greece, Vatopoulos et al. investigated 23 consecutive ampicillin-resistant *Salmonella* isolates from patients with epidemiologically unrelated cases of food poisoning (*144*). One strain was *S. saintpaul*, one was *S. typhimurium,* and the rest were *S. enteritidis* PT 6a. Plasmid analysis further divided the *S. enteritidis* isolates into five groups. Ampicillin resistance was readily transferred to *E. coli* by the 34-MDa plasmid found in four groups and by a 100-MDa plasmid found in the fifth group. All 34-MDa plasmids and the 100-MDa plasmid had a common 6.6-MDa fragment that was the locus of a β-lactamase gene. The authors concluded that in Greece, ampicillin resistance is primarily due to the spread of a limited number of clones of *S. enteritidis* PT 6a that carry related 34-MDa plasmids.

**RISK FACTORS.** *Salmonella* usually causes gastroenteritis, but sometimes causes septicemia, urinary tract infection, infection at other extraintestinal sites, or multiple infections. Persons with AIDS are at increased risk for salmonella infections, particularly septicemia. Gruenewald et al. investigated the relationship between HIV infection and salmonellosis in 20- to 59-year-old residents of New York City (*145*). When septicemia was the sole manifestation of salmonellosis, patients listed in the AIDS registry had an infection rate of 457 per 100,000, whereas the rate for those not listed was 2.3 per 100,000. For patients listed in the AIDS registry, the sex ratios for septicemia and multiple-site infections roughly reflected the sex ratio in the registry. However, among patients not listed there was a substantial excess of men with these infections (2.7:1 for septicemia and 3:1 for multiple-site infections) and a smaller excess for gastroenteritis and urinary tract infection. The authors suggested that men be tested for HIV infection whenever salmonella septicemia or multiple-site infection is diagnosed, particularly in areas with a high incidence of AIDS.

Neal et al. reported that gastric surgery or recent treatment with $H_2$ antagonists and antibiotics predisposes individuals to salmonella infection (*146*). The presumed mechanism is reduced production of gastric acid.

**COMPLICATIONS OF SALMONELLOSIS.** Except for wound infections, the most likely cause of salmonella infection and abscess is generally considered to be hematogenous spread from a primary gastrointestinal infection, even if there is no history of gastroenteritis. Lalitha and John reported that from January 1981 through December 1992, 100 patients at one hospital in India required surgery for unusual manifestations of salmonellosis (*147*). Serotypes most frequently encountered were *S. typhi* (36 cases), *S. typhimurium* (36 cases), and *S. paratyphi* (15 cases). Eighteen patients had wound infections. Of the remaining infections, 31 involved the hepatobiliary system, 10 involved gastrointestinal and other intraabdominal sites, 15 involved bone and joint, 15 involved soft tissue, and 4 involved genital organs. In Denmark, an abscess of the submandibular gland caused by *S. typhimurium* biotype 10 was reported in a man whose occupation was transporting pigs from farms to the slaughterhouse (*148*). Although some of the pigs were salmonella-infected, the patient had no history of skin lesions or abscesses. In the UK, a woman had subcutaneous salmonella infection in both legs (*149*). The lesions ulcerated while she was hospitalized, and *S. enteritidis* PT 4 and *Staphylococcus aureus* were cultured from all swabs. Cummins and Atia reported a case of Bartholin's abscess complicating food poisoning with *S. panama* (*150*). The source of the infection was thought to have been a chicken meal eaten in a restaurant in France 24 h before the onset of gastrointestinal symptoms. In Spain, a 15-year-old patient experienced diarrhea, cramps, vomiting, and fever a few hours after eating a dessert containing chocolate (151). Fecal culture obtained on hospital admission was positive for Salmonella sp. Six days later, the patient experienced abdominal pain and further studies led to a diagnosis of acute cholecystitis. Cholecystitis is a fairly common complication of typhoid fever and other salmonella infections, but it nearly always occurs in the presence of morphologic anomalies of the biliary tract and or gallbladder stones. This patient had neither.

Erythema nodosum and arthropathy developed in the shins and one knee of a 13-year-old boy about one week after he became ill with S. enteritidis enteritis (152). John et al. reported a rare case of septic arthritis due to S. enteritis in a 29-year-old man with Hodgkin's lymphoma (153). Both knees were involved. Thomson et al. studied the secretory immune response and clinical sequelae in 84 patients with S. enteritidis gastroenteritis caused by contaminated turkey eaten at a wedding reception (154). Patients were tested and interviewed 6, 12, and 24 months after the outbreak. An unexposed control group consisted of 18 general rheumatology patients. Compared with controls, the gastroenteritis patients had a prolonged salivary IgA and anti-lipopolysaccharide (anti-LPS) response. Reactive arthritis or reactive enthesitis developed in 11 exposed patients. A ratio of salivary IgA anti-LPS to serum IgA anti-LPS >1 was associated with remission of reactive arthritis, whereas a ratio <1 was associated with chronic disease.

Huppertz and Sandhage reported a case of reactive carditis caused by S. enteritidis in an 11-year-old girl (155). The carditis accompanied reactive arthritis, which had begun 2 weeks after febrile diarrhea and involved the patient's knees, wrists, and several small finger joints. Despite treatment there was permanent damage to the right coronary aortic valve. Mitral valve endocarditis caused by S. enteritidis developed in a 65-year-old woman who had no history of recent gastroenteritis (156). Pericarditis caused by S. enteritidis PT 1 developed in a 45-year-old man, otherwise healthy, who had experienced no gastrointestinal symptoms (157).

Sharma et al. reported a case of S. arizonae peritonitis in a 69-year-old Mexican-American man who was taking rattlesnake capsules to cure his gastric cancer (158). The organism was found in samples of the patient's urine and peritoneal fluid and in rattlesnake capsules from a fresh box from the same Mexican supplier. Two months later the patient was treated for a recurrent

episode of S. arizonae peritonitis, although he denied any further consumption of the capsules.

Perras et al. described a case of S. enteritidis septicemia and spondylodiscitis in a veterinarian (159). The patient had had an attack of bronchopneumonia 4 weeks earlier. The source of the infection was thought to be contact with infected animals.

### SALMONELLA ENTERITIDIS

An interesting paper by Watier et al. reports the use of a simple deterministic compartmental model to analyze the development of the S. enteritidis epidemic in France and the mid-Atlantic region of the USA (160). The model distinguishes only two groups of individuals, susceptible and infected, because S. enteritidis is not known to confer any immunity. A time-dependent transition rate from susceptible to infected is modeled in terms of a baseline transmission rate ($\beta_0$) from the animal reservoir to humans and a seasonal multiplicative factor. Person-to-person contact is not considered because most new cases are related to the animal reservoir through contamination of foods. The French model contains an additional time component in the transmission rate to reflect the important contribution of eggs from nonindustrial free-range hens, whose laying season is April–October. For both France and the USA, predicted transmission rates were remarkably close to observed rates. In France, $\beta_0$ was stable until 1986 but was multiplied by 2.3 in 1987 and by 4.1 in 1988, and has continued to increase linearly. In the mid-Atlantic states, the linear increase began in 1984 and leveled off in 1990, presumably reflecting the effect of preventive measures. (A corollary of this is that preventive measures in France have had less impact.) Nevertheless, the similarity between France and the USA in the rate of increase of $\beta_0$ suggests that common processes, probably connected with egg production, are involved in the S. enteritidis epidemic. Halloran commented on the assumptions underlying this model, emphasizing the distinction between two types of causal statements—the causes of a given effect and the effect of a known cause (161). Despite some questions, she concluded that the model provided a thought-provoking analysis of surveillance data. She suggested greater use of such data for analyzing trends and evaluating the effectiveness of intervention measures, even though it will remain difficult to attribute changes to particular causes.

A special issue of International Journal of Food Microbiology was devoted to S. enteritidis (162). It has become clear that the main sources of S. enteritidis infections are food products of animal origin, which are inadequately prepared before consumption. It is also clear that the organism is perpetuated by environmental cycling, which involves infected humans, infected animal products, infected animal carriers, environmental contamination, and cross-contamination of all types of foods. However, most illness is caused by contaminated eggs and poultry. Papers were solicited for this special issue to provide as broad an overview as possible. Roberts and Sockett reviewed the methodologic issues involved in estimating the economic impact of salmonellosis (*163*). They summarized their own studies of the distribution of costs arising from human salmonellosis, estimating the likely share of *S. enteritidis* to be £224 to £321 million annually. Nearly three-quarters of the costs of *S. enteritidis* infection in England and Wales were direct costs associated with treatment and investigation of cases, and production losses related to absence from work. In Canada, *S. enteritidis* infections in people have increased only slightly in recent years, from 9% of all salmonella isolates to 12% (*164*). The prevalence of *S. enteritidis* in Canadian poultry flocks is still low, and the prevalence of contaminated eggs from two infected flocks was 0.06%. Phage types 8, 13, and 13a are the most prevalent in both poultry and people; Canadian flocks have not yet been infected with PT 4. The rate of antimicrobial resistance is low. In Italy, between 1982 and 1992, the percentage of *S. enteritidis* isolates increased from 2.4 to 57.1% for people and from 0.5 to 22.8% from food (*165*). Phage type 4 accounted for 76.8% of the recent isolates. Antimicrobial resistance has not yet become a problem. Argentina has also seen a significant increase in *S. enteritidis* infections since 1986 (*166*). Poland has witnessed two *S. enteritidis* epidemics (*167*). The first, in 1962–1976, primarily affected young children and was spread in the hospital environment. The second, which began about 1980 and is still going on, also primarily affects young children but involves sporadic food-poisoning outbreaks caused by contaminated ice cream, cream cakes, eggs, mayonnaise, and meat products.

Katouli et al. used the Phene Plate system to study the biochemical fingerprints of 86 clinical *S. enteritidis* strains isolated in Germany between 1980 and 1992 (*168*). Twenty-three biochemical phenotypes were identified, but only two of them accounted for 65% of the isolates. One of these was seen continually throughout the period; the other first appeared in 1988. Phage type 4, representing 39 isolates, was the most common. It was followed by PT 8, with 17 isolates. However, PT 8 was isolated continually, whereas all but one of the PT 4 strains were isolated between 1988 and 1992. Combination of biochemical fingerprinting and phage typing identified 25 phenotypes. Of the two major ones, C2:8

was persistent, whereas C4:4 was recently emerged. The Phene Plate system also provided information about relationships among the strains, which was presented as a dendrogram. Phage typing of *S. enteritidis* isolates from poultry and humans in Denmark, 1980–1990, revealed a peak in the proportion of PT 4 clinical isolates in 1983–1985; the proportion of PT 4 then fell, but increased again in 1990 (*169*). The majority of clinical isolates (62%) were PT 4, as in most other western European countries. However, 17% were PT 1—a much higher incidence than expected. Most poultry isolates (58%) were PT 1; 29% were PT 4. In the sample of isolates surveyed, PT 4 first appeared in 1987. Phage type 8 was found only in poultry imported from Germany. Plasmid profiling further differentiated the large groups obtained by phage typing. Only 3.7% of clinical strains and 1% of poultry strains were resistant to antibiotics and there was no indication that resistance is increasing or multiple resistance is developing.

**OUTBREAKS.** Three outbreaks of egg-associated *S. enteritidis* PT 13a food poisoning were reported in California in 1993 (*170*). An outbreak in Los Angeles County was detected by routine surveillance for salmonellosis, when 4 unrelated persons were identified who had gastroenteritis and *S. enteritidis*–positive stool cultures and had recently eaten egg-based dishes at the same restaurant. Two additional cases were found during the ensuing epidemiologic investigation. Investigation of the restaurant revealed that egg salad was held at 15.5°C, a temperature that permits growth of *Salmonella*; and pooled raw eggs were refrigerated at 10°C, whereas California regulations require refrigeration at 7.2°C. In San Diego County, 23 persons who ate at a local restaurant on February 16 became ill with abdominal cramps and diarrhea. Eighteen of the case-patients had eaten an entree served with hollandaise or bearnaise sauce. The hollandaise sauce was prepared with 12 raw egg yolks and was used as a base for the bearnaise sauce. A new batch was prepared at the beginning of each meal shift and held under a heat lamp for up to 3.5 h at 38–40°C. An outbreak in Santa Clara County in March affected 22 persons who had eaten at a local sandwich shop. They had all eaten sandwiches containing mayonnaise made from raw eggs. Traceback of the eggs implicated in these three outbreaks showed that they had been purchased from the same distributor.

In July 1991, a community outbreak of *S. enteritidis* PT 4 infection affected 144 persons who ate food from the same sandwich bar in Colchester, UK (*171*). The implicated vehicle was mayonnaise used in sandwiches provided for two cricket matches and an office lunch. Isolates of *S. enteritidis* PT 4, indistinguishable by plasmid profile analysis, were obtained from stool samples, food items and egg shells from the sandwich bar, and birds from the farm that supplied the eggs. Warnings against the use of raw eggs in uncooked dishes had not been heeded. An outbreak of *S. enteritidis* PT 4 food poisoning in an Edinburgh restaurant in July 1993 was also due to mayonnaise made with raw egg yolks (*172*). Investigation and correlation of cases and further epidemiologic investigation confirmed a common restaurant site at which 10 of 11 case-subjects had eaten melon and mango salad with strawberry mayonnaise and fresh mint. A chef who had tasted the salad dressing also became ill. Although white vinegar was usually used in preparing the dressing, none was used in the outbreak-associated batch. Other problems were also identified during the investigation. Once prepared, the dressing was left on the work bench for convenience. The ambient kitchen temperature was high, and shell eggs were stored for up to a week on top of the refrigerator in the kitchen.

Mintz et al. assessed the effect of the ingested dose of *S. enteritidis* on the length of the incubation period and the severity and duration of illness (*173*). Subjects were 169 people who became ill after attending a wedding reception in a hotel in Connecticut, at which they ate hollandaise sauce made from shell eggs. The cohort was divided into three groups based on their self-reported amount of sauce eaten. As the dose increased the median incubation period decreased from 37 h in the low-exposure group to 21 h in the medium-exposure group to 17.5 h in the high-exposure group (*p* = .006). The proportion reporting body aches increased with exposure from 71 to 85 to 95% (*p* = .0009) and vomiting increased from 21 to 56 to 57% (*p* = .002). Dose was also directly related to median weight loss (3.2, 4.5, and 5.0 kg, *p* = .0001), maximum daily number of stools (12.5, 15.0, and 20.0, *p* = .02), subjective rating of illness severity (*p* = .0007), and number of days of confinement to bed (3.0, 6.5, and 6.5, *p* = .04). The attack rate in this outbreak was 97%.

An outbreak of *S. enteritidis* PT 4 infection followed a buffet meal at a masonic lodge in the UK (*174*). Forty-five of the 55 who attended became ill. Epidemiologic evidence from the cohort study was limited because most guests ate most foods that were available, and the attack rate was high. However, the descriptive and analytical investigations together suggested that meringue and mayonnaise were the vehicles of infection. The egg whites used in the meringue were separated and left at room temperature for 2 h before being beaten, and the meringue was only lightly cooked. A mixture of commercial salad cream and commercial mayonnaise was then blended in the same mixer bowl—

a clear opportunity for cross-contamination. Leftover coleslaw and potato salad, both containing mayonnaise, were taken home by one of the caterers and eaten within 24 h by three family members, all of whom became ill.

In September 1993, Florida experienced its first reported outbreak of *S. enteritidis* food poisoning due to eggs (*175*). Twelve of 14 attendees at a hospital cookout became ill. Eleven of them had eaten homemade ice cream prepared with raw eggs. No other food was associated with illness. Samples of leftover ice cream and stool samples from 3 patients yielded *S. enteritidis* PT 13a. No food-handling errors were identified at the hospital. The distributor of the incriminated eggs purchased eggs from two suppliers, one of whom bought and mixed eggs from many sources.

In June 1992, an outbreak of *S. enteritidis* PT 1 in southwest Scotland was associated with a catered wedding reception (*176*). The epidemiologic investigation suggested that frozen cooked chicken—a relatively safe form of poultry—was the vehicle. This was not confirmed bacteriologically, but the caterer had defrosted the chicken and stored it at ambient temperature for 13 h before serving. Several other items had also been prepared well in advance and left unrefrigerated. (The caterer had recently completed a basic course in food handling.) Of 145 guests, catering staff, bar staff, and band members who were at the wedding and completed questionnaires, 56 were "unwell" afterward, an attack rate of 39%. The epidemic curve suggested a rather long incubation period, but some people had taken food home and eaten it over the next few days. Anecdotally, these people had significantly more severe symptoms. Although 56 people were affected and some of them had fairly severe symptoms for several days, only 3 (5%) consulted their physicians. Based on this statistic it can be calculated that for an outbreak affecting only 10 people there is a 75% probability than only one person or none will become known. This illustrates the high probability of not detecting an outbreak, particularly a small one.

A self-catered wedding reception in northern England was associated with an outbreak of gastroenteritis in August 1993 (*177*). From 84 completed questionnaires, 60 suspected cases of food poisoning met the clinical definition and infection with *S. enteritidis* PT 4 was confirmed in 41. No food samples were available for testing. There were more than 40 items on the menu, but only one dish, prepared from frozen raw chicken, had a highly significant association with illness. It was assumed that either the poultry was undercooked, permitting survival of salmonellas, or that there was cross-contamination from raw to cooked chicken via hands, surfaces, or utensils. Storage conditions were poor where the food was prepared.

Also in northern England, 8 people who ate a business buffet lunch on 30 July 1992 became severely ill with gastroenteritis (*178*). The caterer and three of his contacts were also ill. *Salmonella enteritidis* PT 4 was isolated from 8 persons who attended the buffet, 3 bakery staff, the caterer and another member of the catering staff, and the caterer's brother and 2 of his mother's friends. Three apple pies had been baked early on the morning of the lunch. The caterer had eaten a slice from one and had taken the rest of it to his mother—who didn't like apple pie but served it to her friends. *Salmonella enteritidis* PT 4 was isolated from leftovers of this pie. Thus apple pie (a very unusual vehicle for food poisoning!) was the only food that could account for illness. The pies were glazed with a raw egg and milk mixture just before baking, but it is difficult to see how salmonellas could have survived the 425°F baking temperature. Of the 16 people whose feces were salmonella-positive, only the bakery staff had not eaten pie. Although the infected staff were not involved directly in preparation of the pies, they may have been exposed to ingredients. As of this report, the mystery had not been solved. Contamination of the pies after baking is a possibility, and several hypotheses about how the organism could have survived baking or grown in the acid pie after baking could be tested.

Gonzalez-Hevia et al. used a combination of serotyping, phage-typing, and molecular genetic techniques to study stool and food isolates of *S. enteritidis* associated with a restaurant outbreak in northern Spain (*179*). All isolates carried a 36-MDa plasmid and showed similar DNA and rRNA restriction patterns. The restriction patterns were indistinguishable from those of an *S. enteritidis* PT A strain that has caused salmonellosis in that part of Spain since 1984 or earlier. Samples of shellfish soup, roast lamb, strawberry syrup, and egg-cream cakes were tested and all except the strawberry syrup contained the organism. However, one of the cakes had a much higher population of *S. enteritidis* than any other food. It is thought that the egg cream was the initial source of contamination and other foods were cross-contaminated.

EPIDEMIOLOGIC AND BIOLOGIC INVESTIGATIONS. Bichler et al. analyzed the plasmids of 138 *S. enteritidis* strains of human, animal, and poultry origin (*180*). The 15 human isolates represented 7 plasmid profiles, 4 of which were also seen in chicken isolates from the northeastern USA. Chicken isolates from Minnesota had no profiles in common with any isolates from any other group. Turkey isolates from Minnesota and most animal

isolates from the National Veterinary Services Laboratory carried only the virulence-associated 54-kilobase plasmid. Plasmid profiling is useful, but not definitive, in establishing epidemiologic relationships. For example, isolates from cat feces and an egg belt taken from one barn both carried plasmids of 54 and 5.0 kilobases, and two isolates from salmonellosis outbreaks in this area carried the same two plasmids. The authors also confirmed that not all PT 14b isolates have the same plasmid profile, indicating that plasmid profiles do not identify a phage type and that PT 14b isolates in the Northeast do not represent a single clone. In another investigation, plasmid and DNA fingerprint analysis of *S. enteritidis* isolates from 2 commercial egg-producing flocks and 5 patients with gastroenteritis showed a match between the case isolates and one of the flocks (*181*). Still another commercial flock was identified as the source of eggs implicated in 4 separate gastroenteritis outbreaks from which clinical isolates were available. In the first example, all isolates carried plasmids of 58, 4.8, 4.0, and ≤3 kilobases. In the second, all carried a single 56-kilobase plasmid.

Although an *S. enteritidis*–positive organ culture from a laying hen indicates risk of producing contaminated eggs, infected hens may lay contaminated eggs for only a short time or not at all. Therefore results of organ culture do not necessarily reflect the actual risk to public health. Henzler et al. cultured eggs from 4 commercial chicken layer houses implicated in 3 outbreaks of *S. enteritidis* infection in humans (*182*). *Salmonella enteritidis* PTs 8, 13a, and 23 were isolated from environmental and organ samples, but only PT 8 was cultured from eggs. This was the phage type of clinical isolates in all three *S. enteritidis* outbreaks. The estimated frequency of contaminated eggs was 0.03–0.90%. However, the authors cautioned against jumping to conclusions from the results of egg culturing from flocks identified through tracebacks. The finding of *S. enteritidis* in eggs from a certain house does not prove that that house produced the eggs that caused a specific outbreak. In fact, one outbreak involved in this study was probably caused by a single mishandled contaminated egg, which could have come from any one of 7 houses associated with the implicated flock.

Stanley and Baquar reviewed the phylogenetics of *S. enteritidis* as revealed by restriction fragment length polymorphism (RFLP) typing of chromosomal DNA, rRNA genes, and insertion sequences and by multilocus enzyme electrophoresis (MEE) (*183*). Human isolates of *S. enteritidis* are highly homogeneous genotypically. However, the divergence of this serovar's electrophoretic types (ETs) is inconsistent with common ancestry, and

MEE therefore defines the serovar as polyphyletic. The ETs of such a serovar occur in two or more divisions of an evolutionary tree derived by MEE. By this analysis, the distance between *S. enteritidis* and *S. dublin* is no greater than distances between types within either of these serovars. This suggests that the chromosomal genotypes of *S. enteritidis* and *S. dublin* differ primarily in the sequence of the *fliC* gene encoding the phase I flagellar antigen—a difference that resides in only three substitutions in the central part of the gene. It has been postulated that the globally predominant *S. enteritidis* ET clone En1 corresponds in its enzyme genotype and *fliC* sequence to an ancestral *Salmonella* from which various ETs of the serovars *S. dublin, S. gallinarum,* and *S. pullorum* evolved. The virulence plasmids of *S. enteritidis* and *S. dublin* are distinct and may help determine the host range and pathogenicity of these genetically closely related serovars. A conserved *Hind*III fragment bearing the Salmonella plasmid virulence gene *spvC* has been found in several contemporary virulence plasmids as well as in plasmids belonging to the same class size in ancestral isolates from the preantibiotic era.

*Salmonella enteritidis* is one of the few invasive salmonella serotypes, and *S. enteritidis* PT 4 is the most common cause of salmonellosis in the UK. Hinton and Bale examined some properties of this phage type to identify factors that could give it a competitive advantage over other salmonellas (*184*). Although it may survive mild cooking, it is no more heat-resistant than most other serotypes that cause food poisoning. In young chicks, it appears to be less invasive than *S. typhimurium,* and there is little evidence that it has a predilection for the genital tract. There is evidence that ascending infection is more important than transovarian infection as a route of egg infection. It is sometimes possible to culture *S. enteritidis* from a mixture of yolk and albumen when separate yolk and albumen samples are negative. This would be expected if the bacteria are on the vitelline membrane, or if they are in the albumen but fail to grow because of iron deficiency or the presence of antibacterial substances such as lysozyme. The authors concluded that *S. enteritidis* PT 4 may deserve the epithet "super bug" because of its impact on human health and attitudes toward food safety, but what confers its apparent super powers has so far defied identification.

Threlfall et al. investigated interrelationships between plasmid possession, ability to express LPS, and phage type in *S. enteritidis* strains of phage types associated with poultry and poultry products (*185*). Earlier work showed that PT 4 may be converted to PT 24 after acquisition of incompatibility group N (Inc N) plasmids coding for multiple antibiotic resistance. In this study,

introduction of the Inc N plasmid pDEP 44 into PT 8 also produced a smooth strain of PT 24. The authors argued that PT 8, as well as PT 4, must now be considered as a possible progenitor of PT 24 in epidemiologic investigations of *S. enteritidis* PT 24 infections where PT 8 is common. In general, acquisition of pDEP 44 by strains of *S. enteritidis* PTs 4, 7, 7a, 8, and 30 reduced their sensitivity to typing phages enough to warrant changes in phage-type designation. After acquiring pDEP 44, all strains of *S. enteritidis* PT 7 and rough strains of *S. enteritidis* PT 7a were converted to rough strains of *S. enteritidis* PT 23. Smooth strains of PT 7a were converted to smooth strains of PT 23, which had not previously been encountered. Introduction of pDEP 44 into PPT13 or 13a did not change the phage type. Its introduction into PT 30 rendered the product untypable by the typing phages.

## OTHER SALMONELLAS

*SALMONELLA TYPHIMURIUM.* In Italy, *S. typhimurium* is still the most frequently identified serovar. It is widely disseminated and is differentiated into phenotypically and genetically distinct clones. Nastasi et al. approached the epidemiologic study of *S. typhimurium* by fingerprinting the rDNA from 457 strains of human and animal origin (*186*). The animal strains were from a wide range of wild and domestic birds and mammals. *Hinc*II rDNA patterns were visually screened for bands between 6.5 and 2.0 kilobases, a similarity coefficient was calculated for each pair of ribotypes, and a dendrogram was constructed from the matrix of similarity coefficients. No clusters or ribotypes specific to humans were recognized, although some ribotypes were characteristic of ducks, pigeons, and pet birds. The rDNA patterns suggest that pigs and cattle are the main source of human infection in Italy.

In the UK, infections caused by *S. typhimurium* DT104 have quadrupled since 1990 (*187*). DT104 was the most common type of *S. typhimurium* reported in 1994. The increase is attributed to a strain resistant to ampicillin, chloramphenicol, streptomycin, sulphonamides, and tetracyclines.

Thornton et al. reported the epidemiologic investigation of an *S. typhimurium* DT193 outbreak to illustrate the problems posed by a geographically widespread outbreak involving a frequently isolated organism and a common food (*188*). During the spring of 1992, an outbreak of *S. typhimurium* infection affecting 39 people spread over 3 regional health authorities, 13 district health authorities, and 17 local authorities in northwest England and northern Wales. It was detected only because of the practice of sending specimens to the national reference laboratory for definitive typing, including phage typing and characterization of antibiotic resistance patterns. This led to identification of a cluster of distinctive isolates of *S. typhimurium* DT193 resistant to sulphonamides, trimethoprim, and furazolidone. The subsequent investigation, which involved 20 health authorities and the Public Health Laboratory Service, showed an association between illness and eating sliced cooked ham (*p* = .004). Traceback of the ham implicated a single small local producer (*p* = .00003) and revealed that a batch of ham distributed one day in early April had been undercooked due to an equipment malfunction.

An outbreak of *S. typhimurium copenhagen* food poisoning followed a traditional feast in a Californian Hmong community (*189*). A beef steer had been purchased from a private farm, where it was slaughtered. It was left unrefrigerated for 11 hours before being cut up and used in the preparation of dishes featuring raw and undercooked beef. Within days, 142 people became ill and a 2-year-old child died. Nearly everyone who had eaten beef became ill; the few who had not remained well. *Salmonella typhimurium copenhagen* was isolated not only from samples of raw and cooked beef, but also from several other foods that were served, indicating rampant cross-contamination.

Thirty-one people became ill after attending a retirement party in a close-knit community on the Ardnamurchan Peninsula, Scotland (*190*). Sixteen of the 26 stool specimens submitted were confirmed positive for *S. typhimurium* PT 110; one was confirmed as *S. typhimurium* PT 104b. The shape of the epidemic curve suggested that some secondary transmission occurred, but this could not be verified. A wide variety of foods for the event were contributed by local hotels and restaurants, but mostly by individuals who prepared the food at home. Food was delivered to the party site in the afternoon and arranged on tables, where it sat at ambient temperature for 3–5 h. This scenario provided an epidemiologist's nightmare. No particular food was implicated, but various salads, chicken dishes, and salmon mousse were suspected. Cross-contamination probably occurred during the course of the function.

Gessner and Beller investigated the extent and source of an outbreak of *S. typhimurium* gastroenteritis that followed a community picnic in Juneau, Alaska, in 1992 (*191*). A case–control study of 54 picnic attendees linked illness with eating roast pork from one of two pigs that had been flown in from a restaurant in Seattle. The restaurant had thawed the frozen pigs for several hours at room temperature, then cooked them in a gas-fired flame broiler. One pig was left unrefrigerated for 17–20 h after cooking. Perhaps the most important

observations came from a cohort study of 60 members of households that had taken home leftover food from the picnic. This study identified 43 people who had eaten roast pork, 21 of whom became ill. Only 1 of 17 cohort members who did not eat pork became ill. Thirty people reheated the meat before eating it. None of the 20 who used a conventional oven or skillet for reheating became ill, but all 10 who used a microwave oven did. Clearly, microwave heating did not prevent illness. The authors recommended that the role of heating methods (and microwave ovens specifically) be considered in investigations of salmonellosis outbreaks or other foodborne illness.

MISCELLANEOUS SEROVARS. In England and Wales, *S. virchow* is the third most common salmonella isolated from humans (*192*). Its major animal reservoir is poultry, and particularly chicken. The number of reported cases of illness due to *S. virchow* PT 26 has been increasing, and in 1993 PT 26 became the second most important phage type in England and Wales. The number of reported and confirmed cases of human infection due to this organism was 83 in 1992, 188 in 1993, and 124 in the first 5 months of 1994. In 1994, the adjacent regions of Yorkshire and Trent reported the largest number of cases. Most isolates are fully sensitive to antimicrobial drugs.

An outbreak of *S. paratyphi* B infection associated with cheese made from unpasteurized goat's milk occurred in southwest France (*193*). An unusual increase in the number of *S. paratyphi* B infections was reported in September 1993, and in October the Department of Veterinary Services confirmed that the organism had been isolated during routine testing of a batch of cheese. A national case–control study identified 95 cases associated with consumption of this cheese. Milk from one goat on one farm that supplied the manufacturer tested positive for *S. paratyphi* B; all samples from other goats, domestic animals, and people on this farm, as well as environmental samples, tested negative. Nearly 29,000 kg of cheese was destroyed. In England and Wales, 28 cases of *S. paratyphi* B infection were reported in the year that began in July 1993. Although 21 of these were imported, none came from France. The only two outbreaks of foodborne *S. paratyphi* B infection in England and Wales in recent years were associated with an India Republic Day celebration in the West Midlands in 1988 (50 cases) and—probably—consumption of cold meats in northern England (12 cases).

Human infection with *S. livingstone* increased sharply in the Tayside and Grampian regions of Scotland during 1989–1991, but not elsewhere in Scotland or the UK (*194*). No cases were reported after September 1991.

As is generally typical of salmonellosis in Scotland, most cases occurred in the summer. Except for an outbreak in a geriatric hospital, most cases were sporadic. Nearly half of the 71 Tayside cases were in patients older than 55 y; many patients were also predisposed to infection by factors other than age. Although *S. livingstone* is usually associated with infected poultry flocks, investigation revealed no clear evidence that poultry, eggs, or poultry-related products were responsible for this outbreak. Nevertheless, the self-limiting pattern is consistent with the idea that some locally produced and regionally distributed food became contaminated and then disappeared from the food supply. The outbreak was recognized and its extent determined mainly because *S. livingstone* was previously an uncommon serotype in Tayside.

An outbreak of *S. javiana* food poisoning in a Michigan elementary school was associated with consumption of watermelon at one or both of two school parties held on consecutive days (*195*). Twenty-one cases met the case definition and 12 were confirmed microbiologically. Five people who ate leftovers from the party also became ill, and 13 secondary cases were identified among household contacts of case-patients. Isolates from the watermelon and 5 representative stool cultures had identical plasmid profiles and cDNA restriction patterns. It is most likely that the watermelon was contaminated in the field. It was not washed prior to cutting, and holding it for several hours at room temperature after cutting undoubtedly facilitated bacterial proliferation.

An outbreak of *S. mikawasima* infection followed two wedding receptions at a hotel in Fife, Scotland, in October 1993 (*196*). There were 25 microbiologically confirmed cases and at least 5 probable cases. Illness was associated with eating tuna sandwiches, sausage rolls, and pizza, but none of these food items were available for study and all environmental samples were culture-negative. Around the same time, 7 sporadic cases of *S. mikawasima* gastroenteritis occurred in the Kirkcaldy district of Scotland. The organism involved contained the same 38-MDa plasmid and had the same restriction enzyme pattern as that from the wedding receptions. The most likely explanation seems to be, as in the *S. livingstone* outbreak (*194*), that some contaminated item was introduced into the food supply and subsequently disappeared. A year earlier, *S. mikawasima* had caused at least 9 cases of food poisoning in England (*197*). This outbreak was associated with eating doner kebabs from a takeaway restaurant. The causative organism contained a single plasmid of ~60 MDa. The source of contamination was not identified, but cooking practices and temperature control at the takeaway were poor.

After the implication of domestic and retail aquaria in two cases of *S. java* gastroenteritis in Scotland, retail aquaria in Edinburgh were surveyed for the presence of salmonellas (*198*). The survey documented the continuing presence of potentially pathogenic salmonellas, including *S. typhimurium* PT 104b, *S. typhimurium* PT RDNC, *S. manhattan, S. urbana, S. hvittingfoss, S. stanley, S. wandsworth, S. bovis-morbificans, S. virchow,* and *S. java* PT Dundee. All were from aquaria containing tropical freshwater fish. Only one retailer in the survey reported routinely disinfecting aquaria, and no salmonellas were isolated from samples from that source. Aquaria in the premises with the highest isolation rate showed evidence of snail infestation, and stock was imported directly from dealers in Singapore. The other retailers were supplied by wholesalers. Although many of the serotypes identified are rarely seen in Scotland, *S. typhimurium* and *S. virchow* are common causes of human salmonellosis. The authors suggested that routine communicable disease interviews include questioning about the keeping of aquatic pets.

## Occurrence, Behavior, and Control in Foods

*Salmonella* has been the pathogen most frequently identified as the cause of foodborne illness associated with airline meals. Hatakka and Asplund collected 2211 samples from flight kitchens in 29 countries and assayed them for salmonellas (*199*). The samples represented salads, cheese plates, desserts, 400 other cold dishes, and 1288 hot dishes. *Salmonella* was isolated from 6 samples. One was a cold ham dish prepared in Bangkok (*S. ohio*), one was a hot beef dish prepared in Mombasa (*S. manchester*), and 4 were hot dishes (chicken, beef, fish, and crepes) prepared during the same week in Beijing (*S. braenderup*). The *S. ohio*–contaminated dish was served on a flight from Bangkok to Helsinki on 15 February 1990 and was associated with a subsequent outbreak in Finland. During the following month 14 confirmed cases of *S. ohio* infection were recorded. The illness of 5 passengers may have been connected with the cold dish served on the flight. No reported illness was associated with the contaminated foods prepared in Mombasa or Beijing. The finding of the same serotype in different foods prepared on different days in Beijing may indicate that there was a carrier among the food handlers or that surfaces and facilities in the kitchen were contaminated.

Kasrazadeh and Genigeorgis evaluated the growth of strains of *S. dublin, S. typhimurium, S. newport,* and *S. enteritidis* in Queso Fresco, a soft Hispanic-type cheese (*200*). The lag time, generation time, and specific growth rate were modeled as a function of temperature. The minimum temperature that permitted growth was 8°C. At this temperature the pathogen started to grow after a lag time of 25 d and reached a maximum number of $8\times10^7$ cfu/mL after 67 days, with a generation time of 83.5 h. Addition of sodium benzoate to the cheese, or of potassium sorbate to cheese made from milk acidified with propionic or acetic acid, prevented or significantly delayed growth.

Pork heads are likely to become highly contaminated during slaughtering. This is of concern because head meat is used in a variety of processed products. Frederick et al. evaluated the ability of acetic acid and temperature to reduce numbers of *S. typhimurium* and other bacteria on pork cheek meat (*201*). Artificially inoculated pork cheeks were sprayed with distilled water or 2% acetic acid at 20 or 40°C. Both acid sprays significantly decreased salmonella counts. The 40°C water spray also reduced counts, but less than the acid. When cheeks were sprayed with 2% acetic acid at 25°C in a commercial pork slaughter facility carcass-wash, the incidence of *Salmonella* decreased by 67%. Aerobic plate counts and total coliforms also decreased significantly. The authors recommend use of a head-wash system in commercial slaughter facilities to reduce the incidence of pathogens and other microorganisms.

Walls et al. investigated the effects of various substances on attachment of *S. typhimurium* to artificial sausage casings (*202*). Incubation with glucose, galactose, hyaluronin, chondroitin sulfate, Tween 20, EDTA, gelatin, glycine, or bovine albumin was ineffective. Attachment decreased slightly as NaCl concentration was increased from 0 to 100 mg/mL. Mannose was not inhibitory, indicating that type 1 fimbriae were not involved. Nor were viability and motility required, as irradiation-killed cells and nonirradiated cells attached at similar rates. However, inhibition of attachment by solubilized collagen suggested involvement of a specific interaction between the microorganism and a binding site on the collagen.

Bergis et al. inoculated ground beef with a mixed inoculum of *S. agona, S. dublin,* and *S. typhimurium* and assessed growth of the organisms at 2–10°C under air and two modified atmospheres (*203*). No growth occurred at ≤6°C. At 8 and 10°C the salmonellas grew quickly for 6 d, then reached a plateau. More growth occurred with storage under air than with storage under either gas mixture (20% $CO_2$–80% $N_2$ or 25% $CO_2$–66% $O_2$–9% $N_2$).

OCCURRENCE AND BEHAVIOR IN EGGS. Of 101 outbreaks of salmonellosis involving 2272 cases in Germany in 1991, 92% were caused by *S. enteritidis* and in ~70% of cases the cause was a food prepared with raw

eggs (*204*). Routine food investigations found contamination rates of 13% in poultry meat and 1% in eggs. All other foods were at or below the mean rate of 0.88%. Data were also presented on the prevalence of *S. enteritidis* and *S. typhimurium* in various categories of food animals, and some implications of these data were discussed briefly.

Gast et al. reviewed the case of "*Salmonella enteritidis* and the table egg," which has received so much recent publicity (*205*). They also discussed salmonella contamination of fertile hatching eggs and its impact on the contamination of raw poultry meat. Topics considered were the history and epidemiology of eggborne *S. enteritidis* infections in the USA and the UK; identification and typing of *S. enteritidis*; the pathogenesis, consequences, and detection of *S. enteritidis* infections in chickens; production of contaminated eggs; growth of *S. enteritidis* in contaminated eggs; and elimination of *S. enteritidis* from eggs and egg products. The last part of the review discussed the importance to human health of the penetration of fertile hatching eggs by a variety of potentially pathogenic salmonella serotypes. The presence of salmonellas in hatching eggs has been identified as a critical control point in the control of colonization of broiler chickens by salmonellas.

Humphrey reviewed salmonella contamination of the egg shell and egg contents (*206*). Shells can be contaminated by feces or as a result of oviduct infections. Fecal contamination is probably more important for serotypes other than Enteritidis and may be responsible for much of the *S. enteritidis* PT 13a contamination. However, infection of reproductive tissue may be more important for *S. enteritidis* PT 4. Survival on egg shells is enhanced by high relative humidity and low temperature during storage. The major sites of contamination of the egg contents are the outside of the vitelline membrane and the albumen surrounding it. Albumen is an iron-restricted environment and little growth occurs in it. However, when storage-related changes alter the permeability of the vitelline membrane, salmonellas invade the yolk and grow rapidly in both yolk and albumen. In relation to this, Humphrey and Whitehead reported their studies of factors influencing the growth of *S. enteritidis* PT 4 in egg contents (*207*). The rate of change in membrane permeability is temperature-dependent. Even at 20°C, yolk invasion is uncommon in eggs stored less than 3 weeks. At 30°C, however, or when temperature fluctuates, the organism grows rapidly after a few days.

During 1991, Public Health Laboratory Service laboratories in England and Wales tested more than 90,000 eggs, in batches of 6, for salmonellas (*208*). About 42,000 were from the UK and ~52,000 were from other European Community countries. No distinction was made between contamination of the shell and contamination of the contents and there was no attempt to determine the number of organisms within an egg. Salmonellas were isolated from 65 of 7045 samples of UK eggs (0.9%) and 138 of 8630 samples of imported eggs (1.6%). Of the UK isolates, 47 were *S. enteritidis* and 33 of these were PT 4. Nineteen imported-egg samples contained *S. enteritidis*, of which 16 were PT 4. There was a striking seasonal variation in degree of contamination of imported eggs, but not of UK eggs. Although this level of contamination represents a small risk to an individual who eats a single egg, it poses a potentially major risk to the population. Rampling discussed the international challenge of *S. enteritidis* infection in terms of these data and others (*209*).

Fehlhaber and Braun studied the penetration of *S. enteritidis* PT 4 from the albumen into the yolk of experimentally contaminated hens' eggs and its inactivation by cooking (*210*). Migration from the albumen into the yolk occurred during storage, and the frequency with which this occurred depended on the size of the inoculum. With low-level contamination, penetration of the yolk was uncommon during cool storage. Depending on the egg's starting temperature, the mean yolk temperature of eggs boiled for 5 min was 33–42°C. Most organisms survived under these conditions. However, the yolk temperature continued to rise after boiling stopped, reaching a peak temperature of 59–62°C. After 4 min of frying on one side, the mean surface temperature of the yolk reached only 43°C. Any *S. enteritidis* in the egg must therefore be expected to survive this type of cooking.

When eggs were experimentally inoculated with 20 cfu/egg of *S. enteritidis* the organisms grew to a stationary phase level of $10^9$ cfu/mL within 2–3 days at 23°C, but little or no growth occurred in eggs refrigerated at 4°C (*211*). None of the common methods of cooking eggs eliminated all *S. enteritidis* organisms in heavily contaminated eggs. Higher mean and median temperatures were reached in omelets and boiled eggs than in fried or scrambled eggs under the conditions tested. An important observation was that a larger proportion of organisms survived cooking when eggs were stored at room temperature than when they were refrigerated, even with no difference in final temperature. Moreover, *Salmonella* frequently survived cooking time–temperature combinations that exceeded conditions for pasteurization. The authors concluded that temperature abuse of eggs during storage increases both the population and the heat resistance of *S. enteritidis* in contaminated eggs.

Warburton et al. evaluated the survival of salmonellas in a homemade chocolate liqueur made with raw eggs and inoculated with pooled cultures of a wide range of salmonella serotypes (*212*). The liqueur contained eggs, cream, condensed milk, Irish whiskey, and chocolate syrup. When the raw eggs were inoculated and blended with the whiskey and this mixture stood at room temperature for at least 15 min, there was more than a 4-$\log_{10}$ reduction in populations of all serotypes except *S. senftenberg*, which underwent at least a 2-$\log_{10}$ reduction. However, when all ingredients of the liqueurs were combined before inoculation the salmonellas survived more than 4 days of storage at 4 or 22°C. The authors concluded that if raw eggs must be used in such preparations, reasonable safety can be assured if the eggs are first blended with enough whiskey or other liquor to achieve a lethal concentration of alcohol and the mixture is kept at room temperature long enough to achieve maximal killing.

**OCCURRENCE AND BEHAVIOR IN POULTRY MEAT.** European investigators tested 104 skin samples from fattened ducks for salmonellas (*213*). Twelve were positive.

Several investigators reported studies of factors that influence the attachment of salmonellas to chicken skin (*214–218*). Kim et al. varied scalding temperatures to determine the least favorable skin surface for attachment (*214*). Breast skins were inoculated with *S. typhimurium* immediately after picking. The skin morphology of birds scalded at 52, 56, and 60°C was monitored by light and electron microscopy throughout processing. Skins scalded at the lower temperatures retained most of the epidermis, although 56°C produced a smoother surface than 52°C. At 60°C skins lost most of the epidermal layers and the dermis was exposed after picking. Scanning electron microscopy showed that the number of salmonellas attached to skins processed at 60°C was 1.1–1.3 $\log_{10}$ higher than the number attached to skins processed at the lower temperatures. Culture studies showed no temperature-related differences in attachment, probably due to the inability of the plating method to distinguish between different strengths of attachment. These results indicate that removal of whole epidermis during processing should be avoided to reduce attachment of salmonellas to the skin. Lillard showed that counts of *S. typhimurium* cells attached to broiler breast skin are reduced by <1 $\log_{10}$ during a chlorine rinse (*215*). Sonication was slightly more effective, reducing counts by 1–1.5 $\log_{10}$. However, when skin was sonicated in a chlorine solution there was a 2.44- to 3.93-$\log_{10}$ reduction. Bianchi et al. evaluated a chlorine-free peroxidase-catalyzed chemical dip for reducing *S. typhimurium* and *S. arizonae* on chicken breast skin (*216*). The buffered mixture of horseradish peroxidase and sodium iodide is safe and effective as a cold disinfectant for contact lenses. In this study, however, a 30-min treatment reduced skin contamination by <1 $\log_{10}$ compared to a water treatment of the same duration, and shorter treatments were no more effective than water. The effectiveness of the treatment may be limited by the presence of organic matter. If the peroxidase-catalyzed dip is to be used for carcass treatment its bactericidal activity must be enhanced. However, as used in this study the process may be suitable for equipment. Lillard evaluated the effect of a trisodium phosphate (TSP) dip on *S. typhimurium* attached to chicken skin inoculated with $10^2$ or $10^8$ cfu (*217*). In one set of experiments, whole-carcass rinses and skin homogenates were tested with and without a flowing-water rinse to remove residual TSP. In another set, results of using 0.1% peptone or buffered peptone for the carcass rinse were compared. The results suggested that low recovery of organisms after a TSP dip may be an artifact of pH, reflecting lethal or sublethal damage by the high pH of the carcass rinse rather than a true reduction of attachment. Li et al. inoculated chicken skins with *S. typhimurium* and subjected them to chemical or electrical treatment to reduce bacterial attachment (*218*). Dipping for 10 min in 1% NaCl, $Na_2CO_3$, or TSP reduced attachment by 34–76%, whereas skins immersed in these solutions and treated with 4 mA/cm² for 10 min showed a 90% reduction in attachment.

OCCURRENCE AND CONTROL OF SALMONELLA IN LIVESTOCK. Meyer et al. discussed measures for *Salmonella* control on the basis of epidemiologic classification of serovars important for humans and animals (*219*). They emphasized sanitation and immunization. Available vaccines were described and their use in cattle, pigs, and poultry was discussed.

Gay et al. surveyed the prevalence of fecal *Salmonella* shedding by cull dairy cattle at four saleyards and one slaughterhouse in Washington (*220*). Salmonellas were isolated from 6 of 1289 animals from rectal swabs. Five isolates were *S. typhimurium* and 1 was *S. dublin*. In the two swab-positive cattle for which mesenteric nodes were also sampled, 1-g node samples were negative. As detected by this methodology, the rate of fecal shedding of cull dairy cattle marketed in the state of Washington is estimated to be 4.6/1000 head (95% CI 1.9–10.6); if larger fecal samples are used the expected rate is no higher than 9.2/1000 head. Based on antibiograms and plasmid profiles, none of the 6 isolates matched any isolates of the same serotypes obtained by the state health department 2 years previously from patients with salmonellosis. Four of the 5 *S. typhimurium* isolates matched 3 of 215 *S. typhimurium* isolates obtained from

bovine submissions to the state animal disease diagnostic laboratory and by a field animal-disease investigation unit. The *S. dublin* isolate matched 17 of 165 isolates of *S. dublin* in those submissions. The authors concluded that in Washington, swab sampling of cull dairy cows at the point of first market concentration is not an efficient way to detect infected herds.

Gay et al. cultured samples from cows, calves, and the environment of a large California dairy two years after an outbreak of clinical salmonellosis in the herd had been controlled (*221*). The dairy used free-stall housing and a flush system for manure handling. Based on mean annual production per cow, the dairy consistently ranked in the top 25% of area dairies. Salmonellas were cultured from 108 of 142 environmental samples (76%) and 639 of 1339 fecal samples (48%). Ninety-seven percent of fecal samples from calves fed nonsalable milk were positive, as were 25% of fecal samples collected from cows at the time of breeding. Eighty-two percent of the isolates were *S. montevideo*. These results show that good herd performance and freedom from clinical salmonellosis do not indicate the absence of salmonellas from the premises, and that hardy infectious agents transmitted fecally can become established in the environment of modern dairies of this type.

OCCURRENCE IN THE ENVIRONMENT. Many pathways are involved in the cycling of salmonellas through wild and domestic animals, people, and the environment. Böhm reviewed the environmental dissemination of *Salmonella* and the behavior of selected *Salmonella* serotypes in the environment (*222*). The kinetics of thermal inactivation was discussed and the factors influencing survival of salmonellas on surfaces, in liquids, and in the soil were summarized.

Köhler assessed the prevalence of salmonellas in disposal sites for refuse from households around Berlin (*223*). Seventy-seven of 511 samples were positive. Most of the isolates were from soil samples contaminated by bird feces. The isolation rate peaked during autumn and winter, when large flocks of birds lived on the disposal sites. The principal serovars found were *S. typhimurium, S. anatum, S. saintpaul*, and *S. enteritidis*. *Salmonella enteritidis* lysotype 17 was isolated for the first time in the area. The source of the organism was household refuse contaminated by infected children in West Berlin. Wild birds became contaminated through the refuse. Salmonellas were also monitored for 51 months in four contaminated feedstuff-yeast and animal-meal plants. The organism was found in 12% of 2047 yeast samples and 6% of 337 animal meal samples. The proportion of positive samples was highest in winter and early spring, and the same serotypes persisted for years due to environmental recontamination.

Bisping reported that the predominant serovars in human epidemics, *S. typhimurium* and *S. enteritidis*, are rarely found in animal feed in Germany (*224*). Predominant serovars in animal feed are *S. livingstone*, *S. agona*, *S. anatum*, and *S. senftenberg*. The proportion of *S. typhimurium*–positive fish-meal samples has been decreasing since 1984; no positive samples were found in 1991. Similarly, *S. typhimurium* contamination of imported and domestic animal meals has decreased to a very low level. The epidemiologic importance of contaminated animal feeds was discussed.

A study in Sweden found that *S. dublin*, *S. senftenberg*, and *S. typhimurium* survived less than a week in composted cattle manure (*225*). In cold (not composted) cattle manure *S. dublin* was found after 183 days but not after 190; *S. senftenberg* survived for 204 days but not for 214. In composted pig manure, *S. senftenberg* and *S. typhimurium* survived less than a week; *S. derby* survived for 14 days but not for 21. Temperatures in uncomposted cattle manure ranged between 1 and 30°C, whereas the temperature exceeded 50°C in both composted manures throughout the first week or longer.

Skanavis and Yanko evaluated soil amendments based on composted sewage sludge as a risk factor for salmonellosis (*226*). Most samples contained high levels of fecal coliforms. Although *Salmonella* was detected in commercial soil amendments it was not found in bulking agents and only low levels were found in the composted sewage sludge used to produce the products. The distribution of serotypes in the soil amendments did not suggest a strong link with salmonellosis in the community, and analysis of exposure showed that the probability of infection is low in most scenarios. Although the products do not pose a major risk they cannot be considered risk-free. Of particular importance may be the predominance of *S. ohio*, a serotype frequently isolated from infected children: 45% of amendment isolates were of this serotype, although it was seldom detected in clinical specimens from the area where the products were marketed. Seven of the 10 most common serotypes identified in human infections were also present in the garden products.

DESTRUCTION OF SALMONELLAS. Following up on their observation that the presence of NaCl in an aqueous model food system is a major determinant of *Salmonella* destruction by microwave heating, Heddleson et al. established the NaCl concentration needed to produce a surface-heating effect and alter the survival of bacteria within the solution, and determined the rela-

tionship of time and temperature to bacterial destruction for other salts (*227*). Sodium chloride concentrations ≥0.75% (wt/vol) in phosphate buffer caused marked surface heating. At 1.25% NaCl the temperature difference between the surface of the solution and a point ~1 cm below the surface was 28°C. This salt concentration significantly reduced bacterial destruction when the system was heated to a mixed mean final temperature of 60°C. Thus, although mixed mean final temperatures may appear sufficient to destroy pathogens, the presence of salt creates sharp enough temperature gradients that subsurface temperatures are inadequate for pathogen destruction. Moreover, mean mixed final temperature varied inversely with salt concentration. When buffered solutions of various salts at a concentration of 1% were heated to a mixed mean final temperature of 60°C, the amount of destruction of *Salmonella* was 56% for NaCl, 71% for KCl, 73% for $CaCl_2$, and 89% for $MgCl_2$. In experiments with microwave ovens designed for home use, Heddleson et al. showed that the volume of medium heated, container shape, and covering or not covering the container had no significant effect on destruction of salmonellas heated to a mixed mean final temperature of 60°C (*228*). Postheating holding times of 2 min or more increased bacterial destruction, and more destruction was achieved with 700-W ovens than with a 450-W oven. The authors stressed that for home use, a single temperature probe cannot measure temperatures adequately.

The lactoperoxidase system (lactoperoxidase, potassium thiocyanate, and $H_2O_2$) has antibacterial activity against strains of *S. typhimurium* in trypticase soy broth (*229*). At 37°C, the system killed bacteria at inoculum levels of $10^2$–$10^5$ cfu/mL and delayed growth for 25 h with inocula of $10^6$–$10^7$. Thermal inactivation was enhanced by the lactoperoxidase system. For example, $D_{50°C}$ values were 60 min in untreated broth and 20 min in activated broth; the corresponding $D_{60°C}$ values were 0.31 and 0.20 min.

Lee et al. described two stationary-phase systems that confer acid resistance on *S. typhimurium*, in addition to the previously described log-phase acid-tolerance response (ATR) (*230*). The pH-dependent log-phase ATR involves major molecular realignment of the cell and induction of more than 40 proteins. The newly described stationary-phase ATR is a distinct pH-dependent system that confers a higher level of acid resistance than the log-phase ATR but involves synthesis of fewer proteins. The third system is not induced by a low pH but seems to be part of a general stress resistance induced by the stationary phase. It requires the alternative sigma factor RpoS, whereas regulation of the two ATR responses is independent of this factor. The three systems are thus distinct, but together they afford maximal acid resistance.

Humphrey et al. studied the effects of a temperature shift on the acid and heat tolerance of *S. enteritidis* PT 4 *(231)*. They found that transfer of cells from 20°C to 37–46°C for 5–15 min markedly increased acid tolerance and this was largely independent of protein synthesis. Induction of increased heat tolerance, in contrast, required >60 min for the maximal effect and was dependent on protein synthesis. Transfer of cells from 20°C to 47–50°C rendered cells more acid-sensitive but did not alter the kinetics of induction of heat tolerance. This shows that different mechanisms are involved in induction of the two types of tolerance.

Li et al. evaluated the ability of electrical stimulation to kill *S. typhimurium* in salt solutions of various concentrations *(232)*. Inocula of $2 \times 10^5$ cfu/mL were treated with a 10-mA/cm$^2$ current at a 1-kH frequency and 50% duty cycle for up to 60 min at 22–24°C. At neutral pH and salt concentrations of 0.015 and 0.15 M, all cells were killed after 5 min in NaCl, 30 min in NaNO$_3$, 45 min in sodium acetate or trisodium phosphate, and 60 min in Na$_2$CO$_3$. At high pH, cells were killed in 45 min by 0.0015 M Na$_3$PO$_4$ and in 60 min by 0.0015 M Na$_2$CO$_3$. A preenrichment culture method detected viable cells when direct plating did not, showing that cells were first injured by electrical stimulation and then killed.

## Epidemiology and Control in Poultry Flocks

Poppe et al. characterized 318 *S. enteritidis* isolates predominantly from Canadian poultry flocks and their environment *(233)*. Failure to ferment rhamnose was sometimes a useful marker for epidemiologically related strains. Twelve phage types were recognized, and phage-typing was the most effective method for grouping *S. enteritidis* strains. PT 13 was occasionally associated with septicemia and mortality in chickens. Fifteen plasmid profiles were distinguished; 97% of strains carried a 36-MDa plasmid, and only this plasmid hybridized with a plasmid-derived virulence sequence probe. All strains were sensitive to ciprofloxicin, but 17% were resistant to one or more of the other antimicrobial agents in the drug-testing panel. Thirty-five of 36 strains had the same outer-membrane protein profile and 36 of 41 contained smooth LPS.

Although 55 serotypes of *Salmonella* were identified by the California Veterinary Diagnostic Laboratory among 1971 turkey company submissions from 1984 through 1989, 9 serotypes accounted for >80%: Reading, Anatum, Broughton, Senftenberg, Sandiego, Heidelberg,

Kotthus, Kentucky, and Agona *(234)*. Only 1.8% were *S. typhimurium* and 1.2% were *S. enteritidis*. The most frequent serotypes identified from 24 California meat-turkey ranches were Kentucky, Anatum, Arizonae, Heidelberg, Reading, and Senftenberg. The majority of these isolates were from ill or dead birds. Except for *S. heidelberg* and *S. agona*, the major serotypes isolated from turkeys are seldom seen in clinical isolates.

Plasmid profiles were determined for 151 salmonella isolates, representing 6 serotypes, collected from broiler chicken farms, hatcheries, and poultry slaughterhouses in northern Germany in 1984 and 1990 *(235)*. The 62-MDa plasmid of *S. typhimurium* and the 36-MDa plasmid of *S. enteritidis* were serovar-specific. Plasmids of <5.0 MDa found in *S. virchow* and *S. blockley* appear useful for epidemiologic studies. The authors claim they are the first to describe the plasmids of *S. saintpaul* isolated from poultry. These plasmids have sizes of 22, 3.1, 2.4, and 1.1 MDa.

Poppe et al. investigated the virulence of strains of *S. enteritidis* PTs 4, 8, and 13, *S. typhimurium*, and *S. heidelberg* for hens, day-old chicks, and mice *(236)*. A major finding was that a strain of *S. enteritidis* PT 4 from the UK was more virulent in chicks than *S. enteritidis* PT 4 and PT 8 strains of Canadian origin. In contrast, the Canadian *S. enteritidis* PT 13 strains and *S. heidelberg* strain were just as virulent as the UK *S. enteritidis* PT 4 strain. The UK PT 4 strain was also more virulent than the Canadian for adult laying hens. For mice, however, the UK PT 4 was less virulent than the Canadian PT 4, and PT 13 and *S. heidelberg* had low virulence. Thus phage type is not the major criterion for virulence. Moreover, UK and Canadian PT 4 strains harbored a single 36-MDa plasmid that hybridized with a probe from the virulence sequence of the *S. typhimurium* 60-MDa plasmid. The authors concluded that differences in the virulence of the two strains are probably encoded chromosomally.

Suzuki discussed how bacterial strain, phage type, age of bird, inoculum size, and route of infection can influence the outcome of experimental infections in poultry *(237)*. Some virulence factors associated with *S. enteritidis* were also reviewed.

### CONTROL

As a featured speaker at the Xth International Congress of the World Veterinary Poultry Association, Barrow discussed the history of salmonella control in poultry, how emphasis has changed as a result of new problems and awareness, and prospects for the future *(238)*. Most countries are increasing their monitoring of problematic serotypes. A few countries have reduced infections in poultry and people to very low levels by rigorous monitoring and slaughter. Improvements can still be made in management, farm hygiene, and feed production. However, the speaker believes that a successful, coordinated approach will require financial support for some of the necessary control measures which, because of their potentially enormous cost, could disrupt the poultry industry. It is therefore necessary to determine the general desire for salmonella control and decide the extent to which control should be undertaken.

*Salmonella enteritidis* infections in poultry are a major problem, whereas infection rates in veal calves and pigs are relatively low. Noordhuizen and Frankena discussed some clinical epidemiologic approaches to the prevention and control of *S. enteritidis* (*239*). They diagrammed the sources and cycles of infection and emphasized the value of quantifying each component by modern epidemiologic methods. They also suggested using infection–disease simulation models as a tool. Such models could indicate where action is needed and estimate the economic consequences of various alternatives. Monitoring and surveillance systems clearly have a role, but appropriate sampling protocols are crucial for their success. Risk analysis, management, and communication are more advanced in toxicology, environmental hygiene, and human medicine than in animal production. The authors believe this discipline should now focus on problems such as *S. enteritidis* infections in egg and poultry production.

Papers in the special *S. enteritidis* issue of the *International Journal of Food Microbiology* discussed basic intervention strategies for poultry flocks based on the cumulative infection curve (*240*), and eradication programs in the Netherlands (*241*) and the USA (*242*). The programs in both countries focused on eliminating infection from breeding stock. So far attempts in the Netherlands have been more successful.

EXPERIMENTAL STUDIES. Gast discussed how experimental infection of laying hens has contributed to understanding interactions between *S. enteritidis* and its avian host (*243*). Information gained in this way is the basis for designing field studies and strategies for *S. enteritidis* control. Experimentally infected chickens were used to devise sampling and analytical strategies for optimizing detection of the organism (*244*). The occurrence of natural *S. enteritidis* infection was then monitored throughout the production period at 15 laying-hen sites and 5 hatcheries in Austria. Environmental samples were also tested.

Cason et al. monitored the location of *S. typhimurium* during incubation and hatching of eggs inoculated by a 15-min immersion in a physiological saline solution containing ~$10^5$ cfu/mL of a nalidixic acid–resistant strain (*245*). All shells and membranes were positive 30 min after inoculation, but only 38% were positive after 17–21 days of incubation. A change in the *Salmonella* status of hatching chicks occurred at pipping. No chick rinses were positive before pipping, whereas 15% were positive afterward. Two percent of yolk samples were positive before pipping and 8% after. These experiments confirm that some chicks acquire *Salmonella* from the shell and membrane of their own egg as they hatch. The authors suggested that the number of salmonella-contaminated chicks in commercial hatchers might be reduced even without total elimination of the organism from each egg if the number of bacterial cells between the shell and the shell membranes could be reduced.

Because some strains of chickens may be genetically more susceptible to *S. enteritidis* infection than others, one component of salmonella control might be the breeding of more resistant birds. Lindell et al. looked for variations in susceptibility and response to *S. enteritidis* PT 8 infection among four strains of Leghorn chickens (*246*). Hens were infected orally with $10^8$ cfu per bird and monitored for the next 10 weeks. For the first 30 days the strains did not differ in isolation rates of *S. enteritidis* from liver and spleen, ovary, and cecal tissue. However, during the first 14 days one strain had a significantly higher isolation rate from eggs and feces. The authors believe that transovarian infection can be a major route by which eggs become infected, and data from this study suggest that there are inherent differences among popular layer strains in the probability of producing culture-positive eggs after experimental infection. Members of the same research group studied the mechanism of transovarian transmission of *S. enteritidis* in laying hens (*247*). Attachment and mannose-resistant attachment of the major *S. enteritidis* phage types to chicken ovarian granulosa cells and HEp-2 cells was studied in vitro. In other studies, birds were orally infected with strains of *S. enteritidis* PTs 8 and 28, and egg contents and preovulatory follicles were cultured. The yolks of 8 laid eggs and the whites of 3 were culture-positive; both yolk and white of one egg were positive. The organism was isolated from preovulatory follicles of 16 birds: from the follicle membrane only in 10, from the yolk only in 4, and from both membrane and yolk in 2. In vitro, *S. enteritidis* exhibited three patterns of attachment to granulosa (local, diffuse, and aggregative) but only local attachment to HEp-2 cells. Most isolates demonstrated the mannose-resistant pattern of attachment, but a few showed mannose-sensitive local attachment. Attachment patterns were similar on granulosa cells from mature and developing follicles, indicating that the organism can colonize preovulatory follicles at different stages of development. Preincubation of the bacteria with a tetrapeptide that mediates the interaction of adhesive proteins with cells prevented local attachment to granulosa cells, indicating that *S. enteritidis* colonizes preovulatory follicles by interaction with ovarian granulosa cells and implicating adhesive proteins in the process.

Holt and Porter examined the effect of induced molting on the recurrence and horizontal transmission of a previous *S. enteritidis* infection in laying hens (*248*). Birds were divided into molt and control groups and infected three weeks before molting was induced in the molt group. More "molted" hens than controls were culture-positive on the 38th postinfection day, and these birds shed more *S. enteritidis* than controls. Horizontal transmission to previously uninfected hens in adjacent cages was also higher in the molted group, and the contact-exposed molted hens shed significantly more *S. enteritidis* than unmolted hens. Molting did not affect serum antibody titers to the organism, but titers in the alimentary tract were lower in molted birds. In the molt group, 3 of 8 directly infected birds and 2 of 8 contact-exposed birds laid contaminated eggs; no control bird laid any contaminated eggs. Nevertheless, the rate of egg contamination was low and the authors consider environmental contamination by shedding during an induced molt to be a more important problem.

Immunologic studies showed that a soluble factor produced by concanavalin A–stimulated T lymphocytes from chickens immune to *S. enteritidis* protected day-old Leghorn chicks against organ invasion by *S. enteritidis* (*249*). A similar factor prepared from stimulated macrophages did not. Further studies of immunoprophylaxis with the factor from stimulated T lymphocytes demonstrated a 51–60% reduction in organ invasion in treated chicks that were subsequently challenged with the organism (*250*). This was associated with a significant increase in thickness of the lamina propria of the cecal mucosa. Thus prophylactic administration of *S. enteritidis*–immune lymphokines is accompanied by a measurable microanatomical change.

Liposomes and immunostimulating complexes are adjuvants that potentiate the immune response to the outer membrane protein component of vaccines. Charles et al. evaluated several adjuvanted subunit vaccines for control of *S. enteritidis* infection in turkeys (*251*). Shedding was reduced by all vaccines in birds orally challenged with $10^7$ cfu of *S. enteritidis*, and no vaccinated birds showed clinical signs of disease. Immunostimulating

complexes and positively and negatively charged liposomes were more effective adjuvants than mineral oil.

A feeding study found that dietary propionic acid was ineffective in reducing salmonella infection in the crops and ceca of broiler chicks (*252*).

COMPETITIVE EXCLUSION. Newly hatched chicks are particularly susceptible to colonization by salmonellas. Their resistance increases as the native gut microflora becomes established, and this is the observational basis for the idea of competitive exclusion and the practice of inoculating young chicks with protective cecal bacterial cultures. An important route of salmonella infection may be anal, through contact of the vent with contaminated surfaces. Spontaneous sucking movements of the vent lips of newly hatched chicks accompanied by retroperistaltic contractions have been observed. Corrier et al. reasoned that this route of infection could also be an effective route of prophylaxis (*253*). They treated chicks with protective cultures of cecal bacteria administered by crop gavage, upper-body spray, or application to the vent lip on the day of hatch. Application of a single 0.05-mL drop of culture to the vent lip produced resistance comparable to crop gavage or spray with 0.5 mL. This showed that cecal bacteria from adult chickens rapidly become established in the ceca of chicks after content with the vent lips.

Species of *Eimeria* cause clinical and subclinical coccidial infections in poultry. Although the pathologic changes that accompany clinical coccidiosis can increase susceptibility to *S. enteritidis* infection, subclinical infections are more common in growing birds. Tellez et al. studied the effect of low doses of the chicken coccidium ($10^1$–$10^3$ sporulated oocysts of *Eimeria tenella*) and high doses of the turkey coccidium ($10^5$–$10^7$ sporulated oocysts of *Eimeria adenoeides*) on resistance to *S. enteritidis* infection in Leghorn chicks (*254*). For both coccidial species, there was a clear inverse relationship between dose and extent of organ invasion by *S. enteritidis*. Moreover, coccidial infection was accompanied by increased thickness of the cecal lamina propria and this was highly correlated with *S. enteritidis* organ invasion ($r = -.98$ for *E. tenella* and $r = -.99$ for *E. adenoeides*). The authors concluded that whether or not subclinical *Eimeria* infection enhances resistance to *S. enteritidis* in the poultry production setting, it is unlikely to contribute to the horizontal transmission of the organism. This was supported by other studies of *S. typhimurium* colonization in broiler chicks (*255*). Infection with $2.5\times10^2$–$2.5\times10^4$ *E. tenella* oocysts increased *S. typhimurium* colonization in control chicks, but had no effect in chicks previously inoculated with a protective culture of anaerobic cecal flora with or without dietary lactose.

Nisbet, Corrier, DeLoach, and their associates have published several reports on the effect of dietary lactose and continuous-flow cultures of cecal bacteria on *S. typhimurium* colonization of broiler chicks (*256–259*). In one set of experiments, chicks treated with a mixed cecal culture alone showed a 1.75-$\log_{10}$ decrease in colonization, chicks fed 5% lactose showed a 2.98-$\log_{10}$ decrease, and combined treatment produced a 4.27-$\log_{10}$ decrease (*256*). Lactose reduced cecal pH and the culture increased cecal propionic acid. There was a significant correlation between the cecal concentration of undissociated propionic acid and protection against *S. typhimurium* colonization ($r = -.78$). In other experiments, a defined bacterial culture was tested (*257*). The culture was a mixture of obligate and facultative anaerobes of the genera *Enterococcus, Lactococcus, Lactobacillus, Citrobacter, Escherichia, Bifidobacterium*, and *Propionibacterium*. Results were similar to those reported in reference *256*. The authors also concluded that continuous-flow cultures can be used to identify bacteria that are antagonistic to *S. typhimurium* in the chick cecum. A mixed bacterial culture, derived from the cecal contents of an adult broiler chicken and maintained in continuous-flow culture, protected not only broiler chicks but also turkey poults against cecal colonization by *S. typhimurium* (*258*). However, the number of salmonellas in cecal contents was 100–1000 times higher in poults than in chicks. Again, protection was enhanced by dietary lactose. These results suggest a species specificity of the protective cecal flora. Another paper reported that inoculating newly hatched broiler chicks by crop gavage with a continuous-flow culture of cecal microflora obtained from adult chickens facilitates early cecal colonization by native cecal microflora, and this increases resistance to *S. typhimurium* (*259*). The level of resistance was significantly associated with counts of cecal bacteria, total volatile fatty acids, and propionic acid concentration in 3-day-old chicks. Two percent dietary lactose enhanced protection.

Defined competitive exclusion cultures have certain practical and theoretical advantages over undefined cultures. Because *S. enteritidis* and most other *Salmonella* serotypes do not metabolize lactose, Behling and Wong reasoned that lactose-utilizing cecal isolates might have a growth advantage over *S. enteritidis* in a lactose-rich cecal environment (*260*). They therefore attempted to identify such isolates and maintain them in aerobic culture. Of 78 cecal isolates screened, 25 utilized lactose. These were apportioned among three mixtures and tested for ability to protect chicks against *S. enteritidis* infection. All mixtures afforded moderate protection (protection factor 1.6–2.2), but only in the presence of dietary

lactose. Two isolates, *Escherichia coli* O75:H10 and *E. coli* O2:H44, inhibited growth of *S. enteritidis* in vitro. Further in vivo testing found that the most effective treatment was treatment with *E. coli* O75:H10 and dietary lactose. The authors concluded that discovery of protective strains is facilitated by preliminary in vitro screening for lactose utilization and inhibition of *S. enteritidis* growth. Corrier et al. used ability to utilize lactose or its fermentation products as a primary carbon source as a criterion for developing a defined protective culture of cecal bacteria (*261*; also see ref. *257*). They showed that a defined mixed continuous-flow culture of 11 such cecal bacteria significantly inhibited *S. enteritidis* cecal and organ colonization of leghorn chicks in conjunction with dietary lactose.

To facilitate delivery of protective cultures to broiler chicks, Hollister et al. tried lyophilizing them in skim milk and encapsulating them in alginate beads (*262*). The lyophilized powder was mixed with feed; the alginate beads were force-fed or top-dressed on the feed. Both treatments were tested with 2% dietary lactose. The positive control treatment was crop gavage with a broth culture. Chicks were challenged on the third day with $10^4$ cfu of *S. typhimurium*. Alginate beads and crop gavage provided equivalent and significant protection against colonization; the powder was less protective.

Bacterial cultures containing only *Veillonella* and lactic acid bacteria can reduce cecal colonization of young chicks by *S. typhimurium*, but undefined mixed cultures are more effective. Hinton et al. reasoned that this is because lactic acid bacteria preferentially colonize the upper digestive tract, whereas *Veillonella* and other volatile fatty acid–producing bacteria colonize the lower digestive tract; the *Veillonella* in the simple culture might not receive enough lactate to produce inhibitory concentrations of volatile fatty acids in the cecum (*263*). They investigated the role of intermediates in the metabolic conversion of lactate to acetate and propionate in the inhibition of *S. typhimurium* and *S. enteritidis* by *Veillonella* sp. by growing *Veillonella* on agar medium containing various intermediates, with pH levels adjusted in increments of 0.2 units within the range of 5.7 to 6.7. This medium was overlaid with fresh medium on which cultures of *S. enteritidis* or *S. typhimurium* were spread. *Veillonella* did not inhibit growth of either salmonella on any control or pyruvate-supplemented medium. It inhibited both salmonellas on lactate medium at pH 5.9–6.3 and succinate medium at pH 5.7. On fumarate medium, it inhibited *S. typhimurium* at pH 5.9–6.7 and *S. enteritidis* at pH 6.1-6.7. Inhibition on lactate agar was correlated with production of acetate and propionate and with residual lactate in the medium;

inhibition on fumarate agar was correlated with production of propionate and lactate; and inhibition on succinate agar was correlated with production of propionate at low pH. The authors concluded that anaerobic bacteria that produce these metabolic intermediates or can convert them to volatile fatty acids may be important components of cultures that reduce salmonella colonization of chicks.

## Detection and Identification

### GENERAL AND CULTURE METHODS

Barnhart et al. studied the influence of procedures for sample collection and preparation on the detection of *Salmonella* in hen ovaries (*264*). Carcasses of spent hens from 19 flocks were obtained at the time of slaughter, packed on ice, and taken to a necropsy laboratory, where they were opened aseptically and one hard-shelled egg, one ovary, and a section of oviduct were collected from each bird. These specimens were placed on ice and taken to a microbiology laboratory, where eggshells and ovarian surfaces were carefully cleaned and aseptic procedures were used throughout preparation of the samples. The initial incubation of the samples began within 12 h of collecting the birds. An untypable *Salmonella* and *S. heidelberg* were the only serotypes found. Six of 407 ovaries (1.5%), 2 oviducts (0.5%), and no eggs were *Salmonella*-positive. Birds with positive oviducts had the same serotype in their ovaries. These results contrast sharply with previous studies by these authors and others, which found a much greater prevalence of salmonellas and as many as 17 serotypes. The authors attribute at least part of the difference to the meticulous procedure for sample collection and preparation used in this study, which ensured that only systemic organisms were reported.

Blackburn reviewed rapid and alternative methods for detecting salmonellas in foods (*265*). Rapid culture techniques, measurements of metabolism, immunoassays, bacteriophage techniques, use of gene probes, and separation and concentration techniques were summarized. Time savings of as much as 5 days over conventional culture techniques have been achieved, but all current methods depend on some form of cultural enrichment and this may be impractical in some laboratories. The time required for repair of sublethally damaged salmonellas makes development of a truly rapid method that relies on cell multiplication unlikely. The type of food to be analyzed may dictate the appropriate method(s). Most commercial kits merely replace the use of plating media and their cost ranges widely. Some methods require capital expenditure. Therefore the higher cost of these methods must be balanced against the savings in time and labor.

Orden et al. found the Wellcolex color test for the most common O serogroups of *Salmonella* and the Vi antigen to be 100% sensitive and specific with colonies taken directly from primary culture plates (*266*). A selenite broth test required modification to achieve satisfactory sensitivity.

The modified impedance method of Di Falco et al. is satisfactory for rapid detection of many but not all serotypes of *Salmonella* in fresh meat (*267*). Pless et al. described a new impedance-splitting method for rapid screening for *Salmonella* in foods (*268*). The method is highly sensitive and selective, and a negative result can be obtained within 38 h.

van der Zee reviewed conventional methods for detection and isolation of *S. enteritidis* (*269*). Use of a semisolid medium in addition to one of the routine selective media is recommended.

Whittemore used a modified most-probable-number (MPN) technique employing a single 10-fold dilution series to enumerate the total aerobes in a whole-carcass poultry rinse (*270*). Subculturing of MPN-positive tubes then permitted identification and enumeration of *Salmonella* and *Enterobacteriaceae*.

Methods normally used to enumerate cells surviving a heat treatment might not detect injured cells. Most of these methods involve aerobic incubation. Based on results with *Listeria monocytogenes*, Xavier and Ingham hypothesized that anaerobic enumeration techniques would enhance recovery of heat-stressed *S. enteritidis* (*271*). They measured *D*-values for *S. enteritidis* ATCC 4931 in skim milk and a broth medium supplemented with yeast extract, at temperatures between 52 and 58°C. Three anaerobic and an aerobic enumeration method were compared. The anaerobic methods gave significantly higher *D*-values. These observations may be relevant for safety evaluation of lightly heated foods packaged under low-oxygen conditions.

PREENRICHMENT AND ENRICHMENT MEDIA. An interlaboratory study validated two methods using refrigerated preenrichment and enrichment broth cultures for detection of *Salmonella* in dry foods (*272*). Results were in complete agreement with those from the standard AOAC/BAM procedure. Refrigeration of cultures for up to 72 h could enhance analytical flexibility and laboratory productivity.

Reissbrodt and Rabsch reported that siderophore supplementation of preenrichment cultures permitted detection of 14 of 18 food-poisoning *Salmonella* strains stored in albumen, whereas only 4 strains were detected without supplementation (*273*). Moreover, *S. enteritidis*

PT 4/6 could be isolated in great numbers from mixed cultures with *E. coli* kept in albumen when ferrioxamines E and G were added to the medium, because *E. coli* is unable to utilize iron from these substances.

Asperger and Pless compared a variety of methods for detecting *Salmonella* in cheese in the presence of competing *Enterobacteriaceae* at population levels ranging from <10² to >10⁷ cfu/g (*274*). The success of gene probe and latex agglutination methods in particular depended on an optimal enrichment step. Effective enrichment was crucial for the standard and alternative methods as well.

Chen et al. studied the ways in which non-*Salmonella* bacteria are inhibited by selenite cystine selective broth (*275*). The authors determined the minimum cell density required for complete inhibition by selenite. This confirmed the insensitivity of *Pseudomonas aeruginosa, Proteus vulgaris*, and *S. typhimurium*. Complete inhibition occurred below 10⁶ cfu/mL for *Staphylococcus aureus*, 10³ cfu/mL for *Bacillus cereus*, 10² cfu/mL for *E. coli*, and 10 cfu/mL for *Citrobacter freundii*. Other experiments indicated that in addition to the specificity and efficiency of killing by selenite, the selective action of selenite is related to the frequency with which resistant variants are generated and to the growth and death rates of these resistant variants in selenite. Since *Salmonella* samples generally contain unknown numbers and types of sensitive bacteria, it is difficult to predict the effectiveness of selenite cystine broth in inhibiting them.

A motility-enrichment step on modified semisolid Rappaport-Vassiliadis (MSRV) medium is frequently employed for detection of *Salmonella*. Joosten et al. evaluated this medium and an automated conductance method for use with naturally and experimentally contaminated environmental samples from a milk-powder factory (*276*). They also tested the diagnostic value of Rambach agar. Compared with the standard culture procedure, the MSRV method detected 82% of positive samples, whereas conductance detected only 66%. Use of Rambach agar increased the efficiency with which salmonellas were isolated from enrichment broths. A collaborative study validated use of MSRV medium for rapid detection of motile salmonellas in cocoa powder and chocolate (*277*). The method was adopted first action by AOAC International. A study in Vienna found a larger number of positive food, fecal, and tissue samples using MSRV medium than with the standard culture method (*278*). When combined with a latex agglutination test, the MSRV method gave positive results in 40 h. O'Donoghue and Winn compared the MSRV method with their in-house conventional culture method for detecting 11 *Salmonella* serotypes in a variety of high-

and low-moisture foods (*279*). Their results indicated that the MSRV method could appropriately replace conventional culture for a wide range of foods. However, MSRV medium, BGA agar, and MLCB agar all failed to detect *S. typhimurium* NCTC 74 and *S. dublin* NCTC 9676. Curtis and Clarke provided evidence suggesting that this was due to the inhibitory effect of the malachite green in MSRV medium and of the brilliant green incorporated into the other two media (*280*).

PLATING MEDIA. A collaborative study among 17 Canadian laboratories compared 6 plating media used for rapid isolation of *Salmonella* (*281*). Quantitatively, the methods yielded results within one log₁₀ of each other. Qualitatively, EF-18 agar recovered the greatest number of isolates and Hektoen enteric agar ranked second. Qualitative results with brilliant green sulpha, bismuth sulfite, xylose lysine deoxycholate, and Rambach agars were similar. Problems encountered with the various media were summarized. The group recommends use of bismuth sulfite agar and at least one other.

Gast evaluated the effectiveness of direct plating of incubated pooled egg contents against several broth-enrichment strategies for detecting *S. enteritidis* (*282*). Although direct plating on a brilliant green agar plate was relatively rapid and inexpensive, more intensive procedures were more sensitive.

A number of authors have evaluated Rambach agar as a selective diagnostic medium for *Salmonella* under various conditions (*283–286*). Garrick and Smith reported that 23 of 25 strains produced typical, easily interpreted reactions and colony forms and only a strain of *Citrobacter freundii*, of 135 other *Enterobacteriaceae* tested, could not be differentiated from *Salmonella* (*283*). Kühn et al. reported that strains of *Salmonella* subspecies IIIa, IIIb, and V produced β-D-galactosidase and blue-green colonies whose color could not be distinguished from that of *E. coli* and other lactose-fermenting *Enterobacteriaceae* (*284*). Most strains of subspecies I, II, IV, and VI produced the expected red colonies. However, the authors urged that not only red but also blue-green colonies be studied further. Abdalla et al. reported that one strain of *Pseudomonas aeruginosa* and one of *Acinetobacter baumannii* produced red colonies on Rambach agar (*285*). Among salmonellas, 44 of 54 fecal isolates and 66 of 82 stock cultures produced bright red colonies after 24 h at 37°C; this number increased to 48/54 and 74/82 after 48 h. Rambach agar gave poor results with *Salmonella typhi* and *Salmonella paratyphi* A, but the 4-methylumbelliferyl caprylate fluorescence test (MUCAP) identified these strains. Using Rambach agar, Monfort et al. were able to shorten the preenrichment period and achieve satisfactory results in isolating and enumerating salmonellas from bivalve shellfish (*286*). The new protocol was more efficient than the reference technique and was also faster and simpler.

Commercial culture plates with extended shelf-life are being developed. Allen et al. tested one of the first of these "stabilized" products, bismuth sulfite agar, and found its performance equivalent to that of bismuth sulfite agar prepared in the laboratory (*287*).

Cox described a new medium, lysine–mannitol–glycerol agar, for isolation of *Salmonella* spp. including *S. typhi* and atypical strains (*288*). The medium combines features of xylose–lysine–deoxycholate agar and mannitol–lysine–crystal violet–brilliant green agar, with glycerol added to differentiate *Salmonella* from *Citrobacter*. It detects *S. typhi* after enrichment.

CULTURE METHODS FOR FECAL SAMPLES. Muñoz et al. tested the MUCAP method for rapid screening of stool cultures for *Salmonella* (*289*). The method had 100% sensitivity (176 of 176) but yielded 8% false-positive results (65 of 800 non-*Salmonella* species). Most of these were *Pseudomonas*. Monnery et al. found Rambach agar and another new chromogenic medium to be 100% sensitive and considerably more specific than conventional media for detecting salmonellas in stool samples (*290*). Cherrington and in't Veld developed a 24-h screen for viable salmonellas in feces (*291*) and compared it with conventional isolation protocols (*292*). Their strategy in developing the method was to study the growth dynamics of salmonellas and competing microflora in various combinations of enrichment media and artificially inoculated pig feces. After enrichment, testing was done by an ELISA. Schlundt and Munch reported the isolation frequencies observed with different methods of isolating salmonellas from biomass samples at animal waste biogas plants (*293*). The broths compared were Rappaport-Vassiliadis, and tetrathionate and selenite with and without preenrichment. Rappaport-Vassiliadis broth revealed a high frequency of *S. typhimurium* and *S. dublin*, whereas tetrathionate broth identified these serotypes with a low frequency regardless of preenrichment.

## TYPING METHODS

Olsen et al. reviewed typing methods applicable in epidemiologic investigations of salmonellosis in livestock and in veterinary public health (*294*). Serotyping and phage typing are the most obvious choices for surveillance. Random amplification of polymorphic DNA, a PCR-based method, can potentially allocate strains into relevant groups faster, and this may become the method of choice in the future. Other methods discussed were biotyping, antimicrobial resistance typing, protein profile determination, and modern genotypic methods.

Threlfall and Chart described methods used for identification and typing of *S. enteritidis* (*295*). They also considered plasmid- and LPS-mediated interrelationships between several phage types associated with poultry and poultry products. Knowledge of these interrelationships has increased understanding of the biology of this serotype. Threlfall et al. also described the use of plasmid profile typing for surveillance of *S. enteritidis* PT 4 (*296*). From 1988 through 1992, plasmids were found in 94% of 1089 drug-sensitive strains from humans, chickens, and eggs in England and Wales. Eleven profile types were identified in strains from humans, 21 from chickens, and 3 from eggs. Eight of the patterns in human isolates also occurred in chicken isolates and 2 occurred in strains from eggs. Strains with a single 38-MDa plasmid predominated, comprising >90% of strains from humans and eggs and 70% from chickens. Thus, although plasmid typing is useful for rapid differentiation within PT 4, methods that discriminate within the predominant profile type are also required.

Stubbs et al. evaluated biochemical tests, antibiotic susceptibility typing, plasmid analysis, and three additional phage-typing systems for differentiating among 30 *S. enteritidis* PT 8 strains (*297*). These included 21 isolates from 18 egg-related outbreaks. Twenty-seven strains contained a 55-kilobase plasmid that is associated with this serotype. Relatively few strains of PT 8 could be further differentiated by phenotypic or molecular techniques. Even though minor phenotypic differences were seen among the egg-related strains, the strains were similar enough that they may represent a single clone.

## IMMUNOLOGIC METHODS

EIAs. Krusall and Skovgaard compared a new automated enzyme immunoassay (EIA), the EiaFoss Salmonella Method, with the Rappaport-Vassiliadis procedure for detection of salmonellas in 170 samples of raw and processed food, food components, and animal feeds (*298*). The EIA identified 27 samples as *Salmonella*-positive, whereas the reference method identified 24. The authors attributed this difference to the superior enrichment procedure used in the EIA. The EIA gave 3 false-positive results, all of them for samples of animal-feed concentrate, one of which was also judged positive by the reference method.

Blais et al. employed O antisera as detecting antibodies for *Salmonella* antigens in an EIA using polymyxin-coated cloth (*299*). Strong cross-reactivity with *Staphylococcus aureus* was eliminated by pregrowing the organisms in the presence of sodium deoxycholate. The O antisera are available commercially and are more economical than monoclonal antibodies (MAbs) or purified polyclonal antibodies.

**ELISAs.** A modified MAb-based colorimetric ELISA (*Salmonella* Bio-EnzaBead) for *Salmonella* detection was validated in a collaborative study (*300*). Samples of artificially contaminated nonfat dry milk, milk chocolate, dried egg, ground black pepper, and soy flour and naturally contaminated raw ground turkey were tested. AOAC International subsequently adopted the method first action.

Flint et al. compared the TECRA immunocapture ELISA with the standard FDA method for detection of *S. typhimurium* in dairy, meat, fish, and vegetable products (*301*). There was close agreement between the methods, but the ELISA results were obtained in 24 h, compared with 96 h for the FDA test.

Kerr et al. compared three sandwich ELISAs (TECRA, LOCATE, and an in-house method) and a 3-step culture method for detecting salmonellas in 1000 veterinary specimens (*302*). Each of the ELISAs indicated that salmonellas were present in 16 samples when none were isolated by initial culture. Eight of these were salmonella-positive when reinvestigated by culture.

House et al. evaluated an indirect ELISA for detecting *S. dublin* carriers at a large drylot dairy (*303*). The ELISA was performed on milk and serum samples; fecal samples were collected for culture. Seropositive cattle were retested by culture and ELISA monthly for 5 months or until antibody titer decreased. No animal remained culture-positive and seronegative. Thirteen animals that maintained a strong serologic response were moved to a research facility for 6 months of intensive monitoring. All of them maintained a high ELISA titer and continued to shed *S. dublin* in milk, feces, or both. They were thus considered *S. dublin* carriers. The organism was isolated from mammary tissue of two calves at necropsy, indicating that bacteremia may be a mode of mammary infection. The authors concluded that serologic screening of milk samples can identify *S. dublin* carriers in the setting of a large dairy.

The Dutch *S. enteritidis* monitoring and eradication program for poultry flocks required periodic examination of all breeding flocks (*304*). During the first years of the program this was done by extensive bacteriologic examination of fecal samples. Subsequent study demonstrated the effectiveness of a flagellar MAb-based ELISA as a flock screening test. Further confirmatory bacteriologic investigation is then conducted in ELISA-positive flocks. Workers in Switzerland developed an ELISA kit for detecting *S. enteritidis* in chicken blood or egg yolk and tracing flock infection (*305*). There were cross-reactions with antibodies against *S. typhimurium*

in 2.5–10% of samples, but none with *S. heidelberg*. Barrow discussed the serologic diagnosis of *S. enteritidis* infection in poultry by ELISA and other tests (*306*). These methods have a considerable advantage over culture methods for routine and preliminary screening of flocks. However, minor problems remain, such as specificity and criteria for determining the cut-off point above which samples are considered positive (*307*).

**LATEX PARTICLE AGGLUTINATION.** Thorns et al. reviewed the development and evaluation of a latex particle agglutination test to identify cultured *S. enteritidis* (*308*). This was the first rapid serotype-specific test for *S. enteritidis* and demonstrates the advantages of fimbrial antigens as diagnostic antigens.

A commercial latex agglutination test kit rapidly detected salmonellas in fecal samples (*309*). It was considerably more sensitive than direct culture and comparable to enriched culture.

**FCIA.** Tsai et al. described a rapid fluorescence concentration immunoassay (FCIA) for detecting salmonellas in chicken-skin rinse water (*310*). When coupled with an 18-h direct enrichment in selenite cystine broth, results were obtained within 24 h.

## MOLECULAR METHODS

Helmuth and Schroeter discussed molecular typing methods for *S. enteritidis* (*311*). The predominance of certain phage types, particularly PT 4, makes further epidemiologic subgrouping necessary. Molecular methods for various species include plasmid profiling, profiling of outer membrane proteins and LPS, ribotyping and fingerprinting of total genomic DNA, and multilocus enzyme electrophoretic typing. When applied to *S. enteritidis* PT 4, these methods reveal a remarkably homogeneous clonal structure in contemporary isolates. They also indicate that today's clone emerged from a preepidemic heterogeneous population.

Doran et al. developed a *Salmonella*-specific DNA probe directed at *agfA*, the structural gene for thin, aggregative fimbriae (*312*). It hybridized strongly with 603 of 604 *Salmonella* isolates but only weakly or not at all with 266 isolates of other *Enterobacteriaceae*. It was a valuable diagnostic tool for isolates arrayed on hydrophobic grid membrane filters.

Most reported *S. enteritidis* outbreaks in the USA are egg-related, and most of these are caused by PT 8. User et al. reported the ribotyping of *S. enteritidis* PT 8 strains from the USA (*313*). The best discrimination was achieved with *Acc*I, which revealed 6 distinct ribotypes. These could be further divided into two additional patterns by using *Sma*I. Epidemiologically related strains had identical patterns. Nevertheless, the results confirm previous conclusions that these strains are closely related.

**PCR.** Aabo et al. developed a set of genus-specific polymerase chain reaction (PCR) primers for *Salmonella* (*314*). Because the targeted 2.3-kilobase fragment shows interserovar diversity, primer selection was based on sequences from 20 different serovars. The specific product of 429 base pairs was formed from 144 of 146 *Salmonella* strains tested, representing 116 of 118 serovars. The two false-negative strains belonged to two serovars of the rare subspecies IIIa (monophasic *S. arizonae*). None of 86 non-*Salmonella Enterobacteriaceae* representing 41 species and 21 genera produced the PCR product. Another *Salmonella*-specific PCR was developed and standardized by Nguyen et al. (*315*). A 2.0-kilobase fragment of chromosomal DNA was amplified by the primer pair.

Because plasmid-associated virulence factors are important determinants of *Salmonella* virulence in BALB/c mice, Rexach et al. developed a PCR for detection of virulence-associated plasmid genes (*316*). This type of search has a place in epidemiologic investigations because it crosses serotype boundaries to detect virulence markers.

Collaborators in Alabama and Kentucky have developed gene probes and PCRs for detecting *Salmonella* in oysters (*317,318*). Another genus-specific PCR was able to detect between 1 and 10 salmonellas per gram of beef, without interference from the endogenous microflora (*319*). Mahon and Lax developed a quantitative PCR method to detect salmonellas carrying the virulence plasmid–associated *spvR* gene (*320*). They used the PCR to estimate the number of salmonella cells in avian feces.

A method combining a PCR and reverse dot-blot hybridization could detect ~$10^4$ salmonellas in fish-meat homogenates in 10 h (*321*). The oligonucleotide probes were designed from the base sequence of the 16S rRNA gene. A PCR combined with fluorescent detection on microwell plates showed promise as a large-scale screening method for salmonellas in foods (*322*). The level of detection was as low as 1–10 cfu.

## Virulence, Pathogenesis, and Molecular Studies

Most strains of *S. typhimurium* harbor a 90-kilobase plasmid (pSTV) that carries a virulence region common to several *Salmonella* serovars. However, pSTV is incompatible with the virulence plasmid of *S. enteritidis* and with the indigenous plasmids of four other serotypes (Choleraesuis, Copenhagen, Dublin, and Sendai). This

indicates their derivation from a common ancestral origin. Because more detailed information on incompatibility could facilitate further characterization of pSTV, Ou mated strains containing the 90-kilobase plasmid or a cointegrate (pWR33) constructed in-house with strains containing the plasmid of 23 of the 27 known incompatibility groups (*323*). Examination of transconjugants selected for the incoming plasmids showed that the 90-kilobase plasmid can coexist for at least 54 generations with plasmids of all of these groups.

*Salmonella typhimurium* ST39 is nonmotile and defective in the *mviS* (mouse virulence Salmonella) locus. Schmitt et al. defined the *mviS* locus and demonstrated its identity to *flgM*, whose product negatively regulates flagellar genes by inhibiting activity of the flagellin-specific sigma factor, FliA (*324*). The attenuated phenotype of an *flgM* mutant was reversed by a mutation in *fliA*. DNA homology studies to determine the prevalence of the *flgM–fliA* system showed that sequences at least moderately homologous to *S. typhimurium*'s *flgM* are confined to *Salmonella* and *Shigella*, whereas sequences related to *fliA* are common throughout the *Enterobacteriaceae*.

McCormick et al. reported studies in an in vitro model of *S. typhimurium* attachment to the intestinal epithelium and transcellular signaling to subepithelial neutrophils (*325*). Although attachment of *S. typhimurium* to apical membranes of T84 cells did not detectably alter the integrity of the monolayer, the organisms physiologically stimulated transepithelial migration of neutrophils placed on the basolateral surface of the membrane. Attachment of a nonpathogenic strain of *E. coli* failed to do this, and the *Salmonella*-induced migration was not attributable to the classical mechanism by which bacteria induce directed migration of neutrophils. The authors further showed that migration required reciprocal protein synthesis by the *Salmonella* and the neutrophils. This interaction stimulated epithelial synthesis of IL-8, but the cytokine was not directly responsible for the neutrophil transmigration.

Although *S. typhimurium* and *Shigella flexneri* differ in most virulence attributes, Groisman and Ochman have identified a chromosomal assemblage of genes responsible for *Salmonella*'s invasiveness that is very similar in arrangement and sequence to the gene cluster on the *Shigella* virulence plasmid that controls the presentation of surface antigens (*326*). In *Salmonella* the complex contains more than 12 genes, and mutations in them destroy the organism's ability to enter epithelial cells. However, a noninvasive mutant of *Salmonella* could be rescued by the *Shigella* homolog. Analysis of *Salmonella* clone RF319, which hybridizes with DNA from plasmid-linked *S. flexneri* sequences, indicated that although the gene cluster promotes equivalent functions in *Shigella* and *Salmonella*, each genus acquired it independently, and it displays motifs used by diverse antigen export systems including those required for flagellar assembly and protein secretion.

Amin et al. developed an in vitro culture system for quantitative studies of invasion by *S. typhimurium (327)*. It maintains the structural and functional integrity of rabbit ileal tissue for up to 4 h. Using this system, the authors studied a number of virulent and avirulent strains and demonstrated a clear correlation between initial mucosal invasion and virulence, defined by clinical origin or ability to induce fluid loss in monkeys or rabbit ileal loops.

Galdiero et al. studied the biological activities of porins isolated from *S. typhimurium (328)*. Their preparation was virtually free of LPS. A dose of 100 ng was lethal to mice sensitized with D-galactosamine, regardless of whether they were LPS responders. Mice were protected by intravenous preadministration of anti-TNFα serum. The porin preparation was also pyrogenic and elicited a local Shwartzman reaction. All activities were also seen when porins were mixed with polymyxin-B in a molar ratio of 1:300. Thus the porins cause immunobiologic effects similar to those of LPS, but the common responses are probably stimulated through mechanisms that are initially different and involve different receptor areas on the affected cells.

*Salmonella typhimurium* is enclosed in membrane-bound vacuoles throughout its intracellular stage, and the ability to replicate within these vacuoles is essential for virulence. Garcia-del Portill et al. demonstrated that replication of *S. typhimurium* within epithelial cells is associated with filamentous structures containing lysosomal-membrane glycoproteins *(329)*. Viable intracellular bacteria were required for formation of these structures, which were not seen in uninfected cells, in HeLa cells infected with *Yersinia enterocolitica*, or in epithelial cells infected with certain *S. typhimurium* mutants defective in ability to replicate intracellularly. Kinetic analysis showed a strict correlation between appearance of the lysosomal-membrane glycoprotein-rich filaments and initiation of intracellular bacterial replication. An intact microtubule network and acidic pH within the vacuole were required for filament formation. The filaments differ structurally and functionally from previously described tubular lysosomes.

Bäumler et al. characterized 30 Tn*10* mutants of *S. typhimurium* having a diminished capacity for survival in murine macrophages and decreased virulence in mice *(330)*. They also mapped the locations of Tn*10* insertions

for 23 of these strains and cloned and sequenced short fragments of DNA flanking the transposon. Seven mutants carried insertions in known genes (*htrA, prc, purD, fliD, nagA,* and *smpB*). Possible roles of these genes in *Salmonella* virulence were discussed. Two insertions were in genes with significant homologies with other species. Fourteen insertions were in genes with no significant homologies to entries in the DNA and protein databases. Thus 16 insertions defined loci (termed *ims* for impaired macrophage survival) that have not yet been described in *S. typhimurium* but are necessary for full virulence in mice. Most of these loci are randomly distributed throughout the chromosome, but one cluster was found between 75 and 78 min.

By screening for hemolysis on blood agar, Libby et al. identified a *Salmonella* gene that encodes a cytolysin required for survival within macrophages *(331)*. The gene *slyA* was found in every strain of *Salmonella* examined and also in *Shigella* and enteroinvasive *E. coli*, but not in other *Enterobacteriaceae*. SlyA (salmonlysin) purified from a derivative of the original clone had hemolytic and cytolytic activity. Its $LD_{50}$ and infection kinetics in mice indicate that SlyA facilitates bacterial survival within macrophages and is required for virulence. The authors located *slyA* between 28.5 and 30 min, a region where few genes have been identified either in *Salmonella* or in the related region of *E. coli*. The gene appears to be duplicated in some serotypes of *Salmonella*.

Buisán et al. constructed a restriction map of the *S. enteritidis* 61-kilobase virulence plasmid and compared it with the map of the *S. typhimurium* 90-kilobase virulence plasmid *(332)*. They found a region homologous to the previously described *S. typhimurium rck* virulence locus but found no homologies with the *traT* locus of *S. typhimurium* or the *vagD/vagC* locus of *S. dublin*.

Spink et al. used a reporter gene linked to the *spvR* promoter from the *S. dublin* virulence plasmid to study regulation of *spvR (333)*. This gene activates downstream *spv* genes and itself. The level of *spvR* expression was affected by the number of copies of the *spv* region within the cell. After remaining constant throughout exponential growth it increased rapidly with the onset of the stationary phase under both aerobic and anaerobic conditions. Activity was also influenced by the availability of iron, being greatest under low-iron conditions in the stationary phase. The gene product SpvA regulated *spvR* expression through a negative feedback mechanism.

Rahman et al. purified and characterized an enterotoxin from culture supernatants of strains of *S. typhimurium* isolated from pigs with diarrhea *(334)*. With

PAGE, it yielded a single protein band of 100 kDa. It had enterotoxic, delayed permeability, and CHO cell elongation activities and was highly immunogenic in rabbits. Antigenically, it was unrelated to cholera toxin, Shiga toxin, and the heat-labile enterotoxin of *E. coli.* It did not bind to the $G_{M1}$ ganglioside. Chary et al. located an enterotoxin gene (*stn*) in *S. typhimurium* and characterized its product (*335*). The gene encoded polypeptides of 25 and 12 kDa. Enterotoxic activity resided in the 25-kDa product, as determined by elongation of CHO cells, fluid accumulation in rabbit intestinal loops, and altered vascular permeability in rabbit skin. The 25-kDa protein also caused an elevation in intracellular cAMP in CHO cells. Activity of this enterotoxin was blocked by $G_{M1}$ ganglioside and neutralized by antibodies against cholera toxin. A subsequent paper reported further molecular characterization of *stn* and its product (*336*). The most unusual feature of *stn* was its unusual TTG initiation codon, in place of the typical ATG. The gene was located opposite the *hydHG* operon that regulates labile hydrogenase activity in *Salmonella* and *E. coli.* The predicted sequence of the 29-kDa enterotoxin was dissimilar to all published sequences, including cholera toxin and other adenylate cyclase–activating proteins. However, a small region showed intriguing similarity to sequences from several other protein toxins that ADP-ribosylate host-cell proteins. The homologous region may represent a conserved motif within the active site that is involved in stimulating adenylate cyclase activity.

Harne et al. purified and partially characterized an enterotoxin in the culture supernatant of *S. newport* (*337*). Its properties were similar to those of the *S. typhimurium* enterotoxin described in reference *334*.

Petter's laboratory has reported that field isolates of *S. enteritidis* may differ in their ability to produce O antigen or to link it to the LPS core in vitro. This linkage is important in pathogenesis because it is associated with an organism's ability to avoid complement inactivation and phagocytosis in vivo. Petter has now reported studies of how heterogeneity in the LPS structure of *S. enteritidis* strains is related to the process of egg contamination (*338*). Isolates from eggs of hens infected with an *S. enteritidis* PT 13a strain that does not usually contaminate eggs exhibited two subtly different phenotypes. One was typically smooth; the other, transiently rough. The phenotypic difference was due to a quantitative difference in O antigen and possibly a qualitative difference in the lipid A core region. Stationary phase cultures of the isolates also differed in opacity at 600 nm. When laying hens were injected with cultures of the two phenotypes, the smooth type was able to contaminate eggs with a significantly greater frequency.

## *SHIGELLA*

### Outbreaks and Epidemiology

After an increase in domestic cases of *Shigella sonnei* infection was noted in Sweden in May 1994, investigators informed collaborators in the European surveillance scheme Salm-Net (*339*). Similar increases had been seen in parts of England during late May and early June. These included sporadic cases, family outbreaks, and larger outbreaks associated with restaurants and hotels. Scotland and Norway also reported several outbreaks. The Swedish investigators concluded that illness was associated with imported iceberg lettuce. Following this clue, inquiries in the UK also implicated imported iceberg lettuce. Investigations are continuing. These outbreaks highlight the importance of thoroughly washing lettuce and other vegetables that are eaten raw.

An outbreak of shigellosis affected more than 600 passengers and crew aboard a Royal Caribbean Cruise Line ship in early September 1994 (*340*). *Shigella flexneri* was identified in stool samples of ill persons. The source of the outbreak had not been identified at the time of the report.

Although there is ample evidence that certain enteric bacterial infections trigger reactive arthritis in genetically susceptible individuals, details of the mechanism remain in question. Certain *S. flexneri* strains responsible for dysentery epidemics associated with reactive arthritis carry a 2-MDa plasmid that encodes a pentapeptide homologous with the polymorphic region of the HLA-B27 1α domain. Stieglitz and Lipsky, who characterized this plasmid (pHS-2), screened additional pathogenic *Shigella* strains for the 2-MDa plasmid and the mimetic epitope (*341*). They consistently found pHS-2 in all *S. flexneri* strains associated with reactive arthritis, including 27 isolates from a rhesus monkey colony in which diarrhea and reactive arthritis-like symptoms had developed. Although not all strains of *S. flexneri* carry this plasmid, the authors previously found it in about 65% of the enteropathogenic isolates screened. They postulate that the putative pHS-2 protein containing the HLA-B27 mimetic peptide acts as the arthritogenic trigger because of its similarity to the host protein HLA-B27. If normal tolerance to the B27-derived peptide is overcome during enteric infection, subsequent disease activity could be propagated by production of the self peptide within the synovium.

There have been many reports of *Shigella*'s increasing resistance to multiple antibiotics. To obtain information on the situation in Germany, investigators tested the resistance of 255 *Shigella* strains to 28 antibiotics *(342)*. All strains were isolated in Germany in 1989–1990 and were associated with shigellosis. The incidence of multiple resistance was 93.5% in imported cases and 62.7% in domestic cases.

## Isolation and Identification

Preston and Borczyk conducted RFLP analysis of 49 Canadian clinical isolates of *S. sonnei* *(343)*. Twenty strains associated with sporadic infections showed 15 distinct RFLP patterns by *Hae*III digestion and 12 by *Rsa*I digestion. RFLP patterns of individual isolates in 6 epidemiologically related groups were identical within each group and distinct from those of unrelated isolates. These patterns could be used to determine the genetic relationships between isolates associated with separate outbreaks of shigellosis.

June et al. evaluated the effectiveness of the FDA's BAM culture method for recovery of *S. sonnei* from potato salad, chicken salad, cooked shrimp, lettuce, raw ground beef, and raw oysters inoculated with unstressed, chill-stressed, or freeze-stressed cells *(344)*. Because the infective dose of *Shigella* can be as few as 10 cells, culture methods must be able to detect this low number. The method was relatively ineffective for recovery of the organism from ground beef and oysters. Moreover, its effectiveness decreased as the degree of stress injury to the inoculum increased. The smallest number of freeze-stressed cells that could be recovered from ground beef and oysters ranged from $7.6 \times 10^2$ to $1.1 \times 10^4$, depending on the food and the *Shigella* strain.

Oberhelman et al. evaluated an alkaline phosphatase–labeled *ipaH* probe for diagnosing *Shigella* infections *(345)*. The *ipaH* gene is a repetitive sequence thought to be present on both the virulence-related plasmid and the chromosome of all strains of *Shigella* and enteroinvasive *E. coli* (EIEC). The probe detected 85% of cases of shigellosis with a specificity of 95%. It also detected three cases of EIEC infection that were not detected by stool culture techniques.

## Pathogenicity and Molecular Studies

*Shigella sonnei* is antigenically homogeneous and is sometimes considered a pathogenic clone of *E. coli*. Karaolis et al. examined the genetic variation among 46 epidemically unassociated strains of *S. sonnei* isolated from patients in different countries between 1950 and 1991 *(346)*. RFLP analysis and DNA sequencing of genes *mglB* and *gnd* in 10 strains identified only one nucleotide substitution in *mglB* in one strain.

Ribotyping of 31 strains from 5 countries detected 8 polymorphic sites, with a worldwide change in the frequency of alleles at one site during the period studied. Thus, although overall variation was low, there was clear evidence for temporal variation in frequency of a particular restriction site. This could be due to either periodic selection or genetic drift. The authors are conducting further studies to test their idea that bacterial clones are adapted to specific niches and can evolve within those niches.

Kozlov et al. purified the Shiga toxin of *S. dysenteriae* and characterized it crystallographically *(347)*. The asymmetric unit of the crystals appears to contain two $AB_5$ units. Haddad et al. determined the minimum sequence of the A subunit required for enzymatic activity *(348)*. The minimum domain that showed enzymatic activity comprised residues 75–268 of the 293-residue A polypeptide.

A chromosomal virulence gene, *vacJ*, required for intercellular spread of *S. flexneri* has been identified by Tn*10* insertion mutagenesis *(349)*. This locus is not involved in either invasion of epithelial cells or intracellular movement. The *vacJ* gene is distributed among both shigella and EIEC strains. It encodes a 28.0-kDa protein, with a signal peptide at the *N*-terminus that contains the motif characteristic of lipoproteins. The product VacJ is exposed on the bacterial surface, but its mechanism of action is not understood. However, several steps in the epithelial cell invasion process (entry, intracellular spread, and passage into adjacent cells) involve bacterial interaction with the host cell's cytoskeleton. Goldberg and Sansonetti reviewed current knowledge about the interaction of *S. flexneri* with the cellular cytoskeleton at various stages of invasion *(350)*.

## ESCHERICHIA COLI

Echeverria et al. described the four groups of *E. coli*—enterotoxigenic (ETEC), enteroinvasive (EIEC), enteropathogenic (EPEC), and enterohemorrhagic (EHEC)—and discussed their transmission via food and water *(351)*. Cattle and pigs are frequently infected with types of *E. coli* that cause illness in humans, and animals and foods of animal origin have been incriminated in ETEC, EIEC, EPEC, and EHEC infections. The toxins, pathogenic mechanisms, and genetic determinants of virulence of these organisms were reviewed.

Investigators in Tasmania compared the bacterial flora of 38 SIDS infants with the fecal flora of 134 healthy control infants (*352*). Toxigenic *E. coli* were isolated from 39% of SIDS infants, but from only 1.5% of controls (*p* <.001). Toxin titers were low. Most toxigenic strains produced either verotoxin (VT) or heat-labile toxin. Some atypical strains of *E. coli*—lactose nonfermenters that were cytotoxic to Vero cells—were also identified from SIDS infants. These were considered questionable VT producers. Rotavirus and adenovirus were found in both SIDS infants and controls, with a nonsignificantly larger percentage of SIDS infants being infected. Other potentially toxigenic bacteria of the genera *Clostridium, Klebsiella, Staphylococcus, Streptococcus,* and *Proteus* were isolated from SIDS infants and controls but were not investigated further.

An interesting survey of enterotoxigenic, verotoxigenic, and necrotoxigenic *E. coli* in diarrhetic and healthy cattle in Spain suggested that some of these pathogens may be part of the normal intestinal microflora (*353*). ETEC was isolated from 1% of calves with diarrhea and 4% of healthy controls. Verotoxigenic *E. coli* (VTEC) was isolated from 9% of diarrhetic calves and 19% of healthy cattle. Necrotoxigenic *E. coli* that produced cytotoxic necrotizing factor 2 was isolated from 20% of ill calves and 34% of controls. Although the VTEC belonged to 18 serogroups, only 4—O26, O103, O113, and O157—accounted for 25 of the 45 strains. Of the 26 serogroups representing the 108 cytotoxic necrotizing factor 2–producing strains, O1, O3, O15, O55, O88, and O123 accounted for 69 strains.

Diarrhea-causing strains of *E. coli* are biochemically indistinguishable from strains characteristic of the normal fecal flora. However, molecular probes for virulence factors permit identification of pathogenic strains. Schmidt et al. screened 98 EPEC strains and 82 EHEC strains by PCR for the presence of *E. coli* attaching and effacing genes (*eae*) (*354*). They also tested for hybridization with the enteropathogenic adherence factor (EAF) probe and for reaction in the fluorescence actin staining assay for the attaching–effacing lesion. All 26 class I EPEC showing localized adherence to HEp-2 cells carried EAF and *eae* genes, whereas only 1 of 72 EPEC strains with no or diffuse adherence was EAF-positive and only 6 were *eae*-positive. The *eae*-PCR also detected 91.5% of EHEC. Interestingly, 15 of 21 EHEC strains that lost their Shiga-like toxin genes (*slt*) during subculture were *eae*-positive. All ETEC, EIEC, and normal flora controls were *eae*-negative. Four strains were positive in the fluorescence actin staining test but *eae*-negative. The authors concluded that *E. coli* strains bearing *eae* are heterogeneous with respect to other virulence determinants and that loss of virulence plasmids and phage-encoded

*slt* genes in the host or during storage may contribute to this.

Tarkka et al. reported that ribotyping can contribute to epidemiologic investigations of *E. coli*, particularly when serotyping methods are not available (*355*). They analyzed RFLP patterns of rRNA genes of 133 *E. coli* strains. Twenty ribotypes were recognized. The distribution of strains among the ribotypes correlated generally with their O:K:H serotypes. The origin of the strains and the presence of virulence-associated factors did not correlate with ribotype.

Members of the Shiga toxin family, which include the Shiga-like toxins (SLT), and of the cholera toxin family, which includes the heat-labile enterotoxins, have important structural similarities—viz., they are composed of a single enzymatic "A" subunit noncovalently associated with 5 receptor-binding "B" subunits. Many structural and sequencing studies of these toxins have been published. Now Haddad and Jackson have identified the residues in the Shiga toxin A subunit that are required for assembly of the holotoxin (*356*). They located a stretch of 9 nonpolar amino acids near the C terminus. Tryptophan and aspartic acid residues at the N-terminal boundary and two arginine residues at the C-terminal boundary stabilize subunit association. The authors postulate that residues 279–287 of the 293-residue A subunit penetrate the pore of the B pentamer while the tryptophan, aspartic acid, and arginine residues named interact with charged or aromatic amino acids outside the pore on the planar surfaces of the B pentamer.

The reason for combining food-preservative treatments is to ensure the microbiological safety of the product without adversely affecting its sensory properties. Sublethal damage by one treatment can render cells more susceptible to killing by another. Fielding et al. determined the effects of electron beam irradiation in conjunction with low pH on survival of *E. coli* in model systems with potential relevance to food systems (*357*). They irradiated an exponential-phase culture with 0–2.4 kGy in enriched nutrient broth at pH values between 7.0 and 4.0. Irradiation caused a dose-related decrease in the number of viable cells. The $D_{90}$ was 0.34 kGy. A 2.4-kGy dose reduced the count by ~5 $\log_{10}$. The lag time of survivors also appeared to be dose-related. By itself, lowering the pH had little effect on the organism's survival although growth rate was progressively decreased. Moreover, between 7.0 and 4.3 pH had little effect on the organism's radiation sensitivity. However, when pH was lowered to 4.13 or 4.0 before radiation treatment, death rate was increased over the whole range of radiation doses.

## Escherichia coli O157:H7 and Other VT-Producing and Enterohemorrhagic E. coli (VTEC and EHEC)

Like all foodborne illness, illness from E. coli O157:H7 is greatly underreported. Based on a CDC literature survey of the history of E. coli O157:H7 infections in the 1980s and early 1990s, Marks and Roberts analyzed the medical and other costs of such infections (358). In the USA, the incidence is estimated to be 3–8 per 100,000 per year, or 7600–20,500 annual cases. From estimates of the USDA's Economic Research Service, E. coli O157:H7 ranks as the fourth most costly agent of foodborne disease, behind Toxoplasma gondii, Salmonella, and Campylobacter. Voelker reflected on the problem of foodborne illness and heightened awareness of it (359). The outbreak of E. coli O157:H7 in four western states certainly triggered this. In recent years the incidence of reported listeriosis has decreased sharply and reports of salmonellas have leveled off or decreased slightly, but reports of E. coli O157:H7 infection have risen sharply. At the same time, cases of hemolytic uremic syndrome (HUS) appear to be increasing and E. coli O157:H7 is its main cause.

OUTBREAKS AND EPIDEMIOLOGY. A great deal has been written about medical and food-safety aspects of the hamburger-related outbreak of E. coli O157:H7 infection in the western USA in 1992–1993. Dorn has now reviewed the literature on this outbreak and related matters that are most pertinent to the veterinary profession (360). He summarized epidemiologic and clinical aspects of E. coli O157:H7 infection, including hemorrhagic colitis and HUS. Serotype O157:H7 is classified as an EHEC because it causes hemorrhagic colitis, produces Shiga-like toxin (verotoxin), does not produce heat-stable or heat-labile enterotoxin, and is not invasive. However, the flagellar antigen (H) of serogroup O157 is critical to the organism's pathogenic potential, and some O157 strains other than O157:H7 have been classified as ETEC because they produce enterotoxin instead of verotoxin. Dorn's review primarily discusses the reservoirs of E. coli O157:H7 and its transmission and control. O'Brien et al. reported the characteristics of the E. coli O157:H7 responsible for the hamburger-related outbreak of hemorrhagic colitis and HUS in Washington (361). Isolates from stool samples of 5 patients were identical in their VT profile, adherence and plasmid traits, virulence for mice, capsule characteristics, and production of enterohemolysin. Their properties were similar to those of E. coli O157:H7 strain EDL933,

which caused a similar hamburger-associated food-poisoning episode in 1982.

Most epidemiologic investigations of E. coli O157:H7 infections have involved restaurant-associated outbreaks. However, in California in 1993, three cases of culture-confirmed E. coli O157:H7 infection were traced to consumption of hamburger purchased at a local grocery store and cooked at home (362). All five family members of one patient also ate hamburgers cooked medium rare and they too reported diarrhea. Two family members of the second patient had nonbloody diarrhea after eating the hamburger. The third patient, an 84-year-old woman, died. A member of her family also had diarrhea. Escherichia coli O157:H7 was isolated from leftover hamburger in the home of the first patient and from 4 of 15 samples of ground beef from the grocery store at which the implicated meat had been purchased. Isolates from the three patients, the leftover meat, and the two samples from the grocery store were of PT 31. An isolate from a grocery store not associated with the cases was PT 4.

Although the incidence of E. coli O157 infection reported in the UK is low compared with that in North America, it is increasing. Sharp et al. reviewed E. coli infections in Scotland, where the majority of laboratories have tested for this organism since 1990 (363). Some parallel data for England and Wales and North America were presented. In Scotland, there were fewer reports in 1992 than in 1991, with no known change in laboratory practice or intervention measures. Isolation rates are considerably higher in the east than in the west of Scotland and again, the reason is not clear. Food or water sources of infection are infrequently identified, but isolations from veterinary sources are providing leads. In 1992, 115 E. coli O157 infections were reported, compared with 202 in 1991 and 165 in 1990 (364). There was a sharp summertime peak; a secondary peak occurred toward the end of the year. The very young and the elderly were most commonly affected.

In the UK, the Laboratory of Enteric Pathogens found evidence of VTEC infection in 232, 428, and 615 individuals in 1989, 1990, and 1991, respectively (365). VT-producing E. coli O157 was the most frequently encountered serogroup, accounting for 1092 of the 1275 isolates. Overall the incidence of VTEC infection increased from 0.41 to 1.07 per 100,000 during this period. In Scotland it increased from 1.37/100,000 in 1989 to 3.97/100,000 in 1991. Twenty-three phage types were identified in the 1092 E. coli O157 isolates (366). The most common were PT 2 (36.1%), PT 49 (29.6%), PT 1 (10.3%), and PT 4 (8.9%). The major phage types did not change from 1989 to 1991, but the proportion belonging to type 2 and 49 increased. PT 49 was associated with 7 of 17 outbreaks. In contrast, this phage type had not been reported in North America as of 1990.

A study in a remote Inuit community in northern Canada evaluated risk factors for childhood HUS and gastroenteritis during an epidemic of *E. coli* O157:H7 infection (*367*). Patients with HUS and patients with uncomplicated gastroenteritis differed only on measures of clinical severity. Eating undercooked ground meat and traditional Inuit foods were not risk factors for infection. However, there was evidence of extensive intrafamilial transmission of infection after it was introduced into the community.

In the UK, a cluster of *E. coli* O157 infections was linked to consumption of untreated milk from a particular farm (*368*). Milk samples were obtained from 10 cows whose rectal swabs were positive for *E. coli* O157; one of these was also positive. Isolates from the patients, the cows, the milk, and the farmyard all harbored a single 92-kilobase plasmid, produced VT2 but not VT1, and were PT 1. This is the first report of *E. coli* O157 infection in the UK in which a suspected food source was confirmed microbiologically. It is not known whether the organism was excreted in the milk or entered the milk from a contaminated udder. In any case, milk is a not infrequent source of infection. Investigators at a pediatric hospital in Argentina reported that consumption of unpasteurized milk is much more common among HUS patients than among control children (*369*).

A locally produced, live, full-fat yogurt made from pasteurized milk caused 16 cases of *E. coli* O157:H7 PT 49 infection in England in autumn 1991 (*370*). Eleven of the case patients were between 1 and 10 years old. Five children had HUS. The organism was not detected in samples of raw or pasteurized milk or in yogurt produced after the suspect batch. However, several opportunities for cross-contamination were identified during examination of the production process. The authors report that this is the first time an outbreak of *E. coli* O157:H7 infection has been linked to the consumption of yogurt.

An epidemiologic investigation suggested that a cluster of infections with VT-producing *E. coli* O157 in spring 1992 were associated with consumption of beef from a particular slaughterhouse in South Yorkshire (*371*). During investigation of the slaughterhouse, bovine rectal swabs, surface swabs from beef carcasses, and samples of meat were examined for the organism. *Escherichia coli* O157 was isolated from 84 (4%) of 2103 rectal swabs; 78 of these produced VT, and the most common phage types were 2 and 8, the types seen in the clinical isolates. The positive cattle came from diverse

farms. The organism was isolated from 7 of 23 carcasses of rectal swab–positive cattle and from 2 of 25 carcasses of rectal swab–negative cattle. This indicates that cattle are a reservoir of VT-producing *E. coli* O157 in England, that carcasses can be contaminated during slaughter and processing, and that the resulting contaminated meat can cause infection in humans. Direct transmission between cattle and humans can also occur. In Canada, a 13-month-old boy became ill after playing in the family's barn and *E. coli* O157:H7 PT 23 was isolated from his stool (*372*). He had repeatedly touched the veal calves, then put his fingers into his mouth. Fecal samples from 3 of the 7 calves were positive for VTEC, and 2 isolates were obtained. One was *E. coli* O157:H7 PT 23, the same type isolated from the child. Two older children in the family subsequently became ill with diarrhea and stomach cramps and VTEC O157:H7 PT 23 was isolated from the stool of one of them. It seems clear that the youngest child was directly infected by contact with the calf or its feces; the older children could have become infected in the same way, or by secondary transmission from their brother. In Scotland, a possible link between cattle and *E. coli* O157 infection in a young child was more complex (*373*). One plausible scenario involved the family dogs romping through the neighboring cow pasture and midden, picking up the organism from a dung pat, and carrying it into the house. Isolates from the child and from a dung pat yielded *E. coli* O157:H7 PT 49, which produced VT2 but not VT1.

In September 1992, several cases of *E. coli* O157:H7 infection occurred in rural Maine (*374*). The first patient was a 39-year-old ovolactovegetarian who lived on a small farm. Her diet was based on vegetables from her own garden, which she fertilized with manure from her cow and calf. Fecal specimens from these animals and milk from the cow tested negative for the pathogen; but both animals had greatly elevated antibody titers to *E. coli* O157 LPS, and *E. coli* O157:H7 was isolated from a swab of manured garden soil. Three contacts of this patient subsequently became ill, with disease onset 6, 9, and 14 days after onset of the first case—a pattern suggesting person-to-person transmission. HUS developed in a 2-year-old patient, who died. It thus appears that the pathogen can survive in manured soil and that illness can be transmitted through handling or eating manured vegetables.

A non-O157 VTEC was responsible for the first outbreak of VTEC infection recognized in Italy (*375*). In spring 1992, 9 children were hospitalized with HUS in Lombardia, where only 14 cases of this syndrome had been recognized in the previous 4 years. Cases were scattered among 5 provinces. The cause was never found, although there was a possible link with eating ground beef prepared at home. Seven children were examined for VTEC; 6 had serum antibodies to the LPS of *E. coli* O111. VTEC were isolated from two patients. One isolate, belonging to serotype O111:NM, produced VT1 and VT2 and was resistant to gentamicin and tetracycline. The other belonged to serogroup O145 and produced only VT1.

Paros et al. compared *E. coli* O157:H7 strains isolated from the bovine reservoir (22 isolates) and sporadic human infections (50 isolates) (*376*). They identified 23 RFLP profiles, 4 verotoxin genotypes, and 8 plasmid profiles. Together the typing methods distinguished 43 strains, of which 3 were isolated from both humans and animals. RFLP analysis using a bacteriophage λ probe proved very useful in identifying strains of *E. coli* O157:H7.

Beutin et al. studied virulence factors and phenotypical traits of clinical VTEC isolates in Germany (*377*). The 54 VTEC strains belonged to 13 serotypes; 46 were *E. coli* serotypes O157:H7, O157:H⁻, O145:H⁻, O111:[H8], and O26:[H11]. Fifty strains hybridized with the VT1 probe, the VT2 probe, or both. The 4 strains that did not hybridize with either probe differed from the positive strains in serotype, did not produce α-hemolysin, and did not contain EHEC plasmids or *eae*-specific DNA sequences. The clinical presentation of the associated cases ranged from uncomplicated diarrhea to hemorrhagic colitis to HUS. The more severe illnesses tended to be associated with the O157 serogroup. Non-O157 VTEC were isolated exclusively from infants. The reasons for this were not clear.

In addition to VT1 and VT2, two verotoxins considered variants of VT2 have been described. One, VTe, is produced by strains causing edema disease in pigs. The other, VT2v, has been associated with illness in humans. Caprioli et al. characterized VTEC isolates from healthy cattle and pigs and diarrheic calves in northern Italy (*378*). The prevalence of VTEC was 8% in pigs, 18% in veal calves, and 11% in dairy cows. Most pig isolates produced only VTe, whereas cattle isolates produced VT1, VT2, or both. No *E. coli* O157:H7 was isolated, but 6 isolates belonged to serogroups associated with human infections, including VTe-producing serogroup O101 isolated from pigs. Pigs appear to be the natural reservoir of O101 strains and pork products may be contaminated with them. Some strains isolated from healthy dairy cows and healthy and diarrheic calves also belonged to non-O157 serogroups associated with human illness.

Rüssman et al. reported that VT2 variants constitute a major component of toxins produced by *E. coli*

O157 isolates from HUS patients in Germany (*379*). Of 38 strains examined, 17 contained sequences for the VT2v product and 4 of them contained only the variant gene sequence (*slt-IIv*). Three strains carried both *slt-I* and *slt-IIv* and 10 carried both *slt-II* and *slt-IIv*. The remaining 21 strains were of genotype *slt-I, slt-II,* or *slt-I/slt-II*. Implications of this considerable toxin diversity within O157 strains were discussed, including the possible usefulness of SLT genotyping. SLT genotype may also have an important influence on the host response.

Takeda et al. tested serum from 44 children with HUS and from 73 healthy Japanese adults for antibodies to VT1 and VT2 (*380*). They found that a single episode of infection is not enough for acquisition of a high enough titer of VT antibodies for serodiagnosis to be useful in diagnosing VTEC infections. The relatively high prevalence of VT antibodies in adults in Japan suggests that many adults have experienced multiple subclinical infections.

**OCCURRENCE AND GROWTH IN FOODS AND FOOD ANIMALS.** Beutin et al. surveyed 720 healthy cattle, sheep, goats, pigs, chickens, dogs, and cats from the Berlin area for VTEC (*381*). VTEC were most frequently isolated from sheep (66%), followed by goats (56%), cattle (21%), and cats (14%). VTEC were infrequently isolated from pigs (8%) and dogs (5%) and were not found in chickens. Forty-one O:H serotypes and 23 untypable O-groups were isolated. More than half of the strains were serotypes O5:H⁻, O91:H⁻, O146:H21, O128:H2, and OX3:H8. Serotypes O5:H⁻, O91:H⁻, O146:H21, O87:H16, and O82:H3 occurred in more than one species. Nearly 60% of the serotypes isolated have been implicated as human pathogens. All except 9 strains from cats hybridized with at least one verotoxin probe (VT1 or VT2). Verotoxin and enterohemolysin production were closely associated in strains of serotypes O5:H⁻, O146:H21, O128:H2, O77:H4, O119:H25, and O123:[H10]. Only 30 of 240 enterohemolysin-positive strains hybridized with a DNA probe specific for this gene, indicating heterogeneity of regulatory or structural *hly* genes in these organisms.

In the USA, it is common practice to slaughter unwanted dairy calves before they are 10 days old. Martin et al. tested rectal swabs from 304 such calves in Washington, California, and Wisconsin for *E. coli* O157:H7 (*382*). Although a 3M test kit gave 21 positive signals, the organism was not isolated from any sample. Three positive signals were caused by sorbitol-positive H7-negative strains of serogroup O157. The cause of the other 18 signals was not determined. The authors concluded that an ELISA or other noncultural method has the best chance of detecting O157:H7 in heavily contaminated samples such as fecal swabs and that failure to isolate the organism merely reinforces the observation that it is not very common and is difficult to isolate when present.

Studies by Rasmussen et al. suggest that well-fed animals are less likely than fasted animals to become reservoirs for pathogenic *E. coli* (*383*). Strains of *E. coli*, including several of O157:H7, grew well in rumen fluid collected from fasted cattle. However, growth was inhibited by rumen fluid from well-fed animals and was also poor in media that simulated the ruminal environment of such animals. The authors concluded that surveys sampling the feces of well-fed cattle may not accurately represent the incidence of *E. coli* O157:H7 infection in cattle at the time of slaughter. Future studies should consider the impact of dietary stress on populations of this foodborne pathogen.

Willshaw et al. examined 310 samples of minced beef, beef sausages, and beefburgers from the London retail market for VTEC (*384*). No sample contained VT-producing *E. coli* O157 when tested by a combination of VT probes and colony immunoblotting with a commercial anti-O157 serum. Five samples were positive for O157 strains that did not produce VT and differed in other respects from O157 VTEC.

Cutter and Siragusa used a pilot-scale model carcass washer to evaluate the efficacy of organic acids against *E. coli* O157:H7 attached to beef carcass tissue (*385*). Tissues were inoculated with *Pseudomonas fluorescens* or 3 strains of *E. coli* O157:H7, sprayed with water or 1, 3, or 5% acetic, lactic, or citric acid at 24°C, and incubated at 4°C for 24 h. Populations of *E. coli* were then enumerated. Spray with 5% acid was most effective in reducing bacterial populations, but reductions were modest. There were no significant differences between acids. Surface data on pH suggested that the population reductions were due to pH rather than to the acid itself. The three strains of *E. coli* O157:H7 differed in their resistance to acid but all were more resistant than *P. fluorescens*. For all strains, population reductions were consistently greater on fat tissue than on lean. Using a different experimental approach, Brackett et al. also evaluated the effect of acetic, citric, and lactic acid sprays on survival of *E. coli* O157:H7 on raw beef (*386*). Warm (20°C) and hot (55°C) sprays of 0, 0.5, 1.0, and 1.5% acid were tested. Population reductions differed by 0.3 $\log_{10}$ cfu/g immediately after treatment and by <0.5 $\log_{10}$ cfu/g after a 13-day incubation. None of the treatments was considered to be of value for practical use.

Abdul-Raouf et al. studied the fate of *E. coli* O157:H7 inoculated into mixtures of ground roasted beef and commercial mayonnaise, and as influenced by time, temperature, pH, and acidulant (*387*). The organism was able to grow in mixtures with a mayonnaise content commonly found in salads. No growth occurred in 24 h at 5°C, but at 21°C populations increased by 1 $\log_{10}$ in mixtures containing 10% mayonnaise and by 2 $\log_{10}$ with 24% mayonnaise. At 30°C populations increased by ~3–4 $\log_{10}$ with up to 32% mayonnaise. No growth occurred in 40% mayonnaise. In acidified beef slurries heated at 30 or 54°C, the order of effectiveness of acidulants in inhibiting growth was acetic acid > lactic acid ≥ citric acid. Citric and lactic acids did not inhibit population increase in 10–24 h of incubation at pH 4.7–5.4 and 30°C, whereas populations decreased in slurries acidified to pH 4.7–5.0 with acetic acid. Choice of recovery medium is important for detection of heat- or acid-stressed cells.

Samadpour et al. analyzed 294 samples of fresh seafood, beef, lamb, pork, and poultry from grocery stores in Seattle for VTEC (*388*). Five samples yielded colonies with sequence homology to *slt-I*, 34 were homologous to *slt-II*, and 12 were positive with both *slt-I* and *slt-II* probes. None were of the O157 serogroup, but comparison of their electrophoretic typing profiles with those of isolates from diseased people and animals revealed close relationships. The extent to which non-O157 serogroups contribute to human illness is not clear. However, 5 serogroups isolated (O6, O91, O113, O153, and O163) have been associated with diarrhea, hemorrhagic colitis, or HUS.

Abdul-Raouf et al. showed that *E. coli* O157:H7 is able to grow on raw salad vegetables, without changing their appearance, under processing and storage conditions similar to those common in commercial practice (*389*). The organism was inoculated onto shredded lettuce, sliced cucumber, and shredded carrot, which were then stored for up to 14 days. Populations declined on vegetables stored at 5°C and increased on vegetables stored at 12 or 21°C. Growth was most rapid on lettuce and cucumber at 21°C. A reduction in pH was correlated with initial increases in populations of *E. coli* O157:H7 and the natural microflora. Later declines in *E. coli* O157:H7 populations were attributed to the toxic effect of accumulated acids. Packaging under an atmosphere of 97% $N_2$ and 3% $O_2$ had no effect on growth of the pathogen.

An outbreak of *E. coli* O157:H7 food poisoning attributed to contaminated apple cider stimulated investigations of the pathogen's survival in this presumably unfriendly medium. Zhao et al. tested the fate of a clinical strain from a cider-related outbreak in 6 lots of unpasteurized apple cider with and without preservatives (*390*). The pH of the ciders ranged from 3.6 to 4.0. Cider was inoculated with $10^2$ or $10^5$ cfu/mL and incubated at 8 or 25°C. At the higher inoculum level and 8°C, the pathogen population increased by ~1 $\log_{10}$ and then remained stable for 12 days. Depending on the lot of cider, the organism survived for 10–31 days at 8°C and for 2–3 days at 25°C. Potassium sorbate at 0.1% had little effect, but 0.1% sodium benzoate permitted survival for only 2–10 days at 8°C. A still greater rate of inactivation was seen when the preservatives were combined. Miller and Kaspar evaluated the survival of *E. coli* O157:H7 strains isolated from hamburger and an HUS patient in apple cider and trypticase soy broth adjusted to low and high pH (*391*). The O157:H7 strains were still detectable in cider after 14–21 days at 4°C, whereas an *E. coli* control strain was undetectable after 5–7 days. The population of the HUS-related strain decreased by ~3 $\log_{10}$ during the first 14 days, whereas the population of the hamburger-related strain remained stable. When the cider contained 0.1% sodium benzoate, populations of the hamburger-related O157:H7 strain decreased by 57% after 21 days at 4°C but ~$10^4$ cfu/mL still remained. In trypticase soy broth adjusted to pH 2, 3, 4, 11, or 12 the hamburger strain was again more resistant than the HUS strain, but both withstood extremes of pH better than the control strain. Survival in broth was greater at 4°C than at 25°C. These results show that *E. coli* O157:H7 is exceptionally acid tolerant.

Murano and Pierson studied the heat-shock response of *E. coli* O157:H7 (*392*). Cells grown at 30°C for 6 h were "heat shocked" at 42°C for 5 min and then held at 55°C for up to 1 hour. Control cells were not treated at 42°C. Heat shock significantly increased the $D_{55°C}$ value while also increasing the number of injured cells. Heat-shocked cells released material absorbing at 260 nm significantly faster than control cells. Heat shocking resulted in lower catalase and superoxide dismutase activities and greater survival after exposure to $H_2O_2$. Recovery of both heat-shocked and control cells was enhanced by anaerobic conditions. The authors concluded that heat shock does not protect the cells from injury but does improve their ability to recover during storage.

Buchanan et al. developed response surface models for the growth of *E. coli* O157:H7 as a function of temperature (10–42°C), initial pH (4.5–8.5), NaCl concentration (5–50 g/L), and aerobic or anaerobic conditions (*393*). Growth kinetics were independent of inoculum size and the maximum population density was insensitive to cultural variables. Because no published data on growth of *E. coli* O157:H7 in foods were available for validation of the models, the organism was cultured in UHT milk, canned tuna, canned chicken broth, and canned dog food and results were compared with the models' predictions. Published data on generation times in beef slices and raw mutton were also used. The predictions more closely matched experimental data at NaCl levels realistic for the product rather than at levels required to achieve the experimentally observed $a_w$'s. The most effective response surface models were based on a logarithmic transformation combined with a quadratic model, rather than square root or cubic models.

**ISOLATION AND IDENTIFICATION.** Zadik et al. assessed the usefulness of adding potassium tellurite to selective media to reduce the number of other sorbitol nonfermenter colonies when *E. coli* O157 is being isolated (*394*). MICs for VT+ *E. coli* O157 were higher than for *Aeromonas* spp. and other strains of *E. coli*. MacConkey medium containing tellurite, sorbitol, and cefixime permitted growth of VT+ *E. coli* and *Shigella sonnei*, but inhibited or prevented growth of two-thirds of other *E. coli* strains and all or most strains of other sorbitol-nonfermenting species tested. When 391 rectal swabs from cattle were screened, tellurite medium yielded 26 isolates of VT+ *E. coli*, whereas MacConkey agar with sorbitol, rhamnose, and cefixime yielded only 9.

Chart et al. used SDS–PAGE to examine 47 strains of *E. coli* O157 for expression of long-chain LPS, and related the LPS profile to production of verotoxin (*395*). The strains belonged to 10 H types or did not express flagella. Nine strains carried genes encoding VT. Three LPS profiles were recognized. One comprised strains belonging to H types 7 and 8, and all VT+ strains belonged to these flagellar types. The authors pointed out that serologic tests would identify all patients infected with *E. coli* O157, regardless of H type or LPS profile.

Samadpour et al. assessed the usefulness of bacteriophage λ RFLP analysis in epidemiologic investigations of *E. coli* O157:H7 (*396*). They tested isolates from a multistate foodborne outbreak, a day-care center cluster, and a set of temporally and geographically unrelated cases. Isolates from 61 of 63 patients and the incriminated meat in the large outbreak had identical λ RFLP profiles. Similarly, profiles in 11 of 12 patients from the day-care center were identical—but different from those in the multistate outbreak. Isolates from 42 sporadic cases were unrelated to either large cluster and were unique except for three paired isolates. The authors concluded that bacteriophage λ DNA is a useful, stable, and discriminatory tool for epidemiologic analysis.

Harsono et al. examined genomic DNA of 22 clinical and food *E. coli* O157:H7 isolates by pulsed-field gel electrophoresis (*397*). A variety of restriction endonucleases were evaluated. *Sfi*I and *Xba*I generated 6 and 10 genomic profiles, respectively. This suggests that the technique has discriminatory potential in epidemiologic investigations. Total genome length was estimated from the sizes and numbers of restriction fragments generated. Differences in the estimates and possible reasons for them were discussed.

Milley and Sekla developed a colony ELISA using the hydrophobic grid membrane filter (HGMF) format, to isolate VTEC from clinical and food samples (*398*). Chart et al. reported a 1-day immunoblotting procedure for detecting *E. coli* O157 LPS-specific antibodies in serum (*399*). Greatorex and Thorne found that ELISAs for serum antibodies against Shiga toxin and verotoxin had limited diagnostic value, but ELISAs for IgM and IgG to *E. coli* LPS were valuable and sensitive adjuncts to culture methods (*400*).

Karmali et al. first determined the prevalence of VT1-neutralizing antibodies in serum of 790 control subjects and then used an ELISA to test for anti-VT1 IgG in controls and patients with VTEC infections or HUS (*401*). The sensitivity, specificity, positive predictive value, and negative predictive value of the ELISA were 95.7, 98.7, 86.3, and 99.6%, respectively. Implications of the anti-VT1 IgG response were discussed.

Law et al. compared an ELISA with a culture technique for diagnosing VTEC infections from stool specimens (*402*). The ELISA was rapid and sensitive, especially when pathogen numbers were low or infection was caused by a non-O157 serogroup. Another potentially useful diagnostic method is a whole-cell EIA for detection of specific fecal IgA (*403*).

Samadpour et al. developed antisense oligonucleotide DNA probes for detecting and genotyping VTEC (*404*). Three probes were constructed, based on the A subunit of published VT1 and VT2 sequences. One probe hybridized with all VT1-producing strains and another with all VT2-producing strains. The third detected all VTEC regardless of toxin genotype. None of the probes hybridized with any of 91 VT-negative strains.

Bialkowska-Hobrzanska et al. developed a sensitive and specific sandwich hybridization assay for VTEC (*405*). Results from the sandwich hybridization, a direct hybridization assay, and a cytotoxicity assay agreed for 64 of 66 *E. coli* strains tested.

Willshaw et al. hybridized 375 clinical, food, and animal strains of *E. coli* O157 with probes derived from the *eaeA* gene of enteropathogenic *E. coli* (EPEC) and from a VTEC homolog of this gene (*406*). Both probes hybridized with all 246 O157:H7 or H⁻ VTEC strains. The probes also hybridized with 10 VT-negative strains,

which were considered naturally occurring derivatives that had lost their VT genes. The remaining 119 strains of *E. coli* O157 were VT-negative and differed in several properties from O157 VTEC. Of these, 101 failed to hybridize with either probe; 18 H8 and H39 strains hybridized with the EPEC probe but not with its VTEC homolog.

A PCR for VTEC was evaluated using 85 strains of VTEC and 5 of *Shigella dysenteriae* type I (*407*). The PCR amplified *slt* gene sequences from whole colonies, and PCR products were identified by spot blot hybridization with a digoxigenin-labeled DNA probe. Sensitivity and specificity were both 99%, as judged against a toxin neutralization technique using SLT-specific MAbs.

A PCR developed to detect *slt* genes in primary fecal cultures was able to detect fewer than 10 VTEC per milliliter of culture, against a background of more than $10^9$ other organisms (*408*).

A direct immunofluorescence antibody stain directly detected *E. coli* O157:H7 in fecal smears in less than 2 hours (*409*). The method detected all isolates of *E. coli* O157 that were recovered by culture, including nonmotile strains and one strain with a flagellar antigen other than H7, as well as O157:H7 strains. The best results were achieved when fecal specimens were pretreated with 5% bleach and centrifuged. No false-negative results were obtained under these conditions. Another fluorescent antibody technique, a modification of the direct epifluorescent filter method, gave specific enumeration of *E. coli* O157:H7 in milk and apple juice in less than 1 hour by epifluorescence microscopy (*410*). For milk, the method was highly specific in the presence of large numbers of indigenous spoilage organisms.

Ogden reported a conductance assay for detection and enumeration of *Escherichia coli*, including hemorrhagic O157 strains (*411*). Some strains of *Salmonella* and *Citrobacter* gave false-positive results, but *Shigella* did not.

**MOLECULAR STUDIES AND PATHOGENICITY.** A brief review discussed the verotoxins produced by EHEC (*412*). Their structure, biological activities, enzymatic activities, cellular receptors, and detection were considered. Hofmann discussed the role of *E. coli* O157:H7 and verotoxins in HUS and thrombotic thrombocytopenic purpura (*413*). HUS develops in 2–7% of symptomatic cases of *E. coli* O157:H7 infection. Although the proportion of thrombotic thrombocytopenic purpura in adults that is attributable to O157:H7 infection is not known, any elderly person in whom this condition is preceded by bloody diarrhea can be assumed to have the infection.

Some studies have suggested that VT2 has a greater role than VT1 in development of microangiopathic sequelae to EHEC infection. Lindgren et al. compared the activities of VT2 and VT2-related toxins of EHEC in Vero cell cytotoxicity and mouse lethality tests (*414*). They wanted to determine whether differences in cytotoxicity of VT2 and related toxins were responsible for the extreme virulence of EHEC strain B2F1 in orally challenged mice. They compared the lethality of orally administered *E. coli* DH5α(Str$^r$) strains that produced different cytotoxic levels of VT2, VT2vha, VT2vhb, and VT2vhc. These strains were lethal for mice and lethality was not related to cytotoxicity. Moreover, the DH5α strains caused renal lesions. Two purified toxins, VT2 and VT2vhb, were equally toxic for mice but VT2 was ~100 times more cytotoxic to Vero cells and had greater binding affinity for the Gb$_3$ glycolipid receptor. Characterization of the B subunits of VT2-related toxins showed that the reduced in vitro cytotoxicity of these toxins was due to substitution of an asparagine residue at position 16. These results do not support the idea that strain B2F1's unique virulence is related to the in vitro toxicity of VT2-related toxins, but they do demonstrate differences in in vitro cytotoxic activity among toxins of the VT2 group.

Sjogren et al. developed a rabbit model of EHEC-induced colitis (*415*). They used a VT1-converting bacteriophage to create *E. coli* strain RDEC-H19A, an isogenic variant of *E. coli* RDEC-1, which is an enteroadherent diarrheal pathogen in rabbits. RDEC-H19A produces high levels of VT1 and causes a serious noninvasive enteroadherent infection characterized by vascular changes, edema, and severe inflammation. Interleukin-1 and platelet-activating factor appear to be inflammatory mediators in this infection. Tarr welcomed the new model as a definitive tool for future studies of the role of VT1 in enteric disease (*416*). It may also be feasible to use RDEC-1 as a carrier to deliver VT2 and its variants at the surface of the rabbit intestinal mucosa.

Fratamico et al. investigated the virulence of a sorbitol-fermenting mutant of *E. coli* O157:H7 strain A9124-1, using an infant rabbit model and several in vitro assays (*417*). The mutant resembled the wild type in all respects except ability to ferment sorbitol. The two had similar total cell lysate protein profiles, outer membrane protein profiles, plasmid profiles, and cytotoxicity for Vero cells. Both adhered to cultured HEp-2 cells and reacted with antiserum against *E. coli* O157:H7. Observations by light and electron microscopy indicated that the mutant and wild type produced similar diarrheal disease in orally challenged rabbits.

The authors concluded that the sorbitol-nonfermenting phenotype is not associated with the pathogenicity of *E. coli* O157:H7.

Pursuing observations that feeding VT2-producing EHEC to mice caused development of acute renal cortical necrosis and death, whereas mice fed VT1-producing EHEC did not die, Tesh et al. examined the histopathologic effects of the purified toxins when they were injected intravenously or intraperitoneally (*418*). Despite their genetic and structural similarities, VT2 had an LD$_{50}$ about 400 times lower than that of VT1. Both toxins bound to renal cortical tubule and medullary duct epithelial cells. Both toxins bound to the Gb$_3$ glycolipid receptor, but VT1 showed affinity higher by an order of magnitude in a solid-phase binding assay. Thus VT1's lesser capacity to cause acute renal tubular necrosis in mice is not due to inability to bind Gb$_3$ in the mouse kidney. No difference in enzyme activity between the toxins was detected. However, VT2 was considerably more heat- and pH-stable, suggesting that it is overall a more stable molecule. The authors postulate that structural or functional differences between the toxins, possibly involving holotoxin stability, contribute to the difference in their LD$_{50}$'s.

To understand how VT1 and VT2 affect the target cell at the cellular level, Takeda et al. evaluated their in vitro cytotoxic effects on human cells (*419*). The cell lines studied were HUVEC (umbilical cord vascular cells), ACHN (renal adenocarcinoma), T84 (colon cancer), and IMR-32 (neuroblastoma), and also Vero cells. ACHN and Vero cells were highly sensitive to both purified toxins; the other human cell lines required a toxin level at least 8 log$_{10}$ higher for a cytotoxic effect. Urinary markers of tubular function indicated severe dysfunction in patients during the acute stage of HUS, but values returned to normal within 2–3 weeks after onset of the disease as tubules regenerated. The authors concluded that tubular impairment by VT is a major factor in the sudden renal failure associated with VTEC infection, that tubular epithelial cells are the primary target sites of VT, and that histopathologic studies done during the convalescent phase could be misleading.

The Shiga-like toxin VT1 is virtually identical to the Shiga toxin of *Shigella dysenteriae*, and both *S. dysenteriae* and EHEC are associated with HUS. Studies in a transgenic mouse model suggested that Shiga toxin induces TNF synthesis in the kidney, at the same time increasing renal sensitivity to the toxic effects of TNF (*420*). Although this model does not strictly mimic the HUS syndrome in people, it does support the idea that local renal synthesis of TNF contributes to the renal injury caused by Shiga toxin.

Austin et al. assessed the contribution of the noncatalytic A$_2$ fragment of the VT1 A subunit to formation of the VT1 holotoxin (*421*). They compared the ability of the purified VT1 B subunit to combine in vitro with the full-length purified VT1 A subunit of 293 amino acid residues and with the purified VT1 A$_1$ catalytic subunit containing residues 1–255. VT1A combined with VT1B to yield a molecule resembling the holotoxin by nondenaturing PAGE and immunoblot analysis and cytotoxicity to Vero cells. The VT1A$_1$ fragment did not have this ability. The authors concluded that VT1A$_2$ is necessary for holotoxin formation and that it stabilizes the interaction between A and B subunits. Burgess and Roberts investigated whether proteolytic nicking of the A subunit into A$_1$ and A$_2$ fragments is necessary for cytotoxicity (*422*). Normally, nicking occurs at arginine residues in the disulfide loop of the A subunit. When these residues were altered to block the specific proteolysis or the A subunit was truncated, the mutants remained effective toxins, having catalytic activity similar to that of the wild type and only marginally reduced cytotoxicity for Vero cells. In similar studies, Samuel and Gordon replaced either or both of the arginine residues in the disulfide loop of the VT2v toxin with glutamic acid or histidine (*423*). Products of glutamic acid substitution were immunoreactive but not cytotoxic, due to inability to assemble into holotoxin. However, products of histidine substitution retained cytotoxic and enzymatic activity and were lethal to mice in doses comparable to lethal doses of the native toxin. Thus again, proteolytic nicking of the A subunit into A$_1$ and A$_2$ fragments was not essential for toxin activity.

VT1 belongs to a family of ribosome-inactivating proteins with common structural and mechanistic features. One suggested model for the active site of the VT1 A subunit places three aromatic residues in the active-site cleft: tyrosine-77, tyrosine-114, and tryptophan-203. The authors of this model now present data on the phenotypes of conservative point-mutants of VT1A in which tyrosine-114 is altered (*424*). Substitution by phenylalanine reduced the activity of the mutant by a factor of ~30, whereas substitution by a serine residue reduced activity by 3 orders of magnitude. When the same mutations were engineered into a truncated *slt*-IA that directs expression of a product corresponding to VT1A$_1$, phenylalanine substitution reduced activity 7-fold; serine substitution, 300-fold. Tryptic digest profiles indicated that the substitutions had not substantially altered conformation. The authors concluded that tyrosine-114 has a significant role in the activity of VT1A, quantitatively similar to that of tyrosine-77, and this role

depends on both the aromatic ring and the weakly acidic phenolic hydroxyl.

Rüssmann et al. sequenced genes for the B subunit of VT2-related toxins from 15 strains of *E. coli* O157 (*425*). They found 100% homology among all 15 VT2B-related genes, and the sequences were identical to that published for VT2cB. It thus appears that the B subunit genes are highly conserved, and differences in the variant toxins reside in the A subunit of O157 strains.

Lin et al. cloned and sequenced two new VT2 variant genes from VTEC isolated from a cow and a person with diarrhea (*426*). The nucleotide and deduced amino acid sequences were distinct from those of the VT2, VT2vha, VT2vhb, VT2vp1, and VT2vp2 genes, although their degree of homology—particularly with VT2vh—was high. The authors suggest that while VT2 variants may not be of great significance in the study of toxins, minor variations could be very useful in developing a toxin typing system for epidemiologic studies. The same research group constructed PCR primers for detecting VT1, VT2, and VT2 variants (*427*). They discussed the application of these primers in diagnostic and epidemiologic studies of VTEC infections.

Workers in Australia used a PCR to amplify variant VT2 operons found in *E. coli* serotypes O111:H⁻ and OX3:H21 (*428*). Fragments of ~1.5 kilobases were cloned, and sequence analysis identified further variations of published VT2 sequences. They also sequenced a variant VT1 operon from an *E. coli* O111:H⁻ strain isolated from a 12-month-old boy with HUS (*429*). This is the first reported VT1 variant. The sequence of the variant VT1 A-subunit gene differed from sequences previously published for VT1 by 5 base pairs, corresponding to two amino acid changes. It differed from the published sequence for Shiga toxin by only 3 base pairs that resulted in one amino acid change. The sequence of the gene encoding the B subunit was identical to that of VT1 and Shiga toxin. An IS element was detected ~2 kilobases upstream from the toxin gene, suggesting involvement of a transposon in the gene's current (apparently chromosomal) location. DNA sequences highly homologous to a portion of bacteriophage λ were detected ~1 kilobase upstream from the toxin gene.

Fratamico et al. examined 17 strains of *E. coli* O157:H7 for plasmids and ability to adhere to HEp-2 and Int407 cells (*430*). The strains had a common 60-MDa plasmid. Parent and plasmid-cured strains both produced pili and adhered equally well to cultured epithelial cells, corroborating other reports that adherence of *E. coli* O157:H7 is not correlated with the presence of the 60-MDa plasmid. DNA of this plasmid encodes ~35 proteins, including a 33-kDa outer membrane protein whose function is not known. Information was also presented on smaller plasmids harbored by these strains.

Dytoc et al. examined the gene products of the 60-MDa plasmid (pO157) and the *eaeA* gene homolog of *E. coli* O157:H7 in relation to a previously reported 94-kDa outer membrane protein and as possible effectors for O157:H7 attachment–effacement (*431*). Sequencing and immunoassay showed that the O157:H7 *eae* gene product is distinct from the 94-kDa protein (also see reference *433*). Parent and pO157 plasmid-cured O157:H7 strains both demonstrated attaching and effacing adhesion to host epithelial cells and reacted equally well to rabbit antiserum raised against the 94-kDa outer membrane protein. However, *E. coli* Hb101 transformed separately with the cloned *eaeA* gene and pO157 did not form attaching and effacing lesions in vitro or in vivo. Further studies suggested that unidentified proteins inactivated in some Tn*phoA* mutants are also required for O157:H7 attachment–effacement. In a different approach to assessing the role of *eae* in EHEC, Donnenberg et al. constructed an *eae* deletion/insertion mutant in a wild-type *E. coli* O157:H7 strain (*432*). The mutant was deficient in inducing F-actin accumulation in HEp-2 cells and was unable to attach intimately to colonic epithelial cells in a newborn piglet model of infection. Intimate attachment was restored when the EHEC *eae* gene or the EPEC *eaeA* gene was introduced into the mutant on a plasmid. Thus *eae* and *eaeA* are functionally homologous and an *eae* gene is necessary for intimate attachment of EHEC in vivo. In EPEC, *eaeA* encodes a 94-kDa outer membrane called intimin, which is necessary to produce the attaching–effacing lesion. Louie et al. characterized the "intimin" specified by the *eae* homolog in *E. coli* O157:H7 and determined its role in adherence (*433*). They concluded that the product of the EHEC *eae* gene is a 97-kDa surface-exposed protein, and designated it intimin$_{O157}$. Intimin$_{O157}$ is necessary but not sufficient to cause actin polymerization and localized recruitment of F-actin to the site of bacterial attachment. Western immunoblotting and indirect fluorescent antibody studies showed that intimin$_{O157}$ is not the same as a previously described 94-kDa outer membrane protein reported to be involved in adherence of *E. coli* O157:H7.

## Enteropathogenic *E. coli* (EPEC)

One characteristic of classical type I EPEC is the production of attaching-effacing lesions. However, none of 39 strains of EPEC serogroup O126 isolated from cases of infantile diarrhea in Hong Kong, 1982–1988, exhibited localized adherence to HEp-2 cells or the attaching-effacing properties of classical EPEC (*434*). Thirty-one strains were serotype O126:H12 and were enterotoxigenic; one was serotype O126:H10 and was enteroaggregative. Six strains of serotype O126:H21 and one of serotype O126:H8 had no known virulence factors for diarrheagenic *E. coli*. Otherwise, the 39 strains showed close genetic relationships between their virulence markers, outer-membrane protein and LPS profiles, and electrophoretic types by MEE. A study in adult volunteers assessed the role of *eaeA* in experimental EPEC infection (*435*). One group ingested a wild-type O127:H6 strain and another ingested an isogenic *eaeA* deletion mutant of this strain. Diarrhea developed in 11 of 11 subjects who received the wild-type and in 4 of 11 who received the mutant. The mutant produced milder symptoms and lower peak titers of serum IgA and IgG. This study demonstrates unambiguously that *eaeA* is an EPEC virulence gene, but indicates that other factors are also involved.

Law comprehensively reviewed the role of adhesion in virulence of EPEC (*436*). He gave an overview of the pathophysiology of EPEC infection and the role of toxins in it. EPEC adherence was considered in terms of the EPEC adherence factor (EAF), its receptor, and EAF-encoding plasmids; adherence to cultured cells; identification of a fimbrial adhesin; the involvement of chromosomal genes in localized adherence; and EAF-negative EPEC showing localized adhesion. The attaching-effacing lesion was discussed in detail and possible invasive mechanisms were described. Overall, EPEC virulence is complex and its determinants are an amalgam of those found in other enteric pathogens as diverse as *Vibrio cholerae, Yersinia enterocolitica,* and *Citrobacter freundii.* Two other types of adhesion, diffuse and enteroaggregative, were mentioned. True diffusely adherent *E. coli* (DAEC) and enteroaggregative *E. coli* (EAggEC) are unequivocally distinct from EPEC, as they do not stain with the fluorescent actin stain and do not hybridize with the EAF probe.

Expression of "bundle-forming pili" is associated with the EAF plasmid and localized adherence to HEp-2 cells. Two additional morphologic types of fimbriae expressed by an O111:NM strain of EPEC have now been described (*437*). Characterization of these fimbriae revealed *N*-terminal sequence homologies with fimbriae of uropathogenic *E. coli* and DAEC. However, they may have a different receptor specificity. Further studies of these structures suggested that they interact with eukaryotic cells and play a role in the pathogenesis of intestinal disease caused by EPEC infection.

Some strains of EPEC belonging to serogroups O26, O55, O111, and O128 produce verotoxin. Scotland et al. tested 122 clinical strains belonging to these serogroups for hybridization with VT probes (*438*). Eighteen strains of serogroups O26 and O128 were VT-positive. However, 90 strains, including 14 VT-positive strains, hybridized with the *eae* probe and 17 hybridized with the EAggEC probe. Tissue culture tests correlated with probe results for 78 *eae*-positive and 9 EAggEC-positive strains.

*Escherichia coli* strains expressing cytolethal distending toxin cause progressive cellular distention and ultimate death in CHO, HeLa, and HEp-2 cells and to a lesser extent in Vero cells. The initial elongation seen in CHO cells is indistinguishable from that caused by *E. coli* heat-labile toxin. Scott et al. cloned and sequenced the genes encoding the *E. coli* cytolethal distending toxin (*439*). The nucleotide and predicted amino acid sequences have no significant homology with any previously reported genes or proteins.

Foubister et al. reported that EPEC triggers release of inositol phosphates after adherence to HeLa cells (*440*). This flux is followed by actin rearrangement and bacterial invasion. Formation of inositol phosphates requires tyrosine phosphorylation of a 90-kDa HeLa cell protein. This suggests that EPEC-induced tyrosine phosphorylation of one or more host cell substrates leads to release of inositol phosphates, which may then trigger rearrangement of the cytoskeleton.

## Enterotoxigenic *E. coli* (ETEC)

Foodborne outbreaks of ETEC infection occurred in Rhode Island and New Hampshire in late March 1993 (*441*). The Rhode Island outbreak was associated with eating a garden salad served on a flight from Charlotte, North Carolina, to Providence. Forty-seven of the 74 passengers interviewed met the case definition and 46 of them had eaten the salad, which was made from shredded carrots and several varieties of lettuce. Nine of 18 passengers later contacted, who had been served the same meal on a different flight, also reported gastrointestinal illness. A caterer had prepared 4000 portions of the salad for 40 flights on that day. All salad ingredients were of U.S. origin. No food handlers reported gastrointestinal illness or recent foreign travel, and no deficiencies in sanitary conditions were identified at the caterer's facilities. The New Hampshire outbreak affected 121 guests and employees at a mountain lodge. Among guests, illness was most strongly associated with consumption of tabouleh, and this was the only food associated with illness in the employees. As in the Rhode Island outbreak, all ingredients were of U.S. origin and all food preparers denied recent gastrointestinal illness or foreign travel. The ETEC O6:NM strains

associated with these outbreaks had identical plasmid profiles, distinct from profiles of ten O6:NM ETEC strains from other sources. Carrots were the only ingredient common to the two salads. The carrots were grown in the same state, but traceback was unable to identify a single source.

Chérifi et al. investigated clonal relationships among 63 ETEC strains of serogroup O78 isolated in Canada and Europe from infections in people, cattle, sheep, pigs, and chickens (*442*). They identified a main group of 55 clonally related strains having a type A outer-membrane protein pattern, H9 or H⁻ flagellar antigen (except for H12 in one strain), and type 1 biotype. The group comprised 52 isolates from septicemia and 3 enterotoxigenic clinical isolates. The remaining 8 strains (4 human, 4 animal) were clonally heterogeneous. The authors concluded that animals are a possible source of serogroup O78 septicemic *E. coli* infections in people.

Ghosh et al. tested ETEC strains known to produce either colonization factor antigen (CFA) I or II for CFA expression on 16 common plating media (*443*). CFA was detected on CFA agar and also on several other commercial media, particularly nutrient agar. However, it was not detected on other commercial media, e.g. MacConkey agar. The authors recommended nutrient agar with MAb-based coagglutination regents as a simple and rapid way to detect *E. coli* that express CFA I or II.

A polynucleotide probe developed for ETEC was based on the gene encoding a major structural subunit of coli surface antigen 6 (CS6) (*444*).

Uesaka et al. reported a simple method for purifying ETEC heat-labile toxin and cholera toxin (*445*). A single run on an immobilized D-galactose column yielded an electrophoretically homogeneous toxin.

Shida et al. studied the binding of heat-labile enterotoxin to lactose-α-lactalbumin (*446*). Binding was abolished by treatment with β-galactosidase, indicating that the terminal galactose is required. Binding was inhibited by galactose, lactose, and—most effectively—by lactulose. Lactulose is a structural analog of the Amadori rearrangement product of the amino carbonyl reaction between lactose and an ε-amino group of lysine. These and other observations suggest that heat-labile enterotoxin recognizes the lactuloselysine in lactose-α-lactalbumin and binds to glycosylated proteins with lactose by the amino carbonyl reaction.

"Longus," a long pilus produced by clinical ETEC strains, has been characterized (*447*). It comprises a repeating 22-kDa subunit whose *N*-terminal sequence shows homology with the toxin-coregulated pilus of *Vibrio cholerae*, the bundle-forming pilus of EPEC, and type IV pilins of some gram-negative pathogens. Its structural gene, *lngA*, is plasmid-encoded. *lngA* was found only in clinical strains, but was widely distributed in such strains independently of their geographic origin, serotype, toxin production, or other pilus antigens. The authors proposed longus as a new member of the type IV pilus family and a highly conserved ETEC factor for intestinal colonization.

Although many CFAs and putative colonization factors have been described for ETEC, many clinical strains do not possess any of the known antigens. To identify CFAs in ETEC lacking known antigens, Viboud et al. exploited the ability of ETEC to adhere to CaCo-2 cells (*448*). By detailed study of an enterotoxin-producing ETEC O20:K27:H⁻ isolate from a child with diarrhea, they identified and described a new fimbrial putative colonization factor, PCFO20.

## Other *E. coli*

Savarino described enteroadherent *E. coli* as a heterogeneous group of diarrheal pathogens comprising groups with distinct adherence patterns to cultured epithelial cells (*449*). "Localized adherence" applies to formation of distinct microcolonies or bacterial clusters adhering to epithelial cells; it characterizes EPEC that cause infantile diarrhea. The diffuse adherence pattern describes adherence of single bacteria (DAEC) dispersed evenly over the epithelial cell surface. In the enteroaggregative pattern, EAggEC adhere to one another, forming a stacked bricklike lattice on cultured cells. The epidemiologic and pathogenic significance of DAEC and EAggEC were discussed in detail. Brook et al. reported a prospective study of EAggEC and DAEC in patients with various types of diarrhea (*450*). Eight of 135 patients with diarrhea and 4 of 46 controls had probe-positive EAggEC in their stools. Seven diarrheic patients and one control had DAEC. Of 10 patients with diarrhea related to another recognized enteric pathogen, 5 also had DAEC in their stools. EAggEC was the only recognized pathogen in 4 cases of traveler's diarrhea and DAEC, in 2. Investigating the role of different enteroadherence patterns in childhood diarrhea, Bhatnagar et al. concluded that EAggEC may be an important cause of diarrhea in children, with a tendency to cause acute and prolonged disease (*451*). Paul et al. reported a new pattern of aggregative adherence, which they described as having a "honey-combed," in contrast to a "stacked-brick," appearance (*452*). The EAggEC strains identified in this study of diarrhea in Calcutta did not produce any classical enterotoxins and were associated with secretory diarrhea rather than invasive diarrhea. Qadri et al. showed that EAggEC represent a heterogeneous group

of organisms with different types of hemagglutinins or adhesins for the intestinal mucosal surface (*453*). Some strains demonstrated mannose-sensitive hemagglutination of erythrocytes, but most showed mannose-resistant hemagglutination of erythrocytes from all species except rabbits. Hemagglutination patterns could be classified into 19 groups.

Matsushita et al. described the biochemical reactions of 10 enteroinvasive strains of *E. coli* belonging to serotype O121:NM (*454*). All strains harbored a plasmid of 120–140 MDa that has been associated with invasiveness and were positive in an ELISA for virulence plasmid–encoded proteins of *Shigella* and EIEC. Although EIEC and shigellas are genotypically nearly identical, the infective dose of EIEC is typically ~10⁴ times higher. Hsia et al. systematically characterized the virulence genes of the EIEC virulence plasmid pSF204 by transposon mutagenesis (*455*). They located and characterized *ipaC, mxiG, mxiJ, mxiM, mxiD,* and a new locus, *invX*, which is required for entry into HEp-2 cells. The results suggested a high degree of genetic, structural, and functional homology between the large invasion plasmids of EIEC and *Shigella flexneri*.

Bratoeva et al. described a case of diarrhea, bacteremia, and fever caused by a novel strain of *E. coli* (*456*). The non-EPEC strain possessed the *eae* gene, was EAF-negative, was invasive in the gentamicin invasion assay, and expressed two types of pili and K1 antigen. Strain O12:K1:NM:Hly⁺ cannot be classified into any previously recognized group of *E. coli* that cause diarrhea.

## *YERSINIA*

### Clinical and Epidemiologic Studies

A prospective case–control study in Norway sought to identify sources and risk factors for sporadic *Yersinia enterocolitica* infections (*457*). Sixty-seven case-patients and 132 controls matched for age, sex, and geographical location were enrolled in the 16-month study. During the two weeks before the interview (controls) or onset of illness (patients), patients were more likely than controls to have eaten pork (3.79 vs. 2.30 meals, $p = .02$) and sausage (2.84 vs. 2.20 meals, $p = .03$); one patient had eaten raw pork. Patients were also more likely to report a preference for raw or rare meat (47 vs. 27%, $p = .01$) and to have drunk untreated water during the two weeks under consideration (39 vs. 25%, $p = .01$). Each of these factors was independently associated with disease.

Questions remain about the modes of transmission of *Yersinia pseudotuberculosis* infections to humans and about genetic relationships of *Y. pseudotuberculosis* in different parts of the world. Fukushima et al. performed restriction endonuclease analysis of virulence plasmid DNA in 687 strains of *Y. pseudotuberculosis* from Japan, Russia, Canada, Europe, New Zealand, and Australia (*458*). The strains were isolated from patients, wild and domesticated animals, food, and the environment. Composite analysis using five restriction enzymes distinguished 29 patterns. Some patterns were confined to one or two regions; others had broader distribution. Europe and eastern Asia appear to be separate foci of origin of *Y. pseudotuberculosis* strains. Within a geographical region, isolates from dogs, cats, pigs, pork, cattle, and people have identical patterns. This confirms that pets, as well as pigs, are a major reservoir of the organism. The finding of *Y. pseudotuberculosis* in wild animals and river water in mountainous regions suggests that environmental reservoirs are also important.

*Yersinia enterocolitica* infection can have a variety of manifestations and sequelae. A case of *Y. enterocolitica* infection masquerading as appendicitis was reported in an 8-year-old boy with hemoglobin E–β-thalassemia disease (*459*). People with diseases resulting in iron overload are particularly susceptible to yersinia infections. The urease β subunit of *Y. enterocolitica* O9 has been identified as a target antigen for human synovial T-lymphocytes in two patients with reactive arthritis (*460*). This 19-kDa protein contains several T-cell epitopes, one of which cross-reacts with other enterobacteria that are not able to induce reactive arthritis. Thus the arthritogenicity of the 19-kDa antigen may depend on its expression in an organism whose other properties enable it to induce reactive arthritis. Saebø et al. presented evidence that *Y. enterocolitica* infection can initiate chronic neurologic disease in some patients (*461*). During 1974–1983, the infection was diagnosed by antibody response in 458 hospitalized patients in Norway. Two patients had acute peripheral nervous system symptoms and 6 had central nervous system symptoms. All 458 patients were followed until 1987. During follow-up, chronic neurologic conditions developed in 6 additional patients. In 1991, 6 patients still had significant antibody responses by ELISA. Saebø et al. further hypothesized that development of malignant mesothelioma might be induced by *Y. enterocolitica* infection (*462*). This malignancy may occur in more than 10% of persons heavily exposed to asbestos, but its normal annual incidence is more likely around 1–2 per million. However, malignant mesothelioma developed in 2 of the 458 patients the investigators were following for yersiniosis

sequelae. Statistically, this is extremely unlikely to be due to chance. The authors suggested that yersinia infection launched chronic immunologic reactions resembling those that occur in asbestos workers.

## Occurrence and Growth

A survey in the Netherlands of 390 samples of poultry products found yersinias in 8% (*463*). Although 26 isolates were *Y. enterocolitica*, none belonged to pathogenic serogroups. Melo Franco and Landgraf examined samples of 126 foods purchased in retail markets in Sao Paulo, Brazil, for yersinias (*464*). The organisms were found in 45% of raw milk, 14% of pasteurized milk, 13% of raw vegetables, and 40% of meat and meat products sampled, an overall prevalence of 28%. The commonest species was *Y. enterocolitica*, which was isolated from 19% of raw milk, 3% of raw vegetables, and 13% of meats; it was not detected in pasteurized milk.

Kleeman and Scheibner examined the behavior of *Y. enterocolitica* in fresh dry sausages (*465*). The number of viable organisms in experimentally contaminated sausages decreased steadily throughout storage. However, depending on the type of sausage, *Y. enterocolitica* was still detectable by direct plating methods after 30–42 days of cold storage and after 55–73 days when an enrichment step was used. With storage at 15–18°C, the organism was detected by enrichment procedures for up to 50 days. In fermented sausages, survival of *Y. enterocolitica* depends on the starter culture and level of nitrite used (*466*). Sausage was inoculated with $1.7 \times 10^5$ cfu/g of *Y. enterocolitica* O3. The pathogen was not detected by direct plating after 28 days in most sausages formulated with ≥80 mg/kg of $NaNO_2$, and was not detected by either direct plating or enrichment procedures in any sausage after 35 days. Sausages manufactured with ≤50 mg/kg of $NaNO_2$ still harbored the pathogen at the end of the 35-day test period. As a starter culture, *Pediococcus acidilactici* permitted the greatest survival and was associated with the smallest pH decrease during ripening (from 5.7 to 5.4). Pathogen survival was poorest and pH decrease greatest (5.6 to 4.9) with *Lactobacillus pentosus* and intermediate with *Lactobacillus plantarum*.

Manu-Tawiah et al. examined the survival and growth of *Y. enterocolitica* and *Listeria monocytogenes* Scott A in pork chops packaged under various gas mixtures, vacuum, and air (*467*). In air, both pathogens grew slower than psychrotrophic spoilage flora. In modified atmospheres, *Y. enterocolitica* grew at the same rate as spoilage flora and *L. monocytogenes* grew slower. Vacuum packaging was no more effective than modified atmospheres in retarding growth. The authors concluded that modified atmospheres provide a package environment that allows growth of *Y. enterocolitica* and could compromise the safety of meat products.

Investigators in Spain evaluated the ability of *Lactobacillus sake* strains isolated from Spanish dry fermented sausages to inhibit growth of *Y. enterocolitica* O3 and O8 in mixed culture (*468*). All *L. sake* strains were inhibitory, and the degree of inhibition was directly related to incubation temperature. The bacteriocinogenic strain *L. sake* 148 was less inhibitory than strain 23, a stronger lactic acid producer.

Little et al. applied a log-logistic model previously used to describe the thermal inactivation of bacteria to predict the survival of *Y. enterocolitica* under conditions of suboptimal temperature and inhibitory pH (*469*). Predicted values were in excellent agreement with observed values for survival of the pathogen in mayonnaise. The model overestimated the pathogen's survival in yogurt, but would fail safe if used for predictive purposes. The model was developed from survival data in a nutritionally favorable medium free from competing microorganisms. The inaccurate predictions for yogurt could be due to milk's greater buffering capacity or to effects of the large populations of lactic acid bacteria.

Lindberg and Borch modeled the effect of inoculum level, temperature, pH, and L-lactate concentration on aerobic growth of *Y. enterocolitica* by fitting the Gompertz equation to conductance response curves (*470*). The system permitted simultaneous study of many combinations of factors. Conductance responses were seen for all combinations of factors that were tested. Rates predicted from the conductance polynomial models agreed well with rates predicted from a published absorbance model. Sutherland and Bayliss studied the effect of pH, temperature, and NaCl concentration on growth of *Y. enterocolitica* in laboratory medium (*471*). Growth curves were fitted using the Gompertz routine and the parameters derived in this way were modeled. This permitted generation of growth curves for any set of conditions within the limits of the matrix studied, and prediction of growth rate, lag time, generation time, and time to 1000-fold increase. When validated against published data, the model gave realistic and consistently fail-safe predictions for growth of *Y. enterocolitica* in a range of foods representing meat and meat products, milk, eggs, fish, and tofu.

## Identification and Typing

Manafi and Holzhammer compared results from the Gene-trak, API 20E, and Vitek systems for identification

of *Y. enterocolitica* (*472*). The methods were tested with 101 strains of known identity and 83 suspected positive isolates from CIN agar. For these suspected strains, API 20E identified 40 as *Y. enterocolitica* after a 24-h incubation at 37°C and 37 as *Y. enterocolitica* after a 48-h incubation at 30°C; Gene-trak gave positive results with 39 strains and Vitek, with 27. Gene-trak detected *Y. enterocolitica* in mixed cultures so long as the population was at least $10^6$ cfu/mL.

Bosi et al. reported that small numbers of *Y. pseudotuberculosis* on frozen, vacuum-packed venison could go undetected if CIN agar is used as a selective medium (*473*). However, it may be necessary to compromise sensitivity in order to avoid overgrowth with other bacteria.

Amirmozafari and Robertson developed a simple defined medium that supports growth of *Y. enterocolitica* and synthesis of heat-stable enterotoxin at levels comparable to those achieved in trypticase soy broth–yeast extract medium (*474*). Four amino acids were included in the medium, and the carbon source was potassium gluconate. A mixture of thymine, cytosine, and uracil stimulated enterotoxin synthesis, whereas a mixture of adenine and guanine was inhibitory. Vigorous aeration was necessary for maximal production of enterotoxin, and no enterotoxin was detected in culture supernatants when the incubation temperature exceeded 30°C.

Exploiting the ability of *Y. pseudotuberculosis,* pathogenic *Y. enterocolitica,* and enteroinvasive *E. coli* to invade cultured cells, Fukushima et al. developed a new procedure for isolating these pathogens from fecal, meat, and water samples heavily contaminated with other bacteria (*475*). HeLa cell preparations were set up in the wells of microtiter plates and exposed to bacterial suspensions. After inoculation, cells were washed with gentamicin and incubated in fresh medium containing gentamicin. The antibiotic killed extracellular bacteria but did not affect the viability of intracellular organisms. This method was used for selective isolation of pathogenic yersinias from samples of retail pork, polluted mountain rivers, and the cecal contents of raccoon dogs.

Makino et al. used random amplified polymorphic DNA (RAPD) fingerprints to distinguish different strains of *Y. pseudotuberculosis* (*476*). Presence or absence of the large *Y. pseudotuberculosis* plasmid had no effect on RAPD patterns. Preliminary results indicated that the method would be highly discriminatory in epidemiologic studies. The method was subsequently used to identify 30 clinical isolates of serotype 5a associated with an outbreak of Izumi fever in Japan. All isolates showed common patterns that were unique to each of the 10 primers used. Restriction digest patterns of the large plasmids were also identical. These tests confirmed that the isolates were from a single source.

Kapperud et al. developed a two-step PCR procedure to identify the common pathogenic serogroups of *Y. enterocolitica* (*477*). It is based on two nested pairs of primers specific for *yadA*. Serogroups O3, O5,27, O8, O13, and O21 were differentiated from *Y. pseudotuberculosis* and a variety of nonpathogenic yersinias representing 25 serogroups and 4 species. Ten to 30 cfu per gram of meat could be detected in a $10^6$-fold excess of indigenous bacteria. With overnight nonselective enrichment, sensitivity was increased to 2 cfu/g. Immunomagnetic separation was a convenient method of preparing samples for the PCR. Gel electrophoresis and a colorimetric method showed complete concordance in detection of PCR products and discrimination between positive and negative samples.

Immunoblotting of *Yersinia* plasmid-encoded released proteins can be used for serodiagnosis (*478*). Released proteins are naturally separated from cross-reacting proteins that are common to pathogenic and nonpathogenic strains of *Y. enterocolitica* and *Y. pseudotuberculosis*. Another new technique also shows promise in situations where extensive cross-reactions reduce specificity. A simple Western blotting procedure aided the selection of antigens most likely to exhibit serotype-specific epitopes (*479*). These proteins were purified and used as immunogens to generate MAbs in mice. The MAbs developed are promising agents for serological identification of *Y. enterocolitica* O8.

CIN agar, which contains crystal violet and about 1 mmol/L calcium, can be used for phenotypic characterization of *Y. enterocolitica* strains carrying a virulence plasmid. Koeppel et al. confirmed the visual interpretation of culture results by a PCR with primers directed at *virF*, a gene present only in pathogenic strains of *Y. enterocolitica* (*480*).

Studies by Tomita et al. indicated that the salting-out test can differentiate strains of *Y. pseudotuberculosis* that carry the virulence plasmid from those that do not (*481*). All strains of *Y. pseudotuberculosis* that aggregated in 0.9% saline carried the virulence plasmid, whereas none of 27 plasmidless strains aggregated. Four plasmid-bearing strains that did not aggregate were unable to survive in the peritoneal cavity of mice or to colonize the ileum.

Bhaduri and Turner-Jones investigated the stability of the *Y. enterocolitica* virulence plasmid under various anaerobic atmospheres (*482*). The plasmid was retained in growth-phase and stationary-phase cells exposed to vacuum or atmospheres of 80% $N_2$–20% $H_2$ or 94% $CO_2$–6% $H_2$ for 24 h at 28°C. A variety of virulence assays indicated that the cells were still virulent.

## Virulence and Molecular Studies

Mantle and Husar investigated interactions between *Y. enterocolitica* and purified intestinal mucins from rabbits and humans (*483*). Plasmid-bearing virulent organisms bound well to both preparations, but plasmid-free nonvirulent organisms did not. Binding did not appear to involve hydrophobic interactions, although there was evidence that mucin could mask hydrophobic adhesins on the bacterial surface. Analysis of binding curves suggested the presence of a single type of receptor for *Y. enterocolitica* with a similar (but not necessarily identical) structure in mucins from rabbits and humans. Further experiments evaluated the ability of plasmid-bearing and plasmid-free *Y. enterocolitica* to grow in purified mucin and degrade it (*484*). At 37°C (but not at 25°C), both virulent and avirulent organisms grew better in mucin-supplemented medium than in unsupplemented medium. However, only plasmid-bearing strains were able to break the mucin down into compounds of lower molecular weight. Again, this activity was expressed at 37°C but not at 25°C. The authors postulate that the ability to grow well in mucin helps the organism to colonize the intestine, and ability to degrade mucin may help pathogenic strains to solubilize and penetrate the mucus layer. Subsequent studies showed that binding of *Y. enterocolitica* to purified native mucins from rabbits and humans involves interactions with the mucin's carbohydrate moiety (*485*), as had been suggested by analysis of binding curves in the earlier study. Pronase digestion of mucin and removal of nonglycosylated or poorly glycosylated peptide regions had no effect on bacterial binding. Nor did periodate oxidation alter binding, indicating that vicinal hydroxyl groups in the mucin sugars are not important. Boiling, reduction of disulfide bonds, and removal of noncovalently associated lipid enhanced adherence, suggesting that these treatments exposed additional domains with which the bacteria could interact. There was evidence that core regions of the sugar side chains are involved in binding. The authors concluded that *Y. enterocolitica* interacts with the carbohydrate moiety of mucin through a plasmid-mediated process and that when the mucin is denatured, binding is enhanced through hydrophobic and nonhydrophobic interactions with other sites, probably on the mucin protein.

Grützkau et al. studied the histopathologic changes that occur in mice during intestinal infection with virulent and avirulent strains of *Y. enterocolitica* O8 (*486*). The isogenic plasmid-cured nonpathogenic strains showed no evidence of interaction with ileal tissue. After 12 h, microcolonies of the pathogenic strain were seen under the follicle-associated epithelium of the Peyer's patches. After 36 h, changes ranged from limited ulceration to total destruction of the gut-associated lymphoid tissue. However, there were no signs of active epithelial invasion, as is observed in cultured epithelial cells. The authors postulated that rather than actively invading, pathogenic *Y. enterocolitica* O8 is transported across the epithelial barrier by M-cells that overlie the lymphoid follicles.

Pathogenic yersinias block phagocytosis by macrophages by a process involving the YopE protein, which disrupts the host cell's actin microfilament structure. Rosqvist et al. showed that YopE is transferred through the target cell's plasma membrane while the bacteria remain at the surface (*487*). YopE is recovered only within the cytosol of the target cell. This suggests that the pathogen recognizes certain cell structures and focuses the transfer of YopE at the zone of interaction with the target cell. Regulation of this process involves the bacterium's surface-located YopN sensor protein.

Studies of the wild-type *Yersinia* invasion gene, *inv*, and a mutant showed that the gene product, invasin, is required for invasion of cultured cells and for efficient penetration of the intestinal epithelium (*488*). Surprisingly, however, the mutant and wild-type strains had similar $LD_{50}$ values for orally and intraperitoneally infected mice. This suggests that invasin promotes entry during the initial stage of infection but is of secondary importance in subsequent establishment of systemic infection. The occasional colonization of Peyer's patches by the *inv* mutant is presumably due to expression of alternative, less efficient invasion pathways. Normally, invasin production is greater at ambient temperatures than at the host temperature of 37°C. This apparent paradox—that production of a critical invasion factor is reduced at a temperature characteristic of the opportunity for invasion—led the same research group to investigate factors that might affect the thermal regulation of the *Y. enterocolitica inv* gene (*489*). They found that in vitro at 23°C, invasin was not produced until cells reached the early stationary phase of growth, and that production was unaffected by pH in the range of 5.5–8.5. Although at 37°C invasin production was much lower throughout most of this range, at pH 5.5 it equaled that at 23°C. The low pH is probably typical of the pathogen's environment during early stages of infection of the animal host. There was evidence that induction of invasin expression at pH 5.5 and 37°C occurred at the transcriptional level, although some form of additional posttranscriptional control was not ruled out. Expression of *inv* at

37°C was not affected by calcium or iron levels, richness of the growth medium, or oxygen availability, although bacteria grown anaerobically at 23°C produced less invasin. In vivo experiments showed that after 45 h in the mouse intestine, *Y. enterocolitica* was still producing invasin at levels produced in vitro at 23°C. From these results and observations on the status of *Y. enterocolitica* living free in the environment, the authors built a plausible argument for the adaptive value of this mode of regulation of *inv*.

The adhesin YadA is also involved in the pathogenesis of *Y. enterocolitica* infection. Skurnik et al. investigated the binding of the organism to frozen sections of human intestine (*490*). They found that YadA-mediated binding occurs primarily at the submucosal layer of the intestinal wall and to a limited extent at the mucosal layer, where binding is mostly to mucin threads. Partially purified YadA bound to frozen sections with a pattern similar to that of intact bacteria. A combination of collagen and laminin inhibited binding, but individually, collagen, laminin, and partially purified YadA only partially inhibited YadA-mediated binding. The authors suggest that YadA is multifunctional and may be involved in interactions with extracellular matrix molecules after invasion of intestinal tissue. Another role of YadA is protection of *Y. enterocolitica* against phagocytosis by polymorphonuclear leukocytes (PMNs), as demonstrated by China et al. (*491*). Pathogenic *Y. enterocolitica* does not induce the chemiluminescence response of PMNs. The authors found no influence of yersinia outer membrane proteins on this phenomenon, but expression of YadA at the bacterial surface was associated with lack of chemiluminescence and reduced phagocytosis by PMNs. Moreover, as indicated by the classical plating method and a new luminometric assay, when confronted with PMNs, YadA⁻ bacteria were killed but YadA⁺ bacteria were not.

Pathogenic *Y. enterocolitica* is also able to survive within phagocytic cells. Reasoning that the internal environment of the phagocyte should be stressful for the pathogen, Yamamoto et al. investigated the induction of stress proteins that might contribute to survival within the phagocyte (*492*). They found that at least 16 proteins are selectively induced in response to phagocytosis. Several of these were also induced by heat shock at 42°C or by oxidative stress in vitro. The authors concluded that phagocytosis induces a global stress response in *Y. enterocolitica*, which facilitates the pathogen's survival in a hostile environment.

The 70-kilobase virulence plasmids, called pYVs, encode essential virulence factors for *Y. enterocolitica*. Bielecki et al. evaluated the relatedness of virulence plasmids of *Y. enterocolitica* strains belonging to serogroups O9 and O4,32, and discussed a possible role of pYV O4,32 in the Ca$^{2+}$-dependent regulation of chromosomal genes (*493*). pYV O4,32 was found in many clinical isolates of *Y. enterocolitica*. Its restriction fragment pattern differed from patterns of plasmids from serogroups O3, O8, and O9, although O9 and O4,32 plasmids were closely related. Kwaga and Iversen studied the outer membrane proteins and restriction fragment patterns of virulence plasmids of *Y. enterocolitica* and related species associated with pigs (*494*). Only *Y. enterocolitica* of serogroups O1,2,3, O3, O5,27, O8, and O9 harbored pYV and expressed the associated outer membrane proteins and YadA. Restriction patterns of pathogenic bioserotypes of the same serogroup were similar regardless of origin—pigs, clinical samples, or reference strains. This observation reinforces the view that pigs are an important reservoir of pathogenic *Y. enterocolitica*. Straley et al. reviewed the yersinia outer membrane proteins encoded by the highly conserved pYV (*495*). These proteins fall into two broad classes: those with purely antihost functions, and those that are predominantly regulatory. Yersinias have evolved a unique and complex mechanism for regulating the synthesis and export of a set of antihost virulence proteins. Although understanding of this mechanism is incomplete, it has already provided tantalizing glimpses of how bacteria sense and respond to environmental cues.

Many bacteria secrete high-affinity iron-binding factors called siderophores to facilitate the acquisition of iron essential for their growth. Chambers and Sokol characterized an ethyl acetate–extractable siderophore produced by *Y. enterocolitica* and named it yersiniophore (*496*). They were not able to confirm the presence of catechol in the purified yersiniophore. All of 16 clinical strains of serotypes O4, O4,32, O8, and O21 and one strain of *Y. pseudotuberculosis* produced yersiniophore. It was not produced by *Y. enterocolitica* serotypes O3, O5, or O9 or by three other species of *Yersinia*. Food and water isolates of *Y. enterocolitica* produced a different, water-soluble siderophore. Studies of utilization of yersiniophore by 62 clinical, animal, food, and water isolates of *Y. enterocolitica* suggested that yersiniophore production and utilization is important in clinical infections, since all clinical isolates of serotype O8 produced yersiniophore. Apparently *Y. enterocolitica* O3 uses siderophores provided by other organisms or has an alternative mechanism of iron acquisition that does not involve siderophores. Haag et al. also reported purification of an ethyl acetate–extractable siderophore, which they named yersiniabactin (*497*). Yersiniabactin has a molecular size of 482 Da and does contain a catechol, as

demonstrated by chemical assays and spectroscopy. Purified yersiniabactin stimulates growth of *Y. enterocolitica* under iron-limiting conditions and appears to serve as an iron carrier. Studies of transport of $^{55}$Fe-yersiniabactin indicated a receptor-mediated uptake across the outer membrane.

## *VIBRIO*

### Studies of the Genus *Vibrio*

*Vibrio* species have developed successful strategies for surviving under conditions of both feast and famine. Östling et al. discussed the diversity of starvation-induced responses in vibrios (*498*). There is evidence for general responses as well as some that are restricted to particular species or strains. The authors reviewed adaptations to limitations of carbon, other single nutrients, and multiple nutrients and discussed stress proteins and the physiological basis for stress resistance of starved cells. Among the many bacteria able to enter a "viable but nonculturable" state are the pathogenic vibrios *V. cholerae, V. mimicus, V. parahaemolyticus,* and *V. vulnificus*. Oliver reviewed this phenomenon, including the relationship between viable-but-nonculturable and starvation states (*499*). In at least some cases, the response is determined by temperature. For example, at 5°C *V. vulnificus* becomes viable but nonculturable, whereas at 20°C it enters the starvation state. Starvation leads to protection against a variety of stresses, so that carbon starvation of *V. vulnificus* at room temperature reduces the rate at which the organism becomes nonculturable when subsequently incubated at 5°C. Although the viable but nonculturable state is not well understood, it is clear that entrance into this state involves numerous morphologic, physiologic, and biochemical changes in the cells and that the environmental factors inducing these changes vary considerably among species. The state appears to be under genetic control. Cells in this state are able to retain plasmids, many of which remain transferable. Although there is still debate over the possibility of resuscitating nonculturable cells in the laboratory, several pathogens have apparently retained their virulence and become culturable after in vivo or in vitro treatments.

Klontz et al. conducted monthly surveys of vibrios in oysters harvested from Apalachicola Bay, Florida, from March 1989 through March 1990 (*500*). The findings were related to the incidence of vibrio illnesses during 1989 and 1990 in people living in counties near the bay, who had eaten raw oysters. Excluding wound infections and one case for which information was insufficient, 33 of 34 patients in the study area with *Vibrio* infections reported from January 1989 through December 1990 had eaten raw oysters during the week before their symptoms began. The median number of oysters eaten was 13 (range 3–60). Infections occurred in all months except April, with no evidence of seasonality except for a cluster of *V. vulnificus* infections from July to October. Two species were identified in two cases. Illness was associated with *V. parahaemolyticus* (9 cases), *V. vulnificus* (5 cases), *V. hollisae* (5 cases), *V. mimicus* (4 cases), *V. fluvialis* (4 cases), *V. cholerae* non-O1 (7 cases), and *V. cholerae* O1 (1 case). All except *V. hollisae* and *V. cholerae* O1 were recovered from retail raw oysters. It was not expected that *V. hollisae* would be found, because this organism does not grow well on conventional *Vibrio* isolation media. Like the infections, recovery of vibrios occurred throughout the year except for *V. vulnificus*, which was found only during July–October. These findings provide further evidence that the "R" rule is not valid—that raw oysters can transmit *Vibrio* infections throughout the year, not only in months whose names are spelled without *r*'s.

Wong et al. evaluated the toxigenic characteristics of 91 vibrios isolated from foods (*501*). The strains tested represented *V. cholerae* (50), *V. parahaemolyticus* (18), *V. fluvialis* I and II (10), *V. mimicus* (9), and other species (4). About one-third of these strains were hemolytic, about half had either cytotonic or cytotoxic activity, and nearly three-quarters killed mice; but only a few hybridized to probes for verotoxin, cholera toxin, or thermostable direct hemolysin. The authors suggested that the extracellular toxins produced by these strains were responsible for mouse lethality, adding that a cell-mediated mouse-lethal factor cannot be excluded. They concluded that vibrios from foods can produce toxins different from and unrelated to the common toxins of *E. coli*, *V. cholerae*, and *V. parahaemolyticus*.

A set of keys was designed for fast presumptive biochemical identification of environmental vibrios, including those causing human infections (*502*). The keys are based on 28 tests, of which no more than 10 are needed for even the most complicated identification. The keys identified all 33 *Vibrio* species tested and showed some intraspecific discrimination as well.

The most widely used *Vibrio* selective agar, which contains thiosulfate, citrate, bile salts, and sucrose and is referred to as TCBS, is variable in sensitivity and specificity and *V. hollisae* grows poorly on it. An alternative bile-free selective medium has been developed in which potassium iodide is the principal inhibitory agent.

Abbott et al. comprehensively evaluated the new thiosulfate–chloride–iodide (TCI) medium, using 102 strains of *Vibrionaceae* representing 14 species of *Vibrio* and 3 other genera (*503*). TCI was much more selective than TCBS. Whereas 23 of 24 strains of *Aeromonas* and *Plesiomonas shigelloides* grew well on TCBS, none grew well on TCI. The authors did note that previous lots of TCBS had not supported growth of *Aeromonas*, but this type of variability is one problem with TCBS. TCBS also supported good growth of 5 strains of saprophytic vibrios and TCI did not. Plating efficiency was generally higher on TCI. However, selected strains of *V. hollisae* and *V. damsela* did not thrive any better on TCI than on TCBS. Colony sizes were strikingly smaller on TCI. The clinical usefulness of the new medium remains to be evaluated.

Comparison of salt–polymyxin B broth and alkaline peptone water as enrichment broths for enumeration of *V. parahaemolyticus* and *V. vulnificus* showed that alkaline peptone water was generally superior (*504*). Samples of crab legs, oysters, shrimp, lobster, and shark were inoculated at three levels with each pathogen and were tested with and without cold stress. Geometric means of cells recovered were consistently higher with alkaline peptone water and estimates of detectable levels were lower by 1–4 orders of magnitude. Alkaline peptone water was also more efficient in recovering cold-stressed cells.

Kaysner et al. developed a DNA–DNA colony hybridization HGMF technique for identifying and enumerating *V. parahaemolyticus* and *V. vulnificus* (*505*). It was effective with samples as diverse as seawater and oysters.

Rodrigues et al. examined seafood and seawater isolates of *V. parahaemolyticus, V. fluvialis,* and *V. mimicus* for virulence factors (*506*). All strains hydrolyzed DNA, starch, gelatin, and chitin. Results for hemolysin, chondroitin, collagen, elastin, and lecithin tests varied. Five of 70 seafood isolates of *V. parahaemolyticus* and 1 of 49 seawater isolates produced thermostable direct hemolysin. All four *V. fluvialis* strains gave positive results in tests for skin permeability factor and three were lethal to mice, but none caused fluid accumulation in suckling mice. All three *V. mimicus* strains produced skin permeability factor and were lethal to mice; two caused fluid accumulation in suckling mice.

As part of their phylogenetic study of the genus *Vibrio*, Coelho et al. analyzed the V1 and V2 variable regions of the 16S rRNA of three strains of *V. cholerae* and one of *V. mimicus* (*507*). A region of 263 base pairs amplified by the PCR included V1 and V2. The *V. cholerae* strains had identical sequences except for one strain's extra G in a 5-G stretch beginning at position 144. The *V. mimicus* strain had T substituted for *V. cholerae*'s C at positions 188 and 219. However, when attempts were made to align these sequences with rDNA sequences for other *Vibrio* species, a dichotomy was seen in the size of the V1 region, which includes helix 6 and its associated loop. *Vibrio cholerae, V. mimicus, V. vulnificus, V. anguillarum,* and *V. diazotrophicus* had a 46-nucleotide V1, whereas other species had 54- or 55-nucleotide V1 regions. A phylogeny of *Vibrio* was constructed on the basis of these observations.

## *Vibrio cholerae*

THE 7TH CHOLERA PANDEMIC: *V. CHOLERAE* O1. Updates on the number and geographical distribution of cases and the mortality associated with the 7th cholera pandemic were published by the World Health Organization (*508–510*). An epidemic of *V. cholerae* O1 Eltor broke out in Peru in 1991 and rapidly spread throughout Central and South America, with the result that the WHO's Region of the Americas far outstripped Africa and Asia in number of cases by 1993. Popovic et al. discussed food-related aspects of cholera in the Americas, including food-related outbreaks, pathophysiology and clinical features, sources and transmission, and isolation and identification of *V. cholerae* from food (*511*). With one exception, no documented cases of reported cholera have resulted from internationally regulated commercial food trade. However, more than 100 cases of cholera in the USA have been associated with seafood eaten in Latin America or brought into the USA from Latin America by tourists. *Vibrio cholerae* persists as a free-living organism in Australian and U.S. Gulf Coast waters, and 65 domestically acquired cases of cholera have been reported in the USA since 1973.

A case–control study determined risk factors for cholera in Guayaquil, Ecuador, an epidemic area (*512*). Risk was increased by drinking unboiled water (OR 4.0, 95% CI 1.8–7.5), drinking a beverage purchased from a street vendor (OR 2.8, 95% CI 1.3–5.9), eating raw seafood (OR 3.4, 95% CI 1.4–11.5), or eating cooked crab (OR 5.1, 95% CI 1.4–19.2). *Vibrio cholerae* O1 biotype Eltor serotype Inaba was recovered from a pooled sample of conch and from 68% of stool samples from case-patients. More than one-third of fecal isolates were resistant to multiple antibiotics. Other investigators also reported emergence of multiple antibiotic resistance in strains of *V. cholerae* O1 Eltor from Guayaquil (*513*).

Two large outbreaks of cholera have occurred recently in Argentina (*514*). More than 90% of isolates from these outbreaks were serotype Ogawa. All strains associated from the first outbreak and most of those from the second were sensitive to all first-line antibiotics. However, during the second outbreak one clinical isolate of *V. cholerae* O1 Eltor serotype Ogawa showed transferable resistance to ampicillin, cephalothin, aztreonam, cefotaxime, sulphisoxazole, gentamicin, and kanamycin.

A case of cholera caused by *V. cholerae* O1 Eltor, serotype Ogawa, was reported in a southern Italian coastal town in October 1994 (*515*). The presumed source of infection was fish contaminated with accidentally infected seawater. Raw fish, especially mullet and cuttlefish purchased from local markets, is the confirmed source of recent cases of cholera in this area.

Colombo et al. reviewed the current cholera pandemic as it has affected Luanda, Angola (*516*). Here too, resistance and multiple resistance to ampicillin, tetracycline, chloramphenicol, sulfonamide, trimethoprim, and erythromycin is growing. The epidemic recurs in a seasonal pattern, peaking in April and May of the hot rainy season that lasts from January to June. In 1992, 56 of 57 O1 isolates were serotype Inaba, whereas Ogawa was the only serotype seen in 1988. Water from the Bengo River appears to be the major source of contamination.

Epstein discussed the possible role of algal blooms in the persistence and spread of cholera (*517*). The marine microbiota is a known reservoir for *V. cholerae*. The distribution of infectious diseases in plants and animals depends on interactions within the entire community of organisms, and global changes are altering marine ecosystems and population compositions on a large scale. Epstein suggests that when *V. cholerae* O1 Eltor arrived in the Americas, perhaps in the bilge water of a foreign ship, it found an algal host in which to survive unfavorable conditions. When algal populations and their associated vibrios grew exponentially, the blooms were consumed by fish, molluscs, and crustaceans, large populations of infected carriers were generated, and the infection was transported into numerous coastal communities.

THE 8TH CHOLERA PANDEMIC: *V. CHOLERAE* O139 (BENGAL). At the same time that the 7th pandemic appeared to be winding down, the 8th may have begun (*508–510*). During 1993 a new serotype of pathogenic *Vibrio cholerae*, different from the 138 serotypes previously known and now identified as *V. cholerae* O139 (Bengal), caused outbreaks of cholera in Bangladesh, India, Pakistan, Nepal, China, and Malaysia and imported cases were reported by several countries. The clinical disease produced by *V. cholerae* O139 and modes of its transmission appear similar to those of *V.*

*cholerae* O1. However, because populations in endemic countries have no immunity to the new serogroup, the attack rate is high and the proportion of cases in adults is abnormally large. A shift in the predominant organism associated with acute diarrhea occurred in the Indian subcontinent in November 1992, when the previously dominant *V. cholerae* O1 was superseded by a non-O1 serogroup in patients admitted to Calcutta's Infectious Diseases Hospital (*518*). A similar change was taking place in Bangladesh. The new strain not only produced cholera toxin copiously; it also hybridized with probes for the newly described zonula occludens toxin. The displacement of *V. cholerae* O1 with a non-O1 strain of such virulence and producing so similar an illness is unprecedented in the history of cholera. Non-O1 strains had previously been called "non-cholera vibrios"; they had been associated with sporadic cases of gastroenteritis in many parts of the world, but were considered incapable of causing epidemics (*519*). Routine methods for detecting *V. cholerae* O1 will not identify O139, and vaccines currently available or under development for O1 are not expected to protect against O139 (*520*). Since the spread of the new organism cannot be predicted (witness the behavior of *V. cholerae* O1 Eltor in the 7th pandemic), unremitting vigilance is necessary in surveillance and in assuring the safety of water supplies and the adequacy of sewage treatment.

The International Centre for Diarrhoeal Diseases Research described the epidemic of cholera-like disease that began in southern Bangladesh in December 1992 (*521*). By the end of March 1993, more than 100,000 cases and 1473 deaths had been reported. The new epidemic strain, *V. cholerae* O139, appears more closely related to Eltor than to classical vibrios, resembling Eltor in its resistance to polymyxin B and its agglutination of chicken erythrocytes. The emergence of O139 as an epidemic serotype raises further questions of its genetic relationship to serotype O1 biotype Eltor. A battery of molecular studies by Hall et al. at the U.S. FDA indicated that the newly emergent *V. cholerae* non-O1 isolate 1837 is an O-antigen mutant of an Eltor strain with an array of virulence determinants typical of serotype O1 biotype Eltor, and is not a non-O1 strain that has acquired virulence genes by genetic transfer (*522*). The O1 antigen can no longer be relied on as an exclusive indicator of the potential significance of an isolate.

Whereas *V. cholerae* O1 is usually isolated from <1% of Bangladeshi surface-water samples even during epidemics, Islam et al. found O139 in 11 of 92 samples they tested (12%) (*523,524*). These isolates had the same properties as clinical isolates of O139. They were unreactive with an MAb specific for the A factor of

*V. cholerae* O1 but reacted with an MAb raised against serogroup O139. All strains generated the expected fragment of the cholera toxin *ctxA* gene by the PCR. The finding of the new organism in a surprisingly large proportion of water samples suggests that it is hardier than O1 and probably has a competitive advantage, in view of the virtual disappearance of disease caused by *V. cholerae* O1 in areas where O139 is found. Meanwhile, the O139 epidemic reached Thailand in April–June 1993 (*525*). This was the first report of dispersion of the organism beyond India and Bangladesh. The authors compared the earlier, relatively slow spread of Eltor from Indonesia through Bangkok to India with the very rapid spread of O139 in the other direction. The organism had also spread west to Pakistan by the end of 1993 (*526*).

Jesudason et al. reported a case of bloodstream invasion by *V. cholerae* 0139 (*527*). Their observations suggest a different view of the pathogen from that of Hall et al. (*522*). Jesudason et al. point out that non-O1 vibrios sometimes cause bacteremia or septicemia in subjects with predisposing factors such as liver disease, and their patient had cirrhosis. They conclude that *V. cholerae* O139 has acquired the ability to produce cholera toxin while retaining the propensity of non-O1 vibrios to invade the bloodstream.

Cheasty et al. identified 5 strains of *V. cholerae* O139 in England during spring and summer of 1993 (*528*). Four were clinical isolates from patients who had recently returned from travel in India or Bangladesh. No history of recent travel could be established for the fifth patient. The authors do not consider O139 to pose a serious threat in countries with safe drinking water and good sanitation, although it is epidemiologically important to test for the organism.

Individuals with blood group O have an increased risk of contracting cholera caused by *V. cholerae* O1 Eltor and they are less well protected by at least one cholera vaccine. Individuals with blood type AB are particularly resistant. However, there is no correlation between blood group and susceptibility to diarrhea caused by non-O1 serogroups or ETEC. Therefore Faruque et al. looked for an association between ABO blood groups and clinical disease caused by the new O139 serogroup (*529*). Patients who had O139-related diarrhea were nearly twice as likely as controls to be of blood group O. None of the 41 case-patients had blood type AB, compared to 8% of controls.

Garg et al. produced a series of MAbs of different isotypes specific for *V. cholerae* O139 (*530*). The antibodies reacted with a reference strain of serotype O139 but not with reference strains of serotypes O1–O138 and

O140. Moreover, they did not react with any rough (R) culture of *V. cholerae*. The intensity of reaction with O139 varied with the strain. Qadri et al. developed a rapid MAb-based coagulation test for detecting O139 in stool samples (*531*).

Waldor and Mekalanos studied transposon insertion mutants to clarify whether synthesis of the O139 antigen is a consequence of deletion of genes involved in synthesis of the O1 antigen or acquisition of new genes encoding an O139-specific LPS or capsular polysaccharide (*532*). O139⁻ transposon mutants lacked both LPS O side chains and the previously described capsule, suggesting that some of the same genes are involved in synthesis of these two structures. A fragment of DNA adjacent to the end of the transposon was amplified and used in hybridization tests with chromosomal DNA from classical O1, Eltor O1, and O139 strains. Only O139 strains hybridized with the probe. An O139⁻ mutant contained the transposon insertion within the O139-specific fragment. The authors concluded that this transposon insertion is in a gene important for O139 antigen synthesis and that *V. cholerae* O139 acquired unique DNA during its evolution.

Other research groups have also studied similarities and differences between *V. cholerae* O139 and *V. cholerae* O1 Eltor (*533–536*). Higa et al. found that 8 randomly selected isolates of O139 from cholera patients in Bangladesh produced large amounts of cholera toxin, agglutinated human group O erythrocytes, were weakly hemolytic, and were resistant to polymyxin B and both classical- and Eltor-specific phages (*533*). Eltor and O139 had closely related electrophoretic profiles as shown by MEE, but Johnson et al. found that O139 strains were encapsulated and portions of the gene complex for synthesis of the O1 antigen were altered or missing (*534*). The presence of the capsule confers resistance to killing by normal human serum and suggests the potential for bloodstream invasion in susceptible hosts (see ref. *527*). Calia et al. compared O139 with classical and Eltor biotypes of *V. cholerae* O1 by classical microbiologic methods, RFLP analysis of three iron-regulated genes of *V. cholerae* O1, and outer-membrane protein profile analysis (*535*). Results for O139 and Eltor were similar except for O139's constitutive expression of a maltose-inducible outer-membrane protein, OmpS. The authors consider their results consistent with the hypothesis that O139 arose from an O1 strain of biotype Eltor by mutation or loss of the O1-antigen gene cluster. The importance of constitutive expression of OmpS for pathogenesis of *V. cholerae* O139 is being examined. Hisatsune et al. analyzed the O-antigenic LPS and lipid A of *V. cholerae* O139 (*536*). The lipid A contained only glucosamine.

Unlike LPS of *V. cholerae* O1, LPS from O139 contained colitose but not perosamine. A very high serological specificity of O139 LPS was demonstrated.

Sengupta et al. found that *V. cholerae* O139 expresses pili that cross-react with the toxin-coregulated pilus of a *V. cholerae* O1 strain of the classical biotype (*537*). The O139 pili were composed of 20-kDa protein subunits antigenically related to the 20-kDa pilus protein of a diarrheagenic *V. cholerae* O34 strain previously isolated. The O139 pili were involved in intestinal colonization and therefore may contribute to the virulence of the O139 epidemic isolates. Other investigators also purified and characterized pili from a strain of *V. cholerae* O139 and reported that they were morphologically, electrophoretically, and immunologically indistinguishable from the 16-kDa subunit protein of *V. cholerae* O1 (*538*). However, the O139 and O1 pili differed in their hemagglutination inhibition patterns.

Yamashiro et al. purified and characterized a new curved, waxy fimbria from a clinical strain of *V. cholerae* O139 (*539*). The organism also produced small numbers of previously reported non-O1 S7-like pili. The molecular size of the fimbrial subunit was <2.5 kDa, and it differed immunologically from the non-O1 S7 pili. The new fimbrial antigen was detected in all gram-negative bacteria tested (182 strains representing 6 genera) but was not found in any gram-positive organism. The authors postulated that this antigen is a primitive antigen possessed by ancestral organisms before the differentiation of *V. cholerae, V. parahaemolyticus, Aeromonas, Escherichia, Klebsiella,* and *Shigella.*

Faruque analyzed RFLP patterns of *ctxA* and rRNA genes in 27 clinical O139 isolates, 48 clinical O1 isolates, and 21 non-O1 environmental isolates including 2 of O139 (*540*). All 29 *V. cholerae* O139 strains had the same ribotype, suggesting that they represent a clone. However, they demonstrated two *ctxA* genotypes and carried three or more copies of this gene; the chromosomal locations of the copies differed from those of Eltor and classical vibrios. The ribotype represented by O139 strains (designated IIB) was distinctly different from ribotypes of the other non-O1 (III–VI) and classical (IA, IB) vibrios but was closely related to that of Eltor vibrios (IIA). An additional 2.6-kilobase band appeared consistently in O139 strains. There were also differences in the RFLPs of *ctxA* between classical, Eltor, and O139 vibrios, suggesting that changes in the serotype-specific genes alone cannot account for the emergence of O139 vibrios. However, the possibility that *V. cholerae* O139 arose from an Eltor strain as a consequence of multiple mutations and genetic exchanges cannot be ruled out. Sutcliffe et al. also studied the cholera toxin gene of *V. cholerae*

O139 (*541*). Their RFLP analysis led to the conclusion that *ctx* is duplicated many times (at least 10) on the chromosome and this enables the organism to produce very large amounts of toxin to elicit a severe pathogenic response. Using a different restriction enzyme, Iida et al. reported two copies of *ctx* in 11 clinical isolates of *V. cholerae* O139 and one copy in one isolate (*542*). Differences in restriction patterns were also seen. However, when sequences covering nearly three-quarters of *ctxB* were amplified and sequenced, the different isolates had identical sequences, which were the same as that reported for Eltor strain 62746. Bhadra et al. found two copies of *ctx*, present in tandem, in most epidemic strains of O139 from India (*543*). Thus questions remain about the origin and relationships of *V. cholerae* O139 and the multiplicity of its cholera toxin gene.

**EPIDEMIOLOGIC AND CLINICAL STUDIES.** Kaysner reviewed the epidemiology, toxicology, and medical aspects of *V. cholerae* O1 and non-O1 cholera and *V. mimicus* infections (*544*). Weber et al. reviewed reports of cholera outbreaks and sporadic cases in the USA, 1965–1991, to identify and assess the risks for cholera among U.S. residents (*545*). Forty-two of the 136 confirmed cases were acquired abroad, 93 were domestic cases, and the source of 1 was unknown. The majority of domestically acquired cases (60%) were related to the endemic Gulf Coast focus of *V. cholerae* O1, and the major food vehicle was shellfish, particularly crabs, harvested from the Gulf of Mexico or nearby estuaries. In 1991, 11 of 26 domestically acquired cases were caused by food from Ecuador; 3 were caused by food from Thailand. Overall in 1991, the rate of cholera among air travelers returning from South America was 0.3 per 100,000, whereas the rate among air travelers returning from Ecuador was 2.6 per 100,000.

Characterization of *V. cholerae* O1 isolated from patients, food, and the environment in Spain indicated that no focus of endemic cholera exists in Spain (*546*). All isolates from the environment and prawns imported from Ecuador were nontoxigenic and were genetically different and more diverse than clinical isolates. A toxigenic isolate from sewage had the same ribotype, electrophoretic type, and pulsed-field gel electrophoresis pattern as the majority of clinical isolates.

Septicemia caused by non-O1 *V. cholerae* is uncommon, but cutaneous involvement is even rarer. A non-O1 strain caused bullous lesions and fatal septicemia in a Texas man with alcoholic cirrhosis who had eaten raw oysters two days before symptoms began (*547*). The pathogen produced a cytotoxic factor that destroyed CHO cells. Another man with a history of diabetes mellitus

and liver cirrhosis became ill in Taiwan, three days after having eaten raw seafood in Manila (*548*). Chills, fever, and general malaise progressed to nausea, vomiting, watery diarrhea, bilateral calf pain, neck stiffness, generalized edema, bullous lesions, septicemia, and meningitis. *Vibrio cholerae* non-O1 grew from four blood cultures.

A case of acute acalculous cholecystitis due to *V. cholerae* O1 biotype Eltor serotype Ogawa was reported in a cholera patient in Ecuador (*549*). The authors postulated that the pathogen reached the gallbladder in a retrograde fashion from the duodenum via the papilla of Vater.

**OCCURRENCE AND SURVIVAL.** Corrales et al. assessed the survival of *V. cholerae* Eltor serotype Inaba in pasteurized milk, freshwater fish, raw beef, and raw chicken at different temperatures (*550*). The organism remained viable in meats for up to 90 d at −5°C and 300 d at −25°C. In milk, it was no longer viable after 34 d at −5°C or 150 d at −25°C. It survived about 32 d in milk at 7°C and 18–20 d in the other foods. At room temperature, survival never exceeded 10 d. It was no longer detectable in chicken or fish after 2 d of incubation at 35°C.

In July 1992, non-O1 *V. cholerae* was isolated from the anus and/or blowhole of five apparently healthy Atlantic bottlenose dolphins (*Tursiops truncatus*) in Matagorda Bay, Texas (*551*). *Vibrio cholerae* non-O1 is commonly found in water, sediment, shellfish, and birds along the northern Gulf Coast. The authors suggest that dolphins provide a continuing source of these bacteria to the environment and that the spread of the bacteria is influenced by the limited home range of the dolphins.

A substance cryoprotective for *V. cholerae* was extracted from the surface of prawn shells from southeast Asia and purified by ammonium sulfate precipitation and gel filtration (*552*). It was a protein of 81 kDa, which the authors dubbed "cryoprotective protein." It binds to the bacterial cell surface in the presence of $Mg^{2+}$ and appears to be a major receptor site for binding to the prawn-shell surface. Adherence is reduced by heat, trypsin treatment, and antiserum against the cryoprotective protein. When $10^8$ cfu/mL of strains of *V. cholerae* or *V. parahaemolyticus* were treated with the protein in buffered saline containing $Mg^{2+}$, more than $10^2$ cfu/mL still survived after 15 d at −20°C whereas none survived without the protein. The protein had no effect on survival of an *E. coli* strain.

**IDENTIFICATION AND TYPING.** Lesmana et al. used a modified CAMP test to identify 973 *V. cholerae* isolates by phenotype (*553*). Eltor and non-O1 strains were

CAMP-positive; classical strains were CAMP-negative. The football-shaped hemolytic zones produced by Eltor strains were easily distinguished from the thin crescent-shaped bands produced by non-O1 strains. For O1 isolates, CAMP phenotyping and conventional biogrouping based on inhibition by polymyxin B were in complete agreement.

Said et al. compared gene probes, a tissue culture assay, an ELISA, and an RPLA kit for detection of cholera toxin in *V. cholerae* non-O1 (*554*). Only 2 of 790 strains gave positive results with the two digoxigenin-labeled polynucleotide probes. The production of one or more other cytotoxins made it impossible to rely on the Y1 cell assay. Cytotoxin production by the probe-positive strains was confirmed by the immunoassays. Of 252 probe-negative strains tested by both cell assay and immunoassay, 90% produced cytotoxin in the cell assay and 37% gave positive results in the cholera toxin ELISA but were negative by RPLA analysis. The authors concluded that many non-O1 strains produce a toxin that binds to $G_{M1}$ and reacts with antisera to cholera toxin, but it is not identical to cholera toxin.

Guglielmetti et al. developed a PCR assay for detection of the *V. cholerae* heat-stable enterotoxin gene using crude DNA preparations from single bacterial colonies (*555*). They also developed a rapid protocol for direct sequence analysis of the amplification product. Analysis of 22 *V. cholerae* non-O1 clinical isolates from Cuba demonstrated a higher prevalence of the heat-stable enterotoxin gene than has been reported for other nonepidemic areas.

A multiplex PCR was reported that rapidly distinguishes cholera from noncholera vibrios by the presence of the virulence genes *ctxA* and *tcpA* (*556*). These genes encode, respectively, the enzymatic subunit of cholera toxin and the major subunit of the colonization factor. Multiplex PCRs could be a valuable tool for improving *V. cholerae* surveillance. Another rapid PCR method was optimized for detection of enterotoxigenic *V. cholerae* in foods (*557*). It could detect a single colony-forming unit per 10 g of oysters, crabmeat, shrimp, or lettuce in amplification reactions from crude bacterial lysates.

A number of methods were reported for use with clinical specimens. PCRs were developed for detection of *V. cholerae* in stools (*558,559*). Two commercial rapid diagnostic MAb kits were highly specific for *V. cholerae* O1 in stools and detected cholera more frequently than did culture (*560*). A coagglutination assay was used for rapid detection of acute cholera in airline passengers (*561*). Two cholera cases were diagnosed using an enzyme-labeled oligonucleotide *ctx* probe in a clinical laboratory at the Osaka Airport Quarantine Station (*562*).

The test gave positive results for the cholera toxin gene in suspicious colonies within 3 h. It could also detect *ctx* directly in stool specimens. Hasan et al. reported development of a colorimetric immunodiagnostic kit, Cholera SMART, for direct detection of *V. cholerae* O1 in clinical specimens (*563*). The kit was successfully field-tested in Bangladesh and Mexico.

Popovic et al. reported a standardized ribotype scheme based on data from 214 clinical and environmental strains of *V. cholerae* O1 isolated in 35 countries during the past 60 years (*564*). The ribotype patterns are reproducible and stable with time. Sixteen strains of the classical biotype demonstrated 7 distinguishable but very similar ribotypes, designated 1a–1g. Twenty ribotypes and subtypes were seen in 198 strains of biotype Eltor; 6 were seen in strains from the 7th pandemic. Ribotype 8 originated only in central Africa and ribotype 3 originated mainly in Asia and the Pacific Islands. Strains of ribotype 5 are the cause of the current Latin American epidemic. This ribotype was also seen in several other geographical locations, but further molecular methods can differentiate these strains from the Latin American strains. Ribotype 6 was the most widely distributed. It was subdivided into three subtypes. Clinical isolates of U.S. Gulf Coast strains were ribotype 2. Strains related to northeast Australian rivers were ribotypes 9 and 10. Nontoxigenic O1 strains from Latin America and the U.S. Gulf Coast did not form a specific cluster of ribotypes.

Choudhury et al. determined the genomic size and RFLP patterns of *V. cholerae* strains of various serovars and biotypes (*565*). Classical strains had a genomic size of 3000–3200 kilobases; for Eltor strains it was ~2500 kilobases. This result was surprising because the two biotypes are generally considered isogenic. Clinical nontoxigenic strains of non-O1 vibrios had genomic sizes of ~2400 kilobases and thus resembled Eltor, whereas toxigenic environmental strains had a genomic size of 3000 kilobases and resembled the classical biotype. However, only a few such strains were examined. RFLP analysis further distinguished among the strains.

**PATHOGENICITY AND MOLECULAR STUDIES.** Tikoo et al. examined 43 strains of *V. cholerae* O1 Eltor isolated from children and adults with diarrhea, sewage, and water from the Ganges River for production of hemolysin and enterotoxin, change in hemolytic activity after passage through rabbit ileal loops, and correlation between hemolysin production and enterotoxic activity (*566*). Most strains were nonhemolytic. All hemolytic strains and the majority of nonhemolytic strains caused fluid accumulation in rabbit ileal loops, but hemolytic strains caused significantly more. Nonhemolytic strains that caused little or no fluid accumulation did so, without change in their hemolytic character, after 1–4 passages through rabbit ileal loops. They did become hemolytic after more passages through rabbit gut. After storage or repeated subculture they reverted to their original non-hemolytic nature but remained enterotoxic. The authors concluded that Eltor hemolysin is not responsible for fluid accumulation in rabbit gut.

Extracellular proteases are thought to be important in the pathogenesis of diarrheal disease caused by *V. cholerae*. Ichinose et al. investigated the effect of a purified *V. cholerae* protease on enterotoxicity by treating rabbit ileal loops with protease and then inoculating them with low-protease-producing strains of live vibrios, cholera toxin, or Eltor hemolysin (*567*). Protease treatment enhanced fluid accumulation in a dose-related manner after challenge with live *V. cholerae* O1 or non-O1, but not after challenge with purified toxins. The authors concluded that the vibrio protease enhances enterotoxicity by degrading the protective epithelial mucosal layer. This facilitates the colonization of the epithelial cell surface by vibrios and affords enterotoxic factors better access to their receptors.

Toxin-coregulated pili are a virulence determinant and protective antigen for classical *V. cholerae* O1, but their importance for the Eltor biotype is less clear. By overexpressing the Eltor *tcpA* gene in *E. coli,* Voss and Attridge prepared a biotype-specific anti-TcpA serum, which was a sensitive indicator of TcpA production in immunoblotting assays (*568*). By immunoelectron microscopy, antiserum against a cell envelope fraction rich in processed Eltor TcpA revealed typical toxin-coregulated pilus bundles on the cell surface of five Eltor strains known to produce TcpA in vitro. In further studies, Attridge et al. used the infant mouse model to evaluate the role of toxin-coregulated pili in the pathogenesis of *V. cholerae* O1 Eltor cholera (*569*). Four Eltor strains bearing insertion mutations in *tcpA* were drastically reduced in virulence and their in vivo persistence was impaired in mixed-infection competition experiments. Virulence was restored by providing a functional *tcp* operon in *trans*, confirming that the pathogenic potential of Eltor strains depends on a product or products of this operon.

Nakasone and Iwanaga showed that in classical *V. cholerae* O1 it is not the pili but a colonization factor located in the outer membrane that is important in intestinal adhesion (*570*). The classical strain 86B3 has at least two types of cell-associated hemagglutinin: one L-fucose-sensitive and associated with the cell wall, and one D-mannose-sensitive and pilus-associated. Pilus-rich and poorly piliated variants adhered equally well to

rabbit intestine. Adhesion was partially inhibited by L-fucose, but not by D-mannose or by an anti-pilus antibody fraction. The incomplete inhibition by L-fucose suggests the presence of one or more L-fucose-resistant colonization factors in the cell wall as well.

*Vibrio cholerae* has a *recA* system analogous to that of *E. coli*, and duplication and amplification of the cholera toxin gene depends on the *recA* product. Kumar et al. tested RecA$^+$ parent strains and mutants defective in *recA* for ability to adhere to isolated rabbit intestine and colonize the intestine of infant mice (*571*). The proportion of mutants adhering to isolated intestine was only about one-third that of wild type. Nor did *recA* mutants colonize the intestine efficiently. The mutant of one strain was eliminated from the gut within 24 h, whereas the parent colonized the gut and showed high viable counts for up to 72 h.

Some strains of *V. cholerae* O1 produce both cholera toxin and a heat-stable enterotoxin analogous to that of ETEC. Yoshino et al. purified and sequenced the heat-stable enterotoxin of *V. cholerae* O1 Eltor serotype Inaba from strain GP156 (*572*). They found four molecular species, all of which contained three disulfide linkages and had the same *C*-terminal 13-residue sequence, but varied in length. Loss of *N*-terminal residues rendered the toxins more potent. Thus the toxin with the shortest chain length (17 residues) was ten times as potent as the longest toxin, with 28 residues.

In *V. cholerae*, the gene *epsE* is essential for extracellular secretion of cholera toxin and protease. To characterize other genes involved in protein secretion, Overbye et al. studied transposon insertion mutants (*573*). They found that *epsM* encodes a 18.5-kDa protein similar to proteins required for extracellular secretion of pullulanase, pectase lyase, or elastase in other gram-negative bacteria. Most of the EpsM protein is in the cytoplasmic membrane fraction. The gene is located on a 15-kilobase DNA fragment that also contains *epsE*. Two partial reading frames showing similarity to *pulL* and *pulN* of *Klebsiella oxytoca* were designated *epsL* and *epsN*. The authors concluded that genes required for extracellular secretion of enterotoxin and other proteins are clustered in *V. cholerae* and that hemagglutinin, protease, chitinase, and heat-labile enterotoxin are transported through the outer membrane by the same general secretion pathway.

A clinical isolate of nontoxigenic *V. cholerae* O1 that caused intestinal fluid accumulation in adult mice also had proteolytic, hemolytic, and cytotoxic activities in vitro (*574*). Transposon mutagenesis studies showed that the fluid-accumulation activity was independent of proteolytic activity but closely associated with cytotoxic and hemolytic activities. These observations confirm those of other investigators who have demonstrated a linkage in toxigenic *V. cholerae* O1 and non-O1 of cytotoxin and hemolysin with fluid accumulation in rabbit ileal loops. Production of cytotoxin and hemolysin may be involved in the pathogenesis of infections by strains of *V. cholerae* O1 that do not produce cholera toxin.

*Vibrio cholerae* persists in different environments by expressing the particular set of genes appropriate for survival under the prevailing conditions. Thus several key determinants of virulence are coordinately regulated. The regulatory gene *hlyU* up-regulates transcription of the gene for the Eltor secreted hemolysin, *hlyA*. Williams et al. sequenced *hlyU* and investigated its importance for virulence (*575*). In addition to HlyA, *hlyU* up-regulates expression of a 28-kDa secreted protein. A 100-fold increase in $LD_{50}$ in the infant mouse cholera model was associated with a mutation in *hlyU*, indicating that this regulator is required in vivo for expression of HlyA and possibly other virulence determinants. Further studies will investigate the possibility that HlyU activity responds to specific environmental signals and that other proteins help mediate the effects of these signals.

Rodrigues et al. analyzed the virulence factors of 188 *V. cholerae* non-O1 isolates from seawater at beaches near Rio de Janeiro (*576*). Forty-three percent of samples were positive in the vascular permeability factor test in guinea pigs; 29% caused intestinal fluid accumulation in suckling mice; and 63% produced hemolysin. However, only 4% gave positive results in all three tests. Ramamurthy et al. emphasized that the clinical significance of *V. cholerae* non-O1 must be evaluated in terms of the complete spectrum of virulence factors (*577*). They studied virulence patterns of 28 clinical isolates from Calcutta, of which 18 were the sole cause of infection and 10 occurred along with *V. cholerae* O1 infection. Serogroups O5, O11, and O34 predominated in the 23 strains that could be serotyped. Serovars O7, O14, O34, O39, and O97 were isolated only from cases in which *V. cholerae* non-O1 was the sole cause of infection. Nearly all strains were cytotoxic for CHO, HeLa, and Vero cells with end-point titers of 4–512. Only a few strains produced a cytotonic effect. Twenty-one strains hemolyzed rabbit and sheep erythrocytes; fewer were active against chicken and human erythrocytes. Ten strains, nine of which were associated with sole infection, agglutinated human blood. The dominant hemagglutination inhibition pattern was inhibition by mannose but not fucose and galactose. The predominant phenotype was one that produced Eltor hemolysin, a cytotoxin, and a cell-associated hemagglutinin.

Zitzer et al. studied the properties and pore-forming activity of an enterocytolysin produced by a strain of *V. cholerae* non-O1 (*578*). The cytolysin was inactivated by heat, induced production of specific antibodies in rabbits, and did not react with a cholera B-subunit antiserum or with nonimmune serum. It caused hemolysis by a colloid–osmotic mechanism resulting from formation of hydrophilic pores 1.8–2.0 nm in diameter in the cell membrane. It also opened anion-selective pores in lipid membranes. The mechanism of action resembles that of the α-hemolysins of *E. coli* and *Staphylococcus aureus*.

A clinical strain of cholera toxin–negative *V. cholerae* O34 produces a 20-kDa pilus protein with hemagglutination and intestinal adherence properties (*579*). It is antigenically and morphologically distinct from the toxin-coregulated pilus and other types of pili expressed by O1 and non-O1 vibrios. Other investigators characterized the pili of non-O1 strain V10 isolated from stream water in Thailand (*580*). These pili were physicochemically and immunologically distinct from pili of non-O1 strain S7, although the *N*-terminal amino acid sequences were identical up to residue 24 (with the possible exception of residues 1 and 5, which were not determined). There was also high sequence homology between V10 and the flexible pili of *V. parahaemolyticus*, *Aeromonas hydrophila*, and *Aeromonas sobria*, but none with TcpA of *V. cholerae* O1. V10 pilus antigen was found in about 30% of clinical and environmental non-O1 strains but in none of 60 Eltor and classical O1 strains examined. In contrast, the S7 antigen was seen in all O1 strains but in only 16% of non-O1 strains.

As in O1 strains, the expression of cholera toxin and TcpA is coordinately regulated by environmental factors in *V. cholerae* O139. Waldor and Mekalanos showed that O139 derivatives containing a *toxR* null mutation did not express cholera toxin, TcpA, and the outer membrane protein OmpU, indicating dependence on ToxR (*581*). Close similarities between Eltor and O139 strains are suggested by their sharing of an RFLP for *tcpA* and by their production of cholera toxin under similar cultural conditions. The authors conclude that although O139 is a new serogroup of *V. cholerae*, it conforms to the fundamental theme seen in O1 strains: ToxR mediates coordinate regulation of virulence gene expression.

## Vibrio vulnificus

EPIDEMIOLOGY. *Vibrio vulnificus* infection is rare in healthy people, but individuals who are immunocompromised or who have achlorhydria, chronic liver disease, or hemochromatosis are at high risk for fatal infection. Raw oysters are the major source of infection via the gastrointestinal tract. Because the groups at risk are well defined and high risk is associated with eating raw oysters, Ross et al. conducted a study to determine whether nutrition education had been available to people in high-risk groups and whether it had influenced their behavior (582). About one-quarter of the study participants recalled having been instructed to avoid eating raw oysters and one-fifth recalled being told to cook oysters before eating them. Only 26% recalled receiving any type of food safety counseling. Thirty-six percent of at-risk subjects reported eating raw oysters. The major reason given for *not* eating them was not liking them (63%); only 21% cited nutrition education as a reason for avoiding raw oysters. These findings underscore the need for nutrition education for people at high risk for *V. vulnificus* infection. Data on *V. vulnificus* infections associated with raw oysters also illustrate the problem (583). From 1981 through 1992, 125 cases of infection and 44 resulting deaths were reported in Florida. These represented 72 cases of primary septicemia, 35 wound infections, and 18 cases of gastroenteritis. Among patients with primary septicemia, 58 (81%) had eaten raw oysters during the week before onset of illness. Fourteen (78%) of patients with gastroenteritis also had eaten raw oysters. Of the 40 deaths caused by septicemia, 35 were associated with consumption of raw oysters. The death rate among patients with preexisting liver disease was twice that in patients not known to have liver disease. The estimated annual rate of oyster-associated *V. vulnificus* infection in adults with liver disease was 72 per million—80 times the rate for adults without liver disease who ate raw oysters.

Investigation of a raw oyster–related death from *V. vulnificus* infection uncovered a possibly fraudulent scheme to circumvent warning requirements for oysters (584). A visitor from Japan who had had hepatitis in his youth ate two raw oysters in a California restaurant. California law requires restaurants serving Gulf Coast oysters to post warnings of the risks to people with a history of liver disease. The restaurant had no such warnings because the oysters were identified as Virginia Blue Point oysters. However, the oysters were from the Gulf Coast. They had been correctly tagged when harvested, but when routed through a distributor in Virginia they were reportedly retagged to indicate an East-coast harvest site.

OCCURRENCE AND BEHAVIOR. Groubert and Oliver reported that the virulence of *V. vulnificus* and conversion

rates between the encapsulated virulent form and the nonencapsulated avirulent form are not changed by passage through oysters (585). They used a transposon mutant in their studies so they could specifically follow the fate of organisms that were fed to oysters in the laboratory. These studies also showed that vibrios fed in the laboratory were readily eliminated by UV-assisted depuration, whereas vibrios residing in the oysters before the laboratory feeding did not depurate. This underscores the lack of a satisfactory model for depuration of laboratory-infected oysters and the inadequacy of depuration for freeing naturally contaminated oysters of the organism.

Studies by Kaspar and Tamplin further defined conditions influencing the survival of *V. vulnificus* in seawater and oysters (586). Survival was poor at temperatures below 8.5°C. When salinity was between 5 and 25‰, populations increased or remained stable during a 6-day incubation at 14°C. Populations decreased by about 60–90% at salinities of 30–38‰. The organism was lysed in deionized water. Endogenous populations of *V. vulnificus* in oyster shellstock increased >100-fold during a 14-day incubation at 30°C but showed a 10-fold reduction after incubation at 2–4°C and a 100-fold reduction at 0°C. Other investigators monitored the survival and viability of *V. vulnificus* in seawater by flow cytometry and with a fluorescent dye that stains only living cells (587). Resuscitation experiments with cells starved for 14 days at 4°C suggested that the viable but nonculturable state is a transient state leading to cell death. The increase in cell numbers after the temperature was raised from 4 to 20°C was due to proliferation of cells that had not entered the nonculturable state.

DePaola et al. used a most-probable-number procedure to determine the densities of *V. vulnificus* in the intestines of finfish, oysters, and crabs, water, and sediment from the U.S. Gulf Coast (588). Densities were low during winter and the organism was isolated more frequently from sheepshead fish than from water or sediment. From April to October, population densities were 2–5 $\log_{10}$ higher in estuarine fish than in water, sediment, crabs, and oysters. The highest densities were in the intestinal contents of bottom-feeding fish that eat molluscs and crustaceans ($10^8$ per 100 g). Densities in fish that feed primarily on plankton and other finfish were similar to those in oysters, crabs, and sediment ($10^5$ per 100 g). The organism was found infrequently in offshore fish. The presence of large populations of *V. vulnificus* in common estuarine fish may provide clues to the pathogen's growth and transport and suggests precautions against food- and wound-related infections.

Veenstra et al. studied seasonal variations in occurrence of *V. vulnificus* along the Dutch North Sea coast, in relation to water temperature and salinity (*589*). In two consecutive years, the organism was isolated from water samples in August, when the water temperature was highest.

**IDENTIFICATION.** Miceli et al. developed a direct plating procedure for enumerating *V. vulnificus* in oyster homogenates and individual oysters (*590*). A seasonal variation was seen in population densities in oysters harvested from the Atlantic and Gulf coasts. The results indicated that people who eat raw oysters ingest millions of cells of this opportunistic pathogen. Since *V. vulnificus*-related illness is rare in healthy people who eat raw oysters and lethal illness is fairly unusual even in health-compromised individuals, the authors concluded that the lethal dose may be quite high.

Brauns and Oliver reported a PCR procedure using whole-cell lysates for detection of *V. vulnificus* (*591*).

Aznar et al. evaluated ribotyping and RAPD analysis as tools for epidemiologic studies of *V. vulnificus* (*592*). They found RAPD analysis faster for identification of biotypes. It also allowed identification of individual strains. The same research group determined seven new 16S RNA gene sequences of pathogenic vibrios and compared them with previously published sequences, confirming that *V. vulnificus* represents a group of organisms not closely related to the core organisms of the genus (*593*). Moreover, their dendrogram showed that *V. vulnificus, V. anguillarum,* and *V. diazotrophicus* branch off separately from the core group. By sequencing the variable regions of the 23S rRNA genes of *V. fluvialis, V. furnissii, V. harveyi, V. cholerae,* and *V. vulnificus* and comparing these sequences with all published bacterial 23S rRNA sequences, the authors were able to synthesize four oligonucleotide probes specific for *V. vulnificus.*

Heidelberg et al. developed a procedure for enumerating *V. vulnificus* on membrane filters after hybridization with a fluorescent oligonucleotide probe for eubacteria (*594*). This method eliminates potential loss of cells when bacterial suspensions are transferred to gelatin-coated slides. It can be adapted for other specific microbial populations.

**VIRULENCE AND PATHOGENICITY.** *Vibrio vulnificus* biotype 1 is an opportunistic human pathogen; biotype 2 has been defined as an obligate eel pathogen. Amaro et al. compared the virulence mechanisms of the two biotypes in mice (*595*). The biotypes shared characteristics of capsule expression, iron uptake, and production of exoproteins with a virulence role in mice. Because bio-

type 2 was at least as virulent for mice as clinical strains of biotype 1, it can be concluded that biotype 2 is potentially pathogenic for humans; and in fact, at least one case of septicemia has been reported, in a man who handled a contaminated eel.

Miyoshi et al. reviewed the exocellular protease, cytolysin, and other toxic factors produced by *V. vulnificus* (*596*).

*Vibrio vulnificus* produces a capsular polysaccharide that is essential for virulence. Hayat et al. analyzed the capsular types of clinical and environmental strains of *V. vulnificus* (*597*). Four of 21 clinical strains but none of 67 environmental strains reacted with antisera raised against the capsular polysaccharide of clinical strain MO6-24. Thirteen other capsular types were identified among 15 strains from which capsular material was extracted.

Oh et al. developed a procedure for purification of a *V. vulnificus* hemolysin by hydrophobic column chromatography in the presence of detergent (*598*). The method provides enough hemolysin to permit pathogenic and mechanistic studies.

One problem in studying *V. vulnificus* has been the difficulty of introducing foreign DNA. McDougald et al. introduced recombinant plasmids into four strains of *V. vulnificus* by electroporation (*599*). Efficiency was improved by use of a defined growth medium containing glucose, glycine, and betaine.

### *Vibrio parahaemolyticus*

Haddock and Cabanero conducted a case–control study to determine the origin of sporadic *V. parahaemolyticus* infections on Guam (*600*). Case-subjects were asked whether they had eaten seafood during the 24 hours preceding the onset of illness; controls were asked whether they had eaten seafood during the 24 hours preceding the interview. Case-subjects were significantly more likely to have eaten seafood (OR 37.6, 95% CI 8.3–220.2).

The first reported case of reactive arthritis induced by *V. parahaemolyticus* occurred in a 35-year-old Japanese woman (*601*). The patient first sought medical attention because of diarrhea and abdominal pain that developed after she ate raw fish. Manifestations of enterocolitis subsided after 8 days, but by this time polyarthritis was so severe that she was unable to walk or stand.

A PCR method was developed for specific detection of the *V. parahaemolyticus* thermostable direct haemolysin gene, *tdh* (*602*). It clearly identifies TDH-producing strains and provides an alternative to conventional methods for TDH detection. A new latex agglutination test allows rapid identification of *V. para-haemolyticus* (603). A few strains of *V. alginolyticus, V. harveyi,* and *V. mimicus* gave false-positive results.

Lin et al. reported that *V. parahaemolyticus* has a homolog of the *V. cholerae toxRS* operon that mediates environmentally induced regulation of *tdh* (604). All clinical and environmental strains tested contained the *V. parahaemolyticus toxRS* genes, which were designated Vp-*toxRS*. The deduced amino acid sequences of the Vp-*toxRS* products contained regions similar to the proposed transmembrane and activity domains of the *V. cholerae toxRS* products. In the presence of Vp-ToxS, Vp-ToxR promoted expression of *tdh*2, one of the two *tdh* genes carried by strains positive for the Kanagawa phenomenon. The promotion of *tdh* expression was at the transcription level. Vp-ToxR was essential for enterotoxic activity in the rabbit ileal loop. Thus the *toxR* homologs share the function of direct stimulation of the gene encoding a major enterotoxin in a *Vibrio* species.

## Other Vibrios

Some strains of *Vibrio mimicus* produce toxins similar to cholera toxin and heat-stable enterotoxin, but their frequency is estimated to be under 10% for both clinical and environmental isolates. Recently *V. mimicus* was found to produce a hemolysin similar to the TDH of *V. parahaemolyticus*, and its gene was homologous to *tdh*. Uchimura et al. compared the frequency of TDH-like toxin production in clinical and environmental strains of *V. mimicus* (605). Sixteen of 17 clinical strains and one of 2 strains isolated from seafood produced the toxin, whereas no environmental strain did. The seafood in which the toxin-positive strain was detected had caused food poisoning. Cholera-like toxin was detected in one environmental strain. Heat-stable enterotoxin–like toxin was not detected in any strain. The *V. mimicus* TDH gene was detected by a DNA primer specific for *V. parahaemolyticus tdh*. Thus both the TDH gene and a TDH-like toxin were frequently detected in *V. mimicus* isolated from patients with diarrhea.

Ramamurthy et al. studied 13 *V. mimicus* strains from clinical and environmental sources (606). One environmental strain produced cholera-like toxin. Five strains produced a hemolysin that cross-reacted with TDH. Two strains hybridized with a DNA probe specific for the heat-stable enterotoxin of *V. cholerae* non-O1. Culture supernatants of all strains produced a factor that was cytotoxic to Vero and CHO cells. This study demonstrates that *V. mimicus* has the genetic potential to produce several types of toxin simultaneously. Nevertheless, in Calcutta, the organism is seldom isolated from

hospitalized patients with diarrhea even when specific efforts are made to find it. This may mean that the organism is not an important pathogen or that better methods are needed to detect it.

Abbot and Janda reported two cases of severe gastroenteritis caused by *Vibrio hollisae* (607). Both patients had eaten raw shellfish. Previous reports of *V. hollisae* infections in the USA were restricted to the Atlantic seaboard and the Gulf Coast. The two new cases were seen in California and Hawaii.

A healthy 70-year-old man acquired a lethal *Vibrio damsela* infection after cutting himself while filleting bluefish at the New Jersey shore (608). He had no known history of diabetes or liver disease. Hansen et al. reported two severe infections caused by *Vibrio metschnikovii* (609). Both were in elderly people, and no source of infection was identified in either case. Magalhães et al. found evidence of pathogenic potential in some strains of *Vibrio furnissii* tested in the laboratory (610).

## *AEROMONAS*

### Public Health Significance

Some strains of *Aeromonas* occurring in food and water can produce enterotoxins, cytotoxins, and/or hemolysins and are able to invade epithelial cells. Kirov discussed species of *Aeromonas* that are found in foods and raised some questions that need to be answered before the public health risk posed by these organisms can be evaluated (611). Most published reports of foodborne *Aeromonas* gastroenteritis have implicated minimally processed or frozen foods, predominantly seafood and oysters, that were inadequately cooked before being eaten. In a few cases the link between clinical illness and consumption of a contaminated food was very strong; but not many cases have been reported and there are many epidemiologic puzzles. The incidence, distribution, and virulence properties of *Aeromonas* species in foods varies regionally. Species naturally present in foods can grow—sometimes competitively—at low temperatures, their populations increasing 10- to 1000-fold during 7–10 days at 5°C. Salt concentration, pH, atmosphere, and competing microflora interactively influence the growth and survival of aeromonads in foods at low temperature. The behavior of the organisms in foods suggests that illness can result both from colonization and in vivo expression of virulence factors and from ingestion of foods containing preformed toxins. However, toxin production in foods seems less efficient than in bacteriological media, and most toxins are heat-labile. Until questions concerning the pathogenicity of *Aeromonas* and the organism's behavior in foods are answered, the presence of large numbers of aeromonads in food should be regarded as a health threat, particularly for immunocompromised persons.

Palumbo reviewed the occurrence and significance of organisms of the *Aeromonas hydrophila* group in food and water (*612*). Although these organisms are widespread in foods and the environment and can be isolated as the sole pathogen from cases of diarrhea in humans, modern molecular identification methods suggest that food and water isolates differ from clinical isolates. It is interesting that expression of virulence-associated factors is enhanced by culture at temperatures below 37°C. Palumbo discussed sources of *A. hydrophila*, its behavior in foods and the environment, and traditional and modern techniques for characterizing isolates. Ribotyping is one of the more promising tools for epidemiologic studies.

The case of a cardiac surgeon at The Mount Sinai Hospital, New York, provides a dramatic exception to the general difficulty of establishing a link between diarrheal disease and contaminated food (*613*). The surgeon complained to the author, who was director of microbiology at the clinical laboratories, that he had diarrhea every time he ate egg salad in the hospital cafeteria. The first episode was acute (and memorable). After a second complaint, the microbiologist obtained a swab sample of the egg salad for culture and snacked on the leftovers. Diarrhea developed in the microbiologist 18 h later. β-Hemolytic colonies from stool and egg salad samples cultured on blood agar were identified as *A. hydrophila*. In the kitchen, eggs were customarily boiled, shelled, and placed in a sinkful of water to remove shell fragments. They were then sliced, mixed with mayonnaise, and refrigerated at 5–7°C. The sink and the water were heavily contaminated with *A. hydrophila*, which was subsequently able to grow in the egg salad.

From a regulatory perspective, it is not feasible for the FDA to take regulatory action on fishery products that contain *A. hydrophila* (*614*). Although the organisms are widespread in fish and fish products, it is still not clear whether they represent a public health hazard. Although the strength of the evidence that *A. hydrophila* is a true enteric pathogen is increasing, there is still no entirely satisfactory animal model or other way in which to demonstrate that a particular isolate from food can cause human illness. Moreover, there have been no well documented outbreaks of gastroenteritis caused by this organism.

Kirov et al. divided 182 food, water, and clinical strains of *A. hydrophila* from Australasia into three groups on the basis of biochemical characteristics and tested them for ability to produce hemolysin, enterotoxin, and cytotoxin (*615*). Most food and water strains fell into one group and most clinical strains into another. The third group had only a few members, mostly from environmental sources, and they produced virulence factors only infrequently. There was no correlation between biochemical group and geographical source, but strains from mainland Australia produced virulence factors more frequently than strains from Tasmania or New Zealand. The preponderance of food and water strains in one group suggests that most strains from these sources are not of major public health significance, even though nearly half of the strains from this group produced at least 2 virulence factors.

## Occurrence and Growth in Foods

Huang and Leung assessed bacterial indicators and *A. hydrophila* in channel catfish grown in cage and pond culture in southern Georgia (*616*). Water for cage culture had significantly higher fecal streptococci and *A. hydrophila* populations than water for pond culture, and this was reflected in the microbial populations in skin rinse fluid from the fish. Heading, gutting, and skinning the fish reduced bacterial populations on the fish surface. After 8 days of storage at 4°C, bacterial populations were lower on fish packaged in vacuum bags than on fish packaged in conventional plastic wrap.

Samples of 829 poultry, meat, shellfish, and fish products commonly eaten in Switzerland were examined for mesophilic *Aeromonas* spp. (*617*). Overall, aeromonads were found in 24.1% of the samples. Raw products were frequently contaminated (32 of 34 minced meat samples, 38 of 45 raw chicken samples, 21 of 33 living shellfish samples, and 46 of 49 fresh fish samples), and colony counts were as high as $6 \times 10^6$/g. Thirteen of 34 cooked ham slices and >10% of mortadella, smoked cooked sausage, smoked fish, and gravid salmon samples were also contaminated, but colony counts were no higher than ~$2 \times 10^3$/g. The high contamination rate of cooked and hot-smoked foods suggests recontamination after cooking or smoking. Of the identified strains, 61.2% were *A. hydrophila*, 22.5% were *A. caviae*, and 16.3% were *A. sobria*.

Stecchini et al. examined the effects of temperature (5, 10, 15°C), NaCl (0, 1.5, 3%), and ascorbic acid (0, 0.1, 0.2 mmol/L) on the growth kinetics of a clinical strain of *A. hydrophila* in buffered peptone water (*618*). At 5°C, 0.1 or 0.2% ascorbic acid prevented bacterial growth regardless of NaCl concentration, and 3% NaCl prevented growth regardless of ascorbic acid concentration. Some growth occurred under all other combinations of conditions. In a similar set of experiments they tested 0–3% NaCl, ascorbic acid at concentrations of 1.0 and 2.0 mmol/L, and a mild heat treatment (10–30 min at 46°C) (*619*). The observed data set was best fit by a hyperbolic function. When coefficients were combined to obtain a "death value," the effects of experimental factors on the death value were best described by a quadratic response-surface model. Ascorbic acid and NaCl interacted to increase mortality. Because this death-value model is inconsistent with biological phenomena that could yield such curves, the authors suggest that the model may not describe all possible survivor curves. Nevertheless, they consider it a useful predictive tool.

Kirov et al. found that a psychrotrophic toxin-producing strain of *A. hydrophila* grew well in refrigerated slurries prepared from scallops, prawns, fish, chicken liver paté, liverwurst, sliced chicken lunch meat, and commercial baby foods (*620*). In all foods except baby food, exotoxins were produced at levels comparable with their production in bacteriological broth media. Moreover, only prawn and fish slurries showed evidence of spoilage after 7 days under these conditions. UHT milk added to toxin-containing broth culture supernatants decreased or removed hemolytic and cytotoxic activities, whereas baby food preparations did not. This suggests that baby foods inhibit toxin production rather than inactivating the toxin as UHT milk appears to do. The authors concluded that *Aeromonas* can produce exotoxins in many refrigerated foods and under some circumstances this might be a health hazard. In other studies, Kirov et al. found that 6 of 61 strains of *A. sobria* isolated from milk, lamb, chicken, and seafood were able to produce at least two exotoxins at 37°C and to grow at 5 and 43°C (*621*). They adhered to HEp-2 cells at both 5 and 37°C and expressed flexible pili, considered possible colonization factors, in greater numbers at the lower temperature. These and other food isolates of *A. sobria* and *A. hydrophila* lacking adhesive ability produced cytotoxins in broth cultures at 5°C. An *A. hydrophila* strain isolated from goat's milk grew particularly rapidly at low temperature and produced hemolysin, enterotoxin, and cytotoxin within 3 days in broth cultures at 5°C.

## Identification

Carnahan summarized current identification methods for clinical *Aeromonas* isolates (*622*). Identification systems have managed to keep pace with the changing taxonomic classification of these organisms. Pin et al. compared several selective agar media for enumeration of *Aeromonas* spp. isolated from foods (*623*). *Aeromonas hydrophila* and *A. caviae* were easily recovered on all three media, although Aeromonas medium gave better results for foods with high levels of background microflora. However, starch–ampicillin agar and starch–glutamate–ampicillin–penicillin agar recovered only 32–33% of *A. sobria* strains, compared to 86% on Aeromonas medium.

Warburton et al. developed a procedure for testing bottled water for *A. hydrophila* (*624*). It includes use of hydrophobic grid membrane filters, a resuscitation step, and selective plating. The organism survived and proliferated in inoculated water for up to 60 days, depending on the other contaminating bacteria. When *Pseudomonas aeruginosa* was present, *A. hydrophila* survived longer than 60 days in bottled water.

Arzese et al. characterized 31 clinical isolates of mesophilic *Aeromonas* spp. by enzymatic activity and computerized analysis of SDS–PAGE protein profiles (*625*). Protein patterns revealed *A. caviae* strains as a homogeneous group, significantly different from *A. sobria* and *A. hydrophila*. In contrast, *Aeromonas sobria* strains fell into two distinct groups with a correlation coefficient of .7, and strains biochemically identified as *A. hydrophila* had a correlation coefficient of .64 in SDS–PAGE analysis. This heterogeneity was emphasized by the finding of two mixed subgroups, both containing strains designated as *A. hydrophila* and *A. sobria* on the basis of biochemical features. The authors recommended further investigation of the taxonomy of *A. hydrophila* and *A. sobria* because of their role as human pathogens, and suggested that computer-assisted numerical analysis of SDS–PAGE protein patterns would be a useful adjunct to data on virulence factors in clinical and epidemiologic studies.

Three commercial identification kits were compared in their ability to confirm the identity of motile aeromonads isolated from foods (*626*). Both API 20NE and Microbact 24E correctly identified 77 of 80 *Aeromonas* strains as *Aeromonas*. At the species level, however, their agreement was only 69%, the major difference being in classification of a strain as *A. hydrophila* or *A. sobria*. API 20E identified only 58 of 80. The 22 misidentifications by API 20E were about equally divided among *Pasteurella* spp., *Flavobacterium* spp., and not identified at all. The authors concluded that the recognition of a motile aeromonad by API 20NE or Microbact 24E is adequate to confirm the presence of a potential pathogen.

Pathogenic *Aeromonas* strains are unpredictable in their susceptibility to antimicrobial agents, and particularly to β-lactam antibiotics. Schadow et al. tested the ability of the Vitek AMS kit to detect β-lactam resistance in 25 *Aeromonas* strains representing 4 species (*627*). They found the AMS kit to be unreliable in testing the resistance of *Aeromonas* to 8 β-lactam agents.

Lucchini reviewed and compared methods commonly used for epidemiologic investigations of *Aeromonas* spp. (*628*). Although extremely sensitive methods are now available for subtyping *Aeromonas* spp., the source for most infections caused by these organisms is rarely identified. This is partly because of the ubiquity and extreme diversity of the organisms and partly because of a lack of background information on the role of environmental reservoirs in human infections.

Millership and Want characterized 68 strains of *A. hydrophila, A. caviae,* and *A. sobria* phenotypically and by whole-cell protein fingerprinting using silver-stained SDS–PAGE (*629*). The protein fingerprints contained 30–40 bands. Protein fingerprints were not correlated with phenotype (see also ref. *625*). However, when phenotype and protein patterns were considered together, clusters of epidemiologically related isolates were seen. Only 9 of 27 strains could be serotyped. In further studies, Mulla and Millership typed 103 environmental and clinical *Aeromonas* isolates by numerical analysis of immunoblotted SDS–PAGE gels (*630*). Again, immunoblot type was not related to biochemical phenotype and attempts to correlate immunoblot type with serotype failed because the majority of strains could not be serotyped. The immunoblotting procedure was satisfactorily reproducible and highly discriminatory, revealing 30 types among the 103 isolates. Computerized analysis eliminated the subjective element and permitted comparisons between gels.

## Virulence and Molecular Studies

Freitas et al. compared the virulence factors produced by a standard strain of *A. hydrophila* and strains isolated from water, pasteurized milk, and urine (*631*). All strains were hemolytic, proteolytic, and staphylolytic. Water, milk, and standard strains had enterotoxin-like activity in suckling mice and were cytotoxic to Vero cells. The milk and standard strains showed autoagglutination in broth culture. The clinical strain was most toxic to mice challenged intraperitoneally. All strains had LPS that was toxic to mice and produced the Shwartzman reaction in rabbits.

Gosling et al. evaluated the phenotypic characteristics of 175 isolates from cases of *Aeromonas*-associated diarrhea to develop a phenotypic basis for assessing the likelihood of an isolate's being enterotoxin-positive (*632*). The cultures represented 23 strains of *A. hydrophila,* 37 of *A. sobria,* 109 of *A. caviae,* and 6 unassignable strains. All of them hydrolyzed arginine and produced acid from glucose and mannitol. None produced acid from inositol, sorbitol, rhamnose, or melibiose. The strains were similar in their ability to utilize various carbon sources. They had nearly identical qualitative enzyme profiles except for production of β-glucosidase, which was characteristic of 70% of *A. hydrophila* strains but only 6% of *A. sobria* and 19% of *A. caviae* strains. Fewer than half of the strains could be serotyped, but 19 different serotypes were represented among those that could. Virtually all strains of *A. hydrophila* and *A. sobria* were enterotoxigenic in the infant mouse assay and completely hemolyzed rabbit erythrocytes. In contrast, only 6% of *A. caviae* strains were enterotoxigenic and none caused complete hemolysis. Phenotypic characteristics associated with toxigenicity were production of acid from arabinose and salicin, utilization of certain compounds as sole sources of carbon, production of gas from glucose, Voges-Proskauer reaction, oxidation of gluconate, hydrolysis of esculin, and production of lecithinase and lysine decarboxylase. The API ZYM system was of little value in identifying species of *Aeromonas* or in predicting enterotoxigenicity. Enterotoxigenicity was highly associated with classification as *A. hydrophila* or *A. sobria.*

Because of uncertainty over the public-health significance of environmental reservoirs of *Aeromonas,* information on the pathogenicity of *Aeromonas* spp. for fish could be important. Esteve et al. showed that *A. hydrophila* and *A. jandaei* are pathogenic to European eels (*Anguilla anguilla*) raised in fresh water (*633*). Epizootics occurred in spring and summer when water temperatures were 17–22°C.

Isolates of *A. hydrophila, A. caviae,* and *A. sobria* were tested for adherence to HEp-2 cells (*634*). Urinary and intestinal tract strains of *A. hydrophila* and *A. sobria* showed "stacked brick" aggregative adherence similar to that shown by enteroaggregative *E. coli.* In contrast, *A. caviae* strains and isolates of *A. hydrophila* from water and a cutaneous infection showed a diffuse adherence pattern. Other studies also supported the idea that adhesive strains of *Aeromonas* are enteropathogenic (*635*). Five of 6 strains that showed mannose-resistant adhesion to Int407 cells also adhered to CaCo-2 cells in the presence of mannose and had cytopathic effects. At least 2, and perhaps 3, strains invaded the CaCo-2 cells.

However, the mechanisms of adhesion and possibly invasion are not clear. No fimbrial structures were seen by transmission electron microscopy. Adhesion of 4 of the 5 strains was inhibited by L-fucose. All strains were negative in the fluorescence actin staining test and failed to hybridize with the *E. coli eae* and *ipaB* probes (associated with attaching–effacing ability and invasion, respectively).

Investigations into the mechanism of adherence in nonpiliated strains of *A. hydrophila* suggested that hydrophobicity is a major factor (*636*). Surface-water isolates showed a diffuse type of adherence to Hep-2, HeLa, CHO, and Vero cells, with >20 adherent bacteria per cell. Clinical isolates showed both diffuse and local adherence, depending on the strain and type of cell. In both clinical and environmental strains, diffuse adherence was correlated with hydrophobicity. Most strains were negative in hemagglutination tests, and there was no correlation between hemagglutination or plasmid profile and adherence pattern.

Majeed and MacRae studied the cytotoxic and hemagglutinating activities of motile strains of *Aeromonas* isolated from slaughtered lambs and processed lamb meat (*637*). Forty-eight of 114 strains were cytotoxic to Vero cells. Cytotoxicity was more common in *A. hydrophila* and *A. sobria* than in *A. caviae*. Hemagglutination activity was seen in about half of the strains of each species. Hemagglutination was inhibited by low concentrations of fucose, galactose, or mannose, and in most cases more than one of these sugars was inhibitory. Certain patterns of hemagglutination inhibition were significantly associated with production of cytotoxin.

Hanes and Chandler showed that a 40-MDa plasmid that codes for antibiotic resistance also regulates certain adherence and hemolytic properties of *A. hydrophila* strain MS-2 (*638*).

Loychern et al. reported a simple method for purification of the *A. hydrophila* β-hemolysin (*639*). The 54-kDa hemolysin was isolated from fish with epizootic ulcerative syndrome and purified by chromatography on DEAE-cellulose. The product yielded a single band on SDS–PAGE.

Parker et al. determined the structure of the *A. hydrophila* toxin proaerolysin by X-ray crystallography at 2.8 Å resolution (*640*). Their models suggested a pathway for biogenesis of the aerolysin channel in which the water-soluble protoxin dimer binds to receptors on the surface of its target cell, where proteolytic nicking leads to oligomerization. This requires dissociation of the dimer and removal of the activation peptide, events which might be promoted by the detergent properties of the lipid bilayer. The resulting exposure of hydrophobic regions on the toxin would create an energetically favorable situation for formation of a transmembrane pore and membrane insertion.

Chopra et al. purified and characterized two types of enterotoxin produced by a diarrheal isolate of *A. hydrophila* (*641*). One is cytolytic; the other, cytotonic. Amino acid residues 245–274 and 361–405 appear to be associated with the cytotoxic and hemolytic function of the cytolytic enterotoxin. It is also possible that the latter domain represents the binding site of the toxin molecule, as it shows significant homology with the binding domain of the *Clostridium perfringens* type A enterotoxin. When the cytotonic enterotoxin gene was cloned in *E. coli*, cell lysates of the clone caused elongation of CHO cells.

## *CAMPYLOBACTER*

### Epidemiologic and Clinical Reports

The UK's Advisory Committee on the Microbiological Safety of Food found the significant properties of most *Campylobacter* spp. to be their failure to grow at room temperature and below and their inability to grow in air (*642*). Campylobacters are sensitive to drying, acidic conditions, and salt concentrations above 2%. They are inactivated at temperatures ≥48°C. They can enter a viable but nonculturable form, probably in response to environmental conditions. It is not clear whether such nonculturable organisms are infectious. In the UK, campylobacteriosis is generally an inflammatory-type disease, different from the secretory type of enteritis common in developing countries, and most cases are sporadic. The infectious dose is small, although some degree of acquired immunity is possible. The relative potential of various *Campylobacter* species and strains of *Campylobacter jejuni* and *Campylobacter coli* to cause disease is poorly understood, and the true incidence of campylobacteriosis is probably underestimated. Other aspects of the epidemiology of campylobacter infection in humans and animals were summarized and recommendations were made for needed studies and actions.

Most *Campylobacter* infections in humans result from contact with infected animals or eating contaminated food. Altekruse et al. reviewed the food sources and animal reservoirs of campylobacters and illustrated cycles of transmission in the environment, wild and domestic animals, and foods (*643*).

To study the environmental cycles of *Campylobacter* in more detail, investigators in the Netherlands monitored three municipal sewage treatment plants and the wastewaters of two poultry slaughterhouses for culturable campylobacters (*644*). The number of campylobacters isolated from the plants was related to the presence of poultry slaughterhouses in the drainage area. The numbers seen in the sewage of the activated sludge system varied seasonally, averaging 1 $\log_{10}$ lower at the end of the summer than during the rest of the year. This difference was not related to water temperature, $pO_2$, pH, rainfall, or amount of sunlight. Purification in an activated sludge tank reduced counts by 1 $\log_{10}$; in a trickling filter system the reduction was 0.6 $\log_{10}$. The authors recommended that disinfection of sewage plant effluents be considered to obstruct the environmental cycles of *Campylobacter*, since the elimination of campylobacters in sewage systems is far from complete.

A study in Mexico showed that breast-fed infants have significantly fewer episodes of campylobacter infection than infants who are not breast fed (*645*). The protective effect of breast milk was associated with the presence of IgA antibodies directed against *C. jejuni* flagellin.

A study in Greece evaluated the antibiotic resistance of 31 strains of *C. jejuni* isolated from children with diarrhea (*646*). Ten strains were resistant to nalidixic acid, and these strains were also relatively resistant to the fluoroquinones ciprofloxacin, norfloxacin, and ofloxacin. In contrast, 8 nalidixic acid–susceptible strains were also sensitive to the fluoroquinones.

The genus *Campylobacter* causes a variety of infections and problems. Steinkraus and Wright reported an unusual case of septic abortion with intact fetal membranes caused by *C. fetus fetus* in an 18-year-old woman (*647*). de Guevara et al. reported 7 cases of *C. jejuni* or *C. coli* bacteremia: 5 in immune-deficient adults, one in a newborn baby, and one in a surgical patient (*648*). They concluded that patients who have diarrhea as a result of *Campylobacter* infection are at risk of subsequent bacteremia. Kruijk et al. described a case of acute encephalopathy in a 13-year-old boy who had had gastroenteritis 6 days earlier (*649*).

**GUILLAIN-BARRÉ SYNDROME (GBS).** The GBS–*Campylobacter* connection has received considerable attention. Griffin et al. briefly reviewed how inquiries into this syndrome of paralysis, areflexia, and elevated spinal fluid protein spawned intensive study of enteric bacteriology and glycoconjugate chemistry nearly three-quarters of a century after the syndrome was first described (*650*). Better understanding of the *Campylobacter* con-

nection should reveal the nature of at least some antigens against which the presumed autoimmune attack is directed and might help explain the variations in clinical manifestations, pathophysiology, and worldwide epidemiology of the syndrome. Rees et al. reviewed *Campylobacter* enteritis, the Guillain-Barré syndrome, and evidence suggesting that a particularly severe form of GBS follows *C. jejuni* infection (*651*). The association between *C. jejuni* and GBS provides an opportunity to learn how a bacterial infection induces an autoimmune disease in susceptible patients. Cross-reactivity between neural antigens and *C. jejuni* may be one mechanism that triggers GBS. Symptoms begin while the autoimmune response is still developing and the causative organism can still be recovered from the stool. In these cases it should be possible to detect antigen, antibody, and target organ damage simultaneously in the same patient. Isolation of *C. jejuni* from stools of GBS patients indicates that the disease is likely to be severe and prolonged, possibly with severe axonal degeneration. The presence of anti-ganglioside-$G_{M1}$ antibodies is another adverse prognostic factor. Mishu and Blaser discussed the role of *C. jejuni* infection in initiating GBS in terms of a specific genetic predisposition in the host and the particular virulence of certain *C. jejuni* clones (*652*). Campylobacter-associated GBS is most common in patients who have the HLA-B35 antigen. Also, at least in Japan, *C. jejuni* strains of Penner serotype O19 are strongly associated with GBS. Observations in one patient suggested that *C. jejuni* antigens stimulate production of antibodies that react with peripheral nerve myelin. A case–control study by Mishu et al. confirmed reports that patients with GBS are more likely than control subjects to have serologic evidence of recent *C. jejuni* infection (*653*). Sixty-nine of 118 case-patients (58%) and 36 of 103 controls (35%) had an optical density ratio $\geq 1$ in the IgA assay; 56% of case patients and 41% of controls had an elevated optical density ratio in the IgG assay; and 61% of case-patients and 42% of controls had an elevated optical density ratio in the IgM assay. When the threshold for defining a positive response was increased to an optical density ratio of $\geq 2$ or $\geq 3$, the strength of the association between *C. jejuni* infection and GBS also increased. Investigators in Germany, using a more sensitive and specific immunoassay, detected anti–*C. jejuni* IgM and/or IgG antibodies in 15 of 38 GBS patients but in only 7 of 39 healthy controls, 3 of 20 MS patients, and 2 of 72 patients with neuroborreliosis (*654*). In GBS patients the antibodies were predominantly directed to outer membrane proteins of the Lior 11 serotype, whereas the most common serotype associated with enteritis in Germany is Lior 4. There was no correlation between severity, type (axonal degeneration or demyelinating), or outcome and the presence of a humoral immune response to *C. jejuni* or glycoconjugates. Thus this study did not support suggestions of a poorer prognosis for patients whose GBS is associated with a preceding *C. jejuni* infection.

Sugita et al. described a case of GBS that followed *C. jejuni* enteritis and was associated with IgM anti-$G_{M1}$ antibody (*655*). The patient was a 4-year-old girl who had the HLA-B35 antigen and had had an acute episode of abdominal pain and bloody diarrhea associated with *C. jejuni* of Penner serotype O19 (see also ref. *652*). Aspinall et al. reported that *C. jejuni* serotypes O4 and O19 have core oligosaccharides with terminal structures resembling human gangliosides $G_{M1}$ and $G_{D1a}$ (*656*). Yuki et al. reported that the LPS fraction of Penner's serotype O4 bears an LPS with a $G_{M1}$ epitope and another with a $G_{D1a}$ epitope (*657*).

## Occurrence and Behavior in Food and Food Animals

Weijtens et al. monitored the prevalence of campylobacters in pigs and feed at 8 pig farms in the Netherlands (*658*). This included examination of the gastric, ileal, and rectal contents of pigs after slaughter. More than 85% of the sampled porkers on all farms were intestinal carriers of campylobacters at all stages of fattening. Contamination was heavy, although fecal populations tended to decrease as pigs got older. Subsequent groups of pigs housed in the same stalls were also carriers. The prevalence of campylobacters was not influenced by the feeding system (wet or dry), and campylobacters were isolated from only 2 feed samples. RFLP typing revealed a high diversity of campylobacter types. There were similarities between types isolated from repeated samplings of the same group of pigs, but not between samplings of successive groups of pigs from the same stall. This suggests that piglets were infected while very young and still on the breeding farm. Although the role of pigs in foodborne campylobacter infection and in direct transmission of infection to other animals has not been clearly established, it seems certain that pig farms and slaughterhouses are a major source of environmental contamination.

A study in Poland assessed the prevalence of campylobacters and salmonellas in poultry at the time of slaughter (*659*). Campylobacters were found in 61% of laying chickens, 63% of broilers, 54% of geese, and 81% of ducks. For salmonellas, these values were 18, 3, 15, and 39%, respectively. Campylobacter infection was associated with pathological changes in the liver. All

birds infected with both campylobacter and salmonella showed such changes.

In Northern Ireland, campylobacters were found in 65% of 153 samples of chicken wings purchased from retail outlets (*660*). Forty-five isolates were *C. jejuni* and 25 were *C. coli*; 21 could not be identified to species by the API Campy method used in this study. Three isolates were identified as *C. jejuni doylei*, 2 as *C. fetus fetus*, and 3 as *C. cryaerophilia*. Because *C. jejuni* and *C. coli* cause similar illness, their differentiation is considered important only for epidemiologic purposes. The infective dose for *C. jejuni* may be as low as 500–800 organisms; therefore good hygiene and cooking practices are essential to prevent illness from the handling or consumption of chicken products.

Slavik et al. evaluated the ability of a 15-s dip in 10% trisodium phosphate at 50°C to reduce populations of campylobacters attached to postchill chicken carcasses (*661*). Immediately after the dip, there was no difference between treated carcasses and controls. After 1 day of storage at 4°C, *Campylobacter* was present on ≥96% of controls and ≤28% of treated carcasses as measured by a nitrocellulose membrane lift method, but reduction was only 4–36% when assessed by culture. When populations were estimated by an MPN method, populations on treated carcasses were 1.5 $\log_{10}$ lower after 1 day of storage and 1.2 $\log_{10}$ lower after 6 days. When the dip was done at 10°C there was only a nonsignificant 0.16-$\log_{10}$ reduction in campylobacters.

Castillo and Escartin assessed the survival of *C. jejuni* inoculated onto the surface of cubes of watermelon and papaya (*662*). From 7.7 to 61.8% of organisms survived for at least 6 h at room temperature. When 0.05 mL of fresh lemon juice per cube was added, 0–14.3% of the organisms survived for 6 h at room temperature. Lemon juice was more destructive to *C. jejuni* on papaya than on watermelon. The authors concluded that *C. jejuni* can survive on these sliced fruits long enough to be a risk for the consumer, and that adding lemon juice reduces but does not completely eliminate this risk.

EPIDEMIOLOGY AND CONTROL IN POULTRY FLOCKS. Humphrey et al. assessed the campylobacter status of 49 broiler flocks from 23 farms in a year-long study in the UK (*663*). The cecal contents of the birds were examined at the time of slaughter. Thirty-seven flocks were positive. The mean prevalence of colonization in positive flocks was 50%; it ranged from less than 10% in 5 flocks to more than 75% in 13. No seasonal variation in carriage was seen, and the prevalence of colonization was not associated with water source, drinker type, floor type, flock size, other farming activities, or standards of farm hygiene. On one farm, the practice of workers dipping their boots in a phenolic disinfectant before entering the broiler houses seemed to delay or prevent colonization.

Hygiene- and husbandry-related risk factors for introduction of *Campylobacter* into broiler flocks were investigated in southeastern Norway (*664*). All 176 broiler farms in the study area participated. Each farm was represented by one randomly selected flock, which was examined at the time of slaughter. *Campylobacter* spp. were recovered from 32 flocks; *C. jejuni* biotype 1 was isolated from 24. Colonized flocks were more likely to have come from the Hedmark region and to have been slaughtered from August through November. Use of nondisinfected drinking water and tending of pigs or other poultry by workers before entering the broiler house were significantly and independently associated with increased risk of colonization; presence of rats on the farm nonsignificantly increased risk. Disinfection of drinking water appeared to be the preventive measure with the greatest potential for reducing risk.

Glünder reviewed the epidemiology and importance of *Campylobacter* infections in poultry (*665*). The organisms can colonize the digestive tract of chickens and turkeys without producing clinical symptoms, or can produce enteritis or enterohepatic disease with accompanying pathologic changes in the liver and kidneys. The period of excretion of the bacteria depends on the age of the bird, and excretion rate varies among campylobacter strains. Hygienic measures on the farm can prevent or reduce transmission of infection to poultry populations at risk, and good hygiene in slaughterhouses and processing plants further reduces risk to consumers.

The avian cecum appears to be the natural environment for *C. jejuni*. In studies of colonization of chickens by the wild type and motility mutants of a clinical strain of *C. jejuni*, Wassenaar et al. evaluated the importance of flagella (*666*). Although flagella were not required for colonization, absence of both flagellin genes (*flaA* and *flaB*) decreased colonization efficiency. However, inactivation of *flaB*, which did not affect motility, enhanced cecal colonization by 3 orders of magnitude. A poorly motile variant with flagella composed of flagellin A also colonized better than the wild type. However, mutants with an inactivated *flaA* gene colonized 100–1000 times less efficiently than the wild type, regardless of their motility (conferred by flagellin B flagella). The authors concluded that it is the presence of flagellin A, rather than motility, that is essential for optimal colonization of the chick cecum.

COMPETITIVE EXCLUSION. Initial attempts to diminish colonization of chickens by administration of competi-

tive microflora were less successful for *Campylobacter* than for *Salmonella*. Stern has attempted to find a better source than the indigenous intestinal flora for flora antagonistic to *C. jejuni*. He developed a procedure for isolating indigenous flora from the cecal mucin and discussed the advantages and limitations of the resulting mucosal competitive exclusion culture (*667*). Somewhat better results were obtained with the mucosal culture than with standard competitive exclusion cultures, although results were still inconsistent. In general, the efficacy of the mucosal culture decreased with time in storage at –80°C.

Schoeni and Wong studied conditions for maximizing the inhibition of *C. jejuni* colonization of chicks by defined competitive exclusion cultures (*668*). Treatment with competitive exclusion culture and/or 2.5% dietary α-lactose, D-mannose, or fructooligosaccharides was administered before, after, or at the time of inoculating chicks with *C. jejuni*. All treatments reduced colonization. The most effective culture was a combination of *Citrobacter diversus, Klebsiella pneumoniae,* and *E. coli*. The most effective preventive treatments were dietary fructooligosaccharides or protective culture plus dietary mannose. Culture plus dietary lactose greatly reduced established infections. Booster treatments with protective culture did not increase effectiveness.

## Isolation and Identification

*Campylobacter upsaliensis* was isolated from dogs in 1983 and later shown to be a new species potentially pathogenic for humans. Common selective media for campylobacters are not satisfactory for *C. upsaliensis*. Aspinall et al. developed a selective supplement for recovery of thermophilic campylobacters including *C. upsaliensis* from feces, using a commercial campylobacter blood-free selective agar as a base for comparison (*669*). Isolation rates of campylobacters other than *C. upsaliensis* were comparable on the two media, but *C. upsaliensis* (4 of 5 strains) was only recovered on the new medium incorporating cefoperazone, amphotericin, and teicoplanin.

Lam reported a 7-h [51]Cr-release cytotoxicity assay for detection of *C. jejuni* toxin in the culture supernatant (*670*). There was no direct correlation between the organism's pathogenicity and the supernatant's toxicity for chicken lymphocytes. The toxin was heat stable.

Nicholson and Patton used the scheme of Lior to biotype 140 genetically identified strains of *Campylobacter* (*671*). Biotyping did not differentiate human from animal and environmental strains or separate them geographically. Typical hippurate-positive strains of *C.*

*jejuni jejuni* were distributed among the four Lior biotypes, but 33 of 37 belonged to biotype I or II. Nalidixic acid–resistant strains of *C. jejuni jejuni* were divided approximately equally between biotypes I and II. All *C. jejuni doylei* strains belonged to biotype I. All hippurate-negative *C. jejuni jejuni* strains and 6 of 35 *C. lari* strains were grouped with *C. coli* biotypes.

The success of immunologic detection methods requires an economical source of antibodies to selected antigens. Chandan et al. reported a simple, efficient method for extracting *C. jejuni* and *C. coli* LPS and protein antigens and producing antibodies to them in yolks of eggs from immunized hens (*672*).

Salt tolerance is a criterion for differentiating *C. laridis* from other thermophilic campylobacters. However, not all *C. laridis* strains grow in 1.5% salt, whereas some strains classified as *C. jejuni* or *C. coli* on the basis of other phenotypic characteristics do grow at this salt concentration. Although acquisition of salt tolerance is independent of other phenotypic characteristics, salt-sensitive parental strains and their salt-tolerant variants have been reported to differ in serological behavior. Glünder adapted campylobacter strains to growth in 3% NaCl and examined them for antigenic changes by immunodot blot, immunoblot, and immunoprecipitation tests (*673*). Both heat-labile and heat-stable antigens of salt-tolerant variants differed from those of salt-sensitive parental strains. The differences suggested alterations in the antigenic structure of flagella and possibly outer membrane proteins.

Kato et al. examined the electrophoretic protein-banding patterns on nondenaturing polyacrylamide gels of 23 strains of *C. jejuni*, *C. coli*, and *C. lari*, including 17 atypical strains of *C. jejuni* and *C. coli* (*674*). Sixteen of the atypical strains showed banding patterns virtually identical to those of typical strains of the same species and distinct from patterns shown by the other two species. One strain originally considered *C. coli* was identified as *C. lari* from its profile.

Birkenhead et al. developed a PCR for detection and typing of campylobacters based on the *flaA* gene (*675*). The selected primers amplified a 1.3-kilobase fragment of the *C. jejuni* and *C. coli* genes and an easily distinguished 1.7-kilobase fragment from *C. upsaliensis*. Other species of campylobacter failed to yield product. The PCR products showed considerable restriction fragment length polymorphism, which should permit development of a new rapid typing scheme that does not require preliminary culture. Owen et al. reported successful use of PCR-based RFLP analysis based on sequence diversity of flagellin genes of *C. jejuni* and allied species (*676*). Twenty-nine strains of *C. jejuni*, *C. coli*, *C. lari*, and

*C. helveticus* were grouped into 10 genotypes on the bases of *fla* restriction site similarities.

Endtz et al. showed the potential usefulness of PCR-mediated DNA typing of *C. jejuni* in a study of strains isolated from patients with recurrent infections (*677*). The PCR-mediated analysis distinguished 14 patterns among 24 strains, whereas combined results of biotyping and serotyping recognized only 9 different types. Giesendorf et al. evaluated PCR-mediated DNA fingerprinting for epidemiologic investigations (*678*). They used primers directed at repetitive extragenic palindromic elements, enterobacterial repetitive intergenic consensus sequences, and an arbitrary DNA motif. A single PCR and simple gel electrophoresis revealed strain-specific banding patterns for *C. jejuni* and *C. upsaliensis*. DNA from multiple strains isolated during an outbreak of *C. jejuni* meningitis generated identical banding patterns and could be distinguished from randomly isolated strains. Strains from a community outbreak of *C. upsaliensis* infection that were identical by conventional typing methods were separated into two genetically different groups.

Stonnet and Guesdon reported a PCR specific for *C. jejuni* (*679*). No amplification product was detected from 9 other campylobacter species or 9 noncampylobacters.

Wegmüller et al. developed a PCR using semi-nested primers for direct detection of *C. jejuni* and *C. coli* in raw milk and dairy products (*680*). After initial studies on artificially contaminated water, milk, and soft cheese samples, 93 samples of dairy products were screened for the presence of these organisms. Six positive samples were identified by the PCR, whereas a conventional culture method found none.

Oyofo and Rollins adapted a PCR assay for *C. jejuni* and *C. coli* that amplified a target region in *flaA* for use with environmental water samples (*681*). In particular, they evaluated various types of filters for use in the assay. No amplification was obtained with cellulose acetate filters. With Fluoropore and Durapore filters, the PCR could be run without removing the filters from the reaction tube. The system was tested on a broiler chicken farm's water supply, which was suspected as the source of *C. jejuni* on the farm despite repeated failure of attempts to culture the organism. The filtration-PCR method detected campylobacter DNA in more than half of the farm water samples examined.

Quentin et al. reported a case of human abortion due to campylobacter infection and described use of nonradioactive DNA probes to identify the causative organism (*682*). Cultural methods revealed two morphologically different colony types. By conventional methods, the large colonies were identified as *C. jejuni* and the small colonies as *C. coli*. However, dot blot hybridization and examination of rDNA restriction fragment patterns showed that both colony types were the same strain of *C. jejuni*.

Suzuki et al. compared the cleavage patterns of the genomic DNA of 42 clinical isolates of *C. jejuni*, as determined by pulsed-field gel electrophoresis, with their Lior and TCK serotypes (*683*). The *Sal*I enzyme produced 13 distinct restriction patterns; *Sma*I produced 22. Patterns from both enzymes were heterogeneously distributed among strains of Lior types 24 and 4, indicating that genomic DNA typing is useful in subclassifying strains of these serotypes. However, strains of TCK type I appeared relatively homogeneous in their restriction fragment patterns. One of the chromosomal patterns was seen in isolates of three different serotypes, posing the question of why isolates with the same genetic pattern have different antigens. Nine strains were further examined for plasmid DNA profiles. However, 5 of them had no distinctive plasmid; and digestion of total DNA by restriction enzymes produced too many bands for practical analysis.

Fayos et al. used rDNA patterns, RAPD profiles, and plasmid profiles to discriminate among strains of *C. jejuni* of Penner serogroups O1 and O2 (*684*). Seven strains were from a school outbreak in the UK and 21 were from sporadic cases of campylobacteriosis in 4 countries. The outbreak strains were homogeneous in most features, but a variety of types was found among the strains from sporadic cases. There were 5 groups of 2 or more strains with identical ribopatterns and within each, all strains had the same serogroup. Results from RAPD profile typing based on numerical analysis were comparable to results from ribotyping. Plasmid profiles were least discriminatory, but were useful in separating some strains that were similar in other respects.

Owen et al. analyzed the ribopatterns of 72 strains of *C. jejuni jejuni*, *C. jejuni doylei*, *C. coli*, *C. upsaliensis*, and *C. lari* (*685*). *Hae*III ribotypes were defined by computer-assisted numerical analysis. For *C. jejuni*, *C. coli*, and *C. lari* these patterns were reproducible, easy to code for numerical analysis, and highly discriminatory. *Pst*I ribotyping revealed further diversity within 3 of the *Hae*III types. *Campylobacter upsaliensis* could also be ribotyped with *Hae*III, but *Hin*dIII, *Pvu*II, and *Pst*I were less satisfactory. In general for these species, *Hin*dIII ribopatterns were complex and difficult to compare, and *Pvu*II profiles were least discriminatory. The authors concluded that choice of restriction enzyme is critical when ribotyping different species of *Campylobacter*.

## Pathogenesis and Molecular Studies

Wallis reviewed the pathogenesis of *C. jejuni* infection (*686*). The infective dose can be as low as 800 cells. The organism penetrates the gastric mucus, aided by its spiral shape and high motility, and adheres to the gut enterocytes. Diarrhea is induced by the release of toxins, which vary from strain to strain of *C. jejuni* but are mainly enterotoxin and cytotoxins. The immune response to *C. jejuni* infection and areas where further research is needed were discussed.

Kaur et al. reported studies on the pathophysiological mechanism of fluid secretion induced by *C. jejuni* in ligated rat ileal loops (*687*). Protein kinase C and $Ca^{2+}$ appear to be important second messengers involved in stimulating intestinal fluid accumulation.

*Campylobacter fetus fetus* has a broad host range, which includes sheep, cattle, and poultry. Although foods are sometimes contaminated with *C. fetus*, this organism generally causes illness only in compromised hosts. Bacteremia is the hallmark of such infections. Blaser discussed the role of S-layer proteins in the serum resistance and antigenic variation of *C. fetus* (*688*). The acidic, high-molecular-weight proteins comprising the paracrystalline S-layer resist binding by the C3b component of complement, which explains their serum and phagocytosis resistance. The size of the protein subunits, crystalline structure, and antigenicity can vary from strain to strain. Several genes with both conserved and divergent sequences encode the S-layer proteins. This permits gene rearrangement and antigenic variation, providing a measure of resistance against host antibodies. Studies of *C. fetus* suggest a model of bacterial pathogenesis relevant to the many bacterial species on which S-layers have been identified.

## *LISTERIA*

## Epidemiology, Outbreaks, and Clinical Features

Czuprynski reviewed research on host resistance to *Listeria monocytogenes* infection, emphasizing pathogenesis in the gastrointestinal tract (*689*). After an overview of the immune system and the virulence mechanisms of *L. monocytogenes*, the author briefly discussed resistance to listeriosis in laboratory animals inoculated by various routes and then considered the host response to gastrointestinal inoculation. Implications for food safety and human health were examined. Many questions remain to be answered about the behavior of *L. monocytogenes* after it is ingested, the relative importance of local and systemic host defense mechanisms, and the importance of the normal intestinal microflora and the food vehicle in which the pathogen is suspended.

RAPD pattern analysis was used to verify the causal relationship between food and clinical isolates of *L. monocytogenes* associated with four outbreaks of foodborne illness (*690*). RAPD profiles were generated for at least one food and one clinical isolate from each outbreak. For two outbreaks, corresponding food and clinical isolates yielded identical profiles for all 20 primers used. Isolates from an outbreak involving alfalfa tablets gave identical patterns for 19 primers, but one produced an additional 1.8-kilobase fragment in the food isolate. This was shown to be due to a deletion of at least 1.8 kilobases in the clinical strain. However, loss of this fragment could not be induced by animal passage or by culturing the organism under selective conditions. For this reason the authors suggested that the alfalfa isolate was not identical to the clinical isolate. This study demonstrated the ability of RAPD analysis to discriminate between strains of the same serotype and MEE type.

Nørrung and Skovgaard reported application of MEE in epidemiologic studies of *L. monocytogenes* in Denmark (*691*). Ten of the 12 enzymes assayed were polymorphic, having 2–4 alleles per locus. The authors identified 33 electrophoretic types among 245 clinical, animal, and food isolates that included all clinical strains isolated in Denmark during 1989 and 1990. The genetic relationships among the 33 types were illustrated by a dendrogram, which shows two distinct clusters separated by a genetic distance of .376. Only two electrophoretic types accounted for nearly three-quarters of the human clinical strains. One of these was also found frequently in animal clinical cases. It was found only sporadically, however, among isolates from foods and food processing plants. This may indicate something distinctive about this clone that makes it particularly pathogenic for humans or that enables it to multiply to infectious levels in foods. The other common electrophoretic type in human clinical isolates was also the type most frequently encountered in food isolates.

Harvey and Gilmour used MEE and RFLP analysis to examine 141 *L. monocytogenes* strains isolated from foods, raw milk, and clinical and veterinary sources (*692*). The 48 electrophoretic types identified by MEE fell into two groups at a genetic distance of .585. All enzymes assayed were polymorphic, with 2–5 alleles at each locus. Milk strains displayed greater genetic diversity than nondairy food strains. Both MEE and RFLP analysis indicated that milk and nondairy foods fre-

quently contain recurring strains, suggesting that the presence of listerias in the product is due to contamination from within the processing environment. Most recurring strains were serogroup 1/2. Some recurrent food strains were closely related to clinical and veterinary strains, suggesting that strains adapted to the food-processing environment retain their pathogenic potential.

Cheese has been the vehicle in some major outbreaks of listeriosis. The pathogen may be present in the raw milk delivered to the dairy, or curd and cheeses may become contaminated by organisms in the processing plant or ripening room. After a case of listeriosis occurred in a goat on a goat farm where cheese was manufactured, Eilertz et al. tested cheese and environmental samples from the farm for *L. monocytogenes* (*693*). Isolates of similar subtype were made from the brain of the infected goat, a fresh cheese that did not contain any milk from that goat, and a shelf of the refrigerator where cheeses were stored. Before the goat became ill a cheese had been made from her milk. The authors postulated that this milk contained listerias and the cheese contaminated the refrigerator, which served as a *L. monocytogenes* reservoir for new cheeses made during the following weeks.

Paul et al. reviewed the epidemiology, clinical features, and outcome of 84 cases of listeriosis seen at four teaching hospitals in Sidney, Australia, during 1983–1992 (*694*). Their findings agreed with other reports. Listeriosis is primarily a disease of the elderly, immunocompromised individuals, pregnant women, and neonates. Nearly one-quarter of the cases occurred in patients who were already hospitalized, suggesting that *L. monocytogenes* may be an important hospital-associated pathogen in immunocompromised patients. Septicemia and central nervous system disease were the major clinical presentations. Eighteen patients (21%) died as a direct consequence of their listerial infection; nine more died of their underlying disease during their hospitalization for listeriosis.

A study in Denmark found that consumption of unpasteurized milk was a risk factor for sporadic listeriosis and an outbreak of a European epidemic strain was clearly linked to cheese (*695*). However, high-risk foods could explain only a minor fraction of sporadic cases. Leukemia, AIDS, and kidney transplantation increased risk more than 1000-fold.

In England, Wales, and Northern Ireland only 108 cases of listeriosis were reported in 1992 (*696*). Clinically and epidemiologically these cases were similar to those in previous years and in other countries. There was a reduction in fatality rate for cases not associated with pregnancy. The cause of an outbreak of at least 33 cases of listeriosis in France was traced to pork rillettes produced by a single plant in Brittany (*697,698*). Two deaths, 2 stillbirths, and 5 abortions were registered.

An 11-month-old girl, hospitalized with fever and gastrointestinal symptoms, was found to have listeria meningitis and bacteremia (*699*). Two days before admission she had been found in the barnyard of her parents' dairy farm, close to the dung heap, with her mouth full of soil. Although the source of infection was not determined, frequent exposure to sources of listeria was possible on the dairy farm.

In pregnant women, listeriosis is usually asymptomatic or very mild, but the mortality rate in infected fetuses and neonates is around 50%. Investigators in the UK determined the prevalence of fecal carriage of listeria in each trimester of pregnancy (*700*). Serial samples from 147 women were cultured. Four of the 348 samples, from 4 different women, were positive for *L. monocytogenes*. Two isolates were serovar 4b and two were 1/2c, the serovars usually associated with listeriosis. The isolations were made during gestational weeks 12, 26, 28, and 36. Three pregnancies were uncomplicated. The woman who was culture-positive at 28 weeks was induced at 38 weeks. Her infant, who weighed only 1.8 kg, had an uncomplicated neonatal course and no evidence of listeria was found in the baby, placenta, cord blood, maternal serum, or peripartum maternal feces. The authors concluded that transient fecal carriage of listeria occurs in at least 1 of 20 pregnant women without adverse effect and that screening fecal samples for listeria during pregnancy cannot identify those at risk of developing listeriosis.

Jensen evaluated the prevalence, level, and duration of *L. monocytogenes* excretion in 74 listeriosis patients (*701*). Her rapid screening method used L-PALCAMY and PALCAM selective media. Sixteen patients (22%) excreted the organism, whereas none of 103 control specimens from ordinary types of diarrhea contained the organism. Early in the infection, specimens contained at least $10^4$ organisms per milliliter of feces. Excretion stopped within 2 weeks, except in one neonate.

A study in Los Angeles County found rates of listeriosis in pregnant women per 100,000 pregnancies (live births plus fetal deaths) to be 19.8 for singleton gestations and 74.9 for multiple gestations (OR 3.8, 95% CI 2.1–6.8) (*702*). The risk for triplet gestations was 38.4 (95% CI 9.6–153.3). The increased risk during multiple-gestation pregnancies was greatest among women ≥35 year old and among Hispanic women. This is the first report of listeriosis as a medical complication in women with multiple gestations.

From the UK, Long et al. reported three cases of *L. monocytogenes* meningitis occurring 4 to 90 months after bone marrow transplantation (*703*). The patients were not receiving prophylactic antibiotics.

Listeria infection sometimes involves the liver. Braun et al. described a case of liver abscess due to *L. monocytogenes* in an elderly diabetic woman and reviewed the literature on hepatic manifestations of listeriosis (*704*). Patients with solitary liver abscesses recovered with antimicrobial therapy and abscess drainage, but 7 of 8 patients with multiple abscesses died. However, these patients with multiple abscesses were symptomatic and far sicker than the patients with a solitary abscess. A reader reported the case of a 67-year-old diabetic man with multiple asymptomatic liver abscesses (*705*). The patient was well 6 months after treatment. The authors concluded that asymptomatic liver infection mimicking a neoplastic process should be added to the list of manifestations of listeriosis. The postulated scenario involved enteric colonization by *L. monocytogenes* followed by portal vein bacteremia and seeding of the liver. From Belgium, Bourgeois et al. described what may be the first reported case of listeria hepatitis in an organ transplant recipient (*706*). The patient, a middle-aged man, had received a liver transplant 8 months earlier. He recovered after antimicrobial therapy.

A relapsed infection due to *L. monocytogenes* was confirmed by RAPD analysis (*707*). Isolates obtained at the time of the initial infection and upon relapse had identical antimicrobial susceptibility profiles and indistinguishable RAPD profiles, which were very similar to a control strain of *L. monocytogenes* serovar 4b. Many strains of *L. monocytogenes* 4b from the UK produce similar RAPD profiles, but very few are identical.

Cummins et al. reported a case of *L. ivanovii* infection in a patient with AIDS (*708*). A gastrointestinal route of infection was suspected and a food vehicle is a possibility, but the source of the infection was not identified.

## Occurrence and Behavior of *Listeria* in Foods and the Food Environment

SOURCES OF LISTERIAL CONTAMINATION. The presence of *L. monocytogenes* on foods subjected to listeriocidal processes could result from postprocessing contamination in the manufacturing environment or from cross-contamination from food handlers, surfaces, or other foods in the storage and preparation environment. Jackson et al. sampled surfaces from 195 residential refrigerators in Texas to determine the presence of *L. mono-*

*cytogenes (709)*. Refrigerator owners were selected at random and were not permitted to clean their refrigerators before samples were taken. No sample from any refrigerator was positive. This result was surprising, in view of the organism's hardiness, ability to grow at refrigeration temperatures, and rather common occurrence on raw foods. The authors suggested that *L. monocytogenes* is only a transient inhabitant of refrigerator surfaces, and long-term colonization of such surfaces is unusual.

From 1988 to 1990, Jacquet et al. examined a French cheese plant for *Listeria* contamination and characterized the strains isolated (*710*). Forty-four isolates of *L. monocytogenes* and 17 of *L. innocua* were obtained from 340 samples. No *L. monocytogenes* was recovered from cheeses until the ripening and rind-washing stages, indicating that contamination occurred at these points. A number of serotypes and phage types were found. Some strains of the same serovar and phagovar were isolated from both cheeses and shelves, indicating that cheese became contaminated during ripening. Both *L. monocytogenes* and *L. innocua* were isolated from some cheeses. Only one rDNA restriction pattern was found upon analysis of 38 *L. monocytogenes* strains with different serovars and phagovars, raising the possibility that all of the dairy plant isolates arose from a single ancestral group. Another study of sources of contamination by *Listeria* during manufacture of semisoft surface-ripened cheese also indicated that contamination occurred at the start of ripening (*711*). Although 22% of milk samples were contaminated, satisfactory curds were produced after pasteurization. Subsequent contamination was principally due to washing with brushing machines.

Sasahara and Zottola evaluated the ability of *L. monocytogenes* serotype 3a to attach to glass coverslips in a continuous-flow slide chamber and then to develop biofilms (*712*). In pure cultures, attachment was sparse. However, when *L. monocytogenes* was grown in mixed culture with *Pseudomonas fragi*, an exopolymer-producing organism, its attachment and formation of microcolonies were enhanced. In flowing systems, the presence of an exopolymer-producing microorganism may be a more important influence than hydrophobicity, surface charge, or flagellar movement on the attachment ability of *L. monocytogenes*. Another study compared results from culture methods and epifluorescence microscopy during biofilm development on stainless steel surfaces (*713*). Biofilms were grown in slime broth inoculated with *L. monocytogenes* or a food-spoilage microbe. For *L. monocytogenes*, the mean area coverage of the biofilm increased from ~1% at 2 days to 20% at 10 days. This biofilm did not produce much slime, and the

cells gathered in crevices on the surface. The organisms could easily be detected by cultivation at all stages of biofilm development. In contrast, biofilms produced by *Bacillus subtilis, Pediococcus pentosaceus,* and *Pseudomonas fragi* covered a greater percentage of the surface area and produced more slime. Although *B. subtilis* and *P. fragi* could easily be cultivated after 2 days they were difficult to detect by cultivation after 10 days, even though growth could be demonstrated by microscopy. The *Pediococcus* strain tested was the strongest slime producer but its total cell count was the lowest.

Vishinsky et al. described a case of listerial udder infection and widespread carcass contamination in an apparently healthy dairy cow (*714*). The cow, which was clinically free of mastitis, was slaughtered because she persistently shed *L. monocytogenes* in her right hind quarter milk and did not respond to antimicrobial therapy. After slaughter, *L. monocytogenes* was isolated from deep portions of tissues sampled aseptically after surface sterilization. The authors postulated that the mammary gland was the original site of infection and that stress-induced bacteremia permitted the organism's spread to other organs. Another possibility is a generalized infection with secondary hematogenous invasion of the udder. For purposes of food safety, the authors recommended that animals with persistent *L. monocytogenes* udder infections be examined bacteriologically after slaughter.

A survey in Germany found *Listeria* species in 30% of tortoises, 12% of lizards, 60% of amphibians, and 1% of snakes kept as pets (*715*). Eight isolates were identified as *L. monocytogenes*, 4 as *L. ivanovii*, 3 as *L. innocua,* and 2 as *L. welshimeri*.

**OCCURRENCE IN FOODS.** In a year-long survey in the UK, MacGowan et al. tested for the presence of listerias in retail foods, human feces, sewage, and urban soils (*716*). Listerias were found in 20% of 822 food samples, 94% of 115 sewage samples, 15% of 136 soil samples, and 1% of 692 fecal samples. For *L. monocytogenes* these values were, respectively, 10%, 60%, 1%, and 1%. There was no seasonal variation in rate of isolation from sewage or foods, and *L. monocytogenes* and *L. innocua* were the commonest species in both. Mutton was the predominant food source of *L. ivanovii*. Poultry had the highest rate of *L. monocytogenes* contamination (21 of 32 samples), but 28–40% of beef, lamb, pork, and sausage samples also contained this species. Although paté and soft cheeses have caused large outbreaks of listeriosis in the past, this study found *L. monocytogenes* in only 1 of 40 paté samples and 1 of 251 samples of soft cheese. The most common species isolated from soil were *L. ivanovii* and *L. seeligeri,* and isolation rates peaked during July–September. Harvey and Gilmour determined the incidence of *Listeria* species in 513 samples of foods produced in Northern Ireland (*717*). The overall incidence of listeria was 35.5%; *L. monocytogenes* was found in 18.3% of samples. Contamination was associated with the extent to which foods were processed. Over time, a distinctive *Listeria* microflora was discernible in products from particular processors. In some cases this was confirmed by MEE and RFLP typing.

Surveys of the contamination of paté by *L. monocytogenes* were made in England and Wales in July 1989 and July 1990 (*718*). Ten percent of 1698 samples were contaminated in 1989, whereas only 4% of 626 samples were contaminated in 1990. The number of samples from which >$10^3$ organisms per gram were recovered also decreased. The higher rate of contamination in 1989 was attributed to an outbreak-related paté from a single manufacturer. This paper presents a more detailed analysis of the 1989 nationwide paté survey than was published previously. In both surveys, paté sold as loose slices had higher rates of contamination than prepackaged paté. In 1989, only 65% of samples were stored at temperatures ≤7°C, whereas 83% of samples were adequately refrigerated in 1990. Although contamination occurred at nearly all temperatures, it was qualitatively and quantitatively greater in samples stored at >7°C. The rate of contamination was also greater in samples with expired sell-by dates. High total viable counts were positively associated with the presence of *L. monocytogenes.*

During the course of a year, Dillon et al. obtained samples of smoked fish products from retail outlets in Newfoundland and tested them for *Listeria* (*719*). Seven of 116 cold-smoked products and 36 of 142 hot-smoked products yielded listerias, for an overall isolation rate of 16.7%. Cod had the highest rate of contamination, 46.7%. Eighteen isolates were *L. innocua*, 13 were *L. welshimeri,* and 12 were *L. monocytogenes.* Isolation rates peaked from October through April.

Wang and Muriana found *L. monocytogenes* in 6 of 20 brands of frankfurters purchased in retail markets in Indiana (*720*). In samples representing 19 of the brands, *Listeria* species were found in 9 of 93 packages. Seven isolates were *L. monocytogenes* and 2 were *L. innocua.* For the remaining brand, 17 of 24 samples (71%) contained *L. monocytogenes* and 81% contained *Listeria* spp. This brand had the highest pH and NaCl levels of 5 brands tested. Listeria was found only in the exudate, indicating that contamination occurred after processing.

Sheridan et al. tested for *Listeria* in 549 samples of fresh, frozen, and ready-to-eat retail meat, fish, and poultry products in the Dublin area (*721*). Cooked meats prepackaged by the manufacturer were negative, but listeria was isolated from 21% of cooked meats sold unpackaged at retail, indicating postprocessing contamination. *Listeria* spp. were most frequently isolated from frozen beefburgers (97%) and fish fingers (95%). For frozen products, a new resuscitation method gave counts up to 2.5 $\log_{10}$ higher than a standard recovery procedure. Sixty-one isolates were *L. monocytogenes,* 210 were *L. innocua,* and 40 were other species (*L. welshimeri, L. seeligeri, L. ivanovii, L. murrayi,* and *L. grayi*).

Although large populations of listerias were found in meats and seafoods purchased from markets in India, no *L. monocytogenes* was seen (*722*). *Listeria innocua* and *L. murrayi* were the major species in meat products, whereas *L. grayi* and *L. seeligeri* predominated in fish.

Moura et al. evaluated the incidence of *Listeria* spp. in raw and pasteurized milk from a dairy plant in Brazil (*723*). Ten samples of each type of milk were collected monthly, except in December, for one year. Thirteen percent of raw milk samples and 1% of pasteurized milk samples were positive for *Listeria.* The corresponding contamination rates for *L. monocytogenes* were 10% and 0%. Besides *L. monocytogenes,* raw milk also contained *L. innocua, L. welshimeri,* and *L. grayi.* Pasteurized milk contained only *L. innocua.*

Investigators in the UK sampled an egg pasteurizing plant's in-line filters that remove solids from raw blended egg, to check for the presence of listerias (*724*). During daily sampling for 5 months, 173 samples were collected. Of these, 125 (72%) were positive. The only species isolated were *L. innocua* (62%) and *L. monocytogenes* (38%). A most-probable-number method was used to estimate the numbers of listerias in the blended raw egg. Samples from 9 successive days' production had a mean level of 1 organism per milliliter. Although listerias were frequently present at low levels in raw egg before pasteurization, none of 500 samples tested positive for listeria after pasteurization.

SURVIVAL AND GROWTH IN FOODS. A survey of 101 retail samples of various types of paté found *L. innocua* in 12 samples, *L. monocytogenes* in 7, and *L. welshimeri* and *L. ivanovii* in one each (*725*). Although *L. monocytogenes* survived in naturally contaminated patés during 3 weeks of storage at 4°C, it grew only in a turkey-based product. The organism also survived but did not grow at 4°C in artificially inoculated patés. Examination of the ingredients in the patés suggested that preservatives, pH, $a_w$, and temperature together secured the microbial stability of these products. Random sampling also detected low numbers (10/g) of *L. monocytogenes* in some samples of wieners, turkey breast, and vacuum-packaged sliced ham. Again, the organism survived but showed virtually no growth in these meats during storage at 4°C. A similar study of the *L. monocytogenes* content of unpackaged sliced lunch meats purchased from supermarkets and small retail shops in Germany found low levels of natural contamination and no growth after 1 week of storage at 2–4°C (*726*). At 7°C, populations increased by 2–4 $\log_{10}$. These investigators concluded that growth of *L. monocytogenes* was inhibited by lactic acid bacteria in the cold-cuts.

Hardin et al. evaluated the survival of *L. monocytogenes* in precooked beef roasts inoculated with $10^9$ cfu before various regimens of postpasteurization and storage (*727*). The postpasteurization conditions tested were 91 and 96°C for 3 and 5 min. Storage was at 4 or 10°C. Although some organisms survived each of the treatments, the lethality of postpasteurization was directly related to time and temperature. Storage temperature had a negligible effect on subsequent growth.

Fang and Lin studied the effect of a system combining modified-atmosphere packaging (MAP) and nisin on the relative growth of *L. monocytogenes* and a spoilage organism, *Pseudomonas fragi*, in cooked pork tenderloins (*728*). The atmospheres tested were air, 100% $CO_2$, and 80% $CO_2$ plus 20% air. In air, *P. fragi* outgrew *L. monocytogenes* with or without nisin at both 4 and 20°C. Treatment with $10^4$ IU/mL of nisin prevented growth of *L. monocytogenes* but had no effect on *P. fragi*, whereas *P. fragi* was inhibited by elevated $CO_2$ concentrations and *L. monocytogenes* was not. Combined treatment with MAP and nisin inhibited both organisms, but the inhibitory effects were greater at 4°C than at 20°C.

Grant et al. studied the growth of two outbreak-related strains of *L. monocytogenes* inoculated into portions of cook–chill roast beef and gravy before irradiation with 2 kGy (*729*). Unirradiated samples were inoculated with $10^2$ cfu/g, and irradiated samples received a large enough inoculum to insure survival of $10^2$/g after irradiation. The pH of the beef and gravy was 6.0, which is optimal for growth of the organism in meat products. Specific growth rates were similar in irradiated and nonirradiated portions. However, irradiation delayed the exponential growth phase by 6–9 days at 5°C and by 3–4 days at 10°C. The corresponding lag periods in unirradiated samples were 1–2 days and 0.1 days. The author concluded that irradiation of cook–chill roast beef and gravy to a level of 2 kGy does not increase risk of listeriosis.

Huang et al. studied the survival and growth of *L. monocytogenes* in chicken gravy during cooling and storage (*730*). After cooking to 70–77°C, different volumes of gravy (1.9, 3.8, or 5.7 L) were refrigerated at 7°C in rectangular pans measuring 17.5 cm by 32.4 cm. When the temperature reached 40°C, the gravy was inoculated with *L. monocytogenes* Scott A to give ~$10^4$ cfu/mL. The time required for the gravy to cool to 40°C ranged from 12 h for 1.9 L to 26 h for 5.7 L. Populations of *L. monocytogenes* ranged from $1.0 \times 10^5$ to $3.2 \times 10^6$ cfu/mL after 24 h of refrigeration, and growth rates in different volumes of gravy were significantly different ($p < .001$). Maximum growth ($\geq 10^8$ cfu/mL) was achieved 4–6 days after inoculation, depending on the volume of gravy. No further change occurred even after extended storage. These data demonstrate the importance of rapid chilling of heated foods.

The most common way for pathogens and spoilage organisms to enter the contents of eggs is thought to be by contamination from the shell when the egg is broken. Bartlett investigated the survival of *L. monocytogenes* inoculated onto shell eggs and its resistance to sodium hypochlorite (*731*). No listerias were recovered from the contents of any inoculated eggs. The number of loosely bound survivors decreased during storage at 10°C, until no more were detected after 11 days. Numbers of cells judged as tightly bound to the shell did not decrease significantly after 11 days. A 30-s application of sodium hypochlorite solution containing 50 or 100 ppm of available chlorine completely eliminated loosely bound cells, whereas there was little or no decrease in numbers of strongly attached cells even after 5 min. The authors concluded that loosely attached cells remain viable long enough to reach the egg-breaking stage of a commercial operation and could contaminate liquid egg during the breaking process. Use of a sanitizing rinse effectively eliminates loosely bound cells and minimizes the risk of contaminating the liquid egg. However, the survival of tightly attached *L. monocytogenes* cells shows the importance of preventing introduction of shell material into the egg product.

Back et al. found that *L. monocytogenes* survived and usually grew when inoculated into the cheese milk of laboratory-made Camembert cheese (*732*). Growth rates were higher at the surface of the cheeses than at the center, possibly because of the greater availability of oxygen at the surface or the proteolysis and higher pH associated with the mold ripening process. Similar results were obtained when Camembert cheeses were surface-inoculated after manufacture. The organism survived on all commercially manufactured soft cheeses tested, but it failed to grow in blue and white Stilton, Mycella, Chaume, and a full-fat soft cheese with garlic and herbs. Significant growth occurred at 5 and 10°C on Cambazola, several kinds of brie, and blue and white Lymeswold, but storage at 3°C severely restricted growth.

Because *L. monocytogenes* frequently contaminates raw vegetables and can survive or grow slowly under refrigeration, it may be a hazard in prepackaged salads with extended shelf-life. The first phase of a Canadian investigation of the potential for *L. monocytogenes* to proliferate in chilled vegetable products has been completed (*733*). A factorial experiment showed the effects of inoculum size, modified atmosphere, and storage temperature on growth of *L. monocytogenes* Scott A in coleslaw. The undressed coleslaw formulation of cabbage plus carrot and the low-barrier polyethylene packaging film conformed to those in typical commercial products. Rates of growth at the two inoculum sizes ($10^3$ and $10^6$ cfu/g) did not differ significantly, indicating that competition from the indigenous flora did not restrict growth. Nor did modification of the package atmosphere affect growth of *Listeria*, but this was not surprising because the low-barrier packaging film required to permit aerobic respiration of the cabbage also permitted rapid equilibration with the ambient atmosphere. Little or no growth occurred at 3°C, but there was significant growth at 8°C. The authors concluded that with mild temperature abuse, high populations of *L. monocytogenes* can develop in coleslaw with no obvious signs of spoilage, regardless of the packaging method. Further studies are examining the competitive ability of *Listeria* inocula within the range of realistic natural contamination levels and the effects of a variety of highly permeable packaging materials.

Omary et al. determined how packaging films with different oxygen-transmission rates affected growth of *Listeria* in shredded cabbage, using *L. innocua* as a surrogate for *L. monocytogenes* (*734*). The oxygen-transmission rates of the four films tested ranged from 5.6 to 1000 cm$^3$/m$^2$ in 24 h. Populations remained stable or dropped slightly after 14 d at 11°C, but increased after 21 d. The greatest decrease at 14 d and the smallest increase at 21 d were seen for the film with the highest oxygen-transmission rate.

Another study determined the fate of *L. monocytogenes* on broad-leaved and curly-leaved endive, butterhead lettuce, and lamb's lettuce stored for 7 days at 10°C (*735*). These types of salad greens are widely sold as ready-to-use products in France. In 4 days, *L. monocytogenes* populations increased by 1.5 $\log_{10}$ on broad-leaved endive and butterhead lettuce and by 0.5 $\log_{10}$ on curly-leaved endive. They decreased by 1 $\log_{10}$ on lamb's lettuce. Little or no additional growth occurred between day 4 and day 7.

Because *L. innocua* is isolated from foods more often than *L. monocytogenes,* Petran and Swanson evaluated the growth of the two species when they were grown separately and simultaneously in several *Listeria* culture media and in cheese sauce (*736*). Growth and population maxima of the two species were similar in cheese sauce and trypticase soy broth plus yeast extract. However, in the more selective Fraser broth and University of Vermont medium, *L. innocua* populations were significantly higher than *L. monocytogenes* populations whether the media were inoculated with only one species or both. The authors concluded that choice of culture media may influence the relative frequency with which these species are isolated from food and environmental samples. Moreover, cultural methods that rely on selective enrichment media for isolation of *L. monocytogenes* may not permit recovery of the organism if significant levels of *L. innocua* are also present.

The resistance of *L. monocytogenes* to osmotic stress, combined with its ability to survive and grow under refrigeration, make it a formidable and insidious threat in foods. Ko et al. showed that the organism's accumulation of exogenous glycine betaine, a ubiquitous and effective osmotic agent, is stimulated by both cold stress and salt stress and confers both cryotolerance and osmotolerance (*737*). Intracellular accumulation is due to transport from the medium rather than to biosynthesis. In terms of kinetics, the cold- and salt-stimulated transport systems are indistinguishable and may be the same. Activation was not blocked by chloramphenicol, indicating that the system or systems are constitutive. The finding of a cold-activated transport system is novel and has implications for the physical state of the cell membrane at low temperatures.

Hefnawy and Marth investigated the growth and survival of *L. monocytogenes* strains Scott A and V7 in tryptose broth at 4 and 13°C in the presence of sublethal concentrations of NaCl (*738*). Storage time, strain of *L. monocytogenes*, and NaCl concentration were individually and interactively significant in determining the bacterium's behavior at the two temperatures. Although a wide range of salt concentrations permitted growth, storage at 4°C enhanced the inhibitory action of NaCl. Strain V7 was more salt-sensitive than Scott A at both temperatures.

Oh and Marshall studied the interactive effects of temperature, pH, and glycerol monolaurate on survival and growth of *L. monocytogenes* Scott A in tryptic soy broth with yeast extract (*739*). Temperature and pH strongly influenced the antilisterial potency of monolaurin. The substance was bactericidal at pH 5.0 but not at pH 5.5 or 7.0. At constant pH, lethal action increased with temperature but sublethal effects decreased with temperature.

Beuchat et al. found that the lethal and inhibitory effects of carrot juice on *L. monocytogenes* were greatest in a pH range of 5.0–6.4 (*740*). Inhibition was greater in 10% carrot juice than in 1% or 100% and was inversely related to temperature in the range of 5–20°C. At concentrations up to 5%, NaCl protected *L. monocytogenes* against inactivation by carrot juice. The effect was greatest in 10% juice at 5 or 12°C. The behavior of background microflora in the carrot juice was not significantly influenced by factors affecting antilisterial activity. The listericidal and listeriostatic effects of carrot juice have not been evaluated in food systems.

A Canadian study evaluated the ability of wieners to support growth of *L. monocytogenes* and the biochemical and microbiological factors that influence the pathogen's survival and growth (*741*). All-beef, poultry, and beef-and-pork wieners from 6 Canadian processing plants were surface-inoculated with a 3-strain mixture of *L. monocytogenes* and stored under vacuum at 5°C for 28 d. Forty of 61 samples supported growth under these conditions. A stepwise multiple regression model was developed from data on 35 samples, based on initial values for pH and counts of lactic acid bacteria and counts of lactic acid bacteria after 14 d. This model explained 48.1% of the variation in *L. monocytogenes* counts after 14 d. The USDA's Pathogen Modelling Program, based on storage temperature, initial pH, and nitrite and salt concentrations, explained only 12.4% of the variation in observed times to a 1-log$_{10}$ increase in the pathogen population. As revealed by scanning electron microscopy, the surface of a skinless wiener consists of a dense layer of coagulated protein with some small cavities, which may provide a different environment from that in the general product formulation. The authors concluded that the ability of some wieners to support growth of *L. monocytogenes* makes them a health hazard if they become contaminated after processing. They also stressed the need for better predictive models to describe the growth of *L. monocytogenes* in ready-to-eat meat products.

Using data from factorial experiments, Hudson developed and tested several response-surface models of the growth of *L. monocytogenes* in tryptose phosphate broth under aerobic conditions with various values of initial pH and NaCl and nitrate concentration (*742*). Cubic models were slightly superior to quadratic equations. The model for strain Scott A was better for predicting lag times, whereas the model for food-derived strain L70 was better for predicting generation times. This was well illustrated in a table comparing predicted values

with measured kinetic data, based on mixed inocula, for growth of *L. monocytogenes* on smoked salmon, paté, cooked beef, and minced mussels. The authors recommend either the construction of models for more than one strain or the use of mixtures of strains.

Sörqvist reported significant differences in heat resistance between serovars and strains of *L. monocytogenes*, as measured in physiological saline solution by a glass capillary tube method (*743*). *D* values were higher when the recovery medium was preincubated. Ranges of *D* values at 58, 60, 62, and 64°C were, respectively, 1.7–3.4, 0.72–3.1, 0.30–1.3, and 0.33–0.68 min. The *z* values ranged from 5.2 to 6.9°C. These results demonstrate the importance of basing guidelines for thermal processing on the more heat-resistant strains of *L. monocytogenes*.

To test the ability of microwave cooking to destroy *L. monocytogenes* and *Aeromonas hydrophila*, catfish fillets were surface-inoculated with a mixed culture to give ≈10$^6$ cfu/cm$^2$ of each organism (*744*). Uncovered fillets and fillets covered with polyvinylidene chloride film were then cooked to internal temperatures of 55, 60, and 70°C. *Listeria monocytogenes* was more heat-resistant than *A. hydrophila*, although cooking covered fillets to an internal temperature of 70°C caused a 6-log$_{10}$ reduction in populations of both organisms. Covering the fillets increased lethality at all temperatures, by increasing the thermal end-point temperature and making heating and cooling more even. Nevertheless, some pathogens survived at temperatures ≤60°C. At 60°C, *L. monocytogenes* populations were reduced by ≈4 log$_{10}$ in covered fillets and ≈2 log$_{10}$ in uncovered fillets.

Palumbo et al. studied the thermal destruction of *L. monocytogenes* Scott A during production of liver sausage (*745*). Liver sausage emulsion was inoculated to give an initial population of ~10$^9$/g, stuffed into large-diameter moisture-proof fibrous casings, and cooked in a smokehouse. As the product reached each predetermined initial temperature, core samples were tested for viable *L. monocytogenes*. Viable counts remained constant up to 140°F (60°C). Fewer viable organisms were detected at 145°F (63°C), and none at 155°F (68°C). The authors concluded that liver sausage and other large-diameter nonfermented sausages should be free of viable *L. monocytogenes* if heated to 155°F.

In the past, *L. monocytogenes* has survived the pasteurization of milk to cause outbreaks of foodborne listeriosis. Because the variable fat content of different milks may affect the effectiveness of pasteurization, MacDonald and Sutherland evaluated the survival of *L. monocytogenes*, *L. innocua*, and gram-negative psychrotrophic spoilage bacteria in heat-treated milk from

sheep, cows, and goats (*746*). When $10^6-10^7$ cfu/mL of
4 *Listeria* strains were inoculated into test tubes with
cow's and sheep's milk containing 1, 5, or 10% homologous fat and heated at 65°C, no organisms were recoverable from cow's milk after 45 min. However, sheep's
milk samples with 5 and 10% fat contained viable listerias
after 45 min. A starting inoculum as low as $9\times10^2$/mL
survived for 30 min in sheep's milk containing 10% fat,
but no viable organisms were recovered after heating
for 45 min. Sheep fat added to skim cow's milk was
protective, whereas the same concentration of cow fat
was not. In whole sheep's milk (7% fat), listerias survived a 30-min heat treatment at 68°C but not a 15-min
treatment at 72°C. However, when whole sheep's milk
containing $10^6$ cfu/mL of *L. monocytogenes* was heated
in a plate pasteurizer at 68–74°C for 15 s, only 10 cfu/mL
survived at 68°C and none were recovered at higher
temperatures. The authors concluded that factors specific to sheep's milk protect bacteria against heating, but
that even high levels of *L. monocytogenes* in whole milk
could not survive the current HTST plate pasteurization
process used in the UK.

Investigators in Denmark evaluated the heat resistance of two *L. monocytogenes* strains in sous-vide
cooked fillets of cod and salmon (*747*). *D*- and *z*-values
were determined from tests of bacterial survival in 5-g
fish sticks at various time–temperature combinations.
Both strains were more heat-resistant in salmon than in
cod, perhaps because of salmon's higher fat content.
*D*-values were within the range published for other
food products: $D_{60}$ ranged between 1.95 and 4.48 min
depending on the listerial strain and the type of fish.
Values for *z* were 5.65 and 6.4°C for the two strains. The
data obtained can be used to predict the heat process
necessary to achieve the desired reduction of listerial
populations in small fish fillets.

Kim et al. studied how heating and storage conditions affect survival of *L. monocytogenes* in ground pork
and the recovery of injured cells (*748*). There were
significantly more survivors when the heating rate was
1.3°C/min than when it was 8.0°C/min. Cells inoculated
into pork that had been stored at –10°C for 3 months
were more sensitive than cells inoculated into freshly
ground pork ($D_{62°C}$ = 5.2 and 7.7 min, respectively).
Aerobic heating permitted more survivors than anaerobic heating, but storage under vacuum at 4 or 30°C
allowed faster recovery than storage under air.

Ergo is a naturally fermented product made from
raw milk and widely consumed in Ethiopia. It is made in
the home by leaving milk at ambient temperature for
about 24 h. In some areas raw milk is kept in a ferment-
ing vessel that is smoked with acacia or olive wood. To
assess the potential listeriosis hazard of Ergo, Ashenafi
monitored the fate of three strains of *L. monocytogenes*
during the souring of raw milk (*749*). When inoculated
into sterile milk at a level of ~$10^3$ cfu/mL, all strains
reached counts >$10^7$/mL within 24 h, after which there
was little change. Smoking of containers decreased the
growth rate slightly. When the strains were inoculated
into Ergo, counts increased by 1.0–1.7 $\log_{10}$ during the
first 12 h, dropped slightly but remained at or above the
initial level at 24 h, and then fell sharply to undetectable
levels by 48–60 h. In smoked containers inactivation was
complete or nearly complete by 36 h. During souring,
the pH dropped from ~6.5 to ~4 within 24 h and then
remained constant. Since Ergo is generally consumed
after about 24 h of fermentation, there is danger of
acquiring listeriosis if the raw milk is contaminated with
*L. monocytogenes.*

Dillon and Patel surface-inoculated cod fillets with
*L. monocytogenes*, cold-smoked and vacuum-packaged
the fillets, and stored them at 4°C for 3 weeks or at –20°C
for 3 months (*750*). At each stage of smoking and
periodically during storage, listerias were enumerated by
the 3-tube MPN method. Counts were relatively stable
throughout smoking. During storage they increased
at 4°C but decreased at –20°C. Substantial growth
occurred during storage when the inoculum level was
high ($10^5-10^6$/g), but growth was very slow when the
inoculum level was only $10^1$/g.

White pickled cheese is a traditional Sudanese
product made from raw milk to which 6–20% salt is
added for control of foodborne pathogens. Abdalla et al.
monitored the chemical composition of the cheese and
the survival of *L. monocytogenes* during cheese making
(*751*). They found that 8% salt inhibited the growth and
acid production of the lactic acid starter culture but did
not inhibit growth of *L. monocytogenes.*

## Control of *Listeria* in Foods

The few reported cases of foodborne listeriosis in otherwise healthy individuals are apparently due to consumption of large numbers of the pathogen. For the old, the
very young, immunosuppressed persons, and pregnant
women, however, the infective dose is considerably
lower—but how low is not known. Certain foods pose a
greater risk than others. Based on this evidence and on
principles laid down by the International Commission
on Microbiological Specifications for Foods (ICMSF),
the ICMSF developed a decision tree to facilitate selection of an appropriate sampling plan and criteria for *L.
monocytogenes* (*752*). The Commission recommends
use of the sampling plan in conjunction with an HACCP

plan, to verify that HACCP is working correctly. It also recommends that guidelines for the selection and safe handling of foods be provided for high-risk individuals.

To identify critical points for introduction of *L. monocytogenes* in meat production, van den Elzen and Snijders monitored animal and environmental samples during slaughter and processing of pork and beef (*753*). For pork, 2–7% of carcasses and 0–10% of environmental samples from the "clean" part of the slaughter line were positive for *L. monocytogenes*. No *L. monocytogenes* was isolated from the anus borer, indicating that feces are not an important source of contamination. The incidence increased after chilling and cutting: 11–36% of primal cuts and 71–100% of environmental samples from the cutting room were positive. Primal cuts and consumer units were still contaminated in the distribution plant. These results indicate that most contamination occurs from environmental sources in the chilling room and cutting room. The incidence of *L. monocytogenes* in carcass and environmental samples from the beef processing line was much lower, 0–60%. This could be explained by different conditions and procedures in the beef slaughterhouse and processing line. Other species of *Listeria* were also isolated in this study.

**CHEMICAL AND PHYSICAL CONTROL AND PACKAGING.** Wederquist et al. assessed the inhibition of *L. monocytogenes* in laboratory-formulated turkey bologna by chemical additives (*754*). After cooking and cooling, the bologna was peeled, sliced, surface-inoculated with ~$10^2$ cfu/g of a 7-strain mixture of *L. monocytogenes*, vacuum-packaged, and stored at 4°C. The six treatments were 0.5% sodium acetate, 1% sodium bicarbonate, 3% sodium lactate, 0.26% potassium sorbate, all four of these combined, and no chemicals. Bologna treated with sodium bicarbonate or all four chemicals had an initial pH of 7.6. The initial pH for the other treatments was 6.6–6.7. Sodium acetate prevented growth of *L. monocytogenes*, although the organism survived throughout the 100-day storage period at its initial inoculum level. The relative effectiveness of the treatments was sodium acetate > sodium lactate = potassium sorbate > combination > sodium bicarbonate = no chemicals.

Sodium diacetate ($CH_3COOH \cdot CH_3COONa$) is used in foods for pH control and flavoring and as an antimicrobial agent. Shelef and Addala evaluated its ability to inhibit *L. monocytogenes* and other bacteria in BHI broth, beef slurry, and ground beef (*755*). In broth, sodium diacetate inhibited *L. monocytogenes* Scott A more effectively than acetic acid in the pH range of 5.0–6.0. Addition of 0.3% diacetate to ground beef or beef slurry suppressed total aerobic counts during refrigerated storage. Although treated samples had a slightly lower pH (5.2 vs. 5.6), most of the effect was attributable to the diacetate itself. Sodium diacetate suppressed growth of *E. coli*, *Pseudomonas fluorescens*, *Salmonella enteritidis*, *Shewanella putrefaciens*, and 4 strains of *L. monocytogenes*. *Pseudomonas fragi*, *Yersinia enterocolitica*, *Enterococcus faecalis*, *Lactobacillus fermentis*, and *Staphylococcus aureus* were insensitive to the compound.

Schlyter et al. monitored the antilisterial activity of sodium diacetate, pediocin, and ALTA™ 2341, a commercial shelf-life extender, in turkey breast-meat slurries held at 25°C (*756*). In control slurries, populations increased by about 5 $\log_{10}$ units in 7 days. Addition of 0.3% diacetate increased the generation time from 1.7 h to 7 h, and 0.5% diacetate caused an 0.4-$\log_{10}$ decrease in counts after 7 days. ALTA and pediocin had similar intrinsic listericidal activity. Concentrations of ALTA ≤0.75%, alone or in combination with 0.1% diacetate, had no effect. However, the combination of 0.25, 0.50, or 0.75% ALTA with 0.3 or 0.5% diacetate had greater antilisterial activity than diacetate alone. These data confirm the utility of diacetate as an antilisterial agent for poultry and document the added (if limited) effect of combining ALTA with diacetate. In similar studies, the same research group evaluated the antilisterial effects of sodium diacetate with nitrite, lactate, or pediocin in turkey slurries (*757*). Again, diacetate alone delayed growth of *L. monocytogenes*. Nitrite and lactate alone had no effect, whereas pediocin had a temporary effect lasting only for the first day. However, combinations of diacetate with lactate or especially pediocin had a synergistic or additive effect, which would provide an additional level of safety.

Glycerol monolaurate (monolaurin), approved in the USA as a food emulsifier, also has broad-spectrum antimicrobial activity. However, the latter property is reduced by many food components. Because monolaurin is insoluble in water, it is frequently dissolved in ethanol. Thus its interactions with ethanol are of interest. Oh and Marshall determined the MICs of monolaurin, ethanol, and lactic acid, alone and in combination, against *L. monocytogenes* in tryptic soy broth (*758*). There was evidence of a small additive effect of ethanol and either monolaurin or lactic acid.

Wang et al. synthesized monoacylglyerols by reacting coconut oil and milk fat with lipase in the presence of unesterified glycerol (*759*). The product was removed by solvent fractionation and tested for antilisterial activity. Activity depended on the fatty acid composition of the preparation. The monoacylglycerol mixture from coconut oil inactivated *L. monocytogenes* at a concentration of 250–400 µg/mL in pasteurized skim milk, 500–750 µg/mL in 2% milk, and 750–100 µg/mL in full-fat milk. It was more effective than monolaurin against *L. monocytogenes* in BHI broth and pasteurized milk. In contrast, the milk-fat preparation did not inhibit the organism in milk. Certain combinations of monoacylglycerols, particularly monolaurin and monocaprin, had synergistic activity against *L. monocytogenes*. Diacylglyerols, triacylglycerols, and certain other food components reduced the antibacterial effectiveness of monoacylglyerols. The precise mechanism of antibacterial action is not known, but some form of action on the cell membrane is likely.

Dorsa et al. evaluated the effect of citric acid and potassium sorbate sprays on growth of *L. monocytogenes* on crawfish tail meat stored at 4°C (*760*). Treatment with 0.3 g/kg of citric acid had no significant effect. Treatment with 0.3 g/kg of potassium sorbate extended the lag phase by 2 days, but had no effect on generation time. The authors concluded that neither treatment would be of practical use in controlling *L. monocytogenes* on crawfish tail meat.

To validate a predictive model developed for broth cultures, Whiting and Masana examined the effects of nitrite and pH on survival of *L. monocytogenes* in a simulated uncooked fermented meat product (*761*). They ground lean beef with salt, adjusted the pH to five values ranging from 4.0 to 5.1, added nitrite at concentrations of 0, 150, or 300 µg/g, and inoculated portions with $10^7$ cfu/g of a 3-strain mixture of *L. monocytogenes*. Survivors were enumerated during 21 days of storage at 37°C. The time to achieve a 4-$\log_{10}$ decline ranged from 21 days at pH 5.0 to less than 1 day at pH 4.0. Some growth occurred at pH 5.1 after a long lag period. Nitrite did not affect survival under these conditions.

Pelroy and her associates have studied the control of *L. monocytogenes* in cold-smoked salmon by chemicals and packaging (*762–764*). At 10°C, with oxygen-permeable packaging, an inoculum of 10 cfu/g grew to $10^6$–$10^8$ cfu/g in 2 weeks (*762*). Sodium chloride at concentrations of 3, 5, or 6% had no effect on growth at 10°C except for an initial lag in samples with 6% salt. Vacuum packaging suppressed growth by 1–2 $\log_{10}$ units in samples with 3 or 5% NaCl. Salt was somewhat more effective at 5°C. At this temperature, 6% NaCl held populations below $10^2$/g for both types of packaging. However, because consumer acceptability limits the amount of NaCl that can be used, additional inhibitors are needed to prevent growth of *L. monocytogenes* if contaminated products are stored at improper temperatures. Two possible inhibitors are sodium nitrite and sodium lactate. The inhibitory concentration of $NaNO_2$

is related to inoculum size, storage time, and temperature (*763*). The greatest inhibition was seen in vacuum-packaged products with 190–200 ppm of $NaNO_2$ and 5% aqueous-phase NaCl stored at 5°C. These conditions prevented any increase in an inoculum of 10 cfu/g during 34 days of storage. At 10°C, however, the inoculum grew to $10^6$ cfu/g in vacuum-packaged fish and $10^8$ cfu/g with permeable-film packaging, regardless of $NaNO_2$ or NaCl concentration. Sodium lactate had a concentration-dependent antilisterial effect that was enhanced by nitrite, high concentrations of NaCl, or both (*764*). At 5°C, total inhibition of *L. monocytogenes* was achieved for 50 days by 2% sodium lactate combined with 3% aqueous-phase NaCl. At 10°C, total inhibition was achieved for at least 35 days by 3% sodium lactate with 3% NaCl or by 2% lactate with 125 ppm $NaNO_2$ and 3% NaCl. Thus sodium lactate appears promising, when used in conjunction with other hurdles, as a means to control the growth of *L. monocytogenes* in smoked fish during refrigerated storage.

In studies of sliced frankfurter-type sausage, Krämer and Baumgart showed that packaging in an atmosphere containing high levels of $CO_2$ can inhibit growth of *L. monocytogenes* for extended periods of storage at 4, 7, or 10°C (*765*). The extent of inhibition is related to $CO_2$ concentration and gas volume, both of which place practical limits on the degree of inhibition that can be achieved. The highest and most effective concentration of $CO_2$ tested, 80%, imparts an unacceptable sour flavor to the product, whereas large gas volumes require a high expenditure on packaging and are also unacceptable to the consumer. Packaging under $CO_2$ also inhibits growth of *L. monocytogenes* on beef striploin steaks of normal ultimate pH (5.3–5.5) stored at 5 or 10°C (*766*). Steaks were vacuum packaged or flushed and packaged with 100% $CO_2$. With vacuum packaging, populations increased by ~3 $\log_{10}$ units in 23 days at 5°C and in 11 days at 10°C, whereas at both temperatures under $CO_2$, populations decreased slightly during 50 days of storage. The authors did not report the sensory quality of steaks stored under $CO_2$, and the volume of gas was rather high—2 L for a packet of 5 steaks.

The lactoperoxidase system is an antimicrobial system naturally present in milk. It is activated by addition of thiocyanate, and its effect is due to intermediates in the lactoperoxidase-catalyzed oxidation of thiocyanate by $H_2O_2$. Zapico et al. evaluated the effects of the goat's milk system on three strains of *L. monocytogenes* during storage of raw goat's milk (*767*). All strains grew in control milk at 4°C, with population increases of 1–2 $\log_{10}$ units in 10 days. With an activated lactoperoxidase system there was slight but significant antilisterial activity for 3–9 days against all strains at 4°C. Strain NCTC 11994 was considerably more resistant than Scott A and 5069. Inhibition lasted 1–7 days at 8°C and only 1 day at 20°C. Lactoperoxidase was more stable in the activated system than in control milk.

A number of spices are bacteriostatic or bactericidal against *L. monocytogenes* when tested in tryptose broth. Hefnawy et al. extended the studies in this system, comparing the effects of numerous spices on *L. monocytogenes* strains Scott A and V7 (*768*). Scott A was the more sensitive strain. At a concentration of 1% spice, the population of Scott A fell from the inoculum level of $10^5$–$10^7$/mL to <10/mL in 1 day with sage, 4 days with allspice, and 7 days with cumin, garlic powder, paprika, or red pepper. Black pepper and mace were less effective, and white pepper enhanced growth. Only sage reduced populations of strain V7 to <10/mL, and 7 days were required. Allspice, mace, and nutmeg had some activity against V7 at concentrations of 3 and 5%. The next step is study of the most active spices in foods, at concentrations likely to be used in foods. One such study was reported by Pandit and Shelef (*769*). In addition to ground rosemary they tested various components of rosemary: its essential oil, four major oil constituents (cineole, borneole, α-pinene, camphor), oleoresin, encapsulated oil, and an antioxidant extract. Testing was done in BHI broth and in ready-to-eat pork-liver sausage. In BHI broth, 0.5% rosemary was listericidal after 48 h at 35°C. Rosemary oil was inhibitory at a concentration of 10 µL per 100 mL. Of the major constituents of rosemary oil, only α-pinene (0.1 µL per 100 mL) delayed growth. Other active constituents were the oleoresin (100 mg per 100 mL), the encapsulated oil (1 g per 100 mL), and the antioxidant extract (0.02 g per 100 mL). The aqueous extract of rosemary was considerably less active than the ethanolic extract or the ground herb. In pork-liver sausage, *L. monocytogenes* counts increased from the inoculum level of $10^2$/g to $10^9$/g after 20 days of refrigerated storage. Addition of 0.5% ground rosemary or 1% rosemary oil to pork-liver sausage before cooking reduced listerial counts by ~1 $\log_{10}$. The encapsulated oil (5%) and the antioxidant extract (0.3–0.5%) reduced counts by ~4.5 $\log_{10}$.

Postpackaging pasteurization effectively controls *L. monocytogenes* in precooked refrigerated beef loin (*770*). Loin chunks were inoculated after cooking. They were then vacuum-packaged, and half of the packages were pasteurized in water at 85°C for 15 min. The internal temperature reached 60°C during pasteurization. Control chunks were not inoculated. Listerial populations increased in all unpasteurized packages, peaking in 7–14 days and then leveling off or falling

slightly and then leveling off. The indigenous listerias in uninoculated loin chunks were mostly *L. welshimeri*. No listerias were detected in the broth or on the surface of any pasteurized loin at any time during 12 weeks of refrigerated storage.

Patterson et al. developed mathematical models to describe the growth of *L. monocytogenes* in irradiated and nonirradiated minced poultry meat stored at temperatures of 6–15°C (*771*). Large inocula (up to $10^7$/g) were used in these experiments. In unirradiated samples, temperatures in this range did not significantly affect lag time. Lag time was longer after irradiation with 2.5 kGy than with 1.0 kGy, but the difference was smaller at higher temperatures. The longest lag time was seen at 6°C after a dose of 2.5 kGy (14.9 days in raw meat and 18.6 days in cooked meat). The authors concluded that even if some *L. monocytogenes* cells survive irradiation, the time needed to recover from radiation damage should delay their growth during the normal shelf-life of the meat.

Lin et al. investigated the antilisterial activity of pressurized $CO_2$ in broth and full-fat, reduced-fat, and nonfat milk (*772*). *Listeria monocytogenes* was inactivated at 35 and 45°C by $CO_2$ under pressures of 70 and 211 kg/cm². Rates of inactivation were temperature- and pressure-sensitive. The pH and moisture content of the medium also influenced the effectiveness of treatment. Bacteria were more difficult to inactivate when the medium contained fat.

**BACTERIOCINS.** Many lactic acid bacteria produce small proteins called bacteriocins that kill or inhibit growth of other bacteria. Héchard et al. discussed the antilisterial bacteriocins produced by *Pediococcus* and *Leuconostoc* (*773*). These bacteriocins are related proteins of 2.7–4.6 kDa encoded by plasmid-linked genes. Three of them for which amino acid sequences are known show strong sequence homology. The authors summarized the purification, characterization, spectrum of inhibition, and mode of action of these bacteriocins.

Benderroum et al. developed two techniques for testing the bactericidal activity of bacteriocins (*774*). Both might be adaptable for testing other antimicrobial substances. The test substance or an inoculum of the bacteriocin-producing organism is placed in a well cut in a lawn of the indicator strain. Lysis of the indicator cells is revealed as a clear zone. The method was developed using a bacteriocin-producing strain of *Lactococcus lactis lactis* and a bacteriocin-negative mutant of it. The indicator organism was *L. monocytogenes* ATCC 7644.

Ryser et al. used a new hydrophobic grid membrane method to screen 105 traditional French cheeses for surface microorganisms inhibitory to *L. mono-cytogenes* V7 (*775*). Fewer than 0.1% of 125,000 colonies produced visible zones of inhibition. Isolates having antilisterial activity were various strains of *Enterococcus faecalis, Staphylococcus xylosus, Staphylococcus warneri*, and coryneform bacteria including one orange coryneform resembling *Brevibacterium linens*. The orange coryneform and all strains of *E. faecalis* that inhibited *L. monocytogenes* V7 were also strongly inhibitory against a panel of *Listeria* strains comprising *L. monocytogenes* (14 strains), *L. innocua* (2 strains), *L. ivanovii* (2 strains), *L. seeligeri* (2 strains), and *L. welshimeri* (1 strain). All inhibitory substances except the one produced by the orange coryneform were sensitive to one or more proteolytic enzymes and were therefore considered to be bacteriocin-like agents.

Raccach and Geshell evaluated the ability of three strains of *Pediococcus acidilactici* (Pa, PAC, PO2) and two of *Pediococcus pentosaceus* (FBB-61, L7230) to inhibit growth of *L. monocytogenes* in milk at 32°C (*776*). Milk was inoculated with $10^5$ cfu/mL of listerias and $10^9$ cfu/mL of pediococci. All pediococci except *P. acidilactici* Pa were known producers of bacteriocins (pediocins), and all except *P. acidilactici* Pa were either listeristatic or listericidal in these experiments. The strain with the least antilisterial activity was *P. acidilactici* PAC. It suppressed growth of *L. monocytogenes* strains V7, OH, and CA for 4 days; the subsequent decline in populations might represent either pediococcal action or a normal loss of viability. With the other pediococcal strains, decline of listerial populations was earlier and steeper.

The production of acid by pediococci can also inhibit listerial growth. Baccus-Taylor et al. compared the effects of pediocin-positive and -negative starter cultures of *P. acidilactici* on the fate of a 5-strain mixture of *L. monocytogenes* during the manufacture of chicken summer sausage (*777*). With the pediocin-negative culture, listerial populations declined between 1 and 2 $\log_{10}$ units by the end of fermentation of batter inoculated with $10^4$ and $10^7$ cfu of listeria per gram. Populations of *P. acidilactici* increased at first, then decreased. Neither organism was recovered after the sausage was cooked and chilled. In sausages fermented with the pediocin-positive strain, listerial populations declined by 2.6 $\log_{10}$ units during fermentation. Again, no listerias were detected after cooking. Although conventional thermal processing eliminates detectable *L. monocytogenes*, use of a pediocin-producing starter culture provides an additional measure of safety. The ability of pediocins to tolerate typical fermentation and cooking suggests that use of pediocin-producing starter cultures could also

lessen the potential for causing listeriosis should postprocess contamination occur.

Liao et al. established the optimal conditions for production of pediocin PO2 by *P. acidilactici* in yeast-supplemented whey permeate and tested the ability of the fermented whey product to control *L. monocytogenes* in milk and liquid whole egg (*778*). In milk, a powder made of the fermented whey permeate delayed growth of *L. monocytogenes* Scott A by 10 h. At the end of the incubation, the listerial count was $5.0\times10^7$ in the untreated control and $5.5\times10^5$ in treated milk. Treating the powder with protease rendered it inactive. For pasteurized liquid whole egg, however, the results were different. The egg itself was listericidal: populations in untreated liquid egg fell to undetectable levels after 10–20 h. Addition of the powdered whey product protected the pathogen from the effects of the egg. However, the whey powder did inhibit growth relative to the protease-treated whey powder, indicating that the pediocin had some effect. This study shows the importance of testing for antagonistic interactions between materials with antilisterial activity.

Screening of 254 strains of lactobacilli isolated from fermented sausages during ripening revealed 56 whose inhibitory effect on one or more of five *Lactobacillus* indicator strains was not related to acid or $H_2O_2$ (*779*). The inhibitory compounds from three strains proved to be bacteriocins with a bactericidal mode of action and a molecular weight exceeding 10,000. *Lactobacillus plantarum* CTC305 and CTC306 and *Lactobacillus sake* CTC372 inhibited *L. monocytogenes*. When *L. sake* was cured of its 84.8- and 41.3-kilobase plasmids it lost its ability to produce bacteriocin and to ferment lactose.

The potential of a bacteriocin-producing starter culture to improve the safety of a product was shown in a study of the effects of various lactic acid starter cultures on behavior of *L. monocytogenes* during the maturation of salami (*780*). The starter cultures tested were the bacteriocin-producing *L. plantarum* MCS, its bacteriocin-nonproducing mutant MCS1, and two commercial starters that had no antilisterial activity in laboratory medium. Comparable populations of lactobacilli were attained after about 10 days whether or not a starter culture was added. Without starter, listerial populations increased for the first 10–14 days and then fell in both naturally and artificially contaminated salami. In salami inoculated with $10^3$–$10^4$ cfu/g of *L. monocytogenes, L. plantarum* MCS and MCS1 prevented listerial growth for about 10 days and then the listerial population declined. MCS had a nonsignificantly greater effect than MCS1. Naturally contaminated salami contained very low numbers of listerias (~6/g). After the first week, when a starter culture was used, the pathogen could be detected only by enrichment. No difference was seen in the effectiveness of the starters until the seventh week, when all samples produced using *L. plantarum* MCS were negative for *L. monocytogenes* even after enrichment, whereas salamis produced using the other cultures still yielded viable listerias after enrichment.

There were reports of the purification and cloning of sakacin 674, a bacteriocin produced by *L. sake* Lb674 (*781*), and of the characterization of a bacteriocin produced by *L. plantarum* C19 (*782*). Strains of *Lactobacillus bavaricus* also produce bacteriocins (*783–784*). Winkowski et al. inoculated packets of minimally heat-treated beef cubes, beef cubes in gravy, and beef cubes in gravy containing glucose with *L. monocytogenes* ($10^2$ cfu/g) and *L. bavaricus* MN ($10^3$ or $10^5$ cfu/g) (*783*). The packets were then vacuum-sealed and tested at intervals for pH, microbial growth, and bacteriocin production. At 4°C, *L. monocytogenes* was inhibited or killed, depending on the inoculum level of *L. bavaricus*. At 10°C pathogen populations were reduced by at least 1 $log_{10}$ in gravy-containing products; the reduction was greater in gravy containing glucose. In beef cubes, *L. bavaricus* caused a transient reduction in listerial growth during the first week of storage but populations reached control levels by the fourth week. Bacteriocin was detected in the samples, and inhibition of *L. monocytogenes* could not be attributed to acidification. Larsen and Nørrung found that 242 of 245 strains of *L. monocytogenes* were sensitive to bavaracin A, a bacteriocin produced by *L. bavaricus* MI401 (*784*). The three resistant strains belonged to three different electrophoretic types and were isolated from diverse sources: smoked salmon, pig feces, and a person with listeriosis.

Nisin is a bacteriocin produced by *Lactococcus lactis lactis*. Abee et al. studied the mode of action of nisin Z, a natural variant of nisin, against *L. monocytogenes* Scott A (*785*). Tests were done in phosphate buffer containing glucose and KCl. Addition of nisin Z to listerial cells caused immediate loss of cell potassium, depolarization of the cytoplasmic membrane, inhibition of respiration, and hydrolysis and partial efflux of ATP. These data indicate that the cytoplasmic membrane is the primary target of nisin Z. The action of nisin Z was maximal at pH 6.0. It was significantly reduced at low temperatures and by divalent and trivalent cations. It was blocked completely by 0.2 mM gadolinium. When cells were grown at 30°C, nisin Z was inactive at temperatures ≤7°C. However, when cells were grown at 4°C there was some nisin-induced leakage of potassium at 4 and 7°C. Studies by Ming and Daeschel also indicated

that nisin acts on the cell membrane (*786*). These authors evaluated the frequency of spontaneous nisin resistance in 8 foodborne spoilage and pathogenic bacteria and produced a nisin-resistant mutant of *L. monocytogenes* Scott A by incrementally increasing nisin exposure. Nisin was not inactivated by growing cells of either the mutant or the parent strain. Compared with the nisin-sensitive parent, the mutant had a higher phase-transition temperature, a higher percentage of straight-chain fatty acids, and a lower percentage of branched-chain fatty acids. The specific growth rate of the mutant was only 41% that of the parent at 20°C, but 88% at 30°C. The authors concluded that nisin resistance is associated with fundamental changes in the structure and function of the cell membrane. In other studies of nisin resistance in *L. monocytogenes*, Davies and Adams compared the sensitive strain NCTC 5105 with the less sensitive strain F6861 (*787*). Mutants with increased nisin resistance could be isolated from F6861 at a frequency of $10^{-7}$–$10^{-6}$. The amount of nisin adsorbed to the cell, as indicated by a nisin-specific ELISA, was directly related to nisin sensitivity. In resistant cells, potassium efflux increased more slowly with increasing concentrations of nisin and had a lower maximum rate. These observations on adsorption behavior and saturation kinetics of potassium efflux suggest that nisin resistance is based on exclusion of nisin and inhibition of nisin binding to the cells. Resistance is acquired by alterations in the cytoplasmic membrane or cell wall that decrease the presence or accessibility of attachment sites. This decreases or prevents the incorporation of nisin into the membrane to produce pores, lysis, and death.

Rekhif et al. selected spontaneous mutants of *L. monocytogenes* ATCC 15313 resistant to bacteriocins produced by *Leuconostoc mesenteroides mesenteroides* FR52 (mesenterocin 52), *Lactobacillus curvatus* SB13 (curvaticin 13), and *L. plantarum* C19 (plantaricin C19) (*788*). They evaluated the frequency and stability of such mutants and conducted preliminary tests on their mode of resistance. The frequency of mutants was in the range of $10^{-4}$–$10^{-3}$. The resistant phenotype was stable throughout 10 subcultures in the presence and absence of the corresponding bacteriocin. Resistance was not due to inactivation of the bacteriocin or to a modification of bacteriocin adsorption onto the target cell. The parent strain and all mutants were sensitive to nisin. However, most mutants selected for resistance to one bacteriocin showed considerable cross-resistance to the other two as well.

Huang et al. compared the inhibition patterns of mesenterocin 5 and organic acids on growth of five pathogenic strains of *Listeria* in broth medium (*789*).

For the first 2 h, mesenterocin was bacteriostatic for one strain and bactericidal for four, causing a 1.0–3.0-$\log_{10}$ drop in viable counts from the initial value of $10^7$. However, after remaining constant for 3–16 h, populations increased and mesenterocin no longer had an important effect on specific growth rate. With lactic and acetic acids, the specific growth rate of all strains decreased as the concentration of acid increased, from the minimal inhibitory concentration to the concentration at which no growth occurred. The strains varied in their sensitivity to acid.

Species of *Enterococcus* produce broad-spectrum bacteriocins active against *L. innocua* and *L. monocytogenes*. Giraffa et al. evaluated the antilisterial activity of a conventional thermophilic starter culture alone and in combination with bacteriocin-producing strains of *Enterococcus faecium* and *Enterococcus faecalis*, under conditions simulating production of Taleggio, an Italian soft cheese (*790*). Satisfactory inhibition of *L. innocua* involved synergism between pH decrease and production of bacteriocin. Large populations of *Enterococcus* developed with the temperature gradient characteristic of Taleggio production. Depending on the size of the enterococcal inoculum, the first antimicrobial activity was detected at the beginning of whey drainage or at the salting step. Incorporation of enterococci into the starter culture sharply reduced the listerial count even before the pH fell to an inhibitory level. The enterococci were effective in the presence of rennet, and the authors recommend their use in conjunction with conventional high-acid-producing starter cultures to enhance product safety.

Two isolates of *E. faecium* from silage produced bacteriocins designated by Kato et al. as enterocins 101 and 102 (*791*). Although the strains that produced these bacteriocins and the previously isolated enterocin 100 were independently isolated, they appeared nearly identical in all bacterial characteristics tested. However, enterocin 101 was considerably different from enterocins 100 and 102 in its antibacterial spectrum, protease sensitivity, heat stability, pH optimum, and molecular size. It strongly inhibited 4 clinical strains of *L. monocytogenes*, and may warrant further investigation as a preserving agent for processed foods. Three other bacteriocins produced by *E. faecium* were characterized by Arihara et al. (*792*). They were stable over a wide pH range and were listericidal without causing cell lysis.

Production of bacteriocins by *Carnobacterium piscicola* was reported by Schillinger et al. (*793*), Stoffels et al. (*794*), and Mathieu et al. (*795*). Strain LV61, isolated from meat, grew and produced piscicolin 61 at refrigeration temperatures (*793*). Piscicolin 61 is a heat-resistant protein larger than 5 kDa and active over a pH range of 2.0–8.0. It was moderately active against strains of 5 listerial species. Loss of the 22-kilobase plasmid resulted in a bacteriocin-negative mutant. Strains of *L. monocytogenes* and *L. innocua* were weakly sensitive to carnocin UI49, produced by a fish isolate of *C. piscicola* (*794*). The same strains were more sensitive to nisin. A *C. piscicola* isolate from a French mold-ripened soft cheese produced a bacteriocin named carnocin CP5 (*795*). Carnocin CP5 reduced initial counts of *L. monocytogenes* in culture broth and skim milk. It was most effective at cold temperatures. In some cases, however, after extended incubations, the *L. monocytogenes* population began to increase. The authors thought this growth came from a subpopulation of resistant cells.

Siragusa and Cutter described brochocin-C, a bacteriocin produced by *Brocothrix campestris* ATCC 43754 (*796*). It inhibits *Listeria* and other gram-positive bacteria.

Villani et al. tested 125 isolates of *Micrococcaceae* from Italian salami for antilisterial activity (*797*). Four isolates of *Staphylococcus xylosus* inhibited growth of all five *L. monocytogenes* strains tested. Two isolates produced antagonistic substances that were inactivated by protease. The antagonistic substances produced by the other two isolates were inactivated only by esterase and lipase.

**SANITIZERS.** The safety of processed foods requires an emphasis on sanitation in the food plant environment. Jacquet and Reynaud evaluated the efficacy of 8 commercial sanitizers, used at concentrations recommended by the manufacturers, against *L. monocytogenes* and *L. innocua* strains from several sources (*798*). Only 2 products, one containing amine and one containing quaternary ammonium and peroxide, were able to cause a 5-$\log_{10}$ reduction in bacterial counts in all tests. A chlorine-based product was effective against all listerial strains isolated from a dairy plant but not against the *L. innocua* type strain or 13 of 31 *L. monocytogenes* strains of human, animal, silage, or food origin. Two other chlorine disinfectants, one aldehyde, and two with acid and peroxide did not give a 5-$\log_{10}$ reduction in counts in any test.

Roy et al. evaluated listeriaphages of the family *Siphoviridae* as a means of disinfecting contaminated stainless steel and polypropylene surfaces (*799*). At concentrations of $3.5 \times 10^8$ plaque-forming units per milliliter, the three phages, individually or combined, were comparable to a 20-ppm solution of the quaternary ammonium compound QUATAL in reducing counts of two strains of *L. monocytogenes*. The largest effect was seen when two or more phages were used in combination or when phages were suspended in QUATAL.

Studies by Tuncan showed that two common sanitizers, an iodophor and a quaternary ammonium compound, were ineffective against *Listeria* at 2°C at concentrations and exposure times effective at 25°C (*800*). However, they were effective if either the concentration or the exposure time was increased. Performance of the chlorine sanitizer was not affected by temperature. The impact of cold temperature varied with the species and strain of *Listeria*.

Because cleaning removes food residues from surfaces, *L. monocytogenes* in the food-processing plant environment is exposed to low-nutrient or starvation conditions that may affect its sensitivity to sanitizers. Ren et al. tested the effect of benzalkonium chloride, a quaternary ammonium sanitizer, on starved planktonic and biofilm *L. monocytogenes* (*801*). For planktonic cells, dilution of the dextrose and hydrolyzed protein components of the medium had little effect on resistance to the sanitizer but dilution of the NaCl or potassium phosphate components, or both, sharply increased resistance. However, starvation had no significant effect on the sanitizer-susceptibility of biofilm *L. monocytogenes*. This observation reinforces previous conclusions that cells growing in biofilms are physiologically different from their free-living counterparts. There were also indications that some cells exposed to benzalkonium chloride remained viable even though they were not detected by the plate-count procedures.

## Detection and Identification

Farber presented an overview of methodology, control, and regulatory aspects of current research on *L. monocytogenes* (*802*). The section on methodology reviewed commercial kits for detection and identification of *Listeria*. Dever et al. reviewed methods for isolation and detection of *L. monocytogenes* used in the USA (*803*). They consider the USDA method the most practical cultural method because negative samples are rapidly recognized. However, isolation methods detect all *Listeria* species, so confirmation at the species level is required after isolation. Although the Listeria-Tek ELISA and the Gene-Trak Listeria Assay are faster and more objective than cultural procedures, they still require an enrichment step. Biochemical test kits provide fairly fast and reliable identification of *Listeria* species. API Listeria identified test strains without a complementary CAMP test.

After a collaborative study evaluated the performance of the AutoMicrobic System Gram-Positive and Gram-Negative test kits, this method was adopted first action by AOAC International for the biochemical characterization of *Listeria* species isolated from food and environmental sources (*804*). Another collaborative study compared the MICRO-ID *Listeria* method with conventional biochemical methods (*805*). MICRO-ID *Listeria* agreed with conventional biochemical identification on 98% of *L. monocytogenes*, 77% of *L. seeligeri*, 90% of *L. ivanovii*, 96% of *L. grayi/L. murrayi*, 74% of *L. welshimeri*, and 100% of *L. innocua* isolates and was adopted first action by AOAC International. Many errors in identifying *L. seeligeri* and *L. ivanovii* cultures were caused by inaccurate reading of the CAMP and hemolysis tests and not by errors in the test strip. The International Dairy Federation (IDF) conducted a collaborative study on the recovery of viable *L. monocytogenes* from milk and dairy products (*806*). The IDF procedure involved enrichment, culture on solid isolation medium, and identification by conventional morphologic, physiologic, and biochemical tests. The calculated 50% detection limit for all products except Limburger cheese was 1.6 cfu per 25 g. The 50% detection limit for Limburger cheese was 4.1 cfu per 25 g. The method was adopted first action by AOAC International. Investigators in Sweden compared a common cold-enrichment procedure with the IDF method for isolating *L. monocytogenes* from animal autopsy material (*807*). For this purpose the IDF method was considerably more sensitive.

Herman and De Ridder found that a DNA colony hybridization method and the classical method (black colonies on Oxford medium identified by biochemical and morphological tests) gave comparable results when used to detect *L. monocytogenes* in dairy products (*808*). The sensitivity of a PCR method applied directly on the enrichment culture depended on the type of dairy sample being investigated. A comparative study of methods for detecting *Listeria* in raw milk found that the Gene-Trak protocol yielded significantly more confirmed positive results than the Listeria-Tek and FDA methods (24 vs. 13) (*809*). Various modifications to the Gene-Trak assay failed to increase the detection rate significantly. Compared with the IDF method, Gene-Trak gave a false-negative rate of 5.9% (*810*). Of 250 naturally contaminated cheese and environmental samples, the IDF method revealed 153 positive samples and Gene-Trak detected 144. False-positive results could not be documented in this study. Oxford agar gave more satisfactory results than LPM agar with Gene-Trak. Extending the enrichment time to 7 d produced a small increase in the number of samples positive by the IDF method but drastically reduced the number of positive samples from Gene-Trak.

Nørrung and Gerner-Smidt compared MEE, ribotyping, restriction enzyme analysis, and a new Danish phage-typing system for typing *L. monocytogenes* and calculated a discriminatory index (DI) for each method (*811*). The DI represents the probability that two epidemiologically unrelated strains will be distinguished and is determined by the number of types defined by the method and the relative frequency of these types. Serotype 1 was best discriminated by the molecular methods, particularly restriction enzyme analysis (DI = .92). Serotype 4 strains were best discriminated by phage typing (DI = .78). Overall, the most discriminatory single method was phage typing (DI = .88). This was followed by restriction enzyme analysis, MEE, and ribotyping, with indexes of .87, .83, and .79, respectively. When combinations of typing methods were tested, the combination of restriction enzyme analysis and MEE was most discriminatory. Phage typing was considered the most suitable method for mass screening.

Wong et al. analyzed DNA digests from selected strains of *L. monocytogenes* isolated in Taiwan (*812*). They characterized the listeriolysin O gene and identified variants that may prove useful in epidemiologic studies. Strains isolated from local foods showed three major patterns, which did not seem to be related to food or geographical source or to serotype.

**CULTURE MEDIA.** Fujisawa and More reported that all *L. monocytogenes* strains tested showed clear hemolysis on blood agar base #2 and on Columbia blood agar base supplemented with 5% horse blood (*813*). These strains could be correctly identified and differentiated from *L. innocua* and other *Listeria* species by the API Listeria system.

Gunasinge et al. found that PALCAM agar was consistently more effective than Oxford agar in suppressing microorganisms other than *Listeria* (*814*). The isolation of listerial species for identification was also easier with PALCAM.

Because of concern that the resuscitation of heat-injured *L. monocytogenes* cells during refrigerated storage of food could lead to underestimation of their heat resistance, Mackey et al. examined the recovery of heat-injured *L. monocytogenes* as a function of incubation temperature and composition of the recovery medium (*815*). They established that cold enrichment does not allow better recovery of heat-injured cells than incubation at higher temperatures and is not optimal for resuscitation of cells unable to grow on selective media. Recovery of heat-injured cells depended on the composition of the recovery medium but was maximal at 20–25°C. The authors concluded that refrigeration

of heat-treated foods does not increase the risk that injured cells will recover from the heat treatment.

Tran and Hitchins determined recovery limits of heat-injured *L. monocytogenes* from enrichment broth and enriched cultures of inoculated Brie cheese and cooked shrimp (*816*). The recovery limit ($RL_{50}$) was the calculated size of inoculum needed to recover the organism on half of the isolation plates after streaking from the enrichment culture. $RL_{50}$ values for injured and uninjured cells were comparable for three selective media after a 48-h incubation in *Listeria* enrichment broth. For food isolates, modified McBride agar gave consistently but nonsignificantly higher $RL_{50}$ values (i.e., poorer recovery) than Oxford or lithium chloride–phenylethanol–moxalactam agars, presumably because of the competing microflora. Addition of lactose or pyruvate to the enrichment broth failed to improve recovery from foods.

**IMMUNOLOGIC AND HYBRIDIZATION METHODS.** In a study by Meier and Terplan, the Listeria-Tek ELISA identified listeria-negative food samples within 2 days (*817*). It gave no false-negative results and only 1 of 32 samples gave a false-positive result. ELISA-positive samples require verification by isolation and by biochemical and hemolysis tests.

Torensma et al. developed 7 MAbs against *Listeria* spp. and characterized their reaction patterns with strains of various serotypes (*818*). Two MAbs were members of the IgM class and 5 were members of the IgG class. Fliss et al. produced 2 IgM MAbs specific for DNA-RNA hybrids (*819*). With one of these they developed an immunoassay for detection of *Listeria* DNA-RNA hybrids. The assay was genus-specific and allowed detection of as little as 2.5 pg of target rRNA. Blais enhanced the sensitivity of an *L. monocytogenes* PCR detection system (*820*). The transcript was detected by hybridization with a DNA probe immobilized in the wells of a microtiter plate and assayed immunoenzymatically with an anti-RNA-DNA hybrid antibody. Reactions were seen with various *L. monocytogenes* isolates but not with other *Listeria* or non-*Listeria* species.

Blais and Phillippe synthesized an RNA probe specific for the *hlyA* gene of *L. monocytogenes* (*821*). The probe hybridized with *hlyA* PCR products on a membrane, producing RNA-DNA hybrids that were detected by an immunoenzymatic assay. This system was more sensitive than conventional agarose gel electrophoresis. The RNA probe reacted with all 62 *L. monocytogenes* strains tested but with no other *Listeria* species. Of species from other genera, only *Enterococcus faecalis* gave a weakly positive reaction, and

>10⁹ cfu/mL were required. Another genus-specific probe, developed by Emond et al., was targeted at the rRNA of *L. monocytogenes* (*822*). The rDNA fragment contained the entire spacer region and partial 16S and 23S sequences. The assay involved aqueous-phase hybridization between *L. monocytogenes* rRNA and the biotinylated rDNA probe, capture of the heteroduplex nucleic acid (HNA) with specific anti-RNA-DNA MAbs, and detection of the complex with an enzyme–streptavidin conjugate. The assay, named the HNA ELISA, could detect as few as 500 listerias in artificially contaminated meat homogenates.

Johnson and Lattuada compared nucleic acid hybridization assays and biochemical tests for the confirmation of *L. monocytogenes* (*823*). Forty-four *Listeria* isolates, representing all 5 species, were tested. All the commercial kits examined were easy to use and could provide results within 24 h. Specific problems with the various kits and biochemical tests were discussed.

Using the OPM-01 primer in the PCR, Lawrence et al. generated RAPD profiles for 91 strains of *L. monocytogenes* from food, veterinary, medical, and food-environment sources (*824*). They identified 33 profiles. The 29 strains from raw milk represented 7 RAPD profiles, which were specific to isolates from this source. The 44 food isolates showed 19 profiles; 15 were found only in food, and one of these was particularly common. The profiles permitted discrimination within serotypes, although 5 profiles were not confined to a single serotype.

Serotyping is of limited usefulness in epidemiologic studies of foodborne listeriosis because some 90% of outbreak strains belong to serotypes 1/2a, 1/2b, and 4b. Fingerprinting of *L. monocytogenes*, using an *Sma*I digest of chromosomal DNA separated by pulsed field gel electrophoresis, gives distinctive banding patterns for strains of these common serotypes (*825*). Matched sets of food and clinical isolates from the same outbreak or case were very similar, and different from strains involved in other episodes.

Bsat and Batt developed a method for detection of *L. monocytogenes* based on a nested PCR and a modified reverse dot-blot assay of the digoxygenin-labeled PCR product (*826*). For environmental sampling, the assay requires an additional overnight enrichment. It then has a sensitivity of 5 cfu per 25 cm² of surface.

Wiedmann et al. modified their previously reported PCR-coupled ligase chain reaction (LCR) assay for *L. monocytogenes* so that the LCR product could be detected nonisotopically (*827*). Detection with the chemiluminescent substrate Lumi-Phos 530 permitted detection of LCR products in less than 3 h. The entire assay could be completed in 10 h. The chromogenic substrate *p*-NPP gave equivalent results.

At the molecular level, it is difficult to distinguish illness-causing strains of *L. monocytogenes* from harmless strains. Chen et al. developed an approach they called subtracter probe hybridization to detect sequences specific to *L. monocytogenes* (*828*). Three sequences that hybridized with virulence-probe DNA but not with a subtracter DNA probe from *L. innocua* represent unique sequences that may also be associated with virulence. Their virulence potential is being assessed, and they are being adapted as probes for detecting *L. monocytogenes* in foods. Different combinations of virulence probes and subtracter probes may be useful in studies of pathogenicity.

Because many foods have components that inhibit the PCR, suitable methods of pretreating samples must be developed before the PCR can find wide application in the food industry. Powell et al. partially characterized an inhibitory factor in cow's milk and suggested ways to prevent this inhibition (*829*). The cow's milk inhibitor appeared to be a proteinase, and from the types of inhibitors that were active against it the authors conclude that it may be plasmin. Its effect could be prevented by adding bovine serum albumin or proteinase inhibitors to the sample before running the PCR.

During an evaluation of the Accuprobe kit for detection of *L. monocytogenes*, Partis et al. found that use of Fraser broth or University of Vermont broth for sample enrichment gave false-negative results (*830*). The high salt concentrations in these enrichment broths protected the cells from lysis, preventing the probe from gaining access to the cellular RNA.

**OTHER METHODS.** Hancock et al. developed a selective medium for detection of *L. monocytogenes, L. innocua,* and *L. welshimeri* by an impedimetric assay (*831*).

Bhunia et al. described an in vitro cell culture model for detecting virulent *L. monocytogenes* strains isolated from food and clinical sources (*832*). Three MAb producing hybridoma cell lines were equally sensitive to pathogenic *Listeria*. Strains V7 and Scott A of *L. monocytogenes* killed ~50% of the hybridoma cells within 2 h and 94–98% within 6 h. Strains of *L. innocua, L. seeligeri, L. welshimeri, L. ivanovii, L. grayi,* and *L. murrayi* killed only 0–2% of cells in 2 h and 6–22% after 8 h. A hemolysin-negative strain of *L. monocytogenes* killed 13% of the hybridoma cells in 8 h, indicating that hemolysin is involved in the killing. In hours, the assay produced results comparable to those from the immunocompromised mouse model, which requires days.

The CAMP reaction is the synergistic lysis of erythrocytes by *L. monocytogenes* and either *Staphylococcus aureus* or *Corynebacterium equi*. Conflicting reports show the subjective nature of this test and cast doubt on its validity as an indicator of virulence. To assess the relationship between the CAMP reaction and virulence of *L. monocytogenes*, McKellar attempted to identify the virulence factors involved in the CAMP reaction (*833*). With *C. equi* the reaction appears to involve cholesterol oxidase from the corynebacterium and listeriolysin O from *L. monocytogenes*. With *S. aureus* it appears to involve the staphylococcal β-lysin and either of the two phospholipase C enzymes produced by *L. monocytogenes*. Mutants deficient in both listeriolysin O and the two phospholipases C did not react with *S. aureus* and reacted only weakly with *C. equi*. McKellar proposed a modified CAMP test, incorporating cholesterol oxidase into sheep blood agar, for rapid identification of *L. monocytogenes*.

## Virulence

MODELS. Comparison of aerosol and intragastric routes of listerial infection revealed that the aerosol route is the more sensitive and consistent (*834*). For aerosol infection, mice were exposed to $10^{10}$ cfu/mL for 5 min. Animals challenged by gastric intubation received $5 \times 10^9$ cfu directly into the stomach. Aerosol infection caused 100% mortality within 4–5 days in immunocompetent mice, whereas fewer deaths occurred from gastric infection, most of them not until day 7. In some cases the $LD_{50}$ could be calculated for the aerosol route, but this was impossible for gastric infection. Bacterial counts in the livers and spleens of aerosol-infected mice were related to the virulence of the infecting strain, and could be used in place of conventional $LD_{50}$ tests to indicate virulence.

Schlech described a rat model of virulence of foodborne *L. monocytogenes* (*835*). Experiments using the model showed the effects of various factors associated with the pathogen (motility, smooth or rough colony form, culture conditions) and the host (pregnancy, immune status, intestinal flora). Thus the model is applicable for studies of virulence and host susceptibility.

ENVIRONMENTAL INFLUENCE ON VIRULENCE. Some evidence suggests that the conditions under which *L. monocytogenes* is grown affect its virulence and the activity of its virulence factors. Listeriolysin O is a known virulence factor, and it is thought that catalase and superoxide dismutase protect the organism against cytotoxic oxidants produced during the respiratory burst in macrophages. Because NaCl and KCl are frequently added to foods to enhance flavor and reduce $a_w$, Myers et al. grew *L. monocytogenes* in culture media with various concentrations of these salts and evaluated the effect on activity of listeriolysin O, catalase, and superoxide dismutase (*836*). A virulent strain and a nonhemolytic mutant were tested. For both strains, catalase activity peaked at a 428-mM concentration of either salt and superoxide dismutase activity peaked at a salt concentration of 1112 mM. The hemolysin titer of the virulent strain also peaked at 428 mM NaCl or KCl, but the effect of KCl was significantly greater. However, growth of the organism in salt-containing medium did not affect its virulence for mice. Further studies with the virulent strain showed that activities of catalase and listeriolysin O were greatest when cells were grown at 37°C in 428-mM NaCl or KCl (*837*). No listeriolysin O activity was detected at 25 or 4°C regardless of salt, and catalase activity was lower at these temperatures. Superoxide dismutase activity also increased with temperature. Thus production of these virulence-related factors appears to be thermoregulated.

Khan et al. determined the effect of temperature and pH on hemolysin production by three strains of *L. monocytogenes* (serotypes 1/2a, 4a, and 4b) and one of *L. seeligeri* (*838*). All strains produced hemolysin in tryptose phosphate broth at both 20 and 32°C and throughout the 5–9 pH range tested. At 32°C, maximal production occurred at pH 7. At 20°C, two strains showed maximal production at pH 7 and two at pH 9.

Datta and Kothary evaluated the effects of glucose (0.0–1.0%), temperature (26 and 37°C), and pH on listeriolysin O production by different serotypes of *L. monocytogenes* (*839*). Expression of listeriolysin O was assessed by a direct hemolysin assay, immunoblotting experiments, and an ELISA. Expression was greater at 37°C and was maximal with 0.2% glucose. No activity was detected with ≥0.5% glucose. The effect of glucose appeared to be due to a change in the pH of the growth medium.

GENETIC REGULATION OF VIRULENCE. Datta reviewed the factors controlling expression of virulence genes in *L. monocytogenes* (*840*). Some known virulence genes and their properties were listed, and their environmental and genetic regulation was summarized.

Freitag et al. are studying regulation of the *prfA* transcriptional activator of *L. monocytogenes* (*841*). The product of this gene, a site-specific DNA-binding protein, controls determinants of pathogenicity. The authors characterized two classes of mutants: those that contain transposon insertions in the *prfA* structural gene and those that contain the insertions in the *prfA* promoter region. Both classes are avirulent and secrete greatly reduced levels of listeriolysin O and phosphatidyl-inositol-specific phospholipase C. Unlike the structural-gene mutant, a mutant of the second type was able to escape from the phagosome and grow in the cytoplasm. However, it was unable to nucleate actin filaments and spread to adjacent cells. Transcription of *prfA* in this mutant was directed from $prfAp_2$, a previously unidentified promoter close to the *prfA* initiation codon. Transcription from the $prfAp_1$ and $prfAp_2$ promoters was increased in the absence of functional PrfA, suggesting that this protein down-regulates its own expression.

Listeriolysin O (encoded by *hly*) and a phosphatidyl-inositol-specific phospholipase C (encoded by *plcA*) are required for invasion of the host cell. Intracellular movement and cell-to-cell spread depend on the bacterial surface protein ActA, and a phosphatidylcholine-specific phospholipase C (encoded by *plcB*) is involved in disrupting the double membrane that forms around the bacterium when it enters a neighboring cell. A zinc-dependent metalloprotease, Mpl, processes PlcB from its precursor to its active form. The chromosomal genes encoding these proteins are arranged in a cluster in the order *plcA, hly, mpl, actA, plcB*; *prfA* is also part of this cluster. Hly, Mpl, ActA, and PlcB are preferentially synthesized in minimal essential medium (MEM) in the presence of 5% $CO_2$. Bohne et al. showed that the preferential synthesis of ActA, PlcB, and listeriolysin O in MEM is caused by transcriptional induction, the long lifetime of the mRNAs for these proteins, or both (*842*). The PrfA-controlled genes appear to be regulated differently in NCTC 7973 and EGD, the two *L. monocytogenes* strains studied. Transcriptional induction of *prfA* and *hly* was seen in strain EGD but not in NCTC 7973. The most interesting observation was that ActA is also highly induced in the phagocytic cell line J774 when the bacterium enters the host cell's cytoplasm. This suggests that a specific cytosolic signal induces transcription of the *actA–plcB* bicistronic mRNA as it does in MEM. Although MEM and the host-cell cytoplasm are two quite different nutrient "media," they may provide the same signal—a low concentration of some component—that results in induction of the PrfA-dependent genes.

VIRULENCE MECHANISMS. Schlech et al. investigated the interaction of listerial species with monolayer cultures of four human cell lines (HeLa, Int407, CaCo-2, 3T6) (*843*). A strongly hemolytic strain of *L. ivanovii* showed the highest degree of internalization in all cell lines; *L. innocua* and a hemolysin-negative strain of *L.*

*monocytogenes* showed the least. Phenotypic changes expressed by roughness or smoothness of colonies did not affect bacterial–monolayer interaction in this model. Studies of bacterial association with Int407 and HeLa cells at 4, 22, and 37°C showed a direct relationship between internalization and temperature and suggested that the cell lines, not the bacteria, had the major role in determining this. At 4°C the cell line was metabolically inactive and little internalization occurred. Nor did bacterial motility have an important influence on bacterial–cell line interaction. The authors speculated on why *L. ivanovii*, which is generally not considered pathogenic in humans, was more invasive than pathogenic *L. monocytogenes* in these studies.

Bunduki et al. examined clinical, animal, food, and environmental strains of five listerial species to see if their potential for attachment to guinea pig intestinal epithelium was related to their behavior toward gut macrophages and peripheral blood phagocytes (*844*). In this model as in the cell culture model (*843*), *L. ivanovii* demonstrated an ability to attach that equaled or surpassed that of pathogenic *L. monocytogenes* strains and *L. innocua* showed the least adherence. All strains of *L. monocytogenes* were detected intracellularly after a 1-h incubation and *L. ivanovii* had also begun to invade. Differences between animals from which the phagocytes were obtained accounted for the major part of variation in phagocytic activity of gut macrophages, although some small but significant differences between bacterial strains and species were seen. This supports the idea that resistance to listeriosis is genetically determined and may explain why some people are more susceptible to listerial infection than others.

The listerial surface-bound protein ActA acts as a nucleator to induce reorganization of the host cell's actin cytoskeleton. To investigate the interaction of ActA with the microfilament system in the absence of other bacterial factors, Pistor et al. expressed *actA* in a kidney epithelial cell line (*845*). ActA, including its *C*-terminal bacterial membrane anchor, was associated with mitochondria in the transfected cells. It recruited actin and α-actinin to these organelles, with concomitant reorganization of the microfilament system. Removal of the proline-rich repeat region of ActA completely abolished interaction with cytoskeletal components. To explore the possibility that the polyproline repeats in ActA serve as binding sites in the actin-regulatory protein, Southwick and Purich synthesized a peptide representing one of these sequences and injected it into *Listeria*-infected kidney epithelial cells (*846*). Over an estimated intracellular concentration range of 80 nM to 0.8 μM, this peptide rapidly blocked formation of actin-filament tails, arrested bacterial motility, and caused retraction of host cell membranes. Injection of poly-L-proline to give an intracellular concentration of 1–20 μM failed to block listerial movement or polar actin-filament assembly but did cause membrane retraction. The authors postulate that a cytoskeletal component sensitive to specific oligoproline peptides participates in the protein–protein interactions essential for actin-associated processes. Their model also predicts the basic features of what may be a class of proline-rich membrane proteins or peptides that control actin-dependent processes. Other studies in cultured kidney epithelial cells indicated that the intact α-actinin molecule is needed for the assembly of actin into bacterial "tails" and the locomotion of *L. monocytogenes* within infected cells (847). Injection of a 53-kDa fragment of α-actinin into listeria-infected cells caused the bacteria to lose their actin tails and their ability to move intracellularly and to form filopodia. Two other α-actinin-binding proteins, vinculin and talin, were demonstrated in the tails, suggesting the similarity of the tails to the attachment plaques normally present in uninfected cells. The authors postulate that the attachment-plaque proteins α-actinin, talin, and vinculin bind and stabilize actin filaments as they polymerize behind the bacteria and perhaps also enable the tails to bind to the cell membrane in the filopodia. This would explain the ability of *L. monocytogenes* to move within the cytoplasm and to push out the surface of the host cell to form filopodia.

During the invasion of epithelial cells by *L. monocytogenes*, two proteins in the host cell become tyrosine phosphorylated. Tang et al. have identified these proteins as 42- and 44-kDa isoforms of mitogen-activated protein kinase (MAP kinase) (848). Activation begins within 5–15 min of bacterial infection. The tyrosine kinase inhibitor genistein blocks both invasion and the tyrosine phosphorylation of the two MAP kinases. The authors demonstrated that attached bacteria or bacteria in the process of invasion, not intracellular bacteria, are required for kinase activation. They postulate that *L. monocytogenes* activates MAP kinase during invasion, and an MAP kinase signal transduction pathway mediates bacterial uptake.

Portnoy et al. (849) and Smith and Portnoy (850) reported studies on the role of the two phospholipases C in the pathogenicity of *L. monocytogenes*. They constructed mutants with in-frame deletions in one or both of the enzymes. Both single mutants had only slightly reduced virulence, but virulence of the double mutant was profoundly reduced. The authors postulate multiple and overlapping roles for the enzymes. However, the phosphatidylinositol-specific phospholipase C appears

to be involved in the bacterium's escape from the host vacuole and the phosphatidylcholine-specific phospholipase C has a role in cell-to-cell spread.

By immunogold labeling of *L. monocytogenes* virulence factors within infected CaCo-2 cells, Quinn et al. showed that listeriolysin O, phospholipases, and other putative virulence-related proteins produced by the bacterium are primarily associated with the cell wall (851). This observation was surprising, because it was thought that many of the *L. monocytogenes* extracellular proteins were secreted and therefore would be observed throughout the cytoplasm of the host. The observations also suggested that there are fundamental structural differences in the listeriolysins made by serotypes 1/2a and 4b, as antibodies made to one reacted poorly with the other. Polyclonal antibodies specific for the p60 protein (the major protein in culture supernatants) reacted poorly with intracellular *Listeria,* suggesting that the protein either is not produced or is not surface-exposed during intracellular growth in CaCo-2 cells. The pseudopod-like projections in the CaCo-2 cells, which contain virulent *L. monocytogenes* and are probably involved in cell-to-cell spread of the organism, had no detectable *Listeria* antigens on their anterior surface or within their structure. From this the authors concluded that the phagocytic process is primarily host-cell-dependent after it has been initiated by the bacterium.

It has been suggested that synthesis of listerial heat-shock proteins is induced during phagocytosis. The observation that expression of virulence genes is thermoregulated strengthens this idea. The research group of Morange, Hévin, and Fauve has studied the synthesis of heat-shock proteins in culture medium (852) and in mouse resident peritoneal macrophages (853). As a first step they analyzed the responses of virulent and avirulent strains and species of *Listeria* to heat, acid, and oxygen stress (852). Differences in synthesis of heat-shock proteins at 37°C were linked to differences in response to acid and oxygen stress. These differences may be correlated with the better survival of virulent strains in phagocytic cells, where they are transiently exposed to reactive oxygen metabolites and to an acid pH in the phagolysosome (853).

## OTHER MICROBIAL PATHOGENS

### *Brucella*

Although brucellosis has been eradicated or controlled in most industrialized countries, occasional outbreaks still occur. During 1992, a county health department in North Carolina reported 18 cases of brucellosis among employees at a pork processing plant (*854*). *Brucella suis* was isolated from the blood of 11 patients at the time of acute illness. All patients were exposed to the kill floor of the plant. Investigation by NIOSH identified 30 employees who met the case definition. Within the kill division, risk was greatest among workers in the head and red offal departments. Risk was also associated with ever having been cut or scratched at work.

The clinical manifestations of brucellosis vary. One form is "undulant fever," which is particularly characteristic of *Brucella melitensis* infection. Radolf notes that there has been an upsurge of *B. melitensis* infections caused by consumption of unpasteurized goat's milk or goat's-milk cheese from Mexico (*855*). He reviewed the microbiology and molecular biology of *B. abortus, B. suis,* and *B. melitensis*; the discovery, epidemiology, and pathogenesis of brucellosis; and diagnosis, clinical manifestations, and treatment, which he illustrated by 4 case histories from a Texas hospital. The onset of illness can be abrupt or insidious, and virtually every organ system can be affected. Case 1 was a case of acute brucellosis caused by *B. abortus*, the only case in the hospital records not due to *B. melitensis*. Case 2 was a typical case of undulant fever in a patient who habitually ate cheese made from unpasteurized goat's milk. The 3rd case was *Brucella* sacroiliitis. Case 4 was suppurative arthritis in a man who had done chores on a farm in Mexico.

Robson et al. discussed the reemergence and changing epidemiology of brucellosis in Queensland, Australia (*856*). Effective eradication programs in cattle have virtually eliminated disease from that source. However, review of 34 cases diagnosed between October 1989 and October 1991 found that all of the patients were involved in the slaughter of feral pigs. Because of cross-reactivity among brucella species in serological tests, species identification was difficult; but in each case where the species could be identified, it was *B. suis*. The clinical and laboratory investigation of these cases was described.

Investigators in Spain made what they believe to be the first report of esophageal brucellosis (*857*). The patient was a young man who came into direct contact with goats and drank unpasteurized goat's milk daily. Brucellosis was diagnosed on the basis of the systemic picture and serology, and *B. melitensis* was subsequently confirmed. The authors conclude that this etiology of lower esophageal tumor should be considered in areas where brucellosis is endemic.

## *Helicobacter pylori*

There is now powerful evidence that *Helicobacter pylori* infection increases risk of gastric cancer. Although it is logical to assume that an organism causing infection in the stomach is swallowed and if it is swallowed it could be transmitted by food, there is little information concerning its source. It has now been reported that raw poultry may be a vector for *H. pylori* infection (*858*). At room temperature, the organism remains viable for 24 h in raw chicken. It survives for several days when the chicken is refrigerated.

Hwang et al. discussed the role of diet, *H. pylori* infection, and food preservation in gastric cancer risk (*859*). *Helicobacter pylori* infection is extraordinarily common. It is estimated that half of North American adults older than 50 y are infected. In some developing and newly industrialized countries virtually all adults are infected. The gastric cancer risk in a population 100% infected with *H. pylori* has been estimated as 6 times that in an uninfected population. Sipponen (*860*) and Veldhuyzen van Zanten and Sherman (*861*) have also reviewed the *H. pylori*–gastric cancer connection. Veldhuyzen van Zanten and Sherman (*861*) also discussed *H. pylori* infection as a cause of dyspepsia, gastritis, and duodenal ulcer.

## Lactic Acid Bacteria

Lactic acid bacteria are common commensals of man's indigenous flora, inhabiting nearly all nonsterile sites of the body. They have long been used worldwide to produce a broad range of fermented foods, and their benefits for health are well documented. However, they occasionally cause infections in humans, particularly patients with other serious illness. Gasser reviewed the clinical infections associated with lactic acid bacteria (*862*). Most cases of bacterial endocarditis involving lactic acid bacteria are due to *Lactobacillus* spp., including *L. rhamnosus, L. plantarum, L. casei, L. salivarius,* and possibly *L. acidophilus*. Bloodstream infections caused by lactic acid bacteria are rare. Most *Lactobacillus* bloodstream infections are secondary; in a few cases the primary infection has been gastrointestinal. Many *Bifidobacterium* bloodstream infections also originate in the digestive tract. Cases of digestive tract infection have been associated with *L. acidophilus, L. rhamnosus,* and unspecified species of *Lactobacillus* and *Leuconostoc*. The virulence factors of lactic acid bacteria were discussed. Gasser concluded that even though lactic acid bacterial infections sometimes occur in debilitated persons, these bacteria have a long history of use and consumption in the general population worldwide and there is insufficient evidence to suggest that their continued use in food fermentation poses any danger.

Donohue et al. discussed the toxicity of lactic acid bacteria from a different perspective (*863*). They believe that even though lactic acid bacteria are considered not only safe but also beneficial for health, the occasional reports linking them with infections warrant study of the pathogenic potential of new strains. In Europe, guidelines for the use of lactic acid bacteria as novel foods, food ingredients, or therapeutic products require traditional toxicity testing. For newer strains, especially those derived by biotechnology, testing in an animal model has been proposed. However, the authors' tests of *Streptococcus thermophilus, Lactobacillus helveticus,* and *L. casei,* three species common in cheeses, revealed no acute toxicity. Data of others also indicate that most lactic acid bacteria do not possess acute toxicity. The authors suggest that for established strains it may be more useful to explore other aspects of toxicity.

### Streptococcus

During February 1991 a foodborne outbreak of streptococcal pharyngitis occurred in an Israeli military unit. Shemesh et al. reported the epidemiologic analysis of this outbreak (*864*). *Streptococcus pyogenes* group A was isolated from 53 patients, including the cook. After preliminary investigation, attention focused on a dinner served 35–48 h before the outbreak began. All case-subjects had eaten cabbage salad at this meal, compared with only 17% of controls. The salad was prepared by the sick cook, whose symptoms began two days before the meal was served. Although no food samples remained for testing, the investigators concluded that the cook was the source of infection and the cabbage salad was the food vehicle.

### Plesiomonas

Sugita et al. used a DNA–DNA microplate hybridization method to examine the distribution of *Plesiomonas shigelloides* in the intestines of 8 species of farmed freshwater fish (*865*). The organism was found in 29 of 51 fish specimens and 4 of 10 water samples. From 73 to 100% of black bass, Japanese eel, ayu, and tilapia samples contained *P. shigelloides* and densities were high ($10^4$–$10^8$ cfu/g). Forty percent of rainbow trout, 33% of goldfish, and 25% of carp harbored the organism in their intestines. It was not found in channel catfish. The authors recommend studies of how *P. shigelloides* be-

comes established in the intestines of freshwater fish, so that food poisoning by this organism can be better understood.

### Pseudomonas

Enhanced resistance to iodinated compounds is reportedly associated with biofilm formation in natural and model systems. Brown and Gauthier assessed the relative importance of growth phase and cell density on iodine resistance in *Pseudomonas aeruginosa* (*866*). In their system, resistance depended on the cell density within the biofilm and was independent of the length of time that cells grew on the membrane. The emergence of resistance during the late log phase of growth demonstrated that cells need not be in the stationary phase before they begin to show resistance.

### Legionella

Marrie et al. investigated the prevalence of *Legionella* spp. in the potable water of hospitals and residences in Halifax and hospitals elsewhere in Nova Scotia (*867*). The water supply of 6 of 7 Halifax hospitals was contaminated, whereas *Legionella* was rarely found in hospitals outside Halifax. The rate of colonization of domestic electric water heaters in Halifax was not significantly different from that of the Halifax hospitals.

Rogers et al. determined the influence of temperature and plumbing material on biofilm formation and growth of *L. pneumophila* in a model potable water system (*868*). Filter-sterilized tap water was used to culture a naturally occurring mixed population of microorganisms including virulent *L. pneumophila*. At 20°C *Legionella* accounted for a low proportion of biofilm flora on polybutylene and chlorinated polyvinyl chloride and was absent from copper surfaces. At 40°C, it accounted for up to 50% of the total biofilm flora on plastics. Copper surfaces inhibited biofilm formation and biofilms included only low numbers of legionellas. *Legionella* survived in biofilms on plastic at 50°C but not at 60°C. Biofilms forming on glass surfaces adjacent to copper surfaces incorporated copper ions, which subsequently inhibited colonization of their surfaces. The authors concluded that use of copper tubing in water systems might help to limit colonization by *L. pneumophila*.

### Mycobacterium

von Reyn et al. reported that institutional hot-water systems may be persistently colonized with *Mycobac-*

*bacterium avium*, making potable water a source of *M. avium* infection in AIDS patients (*869*).

## Acinetobacter

A computer-assisted probabilistic method based on phenotypic tests was used to characterize 253 food, water, and clinical isolates of *Acinetobacter* (*870*). Among hospital strains, *A. calcoaceticus* and *A. baumannii* predominated, whereas *A. johnsonii* and *A. lwoffii* were characteristic of food strains. However, strains producing ropy milk were also identified among clinical strains. Based on ability to grow at both 37°C and environmental temperatures, only a few acinetobacters appear capable of being foodborne pathogens.

## Cyanobacteria

An article in *Scientific American* discussed the neurotoxins, hepatotoxins, and cytotoxins of the cyanobacteria (*871*). Two neurotoxins, anatoxin-a and anatoxin-a(s), seem to be unique to these organisms, whereas two others, saxitoxin and neosaxitoxin, also occur in certain marine algae. The chemistry, mechanism of action, and potentially beneficial uses of these toxins were considered. The possible role of the hepatotoxins in development of cancer was discussed.

Rinehart et al. reviewed the structure and biosynthesis of nodularins and microcystins, cyclic pentapeptide and heptapeptide toxins produced by *Nodularia* and *Microcystis* species, respectively (*872*). Their laboratory has isolated and determined the structure of nearly 30 new microcystins. Acyclic peptides, some of them presumed precursors of nodularins and microcystins, have also been isolated and characterized.

Lin and Chu reported studies of microcystin LR, a potent inhibitor of protein phosphatase 2A (*873*). The dose producing 50% inhibition was as low as 0.1 nM, making microcystin LR roughly 100 times more potent than calcyculin A and okadaic acid. The inhibitory effect was abolished when antibodies against the toxin were included in the assay system. Polyclonal antibodies were more effective than MAbs, and the reaction was specific for microcystin. The same authors studied the kinetics of distribution of microcystin LR in the serum and liver of mice injected with 35 µg/kg of the toxin (*874*). They established an ELISA protocol for these analyses. Fifteen minutes after injection, 7.8 ng/mL of toxin was detected in serum and 45 ng/mL was detected in the hepatic cytosolic fraction. After 24 h, the concentration was 37.5 ng/mL in serum and 228.6 ng/mL in hepatic cytosol. Activity of protein phosphatase 2A in liver cytosol

began to decrease 1–2 h after toxin injection, and the maximum decrease was seen 6–12 h after injection.

It appears that chlorination can be effective in removing cyanobacterial peptide toxins from drinking water (*875*). Toxins were destroyed under conditions that produced a chlorine residual of ≥0.5 mg/L after 30 min contact time. Chloramination was ineffective. Toxin destruction was pH-dependent. At high dose rates, sodium and calcium hypochlorite were less effective because of elevated pH.

## Chlamydia

Epidemiologic investigation of a 1989 outbreak of chlamydiosis at a duck farm and processing plant was reported (*876*). *Chlamydia psittaci* was isolated from the ducks, but they exhibited little evidence of infection. Serologic tests showed that 19 workers had been exposed to infection and 4 had not been exposed. Results for 2 were inconclusive. Thirteen exposed workers reported symptoms typical of chlamydiosis; two unexposed workers also reported mild symptoms. Exposure was strongly associated with years of employment. Epidemiologists are well aware that an increased severity of disease in a new host species, followed by return to a milder or subclinical form, is common. In this outbreak, there was no significant disease in the ducks but several cases of human disease were severe.

# GENERAL (MULTIPLE PATHOGENS)

## Epidemiology and Clinical Features

Gastrointestinal illness appears to be increasing worldwide. Madden reviewed trends in diarrheal illness and possible reasons for them (*877*). He discussed the epidemiology and clinical features of infections caused by the foodborne bacteria most often encountered in the USA: *Vibrio*, *Salmonella*, *Shigella*, and *Yersinia* species and *Escherichia coli*.

The *Salmonella* enterotoxin has been difficult to study because it is produced at very low levels and thus has eluded attempts to isolate and purify it. Chopra et al. cloned and sequenced the *Salmonella typhimurium* enterotoxin gene and used the deduced amino acid sequence of its product to prepare antibodies against synthetic peptides representing *N*- and *C*-terminal fragments (*878*). Cell lysates of all *Salmonella* isolates tested showed a prominent immunoblot band at ~29 kDa, as predicted from the estimated size of the product of the cloned enterotoxin gene. Some isolates also formed proteins of 32–69 kDa that reacted with the anti-enterotoxin antibodies. Interestingly, all isolates of *Klebsiella, Enterobacter,* and *Citrobacter* and 2 of 12 *E. coli* isolates produced a similar-sized protein that reacted strongly with the *Salmonella* enterotoxin antibodies, and some also produced larger reactive proteins. Although the antibodies did not react with cholera toxin, the cloned and native *Salmonella* enterotoxin could be neutralized by antibodies to cholera toxin and residues 127–142 of the enterotoxin show considerable homology with sequences found in the A subunits of cholera toxin, and heat-labile enterotoxin. The *Salmonella* enterotoxin gene is opposite the hydrogenase regulatory genes required for hydrogen metabolism in bacteria. The authors postulate that in some genera of the *Enterobacteriaceae* this DNA sequence has evolved, through point mutations, into expressed genes. Perhaps the products of these genes are a family of *Salmonella* enterotoxin-like enterotoxins. However, the finding of *Salmonella* enterotoxin-like sequences in other genera does not necessarily imply a functional toxin protein.

Pohl et al. characterized the plasmids of apramycin-resistant *Enterobacteriaceae* to assess the level of genetic homology between resistance plasmids in strains of human and animal origin in Belgium (*879*). They used replicon-specific probes derived from incompatibility loci of plasmids, which control the plasmids' replication systems. Apramycin–gentamicin resistance plasmids were also characterized by their electrophoretic profiles and antimicrobial resistance patterns. Most plasmids differed in their DNA electrophoretic patterns; 17 antimicrobial resistance profiles were identified; and there were 6 types of replicons. However, two replication genes predominated, one of which occurred mainly in *E. coli* and the other in *Salmonella typhimurium.* Animal and human strains contained the same replication genes. The epidemic spread of apramycin and gentamicin resistance in *E. coli* and *S. typhimurium* from farm animals in Belgium is carried by a variety of plasmids that also carry resistance determinants to other classes of antimicrobial agents. This suggests that the resistance gene is carried on transposable elements. Resistance to apramycin was not found in other species of *Enterobacteriaceae* except for one clinical strain of *Klebsiella pneumoniae* and two veterinary strains of *Citrobacter freundii.*

Increasingly, chronic sequelae to food poisoning—e.g., rheumatoid disease—are being recognized. Bunning summarized immunopathogenic aspects of foodborne microbial disease (*880*). Smith et al. reviewed the relationship between the reactive arthritides and infection by foodborne bacterial pathogens (*881*). They described

reactive arthritis, Reiter's syndrome, and ankylosing spondylitis and their relationship to the major histocompatibility complex antigen HLA-B27. Reactive arthritis can be triggered by pathogens as diverse as *Campylobacter jejuni, Salmonella typhimurium, Shigella* spp., *Chlamydia* spp., *Borrelia burgdorferi,* and *Giardia lamblia.* Some authors suggest that *Klebsiella* is involved in the etiology of ankylosing spondylitis. Molecular mimicry between certain microbial antigens and HLA-B27 was discussed as an explanation for the etiology of these disorders. The roles of antibodies, lymphocytes, bacterial antigens, and stress proteins in the symptoms of the reactive arthritides were reviewed. Yu and Thomson also reviewed the clinical, epidemiological, and pathogenic aspects of reactive arthritis (*882*). The clinical outcome of this frequent sequela to many common enteric infections is not as benign as once was thought, and although symptoms may be controlled, curative therapies are needed.

Contact with animals and animal products is a possible risk factor for infection. However, a study in Denmark found among slaughterhouse workers and greenhouse workers a similar prevalence of antibodies to *Toxoplasma gondii, Campylobacter jejuni, Yersinia enterocolitica, Yersinia pseudotuberculosis, Borrelia burgdorferi,* and *Salmonella* spp. (*883*). The prevalence of toxoplasma antibodies was very high in both groups.

Investigators in Australia analyzed fecal samples from 123 infants who died of sudden infant death syndrome (SIDS) and from 52 age-matched controls for toxigenic bacteria and their toxins (*884*). Serum samples from SIDS infants were also analyzed. The prevalence of pathogens in SIDS infants and controls, respectively, was *Clostridium perfringens,* 45% vs. 20%; *Clostridium difficile,* 28% vs. 15%; *Staphylococcus aureus,* 27% (total) and 20% (enterotoxigenic) vs. 86% (all non-enterotoxigenic); and *Clostridium botulinum,* 5% vs. 0%. *Vibrio parahaemolyticus, Campylobacter jejuni, Yersinia enterocolitica, Bacillus cereus,* and *Salmonella* spp. were not detected. For toxins, the prevalence in SIDS infants and controls was heat-labile toxin lethal to mice, 27% vs. 11%; cytotoxins, 31% vs. 11%; *C. perfringens* enterotoxin, 34% vs. 0%; *C. perfringens* α-toxin, 18% vs. 0%; and staphylococcal enterotoxins, 20% vs. 0%. In SIDS infants, some pathogens and their toxins were more prevalent in bottle-fed than in breast-fed babies. The incidence of *C. perfringens, S. aureus,* and their toxins was higher in babies who died in autumn and winter than in those who died during spring and summer. These observations provide some support for the idea that intestinal toxins have a pathogenic role in SIDS.

## Pathogens in the Food Environment

Rivault et al. demonstrated that cockroaches can cause bacterial contamination of food (885). They analyzed fresh bread left with groups of 5 wild-caught cockroaches (*Blattella germanica*) in sterile containers for 16 h. No bacteria were found in pieces of bread not exposed to cockroaches. However, one or two bacterial species were identified from each of the 11 samples of bread left with cockroaches. Five were species considered potential pathogens: *Enterobacter cloacae*, *Serratia marcescens*, *Citrobacter freundii*, *Klebsiella pneumoniae*, and *Citrobacter diversus*. Kopanic et al. determined the rate at which cockroaches became contaminated when exposed to food pellets inoculated with *Salmonella typhimurium* (886). They then assessed the ability of contaminated cockroaches to infect noncontaminated colony members, food, and water. They also sampled cockroaches collected in a commercial poultry feed mill and hatchery to determine whether they harbored salmonellas. When exposed to food inoculated with *S. typhimurium*, nearly all American and Oriental cockroaches became contaminated within 24–48 h; contamination of German cockroaches was variable. Contaminated cockroaches rapidly spread the bacterium to their water source and to other cockroaches. It was also passed on in large numbers to shell eggs placed in the experimental chamber. *Salmonella* spp. were found on 5 of 45 cockroaches captured at the feed mill and 8 of 45 captured at the hatchery. These studies demonstrate that cockroaches can rapidly pick up salmonellas from contaminated food and readily infect other objects and each other. Thus there is high probability of cross-contamination wherever there are cockroach infestations.

A comprehensive discussion of dairy microbiology and safety included topics such as the incidence and characteristics of pathogens in milk and milk products, various aspects of dairy and milk microbiology and microbiological analysis, new processing technologies, and assurance of microbiological quality and safety (887). There was also a section on mycotoxins in milk and dairy products.

A biofilm consists of microorganisms and extra-cellular substances in association with a substratum. Formation of biofilms in dairy equipment leads to serious obstruction and corrosion, economic loss, and sanitation and health problems. Criado et al. considered the importance, evaluation, and prevention of bacterial adhesion to surfaces in the dairy industry (888). Carpentier and Cerf provided a more general discussion of biofilms in terms of their importance in the food industry (889). They described the formation and ecology of biofilms, problems they cause, and how they might be avoided or eliminated in the food industry. Although there are too many gaps in the understanding of biofilms for specific recommendations to be made, the authors offered some general suggestions—most of which are common sense—for minimizing the formation and excessive build-up of biofilms.

"Cutting board microbiology" attracted the attention of the media last year when Cliver's research group made some counter-intuitive observations. In one paper they reported studies simulating cross-contamination of foods in home kitchens (890). They cut pieces from new and used cutting boards and inoculated each piece with a bacterial culture. The cutting boards represented many types of materials: four polymers, hard rubber, and nine hardwoods. The bacteria tested were three strains of *Escherichia coli* including O157:H7, *Listeria innocua*, *Listeria monocytogenes*, and *Salmonella typhimurium*. Bacteria were applied to the cutting-board surface in nutrient broth or chicken juice and were recovered by soaking the surface in nutrient broth or pressing the block onto nutrient agar. Bacteria were readily recovered from plastic boards and multiplied on boards held overnight. Recoveries from both new and used wooden boards were generally less than from plastic, and the differences increased as holding time on the boards increased. In most cases, when a new wooden cutting board was exposed to fluids containing the number of bacteria likely to be found in raw meat or poultry, no bacteria could be recovered after they entered the wood (3–10 min after inoculation). Treating the wood surface with mineral oil had little effect on recovery. In a companion paper the authors reported studies of the decontamination of plastic and wooden cutting boards by methods appropriate for the home (891). Basic procedures were as before. The persistence and overnight growth of organisms on plastic depended on the maintenance of humidity. New plastic boards were relatively easy to clean effectively, but extensively scratched plastic boards were difficult to clean manually, especially if they had deposits of chicken fat on them. Again, fewer bacteria were recovered from wooden blocks than from plastic ones. Clean wooden boards rapidly absorbed the entire inoculum; but if the surface was coated with chicken fat, some bacteria could generally be recovered after 12 h at room temperature and high humidity. Cleaning with hot water and detergent removed these bacteria regardless of species, type of wood, or new or used condition of the board. Abrishami et al. also found that bacteria were more readily recovered from plastic cutting boards than from wood (892). Further study of the fate of bacteria on wooden boards revealed that nearly 75% remained viable after 2 h. They resided within the structural xylem fibers and vegetative elements of the wood. Conditioning the wood with water before inoculation interfered with bacterial adherence to the wood matrix. Intrinsically, the cutting boards themselves had neither growth-supporting nor toxic properties.

Gill and Bryant determined the numbers of bacteria in the dehairing equipment at two pig processing plants (*893*). Detritus from machines at both plants yielded $8 \times 10^7$–$9 \times 10^8$ cfu/g of total bacteria, $2 \times 10^3$–$1 \times 10^5$ cfu/g of *Escherichia coli*, and $3 \times 10^3$–$1 \times 10^6$ of *Campylobacter*. *Salmonella* was recovered from about 50% of samples at levels of $3 \times 10^4$–$4 \times 10^5$ cfu/g and $1 \times 10^2$ cfu/g at the two plants. The temperature of water circulating through the dehairing machines was <50°C at one plant and 57°C at the other. Water samples contained from several hundred to several thousand cells per milliliter of *E. coli* and 10–800 cfu/mL of *Campylobacter*. *Salmonella* was recovered in low numbers from about 50% of water samples. Carcasses leaving the dehairing equipment were contaminated with *E. coli* at levels ranging from <100 to $4 \times 10^3$/cm². *Campylobacter* counts were well below 100/cm². No salmonellas were detected. Although bacterial counts were sharply reduced after carcasses were singed and polished, the authors concluded that dehairing equipment at large slaughtering plants is a likely source of the mesophilic enteric pathogens that frequently contaminate pork.

## Occurrence of Pathogens in Foods

Of 480 samples of raw meat and seafoods from retail markets in Trinidad, 28 (5.8%) were positive for *Listeria* spp. (*894*). Nine samples contained *Listeria monocytogenes*. Twenty-eight of 29 chicken samples and 1 of 29 shrimp samples contained campylobacters. Although *E. coli* was recovered from 43 samples, only 2 strains produced verotoxins and 1 produced heat-labile enterotoxin. The antimicrobial resistance of *E. coli* was high, resistance to streptomycin and tetracycline being most prevalent. *Salmonella agona* was found in two samples of goat meat; all other samples were negative for salmonellas. No sample contained *Yersinia*. Although the frequency of contamination of meats and seafoods by these pathogens is low, seafoods pose some risk of listeriosis because of their high consumption and people's habit of eating some of them almost raw.

In New Zealand, 100 cow and 100 sheep carcasses at two slaughterhouses were sampled after dressing for microbiological analysis (*895*). *Yersinia enterocolitica* was not isolated and only two samples contained listerias

(one *L. innocua* and one *L. ivanovii*). However, motile aeromonads were isolated from 81% of sheep and 35% of beef carcasses. *Aeromonas hydrophila* accounted for 26 of 35 beef isolates; all but 9 of the sheep isolates were *A. hydrophila* or *A. caviae*.

A summer survey of retail meat and meat products in Beijing found that 66% of 105 samples had aerobic plate counts $\geq 6 \times 10^{10}$/g (*896*). Eighty-five samples were positive for *Clostridium perfringens*, 29 for *Staphylococcus aureus*, 16 for *Salmonella*, and 5 for *Listeria monocytogenes*. The incidence of pathogens was comparable in fresh and frozen products. Only 5 products met the microbiological standards of the Chinese Department of Hygiene.

Satay is grilled animal muscle and organs, marinated with spices at room temperature and usually eaten with peanut sauce. It is a popular dish in Malaysia. Arumugaswamy et al. analyzed 40 uncooked and 60 ready-to-eat samples of satay for salmonellas and listerias (*897*). Of uncooked samples, 59% were positive for *Salmonella* and 48% were positive for *Listeria*. Each species occurred in about one-quarter of cooked samples. Ninety percent of the *Listeria* isolates were *L. monocytogenes*. The predominant salmonellas were *S. agona*, *S. muenchen*, *S. blockley*, and *S. enteritidis*. *Salmonella muenchen* was isolated from one sample of peanut sauce.

Wastewater discharge restrictions and water shortages have created a need to reduce water consumption in pork processing. Miller et al. found that counts of staphylococci, enterics, fecal streptococci, *Listeria monocytogenes*, coliforms, and *Aeromonas* spp. on hams exposed to properly reconditioned and chlorinated water do not differ significantly from counts on hams exposed to potable water during initial slaughter operations (*898*). They concluded that reused water is satisfactory for scalding, dehairing, and polishing operations.

The U.S. Code of Federal Regulations permits reprocessing of poultry carcasses that are accidently contaminated with digestive tract contents during slaughter. An estimated 0.8–1.0% of broilers require reprocessing. Waldroup et al. assessed the effects of reprocessing on the microbiological quality of commercial prechill broiler carcasses in five commercial facilities (*899*). There was some interplant variation in the effectiveness of reprocessing procedures, but in general they were adequate. Total plate counts and counts of coliforms and *E. coli* were significantly lower on reprocessed carcasses than on inspection-passed carcasses. Campylobacter levels were sometimes significantly lower on reprocessed carcasses, and in no case were they higher. The incidence of salmonellas did not differ significantly in reprocessed and inspection-passed carcasses, although reprocessed carcasses from two plants had higher counts of salmonella.

The predominant bacteria isolated from skin, gills, and intestines of pond-raised hybrid striped bass were *Aeromonas* spp. (27%), coryneforms (14%), *Pseudomonas* spp. (12%), members of the *Flavobacterium/Cytophaga/Sphingobacterium* group (8%), *Plesiomonas shigelloides* (7%), and *Bacillus* spp. and *Enterobacteriaceae* (6%) (*900*). *Listeria monocytogenes, Staphylococcus aureus, Shigella dysenteriae, Yersinia pseudotuberculosis,* and *Vibrio* spp. were also occasionally isolated. Overall, however, bacterial loads were similar to those reported for wild fish and there was no indication that pond-raised fish present a higher risk of foodborne illness than wild fish. In fact, since pond-raised fish can be brought to market more quickly than wild fish they probably pose a considerably lower risk.

Berry et al. determined the counts of *Listeria* and *Vibrio* in raw shrimp imported from China, Ecuador, and Mexico (*901*). Frozen samples were obtained from distributors in the USA and previously frozen samples were obtained from retail markets. All wholesale frozen shrimp from Ecuador and China and most from Mexico were of excellent quality, but contamination levels were higher in previously frozen retail samples. The only two samples positive for *Listeria monocytogenes* were previously frozen retail samples, and 4 of 5 samples positive for *Listeria* spp. had been previously frozen. *Vibrio* spp. were present in more than 60% of samples. They were most often seen in frozen shrimp and shrimp from Mexico. The predominant species were *V. parahaemolyticus* and *V. alginolyticus*. *Vibrio vulnificus* and *V. cholerae* were isolated from ≥10% of samples and *V. fluvialis* from 7%. More than half of the *Vibrio* isolates were resistant to at least one antibiotic. These results document differences in the microbial quality of shrimp between retail and wholesale markets and between products imported from different countries.

A 2-year nationwide survey by the FDA assessed filth, microbiological contamination, and decomposition in fresh and frozen shrimp entering U.S. markets (*902*). *Listeria* spp. were found in 6.8% of samples and *Salmonella* spp. in 8.1%. Except for the USA, each country was represented by too few samples to draw conclusions about the relative prevalence of these pathogens. Most of the data in this report related to insect and other animal contamination.

Adesiyun evaluated the bacteriological quality of preprocessed pooled bulk milk from the 16 milk collection centers in Trinidad (*903*). Of 507 raw milk samples, 454 were positive in the California Mastitis Test. *Staphylococcus aureus* was isolated from 478

samples, and 9 of 117 *S. aureus* strains produced staphylococcal enterotoxins A, B, D, or a combination of these. *Escherichia coli* was isolated from 105 samples. Nearly one-quarter of the strains produced verotoxin, but none produced heat-labile enterotoxin.

Dumoulin and Peretz reported that the contamination level of raw goat's milk in France has improved considerably since a system of paying for goat's milk according to its bacteriological quality was implemented in 1986 (*904*). Now, to meet specifications for public health protection, quality improvement policy is directed toward particular prevention programs to limit contamination by pathogens. Brucellosis remains a problem in a few areas. *Staphylococcus aureus* causes considerable clinical and subclinical mastitis. In a recent survey, 12% of milk samples from one milking at 53 farms contained >2000 cfu/mL of *S. aureus* and 22% of samples contained >100 cfu/mL of *E. coli*.

During 1990 and 1991, Maifreni et al. collected 396 samples of ice cream made by local ice-cream shops in Udine, Italy, and evaluated them microbiologically (*905*). No *Salmonella* spp., *Listeria monocytogenes,* or *Staphylococcus aureus* were found. Numerous species of coliforms and yeasts were randomly distributed. Overall, the ice creams were considered to be of moderately poor quality with respect to coliforms. Roughly one-quarter of the ice creams were not fit for sale according to an Italian Ministry Ordinance. Evaluation of techniques for recovery of freeze-stressed coliforms in artificially contaminated ice cream showed that techniques using both selective and nonselective media are preferable to those using only selective media.

Yamani and Al-Dababseh compared the microbial quality of 60 samples of chickpea dip (hoummos) commercially produced in Jordan with the quality of product they produced under hygienic conditions (*906*). Although the microbial load of commercial hoummos was high, no salmonellas were detected and all counts of *E. coli* and *Staphylococcus aureus* were <10/g. The large populations of lactic acid bacteria in the commercial hoummos probably inhibit growth of pathogens, but they cannot guarantee safety of the product when rules of personal hygiene, sanitation, and safe storage are violated.

Rosenberger and Weber assessed bacterial levels in 118 samples of spices and extracts in Germany and compared these with current guide and warning values (*907*). Counts of *Bacillus cereus* and *E. coli* were safely within the guidelines. Clostridia were found in 3 samples of spices and about 50% of spice mixtures contained levels of 10–100/g, again, within guidelines. At $2.1 \times 10^5$/g, the count of mold spores in green pepper slightly exceeded the guideline value of $1 \times 10^5$/g but was below the warning value. Spice oils and extracts were virtually free of microorganisms.

Anderton discussed the sources and routes of bacterial contamination of enteral feeds and feeding systems and factors affecting the rate of growth of microorganisms in these systems (*908*). The role of such contamination in development of bacteremia, septicemia, pneumonia, diarrhea, and infectious enterocolitis was considered.

## Behavior of Pathogens in Foods During Production and Storage

Fang et al. followed the growth of three lactobacilli and the mastitis pathogens *E. coli* and *Staphylococcus aureus* in normal and mastitic milk and whey using the standard plate count method (*909*). The lactobacilli grew well in normal milk, but less well in mastitic milk. In contrast, *E. coli* and *S. aureus* grew better in mastitic milk than in normal milk. However, the pathogens grew faster than the lactobacilli in both normal and mastitic milk. All the bacteria grew well in whey, particularly mastitic whey. Moreover, preculturing in mastitic whey markedly improved the growth of both pathogenic and nonpathogenic bacteria in mastitic milk.

Barbosa et al. evaluated the behavior of *Staphylococcus aureus* and *E. coli* during production and ripening of Parmesan (*910*) and "Prato" (*911*) cheese. Milk was inoculated after pasteurization to give *S. aureus* counts of $10^6$/mL and *E. coli* counts of $10^7$/mL. To assess injury, counts were made by a traditional method and also by a method permitting recovery of stressed cells. In Parmesan cheese, counts of both organisms fell by 1–3 $\log_{10}$ at the whey removal stage of production. Counts of *S. aureus* were reduced by 4 $\log_{10}$ units during ripening; *E. coli* counts initially increased by a factor of 10, then decreased to ~$10^3$/mL by the end of ripening. There was evidence of sublethal heat and acid injury in both organisms—in *E. coli* more than in *S. aureus*. Counts of both organisms were higher in curd than in whey. In Prato cheese, counts of *S. aureus* increased during production whereas *E. coli* counts remained constant. However, by the end of the 98-day ripening period both organisms were virtually eliminated from the cheese. Again, more sublethal injury was seen in *E. coli* than in *S. aureus*.

In Spain, investigators monitored populations of bacterial pathogens during production of 15 batches of La Serena cheese made from raw sheep's milk (*912*). Overall, the microbiological quality of the cheeses was poor. Seven of the samples had coliform and fecal coliform levels of $10^4$–$10^7$ cfu/g after 60 days of ripening.

However, staphylococci were found in only 2 batches at this time, *Salmonella arizonae* was the only *Salmonella* species detected, and no *Campylobacter jejuni* was found. Two batches contained very low numbers of *Listeria monocytogenes* after 20 days of ripening; in one of them the organism was still detected after 45 days. In no case was *L. monocytogenes* recovered by direct plating.

Gram assessed the antibacterial effects of 209 strains of *Pseudomonas* isolated from spoiled iced fish and newly caught fish (*913*). One-third of the strains inhibited growth of one or more of the organisms tested in cultural bioassays (*E. coli, Shewanella putrefaciens, Aeromonas sobria, Pseudomonas fluorescens, Listeria monocytogenes,* and *Staphylococcus aureus*). *Staphylococcus aureus* and *A. sobria* were the most sensitive. Siderophore-producing pseudomonads were the most inhibitory, and the presence of iron eliminated the antibacterial effect of two-thirds of the strains. Overall the observations suggest that microbial competition and antagonism influence the microbial composition of some chilled food products.

The processing, storage, and hauling of beef and fish could be made more efficient in some tropical countries if the same workers and facilities were used for both. However, temperature abuse and unsanitary practices in these countries might enhance the risk of cross-contamination. To assess this risk, investigators in Louisiana evaluated the ability of beef isolates of *E. coli* and *Clostridium perfringens* and an *Aeromonas hydrophila* isolate from fish to grow on raw beef and fish (*914*). Experiments were conducted at a typical ambient retail display temperature (35°C) and aging/conditioning temperature (15°C). At both temperatures, growth of *A. hydrophila* was significantly greater on fish than on beef and growth of *E. coli* was significantly greater on beef than on fish. *Clostridium perfringens* grew better on beef than on fish at 35°C and failed to grow on either at 15°C. The authors concluded that joint handling of the two types of product in the tropics to save space, labor, and energy is safe, particularly with appropriate use of packaging and sanitizing technologies.

To extend the data for validation of predictive models, Hudson and Mott grew *Listeria monocytogenes, Aeromonas hydrophila,* and *Yersinia enterocolitica* at 5 and 10°C on sliced cooked beef packaged aerobically and under vacuum (*915*). Observed growth rates and rates predicted by the MIRINZ type-strain and Y3 models agreed very well for *Y. enterocolitica*. However, MIRINZ models and the USDA model failed to predict growth rates of *A. hydrophila* and *L. monocytogenes* under most conditions and in many cases the models predicted considerably less growth than actually occurred. The USDA model tended to underestimate generation times, and thus provided "safer" estimates than MIRINZ models. The MIRINZ models could be adjusted, however, to provide a safety margin. All species grew well under all conditions except for *A. hydrophila* in vacuum-packaged beef at 10°C. In further studies of the growth of these pathogens on sliced roast beef, the researchers found that storage under a high-$CO_2$ controlled atmosphere extended the shelf life of the product without increasing risk due to pathogen growth (*916*). At −1.5°C pathogen populations decreased in controlled-atmosphere packs but increased in vacuum packs. Although all pathogens grew under both packaging conditions at 3°C, populations were lower in controlled-atmosphere packs than in vacuum packs at the end of the shelf life.

Van Laack et al. studied the effect of hot and cold processing on survival and growth of *Salmonella, Campylobacter, Listeria monocytogenes, Aeromonas hydrophila,* and *Yersinia enterocolitica* on pork loins (*917*). After inoculation with pathogen-containing feces, loin pieces were left unpackaged, vacuum-packaged immediately after hot-boning, or vacuum-packaged after chilling for 1 day. Pathogen numbers were determined after 0, 1, 2, 5, and 9 days of storage at 1°C. *Campylobacter* populations decreased during storage but the organism could still be recovered at the end of the experiment. Survival was poorest on unpackaged loins. The other pathogens were little affected by packaging treatment. Numbers of *L. monocytogenes* increased by a factor of 10 during storage. Survival and growth of *A. hydrophila* was inconsistent. The authors attribute this to possible differences in the competitive fecal flora, which was not standardized between experiments. *Salmonella* populations decreased during storage, but survival was best in hot-packaged pork. The authors reported difficulties in recovering *Y. enterocolitica* reliably, perhaps due to large populations of competing microflora.

In studies similar to their studies with roast beef (*915*), Hudson and Mott measured the growth of *Listeria monocytogenes, Aeromonas hydrophila,* and *Yersinia enterocolitica* in paté at 4 and 10°C and compared the observed values with values predicted by MIRINZ and USDA models (*918*). The type strain and a food-derived strain of each pathogen were tested. Both strains of *L. monocytogenes* grew at both temperatures. The food strain of *A. hydrophila* grew only at 10°C and the type strain did not grow at either temperature. The food strain of *Y. enterocolitica* grew at both temperatures, whereas the type strain grew at neither. In general, measured values of lag and generation times agreed poorly with

those from the models, which predicted much greater growth than was observed. The authors postulated that the competitive flora restricted pathogen growth.

Radford and Board reviewed the fate of pathogens in home-made mayonnaise and summarized data on outbreaks of illness involving mayonnaise and related products (*919*). The safety of low-calorie mayonnaise was also discussed. Attention was focused on *S. enteritidis* because this pathogen is frequently introduced in eggs. Both pH and choice of acidulant influence the survival of *Salmonella* spp., *Clostridium perfringens,* and *Staphylococcus aureus.* Vinegar (acetic acid) is more bactericidal than lemon juice (citric acid). White wine vinegar and distilled malt vinegar are more inhibitory than malt vinegar. Vegetable material in the mayonnaise absorbs acetic acid and reduces its toxicity. Addition of 0.3–1.5 wt% garlic or mustard increases the death rate of *S. enteritidis.* Salt is protective. The death rate of *S. enteritidis* is also higher in mayonnaise prepared from virgin olive oil, which has a high concentration of phenolic compounds, than in mayonnaise prepared from ordinary olive oil or sunflower seed oil. It is recommended that mayonnaise be prepared with vinegar to a pH of 4.1 or lower. Because refrigerated storage protects *Salmonella* from acidulants, a holding time of 24 h at 18–22°C is recommended before refrigeration. Use of pasteurized liquid egg is advised for catering purposes, and use of commercial mayonnaise is recommended in hospitals and other settings where there are large numbers of persons at risk for infection. Interactions between mayonnaise and other food components, as in salads, must be considered.

Erickson et al. followed the fate of *Salmonella* spp., *Listeria monocytogenes,* and indigenous spoilage organisms in salads prepared with commercial mayonnaise and reduced-calorie mayonnaise (*920*). *Salmonella* grew in temperature-abused chicken salad; *L. monocytogenes* grew in both temperature-abused and refrigerated chicken salad, although growth was inhibited for 7 days at 4°C. The microbiological shelf lives of refrigerated chicken and pasta salads were 5 and 7 days, respectively. Whether salads were made with regular or reduced-calorie mayonnaise had no effect on safety or spoilage.

## Identification

Sharpe reviewed new methods for the rapid detection of foodborne disease agents (*921*). He described streamlined versions of traditional tests, physical and chemical tests based on preformed microbial components, electrical impedance techniques, DNA probes, immunological methods, and genetically engineered luminescent organisms. A table summarized many of the commercial test kits. Suppliers' addresses were provided. In editorial comments, Silley discussed instrumentation and problems associated with automated microbiology, and prospects for the future of rapid instrumental techniques (922).

Bishop summarized collaborative studies, underway and on the horizon, of analytical methods for dairy microbiology (923). A similar summary by Andrews for nondairy food microbiology reported assays for *Listeria, Salmonella, Vibrio vulnificus, Clostridium perfringens, Staphylococcus aureus, E. coli, Bacillus* spp. enterotoxins, total coliforms, and aerobic plate counts (924).

De Ryck et al. described rapid biochemical methods to screen for *Salmonella, Shigella, Yersinia,* and *Aeromonas* among isolates from fecal samples (925).

Spierings et al. described a PCR for specific detection of *E. coli/Shigella* and inclusion of a second primer couple to recognize a broad group of closely related enteric bacteria, including *Salmonella* (926).

In an editorial, Pitt reflected on the rationale underlying bacterial typing systems such as biotyping, serotyping, phage typing, bacteriocin typing, and antimicrobial sensitivity typing (927). Requirements of a typing method and interpretation of results from molecular profiling techniques were considered. The question of how many differences in pattern or profile are necessary for considering two isolates distinct has not been answered. Nevertheless, the new methods have provided evidence of the genetic diversity of strains within species involved in outbreaks, clues to the common ancestry of world-wide epidemic strains, and interrelationships between genotype and phylogenetic origin as indicated by rRNA genes. In practical terms, some laboratories may be tempted to do their own typing in response to their own particular needs. Pitt discourages this because it would generate data of local relevance only; standardization is necessary so data can be integrated regionally and nationally. Traditional phenotypic systems should remain important because they are simple and generally valid. Reference laboratories should continue to monitor regional, national, and international movement of strains and to develop and validate typing systems with reference to established schemes.

## Control

In a critical review, Champagne et al. discussed the incidence and control of pathogenic and nonpathogenic psychrotrophs in dairy products (928). The influence of psychrotrophic bacteria on the quality of raw and pasteurized milk and milk products was examined and technological problems associated with these organisms were mentioned. Health concerns and outbreaks of illness caused by psychrotrophic pathogens in dairy products were summarized.

Li and Torres determined growth parameters of *Pseudomonas fluorescens, Brochothrix thermosphacta, Salmonella typhimurium, Enterococcus faecalis,* and *Staphylococcus aureus* in liquid medium as a function of temperature, $a_w$, and solute type (929). Lag phase increased and growth rate decreased as temperature or $a_w$ was decreased, but the amount of change depended on the $a_w$-controlling solute. In general, sucrose had a greater effect than NaCl, which had a greater effect than glycerol. The specific growth rate was less sensitive than the lag phase to the $a_w$-controlling solute. By a linear extrapolation method the authors estimated the minimum $a_w$ that would permit microbial growth. This study demonstrates that solute effects as well as temperature and $a_w$ must be considered in shelf-life modeling, and particular attention should be given to solute effects on the lag phase.

Lysozyme, EDTA, and apo-lactoferrin, individually or in combinations, had no effect on growth of *Salmonella typhimurium* or *Pseudomonas fluorescens* in UHT pasteurized milk (930). EDTA alone inhibited *E. coli* O157:H7 but the effect was not enhanced by the inclusion of lysozyme. Both EDTA and lysozyme inhibited *L. monocytogenes,* and together they had a synergistic bactericidal effect. A combination of 15 mg/mL of apo-lactoferrin and 150 µg/mL of lysozyme slowed the growth of *L. monocytogenes.* Thus these agents and their combinations have potential for enhancing the microbiological safety of refrigerated foods, but their efficacy depends on the microorganism(s) being targeted and probably also on the storage conditions and the nature of the food product.

ORGANIC ACIDS AND RELATED COMPOUNDS. Pork carcasses were randomly assigned to a control group or to treatment with a sanitizing spray of 1.5% acetic, citric, or lactic acid (931). Loins were vacuum-packaged and stored at 0–2°C. Samples were analyzed microbiologically after 0, 14, 28, 35, and 42 days of storage. After packages were opened for sampling the loins were cut into chops, which were film-wrapped on styrofoam trays and held in a lighted display at 2–4°C until they spoiled. No *Salmonella* spp. were found on any loins or chops. *Yersinia* was found in 6% of samples, *Campylobacter* spp. in 5% of samples, and *Listeria* spp. in 69% of loins and 33% of spoiled chops. Acetic and citric acids decreased aerobic plate counts and coliform counts initially but this effect was no longer apparent after 14 days. None of the treatments had any practical effect for long-term storage. The authors suggest that this was because counts of pathogens and nonpathogens were quite low initially, indicating the effectiveness of normal pig-slaughter operations.

van Netten et al. developed an in vitro model of decontamination of meat by lactic acid (932). It was based on the inactivation kinetics of bacteria in suspensions of fecally contaminated pork-belly skin and suspensions inoculated with *Campylobacter jejuni, Salmonella typhimurium,* or *Listeria monocytogenes.* It takes into account the buffering activity of the meat surface, leaching of organic material from surfaces, and microbial interactions. Comparison of the immediate lethality of lactic acid treatment for bacteria in the model meat suspension with the lethality on pieces of meat showed excellent agreement. However, the immediate lethality seen in the model was up to 10 times less than that reported for comparable experiments involving carcass decontamination at the slaughterhouse. The most sensitive pathogen was *C. jejuni.* The least sensitive was *L. monocytogenes.* This model enables the controlled testing of a variety of factors and could provide an economical alternative to field studies.

*Enterobacteriaceae* are often enumerated as part of monitoring the microbiological quality of processed foods. However, the significance of *Enterobacteriaceae* as index organisms is more often assumed than tested. To validate use of the organisms as a quality index, colony counts of *Enterobacteriaceae* and *E. coli* were made on chicken legs subjected to various treatments (933). Untreated legs and legs sprayed with 10% lactic acid–sodium lactate buffer (pH 3.0) were stored in polyethylene bags or packaged under an atmosphere of 90% $CO_2$ and 10% $O_2$ and stored at 6°C. Enumeration of *Enterobacteriaceae* from plates incubated at 37 or 42°C indicated the hygienic condition of legs immediately after processing, but not after 3 or 6 days of storage. Counts of *E. coli* were a more realistic hygienic index for stored poultry and were also a good indicator of temperature abuse during storage. Decontamination with the lactic acid buffer produced an immediate 1-$\log_{10}$ reduction in *Enterobacteriaceae* colony counts, which was followed by a bacteriostatic effect on the psychrotrophic members of this group that amounted to as much as 3 $\log_{10}$.

The effect of a trisodium phosphate dip on numbers of *E. coli* and *Salmonella typhimurium* attached to fat and fascia surfaces of beef was evaluated by microbiological plating and scanning electron microscopy (934).

Surfaces were exposed to $10^9$ cfu/mL of each inoculum for 15 min, then rinsed with 10% trisodium phosphate for 15 s. The rinse reduced colony counts of *E. coli* by 1.35 $\log_{10}$ on fat and 0.92 $\log_{10}$ on fascia surfaces. The corresponding reductions for *S. typhimurium* were 0.91 and 0.51 $\log_{10}$. By scanning electron microscopy, the rinse reduced counts on fascia surfaces by 1.39 $\log_{10}$ for *E. coli* and 0.86 $\log_{10}$ for *S. typhimurium.* Thus the rinse was more effective on fat than on fascia and for *E. coli* than for *S. typhimurium.*

To extend observations on the antibacterial activity of sodium lactate, Miller and Acuff studied its effects on *Listeria monocytogenes, Staphylococcus aureus, Salmonella typhimurium, Clostridium perfringens,* and *E. coli* O157:H7 in precooked vacuum-packaged beef during storage at 10°C (935). Roasts were injected before cooking to contain 0, 2, 3, or 4% sodium lactate. Noninoculated control samples remained sterile throughout the 28-d experiment. Four percent lactate inhibited growth of *S. typhimurium* by about 2 $\log_{10}$ after 7 days; at 14 and 28 days MPN/cm² counts were about 3 $\log_{10}$ lower with 3 and 4% lactate than with 0 or 2%. Growth of *L. monocytogenes* and *E. coli* O157:H7 was completely prevented by 4% lactate; 3% lactate had a lesser, but significant, effect during later stages of storage. There was no effect on *S. aureus. Clostridium perfringens* was undetectable at 7 days in samples containing 3 or 4% lactate. However, counts had also fallen very low in samples containing 0 or 2%, making it difficult to evaluate the effect of lactate on *C. perfringens* under these conditions. Because sensory evaluations rule out use of 4% lactate, the authors recommend 3% lactate as the best compromise from the joint perspectives of food safety and acceptability.

Other investigators tested the microbiological safety of beef roasts injected before cooking to contain 1.5, 2.5, or 3.5% sodium lactate, glycerol monolaurin, or sodium gluconate (936). Some roasts were also injected with *Clostridium sporogenes* and *Listeria monocytogenes* before cooking. Others were surface-inoculated after cooking. Storage was at typical wholesale, retail, and consumer storage temperatures (2–4, 7, and 10°C) and an abusive temperature (25°C). None of the chemical treatments compromised sensory quality. For both organisms, counts in internally inoculated roasts were low and there were no significant differences between treatments. In surface-inoculated roasts sodium lactate provided the best control and remained effective in temperature-abused samples. Sodium gluconate afforded no significant control. High counts of both organisms were obtained from roasts injected with standard NaCl–phosphate brine. This gives cause for concern, because roasts treated with this brine are typical of products being marketed.

Houtsma et al. determined the MIC of sodium lactate for pathogens and spoilage organisms that occur in meat products (*937*). Tests were done in laboratory media under optimal growth conditions for the organisms. Gram-positive bacteria were generally more sensitive than gram-negative, and bacteria able to grow at $a_w \leq .95$ in the presence of NaCl (e.g., *Staphylococcus aureus, Listeria monocytogenes*) were especially sensitive. These results suggest that addition of lactate to food products with a pH near neutrality is likely to extend their shelf life.

LACTIC ACID BACTERIA. Abdalla et al. assessed the survival of *Listeria monocytogenes, Salmonella typhimurium,* and *Staphylococcus aureus* in white pickled cheese made with a lactic acid bacteria starter culture, nisin, hydrogen peroxide, or potassium sorbate (*938*). The starter culture inhibited all three pathogens, whereas the antimicrobials did not. *Listeria monocytogenes* was no longer detected in the curd on day 50; *S. aureus* and *S. typhimurium* were no longer detected on day 30. The pathogens disappeared from the brine even sooner. The pH of the brine solution dropped below 4.7 when the lactic acid starter culture was used; in all antimicrobial treatments the pH exceeded 5.5. The authors concluded that use of a starter culture is extremely important for safe production of white pickled cheese.

Tested by the agar well diffusion method, neutralized culture filtrates of four strains of *Lactobacillus* and *Lactococcus* isolated from the cultured Indian milk product "dahi" had mild to moderate antimicrobial activity against *Staphylococcus aureus, E. coli,* and a number of *Bacillus* species including *B. cereus* (*939*). The minimum concentration of culture filtrate that completely inhibited an inoculum of $10^3$ cfu/mL was 20–26 vol%. At 10 vol% the filtrate suppressed or retarded growth during a 24-h incubation at 37°C. This study shows the potential antimicrobial activity of dahi and the possible utility of neutralized extracellular culture filtrates of lactic acid bacteria in the biopreservation of foods.

Jeppesen and Huss demonstrated antagonistic effects of *Leuconostoc* sp. V6 and *Lactobacillus plantarum* LKE5, both isolated from fish products, against *Listeria monocytogenes* Scott A and *Yersinia enterocolitica* O3 in sterile shrimp extracts at 5°C (*940*). The pH was adjusted to 6.0 or 5.8 with citric acid. In the second experiment 3% NaCl was also added. Both strains of lactic acid bacteria were inhibitory toward both pathogens. *Listeria monocytogenes* was the more sensitive of the pathogens. However, the extent and duration of

inhibition was also related to the strain of lactic acid bacterium, the size of the initial pathogen population, and the presence of NaCl. Under some circumstances *L. plantarum* was more effective than *Leuconostoc* sp.

PHYTOCHEMICALS. Some phenolic plant constituents have antimicrobial activity and may defend the plant against microbial infections. Chung et al. tested the antimicrobial properties of tannic acid, gallic acid, ellagic acid, and propyl gallate against 15 foodborne bacteria including major pathogens, using the well assay technique (*941*). Tannic acid inhibited growth of all bacteria. Propyl gallate was also inhibitory (12 of 15 strains), but gallic acid and ellagic acid were not. Gallic acid is a hydrolysis product of both tannic acid and propyl gallate; ellagic acid is a hydrolysis product of tannic acid. The authors concluded that the ester linkage between gallic acid and glucose or propanol is necessary for the antimicrobial activity of these compounds. Baumann and Müller tested the effects of suspensions of dried ground leaves from 10 species of tannin-containing tropical plants against *E. coli, Salmonella typhimurium,* and *Clostridium perfringens* (*942*). Leaf suspensions from 8 of the 10 plants inactivated *C. perfringens* but none were active against *E. coli* or *S. typhimurium.* Leaves were analyzed for content of total phenols, tannic phenols, and condensed soluble tannins. The total polyphenol content was not correlated with the in vitro effect.

There have been several reports that carrot extracts have antimicrobial activity. Most recently, Babic et al. tested the effects of purified ethanolic extracts of carrot against a range of foodborne pathogens and spoilage organisms (*943*). Extracts were made from fresh shredded carrots and from shredded carrots stored at 4°C for 7 days in air or under OPP film. The minimum inhibitory concentrations were expressed as milligrams of freeze-dried carrot used for the extraction per milliliter of culture solution. The following MICs were determined: *Leuconostoc mesenteroides,* 27 mg/mL; *Listeria monocytogenes* and *Staphylococcus aureus,* >27 <55 mg/mL; *Pseudomonas fluorescens* and *Candida lambica,* >55 <110 mg/mL; *E. coli,* >110 <220 mg/mL. Dodecanoic acid and methyl esters of dodecanoic and pentadecanoic acids were identified by GC-MS in purified active carrot extracts and could be responsible for the antimicrobial activity. Crude extracts were inactive. Chlorogenic acid and *p*-hydroxybenzoic acid, the most abundant phenolic compounds identified in purified extracts, had little or no activity.

Fungi (*Aspergillus* and *Penicillium* spp.) and yeasts (*Saccharomyces* and *Candida* spp.) are more sensitive than bacteria to the antimicrobial properties of cumin, cumin volatile oil, and cuminaldehyde (944). Among the bacteria tested, *Pseudomonas aeruginosa* and *Staphylococcus aureus* were the least sensitive and *E. coli* and *Bacillus* spp. the most sensitive.

Gundidza et al. studied the antimicrobial activity of the essential oil from the lavender tree (*Heteropyxis natalensis*) (945). The microorganisms tested included animal and plant pathogens, food-poisoning bacteria, and mycotoxigenic fungi. The oil strongly inhibited all test organisms. Its constituents included 1,8-cineole, limonene, β-myrcene, α-phellandrene, and α-pinene.

**SANITIZATION.** Wong's research group has been investigating the development and inactivation of biofilms on stainless steel and Buna-n rubber (946,947). They showed that biofilm formation is influenced by the type of surface, nutrient level, and bacterial strain (946). The 7 *Listeria monocytogenes* strains and one *Salmonella typhimurium* strain tested grew well and developed biofilms on stainless steel under both high- and low-nutrient conditions. Buna-n rubber was strongly bacteriostatic against *L. monocytogenes* and reduced biofilm formation by 4 of the 7 strains under low nutrient conditions. Other types of rubber had less or no effect. The four sanitizers tested reduced populations of suspended bacteria by 7–8 $\log_{10}$. Populations in biofilms on stainless steel were reduced by 3–5 $\log_{10}$, whereas reduction was only 1–2 $\log_{10}$ on Buna-n. Chlorine and anionic sanitizers removed extracellular material more effectively than iodine or quaternary ammonium sanitizers. Another study examined the effects of trisodium phosphate on suspended and biofilm cells of *Campylobacter jejuni*, *L. monocytogenes*, *E. coli* O157:H7, and *S. typhimurium* at room temperature and 10°C (947). All organisms readily formed biofilms on stainless steel, but *C. jejuni* and *E. coli* did not form biofilms on Buna-n. No attached or suspended *E. coli* cells were detected after a 30-s exposure to 1% trisodium phosphate; *C. jejuni* was only slightly less sensitive. In contrast, *L. monocytogenes* populations were reduced by <1 $\log_{10}$ even after a 2-min exposure to 8% trisodium phosphate. *Listeria monocytogenes* was more resistant at 10°C than at room temperature, whereas *S. typhimurium* was more resistant at room temperature. The ability of the pathogens to survive and grow in culture medium containing various concentrations of trisodium phosphate was also evaluated. Trisodium phosphate seems to have considerable potential as a cleaning aid for surfaces, but the optimal concentration, exposure time, and temperature need to be defined for each application.

Restaino et al. compared a buffered organic acid anionic surfactant with 6 traditional sanitizers for ability to reduce populations of *Staphylococcus aureus* on an inoculated Formica surface (948). Immediately after exposure, in the absence of organic matter, traditional sanitizers were no more effective than water, whereas concentrations of the new sanitizer ≥1.2% significantly reduced bacterial populations. Sixty minutes after exposure the new sanitizer was more than 100 times as effective as organic chlorine. Organic matter reduced the efficiency of all sanitizers. A 30-s exposure to the buffered organic acid anionic surfactant at a concentration of 0.6% caused a greater than 5-$\log_{10}$ reduction in counts of *S. aureus*, *Salmonella typhimurium*, *Listeria monocytogenes*, and *Pseudomonas aeruginosa*.

A 0.25% iodine premilking teat disinfectant for prevention of new intramammary infections was evaluated for 14 months in a natural exposure study, using a split-udder design (949). After milking, control and pretreated teats were dipped with the same teat dip. New infections by gram-negative bacteria were significantly fewer in predipped teats. The percentage of pretreated quarters newly infected by major mastitis pathogens was roughly half that of control quarters. However, predipping and postdipping was no more effective against *Staphylococcus aureus* than postdipping only.

## CONTROL

Shapiro and Mercier discussed the new holistic approach to safe food manufacturing (950). They considered biotechnology and the control of residues, contaminants, and nutritional quality as well as microbiological safety and quality. Packaging was discussed in terms of its contributions to food safety (including protection from criminal damage) and the migration of packaging components into the food product. The importance of environmental protection was emphasized, particularly with respect to the recyclability and reusability of packaging materials. Another broad look at food safety and quality was presented by Paulus (951). A thorough approach to quality assurance is not a bureaucratic exercise but a prescription for success. Although Paulus spoke from the viewpoint of the European community, the ideas apply to burgeoning global trade: the key is to transform general quality standards into programs of quality assurance tailored to individual companies. Hazard analysis critical control point (HACCP) systems and the ISO 9000 series of standards were discussed.

## HACCP and Related Procedures for Hazard Analysis

HACCP is a proactive strategy that anticipates hazards and identifies the critical control points at which a hazard can be managed. The book *HACCP Principles and Applications* (*952*) is based on a short course presented by the Continuing Education Committee of the Institute of Food Technologists. Although based on the seven principles recommended by the National Advisory Committee on Microbiological Criteria for Foods (NACMCF), the presentations cover all biological, chemical, and physical hazards. After introductory chapters on principles, definitions, and hazards, each of the HACCP principles is analyzed in depth. One chapter is devoted to control points other than those relating to safety within the context of HACCP. In addition, recognizing that HACCP processes have continued to evolve since they were first described, the NACMCF recently defined the relative roles of regulatory agencies and industry in the development and implementation of HACCP plans (*953*). Agencies are urged to adopt inspection techniques that verify that HACCP plans are adequate and are being followed. Stringer discussed safety and quality management through HACCP and ISO 9000 as a way to harmonize disparate national approaches to trade and commercial requirements within the European community (*954*). The Campden Food and Drink Research Association has introduced computer software for use as a HACCP documentation tool. The key features of this software, which can also be used as part of a training program, were described.

van Schothorst and Jongeneel compared classical methods of inspection and end-product testing with microbiological process control and HACCP systems for assuring food safety (*955*). Line monitoring by physicochemical methods and observation are more reliable than end-product testing. Moreover, the availability of monitoring results to relevant regulatory agencies and enforcement officials promotes trust and mutual understanding, facilitates international trade, and provides a basis for dialogue with consumers.

A survey of meat- and poultry-company executives in the northeastern USA was conducted to learn how well the position on HACCP formally taken by national organizations in the meat and poultry slaughtering and processing industry reflected regional views (*956*). Only 11 of the 105 responding companies had HACCP programs in place when the survey was conducted. More than half of those that did not were "waiting to see what happens at FSIS" (Food Safety and Inspection Service). The majority of companies felt they were inadequately

staffed to implement HACCP. Although the majority of companies understood the HACCP concept and thought they could identify their own critical control points, they were less confident in their ability to implement HACCP. Moreover, nearly 50% of companies thought that traditional inspection programs are adequate and fewer than 25% considered HACCP more reliable than traditional methods. In terms of the importance of benefits associated with HACCP, economic factors (increased sales, decreased costs, etc.) were perceived as most important, whereas confidence in the safety of the product was ranked 5th in a list of 10 benefits. The major concerns related to implementing HACCP were the high costs of laboratory facilities, employee training, and operating the system. However, concern about product safety was ranked as the most important factor that might influence the decision to implement HACCP. Although some employees of most large companies had received formal HACCP training, most small companies had no employees with such training. Only a few companies thought that HACCP should be mandatory. The authors concluded that the main tasks facing FSIS are to educate industry about HACCP and convince it that HACCP is cost-effective.

Australia is a relative newcomer to the HACCP scene, but its problems in applying HACCP principles are much like problems experienced elsewhere. Some of these were summarized at the several levels at which HACCP is now being applied (*957*). Top management still frequently resists shifting its philosophy from detecting failure to preventing failure. However, HACCP cannot succeed even with a committed management if unconvinced operations and production personnel need to be dragged along by edict. Problems associated with developing the HACCP plan, identifying hazards and critical control points, monitoring, verification, and regulatory aspects were reviewed. These problems do not stem from defects in the HACCP concept or its potential performance, but rather are people-problems that can be solved by adequate commitment and training.

The state of Alaska has warned the FDA that the HACCP system does not change inherent problems such as short-cut practices, poor maintenance of facilities and equipment, and poor judgment (*958*). While supporting a mandated HACCP plan for the seafood industry, such a plan does not automatically reduce the need for inspections and active enforcement. Nor is HACCP a cure-all in food service (*959*). Some of the problems a restaurant HACCP program cannot deal with are malicious tampering with foods, guaranteeing the absence of residues and contaminants, and idiosyncratic customer complaints. Rapid staff turnover (~400% per year in fast-food outlets) is a major obstacle to compliance with a HACCP plan. Nevertheless, the author points out that HACCP is a journey, not a destination, and needs to be taken very seriously by the food-service industry.

Longitudinal integrated safety assurance (LISA) is a concept very similar to the HACCP approach and is also based on hazard analysis and identification of critical control points. van Logtestijn et al. presented an overview of LISA and its application to interrupting bacterial cycles in animal production (*960*). This was an introduction to a workshop convened to discuss progress in production of safe foods of animal origin.

Huis in 't Veld et al. discussed the impact of animal husbandry and slaughter technologies on the microbial contamination of meat (*961*). They emphasized that preventive quality assurance along the entire chain from production through processing is the only effective way to control the microbiological safety and quality of meat. This involves identification of hazards and critical control points and choice of procedures for monitoring the microbiological status of both animals and carcasses, since total control is impossible at most critical points. Process-integrated microbiology, microbiological problems associated with meat production, and specific problems of pork and poultry meat production were briefly discussed. New monitoring techniques based on impedimetry, turbidimetry, flow cytometry, bioluminescence, fluorescence, immunoassays, DNA technology, and various biosensors were summarized. The authors believe that creative combinations of immunoassays, DNA technology, and automated instrumental techniques will be the basic microbiological monitoring systems in the future.

Troeger reviewed the hygienic risks and critical control points during the slaughter of pigs and cattle (*962*). Neuber discussed the concept of a microbiologically controlled room, or "clean room," as applied to the meat-processing industry (*963*). Inglefinger discussed criteria for cleaning and disinfection systems in the meat industry (*964*).

The NACMCF proposed a generic HACCP plan for beef "from farm to consumption" (*965*). The epidemiology of foodborne illness associated with raw beef was reviewed and the ecology and microbiology of raw beef were described. Hazard analysis then leads to the conclusion that raw beef can be an important vehicle for transmission of salmonellas and *E. coli* O157:H7—pathogens that are similar in their ability to multiply in the bovine intestinal tract without producing symptoms, their sensitivity to heat, cold, and chemicals, and their potentially low infectious doses. The generic HACCP plan was therefore directed primarily at these

pathogens. Among the topics considered were animal husbandry and farm management practices, the effects of stress on infection and contamination, transportation and marketing, identification of animals, slaughter operations, distribution, retailing, and final preparation. The roles of regulatory agencies and industry in HACCP-based beef processing were delineated. Suggestions were made for decontamination, reducing the potential for contamination, carcass identification, and product coding. Areas where more research is needed were highlighted.

The Microbiology and Food Safety Committee of the National Food Processors Association proposed a generic model for implementing HACCP plans for chilled foods (*966*). Producers of these popular new-generation foods range from large multinational corporations to small family-operated businesses. This model is addressed to products produced at a central location and distributed to retail establishments through refrigerated distribution channels. A hypothetical HACCP description of a food ("XYZ chunky chicken salad"), its distribution, and its intended use were presented. One flow diagram showed the stages of the process and the critical control points from production and processing of raw materials through fabrication and retailing of the product to its purchase by the consumer. Another showed the individual steps in product fabrication beginning with receipt of the raw materials. The distinction between true critical control points and simple control points was emphasized. The remaining HACCP principles—setting critical limits for each critical control point, monitoring, determining corrective actions for deviations, keeping records, and verification procedures—were covered briefly.

Leistner discussed the use of hurdle technology for food preservation in the context of the HACCP concept (*967*). The microbiological stability of foods is determined by many factors, including $a_w$, pH, and preservatives, which can be exploited jointly to maximize the shelf life and safety of foods. Developments in hurdle technology and fundamental issues still under investigation were summarized. The interface between hurdle technology and predictive microbiology was discussed.

## Predictive Modeling

Mathematical models have been developed to evaluate the effects of temperature abuse on the shelf life of refrigerated foods (*968*). The models show that even when the fraction of the total storage time at an abusive temperature is small (e.g., 2–3%), the reduction in shelf life can be relatively large (20–30%). Package size and heat-transfer properties are also important. The models presented here facilitate the types of evaluation needed to reduce product loss during the distribution and display of chilled foods. For example, the benefits of more costly packaging alternatives can be assessed for various temperature scenarios.

A rigorous equation has been derived for calculating the *F*-value in isothermal sterilization processes (*969*). It does not assume that *z* is independent of temperature, as do the simplified equations in common use in the food industry. In this model, equations for *z*- and *F*-values were derived according to kinetic theory and used to predict the level of sterility achieved during isothermal sterilization. *F*-values obtained in this way were always higher than those obtained using the simplifying assumption. Tables of *F*-values were presented.

## Irradiation

A review presented background information on the technology of low-dose irradiation of food, emphasizing the radiation sensitivity of specific pathogens of importance (*970*). Some benefits ascribed to the technology are increased shelf-life, reduced use of chemical preservatives, and increased safety. Some $D_{10}$-values in various substrates were listed for strains of *Listeria monocytogenes, Aeromonas hydrophila, Yersinia enterocolitica, Campylobacter jejuni,* and salmonellas. Factors that influence the effectiveness of irradiation are the temperature at which treatment is carried out, the $a_w$ of the product, bacterial strain, bacterial growth phase, packaging atmosphere, and storage conditions. Another discussion emphasized that hygienic practices alone cannot ensure food safety, but neither can treatment by ionizing radiation replace good manufacturing practices (*971*). Because many factors influence the effectiveness of irradiation, the minimum radiation dose that eliminates pathogens must be determined from food-based data for specific pathogens and defined processing parameters. These data can be used for predictive modeling if they allow prediction of the microbiological consequences of changes in operating conditions. There are abundant data on the sensory and toxicologic properties of irradiated food, but further studies are necessary to determine the sources and nature of risks associated with the inappropriate use of irradiation technology.

In 1993, the FAO, IAEA, and WHO sponsored an international symposium on cost–benefit aspects of food irradiation. A summary of the report and recommendations of the Symposium Working Group was published (*972*). Thirty-seven countries allow use of this technology for treating one or more food items. Spices and dried

vegetable seasonings are the most common commercially irradiated products. Practical applications will probably increase because of increasing international trade and bans or restrictions on several common fumigants. The Working Group states that the safety of irradiated food has been conclusively demonstrated by national and international experts. Benefits of irradiation include control of the morbidity, mortality, and economic loss associated with foodborne illness, reduction of food losses, and expansion of international trade. Successful examples of technology transfer, the advantages of electron beam facilities over conventional γ-irradiation using $^{60}$Co, and the role of contract irradiators were discussed.

Existing and proposed regulations for radiation processing of food in the USA were discussed and compared with regulations in other countries (*973*). Worldwide, more than 40 foods or food groups have been approved for irradiation. Legislation passed by the UK in 1990 permits irradiation of fruits, vegetables, cereals, bulbs and tubers, spices and condiments, fish and shellfish, fresh meat, and poultry. The regulations specify requirements for licensing, process control, dosimetry, record keeping, packaging, microbiological testing, facility safety, and labeling. Recent legislation in the Netherlands stipulates a maximum average absorbed dose of 10 kGy for both food commodities and packaging materials. The longstanding interest of the U.S. Army in radiation processing of food and the more recent involvement of the Department of Energy were reviewed. Issues requiring international harmonization were summarized. Another paper also reviewed the development of regulations for food irradiation and discussed current and potential applications of the technology (*974*). In many cases, irradiation is an effective replacement for fumigation. It can also reduce dependence on refrigeration, which is a boon to developing countries that cannot afford the expensive alternative refrigerants that will replace chlorofluorocarbons in the next century. Furthermore, irradiation requires less energy than canning, refrigeration, and frozen storage. Questions of consumer acceptance and the attitude of industry were mentioned. In France, the transfer of technology from government and universities to industry has resulted in successful commercialization of food irradiation (*975*). The steps in successful technology transfer were discussed. Camembert cheese and mechanically deboned poultry meat were cited as important examples of irradiated foods in France.

Thayer et al. reviewed the effects of ionizing radiation on the microbiological, nutritional, and structural quality of meats (*976*). Treating fresh or frozen meats with ionizing radiation can reduce or eliminate *Salmo-*

*nella, Campylobacter, Listeria, Trichinella,* and *Yersinia.* Some major parasites, especially *Toxoplasma gondii* and cysticerci of *Taenia saginata,* are also highly sensitive to irradiation. Irradiated meat is high quality, shelf-stable, and commercially sterile. Radiation doses up to 3.0 kGy have little effect on vitamin content, enzyme activity, or structure of refrigerated chicken meat. The FDA-approved maximum radiation dose for controlling *Trichinella* in pork has little effect on the pork's thiamin content, but higher doses reduce thiamin content significantly. Losses of thiamin in irradiated chicken are considered nonsignificant because chicken is not an important source of this vitamin. Thayer also reviewed research showing that irradiation extends the shelf life of refrigerated poultry, pork, and beef (*977*). Combined treatment with irradiation and vacuum or modified-atmosphere packaging have produced better-than-predicted results, and additional research on combined processes is recommended.

Naik et al. monitored the microbiological quality of prepackaged buffalo meat nonirradiated or irradiated with a dose of 2.5 kGy and stored at ambient temperature (28–30°C) (*978*). Nonirradiated samples initially contained *Enterobacteriaceae* and *Staphylococcus* spp. These increased during storage. After 12 h, *Clostridium* spp. were seen. Based on microbiological, chemical, and sensory evaluation, the shelf life of nonirradiated samples was 18 h. In irradiated samples, *Staphylococcus* spp. were seen after 12 h, but no clostridia and *Enterobacteriaceae* were detected. The shelf life of irradiated samples was 42 h.

To assess the inactivation of *E. coli* O157:H7, salmonellas, and *Campylobacter jejuni* by γ-irradiation, raw ground beef patties containing 8–14 and 27–28% fat were inoculated with stationary-phase cells and irradiated with 0–2.52 kGy from a $^{60}$Co source (*979*). Some samples were irradiated at −17 to −15°C and some at 3 to 5°C. The observed $D_{10}$ values were 0.175–0.235 kGy for *C. jejuni,* 0.241–0.307 kGy for *E. coli* O157:H7, and 0.618–0.800 kGy for salmonellas. Fat content did not affect $D_{10}$ values significantly, but organisms were generally more resistant when irradiated at the lower temperature. An applied dose of 2.5 kGy would reduce numbers of *E. coli* O157:H7 by 8.1 $\log_{10}$, of salmonellas by 3.1 $\log_{10}$, and of *C. jejuni* by 10.6 $\log_{10}$. Considering the numbers of these organisms likely to occur in ground beef patties, this level of killing would be expected to eliminate these pathogens.

Rowe and Towner examined the effect of irradiation on the detection of bacterial DNA in food samples (*980*). Duplicate portions of suspensions of chicken, prawns, potato, lentils, garlic, onion, tomato, mushroom, flour, rice, and several spices were inoculated with a genetically marked strain of *E. coli* K12 and frozen. Samples to be irradiated were thawed immediately before irradiation with $^{60}$Co. Thyme, marjoram, and cardamom received 10 kGy; all other samples received 2.5 kGy. Samples were then refrozen immediately. In no case were viable bacteria detected after irradiation. Bacterial DNA was detected by DNA hybridization on a nitrocellulose membrane. Although hybridization signals were weaker in irradiated samples than in the corresponding nonirradiated samples, 10$^6$ cfu gave a signal in 12 of the 13 foods in both irradiated and nonirradiated samples. This level of contamination did not give a detectable signal in either chicken sample.

## Lactic Acid Bacteria

**PROBIOTICS.** Because production of safe food begins on the farm, there is considerable interest in the use of probiotics to improve the health of food animals and increase their resistance to infection. A volume on probiotics discusses all aspects of the gut microflora, the selection and development of strains for use as probiotics, and probiotics and their function in chickens, pigs, and ruminants (*981*). Of particular interest are a chapter on probiotics and the immune state, which discusses the humoral immune response and specific and nonspecific cellular responses and protection against enteric infections (*982*), and a chapter discussing nutritional and therapeutic benefits and prospects for future development and applications of probiotics for humans (*983*). A chapter in another volume discussed the gut microflora in pigs and calves and possible modes of action of lactic acid bacteria used as probiotics (*984*). Criteria for selecting lactic acid bacteria for probiotic use were presented and results of trials in pigs and ruminants were summarized.

**BACTERIOCINS.** Several reviews have addressed uses of lactic acid bacteria and bacteriocins for enhancing food safety (*985–990*). Stiles discussed the potential for controlling foodborne pathogens by bacteriocins or bacteriocinogenic strains of bacteria, beginning with a brief history of research on exploiting bacterial competition and interference for microbial control (*985*). He focused on the lactic acid bacteria as competitors and producers of antimicrobial polypeptides known as "bacteriocins." Nisin is the prototype bacteriocin produced by lactic acid bacteria. A member of a group of bacterial compounds containing lanthionine ring structures, it is also classed as a "lantibiotic." Nisin can serve as a model for discovery of other bacteriocins suitable for use as food additives or in production steps. Some of these, and the organisms that synthesize them, were discussed.

Although early widespread interest in nisin gave the impression that lanthionine-related residues are typical of bacteriocins produced by lactic acid bacteria, it now appears that simple polypeptides are more common (*986*). Expression of active bacteriocins has been demonstrated from cloned gene sequences of several bacteriocins, but so far the expression of active nisin has not been achieved. This is attributed to the posttranslational processing that creates the lanthionine structure. Nisin is the only bacteriocin that has attained widespread approval and use as a food additive, even though numerous bacteriocin-producing lactic acid cultures are used in the food industry. It is predicted that heat-stable bacteriocins other than nisin will find application as biopreservatives in thermally processed foods. Although bacteriocins are generally effective only against gram-positive organisms, it is sometimes possible to extend their spectrum of activity by using them in conjunction with chelating agents to bypass the outer membrane of gram-negative organisms. Perhaps the most interesting aspect of this review is its discussion of the antimicrobial peptides produced by frogs (magainins), insects (cecropins), and mammals (defensins). Unlike the bacteriocins of lactic acid bacteria, these compounds inhibit a wide range of gram-positive and -negative bacteria, fungi, and protozoa. Their broad inhibitory spectrum has prompted suggestions for therapeutic applications and use as protective agents in foods. They are also of interest for comparison with bacteriocins in mechanistic and structure–function studies.

Hammes and Tichaczek also reviewed the potential of lactic acid bacteria for enhancing food safety (*987*). The benefits of these organisms are related to their production of lactic acid and some acetic and formic acids, their production of antimicrobial compounds (bacteriocins, $H_2O_2$, fatty acids), and their probiotic effects as live organisms in food and feed. The importance of protective cultures and their metabolic products in the manufacture of dry sausage was discussed by Weber (*988*). He considered $H_2O_2$, bacteriocins, lactic and acetic acids, diacetyl, and reuterin. Davidson and Hoover gave an overview of peptide and nonpeptide antimicrobial products of lactic acid bacteria (*989*). They then discussed specific bacteriocins produced by species of *Lactococcus, Pediococcus, Lactobacillus,* and *Leuconostoc.* Vandenbergh summarized studies of the antimicrobial effects of metabolic products of the lactic acid bacteria (*990*). Specific applications of nisin and pediocin in the food industry were emphasized. Actions of other bacteriocins, diacetyl, acetaldehyde, acids, $H_2O_2$,

and small organic molecules—possibly aromatic—were summarized briefly.

Vaughan et al. examined the ability of isolates of lactic acid bacteria from a variety of foods to inhibit spoilage and pathogenic bacteria in foods (*991*). *Pseudomonas fragi, Staphylococcus aureus, Listeria innocua,* and *Lactobacillus delbrueckii bulgaricus* were chosen as indicator organisms for the examination of approximately 1000 isolates by the deferred antagonism procedure. Isolates from milk, cheese, and meats were most inhibitory to *L. innocua,* whereas isolates from vegetables and silage inhibited only *S. aureus.* Most isolates inhibited only one of the indicator species. None inhibited all four. In similar studies, Garver and Muriana isolated 40 bacteriocin-producing strains of lactic acid bacteria from samples of foods purchased at retail markets (*992*). Only 8 isolates, all *Lactococcus lactis,* inhibited the foodborne pathogens *Listeria monocytogenes, Bacillus cereus, Clostridium perfringens,* and *Staphylococcus aureus* and the model spore-former *Clostridium sporogenes.* Although this activity is characteristic of nisin, the spectrum of inhibition was different from nisin's. It is interesting that levels of lactic acid bacteria found in raw ground beef and ground chicken were similar to those in ready-to-eat meats. This indicates considerable postprocessing contamination or growth and raises the possibility that the sources of these bacteria in raw products and processed products are not the same. In any case, bacteriocin-producing lactic acid bacteria are widespread natural contaminants of foods.

In a comprehensive review with 207 references, Klaenhammer discussed the biochemistry and genetics of bacteriocins produced by lactic acid bacteria (*993*). He cited commonalities among the classes of bacteriocins and briefly covered advances in genetic engineering.

The literature on bacteriocins led Bruno and Montville to postulate a common mode of action for the bacteriocins of lactic acid bacteria, namely, dissipation of the proton motive force (PMF) in sensitive cells (*994*). The PMF drives the synthesis of ATP and accumulation of ions and metabolites. To test the PMF-depletion hypothesis, the authors determined the influence of pediocin PA-1 and leuconocin S on the PMF of *Listeria monocytogenes.* Because lactacin F was ineffective against *L. monocytogenes* they tested it against *Lactobacillus delbrueckii.* Pediocin PA-1 (20 µg/mL) and leuconocin S (48.5 µg/mL) mediated total or major PMF dissipation in energized *L. monocytogenes* Scott A and the effect was concentration-dependent. Lactacin F (13.5 µg/mL) caused 87% PMF depletion in energized *L. delbrueckii* cells and this effect was also concentration-dependent. Using the ionophores nigericin and valinomycin to cause partial and specific deenergization of the target organisms, the authors demonstrated that pediocin PA-1, leuconocin S, and lactacin F have an energy-independent mode of action and confirmed that nisin activity is energy-dependent. Thus bacteriocins of lactic acid bacteria act by the common mechanism of PMF dissipation, resemble other PMF-depleting antimicrobial proteins such as colicins and defensins, and can be subclassified on the basis of their energy requirements for activity.

The antimicrobial spectrum of bacteriocins can frequently be extended by using them in conjunction with chelating agents, which provide access to the bacteriocin's primary target, the cytoplasmic membrane. Schved et al. found that EDTA (and to a lesser extent EGTA) enabled nisin to breach the outer membrane of *E. coli* and gain access to the cytoplasmic membrane, causing subsequent changes in permeability (995). These changes were indicated by an increase in intensity of ANS fluorescence and a shift in its emission maximum. No spectral changes occurred when the EDTA was saturated with $Ca^{2+}$ or $Mg^{2+}$. Pediocin SJ-1 also traversed the EDTA-permeabilized outer membrane but was unable to kill the cell; ANS fluorescence data indicated that it did not perturb the cytoplasmic membrane. Spheroplasts prepared from *E. coli* were lysed by nisin but not by pediocin SJ-1. The authors concluded that pediocin's inactivity against gram-negative bacteria is due not only to its inability to permeate the outer membrane but also to its inability to interact with the cytoplasmic membrane.

Lantibiotics contain the unusual amino acids *meso*-lanthionine, β-methyllanthionine, dehydroalanine, and β-methyldehydroalanine, which may result from the dehydration of serine or threonine and reaction of the dehydro-amino acids with cysteine. Nisin, subtilin, and epidermin (synthesized by *Lactococcus lactis, Bacillus subtilis,* and *Staphylococcus epidermidis*, respectively) are prominent examples of lantibiotics. Entian and Klein illustrated the structures of these compounds and reviewed their synthesis and mode of action (996). The lantibiotics are ribosomally synthesized as prepeptides. Certain amino acid residues are then modified posttranslationally and the modified propeptide is transported through the cell membrane, where a putative protease cleaves the signal sequence from the secreted peptide. Genes thought to encode the relevant biosynthetic enzymes have been identified adjacent to the structural genes for subtilin, nisin, and epidermin. Hansen reviewed the literature on subtilin and nisin, viewing nisin as a model lantibiotic and food preservative (997). He emphasized the genetics of nisin and its natural analog subtilin, and progress in the construction and

biological expression of genetically engineered structural analogs of nisin. The properties of these natural and engineered analogs provide insight into some structure–function relationships in the lantibiotics. Hanson also proposed a model for the rational design and construction of a subtilin mutant with enhanced chemical and antimicrobial properties, and use of *Bacillus subtilis* as an industrial-scale producer of lantibiotics. He discussed the promise and problems of further development of nisin analogs as food preservatives.

De Vuyst reported enormous differences among 27 strains of *Lactococcus lactis lactis* in capacity for nisin production (998). Titers ranged from 0 to 1900 IU per milliliter of culture medium. Transconjugant strains possessing several copies of the relevant genes did not necessarily produce more nisin than the parent strain. The degree of nisin immunity also differed from strain to strain and paralleled the level of nisin production. Low and high producers transcribed the nisin genes and translated the transcript with similar efficiency, as revealed by Northern-blot analysis and SDS-PAGE. Prenisin expression occurred early in logarithmic growth, whereas nisin production was maximal toward the end of the log phase. The level and activity of postprocessing enzymes and nisin-degrading proteases may explain differences in nisin activity. Alternatively, nutritional factors may be involved. Since nisin immunity and production are related, increasing the resistance of a low producer to its own product might enhance its production capacity. Genetic and protein engineering strategies may further improve nisin-producing capacity, but potential overproducing strains must also be modified into fast acid-producing, high proteolytic, phage-resistant forms before they are suitable as improved industrial starter cultures for dairy fermentations.

Engelke et al. reported the identification, sequencing, and mapping of additional genes involved in regulating nisin biosynthesis and immunity in *Lactococcus lactis* 6F3 (999). In order, the genes on the nisin operon are *nisA*, the nisin structural gene; *nisB, nisT,* and *nisC*, which are probably involved in chemical modification and secretion of the prepeptide; *nisI*, which encodes a lipoprotein and causes increased immunity after its transformation into a nisin-sensitive strain; *nisP*, which encodes a subtilisin-like serine protease possibly involved in processing the leader peptide; *nisR*, encoding a regulatory protein; and *nisK*, encoding a histidine kinase. The deduced amino acid sequences of NisR and NisK have marked similarities to SpaR and SpaK, recently identified as the response regulator and histidine kinase of subtilin biosynthesis. Kuipers et al. also briefly described the organization of the nisin gene cluster and the function of the encoded proteins (*1000*). Their scheme for nisin biosynthesis begins with ribosomal synthesis of a 57-amino-acid precursor. Eight serine and threonine residues are then dehydrated and thio-ether bonds are formed. These reactions are probably catalyzed by membrane-bound NisB and NisC. The product is transported across the membrane by NisT. On the outer side of the membrane, NisP cleaves the leader peptide, releasing mature nisin. All of the biosynthetic proteins may be clustered at the membrane.

Lante et al. immobilized nisin on organic and inorganic matrices and assessed the antimicrobial activity of gradually released nisin on the indicator strain *Lactobacillus delbrueckii bulgaricus* in broth medium and skim milk (*1001*). The efficiency with which the matrix adsorbed nisin was inversely related to nisin concentration and ranged from 76% for Amberlyst to 94% for VA-Epoxy. Efficiency was improved by coating Amberlyst and Florisil with polyethylenimine derivatized by glutaraldehyde. The indicator strain remained viable when exposed to nisin bound to coated Florisil. In all other cases, nisin leaked from the support to provide a concentration of ~10 IU/mL, which inhibited the indicator strain. Thus nisin can be immobilized on a variety of matrices but it displays its antimicrobial activity only when in solution.

Several studies of the antimicrobial activity of *Lactobacillus* species were reported (*1002–1005*). When *Lactobacillus casei* and *Lactobacillus acidophilus* were grown in mixed broth culture with *E. coli*, *Klebsiella pneumoniae*, or *Salmonella typhimurium* in a ratio of $10^3$:1, growth of the pathogen was inhibited by 59–97% after 4 h and by 77–98% after 6 h at 37°C (*1002*). The effect was roughly the same whether the lactobacilli were tested individually or in combination. Inhibition of *Shigella sonnei* by the individual lactobacilli was only 35–43% after 6 h, but together they caused 70% inhibition after 6 h. No viable pathogens were recovered from mixed cultures after 24 h, whereas numbers of lactobacilli increased by a factor of 10–100. Growth rates of lactobacilli in mixed cultures with pathogens were higher than in pure cultures. The authors suggested the possibility of using milk products fermented with *L. casei* and *L. acidophilus* for preventing and treating intestinal infections and to reestablish a normal gut flora after prolonged oral antibiotic therapy. In another study, 106 strains of *Lactobacillus plantarum* isolated from foods were screened for antibacterial activity under conditions that ruled out an effect of organic acids and $H_2O_2$ (*1003*). Five strains produced bacteriocins. They were isolated from sausage, fermented cucumbers, soft cheese, Cameroon palm wine, and goat's milk. The five bacteriocins differed from each other in their inhibitory spectra, thermal stability at various pH values, and susceptibility to hydrolytic enzymes.

The purification and partial characterization of plantaricin C, produced by a strain of *L. plantarum* from Cabrales cheese, was reported (*1004*). Plantaricin C is a bactericidal peptide of 3.5 kDa that retains its activity after boiling, storage, and treatment at different pH's. The first 11 *N*-terminal residues were identified, but then the sequence was blocked. A simple explanation is that a disulfide bond was established at this point. Alternatively, plantaricin C may be a lantibiotic. Its spectrum of activity is intermediate between nisin's and those of bacteriocins from other species of *Lactobacillus*.

Sakacin P is a bacteriocin produced by *Lactobacillus sake* LTH 673; *sakP*, the gene encoding it, has been cloned and sequenced (*1005*).

Bhunia et al. used a 2.3-MDa plasmid probe containing the gene for pediocin AcH to test for plasmid-encoded pediocin genes in 13 strains of *Pediococcus acidilactici* and plasmid-cured derivatives (*1006*). The probe hybridized with a 6.2-MDa plasmid that was present in all pediocin-producing strains. It failed to hybridize with two strains that did not produce pediocin and lacked the plasmid. Nor did it hybridize with plasmids from a bacteriocin-producing strain of *Pediococcus pentosaceus*. Pediocin A, produced by *Pediococcus pentosaceus* FBB61, was purified and partially characterized by SDS-PAGE (*1007*). The 80-kDa protein was inhibitory to numerous lactic acid bacteria and staphylococci and to *Bacillus cereus*, *Listeria innocua*, and *Clostridium sporogenes*.

*Leuconostoc carnosum* LA54A, isolated from processed meat, produces a bacteriocin that is sensitive to α-amylases as well as proteases—indicating that it contains both a protein and a carbohydrate moiety (*1008*). The bacteriocin was purified and characterized. SDS-PAGE analysis revealed a molecule of about 4 kDa. Maximal production occurred during the late-logarithmic phase of growth.

Carnobacteriocins BM1 and B2, produced by *Carnobacterium piscicola* LV17B, were purified and analyzed (*1009*). Carnobacteriocin B1, an oxidized form of carnobacteriocin BM1, was also characterized. Probes synthesized using information from the *N*-terminal amino acid sequences of the bacteriocins were used to locate the corresponding structural genes. A 1.9-kilobase *Hin*dIII fragment from the 61-kilobase plasmid pCP40 contained the carnobacteriocin B2 structural gene, and a 4.0-kilobase *Eco*RI–*Pst*I genomic fragment contained the carnobacteriocin BM1 structural gene. These were cloned. The plasmid gene was fully sequenced and the chromosomal gene was partially sequenced. Expression of the chromosomal bacteriocin and its immunity function required the presence of the 61-kilobase plasmid. Both bacteriocins appear to be synthesized as prebacteriocins, from which an *N*-terminal sequence of 18 amino acids is cleaved, yielding the mature carnobacteriocins BM1 (43 amino acids) and B2 (48 amino acids). The two polypeptides showed significant amino acid homology to each other and to other class II bacteriocins containing a Tyr-Gly-Asn-Gly-Val sequence near the *N* terminus.

## Other Chemical Means of Control

The lactoperoxidase system is a natural system discovered in raw milk. Wolfson and Sumner reviewed its antibacterial activity, which stems from the oxidation of essential protein hydroxyl groups by the hypothiocyanite anion (*1010*). The consequences, which are both bacteriostatic and bactericidal for a wide range of bacteria, are pervasive alterations in cell structure and function. Groups of bacteria differ in their sensitivity to the lactoperoxidase system. Sensitivity is also influenced by temperature, pH, incubation time, cell density and growth phase, and other constituents in the growth medium. The strongest arguments against the possibility of undesirable side effects from activation of the lactoperoxidase system are the widespread distribution of all its components in humans and other animals and the failure of the system to damage mammalian cell membranes. Moreover, newborn calves and human infants have their own lactoperoxidase systems: in calves it is provided primarily by the colostrum; in humans, by the saliva. The lactoperoxidase system can delay the growth of psychrotrophs in milk, increasing storage times. It is possible that the system could be exploited to extend the shelf life of other foods.

Razavi-Rohani and Griffiths extensively evaluated the antibacterial activity of monolaurin and triglycerol 1,2 laurate (*1011*). Activity was assessed by the spiral gradient end-point test to determine the MIC. Monolaurin alone was effective against all 7 gram-positive bacteria studied (MICs 8–96 µg/mL). However, it was active against the 9 gram-negative bacteria only in the presence of EDTA, and even then MICs were much higher (90–1500 µg/mL). The chelators monoglyceride citrate and sodium citrate did not enhance monolaurin's inhibitory activity. Inhibition was greatest at low pH and high NaCl concentration. Triglycerol 1,2 laurate, which was tested because it is more water-soluble than monolaurin, was less inhibitory. EDTA enhanced its activity against all bacteria: with EDTA the MICs for gram-positive organisms ranged from 100 to 380 µg/mL and for gram-negative organisms from 170 to >1588 µg/mL.

Sodium lactate is used as a humectant and flavor enhancer in meat and poultry products, but there is substantial evidence that it has antimicrobial properties as well. These were reviewed by Shelef (*1012*). Potassium and calcium lactates are equally effective in controlling growth of aerobes and anaerobes. The lactate anion also has antibotulinal and antilisterial activity. The specific action of lactate is unknown, but it is apparently not associated with lowering of intracellular pH or reduction in $a_w$. Its action is bacteriostatic rather than bactericidal. Lactate can provide an added measure of safety for meat products during extended refrigerated storage.

Sulfhydryl-containing amino acids and peptides are another group of compounds with potential to enhance food safety. Friedman presented an overview of the biological utilization and safety of sulfur amino acids and possible approaches to ameliorating adverse effects of some substances found in foods, based on the reactivity of the sulfhydryl group with electrophilic centers (*1013*). Interactions with aflatoxins, lysinoalanine, and protease inhibitors and control of nonenzymatic food browning were specifically discussed.

## Other Aspects of Control

There is interest in high hydrostatic pressure as a method of food processing because of reported improvements in quality. Lechowich discussed the implications of this process for food safety (*1014*). Spores of *Bacillus* species are highly variable in their resistance to hydrostatic pressure, and published reports on clostridial spores are limited to one study of *Clostridium sporogenes*. *Clostridium botulinum* spores are of particular concern because of their relatively high resistance to radiation. Other safety questions that remain to be dealt with are the effects of high hydrostatic pressure on package and seal integrity, pH, nutrients and enzymes. High pressures may control some pathogens, however. Carlez et al. reported that in minced beef at 20°C, *Citrobacter freundii* was completely inactivated in 20 min by a pressure of 280 MPa and *Listeria innocua* by a pressure of 400 MPa (*1015*). At higher or lower temperatures less pressure was required for inactivation. Decimal reduction times could be calculated for the different combinations of pressure and temperature. After a 10-min pressurization at 150 MPa the minced beef became paler and at 350 MPa it turned gray.

Packaging materials offer a barrier to pathogenic bacteria, but the bacteriologic safety of the materials themselves must be assured. The European Hygienic Equipment Design Group provided guidelines for the hygienic packaging of food products (*1016*). They considered the design of hygienic packing machines, the storage, handling, and transport of packing materials, and the environment and cleaning of packing machines. The importance of knowing which microorganisms are relevant to the product to be packed was emphasized. Kneifel and Kaser examined the microbiological quality of packaging materials used in the dairy industry (*1017*). They tested reusable brown glass bottles, milk carton materials, paper boxes for the transport of cheeses, and yogurt cups and aluminum sealing foil. Materials were obtained from suppliers, dairy farms, and cheese factories in Austria. Results showed that packaging materials for dairy products pose no hazards as sources or vectors of contamination and provide an adequate barrier against environmental contamination.

Berends et al. evaluated current European Community meat inspection procedures and some of their proposed revisions, in relation to their efficacy in assuring the microbiological safety and quality of meat (*1018*). They concluded that neither current nor proposed procedures are adequate without integrated approaches applied at each step of animal and meat production. For a truly effective and flexible long-term system of safety and quality assurance, formal quantitative risk assessment is necessary.

A working group in Scotland has developed guidelines on bacteriological clearance after gastrointestinal infections (*1019*). Criteria were established for food handlers who prepare or serve unwrapped foods not subjected to further heating and for health-care workers who handle food. Pathogens of concern were *Salmonella* spp., *Shigella* spp., verotoxigenic *E. coli*, *Campylobacter* spp., viruses, and *Cryptosporidium*.

## LITERATURE CITED

1. Bryan, R.T., R.W. Pinner, R.P. Gaynes, et al. Addressing emerging infectious disease threats: a prevention strategy for the United States. Executive summary. *Morbid. Mortal. Weekly Rep.* 43(RR-5) (1994).

2. Doyle, M.P. Reducing foodborne disease—what are the priorities? *Nutr. Rev.* 51:346–347 (1993).

3. Doyle, M.P. The emergence of new agents of foodborne disease in the 1980s. *Food Res. Int.* 27:219–226 (1994).

4. Levine, M.M., and O.S. Levine. Changes in human ecology and behavior in relation to the emergence of diarrheal diseases, including cholera. *Proc. Natl. Acad. Sci. USA* 91:2390–2394 (1994).

5. Savarino, S.J., and A.L. Bourgeois. Diarrhoeal disease: current concepts and future challenges. Epidemiology of diarrhoeal diseases in developed countries. *Trans. Roy. Soc. Trop. Med. Hyg.* 87(Suppl. 3):7–11 (1993).

6. Hedberg, C.W., K.L. MacDonald, and M.T. Osterholm. Changing epidemiology of food-borne disease: a Minnesota perspective. *Clin. Infect. Dis.* 18:671–682 (1994).

7. Baird-Parker, A.C. Foods and microbiological risks. *Microbiology* 140:687–695 (1994).

8. Lacey, R.W. Food-borne bacterial infections. *Parasitology* 107:S75–S93 (1993).

9. Bryan, F.L. Public health problems of foodborne diseases and their prevention. In *Food Poisoning*. A.T. Tu (ed.). New York, Marcel Dekker. *Handbook of Natural Toxins* 7:3–22 (1992).

10. Adams, C.E., and L.M. Crawford. Microbial concerns of the North and South American countries and scientific implications for harmonizing free trade. *Dairy Food Environ. Sanit.* 14:471–472 (1994).

11. van Schothorst, M. Microbiological safety of foods in the Europe of the nineties. What does that imply? *Dairy Food Environ. Sanit.* 14:473–476 (1994).

12. Eyles, M.J. Microbial concerns of the Pacific Rim countries and implications for harmonizing free trade. *Dairy Food Environ. Sanit.* 14:467–470 (1994).

13. Notermans, S., and A. Van de Giessen. Foodborne diseases in the 1980s and 1990s. *Food Control* 4:122–124 (1993).

14. Buchanan, R.L., and C.M. Deroever. Limits in assessing microbiological food safety. *J. Food Protect.* 56:725–729 (1993).

15. Sofos, J.N. Current microbiological considerations in food preservation. *Int. J. Food Microbiol.* 19:87–108 (1993).

16. Irbe, R.M. Microbiology of reduced-fat foods. In *Science for the Food Industry of the 21st Century. Biotechnology, Supercritical Fluids, Membranes and Other Advanced Technologies for Low Calorie, Healthy Food Alternatives.* M. Yalpani (ed.). Mount Prospect, IL, ATL Press. *Frontiers in Foods and Food Ingredients* 1:359–382 (1993).

17. Nout, M.J.R. Fermented foods and food safety. *Food Res. Int.* 27:291–298 (1994).

18. Manning, C.K., and O.S. Snider. Temporary public eating places: food safety knowledge, attitudes and practices. *J. Environ. Health* 56(1):24–28 (1993).

19. Corthier, G., M.R. Popoff, F. Lucas, and P. Raibaud. Human diseases due to food-borne bacterial toxins and toxins produced in the digestive tract. In *Intestinal Flora, Immunity, Nutrition and Health*. A.P. Simopoulos et al. (eds.). Basel, Karger. *World Rev. Nutr. Diet.* 74:58–87 (1993).

20. Bergdoll, M.S. Staphylococcal intoxication in mass feeding. In *Food Poisoning*. A.T. Tu (ed.). New York, Marcel Dekker. *Handbook of Natural Toxins* 7:25–47 (1992).

21. Wieneke, A.A., D. Roberts, and R.J. Gilbert. Staphylococcal food poisoning in the United Kingdom, 1969–1990. *Epidemiol. Infect.* 110:519–531 (1993).

22. Umeki, F., G. Otsuka, A. Tosai, et al. Evaluation of biological character and pathogenicity of *Staphylococcus*

*aureus* isolated from healthy persons, patients, poisoned food and cows. *Milchwissenschaft* 48:552–555 (1993).

23. Gangbar, E., L. Schwartz, W. Gold, and I. Salit. Infective endocarditis in a dairy farmer in association with bovine *Staphylococcus aureus* mastitis. *Can. Vet. J.* 34:677–678 (1993).

24. Bowen, D.A., and D.R. Henning. Coliform bacteria and *Staphylococcus aureus* in retail natural cheeses. *J. Food Protect.* 57:253–255 (1994).

25. Masud, T., A.M. Ali, and M.A. Shah. Enterotoxigenicity of *Staphylococcus aureus* isolated from dairy products. *Aust. J. Dairy Technol.* 48:30–32 (1993).

26. Tamime, A.Y., J. Bruce, and D.D. Muir. Ovine milk. 4. Seasonal changes in microbiological quality of raw milk and yogurt. *Milchwissenschaft* 48:560–563 (1993).

27. Sohal, S., G. Blank, and M. Lewis. Survival and growth of selected microorganisms in khoa during preparation and storage. *J. Food Safety* 13:195–208 (1993).

28. Mead, G.C., W.R. Hudson, and M.H. Hinton. Microbiological survey of five poultry processing plants in the UK. *Br. Poultry Sci.* 34:497–503 (1993).

29. Vorster, S.M., R.P. Greebe, and G.L. Nortjé. Incidence of *Staphylococcus aureus* and *Escherichia coli* in ground beef, broilers and processed meats in Pretoria, South Africa. *J. Food Protect.* 57:305–310 (1994).

30. Thayer, D.W., G. Boyd, and R.K. Jenkins. Low-dose gamma irradiation and refrigerated storage *in vacuo* affect microbial flora of fresh pork. *J. Food Sci.* 58:717–719,733 (1993).

31. Ng, D.L.K., and L. Tay. Enterotoxigenic strains of coagulase-positive *Staphylococcus aureus* in drinks and ready-to-eat foods. *Food Microbiol.* 10:317–320 (1993).

32. Valik, L., and F. Görner. Growth of *Staphylococcus aureus* in pasta in relation to its water activity. *Int. J. Food Microbiol.* 20:45–48 (1993).

33. Betley, M.J., and T.O. Harris. Staphylococcal enterotoxins: genetic characterization and relationship between structure and emetic activity. *Food Microbiol.* 11:109–121 (1994).

34. Daugherty, S., and M.G. Low. Cloning, expression, and mutagenesis of phosphatidylinositol-specific phospholipase C from *Staphylococcus aureus*: a potential staphylococcal virulence factor. *Infect. Immun.* 61:5078–5089 (1993).

35. Novick, R.P., H.F. Ross, S.J. Projan, et al. Synthesis of staphylococcal virulence factors is controlled by a regulatory RNA molecule. *EMBO J.* 12:3967–3975 (1993).

36. Borst, D.W., and M.J. Betley. Mutations in the promoter spacer region and early transcribed region increase expression of staphylococcal enterotoxin A. *Infect. Immun.* 61:5421–5425 (1993).

37. Bennett, R.W., and F. McClure. Visual screening with enzyme immunoassay for staphylococcal enterotoxins in foods: collaborative study. *J. AOAC Int.* 77:357–364 (1994).

38. Bergdoll, M.S. The AOAC official methods for detection of staphylococcal enterotoxins in food. (Letter.) *J. AOAC Int.* 77:31A (1994).

39. Becker, H., G. Schaller, and E. Märtlbauer. Nachweis von *Staphylococcus-aureus*-Enterotoxinen in Lebensmitteln mit kommerziellen Enzymimmuntests. *Arch. Lebensmittelhyg.* 45:27–32 (1994).

40. Park, C.E., M. Akhtar, and M.K. Rayman. Evaluation of a commercial enzyme immunoassay kit (RIDASCREEN) for detection of staphylococcal enterotoxins A, B, C, D, and E in foods. *Appl. Environ. Microbiol.* 60:677–681 (1994).

41. Chang, T.C., and S.H. Huang. An enzyme-linked immunosorbent assay for the rapid detection of *Staphylococcus aureus* in processed foods. *J. Food Protect.* 57:184–189 (1994).

42. Chang, T.C., and S.H. Huang. Evaluation of a latex agglutination test for rapid identification of *Staphylococcus aureus* from foods. *J. Food Protect.* 56:759–762 (1993).

43. Tsen, H.-Y., R.-Y. Yang, and F.-Y. Huang. Novel oligonucleotide probes for identification of enterotoxigenic *Staphylococcus aureus*. *J. Ferment. Bioeng.* 76:7–13 (1993).

44. Wilson, I.G., J.E. Cooper, and A. Gilmour. Some factors inhibiting amplification of the *Staphylococcus aureus* enterotoxin $C_1$ gene (*sec⁺*) by PCR. *Int. J. Food Microbiol.* 22:55–62 (1994).

45. Matthews, K.R., and S.P. Oliver. Differentiation of *Staphylococcus* species by polymerase chain reaction–based DNA fingerprinting. *J. Food Protect.* 57:486–489 (1994).

46. Wilson, I.G., A. Gilmour, J.E. Cooper, et al. A non-isotopic DNA hybridisation assay for the identification of *Staphylococcus aureus* isolated from foods. *Int. J. Food Microbiol.* 22:43–54 (1994).

47. Freney, J., H. Meugnier, M. Bes, and J. Fleurette. Identification of *Staphylococcus aureus* using a DNA probe: Accuprobe®. *Ann. Biol. Clin.* 51:637–639 (1993).

48. Sutherland, J.P., A.J. Bayliss, and T.A. Roberts. Predictive modelling of growth of *Staphylococcus aureus*: the effects of temperature, pH and sodium chloride. *Int. J. Food Microbiol.* 21:217–236 (1994).

49. Buchanan, R.L., J.L. Smith, C. McColgan, et al. Response surface models for the effects of temperature, pH, sodium chloride, and sodium nitrite on the aerobic and anaerobic growth of *Staphylococcus aureus* 196E. *J. Food Safety* 13:159–175 (1993).

50. Ballesteros, S.A., J. Chirife, and J.P. Bozzini. Antibacterial effects and cell morphological changes in *Staphylococcus aureus* subjected to low ethanol concentrations. *J. Food Sci.* 58:435–438 (1992).

51. Tassou, C.C., and G.J.E. Nychas. Inhibition of *Staphylococcus aureus* by olive phenolics in broth and in a model food system. *J. Food Protect.* 57:120–124 (1994).

52. Lee, R.M., P.A. Hartman, D.G. Olson, and F.D. Williams. Bactericidal and bacteriolytic effects of selected food-grade phosphates, using *Staphylococcus aureus* as a model system. *J. Food Protect.* 57:276–283 (1994).

53. Lee, R.M., P.A. Hartman, D.G. Olson, and F.D. Williams. Metal ions reverse the inhibitory effects of selected food-grade phosphates in *Staphylococcus aureus*. *J. Food Protect.* 57:284–288 (1994).

54. Lee, R.M., P.A. Hartman, H.M. Stahr, et al. Antibacterial mechanism of long-chain polyphosphates in *Staphylococcus aureus. J. Food Protect.* 57:289–294 (1994).

55. Liao, C.-C., A.E. Yousef, G.W. Chism, and E.R. Richter. Inhibition of *Staphylococcus aureus* in buffer, culture media and foods by lacidin A, a bacteriocin produced by *Lactobacillus acidophilus* OSU133. *J. Food Safety* 14:87–101 (1994).

56. Ballesteros, S.A., J. Chirife, and J.P. Bozzini. Specific solute effects on *Staphylococcus aureus* cells subjected to reduced water activity. *Int. J. Food Microbiol.* 20:51–66 (1993).

57. Gay, M.F., G. Jaubert, and S. Saboureau. Incidence des traitements technologiques sur la qualité hygiénique du lait et des fromages de chèvre à pâte molle. *Lait* 73:499–509 (1993).

58. Sofos, J.N. Botulism in home-processed foods. In *Food Poisoning.* A.T. Tu (ed.). New York, Marcel Dekker. *Handbook of Natural Toxins* 7:171–203 (1992).

59. Gibbs, P.A., A.R. Davies, and R.S. Fletcher. Incidence and growth of psychrotrophic *Clostridium botulinum* in foods. *Food Control* 5:5–7 (1994).

60. Nakano, H., H. Kizaki, and G. Sakaguchi. Multiplication of *Clostridium botulinum* in dead honey-bees and bee pupae, a likely source of heavy contamination of honey. *Int. J. Food Microbiol.* 21:247–252 (1994).

61. Malizio, C.J., J. Harrod, K.M. Kaufman, and E.A. Johnson. Arginine promotes toxin formation in cheddar cheese by *Clostridium botulinum. J. Food Protect.* 56:769–772 (1993).

62. Eckner, K.F., W.A. Dustman, and A.A. Ryś-Rodriguez. Contribution of composition, physicochemical characteristics and polyphosphates to the microbial safety of pasteurized cheese spreads. *J. Food Protect.* 57:295–300 (1994).

63. Meng, J., and C.A. Genigeorgis. Modeling lag phase of nonproteolytic *Clostridium botulinum* toxigenesis in cooked turkey and chicken breast as affected by temperature, sodium lactate, sodium chloride and spore inoculum. *Int. J. Food Microbiol.* 19:109–122 (1993).

64. Whiting, R.C., and J.E. Call. Time of growth model for proteolytic *Clostridium botulinum. Food Microbiol.* 10:295–301 (1993).

65. Raab, C.A., and K.S. Hilderbrand, Jr. Home-canned smoked fish: a new processing recommendation. *J. Food Protect.* 56:619–621 (1993).

66. Miller, A.J., J.E. Call, and R.C. Whiting. Comparison of organic acid salts for *Clostridium botulinum* control in an uncured turkey product. *J. Food Protect.* 56:958–962 (1993).

67. Houtsma, P.C., A. Heuvelink, J. Dufrenne, and S. Notermans. Effect of sodium lactate on toxin production, spore germination and heat resistance of proteolytic *Clostridium botulinum* strains. *J. Food Protect.* 57:327–330 (1994).

68. Rogers, A.M., and T.J. Montville. Quantification of factors which influence nisin's inhibition of *Clostridium botulinum* 56A in a model food system. *J. Food Sci.* 59:663–668,686 (1994).

69. Crandall, A.D., K. Winkowski, and T.J. Montville. Inability of *Pediococcus pentosaceus* to inhibit *Clostridium*

*botulinum* in *sous vide* beef with gravy at 4 and 10°C. *J. Food Protect.* 57:104–107 (1994).

70. Bowles, B.L., and A.J. Miller. Antibotulinal properties of selected aromatic and aliphatic aldehydes. *J. Food Protect.* 56:788–794 (1993).

71. Bowles, B.L., and A.J. Miller. Antibotulinal properties of selected aromatic and aliphatic ketones. *J. Food Protect.* 56:795–800 (1993).

72. Bowles, B.L., and A.J. Miller. Caffeic acid activity against *Clostridium botulinum* spores. *J. Food Sci.* 59:905–908 (1994).

73. Hutson, R.A., M.D. Collins, A.K. East, and D.E. Thompson. Nucleotide sequence of the gene coding for nonproteolytic *Clostridium botulinum* type B neurotoxin: comparison with other clostridial neurotoxins. *Curr. Microbiol.* 28:101–110 (1994).

74. Willems, A., A.K. East, P.A. Lawson, and M.D. Collins. Sequence of the gene coding for the neurotoxin of *Clostridium botulinum* type A associated with infant botulism: comparison with other clostridial neurotoxins. *Res. Microbiol.* 144:547–556 (1993).

75. Campbell, K., M.D. Collins, and A.K. East. Nucleotide sequence of the gene coding for *Clostridium botulinum* (*Clostridium argentinense*) type G neurotoxin: genealogical comparison with other clostridial neurotoxins. *Biochim. Biophys. Acta* 1216:487–491 (1993).

76. Be, X., F.-N. Fu, and B.R. Singh. Hydrophobic moment analysis of amino acid sequences of botulinum and tetanus neurotoxins to identify functional domains. *J. Nat. Toxins* 3:49–68 (1994).

77. Potter, M.D., J. Meng, and P. Kimsey. An ELISA for detection of botulinal toxin types A, B, and E in inoculated food samples. *J. Food Protect.* 56:856–861 (1993).

78. Doellgast, G.J., M.X. Triscott, G.A. Beard, et al. Sensitive enzyme-linked immunosorbent assay for detection of *Clostridium botulinum* neurotoxins A, B, and E using signal amplification via enzyme-linked coagulation assay. *J. Clin. Microbiol.* 31:2402–2409 (1993).

79. Doellgast, G.J., G.A. Beard, J.D. Bottoms, et al. Enzyme-linked immunosorbent assay and enzyme-linked coagulation assay for detection of *Clostridium botulinum* neurotoxins A, B, and E and solution-phase complexes with dual-label antibodies. *J. Clin. Microbiol.* 32:105–111 (1994).

80. Doellgast, G.J., M.X. Triscott, G.A. Beard, and J.D. Bottoms. Enzyme-linked immunosorbent assay–enzyme-linked coagulation assay for detection of antibodies to *Clostridium botulinum* neurotoxins A, B, and E and solution-phase complexes. *J. Clin. Microbiol.* 32:851–853 (1994).

81. Goodnough, M.C., B. Hammer, H. Sugiyama, and E.A. Johnson. Colony immunoblot assay of botulinal toxin. *Appl. Environ. Microbiol.* 59:2339–2342 (1993).

82. McKinney, M.W., P.N. Levett, and R.W. Haylock. Cloning of a DNA sequence unique to *Clostridium botulinum* group I by selective hybridization. *J. Clin. Microbiol.* 31:1845–1849 (1993).

83. Campbell, K.D., M.D. Collins, and A.K. East. Gene probes for identification of the botulinal neurotoxin gene and

specific identification of neurotoxin types B, E, and F. *J. Clin. Microbiol.* 31:2255–2262 (1993).

84. Szabo, E.A., J.M. Pemberton, and P.M. Desmarchelier. Detection of the genes encoding botulinum neurotoxin types A to E by the polymerase chain reaction. *Appl. Environ. Microbiol.* 59:3011–3020 (1993).

85. Fach, P., D. Hauser, J.P. Guillou, and M.R. Popoff. Polymerase chain reaction for the rapid identification of *Clostridium botulinum* type A strains and detection in food samples. *J. Appl. Bacteriol.* 75:234–239 (1993).

86. Dezfulian, M., and J.G. Bartlett. Rapid identification of *Clostridium botulinum* colonies by *in vitro* toxicity and antimicrobial susceptibility testing. *World J. Microbiol. Biotechnol.* 10:27–29 (1994).

87. Fenicia, L., A.M. Ferrini, P. Aureli, and M. Pocecco. A case of infant botulism associated with honey feeding in Italy. *Eur. J. Epidemiol.* 9:671–673 (1993).

88. Labbé, R.G. *Clostridium perfringens* gastroenteritis. In *Food Poisoning.* A.T. Tu (ed.). New York, Marcel Dekker. *Handbook of Natural Toxins* 7:103–118 (1992).

89. Centers for Disease Control. *Clostridium perfringens* gastroenteritis associated with corned beef served at St. Patrick's Day meals—Ohio and Virginia, 1993. *Morbid. Mortal. Weekly Rep.* 43:137,143–144 (1994).

90. Clarke, L.E., B. Diekmann-Guiroy, W. McNamee, et al. Enteritis necroticans with midgut necrosis caused by *Clostridium perfringens. Arch. Surg.* 129:557–560 (1994).

91. Devriese, L.A., G. Daube, J. Hommez, and F. Haesebrouck. *In vitro* susceptibility of *Clostridium perfringens* isolated from farm animals to growth-enhancing antibiotics. *J. Appl. Bacteriol.* 75:55–57 (1993).

92. Lindsay, J.A., A.S. Mach, M.A. Wilkinson, et al. *Clostridium perfringens* type A cytotoxic-enterotoxin(s) as triggers for death in the sudden infant death syndrome: development of a toxico-infection hypothesis. *Curr. Microbiol.* 27:51–59 (1993).

93. Mach, A.S., and J.A. Lindsay. Activation of *Clostridium perfringens* enterotoxin(s) in vivo and in vitro: role in triggers for sudden infant death. *Curr. Microbiol.* 28:261–267 (1994).

94. Moustafa, S.I., and E.H. Marth. Prevalence of *Clostridium perfringens* in bovine milk. *Milchwissenschaft* 48:383–385 (1993).

95. Stolle, A., H. Eisgruber, D. Kerschhofer, and G. Krauße. Döner Kebap. Untersuchungen zur Verkehrsauffassung und mikrobiologisch-hygienischen Beschaffenheit im Raum München. *Fleischwirtschaft* 73:834–837 (1993).

96. Juneja, V.K., B.S. Marmer, and A.J. Miller. Growth and sporulation potential of *Clostridium perfringens* in aerobic and vacuum-packaged cooked beef. *J. Food Protect.* 57:393–398 (1994).

97. Cooksey, K., B.P. Klein, F.K. McKeith, and H.P. Blaschek. Post-packaging pasteurization reduces *Clostridium perfringens* and other bacteria in precooked vacuum-packaged beef loin chunks. *J. Food Sci.* 58:239–241 (1993).

98. Mengert, U., O. Garcia-Suarez, and P. Janetschke. Untersuchungen zur Beeinflussung der serologischen Aktivität

des *Clostridium perfringens*-Enterotoxins. *Fleischwirtschaft* 73:688–690 (1993).

99. Czeczulin, J.R., P.C. Hanna, and B.A. McClane. Cloning, nucleotide sequencing, and expression of the *Clostridium perfringens* enterotoxin gene in *Escherichia coli. Infect. Immun.* 61:3429–3439 (1993).

100. Titball, R.W., A.M. Fearn, and E.D. Williamson. Biochemical and immunological properties of the C-terminal domain of the alpha-toxin of *Clostridium perfringens. FEMS Microbiol. Lett.* 119:45–50 (1993).

101. McClaine, B.A. *Clostridium perfringens* enterotoxin acts by producing small molecule permeability alterations in plasma membranes. *Toxicology* 87:43–67 (1994).

102. Abeyta, C., Jr., and J.H. Wetherington. Iron milk medium method for recovering *Clostridium perfringens* from shellfish: collaborative study. *J. AOAC Int.* 77:351–356 (1994).

103. Hussain, A., and Purnima. A comparison of methods for isolating plasmid DNA from *Clostridium perfringens. Vet. Res. Commun.* 17:335–339 (1993).

104. Galindo, I., R. Rangel-Aldao, and J.L. Ramirez. A combined polymerase chain reaction–colour development hybridization assay in a microtitre format for the detection of *Clostridium* spp. *Appl. Microbiol. Biotechnol.* 39:553–557 (1993).

105. Cigáneková, V., and J. Kallová. Effect of alkyl-dimethylamine oxides on anaerobic sporulating bacteria of genus *Clostridium. Folia Microbiol.* 38:188–192 (1993).

106. Fujii, N., K. Kimura, N. Yokosawa, et al. Similarity in nucleotide sequence of the gene encoding nontoxic component of botulinum toxin produced by toxigenic *Clostridium butyricum* strain BL6340 and *Clostridium botulinum* type E strain Mashike. *Microbiol. Immunol.* 37:395–398 (1993).

107. Zhou, Y., H. Sugiyama, and E.A. Johnson. Transfer of neurotoxigenicity from *Clostridium butyricum* to a non-toxigenic *Clostridium botulinum* type E–like strain. *Appl. Environ. Microbiol.* 59:3825–3831 (1993).

108. Rodrigo, M., A. Martinez, T. Sanchez, et al. Kinetics of *Clostridium sporogenes* PA3679 spore destruction using computer-controlled thermoresistometer. *J. Food Sci.* 58:649–652 (1993).

109. Ocio, M.J., T. Sánchez, P.S. Fernandez, et al. Thermal resistance characteristics of PA 3679 in the temperature range of 100–121°C as affected by pH, type of acidulant and substrate. *Int. J. Food Microbiol.* 22:239–247 (1994).

110. Li, Y., F. Hsieh, M.L. Fields, et al. Thermal inactivation and injury of *Clostridium sporogenes* spores during extrusion of mechanically deboned turkey mixed with white corn flour. *J. Food Process. Preserv.* 17:391–403 (1993).

111. Welt, B.A., C.H. Tong, J.L. Rossen, and D.B. Lund. Effect of microwave radiation on inactivation of *Clostridium sporogenes* (PA 3679) spores. *Appl. Environ. Microbiol.* 60:482–488 (1994).

112. Drobniewski, F.A. *Bacillus cereus* and related species. *Clin. Microbiol. Rev.* 6:324–338 (1993).

113. Kramer, J.M., and R.J. Gilbert. *Bacillus cereus* gastroenteritis. In *Food Poisoning.* A.T. Tu (ed.). New York, Marcel Dekker. *Handbook of Natural Toxins* 7:119–153 (1992).

114. Wilson, I.G., T.S. Wilson, and J.M. Kramer. Increase in *Bacillus* food poisoning in Northern Ireland. *Lancet* 342:928 (1993).

115. Centers for Disease Control. *Bacillus cereus* food poisoning associated with fried rice at two child day care centers—Virginia, 1993. *Morbid. Mortal. Weekly Rep.* 43:177–178 (1994).

116. Sutherland, A.D., and R. Murdoch. Seasonal occurrence of psychrotrophic *Bacillus* species in raw milk, and studies on the interactions with mesophilic *Bacillus* sp. *Int. J. Food Microbiol.* 21:279–292 (1994).

117. Rangasamy, P.N., M. Iyer, and H. Roginski. Isolation and characterisation of *Bacillus cereus* in milk and dairy products manufactured in Victoria. *Aust. J. Dairy Technol.* 48:93–95 (1993).

118. Baker, J.M., and M.W. Griffiths. Predictive modeling of psychrotrophic *Bacillus cereus*. *J. Food Protect.* 56:684–688 (1993).

119. Sutherland, A.D. Toxin production by *Bacillus cereus* in dairy products. *J. Dairy Res.* 60:569–574 (1993).

120. Sutherland, A.D., and A.M. Limond. Influence of pH and sugars on the growth and production of diarrhoeagenic toxin by *Bacillus cereus*. *J. Dairy Res.* 60:575–580 (1993).

121. Olm, S., and G. Scheibner. Einfluß von pH-Wert, NaCl, Nitrit und Temperatur auf die Enterotoxinbildung von *B. cereus*. *Fleischwirtschaft* 73:691–692 (1993).

122. da Silva, S.M., L. Rabinovitch, and P.G. Robbs. Quantification and behavioral characterization of *Bacillus cereus* in formulated infant foods. I – Generation time. *Rev. Microbiol. São Paulo* 24:125–131 (1993).

123. Shinigawa, K. Serology and characterization of toxigenic *Bacillus cereus*. *Neth. Milk Dairy J.* 47:89–103 (1993).

124. Granum, P.E., S. Brynestad, K. O'Sullivan, and H. Nissen. Enterotoxin from *Bacillus cereus*: production and biochemical characterization. *Neth. Milk Dairy J.* 47:63–70 (1993).

125. Notermans, S., and S. Tatini. Characterization of *Bacillus cereus* in relation to toxin production. *Neth. Milk Dairy J.* 47:71–77 (1993).

126. Granum, P.E., and H. Nissen. Sphingomyelinase is part of the 'enterotoxin complex' produced by *Bacillus cereus*. *FEMS Microbiol. Lett.* 110:97–100 (1993).

127. Beecher, D.J., and A.C.L. Wong. Improved purification and characterization of hemolysin BL, a hemolytic dermonecrotic vascular permeability factor from *Bacillus cereus*. *Infect. Immun.* 62:980–986 (1994).

128. Heinrichs, J.H., D.J. Beecher, J.D. MacMillan, and B.A. Zilinskas. Molecular cloning and characterization of the *hblA* gene encoding the B component of hemolysin BL from *Bacillus cereus*. *J. Bacteriol.* 175:6760–6766 (1993).

129. Sakurai, N., K.A. Koike, Y. Irie, and H. Hayashi. The rice culture filtrate of *Bacillus cereus* isolated from emetic-type food poisoning causes mitochondrial swelling in a HEp-2 cell. *Microbiol. Immunol.* 38:337–343 (1994).

130. Hansen, S., L.K. Hansen, and E. Hough. The crystal structure of Tris-inhibited phospholipase C from *Bacillus cereus* at 1.9 Å resolution. *J. Molec. Biol.* 231:870–876 (1993).

131. in 't Veld, P.H., P.S.S. Soentoro, and S.H.W. Notermans. Properties of *Bacillus cereus* spores in reference materials prepared from artificially contaminated spray dried milk. *Int. J. Food Microbiol.* 20:23–36 (1993).

132. Bennett, R.W., G. Murthy, L. Kaylor, et al. Biological characterization and serological identification of *Bacillus cereus* diarrhoeal factor. *Neth. Milk Dairy J.* 47:105–120 (1993).

133. Christiansson, A. Enterotoxin production in milk by *Bacillus cereus*: a comparison of methods for toxin detection. *Neth. Milk Dairy J.* 47:79–87 (1993).

134. Beecher, D.J., and A.C.L. Wong. Identification of hemolysin BL-producing *Bacillus cereus* isolates by a discontinuous hemolytic pattern in blood agar. *Appl. Environ. Microbiol.* 60:1646–1651 (1994).

135. Kühn, H. Vorkommen von Enteritis-Salmonellen beim Menschen. *Dtsch. Tierärztl. Wschr.* 100:255–258 (1993).

136. Krutsch, H.W. Zur Problematik der Salmonellen. *Fleischwirtschaft* 73:1368–1371 (1993).

137. Sander, J. Pathogenese der *Salmonella*-Infektionen des Menschen. *Dtsch. Tierärztl. Wschr.* 100:283–285 (1993).

138. Sharp, J.C.M., W.J. Reilly, and D.S. Munro. Salmonellosis in Scotland, 1992. *Commun. Dis. Environ. Health Scotland Weekly Rep.* 27(40):3–5 (1993).

139. PHLS Communicable Disease Surveillance Centre. *Salmonella* in humans, England and Wales: quarterly report. *Commun. Dis. Rep.* 4:143–146 (1994).

140. Blaha, Th. Die Ausbreitungsdynamik von Salmonellen in Tierbeständen. *Dtsch. Tierärztl. Wschr.* 100:278–280 (1983).

141. Selbitz, H.-J. Die Wirtsanpassung von Salmonellastämmen und ihre Bedeutung für das Zoonosegeschehen. *Prak. Tierarzt* 74:1102–1105 (1993).

142. Wray, C., I.M. McLaren, and Y.E. Beedell. Bacterial resistance monitoring of salmonellas isolated from animals, national experience of surveillance schemes in the United Kingdom. *Vet. Microbiol.* 35:313–319 (1993).

143. Threlfall, E.J., B. Rowe, and L.R. Ward. A comparison of multiple drug resistance in salmonellas from humans and food animals in England and Wales, 1981 and 1990. *Epidemiol. Infect.* 111:189–197 (1993).

144. Vatopoulos, A.C., E. Mainas, E. Balis, et al. Molecular epidemiology of ampicillin-resistant clinical isolates of *Salmonella enteritidis*. *J. Clin. Microbiol.* 32:1322–1325 (1994).

145. Gruenewald, R., S. Blum, and J. Chan. Relationship between human immunodeficiency virus infection and salmonellosis in 20- to 59-year-old residents of New York City. *Clin. Infect. Dis.* 18:358–363 (1994).

146. Neal, K.R., S.O. Brij, R.C.B. Slack, et al. Recent treatment with $H_2$ antagonists and antibiotics and gastric surgery as risk factors for salmonella infection. *Br. Med. J.* 308:176 (1994).

147. Lalitha, M.K., and R. John. Unusual manifestations of salmonellosis—a surgical problem. *Q. J. Med.* 87:301–309 (1994).

148. Heilesen, A.M., and P.-H. Christensen. Abscess of the submandibular gland caused by *Salmonella typhimurium* biotype 10. *Scand. J. Infect. Dis.* 26:223–224 (1994).

149. Nice, C.S., and H. Panigrahi. Cutaneous abscesses caused by *Salmonella enteritidis*: an unusual presentation of salmonellosis. (Letter.) *J. Infect.* 27:204–205 (1993).

150. Cummins, A.J., and W.A. Atia. Bartholin's abscess complicating food poisoning with *Salmonella panama*: a case report. *Genitourinary Med.* 70:46–48 (1994).

151. Garrido-Benedicto, P., E. González-Reimers, F. Santolaria-Fernandez, et al. Acute acalculous cholecystitis due to *Salmonella*. (Letter.) *Dig. Dis. Sci.* 39:442–443 (1994).

152. Shrivastava, A., and D. Thistlethwaite. Erythema nodosum and arthritis with *Salmonella enteritidis* enteritis. (Letter.) *Br. J. Dermatol.* 128:704 (1993).

153. John, R., D. Mathai, A.J. Daniel, and M.K. Lalitha. Bilateral septic arthritis due to *Salmonella enteritidis*. *Diagn. Microbiol. Infect. Dis.* 17:167–169 (1993).

154. Thomson, G.T.D., M. Alfa, K. Orr, et al. Secretory immune response and clinical sequelae of *Salmonella* infection in a point source cohort. *J. Rheumatol.* 21:132–137 (1994).

155. Huppertz, H.-I., and K. Sandhage. *Salmonella enteritidis* in reactive carditis. (Letter.) *Lancet* 342:1488–1489 (1993).

156. Hufnagel, B., F. Saul, H. Rosin, et al. Mitral-klappenendokarditis durch *Salmonella enteritidis*. *Z. Kardiol.* 82:654–657 (1993).

157. Clesham, G.J., and G.J. Davies. Bacterial pericarditis caused by *Salmonella enteritidis* phage type 1. *Int. J. Cardiol.* 41:241–243 (1993).

158. Sharma, J., D.D. Von Hoff, and G.R. Weiss. *Salmonella arizonae* peritonitis secondary to ingestion of rattlesnake capsules for gastric cancer. (Letter.) *J. Clin. Oncol.* 11:2288–2289 (1993).

159. Perras, B., B. Kreft, and G. Wiedemann. Sepsis und Spondylodiszitis durch *Salmonella enteritidis*. *Dtsch. Med. Wschr.* 118:1844–1846 (1993).

160. Watier, S., S. Richardson, and B. Hubert. *Salmonella enteritidis* infections in France and the United States: characterization by a deterministic model. *Am. J. Public Health* 83:1694–1700 (1993).

161. Halloran, M.E. *Salmonella enteritidis* infections in France and the United States: causes vs causal models. *Am. J. Public Health* 83:1667–1669 (1993).

162. Notermans, S. (ed.). *Int. J. Food Microbiol.* 21(1+2) (1994).

163. Roberts, J.A., and P.N. Sockett. The socio-economic impact of human *Salmonella enteritidis* infection. *Int. J. Food Microbiol.* 21:117–129 (1994).

164. Poppe, C. *Salmonella enteritidis* in Canada. *Int. J. Food Microbiol.* 21:1–5 (1994).

165. Fantasia, M., and E. Filetici. *Salmonella enteritidis* in Italy. *Int. J. Food Microbiol.* 21:7–13 (1994).

166. Caffer, M.I., and T. Eiguer. *Salmonella enteritidis* in Argentina. *Int. J. Food Microbiol.* 21:15–19 (1994).

167. Glośnicka, R., and D. Kunikowska. The epidemiological situation of *Salmonella enteritidis* in Poland. *Int. J. Food Microbiol.* 21:21–30 (1994).

168. Katouli, M., R.H. Seuffer, R. Wollin, et al. Variations in biochemical phenotypes and phage types of *Salmonella enteritidis* in Germany 1980–1992. *Epidemiol. Infect.* 111:199–207 (1993).

169. Brown, D.J., D.L. Baggesen, H.B. Hansen, et al. The characterization of Danish isolates of *Salmonella enterica* serovar enteritidis by phage typing and plasmid profiling: 1980–1990. *APMIS* 102:208–214 (1994).

170. Centers for Disease Control. Outbreaks of *Salmonella enteritidis* gastroenteritis—California, 1993. *Morbid. Mortal. Weekly Rep.* 42:793–797 (1993).

171. Irwin, D.J., M. Rao, D.W. Barham, et al. An outbreak of infection with *Salmonella enteritidis* phage type 4 associated with the use of raw shell eggs. *Commun. Dis. Rep.* 3(Rev. 13):R179–R183 (1993).

172. Sibbald, C.J., D. Fitzsimons, and P.A. Upton. Melon and mango mayonnaise malaise. *Commun. Dis. Environ. Health Scotland Weekly Rep.* 28(2):5–6 (1994).

173. Mintz, E.D., M.L. Cartter, J.L. Hadler, et al. Dose–response effects in an outbreak of *Salmonella enteritidis*. *Epidemiol. Infect.* 112:13–23 (1994).

174. Wright, J.P., W.J. Patterson, C. Boffin, and A.W. Anderson. Food poisoning at a masonic lodge. *Commun. Dis. Rep.* 4(Rev. 5):R58–R60 (1994).

175. Centers for Disease Control. Outbreak of *Salmonella enteritidis* associated with homemade ice cream—Florida, 1993. *Morbid. Mortal. Weekly Rep.* 43:669–671 (1994).

176. Friels, M., and J. Chalmers. An outbreak of *Salmonella enteritidis* phage type 1 food poisoning at a wedding. *Commun. Dis. Environ. Health Scotland Weekly Rep.* 27(20):5–9 (1993).

177. Ayres, P., P. Hatton, M. Schweiger, and D. Bonner. Food poisoning associated with a self-catered wedding reception. *Commun. Dis. Rep.* 4(Rev. 5):R62–R63 (1994).

178. Bonner, D., and M. Schweiger. Apple pie: an unusual vehicle for food poisoning. *Commun. Dis. Rep.* 4(Rev. 5):R60–R61 (1994).

179. Gonzalez-Hevia, M.A., J.J. LLaneza, and M.C. Mendoza. Usefulness of molecular genetic markers in the typing of *Salmonella enterica* serovar Enteritidis causing a food-borne outbreak. *Int. J. Food Microbiol.* 22:97–103 (1994).

180. Bichler, L.A., K.V. Nagaraja, and B.S. Pomeroy. Plasmid diversity in *Salmonella enteritidis* of animal, poultry, and human origin. *J. Food Protect.* 57:4–11 (1994).

181. Dorn, C.R., R. Silapanuntakul, E.J. Angrick, and L.C. Shipman. Plasmid analysis of *Salmonella enteritidis* isolated from human gastroenteritis cases and from epidemiologically associated poultry flocks. *Epidemiol. Infect.* 111:239–243 (1993).

182. Henzler, D.J., E. Ebel, J. Sanders, et al. *Salmonella enteritidis* in eggs from commercial chicken layer flocks implicated in human outbreaks. *Avian Dis.* 38:37–43 (1994).

183. Stanley, J., and N. Baquar. Phylogenetics of *Salmonella enteritidis*. *Int. J. Food Microbiol.* 21:79–87 (1994).

184. Hinton, M., and J.A. Bale. Is *Salmonella enteritidis* PT4 a super bug? *Food Res. Int.* 27:233–235 (1994).

185. Threlfall, E.J., H. Chart, L.R. Ward, et al. Interrelationships between strains of *Salmonella enteritidis* belonging to phage types 4, 7, 7a, 8, 13, 13a, 23, 24, and 30. *J. Appl. Bacteriol.* 75:43–48 (1993).

186. Nastasi, A., C. Mammina, and M.R. Villafrate. Epidemiology of *Salmonella typhimurium*: ribosomal DNA analysis of strains from human and animal sources. *Epidemiol. Infect.* 110:553–565 (1993).

187. PHLS Communicable Disease Surveillance Centre. Changing patterns of infectious diseases. *Commun. Dis. Rep.* 4:203 (1994).

188. Thornton, L., S. Gray, P. Bingham, et al. The problems of tracing a geographically widespread outbreak of salmonellosis from a commonly eaten food: *Salmonella typhimurium* DT193 in North West England and North Wales in 1991. *Epidemiol. Infect.* 111:465–471 (1993).

189. Anonymous. Laotian feast in California turns deadly. *Food Protect. Rep.* 10(10):5–6 (1994).

190. McCover, R. Food poisoning incident, retirement party, Acharacle, Argyll. *Commun. Dis. Environ. Health Scotland Weekly Rep.* 27(31):7–8 (1993).

191. Gessner, B.D., and M. Beller. Protective effect of conventional cooking versus use of microwave ovens in an outbreak of salmonellosis. *Am. J. Epidemiol.* 139:903–909 (1994).

192. PHLS Communicable Disease Surveillance Centre. *Salmonella virchow* phage type 26. *Commun. Dis. Rep.* 4:119 (1994).

193. PHLS Communicable Disease Surveillance Centre. An outbreak of *Salmonella paratyphi* B infection in France. *Commun. Dis. Rep.* 4:165 (1994).

194. Old, D.C., M. Porter-Boveri, and D.S. Munro. Human infection in Tayside, Scotland due to *Salmonella* serotype Livingstone. *J. Med. Microbiol.* 40:134–140 (1994).

195. Blostein, J. An outbreak of *Salmonella javiana* associated with consumption of watermelon. *J. Environ. Health* 56(1):29–31 (1993).

196. Ward, H., and M. Roworth. *Salmonella mikawasima* in Fife. *Commun. Dis. Environ. Health Scotland Weekly Rep.* 28(13):4–7 (1994).

197. Synnott, M., D.L. Morse, H. Maguire, et al. An outbreak of *Salmonella mikawasima* associated with doner kebabs. *Epidemiol. Infect.* 111:473–481 (1993).

198. Carson, A., and M.F. Hanson. An investigation of salmonella associated with retail tropical fresh water aquaria. *Commun. Dis. Environ. Health Scotland Weekly Rep.* 27(34):8–10 (1993).

199. Hatakka, M., and K. Asplund. The occurrence of *Salmonella* in airline meals. *Acta Vet. Scand.* 34:391–396 (1993).

200. Kasrazadeh, M., and C. Genigeorgis. Potential growth and control of *Salmonella* in Hispanic type soft cheese. *Int. J. Food Microbiol.* 22:127–140 (1994).

201. Frederick, T.L., M.F. Miller, L.D. Thompson, and C.B. Ramsey. Microbiological properties of pork cheek meat as affected by acetic acid and temperature. *J. Food Sci.* 59:300–302 (1994).

202. Walls, I., P.H. Cooke, R.C. Benedict, and R.L. Buchanan. Factors affecting attachment of *Salmonella typhimurium* to sausage casings. *Food Microbiol.* 10:387–393 (1993).

203. Bergis, H., G. Poumeyrol, and A. Beaufort. Etude du développement de la flore saprophyte et de *Salmonella* dans des viandes hachées conditionnées sous atmosphère modifiée. *Sci. Aliments* 14:217–228 (1994).

204. Hartung, M. Vorkommen von Enteritis-Salmonellen in Lebensmitteln und bei Nutztieren 1991. *Dtsch. Tierärztl. Wschr.* 100:259–261 (1993).

205. Gast, R.K., N.A. Cox, and J.S. Bailey. Salmonellae in eggs. In *Food Poisoning*. A.T. Tu (ed.). New York, Marcel Dekker. *Handbook of Natural Toxins* 7:49–69 (1992).

206. Humphrey, T.J. Contamination of egg shell and contents with *Salmonella enteritidis*: a review. *Int. J. Food Microbiol.* 21:31–40 (1994).

207. Humphrey, T.J., and A. Whitehead. Egg age and the growth of *Salmonella enteritidis* PT4 in egg contents. *Epidemiol. Infect.* 111:209–219 (1993).

208. de Louvois, J. Salmonella contamination of eggs. (Letter.) *Lancet* 342:366–367 (1993).

209. Rampling, A. *Salmonella enteritidis* five years on. *Lancet* 342:317–318 (1993).

210. Fehlhaber, K., and P. Braun. Untersuchungen zum Eindringen von *Salmonella enteritidis* aus dem Eiklar in das Dotter von Hühnereiern und zur Hitzeinaktivierung beim Kochen und Braten. *Arch. Lebensmittelhyg.* 44:59–63 (1993).

211. Saeed, A.M., and C.W. Koons. Growth and heat resistance of *Salmonella enteritidis* in refrigerated and abused eggs. *J. Food Protect.* 56:927–931 (1993).

212. Warburton, D.W., J. Harwig, and B. Bowen. The survival of salmonellae in homemade chocolate and egg liqueur. *Food Microbiol.* 10:405–410 (1993).

213. Benard, G., A. Eckermann, F. Heurteloup, and C. Labie. Oberflächenkontamination des Brustfleisches von Mastenten mit Salmonellen. *Arch. Lebensmittelhyg.* 45:46–47 (1994).

214. Kim, J.-W., M.F. Slavik, C.L. Griffis, and J.T. Walker. Attachment of *Salmonella typhimurium* to skins of chicken scalded at various temperatures. *J. Food Protect.* 56:661–665 (1993).

215. Lillard, H.S. Bactericidal effect of chlorine on attached salmonellae with and without sonification. *J. Food Protect.* 56:716–717 (1993).

216. Bianchi, A., S.C. Ricke, A.L. Cartwright, and F.A. Gardner. A peroxidase catalyzed chemical dip for the reduction of *Salmonella* on chicken breast skin. *J. Food Protect.* 57:301–304 (1994).

217. Lillard, H.S. Effect of trisodium phosphate on salmonellae attached to chicken skin. *J. Food Protect.* 57:465–469 (1994).

218. Li, Y., J.-W. Kim, M.F. Slavik, et al. *Salmonella typhimurium* attached to chicken skin reduced using electrical

stimulation and inorganic salts. *J. Food Sci.* 59:23–25,29 (1994).

219. Meyer, H., G. Steinbach, and U. Methner. Bekämpfung von Salmonella-Infektionen in Tierbeständen—Grundlage der Reduzierung des Salmonelleneintrags in Lebensmitteln. *Dtsch. Tierärztl. Wschr.* 100:292–295 (1993).

220. Gay, J.M., D.H. Rice, and J.H. Steiger. Prevalence of fecal *Salmonella* shedding by cull dairy cattle marketed in Washington State. *J. Food Protect.* 57:195–197 (1994).

221. Gay, J.M., and M.E. Hunsaker. Isolation of multiple *Salmonella* serovars from a dairy two years after a clinical salmonellosis outbreak. *J. Am. Vet. Med. Assoc.* 203:1314–1320 (1993).

222. Böhm, R. Verhalten ausgewählter Salmonellen in der Umwelt. *Dtsch. Tierärztl. Wschr.* 100:275–278 (1993).

223. Köhler, B. Beispiele für die Anreicherung von Salmonellen in der Umwelt. *Dtsch. Tierärztl. Wschr.* 100:264–274 (1993).

224. Bisping, W. Salmonellen in Futtermitteln. *Dtsch. Tierärztl. Wschr.* 100:262–263 (1993).

225. Forshell, L.P., and I. Ekesbo. Survival of salmonellas in composted and not composted solid animal manures. *J. Vet. Med. B* 40:654–658 (1993).

226. Skanavis, C., and W.A. Yanko. Evaluation of composted sewage sludge based soil amendments for potential risks of salmonellosis. *J. Environ. Health* 56(7):19–23 (1994).

227. Heddleson, R.A., S. Doores, R.C. Anantheswaran, and G.D. Kuhn. Destruction of *Salmonella* species heated in aqueous salt solutions by microwave energy. *J. Food Protect.* 56:763–768 (1993).

228. Heddleson, R.A., S. Doores, and R.C. Anantheswaran. Parameters affecting destruction of *Salmonella* spp. by microwave heating. *J. Food Sci.* 59:447–451 (1994).

229. Wolfson, L.M., and S.S. Sumner. Antibacterial activity of the lactoperoxidase system against *Salmonella typhimurium* in trypticase soy broth in the presence and absence of a heat treatment. *J. Food Protect.* 57:365–368 (1994).

230. Lee, I.S., J.L. Slonczewski, and J.W. Foster. A low-pH-inducible stationary-phase acid tolerance response in *Salmonella typhimurium. J. Bacteriol.* 176:1422–1426 (1994).

231. Humphrey, T.J., N.P. Richardson, K.M. Statton, and R.J. Rowbury. Effects of temperature shift on acid and heat tolerance in *Salmonella enteritidis* phage type 4. *Appl. Environ. Microbiol.* 59:3120–3122 (1993).

232. Li, Y., M.F. Slavik, C.I., Griffis and J.W Kim. Effect of electrical stimulation on killing *Salmonella typhimurium* in various salt solutions. *J. Food Safety* 13:241–252 (1993).

233. Poppe, C., K.A. McFadden, A.M. Brouwer, and W. Demczuk. Characterization of *Salmonella enteritidis* strains. *Can. J. Vet. Res.* 57:176–184 (1993).

234. Hird, D.W., H. Kinde, J.T. Case, et al. Serotypes of *Salmonella* isolated from California turkey flocks and their environment in 1984–1989 and comparison with human isolates. *Avian Dis.* 37:715–719 (1993).

235. Atanassova, V., S. Matthes, E. Mühlbauer, et al. Plasmidprofile verschiedener *Salmonella*-Serovare aus Geflügelbeständen in Deutschland. *Berl. Münch. Tierärztl. Wschr.* 106:404–407 (1993).

236. Poppe, C., W. Demczuk, K. McFadden, and R.P. Johnson. Virulence of *Salmonella enteritidis* phagetypes 4, 8 and 13 and other *Salmonella* spp. for day-old chicks, hens and mice. *Can. J. Vet. Res.* 57:281–287 (1993).

237. Suzuki, S. Pathogenicity of *Salmonella enteritidis* in poultry. *Int. J. Food Microbiol.* 21:89–105 (1994).

238. Barrow, P.A. Salmonella control—past, present and future. *Avian Pathol.* 22:651–669 (1993).

239. Noordhuizen, J.P., and K. Frankena. *Salmonella enteritidis:* clinical epidemiological approaches for prevention and control of *S. enteritidis* in poultry. *Int. J. Food Microbiol.* 21:131–143 (1994).

240. van de Giessen, A.W., A.J.H.A. Amett, and S.H.W. Notermans. Intervention strategies for *Salmonella enteritidis* in poultry flocks: a basic approach. *Int. J. Food Microbiol.* 21:145–154 (1994).

241. Edel, W. *Salmonella enteritidis* eradication programme in poultry breeder flocks in The Netherlands. *Int. J. Food Microbiol.* 21:171–178 (1994).

242. Mason, J. *Salmonella enteritidis* control programs in the United States. *Int. J. Food Microbiol.* 21:155–169 (1994).

243. Gast, R.K. Understanding *Salmonella enteritidis* in laying chickens: the contributions of experimental infections. *Int. J. Food Microbiol.* 21:107–116 (1994).

244. Awad-Masalmeh, M., and G. Thiemann. Salmonellen Monitoring unter Beachtung biologischer Parameter in einigen großen Legehühnerbetrieben und Brüterein in Österreich. *Tierärztl. Umschau* 48:706–713 (1993).

245. Cason, J.A., J.S. Bailey, and N.A. Cox. Location of *Salmonella typhimurium* during incubation and hatching of inoculated eggs. *Poultry Sci.* 72:2064–2068 (1993).

246. Lindell, K.A., A.M. Saeed, and G.P. McCabe. Evaluation of resistance of four strains of commercial laying hens to experimental infection with *Salmonella enteritidis* phage type eight. *Poultry Sci.* 73:757–762 (1994).

247. Thiagarajan, D., A.M. Saeed, and E.K. Asem. Mechanism of transovarian transmission of *Salmonella enteritidis* in laying hens. *Poultry Sci.* 73:89–98 (1994).

248. Holt, P.S., and R.E. Porter, Jr. Effect of induced molting on the recurrence of a previous *Salmonella enteritidis* infection. *Poultry Sci.* 72:2069–2078 (1993).

249. McCruder, E.D., P.M. Ray, G.I. Tellez, et al. *Salmonella enteritidis* immune leukocyte-stimulated soluble factors: effects on increased resistance to *Salmonella* organ invasion in day-old leghorn chicks. *Poultry Sci.* 72:2264–2271 (1993).

250. Tellez, G.I., M.H. Kogut, and B.M. Hargis. Immunoprophylaxis of *Salmonella enteritidis* infection by lymphokines in leghorn chicks. *Avian Dis.* 37:1062–1070 (1993).

251. Charles, S.D., I. Hussain, C.-U. Choi, et al. Adjuvanted subunit vaccines for the control of *Salmonella enteritidis* infection in turkeys. *Am. J. Vet. Res.* 55:636–642 (1994).

252. Hume, M.E., D.E. Corrier, S. Ambrus, et al. Effectiveness of dietary propionic acid in controlling *Salmonella typhimurium* colonization in broiler chicks. *Avian Dis.* 37:1051–1056 (1993).

253. Corrier, D.E., D.J. Nisbet, A.G. Hollister, et al. Resistance against *Salmonella enteritidis* cecal colonization in leghorn chicks by vent lip application of cecal bacteria culture. *Poultry Sci.* 73:648–652 (1994).

254. Tellez, G.I., M.H. Kogut, and B.M. Hargis. *Eimeria tenella* or *Eimeria adenoeides*: induction of morphological changes and increased resistance to *Salmonella enteritidis* infection in leghorn chicks. *Poultry Sci.* 73:396–401 (1994).

255. Kogut, M.H., T. Fukata, G. Tellez, et al. Effect of *Eimeria tenella* infection on resistance to *Salmonella typhimurium* colonization in broiler chicks inoculated with anaerobic cecal flora and fed dietary lactose. *Avian Dis.* 38:59–64 (1994).

256. Nisbet, D.J., D.E. Corrier, and J.R. DeLoach. Effect of mixed cecal microflora maintained in continuous culture and of dietary lactose on *Salmonella typhimurium* colonization in broiler chicks. *Avian Dis.* 37:528–535 (1993).

257. Nisbet, D.J., D.E. Corrier, C.M. Scanlan, et al. Effect of a defined continuous-flow derived bacterial culture and dietary lactose on *Salmonella typhimurium* colonization in broiler chickens. *Avian Dis.* 37:1017–1025 (1993).

258. Hollister, A.G., D.E. Corrier, D.J. Nisbet, et al. Comparison of effects of chicken cecal microorganisms maintained in continuous culture and provision of dietary lactose on cecal colonization by *Salmonella typhimurium* in turkey poults and broiler chicks. *Poultry Sci.* 73:640–647 (1994).

259. Nisbet, D.J., S.C. Ricke, C.M. Scanlan, et al. Inoculation of broiler chicks with a continuous-flow derived bacterial culture facilitates early cecal bacterial colonization and increases resistance to *Salmonella typhimurium*. *J. Food Protect.* 57:12–15 (1994).

260. Behling, R.G., and A.C.L. Wong. Competitive exclusion of *Salmonella enteritidis* in chicks by treatment with a single culture plus dietary lactose. *Int. J. Food Microbiol.* 22:1–9 (1994).

261. Corrier, D.E., D.J. Nisbet, C.M. Scanlan, et al. Inhibition of *Salmonella enteritidis* cecal and organ colonization in leghorn chicks by a defined culture of cecal bacteria and dietary lactose. *J. Food Protect.* 56:377–381 (1994).

262. Hollister, A.G., D.E. Corrier, D.J. Nisbet, and J.R. DeLoach. Effect of cecal cultures encapsulated in alginate beads or lyophilized in skim milk and dietary lactose on *Salmonella* colonization in broiler chicks. *Poultry Sci.* 73:99–105 (1994).

263. Hinton, A., Jr., M.E. Hume, and J.R. DeLoach. Role of metabolic intermediates in the inhibition of *Salmonella typhimurium* and *Salmonella enteritidis* by *Veillonella*. *J. Food Protect.* 56:932–937 (1993).

264. Barnhart, H.M., D.W. Dreesen, and J.L. Burke. Isolation of *Salmonella* from ovaries and oviducts from whole carcasses of spent hens. *Avian Dis.* 37:977–980 (1993).

265. Blackburn, C.deW. Rapid and alternative methods for the detection of salmonellas in foods. *J. Appl. Bacteriol.* 75:199–214 (1993).

266. Orden, B., A. Franco, E. Juárez, et al. Evaluation of a colour test for rapid detection of salmonella. *Eur. J. Clin. Microbiol. Infect. Dis.* 12:630–633 (1993).

267. Di Falco, G., V. Giaccone, G.P. Amerio, and E. Parisi. A modified impedance method to detect *Salmonella* spp. in fresh meat. *Food Microbiol.* 10:421–427 (1993).

268. Pless, P., K. Futschik, and E. Schopf. Rapid detection of salmonellae by means of a new impedance-splitting method. *J. Food Protect.* 57:369–376 (1994).

269. van der Zee, H. Conventional methods for the detection and isolation of *Salmonella enteritidis*. *Int. J. Food Microbiol.* 21:41–46 (1994).

270. Whittemore, A.D. A modified most probable number technique to enumerate total aerobes, Enterobacteriaceae, and *Salmonella* on poultry carcasses after the whole carcass rinse procedure. *Poultry Sci.* 72:2353–2357 (1993).

271. Xavier, I.J., and S. Ingham. Increased *D*-values for *Salmonella enteritidis* resulting from the use of anaerobic enumeration methods. *Food Microbiol.* 10:223–228 (1993).

272. D'Aoust, J.-Y., A.M. Sewell, and P. Greco. Detection of *Salmonella* in dry foods using refrigerated preenrichment and enrichment broth cultures: interlaboratory study. *J. AOAC Int.* 76:814–821 (1993).

273. Reissbrodt, R., and W. Rabsch. Selective pre-enrichment of *Salmonella* from eggs by siderophore supplements. *Zbl. Bakteriol.* 279:344–353 (1993).

274. Asperger, H., and P. Pless. Zum Salmonellennachweis in Käse—Methodenvergleich unter besonderer Berücksichtigung der Begleitfloraproblematik. *Wien. Tierärztl. Monatschr.* 81:12–17 (1994).

275. Chen, H., A.D.E. Fraser, and H. Yamazaki. Modes of inhibition of foodborne non-*Salmonella* bacteria by selenite cystine selective broth. *Int. J. Food Microbiol.* 22:217–222 (1994).

276. Joosten, H.M.L.J., W.G.F.M. van Dijck, and F. van der Velde. Evaluation of motility enrichment on modified semisolid Rappaport-Vassiliadis medium (MSRV) and automated conductance in combination with Rambach agar for *Salmonella* detection in environmental samples of a milk powder factory. *Int. J. Food Microbiol.* 22:201–206 (1994).

277. De Smedt, J., and R. Bolderdijk. *Salmonella* detection in cocoa and chocolate by motility enrichment on modified semi-solid Rappaport-Vassiliadis medium: collaborative study. *J. AOAC Int.* 77:365–373 (1994).

278. Pless, P., H. Asperger, M. Scheider, and E. Schopf. Erweiterte Einsatzmöglichkeiten eines modifizierten Beweglichkeitsmediums (MSRV-Medium) für den Salmonellennachweis. *Arch. Lebensmittelhyg.* 44:125–127 (1993).

279. O'Donoghue, D., and E. Winn. Comparison of the MSRV method with an in-house conventional method for the detection of *Salmonella* in various high and low moisture foods. *Lett. Appl. Microbiol.* 17:174–177 (1993).

280. Curtis, G.D.W., and L.A. Clarke. Comparison of the MSRV method with an in-house conventional method for the

detection of *Salmonella* in various high and low moisture foods. (Letter.) *Lett. Appl. Microbiol.* 18:239–240 (1994).

281. Warburton, D.W., B. Bowen, A. Konkle, et al. A comparison of six different plating media used in the isolation of *Salmonella. Int. J. Food Microbiol.* 22:277–289 (1994).

282. Gast, R.K. Evaluation of direct plating for detecting *Salmonella enteritidis* in pools of egg contents. *Poultry Sci.* 72:1611–1614 (1993).

283. Garrick, R.C., and A.D. Smith. Evaluation of Rambach agar for the differentiation of *Salmonella* species from other Enterobacteriaceae. *Lett. Appl. Microbiol.* 18:187–189 (1994).

284. Kühn, H., B. Wonde, W. Rabsch, and R. Reissbrodt. Evaluation of Rambach agar for detection of *Salmonella* subspecies I to VI. *Appl. Environ. Microbiol.* 60:749–751 (1994).

285. Abdalla, S., J. Vila, and M.T.J. de Anta. Identification of *Salmonella* spp. with Rambach agar in conjunction with the 4-methylumbelliferyl caprylate (MUCAP) fluorescence test. *Br. J. Biomed. Sci.* 51:5–8 (1994).

286. Monfort, P., D. Le Gal, J.C. Le Saux, et al. Improved rapid method for isolation and enumeration of salmonella from bivalves using Rambach agar. *J. Microbiol. Meth.* 19:67–79 (1994).

287. Allen, S.B., R. Firstenberg-Eden, D.A. Shingler, et al. Evaluation of stabilized bismuth sulfite agar for detection of *Salmonella* in foods. *J. Food Protect.* 56:666–671 (1993).

288. Cox, J.M. Lysine–mannitol–glycerol agar, a medium for the isolation of *Salmonella* spp., including *S. typhi* and atypical strains. *Appl. Environ. Microbiol.* 59:2602–2606 (1993).

289. Muñoz, P., M.D. Díaz, E. Cercenado, et al. Rapid screening of *Salmonella* species from stool cultures. *Am. J. Clin. Pathol.* 100:404–406 (1993).

290. Monnery, I., A.M. Freydiere, C. Baron, et al. Evaluation of two new chromogenic media for detection of *Salmonella* in stools. *Eur. J. Clin. Microbiol. Infect. Dis.* 13:257–261 (1994).

291. Cherrington, C.A., and J.H.J.H. in't Veld. Development of a 24 h screen to detect viable salmonellas in faeces. *J. Appl. Bacteriol.* 75:58–64 (1993).

292. Cherrington, C.A., and J.H.J.H. in't Veld. Comparison of classical isolation protocols with a 24 h screen to detect viable salmonellas in faeces. *J. Appl. Bacteriol.* 75:65–68 (1993).

293. Schlundt, J., and B. Munch. A comparison of the efficiency of Rappaport-Vassiliadis, tetrathionate and selenite broths with and without pre-enrichment for the isolation of *Salmonella* in animal waste biogas plants. *Zbl. Bakteriol.* 279:336–343 (1993).

294. Olsen, J.E., D.J. Brown, M.N. Skov, and J.P. Christensen. Bacterial typing methods suitable for epidemiological analysis. Applications in investigations of salmonellosis among livestock. *Vet. Q.* 15:125–135 (1993).

295. Threlfall, E.J., and H. Chart. Interrelationships between strains of *Salmonella enteritidis. Epidemiol. Infect.* 111:1–8 (1993).

296. Threlfall, E.J., M.D. Hampton, H. Chart, and B. Rowe. Use of plasmid profile typing for surveillance of *Salmonella enteritidis* phage type 4 from humans, poultry and eggs. *Epidemiol. Infect.* 112:25–31 (1994).

297. Stubbs, A.D., F.W. Hickman-Brenner, D.N. Cameron, and J.J. Farmer III. Differentiation of *Salmonella enteritidis* phage type 8 strains: evaluation of three additional phage typing systems, plasmid profile, antibiotic susceptibility patterns, and biotyping. *J. Clin. Microbiol.* 32:199–201 (1994).

298. Krusell, L., and N. Skovgaard. Evaluation of a new semi-automated screening method for the detection of *Salmonella* in foods within 24 h. *Int. J. Food Microbiol.* 20:123–130 (1993).

299. Blais, B.W., H.Y. Ong, and H. Yamazaki. Use of inexpensive O antisera as the detecting antibodies for *Salmonella* antigens in the polymyxin–cloth enzyme immunoassay. *Int. J. Food Microbiol.* 20:149–158 (1993).

300. Eckner, K.F,. W.A. Dustman, M.S. Curiale, et al. Elevated-temperature, colorimetric, monoclonal, enzyme-linked immunosorbent assay for rapid screening of *Salmonella* in foods: collaborative study. *J. AOAC Int.* 77:374–394 (1994).

301. Flint, S.H., and N.J. Hartley. Evaluation of the TECRA immunocapture ELISA for the detection of *Salmonella typhimurium* in foods. *Lett. Appl. Microbiol.* 17:4–6 (1993).

302. Kerr, S., H.J. Ball, and R. Porter. A comparison of three salmonella antigen-capture ELISAs and culture for veterinary diagnostic specimens. *J. Appl. Bacteriol.* 75:164–167 (1993).

303. House, J.K., G.W. Dilling, and L. Da Roden. Enzyme-linked immunosorbent assay for serologic detection of *Salmonella dublin* carriers on a large dairy. *Am. J. Vet. Res.* 54:1391–1399 (1993).

304. van Zijderveld, F.G., A.M. van Zijderveld-van Bemmel, R.A.M. Brouwers, et al. Serological detection of chicken flocks naturally infected with *Salmonella enteritidis*, using an enzyme-linked immunosorbent assay based on monoclonal antibodies against the flagellar antigen. *Vet. Q.* 15:135–137 (1993).

305. Furrer, B., A. Baumgartner, and W. Bommeli. Enzyme-linked immunosorbent assay (ELISA) for the detection of antibodies against *Salmonella enteritidis* in chicken blood or egg yolk. *Zbl. Bakteriol.* 279:191–200 (1993).

306. Barrow, P.A. Serological diagnosis of *Salmonella* serotype *enteritidis* infections in poultry by ELISA and other tests. *Int. J. Food Microbiol.* 21:55–68 (1994).

307. Barrow, P.A. Use of ELISAs for monitoring salmonella in poultry. (Letter.) *Vet. Rec.* 134:99 (1994).

308. Thorns, C.J., I.M. McLaren, and M.G. Lojka. The use of latex particle agglutination to specifically detect *Salmonella enteritidis. Int. J. Food Microbiol.* 21:47–53 (1994).

309. Bänffer, J.R.J., J.A. van Zwol-Saarloos, and L.J. Broere. Evaluation of a commercial latex agglutination test for rapid detection of *Salmonella* in fecal samples. *Eur. J. Clin. Microbiol. Infect. Dis.* 12:633–636 (1993).

310. Tsai, H.-C.S., and M.F. Slavik. Rapid fluorescence concentration immunoassay for detection of salmonellae in chicken skin rinse water. *J. Food Protect.* 57:190–194 (1994).

311. Helmuth, R., and A. Schroeter. Molecular typing methods for *S. enteritidis. Int. J. Food Microbiol.* 21:69–77 (1994).

312. Doran, J.L., S.K. Collinson, J. Burian, et al. DNA-based diagnostic tests for *Salmonella* species targeting *agfA*, the structural gene for thin, aggregative fimbriae. *J. Clin. Microbiol.* 31:2263–2273 (1993).

313. Usera, M.A., T. Popovic, C.A. Bopp, and N.A. Strockbine. Molecular subtyping of *Salmonella enteritidis* phage type 8 strains from the United States. *J. Clin. Microbiol.* 32:194–198 (1994).

314. Aabo, S., O.F. Rasmussen, L. Rossen, et al. *Salmonella* identification by the polymerase chain reaction. *Molec. Cell. Probes* 7:171–178 (1993).

315. Nguyen, A.V., M.I. Khan, and Z. Lu. Amplification of *Salmonella* chromosomal DNA using the polymerase chain reaction. *Avian Dis.* 38:119–126 (1994).

316. Rexach, L., F. Dilasser, and P. Fach. Polymerase chain reaction for salmonella virulence-associated plasmid genes detection: a new tool in salmonella epidemiology. *Epidemiol. Infect.* 112:33–43 (1994).

317. Jones, D.D., R. Law, and A.K. Bej. Detection of *Salmonella* spp. in oysters using polymerase chain reactions (PCR) and gene probes. *J. Food Sci.* 58:1191–1197 (1993).

318. Bej, A.K., M.H. Mahbubani, M.J. Boyce, and R.M. Atlas. Detection of *Salmonella* spp. in oysters by PCR. *Appl. Environ. Microbiol.* 60:368–373 (1994).

319. Tsen, H.-Y., J.-W. Liou, and C.-K. Lin. Possible use of a polymerase chain reaction method for specific detection of *Salmonella* in beef. *J. Ferment. Bioeng.* 77:137–143 (1994).

320. Mahon, J., and A.J. Lax. A quantitative polymerase chain reaction method for the detection in avian faeces of salmonellas carrying the *spvR* gene. *Epidemiol. Infect.* 111:455–464 (1993).

321. Iida, K., A. Abe, H. Matsui, et al. Rapid and sensitive method for detection of *Salmonella* strains using a combination of polymerase chain reaction and reverse dot-blot hybridization. *FEMS Microbiol. Lett.* 114:167–172 (1993).

322. Cano, R.J., S.R. Rasmussen, G. Sánchez Fraga, and J.C. Palomares. Fluorescent detection–polymerase chain reaction (FD-PCR) assay on microwell plates as a screening test for salmonellas in foods. *J. Appl. Bacteriol.* 75:247–253 (1993).

323. Ou, J.T. The 90 kilobase pair virulence plasmid of *Salmonella* serovar Typhimurium coexists in strains with a plasmid of the 23 incompatibility groups. *Microb. Pathogen.* 15:237–242 (1993).

324. Schmitt, C.K., S.C. Darnell, V.L. Tesh, et al. Mutation of *flgM* attenuates virulence of *Salmonella typhimurium*, and mutation of *fliA* represses the attenuated phenotype. *J. Bacteriol.* 176:368–377 (1994).

325. McCormick, B.A., S.P. Colgan, C. Delp-Archer, et al. *Salmonella typhimurium* attachment to human intestinal epithelial monolayers: transcellular signalling to subepithelial neutrophils. *J. Cell Biol.* 123:895–897 (1993).

326. Groisman, E.A., and H. Ochman. Cognate gene clusters govern invasion of host epithelial cells by *Salmonella typhimurium* and *Shigella flexneri. EMBO J.* 12:3779–3787 (1993).

327. Amin, I.I., G.R. Douce, M.P. Osborne, and J. Stephen. Quantitative studies of invasion of rabbit ileal mucosa by *Salmonella typhimurium* strains which differ in virulence in a model of gastroenteritis. *Infect. Immun.* 62:569–578 (1994).

328. Galdiero, F., L. Sommese, P. Scarfogliero, and M. Galdiero. Biological activities—lethality, Shwartzman reaction and pyrogenicity—of *Salmonella typhimurium* porins. *Microb. Pathogen.* 16:111–119 (1994).

329. Garcia-del Portillo, F., M.B. Zwick, K.Y. Leung, and B.B. Finlay. Intracellular replication of *Salmonella* within epithelial cells is associated with filamentous structures containing lysosomal membrane glycoproteins. *Infect. Agents Dis.* 2:227–231 (1994).

330. Bäumler, A.J., J.G. Kusters, I. Stojiljkovic, and F. Heffron. *Salmonella typhimurium* loci involved in survival within macrophages. *Infect. Immun.* 62:1623–1630 (1994).

331. Libby, S.J., W. Goebel, A. Ludwig, et al. A cytolysin encoded by *Salmonella* is required for survival within macrophages. *Proc. Natl. Acad. Sci. USA* 91:489–493 (1994).

332. Buisán, M., J.M. Rodriguez-Peña, and R. Rotger. Restriction map of the *Salmonella enteritidis* virulence plasmid and its homology with the plasmid of *Salmonella typhimurium. Microb. Pathogen.* 16:165–169 (1994).

333. Spink, J.M., G.D. Pullinger, M.W. Wood, and A.J. Lax. Regulation of *spvR*, the positive regulatory gene of *Salmonella* virulence plasmid virulence genes. *FEMS Microbiol. Lett.* 116:113–121 (1994).

334. Rahman, H., V.B. Singh, and V.D. Sharma. Purification and characterization of enterotoxic moiety present in cell-free culture supernatant of *Salmonella typhimurium. Vet. Microbiol.* 39:245–254 (1994).

335. Chary, P., R. Prasad, A.K. Chopra, and J.W. Peterson. Location of the enterotoxin gene from *Salmonella typhimurium* and characterization of the gene products. *FEMS Microbiol. Lett.* 111:87–92 (1993).

336. Chopra, A.K., J.W. Peterson, P. Chary, and R. Prasad. Molecular characterization of an enterotoxin from *Salmonella typhimurium. Microb. Pathogen.* 16:85–98 (1994).

337. Harne, S.D., V.D. Sharma, and H. Rahman. Purification & antigenicity of *Salmonella newport* enterotoxin. *Indian J. Med. Res.* 99:13–17 (1994).

338. Petter, J.G. Detection of two smooth colony phenotypes in a *Salmonella enteritidis* isolate which vary in their ability to contaminate eggs. *Appl. Environ. Microbiol.* 59:2884–2890 (1993).

339. PHLS Communicable Disease Surveillance Centre. A foodborne outbreak of *Shigella sonnei* infection in Europe. *Commun. Dis. Rep.* 4:115 (1994).

340. Anonymous. Shigellosis sweeps through cruise ship. *Food Protect. Rep.* 10(10):4–5 (1994).

341. Stieglitz, H., and P. Lipsky. Association between reactive arthritis and antecedent infection with *Shigella*

*flexneri* carrying a 2-Md plasmid and encoding an HLA-B27 mimetic epitope. *Arth. Rheum.* 36:1387–1391 (1993).

342. Aleksić, S., A. Katz, V. Aleksić, and J. Bockemühl. Antibiotic resistance of *Shigella* strains isolated in the Federal Republic of Germany 1989–1990. *Zbl. Bakteriol.* 279:484–493 (1993).

343. Preston, M.A., and A.A. Borczyk. Genetic variability and molecular typing of *Shigella sonnei* strains isolated in Canada. *J. Clin. Microbiol.* 32:1427–1430 (1994).

344. June, G.A., P.S. Sherrod, R.M. Amaguana, et al. Effectiveness of the *Bacteriological Analytical Manual* culture method for the recovery of *Shigella sonnei* from selected foods. *J. AOAC Int.* 76:1240–1248 (1993).

345. Oberhelman, R.A., D.J. Kopecko, M.M. Venkatesan, et al. Evaluation of alkaline phosphatase-labelled *ipaH* probe for diagnosis of *Shigella* infections. *J. Clin. Microbiol.* 31:2101–2104 (1993).

346. Karaolis, D.K.R., R. Lan, and P.R. Reeves. Sequence variation in *Shigella sonnei* (Sonnei), a pathogenic clone of *Escherichia*, over four continents and 41 years. *J. Clin. Microbiol.* 32:796–802 (1994).

347. Kozlov, Y.V., M.M. Chernaia, M.E. Fraser, and M.N.G. James. Purification and crystallization of Shiga toxin from *Shigella dysenteriae*. *J. Molec. Biol.* 232:704–706 (1993).

348. Haddad, J.E., A.Y. Al-Jaufy, and M.P. Jackson. Minimum domain of the Shiga toxin A subunit required for enzymatic activity. *J. Bacteriol.* 175:4970–4978 (1993).

349. Suzuki, T., T. Murai, I. Fukuda, et al. Identification and characterization of a chromosomal virulence gene, *vacJ*, required for intercellular spreading of *Shigella flexneri*. *Molec. Microbiol.* 11:31–41 (1994).

350. Goldberg, M.B., and P.J. Sansonetti. *Shigella* subversion of the cellular cytoskeleton: a strategy for epithelial colonization. *Infect. Immun.* 61:4041–4046 (1993).

351. Echeverria, P., O. Serichantalergs, S. Changchawalit, and O. Sethabutr. *Escherichia coli* gastroenteritis: food and waterborne infections. In *Food Poisoning*. A.T. Tu (ed.). New York, Marcel Dekker. *Handbook of Natural Toxins* 7:71–101 (1992).

352. Bettiol, S.S., F.J. Radcliff, A.L.C. Hunt, and J.M. Goldsmid. Bacterial flora of Tasmanian SIDS infants with special reference to pathogenic strains of *Escherichia coli*. *Epidemiol. Infect.* 112:275–284 (1994).

353. Blanco, M., J. Blanco, J.E. Blanco, and J. Ramos. Enterotoxigenic, verotoxigenic, and necrotoxigenic *Escherichia coli* isolated from cattle in Spain *Am. J. Vet. Res.* 54:1446–1451 (1993).

354. Schmidt, H., B. Plaschke, S. Franke, et al. Differentiation in virulence patterns of *Escherichia coli* possessing *eae* genes. *Med. Microbiol. Immunol.* 183:23–31 (1994).

355. Tarkka, E., H. Åhman, and A. Siitonen. Ribotyping as an epidemiologic tool for *Escherichia coli*. *Epidemiol. Infect.* 112:263–274 (1994).

356. Haddad, J.E., and M.P. Jackson. Identification of the Shiga toxin A–subunit residues required for holotoxin assembly. *J. Bacteriol.* 175:7652–7657 (1993).

357. Fielding, L.M., P.E. Cook, and A.S. Grandison. The effect of electron beam irradiation and modified pH on the survival and recovery of *Escherichia coli*. *J. Appl. Bacteriol.* 76:412–416 (1994).

358. Marks, S., and T. Roberts. *E. coli* O157:H7 ranks as the fourth most costly foodborne disease. *Food Rev.* 16(3):51–59 (1993).

359. Voelker, R. Foodborne illness problems more than enteric. *JAMA* 271:8–11 (1994).

360. Dorn, C.R. Review of foodborne outbreak of *Escherichia coli* O157:H7 infection in the western United States. *J. Am. Vet. Med. Assoc.* 203:1583–1587 (1993).

361. O'Brien, A.D., A.R. Melton, C.K. Schmitt, et al. Profile of *Escherichia coli* O157:H7 pathogen responsible for hamburger-borne outbreak of hemorrhagic colitis and hemolytic uremic syndrome in Washington. *J. Clin. Microbiol.* 31:2799–2801 (1993).

362. Centers for Disease Control. *Escherichia coli* O157:H7 outbreak linked to home-cooked hamburger—California, July 1993. *Morbid. Mortal. Weekly Rep.* 43:213–216 (1994).

363. Sharp, J.C.M., J.E. Coia, J. Curnow, and W.J. Reilly. *Escherichia coli* O157 infections in Scotland. *J. Med. Microbiol.* 40:3–9 (1994).

364. Coia, J.E., J. Curnow, and J. Tolland. *Escherichia coli* O157 infections in Scotland, 1992. *Commun. Dis. Environ. Health Scotland Weekly Rep.* 27(38):5–8 (1993).

365. Thomas, A., H. Chart, T. Cheasty, et al. Vero cytotoxin-producing *Escherichia coli*, particularly serogroup O157, associated with human infections in the United Kingdom: 1989–1991. *Epidemiol. Infect.* 110:591–600 (1993).

366. Frost, J.A., T. Cheasty, A. Thomas, and B. Rowe. Phage typing of Vero cytotoxin-producing *Escherichia coli* O157 isolated in the United Kingdom: 1989–1991. *Epidemiol. Infect.* 110:469–475 (1993).

367. Rowe, P.C., E. Orrbine, M. Ogborn, et al. Epidemic *Escherichia coli* O157:H7 gastroenteritis and hemolytic-uremic syndrome in a Canadian Inuit community: intestinal illness in family members as a risk factor. *J. Pediatr.* 124:21–26 (1994).

368. Chapman, P.A., D.J. Wright, and R. Higgins. Untreated milk as a source of verotoxigenic *E coli* O157. (Letter.) *Vet. Rec.* 133:171–172 (1993).

369. Perez, N., R. Rahman, J. Zalba, et al. Haemolytic uraemic syndrome and unpasteurized milk. (Letter.) *Acta Pædiatr.* 83:142 (1994).

370. Morgan, D., C.P. Newman, D.N. Hutchinson, et al. Verotoxin producing *Escherichia coli* O157 infections associated with the consumption of yoghurt. *Epidemiol. Infect.* 111:181–187 (1993).

371. Chapman, P.A., C.A. Siddons, D.J. Wright, et al. Cattle as a possible source of verocytotoxin-producing *Escherichia coli* O157 infections in man. *Epidemiol. Infect.* 111:439–447 (1993).

372. Renwick, S.A., J.B. Wilson, R.C. Clarke, et al. Evidence of direct transmission of *Escherichia coli* O157:H7 infection between calves and a human. (Letter.) *J. Infect. Dis.* 168:792–793 (1993).

373. Synge, B.A., G.F. Hopkins, W.J. Reilly, and J.C.M. Sharp. Possible link between cattle and *E coli* O157 infection in a human. (Letter.) *Vet. Rec.* 133:507 (1993).

374. Cieslak, P.R., T.J. Barrett, P.M. Griffin, et al. *Escherichia coli* O157:H7 infection from a manured garden. (Letter.) *Lancet* 342:367 (1993).

375. Caprioli, A., I. Luzzi, F. Rosmini, et al. Community-wide outbreak of hemolytic-uremic syndrome associated with non-O157 verocytotoxin-producing *Escherichia coli. J. Infect. Dis.* 169:208–211 (1994).

376. Paros, M., P.I. Tarr, H. Kim, et al. A comparison of human and bovine *Escherichia coli* O157:H7 isolates by toxin genotype, plasmid profile, and bacteriophage λ-restriction fragment length polymorphism profile. *J. Infect. Dis.* 168:1300–1303 (1993).

377. Beutin, L., S. Aleksic', S. Zimmermann, and K. Gleier. Virulence factors and phenotypical traits of verotoxigenic strains of *Escherichia coli* isolated from human patients in Germany. *Med. Microbiol. Immunol.* 183:13–21 (1994).

378. Caprioli, A., A. Nigrelli, R. Gatti, et al. Characterisation of verocytotoxin-producing *Escherichia coli* isolated from pigs and cattle in northern Italy. *Vet. Rec.* 133:323–324 (1993).

379. Rüssmann, H., H. Schmidt, J. Heesemann, et al. Variants of Shiga-like toxin II constitute a major toxin component in *Escherichia coli* O157 strains from patients with haemolytic uraemic syndrome. *J. Med. Microbiol.* 40:338–343 (1994).

380. Takeda, T., H. Nakao, T. Yamanaka, et al. High prevalence of serum antibodies to Verotoxins 1 and 2 among healthy adults in Japan. (Letter.) *J. Infect.* 27:211–213 (1993).

381. Beutin, L., D. Geier, H. Steinrück, et al. Prevalence and some properties of verotoxin (Shiga-like toxin)-producing *Escherichia coli* in seven different species of domestic animals. *J. Clin. Microbiol.* 31:2483–2488 (1993).

382. Martin, D.R., P.M. Uhler, A.J.G. Okrend, and J.Y. Chiu. Testing of Bob calf fecal swabs for the presence of *Escherichia coli* O157:H7. *J. Food Protect.* 57:70–72 (1994).

383. Rasmussen, M.A., W.C. Cray, Jr., T.A. Casey, and S.C. Whipp. Rumen contents as a reservoir of entero-hemorrhagic *Escherichia coli. FEMS Microbiol. Lett.* 114:79–84 (1993).

384. Willshaw, G.A., H.R. Smith, D. Roberts, et al. Examination of raw beef products for the presence of Vero cytotoxin producing *Escherichia coli*, particularly those of serogroup O157. *J. Appl. Bacteriol.* 75:420–426 (1993).

385. Cuttler, C.N., and G.R. Siragusa. Efficacy of organic acids against *Escherichia coli* O157:H7 attached to beef carcass tissue using a pilot scale model carcass washer. *J. Food Protect.* 57:97–103 (1994).

386. Brackett, R.E., Y.-Y. Hao, and M.P. Doyle. Ineffectiveness of hot acid sprays to decontaminate *Escherichia coli* O157:H7 on beef. *J. Food Protect.* 57:198–203 (1994).

387. Abdul-Raouf, U.M., L.R. Beuchat, and M.S. Ammar. Survival and growth of *Escherichia coli* O157:H7 in ground, roasted beef as affected by pH, acidulants, and temperature. *Appl. Environ. Microbiol.* 59:2364–2368 (1993).

388. Samadpour, M., J.E. Ongerth, J. Liston, et al. Occurrence of Shiga-like toxin–producing *Escherichia coli* in retail fresh seafood, beef, lamb, pork, and poultry from grocery stores in Seattle, Washington. *Appl. Environ. Microbiol.* 60:1038–1040 (1994).

389. Abdul-Raouf, U.M., L.R. Beuchat, and M.S. Ammar. Survival and growth of *Escherichia coli* O157:H7 on salad vegetables. *Appl. Environ. Microbiol.* 59:1999–2006 (1993).

390. Zhao, T., M.P. Doyle, and R.E. Besser. Fate of enterohemorrhagic *Escherichia coli* O157:H7 in apple cider with and without preservatives. *Appl. Environ. Microbiol.* 59:2526–2530 (1993).

391. Miller, L.G., and C.W. Kaspar. *Escherichia coli* O157:H7 acid tolerance and survival in apple cider. *J. Food Protect.* 57:460–464 (1994).

392. Murano, E.A., and M.D. Pierson. Effect of heat shock and incubation atmosphere on injury and recovery of *Escherichia coli* O157:H7. *J. Food Protect.* 56:568–572 (1993).

393. Buchanan, R.L., L.K. Bagi, R.V. Goins, and J.G. Phillips. Response surface models for the growth kinetics of *Escherichia coli* O157:H7. *Food Microbiol.* 10:303–315 (1993).

394. Zadik, P.M., P.A. Chapman, and C.A. Siddons. Use of tellurite for the selection of verocytotoxigenic *Escherichia coli* O157. *J. Med. Microbiol.* 39:155–158 (1993).

395. Chart, H., B. Said, N. Stokes, and B. Rowe. Heterogeneity in expression of lipopolysaccharides by strains of *Escherichia coli* O157. *J. Infect.* 27:237–241 (1993).

396. Samadpour, M., L.M. Grimm, B. Desai, et al. Molecular epidemiology of *Escherichia coli* O157:H7 strains by bacteriophage λ restriction fragment length polymorphism analysis: application to a multistate foodborne outbreak and a day-care center cluster. *J. Clin. Microbiol.* 31:3179–3183 (1993).

397. Harsono, K.D., C.W. Kaspar, and J.B. Luchansky. Comparison and genomic sizing of *Escherichia coli* O157:H7 isolates by pulsed-field gel electrophoresis. *Appl. Environ. Microbiol.* 59:3141–3144 (1993).

398. Milley, D.G., and L.H. Sekla. An enzyme–linked immunosorbent assay–based isolation procedure for verotoxigenic *Escherichia coli. Appl. Environ. Microbiol.* 59:4223–4229 (1993).

399. Chart, H., S. Montgomery, and B. Rowe. A rapid immunoblotting procedure for detecting serum antibodies to the lipopolysaccharide of *Escherichia coli* O157. *Lett. Appl. Microbiol.* 18:100–101 (1994).

400. Greatorex, J.S., and G.M. Thorne. Humoral immune responses to Shiga-like toxins and *Escherichia coli* O157 lipopolysaccharide in hemolytic-uremic syndrome patients and healthy subjects. *J. Clin. Microbiol.* 32:1172–1178 (1994).

401. Karmali, M.A., M. Petric, M. Winkler, et al. Enzyme-linked immunosorbent assay for detection of immunoglobulin G antibodies to *Escherichia coli* Vero cytotoxin 1. *J. Clin. Microbiol.* 32:1457–1463 (1994).

402. Law, D., A.A. Hamour, D.E.K. Acheson, et al. Diagnosis of infections with Shiga-like toxin–producing *Escherichia coli* by use of enzyme-linked immunosorbent assays for Shiga-

like toxins on cultured stool samples. *J. Med. Microbiol.* 40:241–245 (1994).

403. Siddons, C.A., and P.A. Chapman. Detection of serum and faecal antibodies in haemorrhagic colitis caused by *Escherichia coli* O157. *J. Med. Microbiol.* 39:408–415 (1993).

404. Samadpour, M., J.E. Ongerth, and J. Liston. Development and evaluation of oligonucleotide DNA probes for detection and genotyping of Shiga-like toxin producing *Escherichia coli*. *J. Food Protect.* 57:399–402 (1994).

405. Bialkowska-Hobrzanska, H., R.F. Fletcher, M. Hurley, et al. Development of sandwich hybridization assay for the detection of Shiga-like toxin I and Shiga-like toxin II determinants in *Escherichia coli*. *Med. Microbiol. Lett.* 2:411–418 (1993).

406. Willshaw, G.A., S.M. Scotland, H.R. Smith, et al. Hybridization of strains of *Escherichia coli* O157 with probes derived from the *eaeA* gene of enteropathogenic *E. coli* and the *eaeA* homolog from a Vero cytotoxin–producing strain of *E. coli* O157. *J. Clin. Microbiol.* 32:897–902 (1994).

407. Begum, D., N.A. Strockbine, E.G. Sowers, and M.P. Jackson. Evaluation of a technique for identification of Shiga-like toxin–producing *Escherichia coli* by using a polymerase chain reaction and digoxigenin-labeled probes. *J. Clin. Microbiol.* 31:3153–3156 (1993).

408. Paton, A.W., J.C. Paton, P.N. Goldwater, and P.A. Manning. Direct detection of *Escherichia coli* Shiga-like toxin genes in primary fecal cultures by polymerase chain reaction. *J. Clin. Microbiol.* 31:3063–3067 (1993).

409. Park, C.H., D.L. Hixon, W.L. Morrison, and C.B. Cook. Rapid diagnosis of enterohemorrhagic *Escherichia coli* O157:H7 directly from fecal specimens using immunofluorescence stain. *Am. J. Clin. Pathol.* 101:91–94 (1994).

410. Tortorello, M.L., and S.M. Gendel. Fluorescent antibodies applied to direct epifluorescent filter technique for microscopic enumeration of *Escherichia coli* O157:H7 in milk and juice. *J. Food Protect.* 56:672–677 (1993).

411. Ogden, I.D. A conductance assay for the detection and enumeration of *Escherichia coli*. *Food Microbiol.* 10:321–327 (1993).

412. Takeda, Y., H. Kurazono, and S. Yamasaki. Vero toxins (Shiga-like toxins) produced by enterohemorrhagic *Escherichia coli* (verocytotoxin-producing *E. coli*). *Microbiol. Immunol.* 37:591–599 (1993).

413. Hofmann, S.L. Shiga-like toxins in hemolytic-uremic syndrome and thrombotic thrombocytopenic purpura. *Am. J. Med. Sci.* 306:398–406 (1993).

414. Lindgren, S.W., J.E. Samuel, C.K. Schmitt, and A.D. O'Brien. The specific activities of Shiga-like toxin type II (SLT-II) and SLT-II-related toxins of enterohemorrhagic *Escherichia coli* differ when measured by Vero cell cytotoxicity but not by mouse lethality. *Infect. Immun.* 62:623–631 (1994).

415. Sjogren, R., R. Neill, D. Rachmilewitz, et al. Role of Shiga-like toxin I in bacterial enteritis: comparison between isogenic *Escherichia coli* strains induced in rabbits. *Gastroenterology* 106:306–317 (1994).

416. Tarr, P.I. Enterocolitis associated with Shiga-like toxin production: an appropriate animal model at last? *Gastroenterology* 106:540–543 (1994).

417. Fratamico, P.M., R.L. Buchanan, and P.H. Cooke. Virulence of an *Escherichia coli* O157:H7 sorbitol-positive mutant. *Appl. Environ. Microbiol.* 59:4245–4252 (1993).

418. Tesh, V.L., J.A. Burris, J.W. Owens, et al. Comparison of the relative toxicities of Shiga-like toxins type I and type II for mice. *Infect. Immun.* 61:3392–3402 (1993).

419. Takeda, T., S. Dohi, T. Igarashi, et al. Impairment by Verotoxin of tubular function contributes to the renal damage seen in haemolytic uraemic syndrome. (Letter.) *J. Infect.* 27:339–341 (1993).

420. Harel, Y., M. Silva, B. Giroir, et al. A reported transgene indicates renal-specific induction of tumor necrosis factor (TNF) by Shiga-like toxin. *J. Clin. Invest.* 92:2100–2116 (1993).

421. Austin, P.R., P.E. Jablonski, G.A. Bohach, et al. Evidence that the $A_2$ fragment of Shiga-like toxin type I is required for holotoxin integrity. *Infect. Immun.* 62:1768–1775 (1994).

422. Burgess, B.J., and L.M. Roberts. Proteolytic cleavage at arginine residues within the hydrophilic disulphide loop of the *Escherichia coli* Shiga-like toxin I A subunit is not essential for cytotoxicity. *Molec. Microbiol.* 10:171–179 (1993).

423. Samuel, J.E., and V.M. Gordon. Evidence that proteolytic separation of Shiga-like toxin type IIv A subunit into $A_1$ and $A_2$ subunits is not required for toxin activity. *J. Biol. Chem.* 269:4853–4859 (1994).

424. Deresiewicz, R.L., P.R. Austin, and C.J. Hovde. The role of tyrosine-114 in the enzymatic activity of the Shiga-like toxin I A-chain. *Molec. Gen. Genet.* 241:467–473 (1993).

425. Rüssmann, H., H. Schmidt, A. Caprioli, and H. Karch. Highly conserved B-subunit genes of Shiga-like toxin II variants found in *Escherichia coli* O157:H7 strains. *FEMS Microbiol. Lett.* 118:335–340 (1994).

426. Lin, Z., S. Yamasaki, H. Kurazono, et al. Cloning and sequencing of two new Verotoxin 2 variant genes of *Escherichia coli* isolated from cases of human and bovine diarrhea. *Microbiol. Immunol.* 37:451–459 (1993).

427. Lin, Z., H. Kurazono, S. Yamasaki, and Y. Takeda. Detection of various variant Verotoxin genes in *Escherichia coli* by polymerase chain reaction. *Microbiol. Immunol.* 37:543–548 (1993).

428. Paton, A.W., J.C. Paton, and P.A. Manning. Polymerase chain reaction amplification, cloning and sequencing of variant *Escherichia coli* Shiga-like toxin type II operons. *Microb. Pathogen.* 15:77–82 (1993).

429. Paton, A.W., J.C. Paton, P.N. Goldwater, et al. Sequence of a variant Shiga-like toxin type-I operon of *Escherichia coli* O111:H⁻. *Gene* 129:87–92 (1993).

430. Fratamico, P.M., S. Bhaduri, and R.L. Buchanan. Studies on *Escherichia coli* O157:H7 strains containing a 60-MDa plasmid and on 60-MDa plasmid-cured derivatives. *J. Med. Microbiol.* 39:371–381 (1993).

431. Dytoc, M., R. Soni, F. Cockerill III, et al. Multiple determinants of Verotoxin-producing *Escherichia coli* O157:H7 attachment–effacement. *Infect. Immun.* 61:3382–3391 (1993).

432. Donnenberg, M.S., S. Tzipori, M.L. McKee, et al. The role of the *eae* gene of enterohemorrhagic *Escherichia coli* in intimate attachment in vitro and in a porcine model. *J. Clin. Invest.* 92:1418–1424 (1993).

433. Louie, M., J.C.S. de Azavedo, M.Y.C. Handelsman, et al. Expression and characterization of the *eaeA* gene product of *Escherichia coli* serotype O157:H7. *Infect. Immun.* 61:4085–4092 (1993).

434. Yam, W.C., R.M. Robins-Browne, and M.L. Lung. Genetic relationships and virulence factors among classical enteropathogenic *Escherichia coli* serogroup O126 strains. *J. Med. Microbiol.* 40:229–235 (1994).

435. Donnenberg, M.S., C.O. Tacket, S.P. James, et al. Role of the *eaeA* gene in experimental enteropathogenic *Escherichia coli* infection. *J. Clin. Invest.* 92:1412–1417 (1993).

436. Law, D. Adhesion and its role in the virulence of enteropathogenic *Escherichia coli*. *Clin. Microbiol. Rev.* 7:152–173 (1994).

437. Girón, J.A., A.S.Y. Ho, and G.K. Schoolnik. Characterization of fimbriae produced by enteropathogenic *Escherichia coli*. *J. Bacteriol.* 175:7391–7403 (1993).

438. Scotland, S.M., G.A. Willshaw, H.R. Smith, et al. Virulence properties of *Escherichia coli* strains belonging to serogroups O26, O55, O111 and O128 isolated in the United Kingdom in 1991 from patients with diarrhoea. *Epidemiol. Infect.* 111:429–438 (1993).

439. Scott, D.A., and J.B. Kaper. Cloning and sequencing of the genes encoding *Escherichia coli* cytolethal distending toxin. *Infect. Immun.* 62:244–251 (1994).

440. Foubister, V., I. Rosenshine, and B.B. Finlay. A diarrheal pathogen, enteropathogenic *Escherichia coli* (EPEC), triggers a flux of inositol phosphates in infected epithelial cells. *J. Exp. Med.* 179:993–998 (1994).

441. Centers for Disease Control. Foodborne outbreaks of enterotoxigenic *Escherichia coli*—Rhode Island and New Hampshire, 1993. *Morbid. Mortal. Weekly Rep.* 43:81,87–89 (1994).

442. Chérifi, A., M. Contrepois, B. Picard, et al. Clonal relationships among *Escherichia coli* serogroup O78 isolates from human and animal infections. *J. Clin. Microbiol.* 32:1197–1202 (1994).

443. Ghosh, A.R., D. Sen, D.A. Sack, and A.T.M.S. Hoque. Evaluation of conventional media for detection of colonization factor antigens of enterotoxigenic *Escherichia coli*. *J. Clin. Microbiol.* 31:2163–2166 (1993).

444. Grewal, H.M.S., A. Helander, A.-M. Svennerholm, et al. Genotypic and phenotypic identification of coli surface antigen 6-positive enterotoxigenic *Escherichia coli*. *J. Clin. Microbiol.* 32:1295–1301 (1994).

445. Uesaka, Y., Y. Otsuka, Z. Lin, et al. Simple method of purification of *Escherichia coli* heat-labile enterotoxin and cholera toxin using immobilized galactose. *Microb. Pathogen.* 16:71–76 (1994).

446. Shida, K., K. Takamizawa, M. Nagaoka, et al. *Escherichia coli* heat-labile enterotoxin binds to glycosylated proteins with lactose by amino carbonyl reaction. *Microb. Immunol.* 38:273–279 (1994).

447. Girón, J.A., M.M. Levine, and J.B. Kaper. Longus: a long pilus ultrastructure produced by human enterotoxigenic *Escherichia coli*. *Molec. Microbiol.* 12:71–82 (1994).

448. Viboud, G.I., N. Binsztein, and A.-M. Svennerholm. A new fimbrial putative colonization factor, PCFO20, in human enterotoxigenic *Escherichia coli*. *Infect. Immun.* 61:5190–5197 (1993).

449. Savarino, S.J. Enteroadherent *Escherichia coli*: a heterogeneous group of *E. coli* implicated as diarrhoeal pathogens. *Trans. Roy. Soc. Trop. Med. Hyg.* 87(Suppl. 3):49–53 (1993).

450. Brook, M.G., H.R. Smith, B.A. Bannister, et al. Prospective study of verocytotoxin-producing, enteroaggregative and diffusely adherent *Escherichia coli* in different diarrhoeal states. *Epidemiol. Infect.* 112:63–67 (1994).

451. Bhatnagar, S., M.K. Bhan, H. Sommerfelt, et al. Enteroaggregative *Escherichia coli* may be a new pathogen causing acute and persistent diarrhea. *Scand. J. Infect. Dis.* 25:579–583 (1993).

452. Paul, M., T. Tsukamoto, A.R. Ghosh, et al. The significance of enteroaggregative *Escherichia coli* in the etiology of hospitalized diarrhoea in Calcutta, India and the demonstration of a new honey-combed pattern of aggregative adherence. *FEMS Microbiol. Lett.* 117:319–326 (1994).

453. Qadri, F., A. Haque, S.M. Faruque, et al. Hemagglutinating properties of enteroaggregative *Escherichia coli*. *J. Clin. Microbiol.* 32:510–514 (1994).

454. Matsushita, S., S. Yamada, A. Kai, and Y. Kudoh. Invasive strains of *Escherichia coli* belonging to serotype O121:NM. *J. Clin. Microbiol.* 31:3034–3035 (1993).

455. Hsia, R.-C., P.L.C. Small, and P.M. Bavoil. Characterization of virulence genes of enteroinvasive *Escherichia coli* by Tn*phoA* mutagenesis: identification of *invX*, a gene required for entry into HEp-2 cells. *J. Bacteriol.* 175:4817–4823 (1993).

456. Bratoeva, M.P., M.K. Wolf, J.K. Marks, and J.R. Cantey. A case of diarrhea, bacteremia, and fever caused by a novel strain of *Escherichia coli*. *J. Clin. Microbiol.* 32:1383–1386 (1994).

457. Ostroff, S.M., G. Kapperud, L.C. Hutwagner, et al. Sources of sporadic *Yersinia enterocolitica* infections in Norway: a prospective case-control study. *Epidemiol. Infect.* 112:133–141 (1994).

458. Fukushima, H., M. Gomyoda, S. Kaneko, et al. Restriction endonuclease analysis of virulence plasmids for molecular epidemiology of *Yersinia pseudotuberculosis* infections. *J. Clin. Microbiol.* 32:1410–1413 (1994).

459. Chandler, N.D., and M.T. Parisi. Radiological cases of the month. Case 2. *Arch. Pediatr. Adolesc. Med.* 148:527–528 (1994).

460. Probst, P., E. Hermann, K.-H. Meyer zum Büschenfelde, and B. Fleischer. Identification of the *Yersinia enterocolitica* urease β subunit as a target antigen for human

synovial T lymphocytes in reactive arthritis. *Infect. Immun.* 61:4507–4509 (1993).

461. Saebø, A., H. Nyland, and J. Lassen. *Yersinia enterocolitica* infection—an unrecognized cause of acute and chronic neurological disease? A 10-year follow-up study on 458 hospitalized patients. *Med. Hypoth.* 41:282–286 (1993).

462. Saebø, A., K. Elgjo, and J. Lassen. Could development of malignant mesothelioma be induced by *Yersinia enterocolitica* infection? *Med. Hypoth.* 40:275–277 (1993).

463. de Boer, E. Vorkommen von *Yersinia*-Arten in Geflügelprodukten. *Fleischwirtschaft* 74:329–330 (1994).

464. dos Reis Tassinari, A., B.D.G. de Melo Franco, and M. Landgraf. Incidence of *Yersinia* spp. in food in Sao Paulo, Brazil. *Int. J. Food Microbiol.* 21:263–270 (1994).

465. Kleeman, J., and G. Scheibner. Verhalten von *Yersinia enterocolitica* in frischen Rohwürsten. *Fleischwirtschaft* 73:783–785 (1993).

466. Asplund, K., E. Nurmi, J. Hirn, et al. Survival of *Yersinia enterocolitica* in fermented sausages manufactured with different levels of nitrite and different starter cultures. *J. Food Protect.* 56:710–712 (1993).

467. Manu-Tawiah, W., D.J. Myers, D.G. Olson, and R.A. Molins. Survival and growth of *Listeria monocytogenes* and *Yersinia enterocolitica* in pork chops packaged under modified gas atmospheres. *J. Food Sci.* 58:475–479 (1993).

468. Rodríguez, J.M., O.J. Sobrino, W.L. Moreira, et al. Inhibition of *Yersinia enterocolitica* by *Lactobacillus sake* strains of meat origin. *Meat Sci.* 37:305–313 (1994).

469. Little, C.L., M.R. Adams, W.A. Anderson, and M.B. Cole. Application of a log-logistic model to describe the survival of *Yersinia enterocolitica* at sub-optimal pH and temperature. *Int. J. Food Microbiol.* 22:63–71 (1994).

470. Lindberg, C.W., and E. Borch. Predicting the aerobic growth of *Y. enterocolitica* O:3 at different pH-values, temperatures and L-lactate concentrations using conductance measurements. *Int. J. Food Microbiol.* 22:141–153 (1994).

471. Sutherland, J.P., and A.J. Bayliss. Predictive modelling of growth of *Yersinia enterocolitica*: the effects of temperature, pH and sodium chloride. *Int. J. Food Microbiol.* 21:197–215 (1994).

472. Manafi, M., and E. Holzhammer. Comparison of the Vitek, API 20E and Gene-trak® systems for the identification of *Yersinia enterocolitica*. *Lett. Appl. Microbiol.* 18:90–92 (1994).

473. Bosi, E., P. Madié, and C.R. Wilks. Growth of *Yersinia pseudotuberculosis* on selective media. (Letter.) *N.Z. Vet. J.* 42:35 (1994).

474. Amirmozafari, N., and D.C. Robertson. Nutritional requirements for synthesis of heat-stable enterotoxin by *Yersinia enterocolitica*. *Appl. Environ. Microbiol.* 59:3314–3320 (1993).

475. Fukushima, H., K. Hoshina, and M. Gomyoda. Selective isolation from HeLa cell lines of *Yersinia pseudotuberculosis*, pathogenic *Y. enterocolitica* and enteroinvasive *Escherichia coli*. *Zbl. Bakteriol.* 280:332–337 (1994).

476. Makino, S.-I., Y. Okada, T. Maruyama, et al. PCR-based random amplified polymorphic DNA fingerprinting of *Yersinia pseudotuberculosis* and its practical applications. *J. Clin. Microbiol.* 32:65–69 (1994).

477. Kapperud, G., T. Vardund, E. Skjerve, et al. Detection of pathogenic *Yersinia enterocolitica* in foods and water by immunomagnetic separation, nested polymerase chain reactions, and colorimetric detection of amplified DNA. *Appl. Environ. Microbiol.* 59:2938–2944 (1993).

478. Cremer, J., M. Putzker, M. Faulde, and L. Zöller. Immunoblotting of *Yersinia* plasmid-encoded released proteins: a tool for serodiagnosis. *Electrophoresis* 14:952–959 (1993).

479. Li, Q., and W.E. Magee. An antibody adsorption technique facilitates antigen selection for development of serotype-specific monoclonal antibodies to *Yersinia enterocolitica*. *BioTechniques* 14:962–971 (1993).

480. Koeppel, E., R. Meyer, J. Luethy, and U. Candrian. Recognition of pathogenic *Yersinia enterocolitica* by crystal violet binding and polymerase chain reaction. *Lett. Appl. Microbiol.* 17:231–234 (1993).

481. Tomita, M., S. Matsusaki, A. Katayama, et al. The salting-out test to identify virulent *Yersinia pseudotuberculosis*. *Zbl. Bakteriol.* 279:231–238 (1993).

482. Bhaduri, S., and C. Turner-Jones. The effect of anaerobic atmospheres on the stability of the virulence-related characteristics in *Yersinia enterocolitica*. *Food Microbiol.* 10:239–242 (1993).

483. Mantle, M., and S.D. Husar. Adhesion of *Yersinia enterocolitica* to purified rabbit and human intestinal mucin. *Infect. Immun.* 61:2340–2346 (1993).

484. Mantle, M., and C. Rombough. Growth in and breakdown of purified rabbit small intestinal mucin by *Yersinia enterocolitica*. *Infect. Immun.* 61:4131–4138 (1993).

485. Mantle, M., and S.D. Husar. Binding of *Yersinia enterocolitica* to purified, native small intestinal mucins from rabbits and humans involves interactions with the mucin carbohydrate moiety. *Infect. Immun.* 62:1219–1227 (1994).

486. Grützkau, A., C. Hanski, and M. Naumann. Comparative study of histopathological alterations during intestinal infection of mice with pathogenic and non-pathogenic strains of *Yersinia enterocolitica* serotype O:8. *Virch. Archiv A* 423:97–103 (1993).

487. Rosqvist, R., K.-E. Magnusson, and H. Wolf-Watz. Target cell contact triggers expression and polarized transfer of *Yersinia* YopE cytotoxin into mammalian cells. *EMBO J.* 13:964–972 (1994).

488. Pepe, J.C., and V.L. Miller. *Yersinia enterocolitica* invasin: a primary role in the initiation of infection. *Proc. Natl. Acad. Sci. USA* 90:6473–6477 (1993).

489. Pepe, J.C., J.L. Badger, and V.L. Miller. Growth phase and low pH affect the thermal regulation of the *Yersinia enterocolitica inv* gene. *Molec. Microbiol.* 11:123–135 (1994).

490. Skurnik, M., Y. El Tahir, M. Saarinen, et al. YadA mediates specific binding of enteropathogenic *Yersinia enterocolitica* to human intestinal submucosa. *Infect. Immun.* 62:1252–1261 (1994).

491. China, B., B.T. N'Guyen, M. de Bruyere, and G.R. Cornelis. Role of YadA in resistance of *Yersinia enterocolitica*

to phagocytosis by human polymorphonuclear leukocytes. *Infect. Immun.* 62:1275–1281 (1994).

492. Yamamoto, T., T. Hanawa, and S. Ogata. Induction of *Yersinia enterocolitica* stress proteins by phagocytosis with macrophage. *Microbiol. Immunol.* 38:295–300 (1994).

493. Bielecki, J., I. Hejduk, J. Wiśniewski, and J. Hrebenda. Lack of correlation between the presence of 70 kb plasmid and plasmid-associated determinants of *Yersinia enterocolitica*. *Microbios* 77:87–94 (1994).

494. Kwaga, J., and J.O. Iversen. Plasmids and outer membrane proteins of *Yersinia enterocolitica* and related species of swine origin. *Vet. Microbiol.* 36:205–214 (1993).

495. Straley, S.C., E. Skrzypek, G.V. Plano, and J.B. Bliska. Yops of *Yersinia* spp. pathogenic for humans. *Infect. Immun.* 61:3105–3110 (1993).

496. Chambers, C.E., and P.A. Sokol. Comparison of siderophore production and utilization in pathogenic and environmental isolates of *Yersinia enterocolitica. J. Clin. Microbiol.* 32:32–39 (1994).

497. Haag, H., K. Hantke, H. Drechsel, et al. Purification of yersiniabactin: a siderophore and possible virulence factor of *Yersinia enterocolitica. J. Gen. Microbiol.* 139:2159–2165 (1993).

498. Östling, J., L. Holmquist, K. Flärdh, et al. Starvation and recovery of *Vibrio*. In *Starvation in Bacteria*. S. Kjelleberg (ed.). New York, Plenum Press. Pp. 103–127 (1993).

499. Oliver, J.D. Formation of viable but nonculturable cells. In *Starvation in Bacteria*. S. Kjelleberg (ed.). New York, Plenum Press. Pp. 239–272 (1993).

500. Klontz, K.C., L. Williams, L.M. Baldy, and M. Campos. Raw oyster-associated *Vibrio* infections: linking epidemiologic data with laboratory testing of oysters obtained from a retail outlet. *J. Food Protect.* 56:977–979 (1993).

501. Wong, H.-C., W.-R. Shieh, and Y.-S. Lee. Toxigenic characterization of *Vibrios* isolated from foods available in Taiwan. *J. Food Protect.* 56:980–982 (1993).

502. Alsina, M., and A.R. Blanch. A set of keys for biochemical identification of environmental *Vibrio* species. *J. Appl. Bacteriol.* 76:79–85 (1994).

503. Abbott, S.L., W.W.K.W. Cheung, and J.M. Janda. Evaluation of a new selective agar, thiosulfate-chloride-iodide (TCI), for the growth of pathogenic *Vibrio* species. *Med. Microbiol. Lett.* 2:362–370 (1993).

504. Hagen, C.J., E.M. Sloan, G.A. Lancette, et al. Enumeration of *Vibrio parahaemolyticus* and *Vibrio vulnificus* in various seafoods with two enrichment broths. *J. Food Protect.* 57:403–409 (1994).

505. Kaysner, C.A., C. Abeyta, Jr., K.C. Jinneman, and W.E. Hill. Enumeration and differentiation of *Vibrio parahaemolyticus* and *Vibrio vulnificus* by DNA–DNA colony hybridization using the hydrophobic grid membrane filtration technique for isolation. *J. Food Protect.* 57:163–165 (1994).

506. Rodrigues, D.P., R.V. Ribeiro, R.M. Alves, and E. Hofer. Evaluation of virulence factors in environmental isolates of *Vibrio* species. *Mem. Inst. Oswaldo Cruz* 88:589–592 (1993).

507. Coelho, A., H. Momen, A.C.P. Vicente, and C.A. Salles. An analysis of the V1 and V2 regions of *Vibrio cholerae* and *Vibrio mimicus* 16S rRNA. *Res. Microbiol.* 145:151–156 (1994).

508. World Health Organization. Cholera—update, end of 1993. *Weekly Epidemiol. Rec.* 69:13–17 (1994).

509. World Health Organization. Cholera in 1993—part I. *Weekly Epidemiol. Rec.* 69:205–212 (1994).

510. World Health Organization. Cholera in 1993—part II. *Weekly Epidemiol. Rec.* 69:213–216 (1994).

511. Popovic, T., Ø. Olsvik, P.A. Blake, and K. Wachsmuth. Cholera in the Americas: foodborne aspects. *J. Food Protect.* 56:811–821 (1993).

512. Weber, J.T., E.D. Mintz, R. Cañizares, et al. Epidemic cholera in Ecuador: multidrug-resistance and transmission by water and seafood. *Epidemiol. Infect.* 112:1–11 (1994).

513. Threlfall, E.J., B. Said, and B. Rowe. Emergence of multiple drug resistance in *Vibrio cholerae* O1 El Tor from Ecuador. (Letter.) *Lancet* 342:1173 (1993).

514. Rossi, A., M. Galas, N. Binztein, et al. Unusual multiresistant *Vibrio cholerae* O1 El Tor in Argentina. (Letter.) *Lancet* 342:1172 (1993).

515. World Health Organization. Cholera. *Weekly Epidemiol. Rec.* 69:332 (1994).

516. Colombo, M.M., M. Francisco, B.D. Ferreira, et al. The early stage of the recurrent cholera epidemic in Luanda, Angola. *Eur. J. Epidemiol.* 9:563–565 (1993).

517. Epstein, P.R. Algal blooms in the spread and persistence of cholera. *BioSystems* 31:209–221 (1993).

518. Nair, G.B., and Y. Takeda. *Vibrio cholerae* in disguise—a disturbing entity. *World J. Microbiol. Biotechnol.* 9:399–400 (1993).

519. Mandal, B.K. Epidemic cholera due to a novel strain of *V. cholerae* non-O1—the beginning of a new pandemic? *J. Infect.* 27:115–117 (1993).

520. Swerdlo, D.L., and A.A. Ries. *Vibrio cholerae* non-O1—the eighth pandemic? *Lancet* 342:382–383 (1993).

521. Cholera Working Group, International Centre for Diarrhoeal Diseases Research, Bangladesh. Large epidemic of cholera-like disease in Bangladesh caused by *Vibrio cholerae* O139 synonym bengal. *Lancet* 342:387–390 (1993).

522. Hall, R.H., F.M. Khambaty, M. Kothary, and S.P. Keasler. Non-O1 *Vibrio cholerae*. (Letter.) *Lancet* 342:430 (1993).

523. Islam, M.S., M.K. Hasan, M.A. Miah, et al. Isolation of *Vibrio cholerae* O139 Bengal from water in Bangladesh. (Letter.) *Lancet* 342:430 (1993).

524. Islam, M.S., M.K. Hasan, M.A. Miah, et al. Isolation of *Vibrio cholerae* O139 synonym Bengal from the aquatic environment in Bangladesh: implications for disease transmission. *Appl. Environ. Microbiol.* 60:1684–1686 (1994).

525. Chongsa-nguan, M., W. Chaicumpa, P. Moolasart, et al. *Vibrio cholerae* O139 Bengal in Bangkok. (Letter.) *Lancet* 342:430–431 (1993).

526. Fisher-Hoch, S.P., A. Khan, Inam-ul-Haq, et al. *Vibrio cholerae* O139 in Karachi, Pakistan. (Letter.) *Lancet* 342:1422–1423 (1993).

527. Jesudason, M.V., A.M. Cherian, and T.J. John. Blood stream invasion by *Vibrio cholerae* O139. (Letter.) *Lancet* 342:431 (1993).

528. Cheasty, T., B. Said, B. Rowe, and J. Frost. *Vibrio cholerae* serogroup O139 in England and Wales. (Letter.) *Br. Med. J.* 307:1007 (1993).

529. Faruque, A.S.G., D. Mahalanabis, S.S. Hoque, and M.J. Albert. The relationship between ABO blood groups and susceptibility to diarrhea due to *Vibrio cholerae* O139. (Letter.) *Clin. Infect. Dis.* 18:827–828 (1994).

530. Garg, S., T. Ramamurthy, A.K. Mukhopadhyay, et al. Production and cross-reactivity patterns of a panel of high affinity monoclonal antibodies to *Vibrio cholerae* O139 Bengal. *FEMS Immunol. Med. Microbiol.* 8:293–298 (1994).

531. Qadri, F., A. Chowdhury, J. Hossain, et al. Development and evaluation of rapid monoclonal antibody–based coagglutination test for direct detection of *Vibrio cholerae* O139 synonym Bengal in stool samples. *J. Clin. Microbiol.* 32:1589–1590 (1994).

532. Waldor, M.K., and J.J. Mekalanos. *Vibrio cholerae* O139 specific gene sequences. (Letter.) *Lancet* 343:1366 (1994).

533. Higa, N., Y. Honma, M.J. Albert, and M. Iwanaga. Characterization of *Vibrio cholerae* O139 synonym bengal isolated from patients with cholera-like disease in Bangladesh. *Microbiol. Immunol.* 37:971–974 (1993).

534. Johnson, J.A., C.A. Salles, P. Panigrahi, et al. *Vibrio cholerae* O139 synonym Bengal is closely related to *Vibrio cholerae* El tor but has important differences. *Infect. Immun.* 62:2108–2110 (1994).

535. Calia, K.E., M. Murtagh, M.J. Ferraro, and S.B. Calderwood. Comparison of *Vibrio cholerae* O139 with *V. cholerae* O1 classical and El Tor biotypes. *Infect. Immun.* 62:1504–1506 (1994).

536. Hisatsune, K., S. Kondo, Y. Isshiki, et al. O-antigenic lipopolysaccharide of *Vibrio cholerae* O139 Bengal, a new epidemic strain for recent cholera in the Indian subcontinent. *Biochem. Biophys. Res. Commun.* 196:1309–1315 (1993).

537. Sengupta, T.K., D.K. Sengupta, G.B. Nair, and A.C. Ghose. Epidemic isolates of *Vibrio cholerae* O139 express antigenically distinct types of colonization pili. *FEMS Microbiol. Lett.* 118:265–272 (1994).

538. Nakasone, N., T. Yamashiro, M.J. Albert, and M. Iwanaga. Pili of a *Vibrio cholerae* O139. *Microbiol. Immunol.* 38:225–227 (1994).

539. Yamashiro, T., N. Nakasone, Y. Honma, et al. Purification and characterization of *Vibrio cholerae* O139 fimbriae. *FEMS Microbiol. Lett.* 115:247–252 (1994).

540. Faruque, S.M., A.R.M.A. Alim, S.K. Roy, et al. Molecular analysis of rRNA and cholera toxin genes carried by the new epidemic strain of toxigenic *Vibrio cholerae* O139 synonym Bengal. *J. Clin. Microbiol.* 32:1050–1053 (1994).

541. Das, B., R.K. Ghosh, C. Sharma, et al. Tandem repeats of cholera toxin gene in *Vibrio cholerae* O139. (Letter.) *Lancet* 342:1173–1174 (1993).

542. Iida, T., J. Shrestha, K. Yamamoto, et al. Cholera isolates in relation to the 'Eighth Pandemic'. (Letter.) *Lancet* 342:926 (1993).

543. Bhadra, R.K., S.R. Choudhury, and J. Das. *Vibrio cholerae* O139 El Tor biotype. (Letter.) *Lancet* 343:728 (1994).

544. Kaysner, C.A. Cholera infection and poisoning. In *Food Poisoning*. A.T. Tu (ed.). New York, Marcel Dekker. *Handbook of Natural Toxins* 7:155–170 (1992).

545. Weber, J.T., W.C. Levine, D.P. Hopkins, and R.V. Tauxe. Cholera in the United States, 1965–1991. Risks at home and abroad. *Arch. Intern. Med.* 154:551–556 (1994).

546. Usera, M.A., A. Echeita, Ø. Olsvik, et al. Molecular subtyping of *Vibrio cholerae* O1 strains recently isolated from patient, food and environmental samples in Spain. *Eur. J. Clin. Microbiol. Infect. Dis.* 13:299–303 (1994).

547. Newman, C., M. Shepherd, M.D. Woodard, et al. Fatal septicemia and bullae caused by non-O1 *Vibrio cholerae*. *J. Am. Acad. Dermatol.* 29:909–912 (1993).

548. Chan, H.-L., H.-C. Ho, and T.-t. Kuo. Cutaneous manifestations of non-O1 *Vibrio cholerae* septicemia with gastroenteritis and meningitis. *J. Am. Acad. Dermatol.* 30:626–628 (1994).

549. Gomez, N.A., J. Gutierrez, and C.J. Leon. Acute acalculous cholecystitis due to *Vibrio cholerae*. (Letter.) *Lancet* 343:1156–1157 (1994).

550. Corrales, M.T., A.E. Bainotti, and A.C. Simonetta. Survival of *Vibrio cholerae* O1 in common foodstuffs during storage at different temperatures. *Lett. Appl. Microbiol.* 18:277–280 (1994).

551. Buck, J.D., and S.A. McCarthy. Occurrence of non-O1 *Vibrio cholerae* in Texas Gulf Coast dolphins (*Tursiops truncatus*). *Lett. Appl. Microbiol.* 18:45–46 (1994).

552. Faming, D., S. Shimodori, T. Moriya, et al. Purification and characterization of a protein cryoprotective for *Vibrio cholerae* extracted from the prawn shell surface. *Microbiol. Immunol.* 37:861–868 (1993).

553. Lesmana, M., D. Subekti, P. Tjaniadi, and G. Pazzaglia. Modified CAMP test for biogrouping *Vibrio cholerae* O1 strains and distinguishing them from strains of *V. cholerae* non-O1. *J. Clin. Microbiol.* 32:235–237 (1994).

554. Said, B., S.M. Scotland, and B. Rowe. The use of gene probes, immunoassays and tissue culture for the detection of toxin in *Vibrio cholerae* non-O1. *J. Med. Microbiol.* 40:31–36 (1994).

555. Guglielmetti, P., L. Bravo, A. Zanchi, et al. Detection of the *Vibrio cholerae* heat-stable enterotoxin gene by polymerase chain reaction. *Molec. Cell. Probes* 8:39–44 (1994).

556. Keasler, S.P., and R.H. Hall. Detecting and biotyping *Vibrio cholerae* O1 with multiplex polymerase chain reaction. (Letter.) *Lancet* 341:1661 (1993).

557. Koch, W.H., W.L. Payne, B.A. Wentz, and T.A. Cebula. Rapid polymerase chain reaction method for detection of *Vibrio cholerae* in foods. *Appl. Environ. Microbiol.* 59:556–560 (1993).

558. Varela, P., G.D. Pollevick, M. Rivas, et al. Direct detection of *Vibrio cholerae* in stool samples. *J. Clin. Microbiol.* 32:1246–1248 (1994).

559. Ramamurthy, T., A. Pal, P.K. Bag, et al. Detection of cholera toxin gene in stool specimens by polymerase chain reaction: comparison with bead enzyme-linked immunosorbent

assay and culture method for laboratory diagnosis of cholera. *J. Clin. Microbiol.* 31:3068–3070 (1993).

560. Carillo, L., R.H. Gilman, R.E. Mantle, et al. Rapid detection of *Vibrio cholerae* O1 in stools of Peruvian cholera patients by using monoclonal immunodiagnostic kits. *J. Clin. Microbiol.* 32:856–857 (1994).

561. Abbott, S.L., and J.M. Janda. Rapid detection of acute cholera in airline passengers by coagglutination assay. (Letter.) *J. Infect. Dis.* 168:797–799 (1993).

562. Miyagi, K., Y. Matsumoto, K. Hayashi, et al. Successful application of enzyme-labeled oligonucleotide probe for rapid and accurate cholera diagnosis in a clinical laboratory. *Microbiol. Immunol.* 38:301–304 (1994).

563. Hasan, J.A.K., A. Huq, M.L. Tamplin, et al. A novel kit for rapid detection of *Vibrio cholerae* O1. *J. Clin. Microbiol.* 32:249–252 (1994).

564. Popovic, T., C. Bopp., Ø. Olsvik, and K. Wachsmuth. Epidemiologic application of a standardized ribotype scheme for *Vibrio cholerae* O1. *J. Clin. Microbiol.* 31:2474–2482 (1993).

565. Choudhury, S.R., R.K. Bhadra, and J. Das. Genome size and restriction fragment length polymorphism analysis of *Vibrio cholerae* strains belonging to different serovars and biotypes. *FEMS Microbiol. Lett.* 115:329–334 (1994).

566. Tikoo, A., D.V. Singh, and S.C. Sanyal. Influence of animal passage on haemolysin and enterotoxin production in *Vibrio cholerae* O1 biotype El Tor strains. *J. Med. Microbiol.* 40:246–251 (1994).

567. Ichinose, Y., M. Ehara, T. Honda, and T. Miwatani. The effect on enterotoxicity of protease purified from *V. cholerae* O1. *FEMS Microbiol. Lett.* 115:265–271 (1994).

568. Voss, E., and S.R. Attridge. *In vitro* production of toxin-coregulated pili by *Vibrio cholerae* El Tor. *Microb. Pathogen.* 15:255–268 (1993).

569. Attridge, S.R., E. Voss, and P.A. Manning. The role of toxin-coregulated pili in the pathogenesis of *Vibrio cholerae* O1 El Tor. *Microb. Pathogen.* 15:421–431 (1993).

570. Nakasone, N., and M. Iwanaga. Cell-associated hemagglutinin of classical *Vibrio cholerae* O1 with reference to intestinal adhesion. *FEMS Microbiol. Lett.* 113:67–70 (1993).

571. Kumar, K.K., R. Srivastava, V.B. Sinha, et al. *recA* mutations reduce adherence and colonization by classical and El Tor strains of *Vibrio cholerae*. *Microbiology* 140:1217–1222 (1994).

572. Yoshino, K.-i., M. Miyachi, T. Takao, et al. Purification and sequence determination of heat-stable enterotoxin elaborated by a cholera toxin–producing strain of *Vibrio cholerae* O1. *FEBS Lett.* 326:83–86 (1993).

573. Overbye, L.J., M. Sandkvist, and M. Bagdasarian. Genes required for extracellular secretion of enterotoxin are clustered in *Vibrio cholerae*. *Gene* 132:101–106 (1993).

574. Moyenuddin, M., K. Wachsmuth, J.E. Houghton, and D.G Ahearn. Potential pathogenic factors produced by a clinical nontoxigenic *Vibrio cholerae* O1. *Curr. Microbiol.* 27:329–333 (1993).

575. Williams, S.G., S.R. Attridge, and P.A. Manning. The transcriptional activator HlyU of *Vibrio cholerae*: nucle-

otide sequence and role in virulence gene expression. *Molec. Microbiol.* 9:751–760 (1993).

576. Rodrigues, D.P., R.V. Ribeiro, R.M. Alves, and E. Hofer. Analysis of some factors involved in the virulence mechanism of *Vibrio cholerae* non-O1. *FEMS Immunol. Med. Microbiol.* 7:297–301 (1993).

577. Ramamurthy, T., P.K. Bag, A. Pal, et al. Virulence patterns of *Vibrio cholerae* non-O1 strains isolated from hospitalised patients with acute diarrhoea in Calcutta, India. *J. Med. Microbiol.* 39:310–317 (1993).

578. Zitzer, A.O., N.O. Nakisbekov, A.V. Li, et al. Enterocytolysin (EC) from *Vibrio cholerae* non-O1 (some properties and pore-forming activity). *Zbl. Bakteriol.* 279:494–504 (1993).

579. Sengupta, T.K., D.K. Sengupta, and A.C. Ghose. A 20-kDa pilus protein with haemagglutination and intestinal adherence properties expressed by a clinical isolate of non-O1 *Vibrio cholerae*. *FEMS Microbiol. Lett.* 112:237–242 (1993).

580. Yamashiro, T., N. Nakasone, and M. Iwanaga. Purification and characterization of pili of a *Vibrio cholerae* non-O1 strain. *Infect. Immun.* 61:5398–5400 (1993).

581. Waldor, M.K., and J.J. Mekalanos. ToxR regulate virulence gene expression in non-O1 strains of *Vibrio cholerae* that cause epidemic cholera. *Infect. Immun.* 62:72–78 (1994).

582. Ross, E.E., L. Guyer, J. Varnes, and G. Rodrick. *Vibrio vulnificus* and molluscan shellfish: the necessity of education for high-risk individuals. *J. Am. Diet. Assoc.* 94:312–314 (1994).

583. Hlady, W.G., and R.C. Mullen. *Vibrio vulnificus* infections associated with raw oyster consumption—Florida, 1981–1992 (1993). *Arch. Dermatol.* 129:957–958 (1993).

584. Anonymous. Mislabeled oysters tied to *Vibrio* death. *Food Protect. Rep.* 10(10):3–4 (1994).

585. Groubert, T.N., and J.D. Oliver. Interaction of *Vibrio vulnificus* and the eastern oyster, *Crassostrea virginica*. *J. Food Protect.* 57:224–228 (1994).

586. Kaspar, C.W., and M.L. Tamplin. Effects of temperature and salinity on the survival of *Vibrio vulnificus* in seawater and shellfish. *Appl. Environ. Microbiol.* 59:2425–2429 (1993).

587. Firth, J.R., J.P. Diaper, and C. Edwards. Survival and viability of *Vibrio vulnificus* in seawater monitored by flow cytometry. *Lett. Appl. Microbiol.* 18:268–271 (1994).

588. DePaola, A., G.M. Capers, and D. Alexander. Densities of *Vibrio vulnificus* in the intestines of fish from the U.S. Gulf Coast. *Appl. Environ. Microbiol.* 60:984–988 (1994).

589. Veenstra, J., P.J.G.M. Rietra, J.M. Coster, et al. Seasonal variations in the occurrence of *Vibrio vulnificus* along the Dutch coast. *Epidemiol. Infect.* 112:285–290 (1994).

590. Miceli, G.A., W.D. Watkins, and S.R. Rippey. Direct plating procedure for enumerating *Vibrio vulnificus* in oysters (*Crassostrea virginica*). *Appl. Environ. Microbiol.* 59:3519–3524 (1993).

591. Brauns, L.A., and J.D. Oliver. Polymerase chain reaction of whole cell lysates for the detection of *Vibrio vulnificus*. *Food Biotechnol.* 8:1–6 (1994).

592. Aznar, R., W. Ludwig, and K.-H. Schleifer. Ribotyping and randomly amplified polymorphic DNA analysis of

*Vibrio vulnificus* biotypes. *System. Appl. Microbiol.* 16:303–309 (1993).

593. Aznar, R., W. Ludwig, R.I. Amann, and K.H. Schleifer. Sequence determination of rRNA genes of pathogenic *Vibrio* species and whole-cell identification of *Vibrio vulnificus* with rRNA-targeted oligonucleotide probes. *Int. J. System. Bacteriol.* 44:330–337 (1994).

594. Heldelberg, J.F., K.R. O'Neill, D. Jacobs, and R.R. Colwell. Enumeration of *Vibrio vulnificus* on membrane filters with a fluorescently labeled oligonucleotide probe specific for kingdom-level 16S rRNA sequences. *Appl. Environ. Microbiol.* 59:3474–3476 (1993).

595. Amaro, C., E.G. Biosca, B. Fouz, et al. Role of iron, capsule, and toxins in the pathogenicity of *Vibrio vulnificus* biotype 2 for mice. *Infect. Immun.* 62:759–763 (1994).

596. Miyoshi, S., E.G. Oh, K. Hirata, and S. Shinoda. Exocellular toxic factors produced by *Vibrio vulnificus. J. Toxicol.—Toxin Rev.* 12:253–288 (1993).

597. Hayat, U., G.P. Reddy, C.A. Bush, et al. Capsular types of *Vibrio vulnificus*: an analysis of strains from clinical and environmental sources. *J. Infect. Dis.* 168:758–762 (1993).

598. Oh, E.-G., Y. Tamanoi, A. Toyoda, et al. Simple purification method for a *Vibrio vulnificus* hemolysin by a hydrophobic column chromatography in the presence of a detergent. *Microbiol. Immunol.* 37:975–978 (1993).

599. McDougald, D., L.M. Simpson, J.D. Oliver, and M.C. Hudson. Transformation of *Vibrio vulnificus* by electroporation. *Curr. Microbiol.* 28:289–291 (1994).

600. Haddock, R.L., and A.F. Cabanero. The origin of non-outbreak *Vibrio parahaemolyticus* infections on Guam. *Trop. Geog. Med.* 46:42–43 (1994).

601. Tamura, N., S. Kobayashi, H. Hashimoto, and S.-I. Hirose. Reactive arthritis induced by *Vibrio parahaemolyticus. J. Rheumatol.* 20:1062–1063 (1993).

602. Lee, C., and S.-F. Pan. Rapid and specific detection of the thermostable direct haemolysin gene in *Vibrio parahaemolyticus* by the polymerase chain reaction. *J. Gen. Microbiol.* 139:3225–3231 (1993).

603. Chang, T.C., C.H. Chen, and H.C. Chen. Development of a latex agglutination test for the rapid identification of *Vibrio parahaemolyticus. J. Food Protect.* 57:31–36 (1994).

604. Lin, Z., K. Kumagai, K. Baba, et al. *Vibrio parahaemolyticus* has a homolog of the *Vibrio cholerae toxRS* operon that mediates environmentally induced regulation of the thermostable direct hemolysin gene. *J. Bacteriol.* 175:3844–3855 (1993).

605. Uchimura, M., K. Koiwai, Y. Tsuruoka, and H. Tanaka. High prevalence of thermostable direct hemolysin (TDH)-like toxin in *Vibrio mimicus* strains isolated from diarrhoeal patients. *Epidemiol. Infect.* 111:49–53 (1993).

606. Ramamurthy, T., M.J. Albert, A. Huq, et al. *Vibrio mimicus* with multiple toxin types isolated from human and environmental sources. *J. Med. Microbiol.* 40:194–196 (1994).

607. Abbott, S.L., and J.M. Janda. Severe gastroenteritis associated with *Vibrio hollisae* infection: report of two cases and review. *Clin. Infect. Dis.* 18:310–312 (1994).

608. Perez-Tirse, J., J.F. Levine, and M. Mecca. *Vibrio damsela*. A cause of fulminant septicemia. *Arch. Intern. Med.* 153:1838–1840 (1993).

609. Hansen, W., J. Freney, H. Benyagoub, et al. Severe human infections caused by *Vibrio metschnikovii. J. Clin. Microbiol.* 31:2529–2530 (1993).

610. Magalhães, V., A.C. Filho, M. Magalhães, and T.T. Gomes. Laboratory evaluation on pathogenic potentialities of *Vibrio furnissii. Mem. Inst. Oswaldo Cruz* 88:593–597 (1993).

611. Kirov, S.M. The public health significance of *Aeromonas* spp. in foods. *Int. J. Food Microbiol.* 20:179–198 (1993).

612. Palumbo, S.A. The occurrence and significance of organisms of the *Aeromonas hydrophila* group in food and water. *Med. Microbiol. Lett.* 2:339–346 (1993).

613. Bottone, E.J. Correlation between known exposure to contaminated food or surface water and development of *Aeromonas hydrophila* and *Plesiomonas shigelloides* diarrheas. *Med. Microbiol. Lett.* 2:217–225 (1993).

614. Madden, J.M. Fish as a threat to human health due to the presence of *Aeromonas hydrophila. Med. Microbiol. Lett.* 2:335–338 (1993).

615. Kirov, S.M., J.A. Hudson, L.J. Hayward, and S.J. Mott. Distribution of *Aeromonas hydrophila* hybridization groups and their virulence properties in Australasian clinical and environmental strains. *Lett. Appl. Microbiol.* 18:71–73 (1994).

616. Huang, Y.-W., and C.-K. Leung. Microbiological assessment of channel catfish grown in cage and pond culture. *Food Microbiol.* 10:187–195 (1993).

617. Gobat, P.-F., and T. Jemmi. Distribution of mesophilic *Aeromonas* species in raw and ready-to-eat fish and meat products in Switzerland. *Int. J. Food Microbiol.* 20:117–120 (1993).

618. Stecchini, M.L., I. Sarais, and S. Milani. The effect of incubation temperature, sodium chloride and ascorbic acid on the growth kinetics of *Aeromonas hydrophila. Lett. Appl. Microbiol.* 17:238–241 (1993).

619. Stecchini, M.L., I. Sarais, and A. Giomo. Thermal inactivation of *Aeromonas hydrophila* as affected by sodium chloride and ascorbic acid. *Appl. Environ. Microbiol.* 59:4166–4170 (1993).

620. Kirov, S.M., and F. Brodribb. Exotoxin production by *Aeromonas* spp. in foods. *Lett. Appl. Microbiol.* 17:208–211 (1993).

621. Kirov, S.M., E.K. Ardestani, and L.J. Hayward. The growth and expression of virulence factors at refrigeration temperature by *Aeromonas* strains isolated from foods. *Int. J. Food Microbiol.* 20:159–168 (1993).

622. Carnahan, A.M. Update on current identification methods for clinical *Aeromonas* isolates. *Med. Microbiol. Lett.* 2:212–216 (1993).

623. Pin, C., M.L. Marin, M.L. Garcia, et al. Comparison of different media for the isolation and enumeration of *Aeromonas* spp. in foods. *Lett. Appl. Microbiol.* 18:190–192 (1994).

624. Warburton, D.W., J.K. McCormick, and B. Bowen. Survival and recovery of *Aeromonas hydrophila* in water: development of methodology for testing bottled water in Canada. *Can. J. Microbiol.* 40:145–148 (1994).

625. Arzese, A., C. Pipan, C. Piersimoni, et al. Characterization of mesophilic *Aeromonas* from clinical specimens by computerized analysis of SDS-PAGE protein profiles and by enzymatic activity. *Microbiologica* 16:333–342 (1993).

626. Ogden, I.D., I.G. Millar, A.J. Watt, and L. Wood. A comparison of three identification kits for the confirmation of *Aeromonas* spp. *Lett. Appl. Microbiol.* 18:97–99 (1994).

627. Schadow, K.H., D.K. Giger, and C.C. Sanders. Failure of the Vitek AutoMicrobic system to detect beta-lactam resistance in *Aeromonas* species. *Am. J. Clin. Pathol.* 100:308–310 (1993).

628. Lucchini, G.M. Typing methods as epidemiologic tools in the genus *Aeromonas. Med. Microbiol. Lett.* 2:226–230 (1993).

629. Millership, S.E., and S.V. Want. Characterisation of strains of *Aeromonas* spp. by phenotype and whole-cell protein fingerprint. *J. Med. Microbiol.* 39:107–113 (1993).

630. Mulla, R., and S. Millership. Typing of *Aeromonas* spp. by numerical analysis of immunoblotted SDS-PAGE gels. *J. Med. Microbiol.* 38:325–333 (1993).

631. Freitas, A.C., A.M. Milhomem, M.P. Nunes, and I.D. Ricciardi. Virulence factors produced by *Aeromonas hydrophila* strains isolated from different sources. *Rev. Microbiol. São Paulo* 24:168–174 (1993).

632. Gosling, P.J., P.C.B. Turnbull, N.F. Lightfoot, et al. Phenotypic characteristics of *Aeromonas* species as "markers" of enterotoxigenicity. *Med. Microbiol. Lett.* 2:287–295 (1993).

633. Esteve, C., E.G. Biosca, and C. Amaro. Virulence of *Aeromonas hydrophila* and some other bacteria isolated from European eels *Anguilla anguilla* reared in fresh water. *Dis. Aquatic Org.* 16:15–20 (1993).

634. Neves, M.S., M.P. Nunes, and A.M. Milhomem. *Aeromonas* species exhibit aggregative adherence to HEp-2 cells. *J. Clin. Microbiol.* 32:1130–1131 (1994).

635. Nishikawa, Y., A. Hase, J. Ogawasara, et al. Adhesion to and invasion of human colon carcinoma Caco-2 cells by *Aeromonas* strains. *J. Med. Microbiol.* 40:55–61 (1994).

636. Bartková, G., and I. Čižnár. Adherence pattern of non-piliated *Aeromonas hydrophila* strains to tissue cultures. *Microbios* 77:47–55 (1994).

637. Majeed, K.N., and I.C. MacRae. Cytotoxic and haemagglutinating activities of motile *Aeromonas* species. *J. Med. Microbiol.* 40:188–193 (1994).

638. Hanes, D.E., and D.K.F. Chandler. The role of a 40-megadalton plasmid in the adherence and hemolytic properties of *Aeromonas hydrophila*. *Microb. Pathogen.* 15:313–317 (1993).

639. Loychern, A., K. Charoensiri, and K. Ratanabanangkoon. A simple purification of *Aeromonas hydrophila* hemolysin. *J. Nat. Toxins* 3:1–4 (1994).

640. Parker, M.W., J.T. Buckley, J.P.M. Postma, et al. Structure of the *Aeromonas* toxin proaerolysin in its water-soluble and membrane-channel states. *Nature* 367:292–295 (1994).

641. Chopra, A.K., M.R. Ferguson, and C.W. Houston. Molecular characterization of enterotoxins from *Aeromonas hydrophila*. *Med. Microbiol. Lett.* 2:261–268 (1993).

642. Advisory Committee on the Microbiological Safety of Food. Interim report on *Campylobacter*. Conclusions and recommendations. *Commun. Dis. Environ. Health Scotland Weekly Rep.* 28(8):4–8 (1994).

643. Altekruse, S.F., J.M. Hunt, L.K. Tollefson, and J.M. Madden. Food and animal sources of human *Campylobacter jejuni* infection. *J. Am. Vet. Med. Assoc.* 204:57–61 (1994).

644. Koenraad, P.M.J.F., W.C. Hazeleger, T. van der Laan, et al. Survey of *Campylobacter* spp. in sewage plants in The Netherlands. *Food Microbiol.* 11:65–73 (1994).

645. Nachamkin, I., S.H. Fischer, X.-H. Yang, et al. Immunoglobulin A antibodies directed against *Campylobacter jejuni* flagellin present in breast-milk. *Epidemiol. Infect.* 112:359–365 (1994).

646. Chatzipanagiotou, S., E. Papavasiliou, and E. Malamou-Lada. Isolation of *Campylobacter jejuni* strains resistant to nalidixic acid and fluoroquinolones from children with diarrhea in Athens, Greece. *Eur. J. Clin. Microbiol. Infect. Dis.* 12:566–568 (1993).

647. Steinkraus, G.E., and B.D. Wright. Septic abortion with intact fetal membranes caused by *Campylobacter fetus* subsp. *fetus. J. Clin. Microbiol.* 32:1608–1609 (1994).

648. de Guevara, C.L., J. Gonzalez, and P. Peña. Bacteraemia caused by *Campylobacter* spp. *J. Clin. Pathol.* 47:174–175 (1994).

649. van der Kruijk, R.A., M.J. Affourtit, H.Ph. Endtz, and W.F.M. Arts. *Campylobacter jejuni* gastroenteritis and acute encephalopathy. (Letter.) *J. Infect.* 28:99–100 (1994).

650. Griffin, J.W., and T.W.-H. Ho. The Guillain-Barré syndrome at 75: the *Campylobacter* connection. *Ann. Neurol.* 34:125–127 (1993).

651. Rees, J.H., N.A. Gregson, P.L. Griffiths, and R.A.C. Hughes. *Campylobacter jejuni* and Guillain-Barré syndrome. *Q. J. Med.* 86:623–634 (1993).

652. Mishu, B., and M.J. Blaser. Role of infection due to *Campylobacter jejuni* in the initiation of Guillain-Barré syndrome. *Clin. Infect. Dis.* 17:104–108 (1993).

653. Mishu, B., A.A. Ilyas, C.L. Koski, et al. Serologic evidence of previous *Campylobacter jejuni* infection in patients with Guillain-Barré syndrome. *Ann. Intern. Med.* 118:947–953 (1993).

654. Enders, U., H. Karch, K.V. Toyka, et al. The spectrum of immune responses to *Campylobacter jejuni* and glycoconjugates in Guillain-Barré syndrome and in other neuroimmunological disorders. *Ann. Neurol.* 34:136–144 (1993).

655. Sugita, K., M. Ishii, J. Takanashi, et al. Guillain-Barré syndrome associated with IgM anti-$G_{M1}$ antibody following *Campylobacter jejuni* enteritis. *Eur. J. Pediatr.* 153:181–183 (1994).

656. Aspinall, G.O., S. Fujimoto, A.G. McDonald, et al. Lipopolysaccharides from *Campylobacter jejuni* associated

with Guillain-Barré syndrome patients mimic human gangliosides in structure. *Infect. Immun.* 62:2122–2125 (1994).

657. Yuki, N., T. Taki, M. Takahashi, et al. Penner's serotype 4 of *Campylobacter jejuni* has a lipopolysaccharide that bears a GM1 ganglioside epitope as well as one that bears a GD1a epitope. *Infect. Immun.* 62:2101–2103 (1994).

658. Weijtens, M.J.B.M., P.G.H. Bijker, J. Van der Plas, et al. Prevalence of campylobacter in pigs during fattening; an epidemiological study. *Vet. Q.* 15:138–143 (1993).

659. Wieliczko, A. Vorkommen von Campylobacter und Salmonellen im Zusammenhang mit Leberveränderungen bei Schlachtgeflügel. *Berl. Münch. Tierärztl. Wschr.* 107:115–121 (1994).

660. Flynn, O.M.J., I.S. Blair, and D.A. McDowell. Prevalence of *Campylobacter* species on fresh retail chicken wings in Northern Ireland. *J. Food Protect.* 57:334–336 (1994).

661. Slavik, M.F., J.-W. Kim, M.D. Pharr, et al. Effect of trisodium phosphate on *Campylobacter* attached to post-chill chicken carcasses. *J. Food Protect.* 57:324–326 (1994).

662. Castillo, A., and E.F. Escartin. Survival of *Campylobacter jejuni* on sliced watermelon and papaya. *J. Food Protect.* 57:166–168 (1994).

663. Humphrey, T.J., A. Henley, and D.G. Lanning. The colonization of broiler chickens with *Campylobacter jejuni*: some epidemiological investigations. *Epidemiol. Infect.* 110:601–607 (1993).

664. Kapperud, G., E. Skjerve, L. Vik, et al. Epidemiological investigation of risk factors for campylobacter colonization in Norwegian broiler flocks. *Epidemiol. Infect.* 111:245–255 (1993).

665. Glünder, G. *Campylobacter*-Infektionen beim Geflügel—Epizootiologie, Bedeutung und Bekämpfungsmöglichkeiten. *Arch. Geflügelk.* 57:241–248 (1993).

666. Wassenaar, T.M., B.A.M. van der Zeijst, R. Ayling, and D.G. Newell. Colonization of chicks by motility mutants of *Campylobacter jejuni* demonstrates the importance of flagellin A expression. *J. Gen. Microbiol.* 139:1171–1175 (1993).

668. Stern, N.J. Mucosal competitive exclusion to diminish colonization of chickens by *Campylobacter jejuni*. *Poultry Sci.* 73:402–407 (1994).

668. Schoeni, J.L., and A.C.L. Wong. Inhibition of *Campylobacter jejuni* colonization in chicks by defined competitive exclusion bacteria. *Appl. Environ. Microbiol.* 60:1191–1197 (1994).

669. Aspinall, S.T., D.R.A. Wareing, P.G. Hayward, and D.N. Hutchinson. Selective medium for thermophilic campylobacters including *Campylobacter upsaliensis*. *J. Clin. Pathol.* 46:829–831 (1993).

670. Lam, K.M. A cytotoxicity test for the detection of *Campylobacter jejuni* toxin. *Vet. Microbiol.* 35:133–139 (1993).

671. Nicholson, M.A., and C.M. Patton. Application of Lior biotyping by use of genetically identified *Campylobacter* strains. *J. Clin. Microbiol.* 31:3348–3350 (1993).

672. Chandan, V., A.D.E. Fraser, B.W. Brooks, and H. Yamazaki. Simple extraction of *Campylobacter* lipopolysaccharide and protein antigens and production of their antibodies in egg yolk. *Int. J. Food Microbiol.* 22:189–200 (1994).

673. Glünder, G. Antigenic changes in *Campylobacter* spp. after adaptation to media with increased sodium chloride concentrations. *Berl. Münch. Tierärztl. Wschr.* 107:109–115 (1994).

674. Kato, Y., T. Satoh, C. Kaneuchi, et al. Differentiation of thermophilic species of *Campylobacter*, in particular *C. coli* and *C. jejuni*, with atypical characteristics, by analysis of protein-banding profiles on non-denaturing polyacrylamide gels. *Microbios* 76:153–160 (1993).

675. Birkenhead, D., P.M. Hawkey, J. Heritage, et al. PCR for the detection and typing of campylobacters. *Lett. Appl. Microbiol.* 17:235–237 (1993).

676. Owen, R.J., A. Fayos, J. Hernandez, and A. Lastovica. PCR-based restriction fragment length polymorphism analysis of DNA sequence diversity of flagellin genes of *Campylobacter jejuni* and allied species. *Molec. Cell. Probes* 7:471–480 (1993).

677. Endtz, H.P., B.A.J. Giesendorf, A. van Belkum, et al. PCR-mediated DNA typing of *Campylobacter jejuni* isolated from patients with recurrent infections. *Res. Microbiol.* 144:703–708 (1993).

678. Giesendorf, B.A.J., H. Goossens, H.G.M. Niesters, et al. Polymerase chain reaction–mediated DNA fingerprinting for epidemiological studies on *Campylobacter* spp. *J. Med. Microbiol.* 40:141–147 (1994).

679. Stonnet, V., and J.-L. Guesdon. *Campylobacter jejuni*: specific oligonucleotides and DNA probes for use in polymerase chain reaction–based diagnosis. *FEMS Immunol. Med. Microbiol.* 7:337–344 (1993).

680. Wegmüller, B., J. Lüthy, and U. Candrian. Direct polymerase chain reaction detection of *Campylobacter jejuni* and *Campylobacter coli* in raw milk and dairy products. *Appl. Environ. Microbiol.* 59:2161–2165 (1993).

681. Oyofo, B.A., and D.M. Rollins. Efficacy of filter types for detecting *Campylobacter jejuni* and *Campylobacter coli* in environmental water samples by polymerase chain reaction. *Appl. Environ. Microbiol.* 59:4090–4095 (1993).

682. Quentin, R., D. Chevrier, J.L. Guesdon, et al. Use of nonradioactive DNA probes to identify a *Campylobacter jejuni* strain causing abortion. *Eur. J. Clin. Microbiol. Infect. Dis.* 12:627–630 (1993).

683. Suzuki, Y., M. Ishihara, M. Funabashi, et al. Pulsed-field gel electrophoretic analysis of *Campylobacter jejuni* DNA for use in epidemiological studies. *J. Infect.* 27:39–42 (1993).

684. Fayos, A., R.J. Owen, J. Hernandez, et al. Molecular subtyping by genome and plasmid analysis of *Campylobacter jejuni* serogroups O1 and O2 (Penner) from sporadic and outbreak cases of human diarrhoea. *Epidemiol. Infect.* 111:415–427 (1993).

685. Owen, R.J., M. Desai, and S. Garcia. Molecular typing of thermotolerant species of *Campylobacter* with ribosomal RNA gene patterns. *Res. Microbiol.* 144:709–720 (1993).

686. Wallis, M.R. The pathogenesis of *Campylobacter jejuni*. *Br. J. Biomed. Sci.* 51:57–64 (1994).

687. Kaur, R., N.K. Ganguly, L. Kumar, and B.N.S. Walia. Studies on the pathophysiological mechanism of

*Campylobacter jejuni*-induced fluid secretion in rat ileum. *FEMS Microbiol. Lett.* 111:327–330 (1993).

688. Blaser, M.J. Role of the S-layer proteins of *Campylobacter fetus* in serum-resistance and antigenic variation: a model of bacterial pathogenesis. *Am. J. Med. Sci.* 306:325–329 (1993).

689. Czuprynski, C.J. Host defense against *Listeria monocytogenes:* implications for food safety. *Food Microbiol.* 11:131–147 (1994).

690. Czajka, J., and C.A. Batt. Verification of causal relationships between *Listeria monocytogenes* isolates implicated in food-borne outbreaks of listeriosis by randomly amplified polymorphic DNA patterns. *J. Clin. Microbiol.* 32:1280–1287 (1994).

691. Nørrung, B., and N. Skovgaard. Application of multilocus enzyme electrophoresis in studies of the epidemiology of *Listeria monocytogenes* in Denmark. *Appl. Environ. Microbiol.* 59:2817–2833 (1993).

692. Harvey, J., and A. Gilmour. Application of multilocus enzyme electrophoresis and restriction fragment length polymorphism analysis to the typing of *Listeria monocytogenes* strains isolated from raw milk, nondairy foods, and clinical and veterinary sources. *Appl. Environ. Microbiol.* 60:1547–1553 (1994).

693. Eilertz, I., M.-L. Danielsson-Tham, K.-E. Hammarberg, et al. Isolation of *Listeria monocytogenes* from goat cheese associated with a case of listeriosis in goat. *Acta Vet. Scand.* 34:145–149 (1993).

694. Paul, M.L., D.E. Dwyer, C. Chow, et al. Listeriosis—a review of eighty-four cases. *Med. J. Aust.* 160:489–493 (1994).

695. Jensen, A., W. Frederiksen, and P. Gerner-Smidt. Risk factors for listeriosis in Denmark, 1989–1990. *Scand. J. Infect. Dis.* 26:171–178 (1994).

696. Newton, L., S.M. Hall, and J. McLauchlin. Listeriosis surveillance: 1992. *Commun. Dis. Rep.* 3(Rev. 10):R144–R146 (1993).

697. World Health Organization. Outbreak of listeriosis. *Weekly Epidemiol. Rec.* 68:295 (1993).

698. Bader, J.-M. Listeriosis epidemic. *Lancet* 342:607 (1993).

699. Edelbroek, M.A.L., J.J.E.M. De Nef, and J.R. Rajnherc. Listeria meningitis presenting as enteritis in a previously healthy infant: a case report. *Eur. J. Pediatr.* 153:179–180 (1994).

700. Gray, J.W., J.F.R. Barrett, S.J. Pedler, and T. Lind. Faecal carriage of listeria during pregnancy. *Br. J. Obstet. Gynaecol.* 100:873–874 (1993).

701. Jensen, A. Excretion of *Listeria monocytogenes* in faeces after listeriosis: rate, quantity and duration. *Med. Microbiol. Lett.* 2:176–182 (1993).

702. Mascola, L., D.P. Ewert, and A. Eller. Listeriosis: a previously unreported medical complication in women with multiple gestations. *Am. J. Obstet. Gynecol.* 170:1328–1332 (1994).

703. Long, S.G., M.J. Leyland, and D.W. Milligan. Listeria meningitis after bone marrow transplant. *Bone Marrow Transplant.* 12:537–539 (1993).

704. Braun, T.I., D. Travis, R.R. Dee, and R.E. Nieman. Liver abscess due to *Listeria monocytogenes:* case report and review. *Clin. Infect. Dis.* 17:267–269 (1993).

705. Manian, F.A. Liver abscess due to *Listeria monocytogenes.* (Letter.) *Clin. Infect. Dis.* 18:841–842 (1994).

706. Bourgeois, N., F. Jacobs, M.L. Tavares, et al. *Listeria monocytogenes* hepatitis in a liver transplant recipient: a case report and review of the literature. *J. Hepatol.* 18:284–289 (1993).

707. Levett, P.N., P. Bennett, K. O'Donaghue, et al. Relapsed infection due to *Listeria monocytogenes* confirmed by random amplified polymorphic DNA (RAPD) analysis. *J. Infect.* 27:205–207 (1993).

708. Cummins, A.J., A.K. Fielding, and J. McLauchlin. *Listeria ivanovii* infection in a patient with AIDS. *J. Infect.* 28:89–91 (1994).

709. Jackson, T.C., G.R. Acuff, L.M. Lucia, et al. Survey of residential refrigerators for the presence of *Listeria monocytogenes. J. Food Protect.* 56:874–875 (1993).

710. Jacquet, Ch., J. Rocourt, and A. Reynaud. Study of *Listeria monocytogenes* contamination in a dairy plant and characterization of the strains isolated. *Int. J. Food Microbiol.* 20:13–22 (1993).

711. Canillac, N., and A. Mourey. Sources of contamination by *Listeria* during the making of semi-soft surface-ripened cheese. *Sci. Aliments* 13:533–544 (1993).

712. Sasahara, K.C., and E.A. Zottola. Biofilm formation by *Listeria monocytogenes* utilizes a primary colonizing microorganism in flowing systems. *J. Food Protect.* 56:1022–1028 (1993).

713. Wirtanen, G., and T. Mattila-Sandholm. Epifluorescence image analysis and cultivation of foodborne biofilm bacteria grown on stainless steel surfaces. *J. Food Protect.* 56:678–683 (1993).

714. Vishinsky, Y., A. Grinberg, and R. Ozery. *Listeria monocytogenes* udder infection and carcase contamination. *Vet. Rec.* 133:484 (1993).

715. Weber, A., A. Prell, J. Potel, and R. Schäfer. Vorkommen von *Listeria monocytogenes* bei Schlangen, Schildkröten, Echsen und Amphibien in der Heimtierhaltung. *Berl. Münch. Tierärztl. Wschr.* 106:293–295 (1993).

716. MacGowan, A.P., K. Bowker, J. McLauchlin, et al. The occurrence and seasonal changes in the isolation of *Listeria* spp. in shop bought food stuffs, human feces, sewage and soil from urban sources. *Int. J. Food Microbiol.* 21:325–334 (1994).

717. Harvey, J., and A. Gilmour. Occurrence and characteristics of *Listeria* in foods produced in Northern Ireland. *Int. J. Food Microbiol.* 19:193–205 (1993).

718. Gilbert, R.J., J. McLauchlin, and S.K. Velani. The contamination of paté by *Listeria monocytogenes* in England and Wales in 1989 and 1990. *Epidemiol. Infect.* 110:543–551 (1993).

719. Dillon, R., T. Patel, and S. Ratnam. Occurrence of *Listeria* in hot and cold smoked seafood products. *Int. J. Food Microbiol.* 22:73–77 (1994).

720. Wang, C., and P.M. Muriana. Incidence of *Listeria monocytogenes* in packages of retail franks. *J. Food Protect.* 57:382–386 (1994).

721. Sheridan, J.J., G. Duffy, D.A. McDowell, and I.S. Blair. The occurrence and initial numbers of *Listeria* in Irish meat and fish products and the recovery of injured cells from frozen products. *Int. J. Food Microbiol.* 22:105–113 (1994).

722. Kamat, A.S., and P.M. Nair. Incidence of *Listeria* species in Indian seafoods and meat. *J. Food Safety* 14:117–130 (1994).

723. Moura, S.M., M.T. Destro, and B.D.G.M. Franco. Incidence of *Listeria* species in raw and pasteurized milk produced in São Paulo, Brazil. *Int. J. Food Microbiol.* 19:229–237 (1993).

724. Moore, J., and R.H. Madden. Detection and incidence of *Listeria* species in blended raw egg. *J. Food Protect.* 56:652–654,660 (1993).

725. Farber, J.M., and E. Daley. Presence and growth of *Listeria monocytogenes* in naturally-contaminated meats. *Int. J. Food Microbiol.* 22:33–42 (1994).

726. Schmidt, U., and L. Leistner. Verhalten von *Listeria monocytogenes* bei unverpacktem Brühwurstaufschnitt. *Fleischwirtschaft* 73:733–739 (1993).

727. Hardin, M.D., S.E. Williams, and M.A. Harrison. Survival of *Listeria monocytogenes* in postpasteurized precooked beef roasts. *J. Food Protect.* 56:655–660 (1993).

728. Fang, T.J., and L.-W. Lin. Growth of *Listeria monocytogenes* and *Pseudomonas fragi* on cooked pork in a modified atmosphere packaging/nisin combination system. *J. Food Protect.* 57:479–485 (1994).

729. Grant, I.R., C.R. Nixon, and M.F. Patterson. Comparison of the growth of *Listeria monocytogenes* in unirradiated and irradiated cook–chill roast beef and gravy at refrigeration temperatures. *Lett. Appl. Microbiol.* 17:55–57 (1993).

730. Huang, I-P.D., A.E. Yousef, M.E. Matthews, and E.H. Marth. Growth and survival of *Listeria monocytogenes* in chicken gravy during cooling and refrigerated storage. *J. Foodserv. Sys.* 7:185–192 (1993).

731. Bartlett, F.M. *Listeria monocytogenes* survival on shell eggs and resistance to sodium hypochlorite. *J. Food Safety* 13:253–261 (1993).

732. Back, J.P., S.A. Langford, and R.G. Kroll. Growth of *Listeria monocytogenes* in Camembert and other soft cheeses at refrigeration temperatures. *J. Dairy Res.* 60:421–429 (1993).

733. Jackson, E.D., L. Hiltz, K.B. McRae, and C.R. Bell. Growth of *Listeria monocytogenes* in coleslaw packaged under modified atmosphere. Agriculture and Agri-Food Canada. *Safety Watch. Foodborne Disease Bulletin* 29 (Summer 1993).

734. Omary, M.B., R.F. Testin, S.F. Barefoot, and J.W. Rushing. Packaging effects on growth of *Listeria innocua* in shredded cabbage. *J. Food Sci.* 58:623–626 (1993).

735. Carlin, F., and C. Nguyen-The. Fate of *Listeria monocytogenes* on four types of minimally processed green salads. *Lett. Appl. Microbiol.* 18:222–226 (1994).

736. Petran, R.L., and K.M.J. Swanson. Simultaneous growth of *Listeria monocytogenes* and *Listeria innocua*. *J. Food Protect.* 56:616–618 (1993).

737. Ko, R., L.T. Smith, and G.M. Smith. Glycine betaine confers enhanced osmotolerance and cryotolerance on *Listeria monocytogenes*. *J. Bacteriol.* 176:426–431 (1994).

738. Hefnawy, Y.A., and E.H. Marth. Survival and growth of *Listeria monocytogenes* in broth supplemented with sodium chloride and held at 4 and 13°C. *Lebensm. Wiss. Technol.* 26:388–392 (1993).

739. Oh, D.-H., and D.L. Marshall. Influence of temperature, pH, and glycerol monolaurate on growth and survival of *Listeria monocytogenes*. *J. Food Protect.* 56:744–749 (1993).

740. Beuchat, L.R., R.E. Brackett, and M.P. Doyle. Lethality of carrot juice to *Listeria monocytogenes* as affected by pH, sodium chloride and temperature. *J. Food Protect.* 57:470–474 (1994).

741. McKellar, R.C., R. Moir, and M. Kalab. Factors influencing the survival and growth of *Listeria monocytogenes* on the surface of Canadian retail wieners. *J. Food Protect.* 57:387–392 (1994).

742. Hudson, J.A. Comparison of response surface models for *Listeria monocytogenes* strains under aerobic conditions. *Food Res. Int.* 27:53–59 (1994).

743. Sörqvist, S. Heat resistance of different serovars of *Listeria monocytogenes*. *J. Appl. Bacteriol.* 76:383–388 (1994).

744. Huang, Y.-W., C.-K. Leung, M.A. Harrison, and K.W. Gates. Fate of *Listeria monocytogenes* and *Aeromonas hydrophila* on catfish fillets cooked in a microwave oven. *J. Food Sci.* 58:519–521 (1993).

745. Palumbo, S.A., J.L. Smith, B.S. Marmer, et al. Thermal destruction of *Listeria monocytogenes* during liver sausage processing. *Food Microbiol.* 10:243–247 (1993).

746. MacDonald, F., and A.D. Sutherland. Effect of heat treatment on *Listeria monocytogenes* and Gram-negative bacteria in sheep, cow and goat milks. *J. Appl. Bacteriol.* 75:336–342 (1993).

747. Embarek, P.K.B., and H.H. Huss. Heat resistance of *Listeria monocytogenes* in vacuum packaged pasteurized fish fillets. *Int. J. Food Microbiol.* 20:85–95 (1993).

748. Kim, K.-T., E.A. Murano, and D.G. Olson. Heating and storage conditions affect survival and recovery of *Listeria monocytogenes* in ground pork. *J. Food Sci.* 59:30–32,59 (1994).

749. Ashenafi, M. Fate of *Listeria monocytogenes* during the souring of ergo, a traditional Ethiopian fermented milk. *J. Dairy Sci.* 77:696–702 (1994).

750. Dillon, R., and I. Patel. Effect of cold smoking and storage temperatures on *Listeria monocytogenes* in inoculated cod fillets (*Gadus morhus*). *Food Res. Int.* 26:97–101 (1993).

751. Abdalla, O.M., G.L. Christen, and P.M. Davidson. Chemical composition of and *Listeria monocytogenes* survival in white pickled cheese. *J. Food Protect.* 56:841–846 (1993).

752. International Commission on Microbiological Specifications for Foods. Choice of sampling plan and criteria for *Listeria monocytogenes*. *Int. J. Food Microbiol.* 22:89–96 (1994).

753. van den Elzen, A.M.G., and J.M.A. Snijders. Critical points in meat production lines regarding the introduction of *Listeria monocytogenes*. *Vet. Q.* 15:143–145 (1993).

754. Wederquist, H.J., J.N. Sofos, and G.R. Schmidt. *Listeria monocytogenes* inhibition in refrigerated vacuum packaged turkey bologna by chemical additives. *J. Food Sci.* 59:498–500,516 (1994).

755. Shelef, L.A., and L. Addala. Inhibition of *Listeria monocytogenes* and other bacteria by sodium diacetate. *J. Food Safety* 14:103–115 (1994).

756. Schlyter, J.H., A.J. Degnan, J. Loeffelholz, et al. Evaluation of sodium diacetate and ALTA™ 2341 on viability of *Listeria monocytogenes* in turkey slurries. *J. Food Protect.* 56:808–810 (1993).

757. Schlyter, J.H., K.A. Glass, J. Loeffelholz, et al. The effects of diacetate with nitrite, lactate, or pediocin on the viability of *Listeria monocytogenes* in turkey slurries. *Int. J. Food Microbiol.* 19:271–281 (1993).

758. Oh, D.-H., and D.L. Marshall. Antimicrobial activity of ethanol, glycerol monolaurate or lactic acid against *Listeria monocytogenes*. *Int. J. Food Microbiol.* 20:239–246 (1993).

759. Wang, L.-l., B.-k. Wang, K.L. Parkin, and E.A. Johnson. Inhibition of *Listeria monocytogenes* by monoacylglycerols synthesized from coconut oil and milkfat by lipase-catalyzed glycerolysis. *J. Agric. Food Chem.* 41:1000–1005 (1993).

760. Dorsa, W.J., D.L. Marshall, and M. Semien. Effect of potassium sorbate and citric acid sprays on growth of *Listeria monocytogenes* on cooked crawfish (*Procambarus clarkii*) tail meat at 4°C. *Lebensm. Wiss. Technol.* 26:480–482 (1993).

761. Whiting, R.C., and M.O. Masana. *Listeria monocytogenes* survival model validated in simulated uncooked-fermented meat products for effects of nitrite and pH. *J. Food Sci.* 59:760–762 (1994).

762. Peterson, M.E., G.A. Pelroy, R.N. Paranjpye, et al. Parameters for control of *Listeria monocytogenes* in smoked fishery products: sodium chloride and packaging method. *J. Food Protect.* 56:938–943 (1993).

763. Pelroy, G.A., M.E. Peterson, P.J. Holland, and M.W. Eklund. Inhibition of *Listeria monocytogenes* in cold-process (smoked) salmon by sodium lactate. *J. Food Protect.* 57:108–113 (1994).

764. Pelroy, G., M. Peterson, R. Paranjpye, et al. Inhibition of *Listeria monocytogenes* in cold-process (smoked) salmon by sodium nitrite and packaging method. *J. Food Protect.* 57:114–119 (1994).

765. Krämer, K.H., and J. Baumgart. Sliced frankfurter-type sausage. Inhibiting *Listeria monocytogenes* by means of a modified atmosphere. *Fleischwirtschaft* 73:1279–1280 (1993).

766. Avery, S.M., J.A. Hudson, and N. Penney. Inhibition of *Listeria monocytogenes* in normal ultimate pH beef (pH 5.3–5.5) at abusive storage temperatures by saturated carbon dioxide controlled atmosphere packaging. *J. Food Protect.* 57:331–333,336 (1994).

767. Zapico, P., P. Gaya, M. Nuñez, and M. Medina. Goats' milk lactoperoxidase system against *Listeria monocytogenes*. *J. Food Protect.* 56:988–990 (1993).

768. Hefnawy, Y.A., S.I. Moustafa, and E.H. Marth. Sensitivity of *Listeria monocytogenes* to selected spices. *J. Food Protect.* 56:876–878 (1993).

769. Pandit, V.A., and L.A. Shelef. Sensitivity of *Listeria monocytogenes* to rosemary (*Rosmarinus officinalis* L.). *Food Microbiol.* 11:57–63 (1994).

770. Chichi, D.K., B.P. Klein, F.K. McKeith, and H.P. Blaschek. Reduction of *Listeria monocytogenes* in precooked vacuum-packaged beef using postpackaging pasteurization. *J. Food Protect.* 56:1034–1038 (1993).

771. Patterson, M.F., A.P. Damoglou, and R.K. Buick. Effects of irradiation dose and storage temperature on the growth of *Listeria monocytogenes* on poultry meat. *Food Microbiol.* 10:197–203 (1993).

772. Lin, H.-M., N. Cao, and L.-F. Chen. Antimicrobial effect of pressurized carbon dioxide on *Listeria monocytogenes*. *J. Food Sci.* 59:657–659 (1994).

773. Héchard, Y., D. Renault, Y. Cenatiempo, et al. Les bactériocines contre *Listeria*: une nouvelle famille de protéines? *Lait* 73:207–213 (1993).

774. Benkerroum, N., Y. Ghouati, W.E. Sandine, and A. Tantaoui-Elaraki. Methods to demonstrate the bactericidal activity of bacteriocins. *Lett. Appl. Microbiol.* 17:78–81 (1993).

775. Ryser, E.T., S. Maisnier-Patin, J.J. Gratadoux, and J. Richard. Isolation and identification of cheese-smear bacteria inhibitory to *Listeria* spp. *Int. J. Food Microbiol.* 21:237–246 (1994).

776. Raccach, M., and D.J. Geshell. The inhibition of *Listeria monocytogenes* in milk by pediococci. *Food Microbiol.* 10:181–186 (1993).

777. Baccus-Taylor, G., K.A. Glass, J.B. Luchansky, and A.J. Maurer. Fate of *Listeria monocytogenes* and pediococcal starter cultures during the manufacture of chicken summer sausage. *Poultry Sci.* 72:1772–1778 (1993).

778. Liao, C.-C., A.E. Yousef, E.R. Richter, and G.W. Chism. *Pediococcus acidilactici* PO2 bacteriocin production in whey permeate and inhibition of *Listeria monocytogenes* in foods. *J. Food Sci.* 58:430–434 (1993).

779. Garriga, M., M. Hugas, T. Aymerich, and J.M. Monfort. Bacteriocinogenic activity of lactobacilli from fermented sausages. *J. Appl. Biochem.* 75:142–148 (1993).

780. Campanini, M., I. Pedrazzoni, S. Barbuti, and P. Baldini. Behaviour of *Listeria monocytogenes* during the maturation of naturally and artificially contaminated salami: effect of lactic-acid bacteria starter cultures. *Int. J. Food Microbiol.* 20:169–175 (1993).

781. Holck, A.L., L. Axelsson, K. Hühne, and L. Kröckel. Purification and cloning of sakacin 674, a bacteriocin from *Lactobacillus sake* Lb674. *FEMS Microbiol. Lett.* 115:143–149 (1994).

782. Atrih, A., N. Rekhif, J.B. Milliere, and G. Lefebvre. Detection and characterization of a bacteriocin produced by *Lactobacillus plantarum* C19. *Can. J. Microbiol.* 39:1173–1179 (1993).

783. Winkowski, K., A.D. Crandall, and T.J. Montville. Inhibition of *Listeria monocytogenes* by *Lactobacillus*

*bavaricus* MN in beef systems at refrigeration temperatures. *Appl. Environ. Microbiol.* 59:2552–2557 (1993).

784. Larsen, A.G., and B. Nørrung. Inhibition of *Listeria monocytogenes* by bavaricin A, a bacteriocin produced by *Lactobacillus bavaricus* MI401. *Lett. Appl. Microbiol.* 17:132–134 (1993).

785. Abee, T., F.M. Rombouts, J. Hugenholtz, et al. Mode of action of nisin Z against *Listeria monocytogenes* Scott A grown at high and low temperatures. *Appl. Environ. Microbiol.* 60:1962–1968 (1994).

786. Ming, X., and M.A. Daeschel. Nisin resistance of foodborne bacteria and the specific resistance responses of *Listeria monocytogenes* Scott A. *J. Food Protect.* 56:944–948 (1993).

787. Davies, E.A., and M.R. Adams. Resistance of *Listeria monocytogenes* to the bacteriocin nisin. *Int. J. Food Microbiol.* 21:341–347 (1994).

788. Rekhif, N., A. Atrih, and G. Lefebvre. Selection and properties of spontaneous mutants of *Listeria monocytogenes* ATCC 15313 resistant to different bacteriocins produced by lactic acid bacteria strains. *Curr. Microbiol.* 28:237–241 (1994).

789. Huang, J., C. Lacroix, H. Daba, and R.E. Simard. Inhibition of growth of *Listeria* strains by mesenterocin 5 and organic acids. *Lait* 73:357–370 (1993).

790. Giraffa, G., E. Neviani, and G.T. Tarelli. Antilisterial activity by enterococci in a model predicting the temperature evolution of Taleggio, an Italian soft cheese. *J. Dairy Sci.* 77:1176–1182 (1994).

791. Kato, T., T. Matsuda, Y. Yoneyama, et al. Antibacterial substances produced by *Enterococcus faecium*. *Biosci. Biotechnol. Biochem.* 58:411–412 (1994).

792. Arihara, K., R.G. Cassens, and J.B. Luchansky. Characterization of bacteriocins from *Enterococcus faecium* with activity against *Listeria monocytogenes*. *Int. J. Food Microbiol.* 19:123–134 (1993).

793. Schillinger, U., M.E. Stiles, and W.H. Holzapfel. Bacteriocin production by *Carnobacterium piscicola* LV 61. *Int. J. Food Microbiol.* 20:131–147 (1993).

794. Stoffels, G., H.-G. Sahl, and Á. Gudmundsdóttir. Carnocin UI49, a potential biopreservative produced by *Carnobacterium piscicola*: large scale purification and activity against various Gram-positive bacteria. *Int. J. Food Microbiol.* 20:199–210 (1993).

795. Mathiou, F., M. Michel, A. Lebrihi, and G. Lefebvre. Effect of the bacteriocin carnocin CP5 and of the producing strain *Carnobacterium piscicola* CP5 on the viability of *Listeria monocytogenes* ATCC 15313 in salt solution, broth and skimmed milk, at various incubation temperatures. *Int. J. Food Microbiol.* 22:155–172 (1994).

796. Siragusa, G.R., and C.N. Cutter. Brochocin-C, a new bacteriocin produced by *Brochothrix campestris*. *Appl. Environ. Microbiol.* 59:2326–2328 (1993).

797. Villani, F., O. Pepe, G. Mauriello, et al. Antimicrobial activity of *Staphylococcus xylosus* from Italian sausages against *Listeria monocytogenes*. *Lett. Appl. Microbiol.* 18:159–161 (1994).

798. Jacquet, C., and A. Reynaud. Differences in the sensitivity to eight disinfectants of *Listeria monocytogenes* strains as related to their origin. *Int. J. Food Microbiol.* 22:79–83 (1994).

799. Roy, B., H.-W. Ackermann, S. Pandian, et al. Biological inactivation of adhering *Listeria monocytogenes* by listeriaphages and a quaternary ammonium compound. *Appl. Environ. Microbiol.* 59:2914–2917 (1993).

800. Tuncan, E.U. Effect of cold temperature on germicidal efficacy of quaternary ammonium compound, iodophor, and chlorine on *Listeria*. *J. Food Protect.* 56:1029–1033 (1993).

801. Ren, T.-J., and J.F. Frank. Susceptibility of starved planktonic and biofilm *Listeria monocytogenes* to quaternary ammonium sanitizer as determined by direct viable and agar plate counts. *J. Food Protect.* 56:573–576 (1993).

802. Farber, J.M. Current research on *Listeria monocytogenes* in foods: an overview. *J. Food Protect.* 56:640–643 (1993).

803. Dever, F.P., D.W. Schaffner, and P.J. Slade. Methods for the detection of foodborne *Listeria monocytogenes* in the U.S. *J. Food Safety* 13:263–292 (1993).

804. Harris, L., and J. Humber. AutoMicrobic system for biochemical identification of *Listeria* species isolated from foods: collaborative study. *J. AOAC Int.* 76:822–830 (1993).

805. Higgins, D.L., and B.J. Robison. Comparison of MICRO-ID *Listeria* method with conventional biochemical methods for identification of *Listeria* isolated from food and environmental samples: collaborative study. *J. AOAC Int.* 76:831–838 (1993).

806. Twedt, R.M., and A.D. Hitchins. Determination of the presence of *Listeria monocytogenes* in milk and dairy products: IDF collaborative study. *J. AOAC Int.* 77:395–402 (1994).

807. Eld, K., M.-L. Danielsson-Tham, A. Gunnarsson, and W. Tham. Comparison of a cold enrichment method and the IDF method for isolation of *Listeria monocytogenes* from animal autopsy material. *Vet. Microbiol.* 36:185–189 (1993).

808. Herman, L., and H. De Ridder. Comparison of different methods for detection of *Listeria monocytogenes* in dairy products. *Milchwissenschaft* 48:684–686 (1993).

809. Rodríguez, J.L., P. Gaya, M. Medina, and M. Nuñez. A comparative study of the Gene-Trak Listeria assay, the Listeria-Tek ELISA test and the FDA method for the detection of *Listeria* species in raw milk. *Lett. Appl. Microbiol.* 17:178–181 (1993).

810. Url, B., A. Heitzler, and E. Brandl. Determination of *Listeria* in dairy and environmental samples: comparison of a cultural method and a colorimetric nucleic acid hybridization assay. *J. Food Protect.* 56:581–584 (1993).

811. Nørrung, B., and P. Gerner-Smidt. Comparison of multilocus enzyme electrophoresis (MEE), ribotyping, restriction enzyme analysis (REA) and phage typing for typing of *Listeria monocytogenes*. *Epidemiol. Infect.* 111:71–79 (1993).

812. Wong, H.-C., L.-W. Ku, C.-M. Yu, and W.-L. Chao. Molecular characterization of listeriolysin O gene of *Listeria monocytogenes* isolated in Taiwan. *J. Gen Appl. Microbiol.* 40:63–68 (1994).

813. Fujisawa, T., and M. Mori. Evaluation of media for determining hemolytic activity and that of API Listeria system for identifying strains of *Listeria monocytogenes*. *J. Clin. Microbiol.* 32:1127–1129 (1994).

814. Gunasinghe, C.P.G.L., C. Henderson, and M.A. Rutter. Comparative study of two plating media (PALCAM and Oxford) for detection of *Listeria* species in a range of meat products following a variety of enrichment procedures. *Lett. Appl. Microbiol.* 18:156–158 (1994).

815. Mackey, B.M., E. Boogard, C.M. Hayes, and J. Baranyi. Recovery of heat-injured *Listeria monocytogenes*. *Int. J. Food Microbiol.* 22:227–237 (1994).

816. Tran, T.T., and A.D. Hitchins. Recovery limits of heat-injured *Listeria monocytogenes* from enrichment broth and enriched cultures of inoculated foods. *J. Food Safety* 13:185–193 (1993).

817. Meier, R., and G. Terplan. Investigation of cheese and other foodstuff samples with the Listeria-Tek ELISA. *Lett. Appl. Microbiol.* 17:97–100 (1993).

818. Torensma, R., M.J.C. Visser, C.J.M. Aarsman, et al. Monoclonal antibodies that react with live *Listeria* spp. *Appl. Environ. Microbiol.* 59:2713–2716 (1993).

819. Fliss, I., M. St. Laurent, E. Emond, et al. Production and characterization of anti-DNA-RNA monoclonal antibodies and their application in *Listeria* detection. *Appl. Environ. Microbiol.* 59:2698–2705 (1993).

820. Blais, B.W. Transcriptional enhancement of the *Listeria monocytogenes* PCR and simple immunoenzymatic assay of the product using anti-RNA:DNA antibodies. *Appl. Environ. Microbiol.* 60:348–352 (1994).

821. Blais, B.W., and L.M. Phillippe. A simple RNA probe system for analysis of *Listeria monocytogenes* polymerase chain reaction products. *Appl. Environ. Microbiol.* 59:2795–2800 (1993).

822. Emond, E., I. Fliss, and S. Pandian. A ribosomal DNA fragment of *Listeria monocytogenes* and its use as a genus-specific probe in an aqueous-phase hybridization assay. *Appl. Environ. Microbiol.* 59:2690–2697 (1993).

823. Johnson, J.L., and C.P. Lattuada. Comparison of nucleic acid hybridization assays and biochemical characterization tests for the confirmation of *Listeria monocytogenes*. *J. Food Protect.* 56:834–840 (1993).

824. Lawrence, L.M., J. Harvey, and A. Gilmour. Development of a random amplification of polymorphic DNA typing method for *Listeria monocytogenes*. *Appl. Environ. Microbiol.* 59:3117–3119 (1993).

825. Moore, M.A., and A.R. Datta. DNA fingerprinting of *Listeria monocytogenes* strains by pulsed-field gel electrophoresis. *Food Microbiol.* 11:31–38 (1994).

826. Bsat, N., and C.A. Batt. A combined modified reverse dot-blot and nested PCR assay for the specific nonradioactive detection of *Listeria monocytogenes*. *Molec. Cell. Probes* 7:199–207 (1993).

827. Wiedmann, M., F. Barany, and C.A. Batt. Detection of *Listeria monocytogenes* with a nonisotopic polymerase chain reaction–coupled ligase chain reaction assay. *Appl. Environ. Microbiol.* 59:2743–2745 (1993).

828. Chen, J., R. Brosch, and J.B. Luchansky. Isolation and characterization of *Listeria monocytogenes*–specific nucleotide sequences.*Appl. Environ. Microbiol.* 59:4367–4370 (1993).

829. Powell, H.A., C.M. Gooding, S.D. Garret, et al. Proteinase inhibition of the detection of *Listeria monocytogenes* in milk using the polymerase chain reaction. *Lett. Appl. Microbiol.* 18:59–61 (1994).

830. Partis, L., K. Newton, J. Murby, and R.J. Wells. Inhibitory effects of enrichment media on the Accuprobe test for *Listeria monocytogenes*. *Appl. Environ. Microbiol.* 60:1693–1694 (1994).

831. Hancock, I., B.M. Bointon, and P. McAthey. Rapid detection of *Listeria* species by selective impedimetric assay. *Lett. Appl. Microbiol.* 16:311–314 (1993).

832. Bhunia, A.K., P.J. Steele, D.G. Westbrook, et al. A six-hour *in vitro* virulence assay for *Listeria monocytogenes* using myeloma and hybridoma cells from murine and human sources. *Microb. Pathogen.* 16:99–110 (1994).

833. McKellar, R.C. Identification of the *Listeria monocytogenes* virulence factors involved in the CAMP reaction. *Lett. Appl. Microbiol.* 18:79–81 (1994).

834. Bracegirdle, P., A.A. West, M.S. Lever, et al. A comparison of aerosol and intragastric routes of infection with *Listeria* spp. *Epidemiol. Infect.* 112:69–79 (1994).

835. Schlech, W.F., III. An animal model of foodborne *Listeria monocytogenes* virulence: effect of alterations in local and systemic immunity on invasive infection. *Clin. Invest. Med.* 16:219–225 (1993).

836. Myers, E.R., A.W. Dallmier, and S.E. Martin. Sodium chloride, potassium chloride, and virulence in *Listeria monocytogenes*. *Appl. Environ. Microbiol.* 59:2082–2086 (1993).

837. Myers, E.R., and S.E. Martin. Virulence of *Listeria monocytogenes* propagated in NaCl containing media at 4, 25, and 37°C. *J. Food Protect.* 57:475–478 (1994).

838. Khan, S.A., S.M. Khalid, and R. Siddiqui. The effect of pH and temperature on haemolysin production by *Listeria* species. *Lett. Appl. Microbiol.* 17:14–16 (1993).

839. Datta, A.R., and M.H. Kothary. Effects of glucose, growth temperature, and pH on listeriolysin O production in *Listeria monocytogenes*. *Appl. Environ. Microbiol.* 59:3495–3497 (1993).

840. Datta, A.R. Factors controlling expression of virulence genes in *Listeria monocytogenes*. *Food Microbiol.* 11:123–129 (1994).

841. Freitag, N.E., L. Rong, and D.A. Portnoy. Regulation of the *prfA* transcriptional activator of *Listeria monocytogenes*: multiple promoter elements contribute to intracellular growth and cell-to-cell spread. *Infect. Immun.* 61:2537–2544 (1993).

842. Bohne, J., Z. Sokolovic, and W. Goebel. Transcriptional regulation of *PrfA* and prfA-regulated virulence genes in *Listeria monocytogenes*. *Molec. Microbiol.* 11:1141–1150 (1994).

843. Schlech, W.F., III, Q. Luo, G. Faulkner, and S. Galsworthy. Interaction of *Listeria* species with human cell monolayers. *Clin. Invest. Med.* 17:9–17 (1994).

844. Bunduki, M.C., C.M. Beliveau, and C.W. Donnelly. Examination of attachment and phagocytic uptake of *Listeria* species by mammalian intestinal cells. *Food Microbiol.* 10:507–516 (1993).

845. Pistor, S., T. Chakraborty, K. Niebuhr, et al. The ActA protein of *Listeria monocytogenes* acts as a nucleator inducing reorganization of the actin cytoskeleton. *EMBO J.* 13:758–763 (1994).

846. Southwick, F.S., and D.L. Purich. Arrest of *Listeria* movement in host cells by a bacterial ActA analogue: implications for actin-based motility. *Proc. Natl. Acad. Sci. USA* 91:5168–5172 (1994).

847. Dold, F.G., J.M. Sanger, and J.W. Sanger. Intact alpha-actinin molecules are needed for both the assembly of actin into the tails and the locomotion of *Listeria monocytogenes* inside infected cells. *Cell Motility Cytoskeleton* 28:97–107 (1994).

848. Tang, P., I. Rosenshine, and B.B. Finlay. *Listeria monocytogenes*, an invasive bacterium, stimulates MAP kinase upon attachment to epithelial cells. *Molec. Biol. Cell* 5:455–464 (1994).

849. Portnoy, D.A., G.A. Smith, and H. Goldfine. Phospholipases C and the pathogenesis of *Listeria*. *Brazil. J. Med. Biol. Res.* 27:357–361 (1994).

850. Smith, G.A., and D.A. Portnoy. The role of two phospholipases in the pathogenicity of *Listeria monocytogenes*. *Infect. Agents Dis.* 2:183–185 (1994).

851. Quinn, F., L. Pine, E. White, et al. Immunogold labelling of *Listeria monocytogenes* virulence-related factors within Caco-2 cells. *Res. Microbiol.* 144:597–608 (1993).

852. Morange, M., B. Hévin, and R.M. Fauve. Differential heat-shock protein synthesis and response to stress in three avirulent and virulent *Listeria* species. *Res. Immunol.* 144:667–677 (1993).

853. Hévin, B., M. Morange, and R.M. Fauve. Absence of an early detectable increase in heat-shock protein synthesis by *Listeria monocytogenes* within mouse mononuclear phagocytes. *Res. Immunol.* 144:679–689 (1993).

854. Centers for Disease Control. Brucellosis outbreak at a pork processing plant—North Carolina, 1992. *Morbid. Mortal. Weekly Rep.* 43:113–116 (1994).

855. Radolf, J.D. Brucellosis: don't let it get your goat! *Am. J. Med. Sci.* 307:64–75 (1994).

856. Robson, J.M., M.W. Harrison, R.N. Wood, et al. Brucellosis: re-emergence and changing epidemiology in Queensland. *Med. J. Aust.* 159:153–158 (1993).

857. Laso, F.J., M. Cordero, and J.E. Garcia-Sánchez. Esophageal brucellosis: a new location of *Brucella* infection. *Clin. Invest.* 72:393–395 (1994).

858. Anonymous. Raw poultry may be vector for *Helicobacter pylori* infection. *Food Chem. News* 35(23):38 (1993).

859. Hwang, H., J. Dwyer, and R.M. Russell. Diet, *Helicobacter pylori* infection, food preservation and gastric cancer risk: are there new roles for preventative factors? *Nutr. Rev.* 52:75–83 (1994).

860. Sipponen, P. Gastric cancer—a long-term consequence of *Helicobacter pylori* infection? *Scand. J. Gastroenterol.* 29(Suppl. 201):24–27 (1994).

861. Veldhuyzen van Zanten, S.J.O., and P.M. Sherman. *Helicobacter pylori* infection as a cause of gastritis, duodenal ulcer, gastric cancer and nonulcer dyspepsia: a systematic review. *Can. Med. Assoc. J.* 150:177–185 (1994).

862. Gasser, F. Safety of lactic acid bacteria and their occurrence in human clinical infection. *Bull. Inst. Pasteur* 92:45–67 (1994).

863. Donohue, D.C., M. Deighton, J.T. Ahokas, and S. Salminen. Toxicity of lactic acid bacteria. In *Lactic Acid Bacteria*. S. Salminen and A. von Wright (eds.). New York, Marcel Dekker. *Food Sci. Technol. Ser.* 58:307–313 (1993).

864. Shemesh, E., T. Fischel, N. Goldstein, et al. An outbreak of foodborne streptococcal throat infection. *Isr. J. Med. Sci.* 30:275–278 (1994).

865. Sugita, H., T. Nakamura, and Y. Deguchi. Identification of *Plesiomonas shigelloides* isolated from freshwater fish with the microplate hybridization method. *J. Food Protect.* 56:949–953 (1993).

866. Brown, M.L., and J.J. Gauthier. Cell density and growth phase as factors in the resistance of a biofilm of *Pseudomonas aeruginosa* (ATCC 27853) to iodine. *Appl. Environ. Microbiol.* 59:2320–2322 (1993).

867. Marrie, T., P. Green, S. Burbridge, et al. *Legionellaceae* in the potable water of Nova Scotia hospitals and Halifax residences. *Epidemiol. Infect.* 112:143–150 (1994).

868. Rogers, J., A.B. Dowsett, P.J. Dennis, et al. Influence of temperature and plumbing material selection on biofilm formation and growth of *Legionella pneumophila* in a model potable water system containing complex microbial flora. *Appl. Environ. Microbiol.* 60:1585–1592 (1994).

869. von Reyn, C.F., J.N. Maslow, T.W. Barber, et al. Persistent colonisation of potable water as a source of *Mycobacterium avium* in AIDS. *Lancet* 343:1137–1141 (1994).

870. Gennari, M., and P. Lombardi. Comparative characterization of *Acinetobacter* strains isolated from different foods and clinical sources. *Zbl. Bakteriol.* 279:553–564 (1993).

871. Carmichael, W.W. The toxins of cyanobacteria. *Sci. Am.* 270(1):78–86 (1994).

872. Rinehart, K.L., M. Namikoshi, and B.W. Choi. Structure and biosynthesis of toxins from blue-green algae (cyanobacteria). *J. Appl. Phycol.* 6:159–176 (1994).

873. Lin, J.-R., and F.S. Chu. *In vitro* neutralization of the inhibitory effect of microcystin-LR to protein phosphatase 2A by antibody against the toxin. *Toxicon* 32:605–613 (1994).

874. Lin, J.-R., and F.S. Chu. Kinetics of distribution of microcystin LR in serum and liver cytosol of mice: an immunochemical analysis. *J. Agric. Food Chem.* 42:1035–1040 (1994).

875. Nicholson, B.C., J. Rositano, and M.D. Burch. Destruction of cyanobacterial peptide hepatotoxins by chlorine and chloramine. *Water Res.* 28:1297–1303 (1994).

876. Hinton, D.G., A. Shipley, J.W. Galvin, et al. Chlamydiosis in workers at a duck farm and processing plant. *Aust. Vet. J.* 70:174–176 (1993).

877. Madden, J.M. The enterics as foodborne pathogens. *Food Res. Int.* 27:227–232 (1994).

878. Chopra, A.K., X.-J. Xu, and J.W. Peterson. *Salmonella typhimurium* enterotoxin epitopes shared among bacteria. *FEMS Microbiol. Lett.* 118:237–242 (1994).

879. Pohl, P., Y. Glupczynski, M. Marin, et al. Replicon typing characterization of plasmids encoding resistance to gentamicin and apramycin in *Escherichia coli* and *Salmonella typhimurium* isolated from human and animal sources in Belgium. *Epidemiol. Infect.* 111:229–238 (1993).

880. Bunning, V.K. Immunopathogenic aspects of foodborne microbial disease. *Food Microbiol.* 11:89–95 (1994).

881. Smith, J.L., S.A. Palumbo, and I. Walls. Relationship between foodborne bacterial pathogens and the reactive arthritides. *J. Food Safety* 13:209–236 (1993).

882. Yu, D.T.Y., and G.T.D. Thomson. Clinical, epidemiological and pathogentic [sic] aspects of reactive arthritis. *Food Microbiol.* 11:97–108 (1994).

883. Lings, S., F. Lander, and M. Lebech. Antimicrobial antibodies in Danish slaughterhouse workers and greenhouse workers. *Int. Arch. Occup. Environ. Health* 65:405–409 (1994).

884. Murrell, W.G., B.J. Stewart, C. O'Neill, et al. Enterotoxigenic bacteria in the sudden infant death syndrome. *J. Med. Microbiol.* 39:114–127 (1993).

885. Rivault, C., A. Cloarec, and A. Le Guyader. Bacterial contamination of food by cockroaches. *J. Environ. Health* 55(8):21–22 (1993).

886. Kopanic, R.J., Jr., B.W. Sheldon, and C.G. Wright. Cockroaches as vectors of *Salmonella:* laboratory and field trials. *J. Food Protect.* 57:125–132 (1994).

887. Vasavada, P.C, and M.A. Cousin. Dairy Microbiology and Safety. In *Dairy Science and Technology Handbook. 2. Product Manufacturing.* Y.H. Hui (ed.). New York, VCH Publishers, Inc. Pp. 301–426 (1993).

888. Criado, M.-T., B. Suárez, and C.M. Ferreirós. The importance of bacterial adhesion in the dairy industry. *Food Technol.* 48(2):123–126 (1994).

889. Carpentier, B., and O. Cerf. Biofilms and their consequences, with particular reference to hygiene in the food industry. *J. Appl. Bacteriol.* 75:499–511 (1993).

890. Ak, N.O., D.O. Cliver, and C.W. Kaspar. Cutting boards of plastic and wood contaminated experimentally with bacteria. *J. Food Protect.* 57:16–22 (1994).

891. Ak, N.O., D.O. Cliver, and C.W. Kaspar. Decontamination of plastic and wooden cutting boards for kitchen use. *J. Food Protect.* 57:23–30 (1994).

892. Abrishami, S.H., B.D. Tall, T.J. Bruursema, et al. Bacterial adherence to cutting board surfaces. *J. Food Safety* 14:153–172 (1994).

893. Gill, C.O., and J. Bryant. The presence of *Escherichia coli, Salmonella* and *Campylobacter* in pig carcass dehairing equipment. *Food Microbiol.* 10:337–344 (1993).

894. Adesiyun, A.A. Prevalence of *Listeria* spp., *Campylobacter* spp. *Salmonella* spp. *Yersinia* spp. and toxigenic *Escherichia coli* on meat and seafoods in Trinidad. *Food Microbiol.* 10:395–403 (1993).

895. Hudson, J.A., and S.J. Mott. A survey for *Listeria* species, motile aeromonads and *Yersinia enterocolitica* on bovine and ovine carcasses. *N.Z. Vet. J.* 42:33–34 (1994).

896. Wang, G.-h., and X.-l. Qiao. Fleisch und Fleischprodukte aus dem Einzelhandel in Beijing. *Fleischwirtschaft* 74:326–328 (1994).

897. Arumugaswamy, R.K., G.R.R. Ali, and S.N. Ab Hamid. Satay and salmonella and listeria infection. (Letter.) *Lancet* 342:247 (1993).

898. Miller, A.J., F.J. Schultz, A. Oser, et al. Bacteriological safety of swine carcasses treated with reconditioned water. *J. Food Sci.* 59:739–741,746 (1994).

899. Waldroup, A.L., B.M. Rathgeber, and R.E. Hierholzer. Effects of reprocessing on microbiological quality of commercial prechill broiler carcasses. *J. Appl. Poultry Res.* 2:111–116 (1993).

900. Nedoluha, P.C., and D. Westhoff. Microbiological flora of aquacultured hybrid striped bass. *J. Food Protect.* 56:1054–1060 (1993).

901. Berry, T.M., D.L. Park, and D.V. Lightner. Comparison of the microbial quality of raw shrimp from China, Ecuador, or Mexico at both wholesale and retail levels. *J. Food Protect.* 57:150–153 (1994).

902. Gecan, J.S., R. Bandler, and W.F. Staruszkiewicz. Fresh and frozen shrimp: a profile of filth, microbiological contamination, and decomposition. *J. Food Protect.* 57:154–158,168 (1994).

903. Adesiyun, A.A. Bacteriological quality and associated public health risk of pre-processed bovine milk in Trinidad. *Int. J. Food Microbiol.* 21:253–261 (1994).

904. Dumoulin, E., and G. Peretz. Qualité bactériologique du lait cru de chèvre en France. *Lait* 73:475–483 (1993).

905. Maifreni, M., M. Civilini, C. Domenis, et al. Microbiological quality of artisanal ice cream. *Zbl. Hyg.* 194:553–570 (1994).

906. Yamani, M.I., and B.A. Al-Dababseh. Microbial quality of hoummos (chickpea dip) commercially produced in Jordan. *J. Food Protect.* 57:431–435 (1994).

907. Rosenberger, A., and H. Weber. Keimbelastung von Gewürzproben. Mikrobiologischer Status im Hinblick auf Richt- und Warnwerte. *Fleischwirtschaft* 73:830–833 (1993).

908. Anderton, A. Bacterial contamination of enteral feeds and feeding systems. *Clin. Nutr.* 12(Suppl. 1):S16–S32 (1993).

909. Fang, W., M. Shi, L. Huang, et al. Growth of lactobacilli, *Staphylococcus aureus* and *Escherichia coli* in normal and mastitic milk and whey. *Vet. Microbiol.* 37:115–125 (1993).

910. Barbosa, C.G., P.G. Robbs, and V. Favarin. Behaviour of *Staphylococcus aureus* and of *Escherichia coli* and injury formation during production and storage phases of Parmesan cheese. *Rev. Microbiol. São Paulo* 24:111–117 (1993).

911. Barbosa, C.G., P.G. Robbs, and S.M.daC. Raimundo. Behaviour of *Staphylococcus aureus* and of *Escherichia coli* and injury formation during production and storage phases of "Prato" cheese. *Rev. Microbiol. São Paulo* 24:118–124 (1993).

912. Sanchez-Rey, R., B. Poullet, P. Caceres, and G. Larriba. Microbiological quality and incidence of some patho-

genic microorganisms in La Serena cheese throughout ripening. *J. Food Protect.* 56:879–881 (1993).

913. Gram, L. Inhibitory effect against pathogenic and spoilage bacteria of *Pseudomonas* strains isolated from spoiled and fresh fish.*Appl. Environ. Microbiol.* 59:2197–2203 (1993).

914. Fapohunda, A.O., K.W. McMillin, D.L. Marshall, and W.M. Waites. Growth of selected cross-contaminating bacterial pathogens on beef and fish at 15 and 35°C. *J. Food Protect.* 57:337–340 (1994).

915. Hudson, J.A., and S.J. Mott. Growth of *Listeria monocytogenes, Aeromonas hydrophila* and *Yersinia enterocolitica* on cooked beef under refrigeration and mild temperature abuse. *Food Microbiol.* 10:429–437 (1993).

916. Hudson, J.A., S.J. Mott, and N. Penney. Growth of *Listeria monocytogenes, Aeromonas hydrophila,* and *Yersinia enterocolitica* on vacuum and saturated carbon dioxide controlled atmosphere–packaged sliced roast beef. *J. Food Protect.* 57:204–208 (1994).

917. Van Laack, R.L.J.M., J.L. Johnson, C.J.N.M. Van der Palen, et al. Survival of pathogenic bacteria on pork loins as influenced by hot processing and packaging. *J. Food Protect.* 56:847–851 (1993).

918. Hudson, J.A., and S.J. Mott. Growth of *Listeria monocytogenes, Aeromonas hydrophila* and *Yersinia enterocolitica* in pâté and a comparison with predictive models. *Int. J. Food Microbiol.* 20:1–11 (1993).

919. Radford, S.A., and R.G. Board. Fate of pathogens in home-made mayonnaise and related products.*Food Microbiol.* 10:269–278 (1993).

920. Erickson, J.P., D.N. McKenna, M.A. Woodruff, and J.S. Bloom. Fate of *Salmonella* spp., *Listeria monocytogenes,* and indigenous spoilage microorganisms in home-style salads prepared with commercial real mayonnaise or reduced calorie mayonnaise dressings.*J. Food Protect.* 56:1015–1021 (1993).

921. White, A.N. Methods for rapid detection of foodborne disease agents. In *Science for the Food Industry of the 21st Century. Biotechnology, Supercritical Fluids, Membranes and Other Advanced Technologies for Low Calorie, Healthy Food Alternatives.* M. Yalpani (ed.). Mount Prospect, IL, ATL Press. *Frontiers in Foods and Food Ingredients* 1:343–358 (1993).

922. Silley, P. Rapid microbiology—is there a future? *Biosens. Bioelectron.* 9(2):xv–xxi (1994).

923. Bishop, J.R. Food microbiology (dairy). *J. AOAC Int.* 77:186–187 (1994).

924. Andrews, W.H. Food microbiology (nondairy). *J. AOAC Int.* 77:187–194 (1994).

925. de Ryck, R., M.J. Struelens, and E. Serruys. Rapid biochemical screening for *Salmonella, Shigella, Yersinia,* and *Aeromonas* isolates from stool specimens. *J. Clin. Microbiol.* 32:1583–1585 (1994).

926. Spierings, G., C. Ockhuijsen, H. Hofstra, and J. Tommassen. Polymerase chain reaction for the specific detection of *Escherichia coli/Shigella. Res. Microbiol.* 144:557–564 (1993).

927. Pitt, T.L. Bacterial typing systems: the way ahead. *J. Med. Microbiol.* 40:1–2 (1994).

928. Champagne, C.P., R.R. Laing, D. Roy, and A.A. Mafu. Psychrotrophs in dairy products: their effects and their control. *Crit. Rev. Food Sci. Nutr.* 34:1–30 (1994).

929. Li, K.-Y., and J.A. Torres. Water activity relationships for selected mesophiles and psychrotrophs at refrigeration temperatures. *J. Food Protect.* 56:612–615 (1993).

930. Payne, K.D., S.P. Oliver, and P.M. Davidson. Comparison of EDTA and apo-lactoferrin with lysozyme on the growth of foodborne pathogenic and spoilage bacteria.*J. Food Protect.* 57:62–65 (1994).

931. Fu, A.-H., J.G. Sebranek, and E.A. Murano. Microbial and quality characteristics of pork cuts from carcasses treated with sanitizing sprays. *J. Food Sci.* 59:306–309 (1994).

932. van Netten, P., J.H. In 't Veld, and D.A.A. Mossel. An *in-vitro* meat model for the immediate bactericidal effect of lactic acid decontamination on meat surfaces.*J. Appl. Bacteriol.* 76:49–59 (1994).

933. Zeitoun, A.A.M., J.M. Debevere, and D.A.A. Mossel. Significance of *Enterobacteriaceae* as index organisms for hygiene on fresh untreated poultry, poultry treated with lactic acid and poultry stored in a modified atmosphere. *Food Microbiol.* 11:169–176 (1994).

934. Kim, J.-W., and M.F. Slavik. Trisodium phosphate (TSP) treatment of beef surfaces to reduce *Escherichia coli* O157:H7 and *Salmonella typhimurium. J. Food Sci.* 59:20–22 (1994).

935. Miller, R.K., and R. Acuff. Sodium lactate affects pathogens in cooked beef. *J. Food Sci.* 59:15–19 (1994).

936. Stillmunkes, A.A., G.A. Prabhu, J.G. Sebranek, and R.A. Molins. Microbiological safety of cooked beef roasts treated with lactate, monolaurin or gluconate. *J. Food Sci.* 58:953–958 (1993).

937. Houtsma, P.C., J.C. de Wit, and F.M. Rombouts. Minimum inhibitory concentration (MIC) of sodium lactate for pathogens and spoilage organisms occurring in meat products. *Int. J. Food Microbiol.* 20:247–257 (1993).

938. Abdalla, O.M., P.M. Davidson, and G.L. Christen. Survival of selected pathogenic bacteria in white pickled cheese made with lactic acid bacteria or antimicrobials. *J. Food Protect.* 56:972–976 (1993).

939. Varadaraj, M.C., N. Devi, N. Keshava, and S.P. Manjrekar. Antimicrobial activity of neutralized extracellular culture filtrates of lactic acid bacteria isolated from a cultured Indian milk product ('dahi').*Int. J. Food Microbiol.* 20:259–267 (1993).

940. Jeppesen, V.F., and H.H. Huss. Antagonistic activity of two strains of lactic acid bacteria against *Listeria monocytogenes* and *Yersinia enterocolitica* in a model fish product at 5°C. *Int. J. Food Microbiol.* 19:179–186 (1993).

941. Chung, K.-T., S.E. Stevens, Jr., W.-F. Lin, and C.I. Wei. Growth inhibition of selected food-borne bacteria by tannic acid, propyl gallate and related compounds. *Lett. Appl. Microbiol.* 17:29–32 (1993).

942. Baumann, M., and W. Müller. Wirkung von tanningaltigem Pflanzenmaterial auf pathogene Keim»in vitro«. *Tierärztl. Umschau* 48:738–741 (1993).

943. Babic, I., C. Nguyen-the, M.J. Amiot, and S. Aubert. Antimicrobial activity of shredded carrot extracts on food-borne bacteria and yeast. *J. Appl. Bacteriol.* 76:135–141 (1994).

944. Shetty, R.S., R.S. Singhal, and P.R. Kulkarni. Antimicrobial properties of cumin. *World J. Microbiol. Biotechnol.* 10:232–233 (1994).

945. Gundidza, M., S.G. Deans, A.I. Kennedy, et al. The essential oil from *Heteropyxis natalensis* Harv: its antimicrobial activities and phytoconstituents. *J. Sci. Food Agric.* 63:361–364 (1993).

946. Ronner, A.B., and A.C.L. Wong. Biofilm development and sanitizer inactivation of *Listeria monocytogenes* and *Salmonella typhimurium* on stainless steel and Buna-n rubber. *J. Food Protect.* 56:750–758 (1993).

947. Somers, E.B., J.L. Schoeni, and A.C.L. Wong. Effect of trisodium phosphate on biofilm and planktonic cells of *Campylobacter jejuni, Escherichia coli* O157:H7, *Listeria monocytogenes* and *Salmonella typhimurium. Int. J. Food Microbiol.* 22:269–276 (1994).

948. Restaino, L., E.W. Frampton, R.L. Bluestein, et al. Antimicrobial efficacy of a new organic acid anionic surfactant against various bacterial strains. *J. Food Protect.* 57:496–501 (1994).

949. Oliver, S.P., M.J. Lewis, T.L. Ingle, et al. Premilking teat disinfection for the prevention of environmental pathogen intramammary infections. *J. Food Protect.* 56:852–855 (1993).

950. Shapiro, A., and C. Mercier. Safe food manufacturing. *Sci. Total Environ.* 143:75–92 (1994).

951. Paulus, K. Quality assurance: the strategy for the production of safe food products with high quality. In *Safeguarding Food Quality*. H. Sommer et al. (eds). New York, Springer-Verlag. Pp. 17–27 (1993).

952. Pierson, M.D., and D.A. Corlett, Jr. (eds.). *HACCP Principles and Applications*. New York, AVI. 1992.

953. USDA. National Advisory Committee on Microbiological Criteria for Foods. The role of regulatory agencies and industry in HACCP. *Int. J. Food Microbiol.* 21:187–195 (1994).

954. Stringer, M.F. Safety and quality management through HACCP and ISO 9000. *Dairy Food Environ. Sanit.* 14:478–481 (1994).

955. van Schothorst, M., and S. Jongeneel. Line monitoring, HACCP and food safety. *Food Control* 5:107–110 (1994).

956. Karr, K.J., A.N. Maretzki, and S.J. Knabel. Meat and poultry companies assess USDA's Hazard Analysis and Critical Control Point system. *Food Technol.* 48(2):117–122 (1994).

957. Christian, J.H.B. Problems with HACCP. *Food Aust.* 46:81–83 (1994).

958. Anonymous. HACCP does not lessen need for inspections, Alaska warns. *Food Chem. News* 36(17):13–14 (1994).

959. Clingman, C.D. Where HACCP in food service falls short. *Food Protect. Rep.* 10(10):2A–3A (1994).

960. van Logtestjin, J.G., B.A.P. Urlings, P.G.H. Bijker, and J.H.J. Huis in 't Veld. Interruption of bacterial cycles in animal production: related to veterinary public health. *Vet. Q.* 15:123–125 (1993).

961. Huis in 't Veld, J.H.J., R.W.A.W. Mulder, and J.M.A. Snijders. Impact of animal husbandry and slaughter technologies on microbial contamination of meat: monitoring and control. *Meat Sci.* 36:123–154 (1994).

962. Troeger, K. Gewichtung von Hygienerisiken im Schlachprozeß. *Fleischwirtschaft* 73:1102,1111–1116 (1993).

963. Neuber, A. Mikrobiologisch kontrollierte Räume in der Fleischwarenindustrie. *Fleischwirtschaft* 73:983–990,993 (1993).

964. Ingelfinger, E. Reinigung und Desinfektion in Naßräumen. Kriterien zur Auswahl eines modernen Hygienesystems in der Fleischwarenindustrie. *Fleischwirtschaft* 73:977–978,980 (1993).

965. USDA. National Advisory Committee on Microbiological Criteria for Foods. Generic HACCP for raw beef. *Food Microbiol.* 10:449–488 (1993).

966. The National Food Processor Association. Microbiology and Food Safety Committee. HACCP implementation: a generic model for chilled foods. *J. Food Protect.* 56:1077–1084 (1993).

967. Leistner, L. Further developments in the utilization of hurdle technology for food preservation. *J. Food Engin.* 22:421–432 (1994).

968. Almonacid-Merino, S.F., and J.A. Torres. Mathematical models to evaluate temperature abuse effects during distribution of refrigerated solid foods. *J. Food Engin.* 20:223–245 (1993).

969. Armenante, P.M. Derivation of a rigorous equation for the calculation of the *F*-value in isothermal sterilization processes. *J. Pharm. Sci.* 83:668–673 (1994).

970. Radomyski, T., E.A. Murano, D.G. Olson, and P.S. Murano. Elimination of pathogens of significance in food by low-dose irradiation: a review. *J. Food Protect.* 57:73–86 (1994).

971. Mayer-Miebach, E. Food irradiation—a means of controlling pathogenic microorganisms in food. *Lebensm. Wiss. Technol.* 26:493–497 (1993).

972. Loaharanu, P. Cost/benefit aspects of food irradiation. A summary of the report and recommendations of the Working Group of the FAO/IAEA/WHO International Symposium. *Food Technol.* 48(1):104–108 (1994).

973. Derr, D.D. International regulatory status and harmonization of food irradiation. *J. Food Protect.* 56:882–886 (1993).

974. Loaharanu, P. Status and prospects of food irradiation. *Food Technol.* 48(5):124–131 (1994).

975. Boisseau, P. Irradiation and the food industry in France. *Food Technol.* 48(5):138–140 (1994).

976. Thayer, D.W., J.B. Fox, Jr., and L. Lakritz. Effects of ionizing radiation treatments on the microbiological, nutritional, and structural quality of meats. In *Food Flavor and Safety. Molecular Analysis and Design*. A.M. Spanier et al. (eds.). Washington, DC, American Chemical Society. *ACS Symp. Ser.* 528:293–302 (1993).

977. Thayer, D.W. Extending shelf life of poultry and red meat by irradiation processing. *J. Food Protect.* 56:831–833 (1993).

978. Naik, G.N., P. Paul, S.P. Chawla, et al. Improvement in microbiological quality and shelf-life of buffalo meat at ambient temperature by gamma irradiation. *J. Food Safety* 13:177–183 (1993).

979. Clavero, M.R.S., J.D. Monk, L.R. Beuchat, et al. Inactivation of *Escherichia coli* O157:H7, salmonellae, and *Campylobacter jejuni* in raw ground beef by gamma irradiation. *Appl. Environ. Microbiol.* 60:2069–2075 (1994).

980. Rowe, T.F., and K.J. Towner. Effect of irradiation on the detection of bacterial DNA in contaminated food samples by DNA hybridization. *Lett. Appl. Microbiol.* 18:171–173 (1994).

981. Fuller, R. (ed.). *Probiotics. The Scientific Basis.* New York, Chapman & Hall (1992).

982. Perdigón, G., and S. Alvarez. Probiotics and the immune state. In *Probiotics. The Scientific Basis.* R. Fuller (ed.). New York, Chapman & Hall. Pp. 146–180 (1992).

983. Goldin, B.R., and S.L. Gorbach. Probiotics for humans. In *Probiotics. The Scientific Basis.* R. Fuller (ed.). New York, Chapman & Hall. Pp. 355–376 (1992).

984. Nousiainen, J., and J. Setälä. Lactic acid bacteria as animal probiotics. In *Lactic Acid Bacteria.* S. Salminen and A. von Wright (eds.). New York, Marcel Dekker. *Food Sci. Technol. Ser.* 58:315–356 (1993).

985. Stiles, M.E. Potential for biological control of agents of foodborne disease. *Food Res. Int.* 27:245–250 (1994).

986. Muriana, P.M. Antimicrobial peptides and their relation to food quality. In *Food Flavor and Safety. Molecular Analysis and Design.* A.M. Spanier et al. (eds.). Washington, DC, American Chemical Society. *ACS Symp. Ser.* 528:303–321 (1993).

987. Hammes, W.P., and P.S. Tichaczek. The potential of lactic acid bacteria for the production of safe and wholesome food. *Z. Lebensm. Unters. Forsch.* 198:193–201 (1994).

988. Weber, H. Dry sausage manufacture. The importance of protective cultures and their metabolic products. *Fleischwirtschaft* 74:278–281 (1994).

989. Davidson, P.M., and D.G. Hoover. Antimicrobial components from lactic acid bacteria. In *Lactic Acid Bacteria.* S. Salminen and A. von Wright (eds.). New York, Marcel Dekker. *Food Sci. Technol. Ser.* 58:127–159 (1993).

990. Vandenbergh, P.A. Lactic acid bacteria, their metabolic products and interference with microbial growth. *FEMS Microbiol. Rev.* 12:221–238 (1993).

991. Vaughan, E.E., E. Caplice, R. Looney, et al. Isolation from food sources, of lactic acid bacteria that produced antimicrobials. *J. Appl. Bacteriol.* 76:118–123 (1994).

992. Garver, K.I., and P.M. Muriana. Detection, identification and characterization of bacteriocin-producing lactic acid bacteria from retail food products. *Int. J. Food Microbiol.* 19:241–258 (1993).

993. Klaenhammer, T.R. Genetics of bacteriocins produced by lactic acid bacteria. *FEMS Microbiol. Rev.* 12:39–86 (1993).

994. Bruno, M.E.C., and T.J. Montville. Common mechanistic action of bacteriocins from lactic acid bacteria. *Appl. Environ. Microbiol.* 59:3003–3010 (1993).

995. Schved, F., Y. Henis, and B.J. Juven. Response of spheroplasts and chelator-permeabilized cells of Gram-negative bacteria to the action of the bacteriocins pediocin SF-1 and nisin. *Int. J. Food Microbiol.* 21:305–314 (1994).

996. Entian, K.-D., and C. Klein. Lantibiotika, eine Klasse ribosomal synthetisierter Peptid-Antibiotika. *Naturwissenschaften* 80:454–460 (1993).

997. Hansen, J.N. Nisin as a model food preservative. *Crit. Rev. Food Sci. Nutr.* 34:69–93 (1994).

998. De Vuyst, L. Nisin production variability between natural *Lactococcus lactis* subsp. *lactis* strains. *Biotechnol. Lett.* 16:287–292 (1994).

999. Engelke, G., Z. Gutowski-Eckel, P. Kiesau, et al. Regulation of nisin biosynthesis and immunity in *Lactococcus lactis* 6F3. *Appl. Environ. Microbiol.* 60:814–825 (1994).

1000. Kuipers, O.P., H.S. Rollema, M.M. Beerthuyzen, et al. Biosynthesis and protein engineering of nisin. In *The Lactic Acid Bacteria. Proceedings of the First Lactic Acid Bacteria Computer Conference.* E.-L. Foo et al. (eds.). Norfolk, England, Horizon Scientific Press. Pp. 9–12 (1993).

1001. Lante, A., A. Crapisi, G. Pasini, and P. Scalabrini. Nisin released from immobilization matrices as an antimicrobial agent. *Biotechnol. Lett.* 16:293–298 (1994).

1002. González, S.N., M.C. Apella, N.C. Romero, et al. Inhibition of enteropathogens by lactobacilli strains used in fermented milk. *J. Food Protect.* 56:773–776 (1993).

1003. Atrih, A., N. Rekhif, M. Michel, and G. Lefebvre. Detection of bacteriocins produced by *Lactobacillus plantarum* strains isolated from different foods. *Microbios* 75:117–123 (1993).

1004. González, B., P. Arca, B. Mayo, and J.E. Suárez. Detection, purification, and partial characterization of plantaricin C, a bacteriocin produced by a *Lactobacillus plantarum* strain of dairy origin. *Appl. Environ. Microbiol.* 60:2158–2163 (1994).

1005. Tichaczek, P.S., R.F. Vogel, and W.P. Hammes. Cloning and sequencing of *sakP* encoding sakacin P, the bacteriocin produced by *Lactobacillus sake* LTH 673. *Microbiology* 140:316–367 (1994).

1006. Bhunia, A.K., T.K. Bhowmik, and M.G. Johnson. Determination of bacteriocin-encoding plasmids of *Pediococcus acidilactici* strains by Southern hybridization. *Lett. Appl. Microbiol.* 18:168–170 (1994).

1007. Piva, A., and D.R. Headon. Pediocin A, a bacteriocin produced by *Pediococcus pentosaceus* FBB61. *Microbiology* 140:697–702 (1994).

1008. Keppler, K., R. Geisen, and W.H. Holzapfel. An α-amylase sensitive bacteriocin of *Leuconostoc carnosum*. *Food Microbiol.* 11:39–45 (1994).

1009. Quadri, L.E.N., M. Sailer, K.L. Roy, et al. Chemical and genetic characterization of bacteriocins produced by *Carnobacterium piscicola* LV17B. *J. Biol. Chem.* 269:12204–12211 (1994).

1010. Wolfson, L.M., and S.S. Sumner. Antibacterial activity of the lactoperoxidase system: a review. *J. Food Protect.* 56:887–892 (1993).

1011. Razavi-Rohani, S.M., and M.W. Griffiths. The effect of mono and polyglycerol laurate on spoilage and pathogenic bacteria associated with foods. *J. Food Safety* 14:131–151 (1994).

1012. Shelef, L.A. Antimicrobial effects of lactates: a review. *J. Food Protect.* 57:445–450 (1994).

1013. Friedman, M. Improvement in the safety of foods by SH-containing amino acids and peptides. A review. *J. Agric. Food Chem.* 42:3–20 (1994).

1014. Lechowich, R.V. Food safety implications of high hydrostatic pressure as a food processing method. *Food Technol.* 47(6):170,172 (1993).

1015. Carlez, A., J.-P. Rosec, N. Richard, and J.-C. Cheftel. High pressure inactivation of *Citrobacter freundii, Pseudomonas fluorescens* and *Listeria innocua* in inoculated minced beef muscle. *Lebensm. Wiss. Technol.* 26:357–363 (1993).

1016. Anonymous. Hygienic packing of food products. *Trends Food Sci. Technol.* 4:406–411 (1993).

1017. Kneifel, W., and A. Kaser. Microbiological quality parameters of packaging material used in the dairy industry. *Arch. Lebensmittelhyg.* 45:38–43 (1994).

1018. Berends, B.R., J.M.A. Snijders, and J.G. van Logtestijn. Efficacy of current EC meat inspection procedures and some proposed revisions with respect to microbiological safety: a critical review. *Vet. Rec.* 133:411–415 (1993).

1019. Consultants in Public Health Medicine (Communicable Diseases and Environmental Health) Working Group. Guidelines on bacteriological clearance following gastrointestinal infection. *Commun. Dis. Environ. Health Scotland Weekly Rep.* 28(26):8–12 (1994).

# 12

# Foodborne Parasitic Infections

Jernigan et al. discussed infections of the small intestine caused by protozoa and helminths (*1*). They briefly summarized the morphology, life cycle, and metabolism of intestinal parasites, their susceptibility to chemotherapeutic agents, and the clinical manifestations of the diseases they cause. Parasitic intestinal disease extorts an enormous toll, particularly in developing countries and among the immunosuppressed. Pathogenic protozoa that may be ingested in contaminated food and water include *Cryptosporidium parvum, Toxoplasma gondii, Giardia lamblia, Dientamoeba fragilis, Blastocystis hominis, Balantidium coli, Isospora belli, Entamoeba* spp., *Sarcocystis* spp., and cyanobacterium-like (coccidian-like) bodies (provisionally identified as a species of *Cyclospora*). Pathogenic nematodes (roundworms) that infect flesh foods include *Ascaris lumbricoides, Trichuris trichiura, Capillaria philippinesis, Angiostrongylus costaricensis, Anisakis simplex,* and *Trichinella* spp. Pathogenic trematodes (flukes) include *Fasciolopsis buski,* ingested with contaminated raw water plants; *Heterophyes heterophyes* and *Metagonium yokogawai,* ingested in infected freshwater fish; and *Echinostoma* spp., ingested in raw infected snails, amphibians, or fish. The well-known pathogenic cestodes (tapeworms) belong to the genus *Taenia.*

# PROTOZOA

## *Acanthamoeba*

Pathogenic species of *Acanthamoeba* are common contaminants in municipal sewage wastes. A new pathogen, *Acanthamoeba stevensoni,* was identified in sewage-contaminated hard-clam (*Mercenaria mercenaria*) beds in Raritan Bay, New York (*2*). The organism was recovered from sediments near the shores of Staten Island, in an area designated by the FDA as requiring depuration of harvested clams before sale because of contamination by sewage-associated bacteria. Eight of 12 stations were positive for at least one of the following *Acanthamoeba* species: *A. castellanii, A. comandoni, A. hatchetti, A. lenticulata, A. polyphaga, A. rhysodes,* and two unidentified acanthamoebas. The authors suggest including amoebas as indicator organisms in areas monitored for enteric bacteria, particularly because many bacteria enter a dormant stage in which they fail to grow on standard culture media.

## *Cryptosporidium*

A case–control study was conducted in a semiurban region of Guinea-Bissau, West Africa, to determine risk factors for *Cryptosporidium* diarrhea in young children (*3*). The following factors were significant by multivariate analysis: keeping of pigs (OR 2.5, 95% CI 1.4–4.7, $p = .004$); keeping of dogs (OR 2.1, 95% CI 1.0–4.2, $p = .051$); storage of cooked food for later consumption (OR 1.8, 95% CI 1.0–3.3, $p = .018$); and male sex (OR 1.9, 95% CI 1.0–3.4, $p = .029$). Breast feeding was protective (OR 0.3, 95% CI 0.1–1.1, $p = .048$). Risk was not significantly associated with keeping of goats, sheep, chickens, ducks, or cats or with water source and sanitation. In this setting pigs roam free, frequently sleeping in houses. Oocysts of *Cryptosporidium* were found in ~20% of pig-feces samples, suggesting that cryptosporidiosis is a zoonosis.

A prospective cohort study examined the transmission of *Cryptosporidium parvum* infection in an urban community in northeastern Brazil (*4*). The organism was highly transmissible and infective in the family setting, with a transmission rate similar to rates for other highly infectious enteric pathogens such as *Shigella* spp. Thirty secondary cases were identified in 18 of 31 households (58%), for an overall transmission rate of 19%. In editorial comments on this paper, Current discussed some clinical observations of *Cryptosporidium* infection (*5*). In areas of endemic infection, illness is most severe in young children. However, a student of Current's contracted severe diarrhea while working with infected calves; two subsequent infections, occurring 4 and 10 months later, were mild. From this Current concluded that infection provides temporary immunity, and those who are repeatedly exposed are protected from debilitating bouts of illness. However, secondary transmission would be expected where *C. parvum* is relatively rare—hence the high attack rate seen in day-care centers and in some waterborne outbreaks. This underscores the threat of *C. parvum* for AIDS patients and other immunosuppressed persons living where the infection is endemic.

A failure of a water filtration system in Washington, D.C., prompted concern about contamination of the water supply with *Cryptosporidium* because this parasite is resistant to normal levels of chlorination (*6*). Outbreaks of waterborne cryptosporidiosis have been associated with relatively small increases in water turbidity. For example, in the Milwaukee outbreak of 1993, a peak turbidity reading of 1.7 units was associated with illness in some 400,000 people. Turbidity levels reached 9.0 units in the District of Columbia. Failure to detect increased rates of cryptosporidiosis among D.C. residents probably indicates that only small numbers of oocysts were present at the time the filtration system failed. Smith et al. pointed out that the importance of small numbers of oocysts in treated water cannot be evaluated unless the viability of individual oocysts can be determined (7). They have monitored *C. parvum* in a potable water supply for more than 4 years, and for the last 2 years have used a viability assay they developed. In 20 instances they detected low numbers of oocysts before chlorination. In 10 instances they were unable to assess viability. In 9 instances only nonviable oocysts were detected, and on only 1 occasion were both viable and nonviable oocysts seen. Under conditions prevailing for this water source, therefore, the authors concluded that small numbers of *C. parvum* oocysts pose little or no public health risk.

## *Giardia lamblia*

On multivariate analysis, a case–control study of giardiasis in the East Suffolk region of the UK found significant risk to be associated with contact with farm animals (OR 4.77, 95% CI 1.31–17.38, $p = .01$) and pets (OR 14.55, 95% CI 4.18–50.62, $p < .0001$) (8). No risk was associated with age or water consumption. This apparently confirms the zoonotic transmission of *Giardia lamblia* infection and highlights the risk associated with pets.

## *Toxoplasma gondii*

Although the disease toxoplasmosis is relatively rare, a large proportion of the U.S. population is serologically positive to the parasite. Thus exposure is common. An extensive review by Smith documented incidents of toxoplasmosis to illustrate conditions leading to outbreaks and to show how *Toxoplasma gondii* is transmitted to humans (9). Of 20 outbreaks, 5 were probably caused by consumption of raw goat's milk and 11 by eating raw or undercooked meat (most often lamb). Two probably resulted from geophagy (pica) and one from inhalation; one was associated with creek water. In one study, about 30% of wildlife workers in South Carolina and Georgia who regularly handled deer viscera were seropositive, and among these seropositivity was significantly associated with eating raw or rare venison. Further data on the relationship between eating raw meat and seropositivity for *T. gondii* were discussed and the occurrence of *T. gondii* cysts in tissues of

game animals and domesticated animals was summarized. Smith concluded that pasteurization of goat's milk and freezing, irradiation, or thorough cooking of meat would prevent large numbers of infections. However, the threat from oocysts in the environment would still remain. Because tissue cysts of *T. gondii* can persist throughout the life of an infected individual and no known drug can eradicate the infection, toxoplasmosis is a particular threat to immunocompromised patients, who may suffer reactivation of previous infections.

Lindsay examined the hearts of 16 wild turkeys killed by hunters in Alabama for encysted *T. gondii* (10). The organism was isolated from 8 hearts, and 6 isolates caused fatal infections in mice; one isolate did not cause death, but there were clinical signs of infection. Sera or tissue fluids from 12 of 17 turkeys (71%) were positive for *T. gondii* antibodies at dilutions of 1:50 or higher in a modified direct agglutination test. This high prevalence of the pathogen in wild turkeys indicates that these birds are potential sources of human infection. Common food-preparation practices would kill most encysted bradyzoites, but viscera from wild turkeys should not be fed to household cats and viscera of field-dressed turkeys should be burned or buried to prevent infection in other animals.

A more extensive survey of wild mammals in Kansas found a 16% prevalence of seropositivity to *T. gondii* (11). Fourteen of 20 raccoons (70%), 47 of 106 white-tailed deer (44%), and 9 of 28 Virginia opossums (32%) were seropositive; <8% of rodents and pronghorn antelope were positive. The authors attributed the different rates of seropositivity in deer and antelope to the fact that all samples from antelope were collected in the western part of the state, where human population density is lower and vegetation is less dense.

Dorny et al. determined the seroprevalence of toxoplasmosis among 400 goats from 32 goat farms in peninsular Malaysia and assessed the risk factors for infection (12). The overall prevalence of antibodies was 35.3%. Seropositive animals were found on 26 farms (81%). Seroprevalence was significantly higher on farms owned by Malay farmers than on farms run by Indians or Chinese; this may be because of an association with cats, which are kept mainly by Malay families. Seroprevalence was also higher on farms with 20 or fewer goats; no goats on two large commercial farms were seropositive. Husbandry, climate, and reproductive variables were discussed. As Malaysians eat their meat well cooked they are at little risk of *Toxoplasma* infection from ingestion of contaminated meat, but infection could result from handling fresh meat or drinking unpasteurized goat's milk.

## Cyanobacterium-like (Coccidian-like) Bodies

Hale et al. reported a case of diarrhea associated with cyanobacterium-like bodies (*13*). The patient was an otherwise healthy 69-year-old man who had helped clean his basement after it was flooded with sewage backup. The home was located below a dairy, and the sewage backup consisted of water that looked milky. The patient's wife, who also assisted with the cleaning, had one day of mild diarrhea.

# NEMATODES (ROUNDWORMS)

Karl and Leinemann described a fast, quantitative method for detecting nematodes in fish fillets and fishery products (*14*). It involves a new method of pressing in conjunction with candling under ultraviolet light. All nematodes show a brilliant white-bluish fluorescence and can be counted easily.

## Anisakis

A study of *Anisakis* larvae in North Sea herring found that larvae are present in the flesh of herring when they are caught, and there is no significant migration into the flesh during storage (*15*). Thus immediate on-board gutting cannot eliminate or even reduce the risk of infection from eating raw or inadequately processed herring. The mean numbers of worms in freshly caught herring (one winter and one summer survey) were 0.06 and 0.09 in double fillets, 0.19 and 0.24 in double belly flaps, and 10.4 and 7.8 in viscera.

Angot and Brasseur examined 3700 fillets of Atlantic salmon (*Salmo salar*) from Norwegian and Scottish farms for anisakid larvae using a candling method (*16*). No larvae were found. This contrasts sharply with reports of larvae in the musculature of 39% of wild Atlantic salmon and up to 100% of wild Pacific salmon (*Oncorhynchus* spp.). Although farmed salmon seem relatively safe, the authors recommended that salmon farmers ensure a systematic survey for infection using the more sensitive digestion method whenever possible and evaluating both flesh and viscera; and that salmon processors use an HACCP approach to ensure that farmed salmon are produced within established guidelines.

A survey of sushi and sashimi from 32 Seattle-area restaurants and several specialty grocery stores found anisakid parasites in nearly 10% of pieces of salmon sushi (*17*). The maximum number of parasites per piece was 3. Single parasites were found in 5% of mackerel sushi pieces. No larvae were found in samples of tuna and rockfish sushi. All nematodes were third-stage juveniles of the genus *Anisakis*, and all except 2 were dead, probably because the fish had been frozen. The two living larvae were moribund. No parasites were found in tuna sashimi but one live larva was found in a rockfish sashimi sample. Candling and inspection by ultraviolet light were ineffective for detecting larvae in most types of samples. Levels of *Bacillus cereus* and *Staphylococcus aureus* well within the range considered safe were found in rice samples from 6 restaurants, and in no case were both organisms found in the same sample.

## Trichinella

The epidemiology of trichinosis was reviewed during the 8th International Conference on Trichinellosis held in Italy, 6–10 September 1993 (*18*). Information was summarized by country, including programs for control.

Borowka and Ring discussed progress in detecting the *Trichinella* parasite, from microscopic observation to sensitive digestion methods and ELISAs (*19*). They discussed efforts to establish the Netherlands as a trichinosis-free zone and whether this is a realistic goal for Germany.

Andrews and Webert described control indicators for the examination of pork for *Trichinella spiralis* by the acid-pepsin digestion method (*20*). The indicators are color-coded modified collagen membranes. Digestion of the blue indicator but not the red indicates that the process is within acceptable limits. Use of these indicators is analogous to use of reference materials in chemical and serological determinations.

Whether there is such a disease entity as chronic trichinosis is still debated. Harms et al. conducted a prospective controlled study of trichinosis patients (*21*). Ten years after acute infection, 38% of the 128 originally infected subjects still had IgG antibodies to *T. spiralis*. Although MRI of the brain revealed no abnormalities and no calcifications of residual larvae were detected by mammography or muscle biopsy, the level of performance in psychometric tests was lower in the previously infected population than in noninfected controls. Nevertheless, the authors considered these differences insufficient to support the conclusion that chronic trichinosis is a distinct entity.

# CESTODES (TAPEWORMS)

## *Taenia solium*

Intestinal infection with *Taenia solium* is acquired by eating meat containing *T. solium* cysts (cysticerci). In the intestine, the organism develops into a "tapeworm," whose eggs are shed intermittently in the feces. Ingestion of eggs leads to cysticercosis—or neurocysticercosis, if the cysts form in the brain. Neurocysticercosis, then, stems from contact with human tapeworm carriers, not from contact with infected meat. Shandera et al. reviewed 112 cases of neurocysticercosis diagnosed at Ben Taub General Hospital, Houston, from 1985 through 1991 (*22*). Twenty-two patients had inactive disease, with calcifications apparent on CT scanning; 73 patients had active parenchymal disease. The most common clinical symptom was seizures. (Neurocysticercosis is the most frequently identified cause of seizures in areas where *T. solium* infection is endemic.) Other manifestations were headaches, psychiatric disorders, difficulty speaking, aphasia, hydrocephalus, and cognitive decline. Control of neurocysticercosis requires attention to pork hygiene to prevent taeniasis, and sanitation to prevent infection of pigs and ingestion of eggs by people.

Encysted in tissues, *T. solium* lives for years. Herrera et al. presented evidence from animal and cell-culture experiments that the parasite causes genetic instability in host cells (*23*). Pigs orally inoculated with *T. solium* eggs showed an increase in lymphocyte proliferation for 6–8 weeks after infection; this was followed by impaired proliferation and significant induction of sister-chromatid exchanges. Moreover, a factor secreted by the cysticerci morphologically transformed primary fibroblasts in culture. In vivo, these changes could result in immunosuppression and malignant transformation of target cells.

## *Diphyllobothrium*

*Diphyllobothrium dendriticum* and *Diphyllobothrium latum* were reported for the first time in fishes from Argentina (*24*). Brook trout and rainbow trout harbored both species. Three of 11 brook trout had *D. dendriticum* and 1 had *D. latum*. Of 114 rainbow trout, 41 harbored only *D. dendriticum*, 7 had only *D. latum*, and 25 were infected by both species. Per fish, there were 7.2 *D. dendriticum* plerocercoids but only 1.4 *D. latum*. Perch harbored only *D. latum* (6 of 32 fish). Pejerrey were not infected. Humans are the principal definitive hosts of *D. latum; D. dendriticum* is also able to infect people, but

is often eliminated spontaneously after a few months. Home-smoked brook or rainbow trout could pose a health hazard if too low a processing temperature is used. However, this study found very low numbers of *D. latum* and the only muscle sample to yield a plerocercoid contained *D. dendriticum*. The authors discussed the pattern of distribution of parasites in the rainbow trout in terms of their ecology and their impact on the fish.

## *Echinococcus granulosus*

Echinococcosis is hyperendemic in Israel, where it is frequently transmitted by dogs and has been reportable since 1981. A survey in northern Israel evaluated the prevalence of *Echinococcus granulosus* in dogs and sheep (*25*). Ten percent of 255 sheep slaughtered in a local slaughterhouse contained *Echinococcus* cysts. Seven of 49 dogs examined were infected with *E. granulosus*, but no *Echinococcus* worms were found in the intestines of 5 stray dogs that were shot. No *Echinococcus* parasites were found in 21 dogs examined 3 months after praziquantel treatment. The authors consider echinococcosis to be a very serious public health problem in Israel and recommend high priority for a control program. Almost no data are available on the prevalence of *E. granulosus* in the 63,000 cows and 55,000 sheep that are slaughtered annually in 18 slaughterhouses. Moreover, 75% of sheep are slaughtered illegally, generally at home, and these are the source of infection in dogs.

The prevalence of *E. granulosus* in slaughtered animals was monitored in the Slovak Republic from 1971 through 1990 (*26*). In pigs, the prevalence fell steadily, by as much as 15% per year, from 3.85 to 0.13%. In sheep, significant 12-, 6-, and 3-year periodicities were superimposed on a small, nonsignificant decrease of 1% per year. As a reult, prevalence fluctuated between 0.49 and 3.72%. These differences are attributed to differences in strains of *E. granulosus*. The domestic sheep strain is uniform throughout Europe. The pig strain in the former Czechoslovakia differs from strains found in other domestic animals, but pigs are also susceptible to the sheep strain. From their data, the authors infer that the pig and sheep strains in the Slovak Republic are distinct and that the sheep strain has become more important economically.

# TREMATODES (FLUKES)

Foodborne trematode infections are a serious but neglected public health problem. An estimated 40 million people are infected with one or more species of trematode (*27*). Most of these infections are related to the habit of eating raw, inadequately cooked, or improperly processed food. In Asia and the former Soviet Union, 113 species of freshwater fish are known hosts for *Clonorchis sinensis*. These fish, which are eaten raw, are commonly raised in ponds contaminated with human and animal excrement. Nine species of snail serve as the first intermediate host for *C. sinensis*, and one or more of these species are generally present in fish ponds. An estimated 7 million people are infected. Snails are also the first intermediate hosts for *Opisthorchis viverrini* and *Opisthorchis felineus*. Nearly 9 million people in Thailand and Laos are infected with *O. viverrini*, and more than 2.5 million people in the former Soviet Union are infected with *O. felineus*. Praziquantel can eliminate the infection, but most patients refuse to relinquish their habit of eating raw fish. In Russia, infections are acquired from 22 species of Cyprinidae that are eaten raw, frozen, pickled, or smoked. In Thailand, infection is from 15 species of small freshwater fish eaten raw, pickled, smoked, or fermented; large fish are rarely infected. Nearly 50 species of snails serve as first intermediate hosts for species of *Paragonimus* and at least 53 species of crabs and crayfish are second intermediate hosts. Paragonimiasis is endemic in 39 countries, mostly Asian: *P. westermani, P. heterotremus, P. skrjabini*, and *P. miyazaki* are focally endemic in Asia; *P. mexicanus* in South America; and *P. africanus* and *P. uterobilateralis* in Africa. Crustaceans are eaten raw, roasted, or soaked in wine or soy sauce, and extracted juice is used for seasoning and medicine. The parasites may also be ingested in meat of an alternative intermediate host, such as wild boar. Human fascioliasis, caused by *Fasciola hepatica* or *Fasciola gigantica*, is reported from 56 countries and is gaining importance. Epidemics of fascioliasis have been reported from Cuba and Iran. An estimated 2.4 million people are infected, mostly in Bolivia, Peru, Egypt, Portugal, and China. Snails are intermediate hosts and watercress, mint, lettuce, parsley, and other plants associated with water and eaten raw are the major sources of infection. More than 1 million people are thought to be infected with intestinal flukes, acquired by eating raw fish, snails, clams, frogs, tadpoles, snakes, and aquatic vegetables. The species involved include *Fasciolopsis buski, Heterophyes heterophyes, Metagonimus yokogawai*, and *Nanophyetus salmincola*.

WHO has recently acknowledged the enormous toll on human health exacted by trematodes, particularly the liver fluke *Fasciola hepatica* (*28*). Liver infections are also caused by *Clonorchis sinensis, Opisthorchis viverrini*,

and *Opisthorchis felineus*. More than 12 million people in China and Thailand are thought to be infected. The most recent edition of WHO's leaflet *A Guide on Safe Food for Travellers* contains a specific warning against trematodes in uncooked food. WHO has also published a brief summary of the biology of pathogenic foodborne trematodes and the epidemiology and clinical features of the infections they cause (*29*). The main food vehicles for fascioliasis are watercress and certain herbs; fasciolopsiasis is associated with Chinese water chestnut (*Eleocharis tuberosa*), water chestnut (*Trapa natans*), and water fern (*Salvinia natans*). Clonorchiasis is associated with eating crustaceans and fish of 9 families, especially Cyprinidae. Opisthorchiasis is mainly associated with eating fish of the family Cyprinidae. *Echinostoma* infections are caused by eating infected land snails, clams, and tadpoles. Mullet is a host for *Haplorchis, Heterophyes,* and *Phagicola*. *Tilapia* is also a host for *Heterophyes*. Frogs and snakes carry *Fibricola*, trout carry *Metagonimus*, snails and aquatic insects carry *Plagiorchis*, oysters carry *Gymnophalloides*, and salmon of the genus *Salmo* carry *Nanophyetus*. *Nanophyetus* infection was at first limited to Siberia, but has now been reported in Washington and Oregon.

Ohshima, Bartsch, and their collaborators have been studying the mechanisms by which chronic infections with such organisms as liver flukes increase cancer risk. Their studies implicate nitric oxide and other oxygen radicals produced in infected and inflamed tissue (*30,31*). This mechanism could apply to other agents including *Helicobacter pylori* and asbestos. Haswell-Elkins et al. also presented a model of endogenous nitric oxide production and extragastric nitrosation to explain the association between liver-fluke infection and cholangiocarcinoma in humans (*32*).

## LITERATURE CITED

1. Jernigan, J., R.L. Guerrant, and R.D. Pearson. Parasitic infections of the small intestine. *Gut* 35:289–293 (1994).

2. Sawyer, T.K., T.A. Nerad, E.J. Lewis, and S.M. McLaughlin. *Acanthamoeba stevensoni* n. sp. (Protozoa: Amoebida) from sewage-contaminated shellfish beds in Raritan Bay, New York. *J. Eukaryotic Microbiol.* 40:742–746 (1993).

3. Mølbak, K., P. Aaby, N. Højlyng, and A.P.J. da Silva. Risk factors for *Cryptosporidium* diarrhea in early childhood: a case–control study from Guinea-Bissau, West Africa. *Am. J. Epidemiol.* 139:734–740 (1994).

4. Newman, R.D., S.-X. Zu, T. Wuhib, et al. Household epidemiology of *Cryptosporidium parvum* infection in an urban community in northeast Brazil. *Ann. Intern. Med.* 120:500–505 (1994).

5. Current, W.L. *Cryptosporidium parvum*: household transmission. *Ann. Intern. Med.* 120:518–519 (1994).

6. Centers for Disease Control. Assessment of inadequately filtered public drinking water—Washington, D.C., December 1993.*Morbid. Mortal. Weekly Rep.* 43:661–663,669 (1994).

7. Smith, H.V., J.F.W. Parker, Z. Bukhari, et al. Significance of small numbers of *Cryptosporidium* sp oocysts in water. (Letter.) *Lancet* 342:312–313 (1993).

8. Warburton, A.R.E., P.H. Jones, and J. Bruce. Zoonotic transmission of giardiasis: a case control study. *Commun. Dis. Rep.* 4(Rev. 3):R32–R36 (1994).

9. Smith, J.L. Documented outbreaks of toxoplasmosis: transmission of *Toxoplasma gondii* to humans. *J. Food Protect.* 56:630–639 (1993).

10. Lindsay, D.S., P.C. Smith, and B.L. Balgburn. Prevalence and isolation of *Toxoplasma gondii* from wild turkeys in Alabama.*J. Helminthol. Soc. Wash.* 61:115–117 (1994).

11. Brillhart, D.B., L.B. Fox, J.P. Dubey, and S.J. Upton. Seroprevalence of *Toxoplasma gondii* in wild mammals in Kansas. *J. Helminthol. Soc. Wash.* 61:117–121 (1994).

12. Dorny, P., C. Casman, R. Sani, and J. Vercruysse. Toxoplasmosis in goats: a sero-epidemiological study in Peninsular Malaysia. *Ann. Trop. Med. Parasitol.* 87:407–410 (1993).

13. Hale, D., W. Aldeen, and K. Carroll. Diarrhea associated with cyanobacterialike bodies in an immunocompetent host. An unusual epidemiological source. *JAMA* 271:144–145 (1994).

14. Karl, H., and M. Leinemann. A fast and quantitative detection method for nematodes in fish fillets and fishery products. *Arch. Lebensmittelhyg.* 44:124–125 (1993).

15. Roepstorff, A., H. Karl, B. Bloemsma, and H.H. Huss. Catch handling and the possible migration of *Anisakis* larvae in herring,*Clupea harengus. J. Food Protect.* 56:783–787 (1993).

16. Angot, V., and P. Brasseur. European farmed Atlantic salmon (*Salmo salar* L.) are safe from anisakid larvae. *Aquaculture* 118:339–344 (1993).

17. Adams, A.M., L.L. Leja, K. Jinneman, et al. Anisakid parasites, *Staphylococcus aureus* and *Bacillus cereus* in sushi and sashimi from Seattle area restaurants. *J. Food Protect.* 57:311–317 (1994).

18. World Health Organization. Veterinary public health: trichinellosis. *Weekly Epidemiol. Rec.* 69:61–63 (1994).

19. Borowka, H.-J., and C. Ring. Trichinenfreie Region—eine realistische Prämisse für den Verbraucherschutz? *Fleischwirtschaft* 73:1362–1366 (1993).

20. Andrews, C.D., and D.W. Webert. Control indicators for the examination of pork for *Trichinella spiralis* by the acid-pepsin digestion method. *J. Food Protect.* 57:173–175 (1994).

21. Harms, G., P. Binz, H. Feldmeier, et al. Trichinosis: a prospective controlled study of patients ten years after acute infection. *Clin. Infect. Dis.* 17:637–632 (1993).

22. Shandera, W.X., A.C. White, Jr., J.C. Chen, et al. Neurocysticercosis in Houston, Texas. *Medicine* 73:37–52 (1994).

23. Herrera, L.A., P. Santiago, G. Rojas, et al. Immune response impairment, genotoxicity and morphological transformation induced by *Taenia solium* metacestode. *Mutat. Res.* 305:223–228 (1994).

24. Revenga, J.E. *Diphyllobothrium dendriticum* and *Diphyllobothrium latum* in fishes from southern Argentina: association, abundance, distribution, pathological effects, and risk of human infection. *J. Parasitol.* 79:379–383 (1993).

25. Furth, M., G. Hoida, J. Nahmias, et al. The development of new foci of echinococcosis in northern Israel: prevalence in domestic animals. *J. Helminthol.* 68:45–47 (1994).

26. Dubinský, P., M. Mikulecký, P. Ondrejka, and A. Štefančíková. Prevalence of echinococcosis in pigs and sheep in the Slovak Republic. *Vet. Parasitol.* 51:149–154 (1993).

27. Rim, H.-J., H.F. Farag, S. Sornmani, and J.H. Cross. Food-borne trematodes: ignored or emerging? *Parasitol. Today* 10:207–209 (1994).

28. McGregor, A. Control of trematode infection.*Lancet* 343:411 (1994).

29. Anonymous. Food borne trematode infections. *Commun. Dis. Environ. Health Scotland Weekly Rep.* 27(47):4–7 (1993). Reprinted from *In Point of Fact* No. 80, Office of Information, WHO, Geneva, October 1993.

30. Ohshima, H., and H. Bartsch. Chronic infections and inflammatory processes as cancer risk factors: possible role of nitric oxide in carcinogenesis.*Mutat. Res.* 305:253–264 (1994).

31. Ohshima, H., T.Y. Bandaletova, I. Brouet, H. Bartsch, et al. Increased nitrosamine and nitrate biosynthesis mediated by nitric oxide synthase induced in hamsters infected with liver fluke (*Opisthorchis viverrini*).*Carcinogenesis* 15:271–275 (1994).

32. Haswell-Elkins, M.R., S. Satarug, M. Tsuda, et al. Liver fluke infection and cholangiocarcinoma: model of endogenous nitric oxide and extragastric nitrosation in human carcinogenesis. *Mutat. Res.* 305:241–252 (1994).

# Appendix

# Food- and Water-Associated Viruses

*Contributed by Dean O. Cliver*

# FOOD VIROLOGY

1994 was an exceptional year in food virology, in that a new, three-volume compilation of foodborne disease knowledge includes eight chapters concerning viruses. Discussed are: hepatitis A and E viruses (*1*); small round viruses causing gastroenteritis (*2*); rotaviruses (*3*); tick-borne encephalitis viruses (*4*); other foodborne viral diseases (*5*); medical management of foodborne viral diseases (*6*); epidemiology of foodborne viruses (*7*); and laboratory methods in food virology (*8*). Brief reviews of viruses transmitted via foods (*9*) and of the epidemiology of foodborne viral disease also appeared as journal publications (*10*).

## Foodborne Viral Disease

The reported incidence of hepatitis A in the United States has ranged downward from ca. 31,000 cases in 1990 to ca. 23,000 cases in 1992 (*11*). Suspected food- or waterborne outbreaks were cited as potential sources of these infections at crude rates of 9.4, 6.0, and 8.0 % in 1990, 1991, and 1992, respectively. When sources were assessed on a mutually exclusive basis (i.e., only one possible source was recorded per infection), the suspected food- or waterborne outbreak rates dropped to 4.4, 3.0, and 4.7 %, respectively, for these 3 years. Another recent report cites estimates of 4,800 and 35,000 cases of food-associated hepatitis A and of 181,000 cases of gastroenteritis due to small, round viruses annually in the USA (*12*). Finally, a report summarizes 12 years of foodborne outbreaks recorded in New York State, including outbreaks of viral gastroenteritis and hepatitis A, showing how the data can be used in risk assessment when preparing hazard analysis–critical control point plans (*13*).

An outbreak of hepatitis A in Denmark affected four people who had eaten Russian caviar illegally imported from Latvia (*14*).

Outbreaks of viral gastroenteritis that occurred at various times were reported in 1994. A virus related antigenically to the Norwalk virus caused an outbreak of gastroenteritis involving at least 217 passengers and 21 crew members on a Hawaiian cruise ship in 1990 (*15*). A smaller outbreak had occurred on the previous cruise of the same ship. At least some of the crew members affected were food service workers; the most probable vehicle appeared to have been fresh-cut fruit. A small, round, structured virus was the cause of a UK outbreak affecting 81 patients and 114 staff of four hospitals served by a common kitchen (*16*). The source

of the virus in turkey salad and tuna salad sandwiches may have been a worker who did not become ill herself until after the food had been contaminated. A sandwich bar, but no single food, was the probable source of a small, round, structured virus that caused gastroenteritis in at least 47 employees of a bank and an insurance company during February of 1993 in the UK (*17*). An outbreak of gastroenteritis associated with raw oyster consumption in Florida in November of 1993, caused by small, round, structured viruses, involved at least 45 persons (*18*). Other outbreaks of gastroenteritis due to small, round, structured viruses are frequently recorded in the UK, but are reported without sufficient detail to be included in this summary (*19*). Norwalk virus coat protein, produced with a recombinant baculovirus, is being used in serologic tests; people who have been infected with the Norwalk virus respond with antibody that reacts demonstrably with the viral protein in an enzyme immunoassay (*20*). Serum samples from persons involved in various outbreaks (at least three of which were food-associated) contained antibody (IgA) against the Norwalk virus in some outbreaks but not in others; at least one oyster-associated outbreak may have involved more than one serotype of virus.

Astrovirus was implicated in an outbreak of gastroenteritis in Katano City, Osaka, Japan (*21*). Food from a common supplier, served to students and teachers at 10 primary and 4 junior high schools, was believed to have transmitted the virus to upwards of 4700 persons. In addition to electron microscopy and other serologic and molecular methods, diagnosis was confirmed by cell-culture isolation of the virus from patients' stools.

Tick-borne encephalitis virus, apparently contracted by drinking raw goat's milk, affected seven persons in central Slovakia during September of 1993 (*22*). Although transmission of this virus via milk occurs infrequently, the problem has been well documented in the past (*4*).

## Detection

Most information about food-associated virus disease has been derived from improved diagnostic tests of ill persons, rather than detection of viruses in foods. Although methods for detecting foodborne viruses have, for many years, been based on infectivity of the viruses in cell cultures, it is now generally recognized that the most important foodborne viruses cannot be detected in this way (*8,23,24*). Emphasis has shifted to detection of viral antigen by radioimmunoassay or enzyme immunoassay, or of viral nucleic acid by probe methods or polymerase chain reaction.

Tests on the efficiency of extracting and concentrating virus from Moroccan shellfish were done with vaccine poliovirus so that quantitative comparisons could be made in cell culture (*25*). Elution–acid precipitation methods were judged possibly satisfactory for recovery of the virus from clams and mussels, but none of the tested methods was thought adequate for oysters. In another model study with poliovirus, the polymerase chain reaction was used to test concentrated extracts of oysters (*Crassostrea gigas* and *Ostrea edulis*) and mussels (*Mytilus edulis*) (*26*). Virus recoveries of 31% for oyster extracts and 17% for mussel extracts, with a sensitivity of 1 viral plaque-forming unit for the reverse transcription–polymerase chain reaction, resulted in an estimated limit of sensitivity of <10 plaque-forming units in up to 5 g of shellfish.

An extraction method followed by precipitation of virus with polyethylene glycol 6000 was used to recover viruses from cockles (*Cerastoderma edule*), mussels (*Mytilus edulis*), oysters (*Crassostrea gigas*), and clams (*Ruditapes philippinarum*) in Brittany, France (*27*). Viral RNA was extracted and, after reverse transcription, tested for hepatitis A virus, rotavirus, and enterovirus with a seminested polymerase chain reaction, verified with digoxigenin-labeled oligoprobes. Various special treatments were used to surmount interference by substances in samples with the reverse transcription and polymerase chain reaction; the three viruses were detected in 14, 20, and 22%, respectively, of field samples of shellfish. RNA of hepatitis A virus and of enterovirus was detected in some sediment samples, in which cases corresponding shellfish samples were also positive.

Another reported procedure captures hepatitis A virus with homologous antibody adhered to the insides of microcentrifuge tubes (*28*). Samples tested included experimentally contaminated clams and oysters. While the virus was captured on the antibody, substances that might interfere with reverse transcription and the polymerase chain reaction could be washed out of the tube. Viral RNA was then liberated by incubation of the tubes at 95°C for 5 min, followed by reverse transcription, amplification by the polymerase chain reaction, etc. The limit of detection was estimated to be four virus particles.

Shellfish (oysters and clams) and other foods (orange juice, milk, cole slaw, melon, and lettuce) experimentally contaminated with Norwalk virus were extracted and tested for the viral RNA by a reverse transcription, nested polymerase chain reaction procedure (*29*). The method was adapted from one developed earlier for rotavirus detection, involving virus adsorption to and elution from a solid matrix, as well as precipitation of the viral RNA with cetyltrimethylammonium bromide.

The limit of detection was estimated at 20 to 200 particles of Norwalk virus.

## Prevention of Foodborne Viral Disease

Shellfish are a continuing concern as potential vehicles for viruses. Fecal bacteria, somatic and F-specific coliphages, and bacteriophages that infect *Bacteroides fragilis* were compared as indicators of probable viral contamination of black mussels (*Mytilus edulis*) (*30*). The bacteriophages of *B. fragilis* were found at the greatest distances from source of pollution near Barcelona, Spain, and were present in greater numbers than enteroviruses in samples containing the latter. Mussels that met European Union standards for contamination with fecal bacteria were often found to contain rotaviruses and hepatitis A virus (*31*). Depuration in ozone-disinfected marine water removed 97 to 100% of experimental virus contaminants from mussels within 96 h.

Inactivation of viruses on porous (paper and cotton cloth) and nonporous (aluminum, china, glazed tile, latex, and polystyrene) surfaces was studied as a function of temperature and relative humidity (*32*). In general, hepatitis A virus and a human rotavirus were more stable than enteric adenovirus and poliovirus and were more resistant to drying. The latter viruses showed some protection when in fecal suspension. A bacteriophage of *B. fragilis* was similar to the more resistant viruses, persisting for at least 60 days at 20°C under many conditions. The stability of hepatitis A virus has also been studied as related to the manufacture of coagulation factor VIII from blood. In the presence of stabilizers added to the product, poliovirus, but not hepatitis A virus, was completely inactivated within 10 h at 60°C (*33*). A reduction of approximately 2 $\log_{10}$ in hepatitis A virus infectivity was observed during freeze-drying of the product, and reductions of ≥4.3 $\log_{10}$ resulted from heating the dried product for 24 h at 80°C or 6 h at 90°C (*34*). Similar results were reported with high-purity factor IX concentrate.

Usefulness of available and contemplated hepatitis A vaccines in preventing the disease is probably significant, even though no hepatitis A vaccine is yet licensed in the USA. (*35*). An inactivated virus vaccine for hepatitis A that is available in Scotland is said to offer a year's protection from a single dose and up to 10 years' immunity if a booster is given 6 to 12 months after the primary dose (*36*).

Immunoglobulin concentrate produced from colostrum milk of rotavirus-immunized cows is being evaluated for peroral prophylaxis against rotavirus gastroenteritis in infants and children (*37*). In vitro digestion studies indicated that antiviral potency was greatly reduced by pH 2 (as might occur in the stomach) and by trypsin, but not by pepsin nor by pancreatic proteases other than trypsin. Protection of the antibody from these adverse effects is suggested.

# WATER AND SOIL VIROLOGY

## Drinking Water

An apparently waterborne outbreak of hepatitis E took place in Somalia in 1988, with 11,413 recorded icteric cases and 346 deaths (*38*). A higher incidence was seen in communities using river water, rather than well or pond water; but severity appeared greater among well-water users. As is usual with hepatitis E, there was a high fatality rate (13.8%) among pregnant women.

A prospective epidemiologic study of the role of tap water in dissemination of Norwalk virus was done in the area of Montreal, Canada, in 1988 and 1989 (*39*). Antibodies against the Norwalk virus were present in most of the subjects, yet Norwalk infections apparently occurred in 33% of these people during the course of the study, with the highest rate during the summer of 1988. Attack rates did not differ significantly between those drinking tap water and those drinking water treated by reverse osmosis, suggesting that tap water was not an important source of the virus in this community.

Ice, but not water, consumed aboard a Hawaiian cruise ship was implicated as the source of Norwalk virus in a 1992 outbreak of gastroenteritis (*40*). Illnesses began within 36 h of embarkation and eventually included 30% of the 672 passengers and crew. Although the virus was detectable by polymerase chain reaction with primers for the reference strain of Norwalk virus, there was only an 81% homology in the amplified sequence between the reference and outbreak strains.

Properties of the hepatitis A virus that relate to its transmission via water have been reviewed (*41*). Although the virus persists for a least a month in water at temperatures of 20 to 25°C, the author concludes that complete drinking water treatment (coagulation, rapid filtration, and disinfection) are effective in removing the virus. Combining copper and silver ions with low levels of chlorine was found not to be an effective approach to disinfecting drinking water contaminated experimentally with hepatitis A virus, human rotaviruses and adenoviruses, and poliovirus (*42*).

A broad review addresses, among other things, the reported incidence of a variety of viruses in several types of water including drinking water, and published detection methods based on infectivity, gene probes, and immunoassay (*43*).

## Wastewater and Surface Waters

New detection methods for viruses in wastewater and water contaminated with wastewater are largely based on the polymerase chain reaction, with the strongest focus on detection of hepatitis A virus. A test intended to detect poliovirus, hepatitis A virus, and rotavirus simultaneously in sewage and ocean water is described as a triplex reverse transcriptase polymerase chain reaction (*44*). The sensitivity of the test to hepatitis A virus and rotavirus was found comparable to individual tests, but sensitivity to poliovirus was somewhat less than the "monoplex" version. Concentrated samples of polluted water can be tested for both adenoviruses and enteroviruses, using nested primers in a polymerase chain reaction (*45*). Because the adenoviruses contain DNA, reverse transcription is not necessary, as it is with the enteroviruses, to permit amplification by the polymerase chain reaction. The method yielded more positive results, in testing environmental samples, than were obtained by testing for viral infectivity in cell cultures. Samples of undigested and anaerobically digested sewage sludge were processed with Sephadex G-50 and Chelex 100 before being tested by the polymerase chain reaction for enteroviruses (seminested procedure) and hepatitis A virus (double procedure) (*46*). The method was apparently more sensitive than infectivity tests in cell cultures, but the authors voice the concern that they may at times have been detecting virus that had already been inactivated. Hepatitis A virus in mixtures of septic tank effluent with animal manure slurry were detected by capture with homologous antibody, followed by reverse transcription and amplification by the polymerase chain reaction (*28*). Because the virus that was inoculated experimentally was the strain that forms plaques in cell culture, it was possible to demonstrate that virus which had been inactivated, apparently by biological degradation, was no longer detectable by the antigen capture–polymerase chain reaction test. Another antibody capture method for detection of hepatitis A virus uses magnetic beads as the vehicle for the antibody, so that the virus can be collected from dilute suspensions before reverse transcription and amplification by the polymerase chain reaction (*47*). The method detected a laboratory strain of hepatitis A virus added experimentally to polluted river water, sea water, and fecal extracts.

Anaerobically digested urban sewage sludge showed most probable number levels of <6.25 to $2.52 \times 10^5$

cell culture infectious units of enteroviruses in a 14-month study, for a removal rate ranging from 68% to >99.94% (48). An anaerobic mixture of septic tank effluent and either dairy cattle manure or swine manure slurry inactivated 90% of hepatitis A virus in approximately 20 days at 22°C, compared to 90 days in phosphate buffered saline (49). Biological degradation by bacteria from the manure appeared to play an important role in the virus inactivation.

A group of military diving trainees who wore wet suits, but usually no breathing apparatus, were monitored biologically and serologically for evidence of infection with enteroviruses and hepatitis A virus (50). Despite detection of enteroviruses, by cell culture and molecular hybridization tests of samples of some of the waters in which they dived, there was no evidence of greater exposure of the divers than of a control group that did not enter the water.

A study of aerosols from wastewater treatment plants revealed viruses, principally coxsackieviruses B and echoviruses, that were infectious in BGM cell cultures (51). Aerosol sampling devices were an electro-precipitator and an impinger, of which the former appeared to be more effective. The author points out that the epidemiologic significance of viruses in sewage plant aerosols has yet to be demonstrated.

## Soil and Groundwater

Poliovirus and coliphages MS2 (25 nm diameter) and PRD1 (62 nm diameter) were inoculated experimentally into secondary and tertiary treated sewage and passed through columns of sandy alluvial soil (52). Effluent type had no effect on virus removal, whereas saturated flow was much less effective than unsaturated flow through the soil. The coliphages moved faster than the poliovirus, and all moved much faster than had been predicted on the basis of batch adsorption studies with the same soil material.

Small, round, F-positive RNA coliphages have been tested in laboratory and field studies with a view to using them as indicators of fecal or viral contamination of groundwater (53). The coliphages met some of the criteria to be useful indicators, in that they were regularly associated with urban wastewater and evidently did not replicate under conditions representative of the environment in Wisconsin. However, the FRNA coliphages were not detected in a significant proportion of on-site wastewater treatment (septic tank) systems, and were rarely present in soil and groundwater samples, even if coliform bacteria were present. It was concluded that FRNA coliphages are unlikely to supplant the inadequate coliform

bacteria as indicators in these contexts, but that the FRNA coliphages might be useful as harmless indicators of virus containment in field studies. Other investigators have suggested that some bacteriophages persist best in soil when in the lysogenic state (54).

Disposable diapers were collected from three landfills in which they had resided for at least 2 years (55). Poliovirus RNA, but not rotavirus or hepatitis A virus RNA, was detected in some of the 110 diapers tested, but no viral infectivity was found.

# VIRAL HEPATITIS

## Detection of Hepatitis A Virus

The organizations of the genomes of hepatitis A, B, and D viruses have been reviewed, with a view to how these affect the selection of primers for the polymerase chain reaction (56). In the case of hepatitis A virus, the fact that infectivity depends on the function of an RNA-dependent RNA polymerase points to one highly conserved region of the genome, in addition to those that code for the structural proteins of the virus. A reverse transcription–semi-nested polymerase chain reaction test has been studied and is recommended as a diagnostic adjunct to testing for antiviral serum IgM in hepatitis A epidemics (57). A competitor template RNA has also been developed, to allow monitoring for accidental contamination of test samples with wild type virus when the polymerase chain reaction is being evaluated (58).

## Hepatitis A Virus in Cell Culture

Translation of the hepatitis A viral genome is known to depend on action of the 5' nontranslated region to afford an internal ribosomal entry site, in that the usual cap at which translation begins is absent. Using a specially developed, permissive line of monkey kidney cells and strain HM175/P16 of the hepatitis A virus, it has been shown that this alternative acts relatively inefficiently, which is thought to contribute to the slowness with which the virus replicates in cell cultures (59). An in situ enzyme immunoassay and a cytopathic effect test in cell culture were shown to provide equally reliable infectivity assays of another hepatitis A virus strain, HM175A.2 (60).

Because hepatitis A virus is inefficiently released from the cultured cells it infects, the cells can be collected from the culture, and the supernatant medium discarded, as a first step in concentrating the virus (61).

Detergent treatments eliminate host cell components, allowing collection of the progeny virus in a single centrifugation step. The authors believe that this simple procedure, which yields up to $10^{10}$ infectious particles per milliliter, will be of value in vaccine production.

## Hepatitis E Virus

Like hepatitis A virus, the virus of hepatitis E contains a single (+) strand of RNA and must be reverse-translated before being amplified by the polymerase chain reaction (62). Several primers for use with hepatitis E virus have been devised and published.

The distribution of hepatitis E virus in the world is still being characterized. It has been shown that French soldiers deployed in Chad in 1983 and in Somalia in 1993 experienced outbreaks of serologically confirmed hepatitis E, although they consumed only food and bottled water shipped from France (63). A serologic survey in Venezuela showed a significant frequency of previous hepatitis E infection, ranging from 1.6 to 5.4% in different subject populations (64).

## VIRAL GASTROENTERITIS

Most recent development of knowledge of viral gastroenteritis has emphasized the Norwalk-like, small, round, structured viruses that are now assigned to the calicivirus group. A study with 50 human volunteers used the latest methods to monitor antibody responses and the presence of Norwalk virus in stools (65). Many, but not all, of those who were infected had preexisting antibody. Not all of those infected became ill (e.g., showing vomiting and diarrhea). Most important, from the standpoint of the potential for contamination if these had been food handlers, the new, more sensitive methods detected virus in stools of some infected persons for 7 days, which was the limit of the sampling period. People with preexisting antibody responded with increased levels of IgM, as well as IgG and IgA, antibodies against the Norwalk virus (66).

A gastroenteritis virus isolated from U.S. troops stationed in Saudi Arabia in 1990 ("Desert Shield virus") is partly reactive in serologic tests with the prototype Norwalk virus (67). A reverse transcription–polymerase chain reaction method, using primers from the region of the genome coding for the RNA-dependent RNA polymerase and from near the 3' end showed that there were significant differences even in the sequence for the polymerase gene, which might have been expected to be

highly conserved (68). Groupings based on earlier serologic comparisons are reflected in homologies and differences both in the polymerase sequence and in the genetic sequence that codes the (antigenic) viral coat protein; at least two major serologic groups are thus defined (69,70,71).

## LITERATURE CITED

1. Cromeans, T., O.V. Nainan, H.A. Fields, et al. Hepatitis A and E viruses. In *Foodborne Disease Handbook: Vol. 2. Diseases Caused by Viruses, Parasites, and Fungi.* Y.H. Hui, et al. (eds.). New York, Marcel Dekker, Inc. Pp. 1–56 (1994).

2. Appleton, H. Norwalk virus and the small round viruses causing foodborne gastroenteritis. In *Foodborne Disease Handbook: Vol. 2. Diseases Caused by Viruses, Parasites, and Fungi.* Y.H. Hui, et al. (eds.). New York, Marcel Dekker, Inc. Pp. 57–79 (1994).

3. Sattar, S. A., V.S. Springthorpe, and S.A. Ansari. Rotavirus. In *Foodborne Disease Handbook: Vol. 2. Diseases Caused by Viruses, Parasites, and Fungi.* Y.H. Hui, et al. (eds.). New York, Marcel Dekker, Inc. Pp. 81–111 (1994).

4. Grešíková, M. Tickborne encephalitis. In *Foodborne Disease Handbook: Vol. 2. Diseases Caused by Viruses, Parasites, and Fungi.* Y.H. Hui, et al. (eds.). New York, Marcel Dekker, Inc. Pp. 113–135 (1994).

5. Cliver, D.O. Other foodborne viral diseases. In *Foodborne Disease Handbook: Vol. 2. Diseases Caused by Viruses, Parasites, and Fungi.* Y.H. Hui, et al. (eds.). New York, Marcel Dekker, Inc. Pp. 137–143 (1994).

6. Matsui, S.M., and H.B. Greenberg. Medical management of foodborne viral gastroenteritis. In *Foodborne Disease Handbook: Vol. 2. Diseases Caused by Viruses, Parasites, and Fungi.* Y.H. Hui, et al. (eds.). New York, Marcel Dekker, Inc. Pp. 145–158 (1994).

7. Cliver, D.O. Epidemiology of foodborne viruses. In *Foodborne Disease Handbook: Vol. 2. Diseases Caused by Viruses, Parasites, and Fungi.* Y.H. Hui, et al. (eds.). New York, Marcel Dekker, Inc. Pp. 159–175 (1994).

8. Herrmann, J.E. Laboratory methodology. In *Foodborne Disease Handbook: Vol. 2. Diseases Caused by Viruses, Parasites, and Fungi.* Y.H. Hui, et al. (eds.). New York, Marcel Dekker, Inc. Pp. 177–197 (1994).

9. Cliver, D.O. Viral foodborne disease agents of concern. *J. Food Protect.* 57:176–178 (1994).

10. Cliver, D.O. Epidemiology of viral foodborne disease. *J. Food Protect.* 57:263–266 (1994).

11. Centers for Disease Control and Prevention. Viral hepatitis surveillance program, 1990–1992. Hepatitis Surveillance Report No. 55. Atlanta, Georgia, Centers for Disease Control and Prevention. Pp. 19–34 (1994).

12. Council for Agricultural Science and Technology. Foodborne pathogens: risks and consequences. Task Force Report No. 122, September 1994. CAST, Ames, IA.

13.    Weingold, S.E., J.J. Guzewich, and J.K. Fudala. Use of foodborne disease data for HACCP risk assessment. *J. Food Protect.* 57:820–830 (1994).

14.    Glerup, H., H.T. Sorensen, A. Flyvbjerg, et al. A "mini epidemic" of hepatitis A after eating Russian caviar. *J. Hepatol.* 21:479 (1994).

15.    Herwaldt, B.L. J.F. Lew, C.L. Moe, et al. Characterization of a variant strain of Norwalk virus from a food-borne outbreak of gastroenteritis on a cruise ship in Hawaii. *J. Clin. Microbiol.* 32:861–866 (1994).

16.    Lo, S.V., A.M. Connolly, S.R. Palmer, et al. The role of the pre-symptomatic food handler in a common source outbreak of food-borne SRSV gastroenteritis in a group of hospitals. *Epidemiol. Infect.* 113:513–522 (1994).

17.    Morgan, D., M.E. Black, A. Charlett, and H. John. Viral gastroenteritis associated with a sandwich bar. *Commun. Dis. Rep.* 4(8) ISSN: R91–R92 (1994).

18.    Centers for Disease Control and Prevention. Viral gastroenteritis associated with consumption of raw oysters—Florida, 1993. *Morbid. Mortal. Weekly Rep.* 43:446–449 (1994).

19.    Public Health Laboratory Service, U.K. Gastrointestinal virus infections, England and Wales: laboratory reports, weeks 94/22-25. *Commun. Dis. Rep.* 4(26):120 (1994).

20.    Parker, S.P., and W.D. Cubitt. Measurement of IgA responses following Norwalk virus infection and other human caliciviruses using a recombinant Norwalk virus protein EIA. *Epidemiol. Infect.* 113:143–151 (1994).

21.    Oishi, I., K. Yamazaki, T. Kimoto, et al. A large outbreak of acute gastroenteritis associated with astrovirus among students and teachers in Osaka, Japan. *J. Infect. Dis.* 170:439–443 (1994).

22.    World Health Organization. Outbreak of tick-borne encephalitis, presumably milk-borne. *WHO Weekly Epidemiol. Rec.* No. 19, 13 May 1994, pp. 140–141.

23.    Fries, R. Viruses in foods: a review. *Fleischwirtschaft* 74:740–742 (1994).

24.    Greiser-Wilke, I., and R. Fries. Methods for detection of viral contaminations in food of animal origin. *Dtsch. Tierärztl. Wschr.* 101:284–290 (1994).

25.    Bouchriti, N., S.M. Goyal, A. El Marrakchi, and M. Jellal. Comparison of three methods for the concentration of poliovirus from Moroccan shellfish. *J. Food Protect.* 57:996–1000 (1994).

26.    Lees, D.N., K. Henshilwood, and W.J. Dore. Development of a method for detection of enteroviruses in shellfish by PCR with poliovirus as a model. *Appl. Environ. Microbiol.* 60:2999–3005 (1994).

27.    Le Guyader, F., E. Dubois, D. Menard, and M. Pommepuy. Detection of hepatitis A virus, rotavirus, and enterovirus in naturally contaminated shellfish and sediment by reverse transcription-seminested PCR. *Appl. Environ. Microbiol.* 60:3665–3671 (1994).

28.    Deng, M.Y., S.P. Day, and D.O. Cliver. Detection of hepatitis A virus in environmental samples by antigen-capture PCR. *Appl. Environ. Microbiol.* 60:1927–1933 (1994).

29.    Gouvea, V., N. Santos, M.D. Timenetsky, and M.K. Estes. Identification of Norwalk virus in artificially seeded shellfish and selected foods. *J. Virol. Meth.* 48:177–187 (1994).

30.    Lucena, F., J. Lasobras, D. McIntosh, et al. Effect of distance from the polluting focus on relative concentrations of *Bacteroides fragilis* phages and coliphages in mussels. *Appl. Environ. Microbiol.* 60:2272–2277 (1994).

31.    Bosch, A., F.X. Abad, R. Gajardo, and R.M. Pintó. Should shellfish be purified before public consumption? *Lancet* 344:1024–1025 (1994).

32.    Abad, F.X., R.M. Pinto, and A. Bosch. Survival of enteric viruses on environmental fomites. *Appl. Environ. Microbiol.* 60:3704–3710 (1994).

33.    Hilfenhaus, J., T. Nowak, F. Feldman, and D. Shouval. Inactivation of hepatitis A virus by pasteurization and elimination of picornaviruses during manufacture of factor VIII concentrate. *Vox Sanguinis* 67(Suppl. 1):62–66 (1994).

34.    Hart, H.F., W.G. Hart, J. Crossley, et al. Effect of terminal (dry) heat treatment on non-enveloped viruses in coagulation factor concentrates. *Vox Sanguinis* 67:345–350 (1994).

35.    Centers for Disease Control and Prevention. New horizons: hepatitis A vaccine. Hepatitis Surveillance Report No. 55. Atlanta, Georgia, Centers for Disease Control and Prevention. Pp. 9–11 (1994).

36.    Anonymous. Hepatitis A vaccine: "Havrix Mono-dose". *Commun. Dis. Environ. Health Scotland Weekly Rep.* 28(94/21):3 (1994).

37.    Petschow, B.W., and R.D. Talbott. Reduction in virus-neutralizing activity of a bovine colostrum immuno-globulin concentrate by gastric acid and digestive enzymes. *J. Pediat. Gastroenterol. Nutr.* 19:228–235 (1994).

38.    Bile, K., A. Isse, O. Mohamud, et al. Contrasting roles of rivers and wells as sources of drinking water on attack and fatality rates in a hepatitis E epidemic in Somalia. *Am. J. Trop. Med. Hyg.* 51:466–474 (1994).

39.    Payment, P., E. Franco, and G.S. Fout. Incidence of Norwalk virus infections during a prospective epidemiological study of drinking water related gastrointestinal illness. *Can. J. Microbiol.* 40:805–809 (1994).

40.    Khan, A.S., C.K. Moe, R.I. Glass, et al. Norwalk virus-associated gastroenteritis traced to ice consumption aboard a cruise ship in Hawaii: comparison and application of molecular method-based assays. *J. Clin. Microbiol.* 32:318–322 (1994).

41.    Nasser, A.M. Prevalence and fate of hepatitis A virus in water. *Crit. Rev. Environ. Sci. Technol.* 24:281–323 (1994).

42.    Abad, F.X., R.M. Pinto, J.M. Diez, and A. Bosch. Disinfection of human enteric viruses in water by copper and silver in combination with low levels of chlorine. *Appl. Environ. Microbiol.* 60:2377–2383 (1994).

43.    Black, E.K., and G.R. Finch. Detection and occurrence of waterborne bacterial and viral pathogens. *Water Environ. Res.* 66:292–298 (1994).

44.    Tsai, Y.L., B. Tran, L.R. Sangermano, and C.J. Palmer. Detection of poliovirus, hepatitis A virus, and rotavirus

from sewage and ocean water by triplex reverse transcriptase PCR. *Appl. Environ. Microbiol.* 60:2400–2407 (1994).

45. Puig, M., J. Jofre, F. Lucena, et al. Detection of adenoviruses and enteroviruses in polluted waters by nested PCR amplification. *Appl. Environ. Microbiol.* 60:2963–2970 (1994).

46. Straub, T.M., I.L. Pepper, and C.P. Gerba. Detection of naturally occurring enteroviruses and hepatitis A virus in undigested and anaerobically digested sludge using the polymerase chain reaction. *Can. J. Microbiol.* 40:884–888 (1994).

47. Monceyron, C., and B. Grinde. Detection of hepatitis A virus in clinical and environmental samples by immuno-magnetic separation and PCR. *J. Virol. Meth.* 46:157–166 (1994).

48. Soares, A.C., T.M. Straub, I.L. Pepper, and C.P. Gerba. Effect of anaerobic digestion on the occurrence of enteroviruses and Giardia cysts in sewage sludge. *J. Environ. Sci. Health Part A - Environ. Sci. Eng.* 29:1887–1897 (1994).

49. Deng, M.Y., and D.O. Cliver. Mixed waste studies with viruses and *Giardia*. In *On-Site Wastewater Treatment.* E. Collins (ed.). Proceedings of the Seventh International Symposium on Individual and Small Community Sewage Systems. Dec. 11–13, 1994. Atlanta, GA. Pp. 573–578 (1994).

50. Garin, D., F. Fuchs, J.M. Crance, et al. Exposure to enteroviruses and hepatitis A virus among divers in environmental waters in France, first biological and serological survey of a controlled cohort. *Epidemiol. Infect.* 113:541–549 (1994).

51. Pfirrmann, A., and G. Vanden Bossche. Occurrence and isolation of airborne human enteroviruses from waste disposal and utilization plants. *Zbl. Hyg. Umweltmedizin* 196:38–51 (1994).

52. Powelson, D.K., and C.P. Gerba. Virus removal from sewage effluents during saturated and unsaturated flow through soil columns. *Water Res.* 28:2175–2181 (1994).

53. Woody, M.A., and D.O. Cliver. FRNA coliphages for monitoring groundwater near on-site systems. In *On-Site Wastewater Treatment.* E. Collins (ed.). Proceedings of the Seventh International Symposium on Individual and Small Community Sewage Systems. Dec. 11–13, 1994. Atlanta, GA. Pp. 551–558 (1994).

54. Marsh, P., and E.M.H. Wellington. Phage-host interactions in soil. *FEMS Microbiol. Ecol.* 15:99–107 (1994).

55. Huber, M.S., C.P. Gerba, M. Abbaszadegan, et al. Study of persistence of enteric viruses in landfilled disposable diapers. *Environ. Sci. Technol.* 28:1767–1772 (1994).

56. Birkenmeyer, L.G., and I.K. Mushahwar. Detection of hepatitis A, B and D virus by the polymerase chain reaction. *J. Virol. Meth.* 49:101–112 (1994).

57. Apaire-Marchais, V., V. Ferre-Aubineau, F. Colonna, et al. Development of RT-semi-nested PCR for detection of hepatitis A virus in stool in epidemic conditions. *Molec. Cell. Probes* 8:117–124 (1994).

58. Goswami, B.B., W.H. Koch, and T.A. Cebula. Competitor template RNA for detection and quantitation of hepatitis A virus by PCR. *BioTechniques* 16(1):114–122 (1994).

59. Whetter, L.E., S.P. Day, O. Elroystein, et al. Low efficiency of the 5' nontranslated region of hepatitis A virus RNA in directing cap-independent translation in permissive monkey kidney cells. *J. Virol.* 68:5253–5263 (1994).

60. Yap, K.L., and S.K. Lam. Infectivity titration of the fast-replicating and cytopathic hepatitis a [sic] virus strain HM175A.2 by an in situ enzyme immunoassay. *J. Virol. Meth.* 47:217–226 (1994).

61. Bishop, N.E., D.L. Hugo, S.V. Borovec, and D.A. Anderson. Rapid and efficient purification of hepatitis A virus from cell culture. *J. Virol. Meth.* 47:203–216 (1994).

62. Schlauder, G.G., and I.K. Mushahwar. Detection of hepatitis C and E virus by the polymerase chain reaction. *J. Virol. Meth.* 47:243–253 (1994).

63. Buisson, Y., P. Coursaget, R. Bercion, et al. Hepatitis E virus infection in soldiers sent to endemic regions. *Lancet* 344:1165–1166 (1994).

64. Pujol, F.H., M.O. Favorov, T. Marcano, et al. Prevalence of antibodies against hepatitis E virus among urban and rural populations in Venezuela. *J. Med. Virol.* 42:234–236 (1994).

65. Graham, D.Y., X. Jiang, T. Tanaka, et al. Norwalk virus infection of volunteers: New insights based on improved assays. *J. Infect. Dis.* 170:34–43 (1994).

66. Gray, J.J., C. Cunliffe, J. Ball, et al. Detection of immunoglobulin M (IgM), IgA, and IgG Norwalk virus-specific antibodies by indirect enzyme-linked immunosorbent assay with baculovirus-expressed Norwalk virus capsid antigen in adult volunteers challenged with Norwalk virus. *J. Clin. Microbiol.* 32:3059–3063 (1994).

67. Lew, J.F., A.Z. Kapikian, X. Jiang, et al. Molecular characterization and expression of the capsid protein of a Norwalk-like virus recovered from a Desert Shield troop with gastroenteritis. *Virology* 200:319–325 (1994).

68. Moe, C.L., T.J. Gentsch, T. Ando, et al. Application of PCR to detect Norwalk virus in fecal specimens from outbreaks of gastroenteritis. *J. Clin. Microbiol.* 32:642–648 (1994).

69. Ando, T., M.N. Mulders, D.C. Lewis, et al. Comparison of the polymerase region of small round structured virus strains previously classified in three antigenic types by solid-phase immune electron microscopy. *Arch. Virol.* 135:217–226 (1994).

70. Lew, J.F., A.Z. Kapikian, J. Valdesuso, and K.Y. Green. Molecular characterization of Hawaii virus and other Norwalk-like viruses: Evidence for genetic polymorphism among human caliciviruses. *J. Infect. Dis.* 170:535–542 (1994).

71. Wang, J.X., X. Jiang, H.P. Madore, et al. Sequence diversity of small, round-structured viruses in the Norwalk virus group. *J. Virol.* 68:5982–5990 (1994).

# Index